4 AUSTRALIA -
NEW ZEALAND
EDITION

Pauline Calleja | Karen Theobald | Theresa Harvey

Estes Health Assessment
& Physical Examination

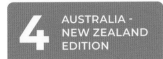

AUSTRALIA -
NEW ZEALAND
EDITION

Pauline Calleja | Karen Theobald | Theresa Harvey

Estes Health Assessment
& Physical Examination

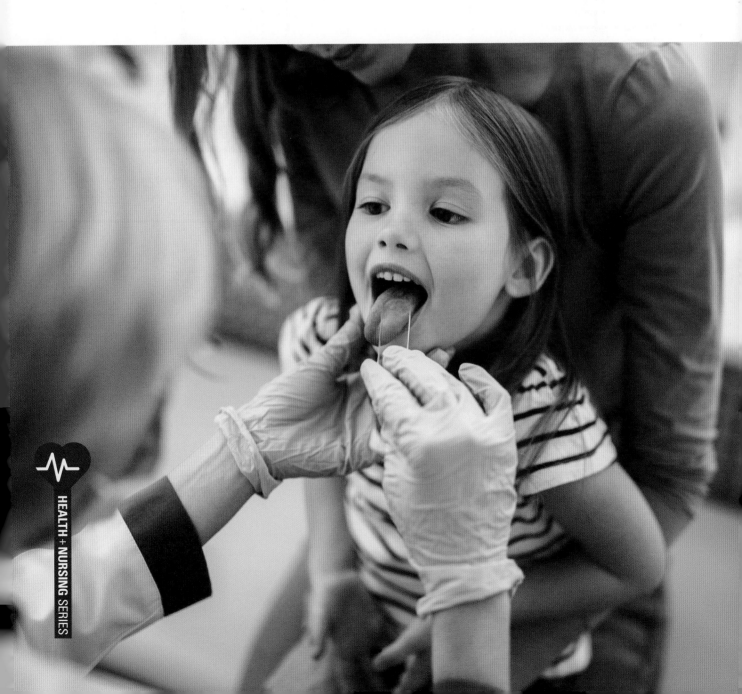

HEALTH + NURSING SERIES

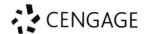

Health Assessment and Physical Examination
4th Edition
Pauline Calleja
Karen Theobald
Theresa Harvey
Mary Ellen Zator Estes

Portfolio manager: Fiona Hammond
Senior product manager: Michelle Aarons
Senior content developer: Margie Asmus/Stephanie Davis
Senior project editor: Nathan Katz
Cover designer: Danielle Maccarone
Text designer: Cengage Creative Studio
Permissions/Photo researcher: Catherine Kerstjens
Editor: Marta Veroni
Proofreader: Paul Smitz
Indexer: KnowledgeWorks Global Ltd.
Art direction: Mariana Maccarini
Cover: Courtesy stock.adobe.com/Yakobchuk Olena
Typeset by KnowledgeWorks Global Ltd.

Any URLs contained in this publication were checked for currency during the production process. Note, however, that the publisher cannot vouch for the ongoing currency of URLs.

Authorised adaptation of *Health Assessment and Physical Examination*, Fifth edition, by Mary Ellen Zator Estes ©2014, Cengage Learning [9781133610939]

This fourth edition published in 2024

Notice to the Reader
Every effort has been made to review and confirm the accuracy of content in this publication. By following the instructions contained herein the reader willingly assumes all risks in connection with such instructions. The reader should review procedures, treatments, drug dosages or legal content. Neither the authors nor the publisher assume any liability for injury or damage to persons or property arising from any error or omission. Inclusion of proprietary names for any drugs or devices should not be interpreted as a recommendation.

Acknowledgements
Cengage acknowledges the Traditional Owners and Custodians of the lands of all First Nations Peoples of Australia. We pay respect to Elders past and present. We recognise the continuing connection of First Nations Peoples to the land, air and waters, and thank them for protecting these lands, waters and ecosystems since time immemorial. Warning – First Nations Australians are advised that this book and associated learning materials may contain images, videos or voices of deceased persons.

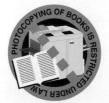

© 2024 Cengage Learning Australia Pty Limited

Copyright Notice
This Work is copyright. No part of this Work may be reproduced, stored in a retrieval system, or transmitted in any form or by any means without prior written permission of the Publisher. Except as permitted under the *Copyright Act 1968,* for example any fair dealing for the purposes of private study, research, criticism or review, subject to certain limitations. These limitations include: Restricting the copying to a maximum of one chapter or 10% of this book, whichever is greater; providing an appropriate notice and warning with the copies of the Work disseminated; taking all reasonable steps to limit access to these copies to people authorised to receive these copies; ensuring you hold the appropriate Licences issued by the Copyright Agency Limited ("CAL"), supply a remuneration notice to CAL and pay any required fees. For details of CAL licences and remuneration notices please contact CAL at Level 11, 66 Goulburn Street, Sydney NSW 2000, Tel: (02) 9394 7600, Fax: (02) 9394 7601
Email: info@copyright.com.au
Website: www.copyright.com.au

For product information and technology assistance,
in Australia call **1300 790 853**;
in New Zealand call **0800 449 725**

For permission to use material from this text or product, please email
aust.permissions@cengage.com

National Library of Australia Cataloguing-in-Publication Data
ISBN: 9780170463140
A catalogue record for this book is available from the National Library of Australia.

Cengage Learning Australia
Level 5, 80 Dorcas Street
Southbank VIC 3006 Australia

For learning solutions, visit **cengage.com.au**

Printed in China by 1010 Printing International Limited.
1 2 3 4 5 6 7 27 26 25 24 23

BRIEF CONTENTS

CONTENTS

Guide to the text

As you read this text you will find a number of features in every chapter to enhance your study of health assessment and physical examination and help you understand how the theory is applied in the real world.

CHAPTER-OPENING FEATURES

349

CHAPTER **11**

EARS, NOSE, MOUTH AND THROAT

LEARNING OUTCOMES
By the end of this chapter you should be able to:
1 identify the structures of the ears, nose, mouth and throat
2 describe system-specific history and normal findings in the physical examination of the ears, nose, mouth and throat
3 describe common abnormalities with pathophysiology found in the physical examination of the ears, nose, mouth and throat
4 identify health education opportunities for consumers with specific conditions
5 perform the physical examination of the ears, nose, mouth and throat
6 discuss the clinical reasoning in evaluating outcomes of health assessment and physical examination including documentation requirements for recording information, health education given and relevant health referral.

Identify the key concepts that the chapter will cover with the **Learning outcomes** at the start of each chapter.

BACKGROUND
Health assessment and physical examination of the ears, nose, sinuses, mouth and throat can be linked to assessment of the neurological, respiratory, endocrine, gastrointestinal, musculoskeletal and cardiovascular systems.
Ear-related conditions include:
> *infections* (either bacterial or viral) such as otitis media (middle ear infection) and otitis externa ('tropical ear' or 'swimmer's ear'). In Australia there are between 900 000 and 2.4 million cases per year of otitis media (Veivers et al., 2022), one of the leading causes of disease in Aboriginal and Torres Strait Islander children, and a significant contributor to hearing loss (De Lacey, Dune & Macdonald, 2020). In 2018–19, 43% of Aboriginal and Torres Strait Islander children aged seven and older had measured hearing loss in one or both ears (AIHW, 2020a). Clinical presentation differs for this cohort, in that they are, on average, younger in age for first infection, have a higher frequency of infection and experience infections of greater severity and persistence, compared with non-Indigenous children (Jervis-Bardy, Carney, Duguid & Leach, 2017). In New Zealand, approximately 60% of children have experienced at least one episode of acute otitis media by age four, and 27% of children aged 0 to 4 years are affected each year (BPAC, 2022). Research indicates Māori and Pasifika children experience higher rates of middle ear infection and subsequent hearing loss than the broader New Zealand population (EMC, 2021).
> *hearing loss*, which may be due to disease processes such as Ménière's disease, age-related changes, drug-related conditions, acoustic neuroma and trauma. Hearing loss in children is significantly correlated with ear disease and infection,

THE HEALTH ASSESSMENT AND PHYSICAL EXAMINATION PROCESS

HEALTH HISTORY

CONSUMER PROFILE	The ears, nose, mouth and throat health history provides insight into the link between a consumer's life and lifestyle and ears, nose and sinuses, mouth and throat information and pathology. Diseases or changes that are age-, sex- and race-specific for the ears, nose, mouth and throat are listed.		
	AGE	EARS	> Elderly consumers: • Hearing loss related to presbycusis, sensorineural degeneration or otosclerosis • Excessive or impacted cerumen
		NOSE	> Elderly consumers: • Decrease in ability to smell
		MOUTH AND THROAT	Orthodonture > Elderly consumers: • Tooth loss and gum disease • Candidiasis related to immunosuppression • Decrease in ability to taste

In each of the examination chapters in Part 2, a **Health History** table details consumer profiles, descriptions of common complaints, important past health history information and relevant family and social history information related to the body system covered in that chapter.

THE HEALTH ASSESSMENT AND PHYSICAL EXAMINATION PROCESS

An **Examination in Brief** box gives a concise summary of key elements in the physical examination process.

EXAMINATION IN BRIEF: EARS, NOSE AND SINUSES, MOUTH AND THROAT

Examination of the ear

Auditory screening
> Voice-whisper test
> Tuning fork tests
  • Weber test
  • Rinne test

Inspection
> External ear

Palpation
> Otoscopic examination

Examination of the nose

Inspection

Palpation and percussion

Transillumination of the sinuses

Examination of the mouth and thro[at]

Examination of the breath

Examination of the lips

Inspection

Palpation

Examination of the tongue

Examination of the buccal mucosa

Examination of the gums

The full IPPA method of physical examination is then outlined for each body system, clearly colour-coded and presented in the **ENAP format**, ensuring a complete, detailed physical examination.

Voice-whisper test

E 1. Instruct the consumer to occlude one ear with a finger.
2. Stand 60 cm behind the consumer's other ear and whisper a two-syllable word or phrase that is evenly accented.
3. Ask the consumer to repeat the word or phrase.
4. Repeat the test with the other ear.

N The consumer should be able to repeat words whispered from a distance of 60 cm.

A The consumer is unable to repeat the words correctly or states that he or she was unable to hear anything.

P This indicates a hearing loss in the high-frequency range that may be caused by excessive exposure to loud noises.

E Examination

N Normal findings

A Abnormal findings

P Pathophysiology

A full **Case Study** at the end of each examination chapter brings everything together – including a complete consumer profile and health history, and demonstrating the process of approaching the case – using the **evaluation and clinical reasoning cycle** (explained in more detail in Chapter 1).

UNIT 2

CASE STUDY

THE CONSUMER WITH ACUTE RHINOSINUSITIS

This case study illustrates the application and the objective documentation of the ears, nose, mouth and throat assessment.

Lianna Potter is a 61-year-old nurse who presents to the health clinic complaining of facial pain and frontal headache.

HEALTH HISTORY

CONSUMER PROFILE	61-year-old Caucasian female	
CHIEF COMPLAINT	'I have had a headache and facial pressure for over 10 days.'	
HISTORY OF THE PRESENT ILLNESS	Consumer was in her usual state of health until 10 days ago, when she developed an upper respiratory infection that seems to have become worse. Her symptoms started with nasal congestion, purulent nasal discharge and mild facial pressure. After 5 days, she developed thick, green, purulent nasal discharge, bilateral frontal headache (4/10 intensity), maxillary facial pain (6/10 intensity), and bilateral maxillary toothache. She has had a low-grade fever (37.4°C) without chills, sweats, ear pain, sore throat, chest congestion, wheezing or dyspnoea. The symptoms seem to get worse when she leans over. She has been taking decongestants every 6 hours and ibuprofen 400 mg at bedtime without relief for 3 days. Consumer has been renovating downstairs bathroom and guest bedroom for the past two weeks.	
PAST HEALTH HISTORY	**MEDICAL HISTORY**	Hypertension since age 40
	SURGICAL HISTORY	Hysterectomy, age 54
	ALLERGIES	Bees – anaphylaxis
	MEDICATIONS	> Hydrochlorothiazide 25 mg every morning > Ibuprofen for headaches 200–600 mg BD PRN > Demazin Cold and Flu – paracetamol (500 mg) and phenylephrine PRN for nasal congestion (5 mg)
	COMMUNICABLE DISEASES	Has had COVID-19 in past three months
	INJURIES AND ACCIDENTS	Denies
	SPECIAL NEEDS	Denies
	BLOOD TRANSFUSIONS	Denies
	CHILDHOOD ILLNESSES	Chickenpox, age 5, without sequelae
	IMMUNISATIONS	All up to date as per employment requirements
FAMILY HEALTH HISTORY		
SOCIAL HISTORY	**ALCOHOL USE**	1–2 glasses of wine per week
	TOBACCO USE	Never smoked
	DRUG USE	Denies
	DOMESTIC AND INTIMATE PARTNER VIOLENCE	Denies
	SEXUAL PRACTICE	Monogamous relationship with husband
	TRAVEL HISTORY	Denies recent travel more than 100 km from home in past month
	WORK ENVIRONMENT	Is a nurse manager at local health service
	HOME ENVIRONMENT	Lives with husband and adult daughter and grandchild in a single-family home. Recent renovation of downstairs area to allow for Airbnb rental to supplement income, as getting ready for retirement
	HOBBIES AND LEISURE ACTIVITIES	Music, playing golf, caravanning

OTHER CHAPTER FEATURES

Other boxed features appear across the text, highlighting important information and helping you build your understanding of key concepts.

Identify and learn how to respond to serious or life-threatening clinical assessment findings that need immediate attention with the **Urgent Finding** alerts.

URGENT FINDING

Cerebrospinal fluid (CSF) drainage from the ear
If the consumer has cerebrospinal fluid (clear liquid that tests positive for glucose on Dextrostix) leaking from the ear, be sure to use good hand washing technique and avoid placing any objects into the ear canal in order to prevent the development of meningitis. A consumer with this finding needs immediate referral to a qualified specialist for emergency assessment.

Understand the decision-making process and develop your clinical judgement skills with the **Clinical Reasoning** boxes.

CLINICAL **REASONING**

Practice tip: Risk factors for hearing loss
Consumers who fit any of the following hearing loss risk factors should be assessed for hearing damage. This is also an opportunity to provide person-centred health education about possible ways to avoid hearing loss based on the risk factor that are identified.

> Noise exposure
> Smoking
> Ototoxic drugs
> Congenital or heredity

> Trauma
> Chronic infection
> Systemic disease
> Tympanic membrane perforation

Explore the application of health assessment and physical examination theory in different real-world clinical situations with the **Putting it in Context** boxes.

PUTTING IT IN CONTEXT

Allergy assessment
Jenny Adams is a 13-year-old Caucasian female attending high school. She presents to the general practice with her mother complaining of hay fever symptoms that have been worsening over the past 6 months. Mum states she notices Jenny is increasingly restless when sleeping, becoming cranky and easily upset, unable to concentrate for long, has watery eyes, sneezes up to 17 times in a row, and normal doses of antihistamines are not helping. Jenny states that sometimes her eyes are so itchy and watery that she has trouble with her vision from rubbing them so hard; she wakes up with a dry mouth and bad breath and mum reports she has been snoring lately.

On examination Jenny's visual acuity is normal, her eyes are slightly reddened, she has a small amount of periorbital oedema, and you observe her sneeze 12 times in a row. Her tonsils are normal size, with no redness or swelling in her mouth or throat. She has had a Claratyne this morning along with ibuprofen for her headache, which she states is in her

Think about your own practice with **Reflection in Practice** boxes, which introduce realistic clinical situations and ethical controversies. These allow you to relate to the issues in a personal way, and to develop critical thinking, effective decision making and problem-solving skills.

REFLECTION IN PRACTICE

The consumer with poor oral hygiene
Mary is a 78-year-old widow who lives alone. She attends the clinic for a blood pressure check-up, but you notice that she has left her dentures out. When you ask her where her teeth are she states they are hurting her. On inspection you note multiple ulcers in her gums, remains of food particles in her gum and cheek margins and a foul smell. On further investigation you find out that she brushes her dentures every few days but does not have a cleaning regimen for her gums and mucous membranes.
> What type of education would you recommend and why?
> Would you refer Mary to anyone?
> What type of treatment may she require and why?

Get guidance on educating for healthy consumer outcomes and emphasising assessment of the whole person with **Health Education** boxes.

HEALTH EDUCATION

Making connections – oral cancer
Oral cancer risk factors are important to consider for long-term health promotion and harm minimisation, especially for factors that are modifiable by a change in lifestyle choices. Consider which of these factors are modifiable and would influence your opportunistic education approaches.
> Male sex
  • Aboriginal and Torres Strait Islander peoples are 1.4 times more likely to die from cancer and have a lower five-year relative survival rate compared to non-Aboriginal and Torres Strait Islander peoples (AIHW, 2018).
> Age > 40 years
> Tobacco use (pipes, cigars, cigarettes)
> Excessive alcohol use
> Sun exposure (lips)
> History of leukoplakia
> History of erythroplasia

Advanced practice material is highlighted throughout the text, to extend your understanding beyond basic assessment.

Transillumination of the sinuses
If palpation and percussion of the sinuses suggest sinusitis, transillumination of the frontal and maxillary sinuses may be performed by the advanced practitioner.
To evaluate the frontal sinuses:
1. Place the consumer in a sitting position facing you in a dark room.
2. Place a strong light source such as a transilluminator, penlight, or tip of an otoscope with the speculum under the bony ridge of the upper orbits (Figure 11.38A).
3. Observe the red glow over the sinuses and compare the symmetry of the two sides.
To evaluate the maxillary sinuses:
1. Place the consumer in a sitting position facing you in a dark room.
2. Place the light source firmly under each eye and just above the infraorbital ridge (Figure 11.38B).
3. Ask the consumer to open the mouth; observe the red glow on the hard palate.
4. Compare the two sides.

E Examination **N** Normal findings **A** Abnormal findings **P** Pathophysiology ▨ Advanced Assessment

END-OF-CHAPTER FEATURES

At the end of each chapter you will find several tools to help you to review, practise and extend your knowledge of the key learning outcomes.

Test your knowledge and consolidate your learning with the **Review Questions**.

CHAPTER RESOURCES

REVIEW QUESTIONS

For answers to these questions, see Answer section at the end of the book.

1. On examination of a 44-year-old man's inner ear, you notice a darkened area or hole in his left tympanic membrane. This is likely to be:
   a. A perforated ear drum
   b. A fungal infection on the ear drum
   c. A bacterial infection on the ear drum
   d. A tumour or ear cancer

Link theory to key skills by reading about the relevant clinical skill, such as in Tollefson & Hillman, *Clinical Psychomotor Skills* 7th edition, and by watching its accompanying **clinical skills videos**.

CS CLINICAL SKILLS

The following Clinical Skill is relevant to this chapter and can be found in Tollefson & Hillman, *Clinical Psychomotor Skills*, 8th edition:
> 27 Healthcare teaching.

Extend your understanding through the suggested **Further Resources** relevant to each chapter.

FURTHER RESOURCES

UNIT 2

> Australasian Sleep Association: http://www.sleep.org.au
> Australian and New Zealand Academy of Periodontists: http://www.perio.org.au/
> Australian Dental Association Incorporated: http://www.ada.org.au/
> Australian Hearing: http://www.hearing.com.au/
> Australian Society of Otolaryngology – Head and neck surgery: http://www.asohns.org.au/
> Health Direct Australia: http://www.healthdirect.gov.au/ear-disorders

Guide to the online resources

FOR THE INSTRUCTOR

Cengage is pleased to provide you with a selection of resources that will help you prepare your lectures and assessments. These teaching tools are accessible via cengage.com.au/instructors for Australia or cengage.co.nz/instructors for New Zealand.

MINDTAP

Premium online teaching and learning tools are available on the *MindTap* platform – the personalised eLearning solution. *MindTap* is a flexible and easy-to-use platform that helps build student confidence and gives you a clear picture of their progress. We partner with you to ease the transition to digital – we're with you every step of the way.

MindTap for *Health Assessment and Physical Examination 4th edition* is full of innovative resources to support critical thinking, and help your students move from memorisation to mastery! Includes:

- *Health Assessment and Physical Examination* 4th edition eBook
- Polling Questions
- Revision Quizzes
- Case Study Quizzes
- Media Quizzes
- Animations and Clinical Skills Videos.

MindTap is a premium purchasable eLearning tool. Contact your Cengage learning consultant to find out how *MindTap* can transform your course.

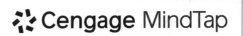

INSTRUCTOR'S MANUAL

The Instructor's manual includes:

- Learning objectives and key terms
- Chapter outlines
- Theory application activities

- Teaching exercises
- Individual exercises and group activities
- Clinical application activities
- Chapter checklists.

TEST BANK

This bank of questions has been developed in conjunction with the text for creating quizzes, tests and exams for your students. Deliver these through your LMS and in your classroom.

POWERPOINT™ PRESENTATIONS

Use the chapter-by-chapter PowerPoint slides to enhance your lecture presentations and handouts by reinforcing the key principles of your subject.

ARTWORK FROM THE TEXT
Add the digital files of graphs, pictures and flow charts into your course management system, use them in student handouts, or copy them into your lecture presentations.

FOR THE STUDENT

MindTap is the next-level online learning tool that helps you get better grades!

MindTap gives you the resources you need to study – all in one place and available when you need them. In the *MindTap Reader*, you can make notes, highlight text and even find a definition directly from the page.

If your instructor has chosen *MindTap* for your subject this semester, log in to *MindTap* to:

- Get better grades
- Save time and get organised
- Connect with your instructor and peers
- Study when and where you want, online and mobile
- Complete assessment tasks as set by your instructor.

When your instructor creates a course using *MindTap*, they will let you know your course key so you can access the content. Please purchase *MindTap* only when directed by your instructor. Course length is set by your instructor.

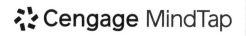

PREFACE TO THIS EDITION

Health assessment forms the foundation of all health care. Assessment is an ongoing process that is person-centred and considers the whole person as a physical, psychosocial and functional being, whether they are young or old, well or ill. *Health Assessment and Physical Examination,* 4th edition for Australia and New Zealand, provides a well-illustrated approach to the process of holistic assessment, including health history interview, physical examination techniques and health education.

The text presents knowledge from foundation to advanced health assessment, and physical examination for commencing students to advanced healthcare practitioners, using a scaffolded approach. This moves the learner through the comprehensive contextual information, including health assessment and physical examination techniques supported by evidence. Through this process abnormal findings are highlighted, and the chapter concludes with assessment applied to practice through an applied case study exemplar.

CONCEPTUAL APPROACH

This text is designed to support learners to holistically assess a consumer as a foundation of health practice. The skills of interviewing, inspection, palpation, percussion, auscultation and documentation enable the reader to make accurate clinical judgements and promote healthy consumer outcomes.

The concept for *Health Assessment and Physical Examination* is based on an organised assessment approach that can be easily applied into clinical practice. Further, this text focuses the reader on a transparent clinical reasoning cycle for ongoing care of the consumer based on the health assessment. The text is organised according to a well-known and applied quality framework called APIE (Assess, Plan, Implement, Evaluate).

Health Assessment and Physical Examination, 4th edition, emphasises the underpinning knowledge of anatomy, physiology and assessment, while highlighting clinically relevant information. This is achieved by taking a person-centred care approach that is displayed through the themes of assessment: cultural, familial, environmental considerations, patient dignity, and health education, including a specialist chapter on Aboriginal and Torres Strait Islander Peoples' health.

This text's consistent, easy-to-follow format with recurring pedagogical features is based on two formats:

1. The IPPA method of physical examination (Inspection, Palpation, Percussion, Auscultation) is consistently applied to body systems for a complete, detailed physical assessment.
2. The ENAP format (Examination, Normal findings, Abnormal findings, Pathophysiology) is followed for every IPPA examination, providing a useful and valuable collection of information. Pathophysiology is included to support understanding of each abnormal finding, acknowledging that nurses' clinical decisions need to be based on scientific rationale. It also enables the reader to study the content specifically relevant to his or her own healthcare practice.

ORGANISATION

Health Assessment and Physical Examination, 4th edition, consists of 22 chapters, which are organised into four units.

Unit 1 lays the foundation for the entire assessment process by guiding the reader through the nursing process, the critical thinking and clinical reasoning cycle, the patient interview including developmental considerations, the health history including documentation, physical assessment techniques, and cultural considerations. Specific tips on professionalism, approaching consumers, and discussing sensitive topics help the reader understand the importance of the nurse–patient relationship in the assessment process.

Unit 2 details assessment procedures and findings for specific body systems. The format used for all applicable systems-focused health assessment and physical examination chapters in this unit includes:

> Background
  • Anatomy and physiology
> Assessment: Taking the patient's health history
> Person-centred health education
> Planning for physical examination
  • Evaluation of subjective data to focus physical examination
  • Environment
  • Equipment
> Implementation: Conducting the physical examination
  • Inspection
  • Palpation
  • Percussion
  • Auscultation
> Evaluation of health assessment and physical examination findings
  • Case study.

The physical examination techniques presented are described for adults.

Unit 3 focuses on assessment techniques and findings for specific lifespan populations including pregnant women, children and the older adult.

Unit 4 helps the reader pull all the core concepts together to perform a thorough, accurate and efficient health assessment and physical examination.

ACKNOWLEDGEMENTS

We would like to acknowledge and sincerely thank our families and friends who have shared 'us' on the weekends, and many evenings, to enable us to complete this fourth edition.

We would like to sincerely thank all expert chapter contributors who provided critical review and input:

> Dr Leanne Brown, PhD, MNSc (NP), Grad DipApplSc (Nephrology, Grad Appl Sc, Grad Dip Appl Sc (Nsg) Grad Cert HMgt, BSc, RN, Nurse Practitioner Cape York Kidney Care.
> Dr Helen Donovan, PhD, RN/RM/CHN, MEd (l'ship); MEd (IncEd) FRCNA, SFHEA. School of Nursing, Queensland University of Technology
> Genevieve Edwards, RN, BN, Nurse Immuniser, Cert. Sex. & Rep. Health, GC Comm. & Public Health, GCHE, MPH, School of Nursing, Midwifery and Paramedicine, Australian Catholic University
> Nicole Hewlett, a proud palawa woman from lutruwita (Tasmania) Project Manager, The First Nations Cancer & Wellbeing Research Program, School of Public Health, Faculty of Medicine, The University of Queensland for developing Chapter 4, Aboriginal and Torres Strait Islander people's health
> Sandra Leathwick, RN, BHealth (Nursing), MEd (Adult), SFHEA, MACORN, MCATSINaM, School of Nursing, Midwifery and Paramedicine, Australian Catholic University
> Kate Lowe, MN (Management), GC (Paed Nursing), BN, LLB, School of Nursing, Midwifery & Paramedicine, Australian Catholic University
> Associate Professor Margaret MacAndrew, PhD, RN, BN, G.Cert (Ageing & Dementia), GCAP (FHEA), School of Nursing, Queensland University of Technology
> Joclyn Neal RM, RN, Master Midwifery, G.Cert (Neonates) School of Nursing, Midwifery and Paramedicine Australian Catholic University (QLD)
> Dr Christina Parker BHlthSci (Nursing) Grad Cert. PhD. Distinguished Educator in Gerontological Nursing (SFHEA), School of Nursing, Queensland University of Technology
> Sharyn Plath, RN, BN (Hons), Grad Cert Intercultural Studies, MNP, School of Nursing, Queensland University of Technology.

Thank you to the following people who contributed to the digital resources that accompany this text:

> Kristy Griffith (Australian Catholic University)
> Victoria Kain (Griffith University).

We would also like to thank everyone who so enthusiastically contributed to previous editions of this text, whose input we benefit from still. Thanks also go to the reviewers from universities in Australia and New Zealand who provided valuable feedback on the chapter drafts. A final thank you goes to the Cengage Content and Production teams, specifically Michelle Aarons and Margie Asmus, Stephanie Davis, Marta Veroni and Nathan Katz for their continued support.

The authors and Cengage Learning would like to thank the following reviewers for their incisive and helpful feedback:

> Amanda Kiernan (Australian Catholic University)
> Anthea Fagan (University of New England)

> Benjamin Hay (The University of Notre Dame Australia)
> Caroline Borzdynski (La Trobe University)
> Charlotte George (EmployEase)
> Courtney Hayes (University of Canberra)
> Dr Mark Lock (Ngiyampaa), Chief Editor at Cultural Safety Editing Service
> Lori Delaney (Queensland University of Technology)
> Mary Huynh (Australian Catholic University)
> Melissa Slattery (EQUALS International)
> Michelle Freeling (Flinders University)
> Paul Jarrett (Queensland University of Technology)
> Rachel Gilder (Swinburne University of Technology)
> Rita Eramo (Victoria University).

Every effort has been made to trace and acknowledge copyright. However, if any infringement has occurred, the publishers tender their apologies and invite the copyright holders to contact them.

Cengage acknowledges the Traditional Owners and Custodians of the lands of all First Nations Peoples of Australia. We pay respect to Elders past and present. We recognise the continuing connection of First Nations Peoples to the land, air and waters, and thank them for protecting these lands, waters and ecosystems since time immemorial.

Warning – First Nations Australians are advised that this book and associated learning materials may contain images, videos or voices of deceased persons.

ABOUT THE AUTHORS

Pauline Calleja
CQUniversity
RN, PhD, BNSc, MANP, GCert HigherEd, BNSc, DipManagement, FCENA, MACN
Associate Professor, CQUniversity, Committee member – Association of Queensland Nursing and Midwifery Leaders, Relieving Director of Nursing, Central West Hospital and Health Service, Registered Nurse, Emergency Department, Innisfail Hospital, Cairns and Hinterland Hospital and Health Service.

Pauline's nursing background has spanned many specialty areas and has included teaching health assessment, physical examination and clinical reasoning in clinical and academic settings. Pauline is an Associate Professor in the School of Nursing, Midwifery and Social Science at CQUniversity. Her experience in special projects includes developing and implementing a support program for rural and remote clinicians, teaching Indigenous primary healthcare workers, developing capacity for clinical teaching, and developing leadership skills in clinical teachers. Pauline has also taught at Griffith University, Queensland University of Technology, University of the Sunshine Coast, James Cook University and within various clinical and vocational education settings and has senior management experience in a remote setting. Pauline is a Fellow of professional associations including College of Emergency Nursing Australasia, and member of CRANAplus, Association of Nursing and Midwifery Leaders and the Australian College of Nursing.

Karen Theobald
Queensland University of Technology (QUT)
RN, PhD (Griff), MHSc (Nursing), GCert (HigherEd), BAppSc (QUT) PFHEA AFHEA (Indigenous)
Associate Professor, Academic Lead Education, School of Nursing QUT, Postgraduate Study Area Coordinator for Health Professional Education in the School of Nursing, Queensland University of Technology; Principal Fellow and Associate Fellow (Indigenous), Higher Education Academy (UK) and Honorary Senior Visiting Fellow of Nursing and Midwifery, Metro North Health.

Karen is an experienced nursing academic and clinician, teaching across a variety of settings, which include healthcare contexts, undergraduate and postgraduate tertiary courses. Most of Karen's teaching is in the areas of acute care nursing, health assessment, advanced life support and developing teachers' capacity to enhance learning. A strong focus in her teaching is a commitment to learning through industry collaboration and work-integrated learning.

In her present role Karen oversees policy and the strategic direction of teaching and learning for the six nursing courses. She is responsible for ensuring ongoing internal and professional accreditation for these courses. Her research focuses on workforce preparation, including co-design and delivery of curricula with industry, transfer of clinical reasoning capability; simulation; peer learning and interprofessional education. Karen also serves in leadership and advisory capacities with professional organisations such as the Australian College of Critical Care Nurses and the Australian Resuscitation Council (Queensland Branch).

Theresa Harvey
Australian Catholic University (ACU)
RN, RM, PhD (CQU) MN (Women's Health), Grad Dip (FurtherEdTraining),
BHlthSc (Nurs), FACN, SFHEA
Senior Lecturer, International Coordinator, Course Coordinator Master of
Leadership and Management in Healthcare, School of Nursing, Midwifery and
Paramedicine, Australian Catholic University (ACU).

Theresa has extensive and varied clinical and nursing education experience
including tertiary and clinical education, clinical expertise in high-dependency,
community and midwifery practice. Theresa's research and teaching focus
incorporates health assessment and physical examination, including development
of clinical reasoning and supporting undergraduate students' clinical learning for
transition to practice, clinical leadership, simulation, developing clinical teaching
skills and developing a global perspective for clinical care. As the School of Nursing
Midwifery and Paramedicine International Coordinator at ACU, Theresa assists
with the globalisation of the curriculum and learning opportunities and facilitates
students' learning experiences in short-term study abroad programs. Theresa has led
professional development of clinical teachers from multidisciplinary health areas
to enhance their support of students on practicum both in Australia and Vietnam.
She has also taught at Queensland University of Technology and Northern Sydney
Area Midwifery School/Ryde Hospital. Theresa is a Fellow of the Australian College
of Nursing and Senior Fellow, Higher Education Academy (UK).

Mary Ellen Zator Estes
Ball State University, Muncie, Indiana
RN, MSN, FNP, APRN-BC, NP-C
Family Nurse Practitioner in Internal Medicine, Fairfax, Virginia Clinical Faculty,
Nurse Practitioner Track, School of Nursing, Ball State University, Muncie, Indiana.

With nearly 30 years' experience as a clinician and academician, Ms. Estes has
taught health assessment and physical examination courses to nurses and nursing
students from a variety of backgrounds. Her hands-on approach in the classroom,
clinical laboratory and healthcare setting has consistently led to positive learning
experiences for her students. She has taught at the University of Virginia,
Marymount University, Northern Virginia Community College, and the George
Washington University Medical Center. She has also served as Clinical Faculty for
Ball State University. Ms. Estes originated and developed the original US edition
of this text.

UNIT 1

LAYING THE FOUNDATION

CHAPTER 1

THE NURSING ROLE IN HEALTH ASSESSMENT AND PHYSICAL EXAMINATION

LEARNING OUTCOMES

By the end of this chapter you should be able to:

1 describe how nurses have a valued role in health assessment for planning, implementing and evaluating culturally safe care
2 discuss components of critical thinking applied to health care
3 discuss the clinical reasoning cycle
4 apply the Universal Intellectual Standards to the clinical reasoning cycle
5 describe the nursing process and applying this when undertaking health assessment and physical examination
6 describe the concept of cultural competence compared with cultural safety.

BACKGROUND

Health assessment and physical examination are two essential skills on which an effective and safe practitioner bases every consumer interaction. Every interaction is an opportunity for nurses to assess the consumer. Critical thinking and following the **nursing process** is what allows nurses to make informed and at times life-saving **interventions** for the consumer. Critical thinking is an essential component of clinical reasoning, which combines nursing knowledge and practice. This text highlights the application of knowledge to practice emphasising the critical thinking and clinical reasoning underpinning care decisions based on health assessment and physical examination findings.

Nursing is a profession with a distinct body of knowledge. Over time, nurses build a repertoire of professional experience that they take into each healthcare encounter, which assists decision making and often informs instinctive responses to certain situations; for example, feeling worried for a consumer and this triggers a medical emergency call (Raymond, Porter, Missen, Larkins, de Vent & Redpath, 2018). In this way, experienced nurses make intuitive links that are not usually made by beginners because they can select strategies that have been successful in the past, and all forms of knowledge can positively impact on the decision-making process (Miller & Hill, 2018). To develop their own body of knowledge, including intuition, nurses must cultivate the skill of professional reflection and critical thinking to ensure that these opportunities for development are realised.

Professional intuition develops over time as nurses begin to link certain patterns or events to specific health outcomes (Hassani, Abdi, Jalali & Salari, 2020). Experienced nurses seem to do this with little conscious effort. The beginner, however, may need guidance to perceive links intuitively recognised by the experienced nurse (Turan et al., 2016). For example, a critical care nurse may feel that the consumer is 'going downhill' even though their vital **signs** are stable. The experienced nurse has a 'feel' for the person and their situation. A few hours later the person has a cardiopulmonary arrest.

How did the experienced nurse know this? That is part of the critical thinking and clinical reasoning that has developed in the experienced nurse (Hassani, Abdi, Jalali & Salari, 2020). The health history findings will inform what the nurse chooses to focus on in the physical examination, and the findings will give the nurse direction for other things to investigate. In this way critical thinking and clinical reasoning link both health history and physical assessment. As such, this will effectively and efficiently guide the nurse in the 'right' direction to assess the person and collaboratively decide on the priorities to be managed.

Expert nursing involves the use of analytical thinking, also known as clinical reasoning. Clinical reasoning is an integral part of professional reflection that every nurse needs to develop (Gonzalez, 2018). In analytical thinking, information is studied and broken into its constituent parts, and relationships and patterns are identified. Causation, key factors, and possible outcomes to a situation are identified where possible and then evidence should be used in decision making.

CRITICAL THINKING AND CLINICAL REASONING

Critical thinking is a purposeful, goal-directed thinking process applied to problem-solve issues using clinical reasoning. It combines logic, intuition and creativity. **Clinical reasoning** is a disciplined, creative and reflective approach that, combined with critical thinking, is used to establish potential strategies to assist people in reaching their desired health goals. For example, a consumer in the cardiac care unit complains of chest pain at rest. The consumer had been lying down after lunch. Your critical-thinking skills lead you to assess all aspects of the person's condition to determine the cause of this episode of pain and treat it accordingly. You recognise that, in addition to the person's diagnosis of angina, they also have a history of gastro-oesophageal reflux disease and a hiatal hernia, for which they take pantoprazole 40 mg each morning. You pursue a line of questioning that uncovers more information about the consumer's pain. You use clinical reasoning skills to determine that their pain is most likely gastrointestinal in nature because the pain is located in the epigastric area, whereas their recent chest pain was located in the substernal region. In addition, there are no ECG changes with the pain (which had previously been present), and the pain was relieved when they sat up in a semi-Fowler's position. The use of reasoning, applying knowledge and information gathering are combined to direct the nurse's action. Therefore, critical-thinking skills are needed to enable the process of clinical reasoning.

Guidelines outlined by the Foundation for Critical Thinking address some of the underpinning key elements of clinical reasoning (**Table 1.1**) and assist in applying the Universal Intellectual Standards for critical thinking. Knowing and understanding these guidelines helps both the novice and the advanced nurse master the clinical reasoning process. The time frame in which this mastery occurs differs for every person. Like most skills, the more clinical reasoning is practised, the more natural and easier it becomes.

TABLE 1.1 Key elements of critical thinking and clinical reasoning

ELEMENTS THAT UNDERPIN CLINICAL REASONING AND CRITICAL THINKING	UNIVERSAL INTELLECTUAL STANDARDS FOR CRITICAL THINKING
> All reasoning has a purpose. > All reasoning is an attempt to figure something out, to settle some question, or to solve a problem. > All reasoning is based on assumptions. > All reasoning is done from a specific point of view. > All reasoning is based on data, information and evidence. > All reasoning is expressed through, and shaped by, concepts and ideas. > All reasoning contains inferences by which we draw conclusions and give meaning to data. > All reasoning leads somewhere, and has implications and consequences.	> Clarity: understandable, the meaning can be grasped > Accuracy: free from errors or distortion, true > Precision: exact to the necessary level of detail > Relevance: relating to the matter at hand > Depth: containing complexities and multiple interrelationships > Breadth: encompassing multiple viewpoints > Logic: the parts make sense together > Significance: focusing on the important not trivial > Fairness: justifiable, not self-serving or one-sided

SOURCE: *HELPING STUDENTS ASSESS THEIR THINKING*, BY R. PAUL AND L. ELDER, 1997. HTTPS://WWW.CRITICALTHINKING.ORG/PAGES/OPEN-MINDED-INQUIRY/579; ELDER AND PAUL (2013)

Applying standards for critical thinking

The quality of critical thinking can be evaluated by applying the nine Universal Intellectual Standards (UIS) proposed by Elder and Paul (2013). These standards are outlined in **Table 1.1** and applied to a clinical example in **Table 1.2**.

Consistent application of these standards to critical thinking leads to refinement and sophistication of clinical reasoning.

TABLE 1.2 Application of critical thinking to clinical example

STANDARD	QUESTIONS TO CONSIDER	CLINICAL REASONING EXAMPLE
Clarity	Could you elaborate further on that point? Could you give me an example? Could you illustrate what you mean?	A 70-year-old consumer may report a breathing difficulty. The nurse would use critical thinking to assist them to specify when and under what conditions the breathing difficulty occurs. Shortness of breath at rest with no provocation will be different from shortness of breath when walking.
Accuracy	Is that really true? How could we check/verify this piece of information?	Thinking that this person is always short of breath every time they mobilise may be an inaccurate fact. This individual may be able to breathe normally when walking on flat surfaces but becomes short of breath walking up six stairs. The nurse would need to ask questions to ensure accurate understanding of information.
Precision	What is the specific or precise information here?	To state that a consumer is 'short of breath' is not precise, especially if they are not short of breath when you are looking at them. The statement 'The consumer reports becoming short of breath on uphill exertion – more than five steps' is precise.
Relevance	How are these connected? Do these topics/issues impact on each other? How does this help us with the issue?	If the consumer presents with urinary frequency and then you discover that they also experience shortness of breath when walking, these issues, while problems for the individual, are not likely to be connected. However, if the person reports shortness of breath on walking, along with dizziness, loss of balance, and urinary frequency and stinging pain on urination, the nurse may suspect that because the person is older, a urinary infection may be causing some systemic issues such as dizziness and loss of balance and thus they become short of breath because they are systemically unwell.
Depth	What are the factors that makes this situation complex? How are the complexities in the situation being considered? Are we dealing with the most significant factors in the situation?	As noted in the above information, relevance and depth really work together, along with precision of information. The factors that make this situation complex include the symptoms that group together to make meaning. The fact that this person is elderly and that urinary infections can cause systemic problems in the older adult means the nurse needs to ensure the significant factors are identified and precise.

>> **TABLE 1.2** *continued*

STANDARD	QUESTIONS TO CONSIDER	CLINICAL REASONING EXAMPLE
Breadth	Do we need to consider various points of view? What would this look like from the point of view of the patient/family member/allied health professional?	Is the consumer's story simplified when relayed to the nurse? Is there a need to consider the views of another person such as a spouse, parent, relative, friend or significant other? Is there additional data that needs to be obtained in order to gain an accurate impression of the consumer's situation? In this situation, if a family member relays to you that the consumer has also been confused over the last two days, and has a history of urinary infections, this will paint a broader picture that the person's urinary symptoms are probably causing these systemic symptoms.
Logic	Does this make sense? Does all of this make sense together?	Does the consumer's or family member's story seem logical? If the consumer stated that they have recently been travelling and therefore have not been able to drink as much water as usual, this would make sense as another contributing factor to the individual's likelihood of having developed a urinary tract infection. Another way to think logically is to attribute signs and **symptoms** to disease entities. The consumer experiences shortness of breath – is this due to heart problems or the systemic issues associated with the urinary tract infection? Logical thinking would seem to point to the latter aetiology, unless a cardiac or respiratory history or other symptoms relevant to heart/lung disease need to be ruled out as contributing factors to the shortness of breath.
Significance	Is this the most important problem to consider? Which of these facts are most important?	For this individual, we would need to consider the underlying probable cause for their problem; in this case we would need to ensure the person is treated for the urinary tract infection, and also rule out other cardiac and respiratory issues simultaneously (for example, we may take an electrocardiogram of the heart, and a peak flow reading of the patient's tidal volume). If the shortness of breath persists after treatment for the infection is complete and no immediate cardiac or respiratory issues are identified, then further testing would be relevant.
Fairness	Do I have a vested interest in this issue? Am I representing the viewpoints of others?	Although we may not always consider the issue of 'fairness' in health care, at times the decisions we make about the amount, type and timing of information we give consumers, and choices in their health care, could be considered in this way. For example, when assessing how to manage your day, do you allow individuals a choice of when to shower or not give them a choice so it is easier for your time management?

Components of critical thinking and clinical reasoning

According to Wilkinson (2007), critical thinking encompasses many skills, including interpretation, analysis, inference, explanation, evaluation and self-regulation. Levett-Jones et al. (2010) have adapted many of these skills into a clinical reasoning cycle specifically derived from nurses' practice. These skills will be discussed to show their relationship with health assessment and physical examination. First, we will discuss what critical thinking is within a clinical context.

Interpretation of a situation requires the nurse to decode hidden messages, clarify meaning and then categorise the information. For example, a consumer may claim to be seeking health care for a bad cough and cold, but actually is concerned about whether the cough is a sign of lung cancer.

During analysis, the nurse examines the ideas and data that were presented, identifies discrepancies, and reflects on possible reasons for these. The nurse can then begin to frame the main points of the consumer's story. For instance, an individual may complain of insomnia but upon questioning reveals that they sleep six hours at night and take a two-hour nap each afternoon. Often, investigating discrepancies for clarity and accuracy leads to a clearer picture of the person's overall situation and reduces the chance of misinterpreting information.

Information and assumptions obtained from the person about their health are analysed using inference and reasoning to create specific premises about the health problems identified. Inference can be a challenging skill for the beginner nurse because they must possess a certain level of knowledge and experience in order to draw conclusions and provide alternatives in any given scenario. Explanation requires that the conclusions drawn from the inferences are correct and can be justified. The use of scientific and nursing literature constitutes the basis for clinical justification. For example, if a person complains of increased incidences of asthma in the mornings, the nurse should inquire about a history of heartburn, also known as gastro-oesophageal reflux disease (GORD). There is a documented scientific link between GORD and asthma, in that many consumers who have one condition are likely to have the other, and GORD may make asthma worse.

The **evaluation** process examines the validity of the information and hypothesis to allow the nurse to develop a judgement of the issue. For example, the nurse assesses the incidences of GORD for the individual, and finds that when the GORD is well controlled, their asthma is also less active. Therefore, a goal in controlling their asthma will be to control their GORD as well.

Self-regulation via reflective practice is a key component of the critical-thinking process. During this process, the nurse reflects on the critical-thinking skills that were used and then determines which techniques were effective and which were problematic. After interviewing a consumer, the nurse reflects on whether leading, biased or judgemental questions were asked. The nurse might also reflect on the use of open-ended questions and the effectiveness of an interpreter. The recognition of both positive and negative outcomes is crucial to developing higher-level thinking skills and professional expertise, but is often the most difficult skill to develop without assistance. This is why most professional nursing programs require students to engage with the reflective process and to demonstrate a base level of competency for this skill.

CRITICAL THINKING AND THE NURSING PROCESS

Critical thinking and clinical reasoning are essential for nurses in contemporary health environments. In practice, these skills direct nurses to intervene effectively and at the right time to keep consumers from deteriorating. In most cases, people will have different levels of complexity requiring management; the nurse will need to be able to decide which health problems must be prioritised. In order to do this, the nurse must use critical thinking and clinical reasoning skills to enable safe and effective assessment and prioritisation of health problems. In health care, using frameworks helps standardise this type of thinking and guides decision making to focus on consumer safety.

There are many frameworks for critical thinking used by the healthcare professions. The nursing profession has developed its own unique tool to frame critical thinking: **the nursing process**. The nursing process is described in different ways, such as a four-, five- or six-phased process:

> APIE: Assessment, Planning, Implementation and Evaluation
> ADPIE: Assessment, Diagnosis, Planning, Implementation and Evaluation
> APOPIE: Assessment, Patient problem, Outcomes identification, Planning, Implementation and Evaluation.

In Australia and New Zealand these frameworks are also referred to as clinical reasoning, as they assist practitioners with their critical thinking to apply knowledge for clinical purposes. In this text we are using a simplified process of Assess (including problem identification), Plan, Implement and Evaluate (APIE) as the overarching organising structure to undertake physical examination. Once a beginner nurse has a good understanding of this basic skills framework to assist in the clinical reasoning process, a similar but more advanced approach to explain how clinical reasoning should be approached is useful (see **Figure 1.1**). Decision making, however, is also tied to scope of practice, so please refer to your national competency standards (web links below) as well as your employer's local regulations on scope of practice within the organisation.

> Australia: http://www.nursingmidwiferyboard.gov.au/Codes-Guidelines-Statements.aspx
> New Zealand: http://www.nursingcouncil.org.nz/Nurses/Scopes-of-practice/Registered-nurse

Regardless of which nursing process framework is used, it remains dynamic and uses information in a meaningful way through problem-solving strategies to place the person, family or community in an optimal health state. The primary focus of this text is assessment and what to do with that assessment. Physical, emotional, mental, developmental, **spiritual** and cultural assessments provide the foundation for the other phases of the nursing process.

APIE has been used in this text for the layout of each chapter. It is used to organise the knowledge required and the processes that the nurse will need to apply to implement and evaluate the health assessment and physical examination of patients across the life span. Health assessment and physical examination are the basis for identifying health problems and deciding what nursing actions need to be taken. Levett-Jones et al. (2010) have researched and refined a process that assists nurses to extrapolate the critical thinking and clinical reasoning inherent in the nursing process for applied nursing practice (see **Figure 1.1**).

The clinical reasoning cycle (**Figure 1.1**) is presented here in the broader view, and the APIE way of organising information in each chapter forms the first four parts of the clinical reasoning cycle (e.g. consider the consumer's situation, collect cues/information, process information, identify problems/issues) used in caring for the person. We have used the APIE process to present most of the content in this text, and the clinical reasoning cycle is specifically applied in each chapter that has a consumer case study so you can see application to practice.

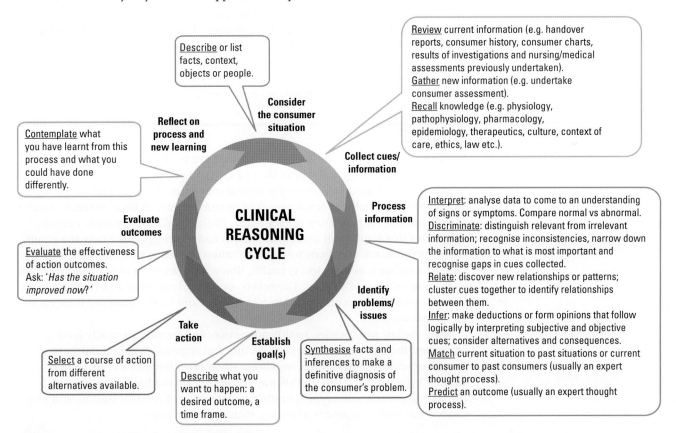

FIGURE 1.1 The clinical reasoning process with descriptors

LEVETT-JONES, T., HOFFMAN, K., DEMPSEY, J., JEONG, S.Y., NOBLE, D., NORTON, C.A., ROCHE, J. & HICKEY, N. (2010). THE 'FIVE RIGHTS' OF CLINICAL REASONING: AN EDUCATIONAL MODEL TO ENHANCE NURSING STUDENTS' ABILITY TO IDENTIFY AND MANAGE CLINICALLY 'AT RISK' PATIENTS. *NURSE EDUCATION TODAY*, 30, 515–20.

CRITICAL THINKING, CULTURAL CONSIDERATIONS FOR HEALTHCARE PRACTICE

Australia and New Zealand have diverse populations; therefore, nurses must be able to apply cultural safety and cultural competence when undertaking health history and physical examination. You will need to apply critical-thinking skills to effectively embed cultural safety in caring for diverse populations, and examine your own cultural identity to cognitively and actively provide culturally safe and appropriate person-centred care. The cultural background of consumers has a significant influence on beliefs about illness and death, and how illness and pain are experienced and expressed. In the health system, it is important that healthcare providers recognise that they hold power over consumers by the very nature of the structure and practice of their roles (Shephard et al., 2019). Being aware of this power helps to mediate the way providers interact with people in their care. Every consumer has the right to safe healthcare provisions that respect their cultural worldview, linguistic diversity, cultural practices and ways of viewing health (Jongen, McCalman & Bainbridge, 2018). This means we need to be aware of and mediate for racial bias.

Racial bias exhibited by health professionals affects the health care of consumers in multiple ways. The research shows 'racial bias at structural, institutional and interpersonal levels' produces healthcare disparities through multiple pathways (Yearby in Jongen et al., 2018: 24). Racial bias occurs in policies, legislation and the allocation of resources within and between institutions, as well as the individual behaviour of health professionals. It affects how people are treated, regarded and even believed. A negative influence of a health provider's racial bias also affects communication and therefore all consumer interactions (Shen et al., 2017). Therefore, there are serious implications not only for consumer–provider interactions but also for treatment decisions and the individual's health outcomes when racial bias goes unexamined and unchecked.

CULTURE

In this textbook we take the approach that **culture** is a learned and socially transmitted orientation and way of life of a group of people. Culture enables members of large groupings of people to find coherence and to survive in the world around them through the development of unique patterns of basic assumptions and shared meanings (Chao, Kung & Yao, 2015). The cultural beliefs, values, customs and norms that result from these assumptions and meanings shape how the group members think, act, and relate to and with others, as well as how they perceive aspects of life such as time, space, health, illness, and family, spousal, parental, work and community-member roles. The beliefs, values and norms of a cultural group are passed informally from one generation to another and exert a powerful force on all group members.

Over the last five decades, healthcare services and providers globally have recognised the vital importance of respecting and responding appropriately to a consumer's culture and cultural worldview when providing health care (World Health Organization, 2020). In this way consumers are not harmed or injured through ignorance, stereotyping or discrimination based on their culture, and they can feel safe and comfortable to engage with and receive care.

Defining cultural competence and cultural safety

In the Australian and New Zealand health contexts, two key approaches that relate to the provision of culturally appropriate person-centred care are cultural competence and cultural safety. These are acknowledged as guides to the provision of safe and equitable healthcare practice and are expanded on in this chapter.

Cultural competence is best defined by Cross et al. (in Jongen et al., 2018: 1) as 'a set of congruent behaviours, attitudes and policies that come together in a system, agency or among professionals that enable the system, agency or profession to work effectively in cross-cultural situations'. This definition is well recognised and applied across the world, as it is inclusive of marginalised minority groups and goes beyond ethnicity and race to encompass the diversity profile. This profile includes gender, age, ability and sexual orientation, as these are all variables that influence a person's culture, worldview and the way they view health and wellbeing. Recent research regarding health differences also recommends that the diversity profile incorporates different language groups and social cultural differences, such as status of education levels (Jongen et al., 2018).

The approach of **cultural safety** as defined by Williams (1999) is the provision of a safe environment that is free from assault and challenge, and accepts an individual's identity and needs. This includes consideration of the physical, mental, social, spiritual and cultural aspects of an individual's wellbeing. The main aim of cultural safety is to respect every individual's culture and beliefs, and to ensure that it is free from discrimination (Australian Human Rights Commission, 2011; CATSINaM, 2016; McGough, Wynaden, Gower, Duggan & Wilson, 2022). The concept of cultural safety is implemented widely in the Australian and New Zealand healthcare sectors, in response to improving the provision of appropriate health care and improved health status of our First Nations peoples. Chapter 4, 'Aboriginal and Torres Strait Islander peoples' health', provides historical and cultural considerations that impact the health and wellbeing of Australian Aboriginal and Torres Strait Islander people today. Providing culturally safe health care is relevant when caring for any person, and means the focus of care is person-centred.

Given these two definitions, providing culturally competent care means to take a culturally safe approach to healthcare provision to ensure that everyone has equitable access to safe and respectful health care, while cultural safety encompasses the approach that a health practitioner should take to each consumer care interaction. What this means, in practice, is to create an environment that is composed of trust, equal power and a genuine partnership. In the next section these two approaches will be explored in more detail and related to the healthcare context and the role of the healthcare professional.

Cultural competence

The approach to cultural competence has shifted and merged to encompass many things over the last five decades. It was originally developed and became a model of social justice born out of the civil rights movement in the USA (Rosenjack Burchum, 2002). This was part of a response to improve health care in minority population groups, who were marginalised through discriminatory policy that created processes and procedures that limited access to basic rights and health care.

In today's society, we continue to witness through popular media the atrocities being carried out by extremist groups or individuals who seek to punish and harm others because of their culture. This portrays a lack of respect for differences in culture, language, faith, geographical location, laws and practices. In Australia and New Zealand, we have diverse individuals from different cultures, who may have fled their homes and nations because of acts of genocide, poverty and more. As a result, they often arrive traumatised, impoverished, and in poor health care (Department of Health, Victoria, 2022). Although it can be challenging, it is important to understand and acknowledge the significance of the impact that discrimination has, particularly if you have not been exposed to being penalised as a consequence of your culture. How we as health professionals care for people in these situations can either extend the trauma and harm they have experienced, or it can make a positive difference and provide a safe healthcare encounter.

Over time, there has been an increased recognition of the need to address issues that go beyond those associated with cultural differences. As a result, the concept of cultural competence has developed to encompass a more inclusive focus on diversity in population groups, with healthcare providers striving to identify and respond to all forms of bias and stereotyping. Identifying biases, redressing historical and ongoing experiences of racism and discrimination, and focusing on the social determinants of health, have all come to be included within the scope of cultural competence (Jongen et al., 2018).

In Australia and New Zealand, cultural competence is a key priority in addressing healthcare inequalities related to access and quality of care for cultural groups (AIHW, 2015). An important point here is that cultural competence cannot be achieved in the short term, or by an individual. Creating a culturally competent healthcare system is a cumulative process: there is not one single step or action that can be taken to accomplish overall cultural competence, nor can a single person's behaviour change the entire system. It requires commitment at all levels – systemic, professional and consumer-care – to change processes and behaviour, in order to create improved healthcare outcomes for everyone (Sherwood & Russell-Mundine, 2017).

Cultural safety

Cultural safety is a concept that builds on cultural competence, with specific relevance for Australia and New Zealand. It was developed in the 1990s from the work of Māori nurse and scholar Irihapeti Ramsden. In cultural safety, the term 'safety' is used because the concept is about preventing the injury that often occurs when a health professional is racist, discriminatory or rude to a consumer. 'Unsafe cultural practice comprises any action that diminishes, demeans or disempowers the cultural identity and wellbeing of an individual' (Nursing Council of New Zealand, 2020). Extreme, but unfortunately not uncommon, examples include cases of Aboriginal people who have died unnecessarily in mainstream healthcare settings, as a result of culturally unsafe health care.

The concept of cultural safety goes beyond the recognition of cultural differences, to acknowledge the circumstances that have historically led to some individuals and groups being marginalised, and aims to recognise the social determinants that affect their health outcomes. This includes, notably, First Nations peoples in both New Zealand and Australia, who suffered personal and institutional marginalisation by new settlers to their countries, but also people with disabilities or mental illness, LGBTQI+ people, and older adults. These are all groups who have been, and in many cases continue to be, marginalised by social institutions. People in these groups have historically not been allowed to fully participate in decision-making processes that affect all aspects of their lives (Richardson, 2015).

Unlike cultural competence, cultural safety is an approach that can be practised by an individual. The pathway to culturally safe person-centred care involves six phases (Dementia Training Australia, 2017; see **Figure 1.2**), and starts with developing personal cultural awareness at an individual level, recognising that there are differences between your own and other cultures, and reflecting on the effects of those differences. It also includes gaining an understanding of another culture, and learning to respond respectfully, with cultural safety the overall aim (National Aboriginal Community Controlled Health Organisation, 2011).

It is important to note that cultural competence and cultural safety go hand in hand. This means that for a consumer to feel culturally safe is also dependent on the nurse being culturally competent (AIDA, 2018). To provide culturally safe and culturally competent nursing care, the nurse must first be willing and able to confront their own cultural biases, or **ethnocentrism**, and stereotyping, to whatever extent they exist. Nurses then need to examine the impact these biases may have on the consumer, with an intention to adjust their future interactions and practice.

Five essential elements contribute to your ability to become more culturally safe:

1. Reflect on your own practice.
2. Seek to minimise power differentials.
3. Engage in discourse with the patient.

4. Undertake a process of decolonisation.
5. Ensure that you do not diminish, demean or disempower others through your actions (Best, 2018).

It is also important to note that whether nursing practice is culturally safe or unsafe is determined by the person or family who is receiving care. Knowing how to deal with one individual or group in a culturally safe manner does not mean you are automatically able to do so with another group or in another context; it needs to be taken on a case-by-case basis, with awareness of the specific needs of the person/group you are providing care for. These considerations for cultural safety and how this impacts the nurses' behaviours are very important for comprehensive and effective health assessment and physical examination.

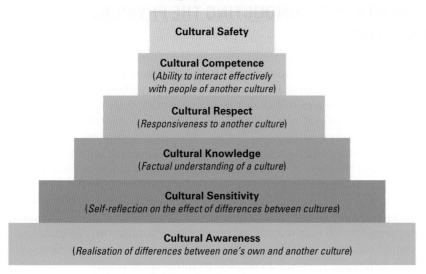

FIGURE 1.2 The pathway to culturally safe person-centred care

DTA (FEBRUARY 2017). CULTURAL ASSESSMENT FOR ABORIGINAL AND TORRES STRAIT ISLANDER PEOPLE WITH DEMENTIA GUIDE FOR HEALTH PROFESSIONALS. DEMENTIA TRAINING AUSTRALIA. RETRIEVED FROM: WWW.DEMENTIATRAININGAUSTRALIA.COM.AU.

ASSESSMENT: TAKING THE PATIENT'S HEALTH HISTORY

Assessment is the first phase of the nursing process, and in this text also includes identifying consumer problem areas to focus on. It is the orderly collection of information concerning the individual's health status using the health history and identifying areas for opportunistic health promotion.

The health history interview is a means of gathering **subjective data**, usually from the individual or, in the case of children (or adults unable to answer questions), close family members. This data is subjective in that it cannot always be verified by an independent observer. Subjective data includes what the person says, and is regarded as the person's attitudes and beliefs. In some instances, however, this information can be validated during the physical examination; for instance, the existence of an individual's self-reported breast lump may be confirmed through palpation.

The health history can also be obtained from sources other than the person. Relatives and friends can provide insightful data for the health history. In some instances, bystanders may be the only source of information; for example, in the case of a severe trauma in which the individual is unconscious. The consumer's old charts or medical records are additional sources of information, as are healthcare colleagues. The nurse can and should use every available medium to gather as much information about the person as possible. The health history is further discussed in Chapter 3. However, you must remember that in most cases the consumer is the primary source of information for good reason, as others around them will only be able to provide information through their own biases, perceptions and motivations, which can at times not be as accurate as consumer-held data.

PLANNING FOR PHYSICAL EXAMINATION

Planning (including goal setting) is the second phase in the nursing process and in this text refers to evaluating subjective data collected during the health history in order to narrow the focus for the collection of physical examination data. Within the planning phase, the nurse considers what additional objective data needs to be collected or validated. Planning for a successful physical examination requires consideration of the environment and equipment required. Throughout the text you will find checklists to use in planning for the physical examination specific to the body system focused on in each chapter.

IMPLEMENTATION: CONDUCTING THE PHYSICAL EXAMINATION

The third phase in the nursing process is **implementation**. In this phase, the nurse executes physical examination based on the health history, using clinical reasoning to progress through the assessment. Within this section of the text, skills for physical examination are outlined within a framework specific to the chapter focus (e.g. inspection, palpation, percussion, auscultation), along with normal and abnormal findings. Where appropriate, further information to support advanced examination is provided and highlighted. As some techniques fall outside the scope of many Registered Nurses (e.g. anal Pap testing) in Australia and New Zealand, they are included as online resources.

Implementation is a dynamic process. The nurse is continually interacting with the consumer or family, during the examination. During this time, new information may be uncovered which may reshape the focus of the examination. The nurse will use clinical reasoning to determine the inclusion or exclusion of specific examination techniques to ensure a complete picture is constructed.

Physical examination findings

Physical examination findings constitute the second means of obtaining information (or collecting cues/information) used in the clinical reasoning cycle. Physical examination findings constitute **objective data**, or information that is observable and measurable and can be verified by more than one person. This data is obtained using the senses of smell, touch, sight and hearing. This text describes the systematic approach and level of foundation to advanced physical examination techniques that will elicit this data (see Chapters 6–20).

Physical examination data can be obtained in a body system or head-to-toe approach. Table 1.3 lists the body systems that are examined. Other approaches to physical examination exist, such as Gordon's Functional Health Patterns, which group human behaviours into 11 patterns that facilitate nursing care (Gordon, 2006). Table 1.4 lists the **functional health patterns**. This text, however, uses the head-to-toe, body systems approach for physical examination, as this is a very common approach in most clinical contexts.

Diagnostic and laboratory data

The final information that needs to be gathered in collecting data/information is any diagnostic and laboratory data that is relevant to the consumer's complaint. Results of blood and urine samples, cultures, X-rays, and various diagnostic procedures constitute objective data, which further contribute to understanding the consumer's overall health status. The collection of some of this data cannot be initiated by the nurse and may require an order by the medical officer (depending on the scope of practice of the nurse).

It is imperative that the nurse documents all the examination findings. The written record is a legal requirement used to chart the consumer's current health status. Chapters 3 and 22 discuss documentation and cover the legal issues of the

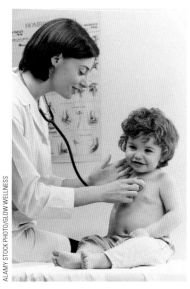

FIGURE 1.3 Physical examination is one component of building a comprehensive picture of the patient's health status.

TABLE 1.3 Body system examination

1.	General survey, vital signs and pain
2.	Mental status and neurological techniques
3.	Integumentary
4.	Head, neck and regional lymphatics
5.	Eyes
6.	Ears, nose, mouth and throat
7.	Breasts and regional nodes
8.	Respiratory
9.	Cardiovascular
10.	Gastrointestinal
11.	Musculoskeletal
12.	Genitourinary

TABLE 1.4 Gordon's Functional Health Patterns

1.	Health perception–health management pattern
2.	Nutritional–metabolic pattern
3.	Elimination pattern
4.	Activity–exercise pattern
5.	Sleep–rest pattern
6.	Cognitive–perceptual pattern
7.	Self-perception–self-concept pattern
8.	Role–relationship pattern
9.	Sexuality–reproductive pattern
10.	Coping–stress-tolerance pattern
11.	Value–belief pattern

SOURCE: *MANUAL OF NURSING DIAGNOSIS* (11TH ED.), BY M. GORDON, 2006, SUDBURY, MA: JONES AND BARTLETT.

health record. The documented health assessment and physical examination also serves as a means of communicating information to other healthcare colleagues. It is often valued over other forms of communication by clinicians and is a key contributor to safety.

EVALUATION OF HEALTH ASSESSMENT AND PHYSICAL EXAMINATION FINDINGS

Evaluation is the final phase of the nursing process. In this text we have used evaluation to draw together all information collected during the health assessment and physical examination to identify what needs to occur next. Within Chapters 6–20, the documentation and evaluation of a consumer case study pertinent to the chapter content is provided to enable you to determine how information can be grouped and documented. At the end of the case study, documented information is presented in a section titled 'Evaluation and clinical reasoning for case study'. Within this section the specific data is linked to processing information as described in the clinical reasoning cycle (see **Figure 1.1**) by interpreting, discriminating, relating, inferring, matching and at times predicting. The synthesis of the data that informs clinical reasoning specific to the consumer and their context is then discussed.

Putting it all together

It is here that we highlight the clinical reasoning that would accompany the collection of information and possible actions required, in order to address priority patient needs or prepare goals for consumers and health teams to achieve. These phases are indicated with the headings of Consider the consumer situation, Collect cues/information, Process information and Identify problems/issues in these consumer case studies. Examples of what the nurse would 'do' with this information next are listed and prioritised.

A **nursing-related consumer problem** requires the nurse to work with the consumer to develop and implement interventions that do not need other disciplines. The nurse needs to ensure they remain within their scope of practice in undertaking interventions that are nursing initiated.

A **collaborative consumer problem** requires the nurse to work jointly with the specialist doctor and other healthcare workers in monitoring, planning and implementing person-centred care (**Figure 1.4**). Some consumer problems are not

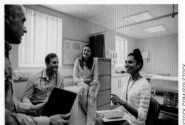

ISTOCK.COM/SOLSTOCK

FIGURE 1.4 Nurses may collaborate with social workers, specialist doctors and other members of the healthcare team to maximise person-centred care.

completely within the domain of the nurse's scope of practice and therefore require the nurse to collaborate with other healthcare team members. For instance, the consumer experiencing cardiac tamponade (medical level problem) with decreased cardiac output and anxiety (nursing level problem) needs immediate nursing and medical attention. The nurse is not ethically or legally permitted to do all that the situation requires to alleviate the tamponade; the nurse, specialist doctor/nurse practitioner, and healthcare team will work collaboratively to relieve the problem.

Prioritisation for consumer acuity

The nurse identifies actual and potential patient problems and opportunities for health promotion that are derived from the **clustering** of data. When there is more than one health problem, the nurse must determine which problem(s) is/are the most vital to the individual's wellbeing at that particular time; this is called prioritisation. It is necessary to **prioritise**, or rank, the importance of each health problem and to do this accurately over time. Critical-thinking and clinical-reasoning skills must be applied systematically. When possible, the patient should assist the nurse with the prioritisation of needs. Individuals who are actively involved with the decision-making process are more likely to be amenable to nursing care, to assist with their care, and to be agreeable to the plan of care.

A theoretical framework that can be used to prioritise nursing diagnoses is Maslow's Hierarchy of Needs (**Figure 1.5**). According to Maslow, basic needs such as food and oxygen take priority over all other issues. **Consumer acuity** is a term used to describe how unwell a person is or how urgent their healthcare needs are: the sicker the person, the higher their acuity (it is also used to predict how many people are needed to be able to provide safe care for the person's acuity level) (DiClemente, 2018). For example, the person experiencing a myocardial infarction is seen as high acuity and must have their physiological needs met before safety needs are attended to. In some instances, however, a person's needs may not follow Maslow's hierarchy, or they may change over time, requiring reprioritisation of the health problem. The person with terminal breast cancer may be more concerned with playing with their children than staying well hydrated. Some problems are equally important and can be prioritised at the same level. The nurse, in conjunction with the consumer and their family, is continually re-evaluating and revising the priority of the problems.

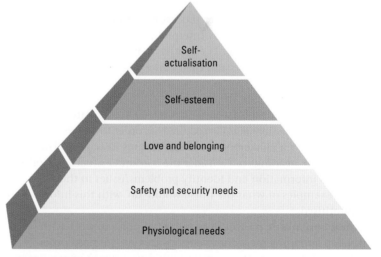

FIGURE 1.5 Maslow's Hierarchy of Needs
ADAPTATION BASED ON MASLOW'S HIERARCHY OF NEEDS.

Evidence-based practice

There is an imperative in health care for evidence-based practice. No longer are healthcare practices being implemented 'because they have always been done that way'; nor are they being enacted intuitively. Rather, evidence-based practice uses the outcomes of well-designed and well-executed scientific studies to guide clinical decision making and clinical care. For example, the use of wound-care dressings and interventions for chronic wounds in people with peripheral arterial disease has undergone drastic changes in the last 10 years. Within the health assessment and physical examination, an example of using evidence to guide practice may be that we now ask individuals about their intention to quit smoking instead of just advising them that they should. Research into behaviour changes identifies that linking consumer intentions to desired behaviour engages individuals in their care more than just providing information or advice. The ultimate goal of evidence-based practice is to assist the person's quality of life by improving outcomes. It remains the nurse's own responsibility to ensure currency with evidence.

CLINICAL (OR CRITICAL) PATHWAYS

Clinical pathways affect how and when we assess a consumer's health status. Clinical pathways are used as a cost-effective, high-quality patient care delivery system. Clinical pathways or maps show the outcome of predetermined consumer health goals over a period of time; that is, they state what activity the person should be capable of performing daily, on the basis of the consumer's Diagnostic-Related Grouping (DRG). The critical incidents, or most crucial nursing interventions for each step of the pathway, are delineated.

One of the advantages of clinical pathways is the early recognition of variances from expected health outcomes. Once the variance is identified, nurses, in collaboration with other healthcare team members, plan and implement specific interventions to deal with the variance. Evaluation is performed daily and, although the terminology is different, clinical pathways incorporate the assessment, planning, implementation and evaluation phases of the nursing process.

CHAPTER RESOURCES

REFERENCES

Australian Human Rights Commission. (2011). Social Justice report 2011. Chapter 4: Cultural safety and security: Tools to address lateral violence. Retrieved from https://humanrights.gov.au/our-work/chapter-4-cultural-safety-and-security-tools-address-lateral-violence-social-justice

Australian Indigenous Doctors' Association (AIDA). (2018). Cultural Safety Factsheet. Retrieved from https://www.aida.org.au/wp-content/uploads/2015/03/Cultural-Safety-Factsheet1.pdf

Australian Institute of Health and Welfare (AIHW). (2015). Cultural competency in the delivery of health services for Indigenous people. Retrieved 26 March 2018 from https://www.aihw.gov.au/reports/indigenous-australians/cultural-competency-in-the-delivery-ofhealth-services-for-indigenous-people/contents/table-of-contents

Best, O. (2018). Chapter 3 The cultural safety journey: An Aboriginal Australian nursing and midwifery context. In O. Best & B. Fredericks (Eds.). *Yatdjuligin: Aboriginal and Torres Strait Islander Nursing and Midwifery Care*, (2nd ed), pp. 58–61. Cambridge University Press.

CATSINaM. (2016). Congress of Aboriginal and Torres Strait Islander Nurses and Midwives: https://www.catsinam.org.au/

Chao, M. M., Kung, F. Y. H., & Yao, D. J. (2015). Understanding the divergent effects of multicultural exposure. *International Journal of Intercultural Relations*, 47, 78–88. doi: 10.1016/j.ijintrel.2015.03.032

Cross, T. L., Bazron, B. J., Dennis, K. W., & Isaacs, M. R. (1989). Towards a culturally competent system of care: A monograph on effective service for minority children who are severely emotionally disturbed. Georgetown University, Child Development Center, Washington, DC.

Dementia Training Australia. (2017). Cultural Assessment for Aboriginal and Torres Strait Islander People with Dementia Guide for Health Professionals. Retrieved from https//:www.dementiatrainingaustralia.com.au

Department of Health, Victoria. (2022). Refugee and asylum seeker health and wellbeing. https://www.health.vic.gov.au/populations/refugee-and-asylum-seeker-health-and-wellbeing

DiClemente, K. (2018). Standardizing patient acuity: A project on a medical-surgical/cancer care unit. *Medsurg Nursing, 27*(6), 355. Retrieved from https://ezproxy.cqu.edu.au/login?url=https://www.proquest.com/

scholarly-journals/standardizing-patient-acuity-project-on-medical/docview/2159928006/se-2?accountid=10016

Elder, L., & Paul, R. (2010). *Universal intellectual standards*. Retrieved 31 October 2011 from http://www.criticalthinking.org

Elder, L., & Paul, R. (2013). Critical thinking: Intellectual standards essential to reasoning well within every domain of thought. *Journal of Developmental Education, 36*(3), 34–5.

Gonzalez, L. (2018). Teaching clinical reasoning piece by piece: A clinical reasoning concept-based learning method. *Journal of Nursing Education, 57*(12), 727–35. doi:10.3928/01484834-20181119-05

Gordon, M. (2006). *Manual of nursing diagnosis* (11th ed.). Sudbury, MA: Jones and Bartlett.

Hassani, P., Abdi, A., Jalali, R., & Salari, N. (2020). The perception of intuition in clinical practice by Iranian critical care nurses: a phenomenological study. *Psychology Research and Behavior Management*, 31–9. http://dx.doi.org.ezproxy.cqu.edu.au/10.2147/PRBM.S101040

Jongen, C., McCalman, J., & Bainbridge, R. (2018). Health workforce cultural competency interventions: a systematic scoping review. *BMC Health Services Research, 18*(1), 232. https://doi.org/10.1186/s12913-018-3001-5

Levett-Jones, T., Hoffman, K., Dempsey, J., Jeong, S. Y., Noble, D., Norton, C. A., Roche, J., & Hickey, N. (2010). The 'five rights' of clinical reasoning: An educational model to enhance nursing students' ability to identify and manage clinically 'at risk' patients. *Nurse Education Today, 30*, 515–20. https://doi: 10.1016/j.nedt.2009.10.020

McGough, S., Wynaden, D., Gower, S., Duggan, R., & Wilson, R. (2022). There is no health without cultural safety: why cultural safety matters. *Contemporary Nurse*. doi: 10.1080/10376178.2022.2027254

Miller, E. M., & Hill, P. D. (2018). Intuition in clinical decision making. Differences among practicing nurses. *Journal of Holistic Nursing, 36*(4), 318–29. doi: 10.1177/0898010117725428

National Aboriginal Community Controlled Health Organisation (NACCHO). (2011). Creating the NACCHO Cultural Safety Training Standards: A background paper. 2011. Retrieved from http://www.naccho.org.au/promote-health/cultural-safety/

Nursing Council of New Zealand. (2020). https://www.nursingcouncil.org.nz/Public/Treaty_of_Waitangi/NCNZ/About-section/Te_Tiriti_o_Waitangi.aspx?hkey=36e3b0b6-da14-4186-bf0a-720446b56c52

Paul, R., & Elder, L. (1997, March 1). *Helping students assess their thinking*. Retrieved 31 March 2023 from https://www.criticalthinking.org/pages/open-minded-inquiry/579

Raymond, A., Porter, J. E., Missen, K., Larkins, J., de Vent, K., & Redpath, S. (2018). The meaning of 'worried' in MET call activations: A regional hospital examination of the clinical indicator. *Collegian, 26*, 378–82. https://doi.org/10.1016/j.colegn.2018.11.002

Richardson, F. (2015). An introduction to inclusive practice. In *Inclusive practice for health professionals* (pp. 2–22). Oxford University Press. https://global.oup.com/academic/product/inclusive-practice-for-health-professionals-9780195593952?cc=au&lang=en&

Rosenjack Burchum, J. L. (2002). Cultural competence: an evolutionary perspective. *Nursing Forum, 37*(4), 5–15. doi:10.1111/j.1744-6198.2002.tb01287.x

Shen, M. J., Peterson, E. B., Costas-Muñiz, R., Hernandez, M. H., Jewell, S. T., Matsoukas, K., & Bylund, C, L. (2018). The effects of race and racial concordance on patient-physician communication: A systematic review of the literature. *Journal of Racial and Ethnic Health Disparities, 5*, 117–40. https://doi.org/10.1007/s40615-017-0350-4

Shepherd, S. M., Willis-Esqueda, C., Newton, D., Sivasubramaniam, D., & Paradies, Y. (2019). The challenge of cultural competence in the workplace: perspectives of healthcare providers. *BMC Health Services Research, 19*, 135. https://doi.org/10.1186/s12913-019-3959-7

Sherwood, J., & Russell-Mundine, G. (2017). How we do business: Setting the agenda for cultural competence at the University of Sydney. In J. Frawley, S. Larkin, & J. A. Smith (Eds.), *Indigenous pathways, Transitions and participation in higher education: from policy to practice* (pp. 133–50). Singapore: Springer.

Turan, N., Özdemir Aydın, G., Özsaban, A., Kaya, H., Aksel, G., Yılmaz, A., Hasmaden, E., & Akkuş, Y. (2019). Intuition and emotional intelligence: A study in nursing students. *Cogent Psychology, 6*(1). https://doi.org/10.1080/23311908.2019.1633077

Wilkinson, J. M. (2007). *Nursing process and critical thinking* (4th ed.). Upper Saddle River, NJ: Pearson Prentice Hall.

World Health Organization. (2020). WHO recommends considering cultural factors to develop more inclusive health systems. Retrieved 20 June 2022 from https://www.who.int/news-room/feature-stories/detail/who-recommends-considering-cultural-factors-to-develop-more-inclusive-health-systems

CHAPTER **2**

CHAPTER **2**

THE HEALTH CONSUMER INTERVIEW APPROACHES INCORPORATING DEVELOPMENTAL CONSIDERATIONS

LEARNING OUTCOMES

By the end of this chapter you should be able to:

1 identify key considerations required for undertaking a consumer health assessment interview
2 explain the nurse's role in assessing spiritual needs during the health interview and care encounters
3 describe personal perceptions that facilitate or hinder the interview process
4 describe effective and ineffective interviewing techniques to use in the consumer interview
5 explain key considerations for undertaking the health assessment interview for the consumer with special needs
6 incorporate appropriate developmental theories and developmental tools associated with each life stage into a consumer's health assessment.

BACKGROUND

The nursing health assessment interview is a purposeful, time-limited verbal interaction between the nurse and the consumer, completed on admission or first contact and updated with any consumer change. It is initiated to collect specific information regarding the consumer and to explore health status. Other purposes include validating appropriate health and illness information presented by the consumer, and identifying the individual's knowledge of personal health. The nurse should also take into consideration the consumer's culture, inclusive of spiritual and religious orientation, to deliver appropriate person-centred care. Accurate and complete information gained from the health assessment interview, serves as a foundation for subsequent interactions and nursing and medical interventions. The nurse–consumer interaction requires skill in interviewing techniques, which the nurse learns and refines over time.

Assessing the growth and development status of consumers, adults as well as children, is an integral part of the health assessment. All individuals, from birth to death, pass through identifiable, cyclical stages of growth and development that determine who they are. **Growth** refers to an increase in body size and function to the point of optimum maturity. **Development** refers to patterned and predictable increases in the physical, cognitive, psychosocial and moral capacities of individuals that enable them to successfully adapt to their environment. It must be noted that although most development is patterned and predictable, you should not impose expected patterns on a particular consumer; it is important to assess them as an individual (Lissauer & Carroll, 2022).

THE CONSUMER INTERVIEW

The nursing health assessment interview can be differentiated from the more traditional medically orientated interview. The medical interview typically focuses on the physical or emotional state, while the nursing interview is more holistic in nature and includes comprehensive information about the person. The nursing interview includes an assessment of the physical, mental, emotional, developmental, social, cultural and spiritual aspects of the person. Data is collected about the person's present and past states of health, including their family status and relationships, cultural background, lifestyle preferences and developmental level. Other factors considered in data collection are the person's self-concept, spiritual and religious affiliation, social supports, burden of care, sexuality and reproductive processes. Remember, the health assessment interview is a goal-directed interview. It is not a social interaction.

The nurse

The nurse is often the first person from the healthcare team to interact with the consumer and assumes the role of intermediary to the larger healthcare system. The nurse sets the stage for the interview and can affect the individual's healthcare experience and outcome. First impressions of individuals are important and imprint long-lasting thoughts and feelings.

The nurse is the facilitator of the interview and thus collaborates with the consumer in establishing a mutually respectful dialogue. Encouraging the consumer to speak freely and express any concerns is essential in this process. For example, if the consumer thinks that no one in the healthcare setting understands their concerns and feelings, they will likely say very little. The consumer must feel comfortable and safe enough to provide information, to ask questions, and to express fears or concerns. Accurate data collection is the primary purpose of the health assessment interview. The nurse can foster an atmosphere of safety and comfort by approaching each consumer with an accepting, respectful and non-judgemental attitude.

REFLECTION IN PRACTICE

Initial consumer impression
An 18-year-old mother with her 12-month-old child comes to the community health clinic. You are the nurse caring for them and note they are dishevelled, their clothes are dirty, and both have offensive-smelling body odour. What might your initial perception of the mother and child be? How might this affect the consumer interview?

The consumer

The consumer should be an active and equal participant in the health interview process and should feel free to openly communicate thoughts, feelings, perceptions and factual information. Most consumers possess previous knowledge of or experience with healthcare interactions that influences their current perceptions and behaviour. Understanding how individuals see their role in healthcare contexts is vital to the successful completion of any health interview. In today's healthcare context, consumers are more active in their care and healthcare decisions. Consumers are much more apt to question healthcare providers, to treat themselves, and to demand an active role in decision making.

In some situations, an individual's passivity is the norm in health care, and exploring and understanding their culture (Chapters 1 and 4), spiritual and religious orientation will assist in encouraging involvement in the interview, to ensure provision of person-centred care. A consumer's spiritual and religious beliefs can influence whether or not they will accept or decline health care (e.g. whether a consumer will agree to take medication, surgery, follow a special diet or execute an advanced health directive) and this may also impact on their healthcare outcomes. Nurses should seek to identify what the consumer's religious and spiritual beliefs are so that a comprehensive understanding of their perspective is attained. Ignorance of a consumer's spiritual and religious beliefs and practices will hamper complete, **holistic nursing** that is person-centred care.

In Australia and New Zealand, people are free to practise any religion they choose, or they may choose to have no religious affiliation. Australia is considered a religious country, with 60% of the population belonging to an organised religion (Australian Bureau of Statistics, 2021). In New Zealand almost 52% of the population identifies with an organised religion (Statistics New Zealand, 2020). First Nations peoples in Australia and New Zealand have their own spiritual belief systems; however, with European settlement and the presence of Christian missionaries in these communities, many Indigenous people converted to Christianity. However, it is important to recognise that many Aboriginal and Torres Strait Islander peoples often practise both belief systems simultaneously (Skye, 2006).

CLINICAL REASONING

Practice tip: Belief systems that may pose a risk to consumer care

> When a consumer's spiritual or religious beliefs are assessed as possibly harmful, the healthcare provider needs to employ a careful and considered approach. Showing respect for the consumer's right to his or her own belief system is still appropriate.

> Consumers should not be separated from visitors who support these difficult beliefs, although visitors, even families, may need to be separated and have selected visiting times in order to decrease conflict.

> Nurses should avoid becoming upset with consumers and visitors who hold different beliefs that may interrupt or require care to be adjusted, or who may even refuse certain aspects of care. A hospital chaplain may help to mediate and assist the consumer and healthcare team to work through the concerns.

> If the consumer has religious or spiritual beliefs that may pose a risk to them, it is appropriate to notify the nursing supervisor or treating medical doctor, and possibly obtain an ethics committee consultation to discuss the treatment plan.

> When a child's health is being harmed by the parents' religious and spiritual beliefs, it is appropriate to invoke the overarching requirements in your area about mandatory reporting of possible child abuse. Such reporting will ensure legal representation for the child and move the discussion to the legal realm.

REFLECTION IN PRACTICE

Religious practices influencing care provided to a young child

A 3-year-old child arrives at the emergency department by ambulance. The child was involved in a car accident, and has sustained extensive trauma to the face, as a result of being thrown through the windscreen. The father accompanies the child in the ambulance, and informs the paramedics that they are Jehovah's Witnesses and, thus, do not permit blood transfusions. You are given this information on the consumer's arrival. The child's blood pressure drops from 80/40 to 50/20. You are asked to call the blood bank for two units of blood.

> How would you respond to this request?
> Do your religious beliefs conflict with this family's beliefs?
> If you feel you cannot assist with the blood resuscitation against the wishes of the father, would you feel comfortable asking a co-worker to step in for you?
> What is your institution's policy?

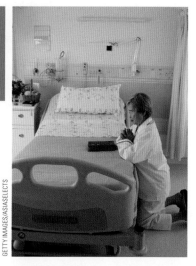

FIGURE 2.1 Religion in a hospital setting

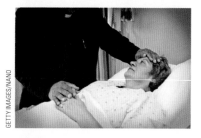

FIGURE 2.2 Rituals such as the sacrament of the Anointing of the Sick are important expressions of religious belief.

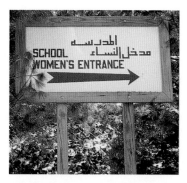

FIGURE 2.3 Awareness of cultural and religious norms and customs will help you deliver appropriate nursing care. Islam separates the sexes in many aspects of public life, as illustrated here.

REFLECTION IN PRACTICE

Refusal of health care – Organ donation recipient
A consumer has end-stage heart disease and will die unless she receives a heart transplant. However, your consumer's religious beliefs forbid her from accepting any blood or organ donation. The consumer tells you she would rather go home once she is stable.
> What are your thoughts about this consumer's decision and situation?
> How would you respond to this consumer's request?

The nurse's role in assessing a consumer's spiritual needs

Almost all religions attempt to explain why human beings suffer from illness and death, and how a higher power can affect healing (**Figure 2.1**). Nurses have a responsibility to attempt to understand various religious and spiritual practices, so they can provide competent person-centred care. For example, a Muslim consumer may ask which direction is west, in order to pray facing Mecca. A Catholic may refuse to enter the operating room, even for life-saving surgery, until they have received the rite of Anointing of the Sick (**Figure 2.2**). A Buddhist may pace and pray. An Orthodox consumer may wish to be able to see an icon from her bed.

When assessing health history, keep in mind that the consumer's lifestyle may raise spiritual and religious issues for the person. For example, the consumer may reveal a requirement for a vegetarian diet (Hindu, New Age), or a history of circumcision (Jews), or the fact that his or her hair has never been cut (women: Orthodox Jews; men: Sikhs). Another consumer may reveal that he or she is estranged from family, due to conversion to a different, even conflicting, religious or spiritual belief, or a rejection of the religious or spiritual belief of the family of origin.

The nurse must be aware of not stereotyping a consumer or jumping to conclusions, based on their past experiences. Don't assume that a holy book on the table means that the consumer is a devout believer. The book may have been left there by a family member or friend, distributed by a missionary group, or donated by a well-meaning volunteer. Additionally, the absence of a holy book does not mean the consumer is not spiritual or religious, as some religions (Unitarian, New Age) do not have holy books. Furthermore, many self-identified members of religious faiths do not follow the teachings of their own religions. A Jew may eat pork, for example; a Jehovah's Witness may accept a blood transfusion, and a Catholic may request birth control. Some consumers who are **atheists** may want to return to the religion of their youth in a time of crisis. Many consumers may blend elements of one religion with those of another religion or spiritual belief. A good understanding of religious and spiritual practices is important, and an understanding of your consumer's specific beliefs is crucial when undertaking the health assessment interview (**Figure 2.3**).

It is important that nurses make their consumers feel comfortable to practise their religion and spirituality, as appropriate. Without overt permission, some reluctant consumers can feel overwhelmed by unfamiliar healthcare environments or by their medical treatment regimen, and may forgo prayers or rituals that might bring them profound relief at a time of crisis. Giving permission also shows respect for consumers' beliefs. However, due to real obstacles to religious and spiritual practices in the healthcare context, the nurse may need to be creative about finding ways to provide the most appropriate care to the consumer while still respecting their religious and spiritual needs.

CLINICAL **REASONING**

Ensuring respect for individuals' beliefs – Actions to avoid

It is important to show respect for your consumers' religious and spiritual beliefs. The following actions are considered disrespectful and should be avoided.

> Do not publicise your own spiritual beliefs. You may share beliefs if the issue comes up, but it is never appropriate to try to convert the consumer to another set of beliefs.

> Do not instruct the consumer in religious or spiritual doctrine. In a time of spiritual distress, a consumer needs support, not instruction. Let the religious or spiritual leader take the lead in any instruction that is required, and follow nursing interventions that will enhance spiritual wellbeing.

> Do not perform the function of a spiritual adviser for the consumer. You and the consumer may become confused about your role.

> Do not respond to the consumer with clichés. Well-known and overused clichés such as 'no sense crying over spilt milk' or 'there's always someone else around who's worse off than you' are inappropriate because they tend to blame or diminish the anguish of the consumer. Clichés about religion, such as 'God helps those who help themselves' or 'it was God's will', are just as inappropriate, because they are patronising and tend to trivialise both the sufferer's problems and the sufferer's religion. Additionally, most well-known religious clichés are based on Western Judaeo-Christian culture and have no bearing on those with other religious or spiritual beliefs. Respond instead with real, heartfelt words or, in some cases, with silence or with touch, if appropriate.

> Avoid taking on the role of spiritual adviser, spiritual healer, minister, priest, teacher, guru and so on. Utilise instead the consumer's pastor, imam, priest or minister, or spiritual support systems, family or the healthcare institutional chaplain to fill that role.

General approach to planning for the health assessment interview

Preparing for the interview

1. Gather all available consumer information.
2. Seek out an appropriate setting for the interview.
3. Set aside a block of time for the interview.
4. Assess your emotional readiness in preparation for undertaking the interview.
5. Begin the interview with a friendly introduction.
   - Introduce yourself by name and title.
   - Call the consumer by formal name, for example 'Mr' or 'Mrs Adams', unless you are asked otherwise. If asked to call the consumer by their first name, you should comply as this will assist in helping the consumer feel less awkward and improve the building of rapport, as long as the nurse continues to respect cultural, spiritual, personal and professional boundaries.

ASSESSMENT **IN BRIEF**

Interviewing considerations

> Be aware of personal beliefs (including cultural and spiritual) and how these were acquired.

> Avoid imposing your beliefs on those you interview and practise a culturally safe approach.

> Listen and observe. Attend to verbal and affective content as well as to nonverbal cues.

> Keep your attention focused on the consumer and use active listening skills.

> Maintain eye contact with the consumer as is appropriate for the consumer's culture.

> Notice the consumer's speech patterns and any recurring themes or issues. Note any extra emphasis that the consumer places on certain words or topics.

> Do not assume that you understand the meaning of all consumer communications. Clarify frequently.

> Paraphrase and summarise occasionally to help consumers organise their thinking, clarify issues, and begin to explore specific concerns more deeply.

> Allow for periods of silence.

> Remember that attitudes and feelings may be conveyed nonverbally.

> Consistently monitor your reactions to the consumer's verbal and nonverbal messages.

> Avoid being judgemental or critical.

> Avoid the use of nontherapeutic interviewing techniques.

Considerations for interviewing

Considerations that need to be recognised prior to the interview commencing are discussed in the next section. Establishing and addressing the consumer's comfort level is a key consideration before commencing.

Environment

The setting for the interview has a direct influence on the amount and quality of information gathered (see **Figure 2.4**). Whenever possible, the interview should be conducted in a private room with controlled lighting and temperature. When a private setting is impossible, control the environment to minimise distractions and interruptions, and to increase the comfort level of the consumer. Utilise any physical barriers available in the room to provide as much privacy as possible. When all efforts to ensure even minimal privacy fail, conduct a shortened interview to gather only immediately pertinent information. Defer the complete interview until a later time (if possible) when privacy can be ensured.

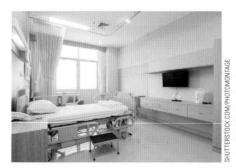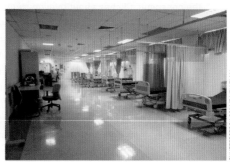

SHUTTERSTOCK.COM/PHOTOMONTAGE

SHUTTERSTOCK.COM/ZAIRIAZMAL

FIGURE 2.4 Environment can have an impact on the consumer interview

Commencing an interview

Prior to approaching the consumer, gather all available consumer information, admission data and past medical records, as this will significantly influence the time needed for the interview. Begin the interview with an introduction, including your name and position. Initially call the consumer by his or her formal name and ask how they would prefer to be addressed. Simple communication utilising appropriate names is respectful, and helps identify individuals as unique persons at a time when they may be feeling quite anxious and vulnerable.

Providing the consumer with an explanation of what is to follow and an approximate time frame for the interview helps in establishing trust. This information also helps to increase the consumer's feeling of control. The more effective you are in establishing trust, the easier it will be to obtain information from the consumer (Stein-Parbury, 2021), for example: 'Good morning, Mrs Liddle, my name is Erin Little. I'm a registered nurse. I'd like to ask you some questions about your health situation today.'

Confidentiality

Confidentiality is essential in developing trust between the nurse and the consumer. The consumer's willingness to communicate private and personal information is predicated on the assumption that this information will be used with discretion and for their benefit (Stein-Parbury, 2021). Your verbal assurance of confidentiality often eases the consumer's concerns, and fosters trust in the relationship. In practice, there are certain exceptions to maintaining absolute confidentiality. (Refer to Chapter 3 for further details.)

For example, in a teaching hospital in which a team approach is used, information must be shared. Another important reason for sharing confidential information is when the consumer is at risk to self or others. Nurses need to be familiar with the policies of their institution, as well as legal statutes on consumer confidentiality and the consequences of not adhering to them. It is essential to inform the consumer prior to the interview when information will be shared with others. Frequently, consumers may have friends or family members with them. To ensure consumer comfort and confidentiality, ask the consumer whether these people should remain in the room for the interview, although you should try not to do this in front of these people where possible as the consumer may feel pressured to elect to allow them to stay. Be sure to review your professional code of conduct and code of ethics, as consumer confidentiality and privacy are outlined in these regulations.

Further information about confidentiality is available from the Australian Commission on Safety and Quality in Health Care, the Human Rights Commission in New Zealand, and the Nursing and Midwifery Board Australia (including the endorsed International Council of Nurses code of ethics for nurses) and Nursing Council of New Zealand (code of conduct).

REFLECTION IN PRACTICE

Breaking confidentiality in the emergency department (ED)

A 22-year-old male presents to the ED and reveals to you that his extensive physical injuries are the result of an assault. He asks you not to share this information with anyone because he is fearful of retribution. A police officer attends and requests information from you about the consumer and his injuries. What is your immediate reaction to this disclosure? What is your institution's policy concerning confidentiality? What are your responsibilities in this situation?

Strategies to support accurate and timely documentation

During the health assessment interview, it is advisable to jot down (or enter into the electronic health record) information as you proceed, although you should be aware that the simple act of noting what the consumer says may cause some discomfort (Figure 2.5). Early in the interview, explain the necessity of noting pertinent information and where this will be stored. Frequently, the consumer will lead the interview or discuss sensitive issues. When this occurs, give full attention to them and defer formal recording of information. Ensure you review Chapter 3 for more information about documentation.

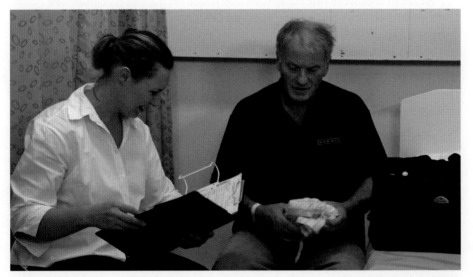

FIGURE 2.5 The consumer interview often requires note taking. Maintain rapport and eye contact as much as possible.

UNIT 1

Time, length, duration

To become fully involved with the consumer, enough time must be set aside for the interview. When scheduling an interview for the consumer, consider their individual daily activities, and select a block of time for the interview that does not conflict with other planned activities. Also, ask the consumer what interview times would be least disruptive to their daily routine, and try to accommodate this.

Biases and preconceptions

Personal beliefs and value systems (inclusive of cultural, spiritual and religious practices), attitudes, biases and preconceptions of both the nurse and the consumer influence the sending and receiving of messages. The cultural and family contexts of each serve as a lens for interpreting societal views on ethnicity, gender, sexual orientation, socioeconomic status, religion and health care. Nurses' and consumers' views of themselves as cultured and gendered beings are highly influential in how they think and feel about health and illness, and have an impact on how they respond to different clinical situations. The nurse must be sensitive to personal as well as individual contexts in order to treat all consumers fairly and respectfully.

The nurse's subjective impressions of the consumer may lead to incorrect assumptions about their situation. For example, a nurse may view a consumer who appears thin and frail as seriously ill or unable to participate in activities of daily living when, in fact, this person may not be seriously ill or incapacitated in any way. To counter incorrect assumptions, biases and preconceptions, continually validate information and personal impressions through the use of careful data gathering and effective interviewing techniques.

CLINICAL **REASONING**

Communicating for safety

Interviewing consumers in a safe manner recognises the importance of always maintaining a person-centred approach and that communicating for safety is paramount. This is reflected in the Australian National Safety and Quality Health Service Standards, which identifies that effective communication is required in supporting continuous, coordinated and safe patient care.

For further information visit: https://www.safetyandquality.gov.au/sites/default/files/2021-05/national_safety_and_quality_health_service_nsqhs_standards_second_edition_-_updated_may_2021.pdf

Stages of the interview process

There are three stages in the interview process: the introduction or joining stage, the working stage, and the termination stage.

Stage I

The **joining stage** is the introduction or first stage of the interview process, during which the nurse and the consumer establish trust and get to know one another. During this stage, work with the individual to identify the relationship and establish goals for this and any subsequent interactions.

Stage II

The **working stage** of the interview process is the time during which most of the consumer data is collected. It is a nursing responsibility to keep the interview goal directed, including refocusing the individual and redefining the goals established in the joining stage.

Stage III

The **termination stage** is the last stage of the interview process, during which information is summarised and validated. During this stage, give the consumer an indication of the amount of time left in the interview, and allow them the opportunity to give additional information and make comments or statements. For example, 'We have about 5 minutes more, Mrs Taylor, is there anything else you would like to add or mention?' Another important step in the termination stage is planning for future interviews.

REFLECTION IN PRACTICE

Decreasing anxiety in the interview
Remember the last time that you cared for an anxious person/family member or friend. What did you do that helped to calm them down?

Now identify some specific actions you might take to decrease a consumer's anxiety during the joining stage of the interview process (Stage 1). It is important to recognise that each person-centred encounter will be different, as individuals display or cope with anxiety in different ways.

Factors affecting communication

Elements that can affect the sending and receiving of messages are discussed in the following sections.

REFLECTION IN PRACTICE

Encouraging active listening
Think of a time when you attempted to talk with someone who didn't appear to be listening. How did that make you feel? What kind of things did you do to get your message across? How many times have you listened to a person/family member or friend with 'half an ear'? What caused you to do this? Identify some specific actions that you might take to ensure that your consumers feel heard.

Listening

Active listening, or the act of perceiving what is said both verbally and nonverbally, is a critical factor in conducting a successful health assessment interview. According to Stein-Parbury (2021), active listening allows the nurse to understand all aspects of what the consumer is communicating, and is an excellent way to build trust. Be aware of how personal characteristics, choice of communication techniques, and the manner and timing of their use can affect communication.

REFLECTION IN PRACTICE

Nonverbal communication
Look at the nurse–consumer encounters in **Figures 2.6** and **2.7**. Describe the nonverbal communication that you see in each.

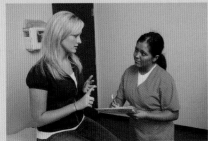
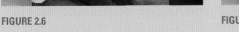

FIGURE 2.6

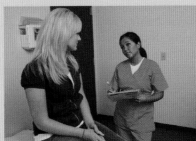

FIGURE 2.7

UNIT 1

Nonverbal cues

Nonverbal communication is communicating a message without words. Nonverbal behaviour effectively supplements the spoken word and provides information about both nurse and consumer. These behaviours can provide insight into the individual's cultural expectations, current physical and emotional states, and perceived self-image. Nonverbal cues such as body position, nervous repetitive movements of the hands or legs, rapid blinking, lack of eye contact, yawning, fidgeting, excessive smiling or frowning, and repetitive clearing of the throat may be indications of the consumer's health and feelings that they may not be comfortable expressing verbally (Stein-Parbury, 2021). Be aware of cultural differences (see Chapters 1 and 4 for more information).

Healthcare environments often evoke a great deal of anxiety, uncertainty or fear in consumers. Loss of personal control is a major obstacle confronting consumers in healthcare settings, whether they are seriously ill or not. In an attempt to maintain some control in unfamiliar circumstances and to decrease anxiety, consumers frequently look to nurses for cues on how to behave or how to respond to questions. Nonverbal acts by the nurse can indicate empathy and attention or indifference and inattention (Stein-Parbury, 2021). Such behaviour powerfully influences consumer comfort levels, feelings of control, and willingness to share information. Because of this, nurses need to continuously monitor their own nonverbal behaviours.

Personal space

Personal space can be defined as the space over which a person claims ownership. In an acute care facility, the consumer's hospital room and bathroom are considered the individual's personal space. The consumer may be very protective of this space and consider unauthorised use of it as an invasion of privacy.

REFLECTION IN PRACTICE

Assessing communication

Record a short video (use a smartphone or other device) of yourself and a colleague role-playing taking a health history. Review the video.
> What nonverbal communication did you identify in yourself? Your colleague?
> What communication techniques did you employ? Were they effective?
> What have you learnt about communication from this exercise?

Distance

Personal space includes distance or the amount of space a person considers appropriate for interaction with another or others. Distance is a significant factor in the interview process and is determined in part by cultural influences. In Western communities, distances are generally categorised as follows, although this can be affected by regional context as well (personal distance in rural and remote areas is often up to double that which is acceptable in metropolitan areas):
> Intimate distance is from the consumer to approximately 40–50 cm.
> Personal distance is approximately 50 cm to 1.2 metres.
> Social distance is approximately 1.2–3.5 metres.
> Public distance is approximately 3.5 metres or more.

Intimate distance is the closest and involves some touching or physical contact. Personal distance may also involve some touching or physical contact, and it may ease communication in some instances, such as for consumers with hearing impairment. In other instances, personal distance may be threatening or invasive to the individual. Social distance is considered appropriate for the interview process because it allows for good eye contact and for ease in hearing and in seeing the consumer's nonverbal cues. Other considerations of social distance must be reviewed and adhered to as required. A good example of this occurred during the

COVID-19 pandemic, where social distance was required in all public spaces. Public distance is usually used in formal settings such as in a classroom where the teacher stands in front of the class. It is not considered appropriate for an interview.

CLINICAL **REASONING**

Practice tip: The use of touch in the consumer interview
You must be mindful of the use of touch during the consumer interview. While a caring touch, a pat on the hand or other gesture may send a message of empathy to a crying individual, it may not be appropriate in all situations. The individual's cultural background may dictate what is or is not appropriate. Also, if a consumer has a history of physical abuse or neglect, or is recovering from a skin disorder such as a burn, a well-meaning touch may be interpreted in a hostile manner.

EFFECTIVE COMMUNICATION TECHNIQUES

Effective communication techniques facilitate or support interactions between the nurse and the consumer and foster their continuation. These techniques encompass both verbal and nonverbal approaches. The more skilled you are in understanding the communication process, the more effectively you can use it in a purposeful, goal-directed manner to meet your need for information and the consumer's need for attention to health concerns or problems (Stein-Parbury, 2021). Because individuals who come to a healthcare provider are frequently anxious, effectively communicating your interest and concern greatly enhances the interview and interaction.

Certain specific verbal communication techniques are available to help you facilitate this interaction. The effectiveness of these techniques will vary from individual to individual. At first, these techniques may feel awkward, stilted or forced; keep in mind that communicating effectively in the healthcare context is a learnt skill (similar to other nursing skills) and, as such, improves with practice.

Using open-ended questions

Open-ended questions encourage the consumer to provide general rather than more focused information (see **Figure 2.8**). Beginning the health assessment interview with open-ended questions provides the individual with a sense of control, leaving the choice of what to say, how much to say, and how to say it up to them. These questions indicate respect for the consumer's ability to articulate important or pressing health concerns and, therefore, to help set priorities.

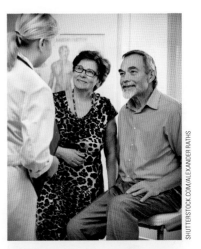

FIGURE 2.8 The nurse uses open-ended questions to gather general information in the consumer interview.

EXAMPLES OF OPEN-ENDED QUESTIONS
> 'What are some of your concerns about caring for your grandmother at home?'
> 'How do you usually manage a hypoglycaemic episode at home?'

Open-ended questions that begin with the words *how, what, where, when* and *who* are usually more effective in eliciting the maximum amount of information than those that begin with the word *why* (Stein-Parbury, 2021). 'Why' questions can cause consumers to become defensive and feel the need to somehow explain or defend their ideas and behaviour, thus setting up an adversarial relationship between the nurse and the individual. Although open-ended questions are quite helpful in the health assessment interview, they can be time-consuming and may not be appropriate in situations requiring rapid access to information and rapid response by healthcare providers. Overuse of this type of question, especially with the consumer who is confused, vague in his or her responses, or extremely talkative, can cause the nurse to miss important information.

In some situations, for example, when a person is anxious and unfamiliar with the healthcare system, they may attempt to ascertain what answers the nurse wants and what areas the nurse seems to feel are important. The consumer will then focus on those, rather than on areas that are most important to them. With open-ended questions, you can encourage the individual to identify what is important. When eliciting the health history, it is usually best to let the consumer speak uninterrupted, allowing them to complete their answer. You should then proceed with questions or clarification.

Using closed questions

Closed questions are those that regulate or restrict consumer response. They can frequently be answered with a 'yes' or a 'no'. Closed questions can be used to focus the interview, pinpoint specific areas of concern, and elicit valuable information quickly and efficiently.

> **EXAMPLES OF EFFECTIVE CLOSED QUESTIONS**
> >   'Are you thinking of harming yourself?'
> >   'Do you use hearing aids??'

If used too frequently, closed questions can disrupt communication because they limit consumer responses and interaction. Even well-directed closed questions may take the initiative away from the consumer, giving them the impression that the nurse is in charge of the interview, does most of the work, often knows the answer to the question asked, and is directing the consumer's response.

> **EXAMPLES OF INEFFECTIVE CLOSED QUESTIONS**
> >   'Do you still feel upset and depressed?'
> >   'Are you afraid to tell your parents that you are sexually active?'

Facilitating

Once the health assessment interview has started, there may be periods when consumers stop talking because of anxiety, uncertainty or embarrassment. You can use a variety of both verbal and nonverbal means to encourage individuals to continue talking. Phrases such as 'go on' or 'uh-huh', the simple repetition of key words the consumer has spoken, or even head nods or a touch on the hand prompt the individual to resume speaking and also indicate your continued interest and attention.

Using silence

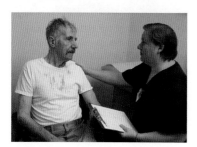

FIGURE 2.9 The nurse remains silent, giving the consumer time to reflect and respond.

Silence, too, has its place in the health assessment interview. Understood and used effectively by the nurse, periods of silence can help structure and pace the interview, convey respect and acceptance, and, in many cases, prompt additional data from the consumer (Stein-Parbury, 2021). Silence on the part of the consumer may indicate feelings of anxiety, confusion or embarrassment, or simply a lack of understanding about the question asked, or an inability to speak English. Nonverbal cues such as these are often lost if the nurse is a persistent talker. Conversely, if overused, silence can contribute to an awkward, disjointed interview that provides minimal structure or direction for the consumer and little helpful data for the nurse.

Using silence effectively may seem like a difficult skill to master (see **Figure 2.9**). Frequently, silences seem longer than they actually are. When silences occur, you may feel discomfort and pressure to speak in order to be actually 'doing' something therapeutic; instead, handle silences by being quiet and observing the consumer's behaviour for what is not being said verbally.

Grouping communication techniques

Communication techniques often seem mechanical and artificial to the beginning nurse. One way to make them less so is to group or cluster them according to their primary purposes. Grouping communication strategies on the basis of purpose helps to clarify the intent of each communication response and indicate when in the assessment interview its use might be helpful. One simple way to group interview techniques is to divide them into two groups: listening responses and action responses.

Listening responses

Listening responses are attempts made by the nurse to accurately receive, process and then respond to consumer messages (Stein-Parbury, 2021). They provide one way for the nurse to communicate empathy, concern and attentiveness. Listening responses provide the nurse with a means to understand the individual's perspective. Consumers realise they have been heard and that the nurse is working with them to elicit and clarify health concerns. Listening responses include making observations, restating, reflecting, clarifying, interpreting, sequencing, encouraging comparisons and summarising.

Making observations

When making observations, the nurse verbalises their perceptions about the consumer's behaviour, and shares them with the individual. Sharing observations is also a way to validate consumer competency and sense of control in an environment or situation where the consumer often feels out of control, uncertain or overwhelmed.

EXAMPLES OF MAKING OBSERVATIONS
> 'Speaking about the symptoms you are experiencing seems to make you upset. I notice that you are clenching your jaw and grimacing.'
> 'I notice that each time you've been exposed to that particular problem, you've known how to handle it well.'

Restating

Restating involves repeating or rephrasing the main idea expressed by the consumer and lets the them know that you are paying attention. It promotes further dialogue and provides the individual with an opportunity to explain or elaborate on an issue or concern.

EXAMPLES OF RESTATING
> *Consumer*: I don't sleep well anymore and I find myself waking up frequently at night.
> *Nurse*: So, you're having difficulty sleeping?

Reflecting

Reflecting is another listening response. It focuses on the content of the consumer's message as well as their feelings. In reflecting, the nurse directs the individual's own questions, feelings and ideas back to them and provides an opportunity for the consumer to reconsider or expand on what was just said. The consumer's point of view is given value, and the nurse, although indicating an interest in what the individual has to say, refrains from giving advice, passing judgement or assuming responsibility for the person's thoughts or feelings.

EXAMPLES OF REFLECTING
> *Consumer*: Do you think I should tell the doctor I stopped taking my medication?
> *Nurse*: Well, do you feel comfortable to tell them? Are you okay to do so?
> *Consumer*: Well, yes; I think that I probably should. Not taking my medication could be one of the reasons I'm feeling so run-down. But that medication just makes me so lethargic and emotional.
> *Nurse*: You sound a bit emotional now. It appears that you have been thinking about this quite a lot.
> *Consumer*: I did tell that young doctor that I had problems with this medication, but he did not listen to me.
> *Nurse*: It sounds as if you are annoyed with him.

Clarifying

Clarifying is a communication technique used by the nurse to make clear something the consumer has said or to pinpoint the message when the person's words and nonverbal behaviour do not agree. Be sure you understand exactly what the consumer means before continuing, because communication may stop if the individual feels misunderstood or not heard. Distortions or misunderstandings about a consumer's data can occur if the nurse interprets the individual's statements using only personal experiences and perceptions. Even more crucial is the fact that making assumptions may cause the interviewer to proceed from a faulty database.

> **EXAMPLE OF A CLARIFYING RESPONSE**
> > *Consumer*: During certain activities, I have the most awful pain in my back.
> > *Nurse*: Tell me what you mean about this pain; **or** I'm not sure that I understand what you mean about your pain. Can you describe what your pain feels like (e.g. stabbing, throbbing, aching).

Interpreting

With interpreting, the nurse has the opportunity to share the inferences or conclusions gathered from the consumer's interview. Although there is always the risk that their interpretation of the facts is incorrect, the nurse is well poised to link events that perhaps the consumer was not able to piece together.

> **EXAMPLES OF INTERPRETING**
> > *Nurse*: Your painful legs seem to occur when you are in bed.
> > *Nurse*: From what you have just told me, do you think that the stress you experience relates to your teaching job and this is causing your headaches?

Sequencing

To effectively assess consumer needs, the nurse often requires knowledge of a time frame within which symptoms or problems developed or occurred. One way to acquire this information involves asking the consumer to place a symptom, problem or event in its proper sequence. Sequencing also helps both consumer and nurse become aware of any patterns in the individual's behaviour that might indicate recurring problems or issues. These can relate to feelings (depression or anxiety), behaviour (refusal to take appropriate medications, consistently putting self in risky situations) or experiences (being physically or verbally abused, being hurt, being misunderstood by healthcare providers). Pattern identification provides the nurse with clues for further assessment focus.

Encouraging comparisons

Encouraging comparisons is a technique that enables both participants in the health assessment interview to become more aware of patterns, issues/themes, or specific symptomatology in the consumer's life. It also helps the consumer to deal more effectively with unfamiliar situations by placing the symptoms or problems in the context of something else that is familiar and, therefore, more comfortable to them. Often an awareness of successful prior dealings with similar situations increases consumer confidence levels.

> **EXAMPLES OF ENCOURAGING COMPARISONS**
> > 'Have you had similar experiences?'
> > 'In what way was this allergy episode different from or the same as your previous ones?'
> > 'In what way was your reaction to this medication similar or different from your reaction to other antibiotics you've had?'

Summarising

Summarising is a communication technique that helps consumers to organise their thinking. As such, summarising is a communication technique that is especially useful at the end of the health assessment interview. A brief, concise review of the important points covered helps the consumer identify anything that has been left out and provides the nurse with an opportunity to make sure that what he or she understood the individual to say, is what was said. In addition, summarising indicates both interest and concern, so the consumer feels they have been heard.

EXAMPLE OF SUMMARISING

> *Nurse*: You have shared with me several health concerns such as a painful left calf, difficulty in losing weight and sleeplessness. The one that is most challenging for you seems to be your difficulty in losing weight. Is this correct?

Summarising also provides a means of smoothly transitioning to a new topic or section of the health assessment interview.

EXAMPLE OF TRANSITIONING

> *Nurse*: You talked about your past experience with diabetes and what happened to you yesterday; now let's talk about why you came in today.

CLINICAL **REASONING**

Practice tip: The use of humour in the consumer interview
Humour can be an effective communication technique in the consumer interview. It can make an anxious person more at ease, diffuse tension, and make it easier for an individual to discuss sensitive issues. However, ill-timed humour or the use of inappropriate humour can offend individuals and make them distrustful of you. It is also important to be aware that humour can be very different for people from various cultural backgrounds who may not share your humorous view or perspective.

Action responses
Action responses are the second group of effective interviewing techniques. These responses stimulate consumers to make some change in their thinking and behaviour. Action responses include such communication techniques as focusing, exploring, presenting reality, confronting, informing, collaborating, limit-setting and normalising.

Focusing
Focusing allows the nurse to concentrate on or 'track' a specific point the consumer has made. This technique is particularly useful with individuals whose heightened anxiety level causes increased confusion, altered concentration, or jumping from topic to topic. With the nurse's assistance in focusing, the individual is able to proceed with the health history interview in a clearer, more organised, thoughtful and thorough manner.

EXAMPLES OF FOCUSING

> 'Tell me more about the chest pain you experience when you begin to exercise.'
> 'You've mentioned several times that your wife is concerned about your smoking. Can we talk about your smoking habit?'

Exploring
In exploring, the nurse is attempting to develop, in more detail, a specific area of content or consumer concern. The purpose of exploring is to identify patterns or themes in symptom presentation or in the way the person handles problems or health concerns.

EXAMPLES OF EXPLORING
> 'Tell me more about how you feel when you do not take your medication.'
> 'Could you describe for me how you handle those periods in your life when you feel out of control?'

Presenting reality

This technique, while typically used with consumers with mental health issues or individuals who are confused, is also useful in the health assessment interview when the nurse is confronted with a consumer who exaggerates or makes grandiose statements. Presenting reality, when done in a non-argumentative way, encourages the individual to rethink a statement and perhaps modify it.

EXAMPLE OF PRESENTING REALITY
> *Consumer:* I can never get an appointment at this clinic.
> *Nurse:* Mr Jasper, could you explain what you mean, as I've seen you several times in the past four months.
> *Consumer:* Well, yes, but I can never get an appointment at a time that is convenient for me.

Confronting

Confronting is a verbal response that the nurse makes to some perceived discrepancy or incongruence in the consumer's thoughts, feelings or behaviour. Gently challenging an incongruence can help the individual reframe a situation in order to see things differently. Focusing the consumer's attention on a behaviour or feeling that could be modified may lead to a more positive outcome in the situation. When confronting is used in a caring, empathetic manner, rather than in a critical or accusatory one, the person can feel encouraged to view themselves as effective individuals.

EXAMPLE OF CONFRONTING
> *Consumer:* I have been working on lowering my risk for heart disease. I have been taking my blood pressure medication and have been watching my diet.
> *Nurse:* Well it's great that you have been taking your medication and being mindful of your diet. There are, however, other factors that significantly increase your cardiovascular risk. For example, you smoke two packs of cigarettes a day and your blood results indicate that your triglyceride level has doubled in the past 3 months. Let's review your heart-health management plan and see where you may need some further assistance.

Informing

Providing the consumer with needed information, such as explaining the nature of or the reasons for any necessary tests or procedures, is a nursing action that can help build trust and decrease a person's anxiety. Giving consumers information is appropriate when trying to assist them to navigate the options to make the best choice for their situation.

EXAMPLE OF INFORMING:
> *Consumer:* Dr Leathwick told me that I need to have my gall bladder taken out.
> *Nurse:* Can you tell me what Dr Leathwick told you about your gall bladder surgery?
> *Consumer:* I didn't understand what he said about the new technique. He said something about a tube.
> *Nurse:* The technique he is going to use is laparoscopic surgery. This is where the surgeon inserts a small scope in your abdomen to remove the gall bladder rather than making a large incision.
> *Consumer:* Yes, that was it, please tell me more about that.

Collaborating

In collaborating, the consumer is offered a relationship in which the nurse and individual work together, rather than one in which the nurse is in total control of the interaction. Use of this technique conveys the message that the consumer has important personal knowledge and information to share. Collaborating provides a respectful, person-centred approach the nurse can use to encourage consumers' active involvement in their own health care in setting goals, in gathering information and in problem solving.

EXAMPLE OF COLLABORATING
> 'Perhaps you and I can talk further about your heart-health management plan and discover what specifically you think you can do to reduce your cardiovascular risk.'

Limit setting

During the interview with a seductive, hostile or talkative consumer, the nurse may find it necessary to set specific limits on the individual's behaviour. If, for example, the consumer persists in asking the nurse personal questions or continues to divert the conversation, despite frequent attempts by the nurse to focus it, it will be difficult to obtain the information needed. This consumer behaviour may be a manifestation of stress produced by the interview situation itself or simply a characteristic specific to that individual. In such situations, consumers may require some direction on how to behave. Provide guidance by calmly, clearly and respectfully telling the consumer what behaviour is expected. Limit only the behaviour that is problematic or detrimental to the purpose of the interview and avoid making a 'big issue' about whatever it is that the consumer is doing. When limit setting, do not argue or use empty threats or promises, but do offer the individual alternatives.

EXAMPLE OF INEFFECTIVE LIMIT SETTING
> *Nurse*: If you don't start answering my questions about your health problems, we'll never finish, and you'll never get to see the nurse practitioner.

EXAMPLE OF APPROPRIATE LIMIT SETTING
> *Nurse*: My role here today is to assist you with your health concerns. It appears that you are feeling pretty unsure of talking about your personal health problems.
> *Consumer*: What do you mean?
> *Nurse*: Well, as you are asking me a lot of personal questions, I am finding it difficult to get you back on track to talk about your health problems. So, can we focus on you and find out what has brought you here to the emergency department today?

CLINICAL **REASONING**

Practice tip: Professional boundaries and answering personal questions
The nurse brings a lifetime of experiences and emotions to each consumer encounter; so too does the consumer. It is only natural for the consumer to be curious about the nurse as the healthcare provider. Sharing personal experiences makes the nurse a real person to the consumer and helps to develop a respectful nurse–consumer interaction. The nurse needs to be certain, however, that the information divulged to the consumer remains generic so that they do not cross the professional boundary to form a more social interaction. Also, remember that the consumer may ask personal questions in order to divert the interview to avoid uncomfortable or sensitive issues.

Normalising

Very often, individuals faced with unexpected or life-threatening illnesses, or surgeries, respond in ways that seem extreme or out of the ordinary (e.g. becoming depressed or overly tearful). Normalising allows the nurse to offer appropriate reassurance that their response may be quite common for this situation. This helps to decrease consumers' anxiety and encourages them to share thoughts and feelings they might otherwise keep to themselves for fear of being judged or misunderstood. However, if used inappropriately or out of context, normalising may give false reassurance.

> **EXAMPLE OF NORMALISING**
> > 'It is no wonder that you've been feeling shocked and overwhelmed since you first found that lump in your breast. Most women who have that experience react in a similar way.'

COMMUNICATION: TECHNIQUES TO AVOID

Just as there are certain communication techniques that facilitate communication between nurse and consumer, there are also some techniques that change, distort or block communication and should be avoided. Verbal and nonverbal behaviours that involve inattentiveness, imposition of values, judgement, lack of interest or an 'I know what's best for you' attitude hinder communication by creating distance rather than connection. Consumers on the receiving end of these behaviours can feel angry, defensive or incompetent, and may refuse to actively participate. Such ineffective techniques include requesting an explanation, probing, offering false reassurance, giving approval or disapproval, defending and advising.

Requesting an explanation

Consumers often perceive questions that begin with 'why' as challenging or threatening. Such questions ask the consumer to provide a reason or justification for personal beliefs, feelings, thoughts and behaviours and imply criticism. If consumers are unable to provide these answers, either from lack of enough knowledge or because the answer is not known to the individual, he or she can feel inadequate, defensive or angry. Some questions are unanswerable and individuals are frequently unaware of why they do some things. Asking the consumer to describe beliefs, feelings or behaviours is preferable to asking 'why'. Providing a description about what happened often helps the consumer elaborate. Enlarging the context provides opportunities for the consumer to increase self-awareness and for the nurse to increase the store of relevant information.

> **EXAMPLES OF REQUESTING AN EXPLANATION**
> **EXAMPLE 1**
> > *Consumer*. I guess I drink two or three six-packs of beer a weekend.
> > *Nurse*: Thank you for sharing this with me. So you enjoy a good time on the weekend. Is there any reason why this includes drinking that much beer? (judgemental)
> > *Consumer*. That's not very much; all my friends drink the same amount.
> A more appropriate response in the preceding example might be:
> > *Nurse*: It sounds as if you might be concerned about the amount of beer you drink. (reflecting)
>
> **EXAMPLE 2**
> > *Consumer*. I'm not sure why I came to the clinic today; I just feel miserable. I don't want to see anyone. I just want to stay in bed with the covers pulled over my head.
> > *Nurse*: Why do you feel that way?
> > *Consumer*. I don't know.
> A more effective response would be:
> > *Nurse*: 'What happened that caused you to feel so miserable?' (clarifying) or 'It sounds as if you are feeling rather overwhelmed today.' (reflecting)

Probing

Repeated or persistent questioning of the consumer about a statement or a behaviour increases their anxiety and can cause confusion, hostility and a tendency to withdraw from the interaction. This consumer withdrawal and the increasing periods of silence resulting from it can escalate the nurse's anxiety. Anxious nurses tend to become more active and more directive in the interview. The consumer's unwillingness or hesitation to discuss a certain event or health concern may indicate the consumer's misunderstanding, misinformation, or a major problem area that needs further clarification or exploration.

A helpful rule of thumb for nurses to use in identifying probing is to pay attention to their own behaviour and feelings. If, in attempting to gather information, nurses feel frustrated or irritated, or that they have become involved in a verbal tug of war with the consumer, then they are most likely probing. More useful responses may include going on to the next part of the health assessment interview, asking the consumer's permission to return to this subject later if it seems likely that more information will be needed, or just sitting quietly until the consumer begins to speak.

EXAMPLE OF AN APPROPRIATE PROBING QUESTION

> *Nurse*: What makes you think that you have arthritis?
> *Consumer*: I'm not sure, I just think I do. It just seems like I have the same health problems as my mother and she had arthritis.
> *Nurse*: Well, do you have pain?
> *Consumer*: Yes. (pause)
> *Nurse*: What makes you think the pain is arthritis pain?

If nurses can be patient, identify and manage their own anxiety, and allow silences, useful discussion usually ensues.

Offering false reassurance

False reassurances are vague and simplistic responses that question the consumer's judgement, devalue and block the individual's feelings, and communicate a lack of understanding and sensitivity on the part of the nurse. The impulse to provide false reassurance typically originates in the nurse's own feelings of helplessness. Giving false reassurance is an attempt by the nurse to take care of themselves rather than the consumer and to relieve personal feelings of anxiety. This behaviour often increases consumer anxiety. A more valuable nursing response would be to first acknowledge personal feelings of anxiety and then to acknowledge the consumer's feelings.

EXAMPLES OF FALSE REASSURANCE

> 'Everything will be fine.'
> 'I wouldn't worry about that.'

EXAMPLE OF AN APPROPRIATE RESPONSE

> 'It must be frightening to think about the possibility of surgery.'

REFLECTION IN PRACTICE

False reassurance

Consider the following example of false reassurance.

Mr and Mrs Temple are awaiting results of diagnostic testing that will confirm or deny a diagnosis of fetal neurological impairment. Mrs Temple says to the nurse, 'It's taking so long to get the results, I'm sure that there must be something wrong with the baby.' The nurse replies, 'Oh, no, you don't need to worry. Everything will be just fine!'

> What do you believe motivated the nurse's response?
> What impact will the nurse's response have on the Temples?

Giving approval

During the health assessment interview, nurses can feel pressured to comment judgementally on a consumer's statements, feelings or behaviours, especially if these contradict the nurse's personal beliefs or feelings. Telling a consumer what is right or wrong is moralising. This may limit the consumer's freedom to verbalise or behave in certain ways that might not please the nurse. Comments such as 'What a good idea,' 'You shouldn't feel that way,' or 'That is bad,' hinder the nurse's attempts to establish rapport, support consumer competence and facilitate communication. When there is concern that the consumer's expressed beliefs or personal behaviours are ill-informed, harmful or destructive, the nurse might more effectively explore the source of the belief or the impact of the consumer's behaviour on others.

> **EXAMPLES OF EFFECTIVE APPROVAL RESPONSES**
> > 'What made you come to that conclusion?'
> > 'What do you think the consequences will be if you continue to keep your illness from your wife?'

Defending

Occasionally, consumers who have had previous stressful or unpleasant experiences (or seen relatives have these) with doctors, specialists or other agents in the healthcare setting will engage in criticism or verbal attack. It is not helpful for the nurse to defend the object of the attack. Defending implies that the consumer has neither the right to hold such opinions or feelings nor the right to express them, especially if they are hostile or angry. The nurse will not be able to change the consumer's opinions or feelings by defending the individual or the object attacked. Rather, deflection or criticism of consumer feelings more often either blocks expression of these feelings or reinforces them. Defending is not therapeutic because it requires the nurse to speak not just for themselves but for others, something that nurses truthfully and realistically are not able to do.

> **EXAMPLES OF INAPPROPRIATE DEFENDING RESPONSES**
> > 'This hospital has an excellent reputation. I'm sure that if you were kept waiting as long as you say, there was a good reason.'
> > 'No one here would hide the truth from you.'

It is more respectful and useful to accept and support consumers' rights to feel as they do and to express those feelings. The nurse can do this without agreeing with the expressed feelings. This empathetic behaviour defuses any antagonism and minimises consumer resistance to the continued interaction.

> **EXAMPLES OF APPROPRIATE DEFENDING RESPONSES**
> > *Nurse:* You sound pretty angry about your previous experiences in this hospital.
> > *Consumer:* Of course I am. Wouldn't you be upset if no one ever told you what was going on and no one answered your call bell?
> > *Nurse:* I guess I'd be pretty upset if I thought people were not treating me respectfully.

Advising

Consistently telling a consumer what to do does not foster competence. Advising encourages consumers to look to others for answers, deprives them of the opportunity to learn from past mistakes, and discourages independent judgement. As some consumers may resort to dependent, passive behaviour when faced with illness, it is important that the nurse does not reinforce this dependence, but rather supports the consumer's healthy functioning as much as possible.

EXAMPLE OF INEFFECTIVE ADVISING RESPONSES
> *Consumer*: Do you think that I should have an abortion?
> *Nurse*: Well, if I were you, I'd certainly think long and hard before I'd have another child. **Or** No, I think you should continue the pregnancy. Abortion is never the answer.

A more helpful response would be for the nurse to support the consumer's own problem-solving ability using therapeutic communication techniques such as exploring or reflection.

EXAMPLES OF EXPLORING
> 'Tell me more about what made you consider an abortion.'
> 'What other alternatives have you considered?'

EXAMPLES OF REFLECTION
> 'Do you think you should?'
> 'How would you feel about having the abortion?'

Questioning techniques which may be problematic

Experienced nurses as well as beginners will find themselves occasionally feeling nervous and perhaps unsure of how to proceed during the health assessment interview. This anxiety can lead to the use of questioning techniques and interviewing responses that, although not specifically identified as nontherapeutic, are potentially problematic. Such techniques increase consumer anxiety, decrease the flow of needed information and have the potential to provide the nurse with irrelevant data. The following are several examples of problematic interviewing techniques the nurse should keep in mind and work hard to avoid. It is a good idea to practise interview questioning with a peer or friend and note areas that you should work on to improve in the future.

Posing leading questions

Leading questions may indicate to the consumer that the nurse already has a certain answer in mind. Their use can be intimidating to the consumer and curtail further communication. This is especially true if these leading questions concern topics that the consumer perceives as sensitive or as possible sources of anxiety.

EXAMPLES OF POSING LEADING QUESTIONS
> 'You've never had any type of sexually transmitted infections, have you, Miss Jenkins?'
> 'Of course, you've told your daughter that her smoking really bothers you, Mr Talbott, isn't that correct?'

Interrupting the consumer

Changing the subject or interrupting the consumer prevents completion of a thought or idea and introduces a new focus. Such behaviour may ease the nurse's discomfort, but it shows a lack of respect, and often just confuses or irritates the consumer. Questions should focus on one topic until all relevant data has been collected and the consumer feels finished. Changing the subject or interrupting cuts off the flow of ideas and communicates the message that whatever the consumer was addressing is not as important as what the nurse wants to discuss next.

Neglecting to ask pertinent questions

It is easy to become complacent when conducting consumer interviews. Do not let a consumer's outward physical appearance, personality or social standing distract you from ascertaining pertinent information. Do not assume that, because an individual is well dressed and talks about a luxury car, he or she is well off. Likewise, do not presume that a poorly dressed and ill-mannered person is poor and uneducated. All consumers deserve to be treated respectfully during the consumer interview.

Using multiple questions

Consumers can become confused if a nurse asks several questions at once. Too many questions may put consumers on the defensive, minimising an individual's participation and impeding the flow of necessary information.

REFLECTION IN PRACTICE

Asking essential information

A 15-year-old female presents to the emergency department with acute abdominal pain. You are asked by the nurse manager to conduct a health assessment with the consumer and her parents. Later you discover that the consumer is experiencing a miscarriage. You tell your nurse manager that you did not inquire about the consumer's sexual activity. What variables in this scenario do you think led you to neglect this part of the interview?

Using medical jargon

The use of medical jargon or slang can make a consumer quite anxious or confused. Nurses who are part of the wider healthcare system, which has its own culture and language, frequently use medical jargon. Consumers who may feel frightened and powerless in this unfamiliar environment may be further disadvantaged by their lack of comprehension and any perceived language barrier. The use of medical jargon can be seen by the consumer as unwillingness to share or attempts to hide information. It can also give the impression that the nurse feels superior to the consumer and is unwilling to engage in collaboration or mutual problem solving. Conduct the health assessment interview in a language that is common to both participants, and check periodically with the consumer as to clarity. This will indicate an interest in the consumer's perspective and a desire to work collaboratively. It may require the nurse to call on an authorised interpreter.

Being authoritative

The use of authority as a healthcare professional can be a problematic technique. It reinforces a patriarchal nurse–consumer relationship and can limit the cooperation of the consumer.

EXAMPLE OF NEGATIVE USE OF AUTHORITY

> 'I've been a nurse, Mr McMahon, for over 15 years, and I think I know what is best for you.'

In a few situations, the use of authority can be an effective communication technique.

EXAMPLE OF POSITIVE USE OF AUTHORITY

> 'As your healthcare provider, knowing about your previous heart attack, history of high blood pressure, and family history of stroke, I would suggest you consider what options you have to assist you to stop smoking.'

Having hidden agendas

Frequently, consumers seek health care for one problem but are concerned about other problems. The consumer may believe that the overriding concern is embarrassing, private or insignificant. Once in the presence of a healthcare provider, the consumer may open up and discuss concerns. For example, a consumer may seek care for a sore throat, then ask for blood tests for HIV. The nurse should deal with the consumer's concerns in the best way possible, then follow up when indicated.

INTERVIEWING THE CONSUMER WITH SPECIAL NEEDS

Consumers with special needs require more consideration by the nurse during the interview. Although the goal of the interview and the specific interviewing techniques remain the same, the process differs according to the consumer's special needs. Conducting a successful assessment interview with the consumer with special needs may require more time and effort than usual, and often requires the help of an intermediary, such as a family member or a friend of the consumer. Remember that consumer privacy and confidentiality laws require consumer consent when an interpreter or other assisting individual is used.

The consumer with impaired hearing

Often, consumers with impaired hearing will read lips, so it is important to remain within sight of the consumer and face the individual when talking. When working with such a consumer, ensure that the hearing aid is in working order and turned on. Background noise should be at a minimum, because noise can be distracting to the consumer with a hearing aid. Even if an **intermediary** (an individual who is a liaison between the consumer and a member of the healthcare team) is with the consumer to assist in communication, always face the consumer and direct all communication to that individual (**Figure 2.10**). It is common for those speaking to a consumer with impaired hearing to speak loudly or slowly; however, though well intentioned, such acts detract from the consumer's ability to read lips. Tone and inflection of voice are lost to the consumer with impaired hearing. However, other nonverbal cues such as facial expression and body movements can be used to convey the meaning of what is said.

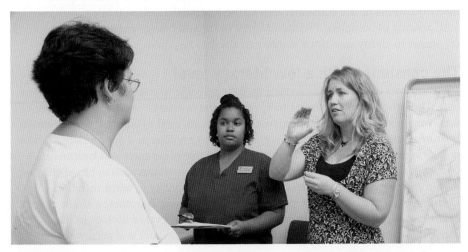

FIGURE 2.10 When working with a consumer with impaired hearing, the interpreter needs to direct questions to the consumer.

Consumers who have never had the ability to hear and those who have not heard for a long time may have speech that is difficult to understand. Often, the best approach to interviewing these consumers is to allow additional time, and to use a written form for gathering data if applicable. When communicating through writing, always remain with the consumer to clarify questions and answers. Information can be reinforced with written instructions.

The consumer with impaired vision

When interviewing a consumer with a visual impairment, always look directly at the consumer as if the individual were sighted. Because they cannot rely on visual cues, voice intonation, volume and inflection are important to the visually impaired. It is common for those speaking to a visually impaired consumer to speak loudly; this is insulting and can hinder communication.

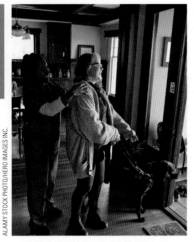

ALAMY STOCK PHOTO/HERO IMAGES INC.

FIGURE 2.11 The nurse needs to inform the consumer with impaired vision when a touch is to occur and ask permission.

Touch is especially important to those with impaired vision; however, an unanticipated touch can be frightening. Before touching the consumer, be certain to inform the consumer and ask permission to touch (**Figure 2.11**). Advise the consumer when you are entering or leaving the room and orientate the individual to the immediate environment. Use clock hours to indicate the position of items in relation to the consumer. Those consumers who are partially sighted may cling to the independence that their limited vision allows; offer assistance to the partially sighted and follow their cues or responses.

The consumer with impaired speech or aphasia

When interviewing the consumer who has impaired speech, ask simple questions that require 'yes' and 'no' answers and allow additional time for consumer responses. Using this technique, it is often necessary to convert open-ended questions such as 'How are you today?' to closed questions such as 'Are you feeling well now?' You may need to repeat or rephrase the question if the consumer did not understand. If you are unable to understand the consumer's responses, use a written interview format, letter boards or 'yes' and 'no' cards. Health settings have technologies with adaptive mechanisms that can aid communication. Also pay close attention to the consumer's nonverbal cues, such as blinking, clicking, or other gestures.

Even when all questions in the interview are asked and answered using closed questions, allow the consumer the opportunity to contribute to the information gathering; for example, 'I have asked all the questions I have to ask you for now, would you like to tell me anything related to any of the questions I have asked?' then continue with, 'Would you like to say anything else before we conclude the interview?'

When someone else is speaking for the consumer, the nurse should speak and direct questions to the consumer, not to the intermediary. If you ask a consumer with aphasia to complete a written format of the interview, remain with the consumer to clarify questions and to explain data requirements.

The consumer with a low literacy level

The consumer who has a low level of literacy is unable to complete or verify written data. Thus, this must be done verbally or with the assistance of a trusted friend or family member. In addition, alternative strategies are used to ensure that appropriate treatment and follow-up are clear. For example, technology and appropriate software programs or illustrated charts can be used to describe procedures and treatments. A picture of a clock can be used to illustrate time for procedures such as blood glucose monitoring. Medications can be colour coded for simplicity in administration. Consumers should be able to repeat all instructions to verify accuracy. Home healthcare clinicians can follow a consumer with a low level of literacy in the consumer's home environment to assess treatment adherence and accuracy.

REFLECTION IN PRACTICE

Caring for the consumer with low literacy

The 22-year-old consumer has just moved to your community and has told you he has trouble with reading and writing and is not able to write more than his name and address. How will you provide education for his follow-up care required after discharge?

The consumer with low literacy is unable to complete or verify written assessment data. Therefore, alternative strategies are used when caring for them to ensure that education on treatment and follow-up is simple and clear. Some strategies to use include:

> illustrated charts to describe procedures and treatments
> technology and software programs
> a picture of a clock to illustrate time
> colour-coded medications
> consumer recall on instructions to double-check accuracy
> follow-up with home healthcare agency when indicated to ensure appropriate care.

The consumer who is culturally or linguistically diverse

Interviewing consumers from diverse cultural or linguistic backgrounds may require the assistance of an interpreter. Most healthcare agencies have a register of interpreters available. Sometimes the consumer will bring a translator to the interview. Often this translator is a friend or family member. The nurse should not assume that the translator can answer questions for the consumer. It is important to direct interview questions to the consumer and not to the interpreter.

Remember that pure translation from one language to another does not consider dialects or **colloquialisms** (words and phrases particular to a community), which have the potential to offend someone. For example, the question 'Are you pregnant?' when translated without considering colloquialisms may mean 'Do you have intercourse outside marriage?'

CLINICAL **REASONING**

Practice tip: Using an interpreter

One of the most common difficulties with communication is when the consumer has English as a second language. The use of an interpreter is an excellent way to overcome these difficulties. The following are some tips to consider when you are using an interpreter to improve communication outcomes.

1. Use a trained medical interpreter whenever possible.
2. When possible, allow the interpreter and consumer a few minutes to converse before initiating the interview.
3. Instruct the interpreter to translate the consumer's replies sentence by sentence, thus avoiding summarisation. This will ensure that important information is not omitted.
4. Keep your questions brief. Inform the interpreter what information you are trying to obtain.
5. Maintain eye contact with the consumer, not the interpreter, during the questioning and translating.
6. Observe the consumer's nonverbal communication, being sensitive to cultural influences.
7. Be patient! Extra time needs to be allotted for this interview exchange.
8. When available, use pre-printed questions and healthcare instructions in the consumer's native language.

Pay special attention to the consumer's nonverbal cues, especially facial expressions and body movements. Often, information that is lost in the translation to English can be gained through nonverbal cues. The use of signs, such as pointing, can be helpful in an emergency situation; however, a more complete interview should be deferred until an interpreter is present.

The consumer who has a low level of understanding

Interviewing the consumer with a low IQ requires time and patience because the consumer may require time to process questions and to formulate answers, and may need clarification of the meaning or intent of questions. Hurrying may cause the consumer to become confused, lose concentration or to refuse to answer. It may be necessary to interview the consumer's family or caregiver for supplemental information. Request permission from the consumer to speak to someone else and respect the consumer's right to be present during all phases of the interview. Always direct interview questions to the consumer and allow the consumer to request assistance from family members or a caregiver. Observe the interaction between the consumer and the family or caregiver, because nonverbal communication can provide valuable information about the consumer's present health or illness state as well as about the relationship between the consumer and the family member or primary caregiver.

UNIT 1

The consumer who is emotional and upset

Consumers may cry during the interview. On some occasions crying can be anticipated, such as when parents relate events that led to their child's death. At other times a consumer may cry unexpectedly. The latter example affords an opportunity for you to gain information about something of importance to the consumer by gently asking what is causing the emotional response. It is important to show empathy and to allow the consumer to cry. Offering tissues indicates to the consumer that it is OK to cry and conveys a message of thoughtfulness. When the consumer has regained composure, proceed with the interview.

Consumers and those who are speaking on behalf of individuals in healthcare settings can become emotionally upset. For example, the parent of a sick child may be overwhelmed by events that led to the child's hospitalisation. Emotional outbursts and crying are often the result of such stress. Allow the consumer, family member or significant other to express emotions. If it is obvious that the person being interviewed is holding back tears, give permission to express emotion with a simple statement such as, 'I can see that you are upset; it's OK to cry.'

When interviewing an obviously angry person, recognise and acknowledge the emotion. A natural instinct is to personalise the anger and become angry in return (Stein-Parbury, 2021); instead, recognise the emotion and bring it to the consumer's attention. 'You appear very angry about something. Before we continue with the interview, please tell me about your feelings.' Avoid statements such as 'Take a moment to get hold of yourself,' because this directive implies that the consumer's feelings are not appropriate and should not be expressed. Acknowledging an individual's emotions and giving them permission to express feelings will convey respect and enhance genuine communication and enacts person-centred care.

Behaviour that may be sexually inappropriate or threatening

A consumer who displays sexually inappropriate behaviour may act out during the interview. For example, the consumer may stand very close to the nurse and say, 'You have been so nice to me, I would like the chance to be nice to you.' The nurse may counter this behaviour by defining appropriate boundaries, sharing personal reactions and refocusing the consumer; for example, stating, 'It makes me feel very uncomfortable when you stand this close to me. Let's get back to getting information to assist in your healthcare needs.' It is important to set limits and to focus on tasks when dealing with a consumer who is behaving in a sexually inappropriate manner. Healthcare professionals need to be cognisant of the power imbalance between them and consumers and employ de-escalation strategies in these situations.

Before they begin the interview, it is important that nurses recognise that they are required to work within their scope of practice, code of conduct and the healthcare organisation's national safety and quality health service standards (NSQHSS, 2017). This includes following policy to ensure your personal safety. In some situations, there may be a history of a consumer's inappropriate behaviour, such as violence or poor impulse control, and the nurse should follow policy to ensure their safety. Keep in mind that sometimes consumers may use hostile behaviour because it may get them what they want. Take care not to respond with anger and hostility, rather focus on what the consumer is communicating (Stein-Parbury, 2020).

You can minimise the risk of aggression through nonthreatening interventions such as limit setting and refocusing. Position yourself near an easily accessible exit. Do not turn your back on the consumer and never allow the consumer to walk behind you or come between you and the exit. Watch for signs of increasing tension in the consumer (e.g. clenched fists, loud voice, angry tone of voice, narrowed eyes). Alert a colleague and security if the consumer makes you nervous or anxious. Always follow your institution's health and safety policies. Trust your instincts and remove yourself from potentially threatening and dangerous situations when necessary.

REFLECTION IN PRACTICE

Inappropriate behaviour
You are undertaking a health assessment on a female consumer just admitted to your ward. She is dressed in a very short skirt and a low-cut, see-through blouse. During the assessment she leans over and exposes her breasts to you. She asks you if you have a partner and says you have sexy eyes. What would you say to this consumer? How would you be sure that your non-verbal communication matches your verbal response?

The consumer who is under the influence of alcohol or drugs

The consumer who is under the influence of alcohol or drugs presents a challenge to the nurse. Depending on the quantity of alcohol consumed and the type of drugs ingested, the consumer can have central nervous system (CNS) depression, or the individual can be very disruptive with CNS stimulation. The consumer's judgement may be impaired, which can lead to physical harm to those in the immediate environment. For this reason, when you have a violent or agitated consumer, security personnel should be alerted and stationed nearby. Always follow your institution's health and safety policies.

Consumers under the influence of some drugs have been known to exhibit profound strength and are capable of inflicting serious physical harm on themselves and others. To care for this person, place yourself at a safe distance, remain calm, and provide care in a nonthreatening manner.

CLINICAL REASONING

Assessing alcohol withdrawal
Regular excessive alcohol consumption is a prominent health issue. Alcohol and drug misuse in consumers presenting to healthcare settings, particularly to emergency departments, is an ongoing issue with only a slight decline reported (AIHW, 2020). To assist in prevention and minimise alcohol-related harm within Australian communities, a national alcohol strategy 2019–2028 was released in 2019 with the aim of reducing harmful alcohol consumption by 10% (Commonwealth of Australia, 2019). Assessing alcohol withdrawal is essential for consumers newly admitted to a healthcare setting, not only for the consumer's outcome but to assist the healthcare provider to ensure consumer safely. A well-known assessment tool is the Clinical Institute Withdrawal Assessment for Alcohol–Revised (CIWA-Ar), which is sensitive to a person experiencing alcohol withdrawal. Reoux and Miller revised the CIWA-Ar in 2000 (Knight & Lappalainen, 2017). The tool contains 10 symptom criteria that the health practitioner uses to calculate an overall score to guide consumer management. Policies will vary among individual healthcare agencies; however, interventions are usually based on the final score calculated for the consumer.

For further information about assessing and managing alcohol withdrawal, refer to Quigley, Connolly, Palmer and Helfgott (2015), who provide a brief guide to the assessment and treatment of alcohol dependence.

DEVELOPMENTAL THEORIES

While the basic interview techniques give you a general understanding of how to undertake a health assessment, you will need to consider the developmental age and stage of the consumer prior to commencing any data collection. Having this fundamental knowledge and understanding of the consumer will enable you to adapt your interview techniques to ensure the consumer is safe, and feels safe and understood during the assessment. It will also help you gather accurate and relevant data for your health assessment.

A variety of theories have been developed that depict and predict growth and development. The theories most widely used for clinical assessment of consumers are the 'ages and stages' theories of Piaget (1952), Freud (1946), Erikson (1974) and Kohlberg (1981). The **ages and stages developmental theories** are based on the premise that individuals experience similar sequential physical, cognitive, psychosocial and moral changes during the same age periods, each of which is termed a **developmental stage**. During each developmental stage, there are specific physical and psychosocial skills known as **developmental tasks/milestones** that are expected. An individual's readiness for each new developmental task is generally considered to be dependent on success in achieving prior developmental tasks and is also known to be influenced by the presence of environmental opportunities in which to develop the new skills. If prior developmental tasks have been delayed, or have occurred in a defective way, the individual's capacity to successfully adapt to their environment can be impacted. A key nursing role in assessment is to identify areas of differentiation or deficit and then develop a plan of care in collaboration with the patient to address their needs.

Transitional developmental theories

A second group of theories include **life events** or **transitional developmental theories**, which are based on the premise that a change in development occurs in response to specific events such as new roles (e.g. parenthood) and life transitions (e.g. career changes). Life events and transitions require adaptive coping behaviour as well as significant changes in an individual's life patterns. Each of these events, which can occur singly or together and may be positively or negatively stressful, is not tied to a specific time or stage in the life span. Each event, however, does have certain tasks associated with it that must be achieved. The degree of success or failure with these tasks influences the individual's potential for success with concurrent and subsequent developmental tasks that occur in response to any other life events. A variety of factors have been found to affect how an individual responds to life events (Kozlowska, Scher & Helgeland, 2020). These factors include biological status, personality, cultural orientation, socioeconomic status, interpersonal support systems, number and intensity of life events, and orientation to life (Kozlowska, Scher & Helgeland, 2020). Although the stress associated with each life event or transition can serve as an impetus for growth, excessive stress can disrupt the individual's equilibrium and lead to a variety of physical and psychological health problems (Kozlowska, Scher & Helgeland, 2020; Saxon, Etten & Perkins, 2015). In identifying life events and stressors, nurses can play a critical role in helping consumers maintain health and control stress.

Ages and stages developmental theories

There are many developmental theories that describe human development across the entire life span. By categorising development into specific stages/ages, the healthcare professional is then provided with a predictable range of expected developmental changes. This predictability allows for an anticipated preparation for the changes and for the healthcare professional to be alert when development may be delayed or interrupted. For the purposes of this text, information about developmental events or tasks is provided in stages for chronological (increasing) age. A summary of the work of four of the most influential developmental theorists (Piaget, Freud, Erikson and Kohlberg) can be accessed from the online resource section of this text.

DEVELOPMENTAL STAGES, TASKS AND LIFE EVENTS

Developmental stages and milestones can be influenced by many factors. These include inherited factors such as physical height and chromosomal anomalies, constitutional factors such as illness, levels of intelligence and the ability to learn, as well as a person's ability to engage socially and emotionally with others (Hayes, 2020). Also, factors such as improved **nutrition**, medical advances and healthier lifestyles can influence growth rates and longevity and hence developmental expectations in Australia and New Zealand. Although there may be developmental changes in the future, for this text the human developmental stages will use the following chronological developmental terms of reference:

> Stage 1 Infancy (birth to 1 year)
> Stage 2 Toddler (1 to 3 years)
> Stage 3 Pre-schooler (3 to 5 years)
> Stage 4 School-age child (5 to 12 years)
> Stage 5 Adolescence (12 to 18 years)
> Stage 6 Young adulthood (18 to 30 years)
> Stage 7 Early middle adulthood (30 to 50 years)
> Stage 8 Late middle adulthood (50 to 70 years)
> Stage 9 Late adulthood (70 years to death).

To enable a holistic view of development, the following section will combine the developmental tasks, life events and transitions from each major theory of development. Although the lists of tasks for each stage are not exhaustive, and do not reflect all the tasks facing the full range of normal human conditions and circumstances, they do provide an overview of parameters with which the healthcare professional can gauge their assessment data. Generally, ask yourself whether the individual's overall development seems consistent with the tasks usually associated with their chronological age. Remember that failure to meet tasks in one area does not always indicate abnormal development. Information presented should therefore form a general approach on which you can base your assessment of an individual's growth and development. If you would like further information about developmental stages of the paediatric consumer, refer to a current paediatric textbook (e.g. Lissauer & Carroll, 2022).

Developmental tasks of infants (birth to 1 year)

Infancy is a period of dramatic and rapid physical, motor, cognitive, emotional and social growth. It is a time of critical growth and development. During the first year of life, infants change from being dependent on others for all levels of activities of daily living to an individual who can interact with their environment and form meaningful relationships with significant others. A list of key gross and fine motor, language and sensory milestones associated with this period can be found in Table 2.1.

TABLE 2.1 Growth and development during infancy

AGE	GROSS MOTOR	FINE MOTOR	LANGUAGE	SENSORY
Birth to 2 months	> Assumes tonic neck posture > When prone, lifts and turns head	> Rooting reflex to feed > Grasp reflex (not fisted) > Draws arms and legs to body	> Vocalises as cry	> Comforts with touch, being held and swaddling > Looks at faces (6 weeks) > Follows objects when in line of vision > Responds to high-pitched voices > Smiles
2 to 4 months	> Can raise head and shoulders when prone to 45°–90°; supports self on forearms > Rolls from front to back	> Looks at and plays with fingers > Grasps and tries to reach objects > Bats objects with their hand	> Vocalises when talked to; coos, babbles > Squeals	> Smiles > Follows objects 180° > Turns head when hears voices or sounds (12 weeks)

>>

>> **TABLE 2.1** *continued*

AGE	GROSS MOTOR	FINE MOTOR	LANGUAGE	SENSORY
4 to 6 months	> Turns from back to stomach > When pulled to sitting, almost no head lag > By 6 months, can sit on floor with hands forward for support	> Can hold feet and put in mouth > Puts objects in mouth	> Squeals > Laughs out loud > Takes turns in 'talking'	> Watches a falling object > Object permanence; will look for the object when it is taken away
6 to 8 months	> Puts full weight on legs when held in standing position > Can sit without support > Bounces when held in a standing position > Creeping on tummy	> Can feed self a biscuit > Can bang two objects together	> Babbles vowel-like sounds, 'ooh' or 'aah' > Imitation of speech sounds ('mummy', 'daddy') beginning > Laughs aloud	> Responds by looking and smiling > Recognises own name > Knows people
8 to 10 months	> Crawls on all fours or uses arms to pull body along floor > Can pull self to sitting > Can pull self to standing > Cruising furniture (9 months)	> Pincer grip thumb–finger grasp > Symmetrical hand use > Has good hand–mouth coordination > Transfers objects from one hand to the other > Copies gestures	> Responds to verbal commands > May say one word in addition to 'mumum' and 'dadad'	> Recognises sounds > Withdraws from strangers > Raises arms to be picked up
10 to 12 months	> Can sit down from standing > Can stand alone and steps forward > Protective reflex actions to prevent falling	> Picks up and drops objects > Can put small objects into toys or containers through holes > Turns many pages in a book at one time > Picks up small objects	> Understands 'no' and other simple commands > Says 3 words > Imitates speech sounds > Babbles loudly > Shakes head for no and nod for yes	> Follows fast-moving objects > Indicates wants > Likes to play imitative games such as patty cake and peek-a-boo > Knows their own name

Nutrition in the first year

Nutrition in the first year of life moves from the infant being totally dependent on liquid feeds of breast milk and/or replacement milk products, to soft foods taken from a spoon at around 6 months of age (e.g. rice cereal, pureed vegetables) and water from a cup. Finger foods at 9 months of age allow independent eating, and then by 12 months of age the toddler will have at least 8 teeth and will enjoy joining in with the social activities of family meals (Australian Government Department of Health, 2022; American Academy of Pediatrics, 2020).

SHUTTERSTOCK.COM/OKSANA KUZMINA

FIGURE 2.12 This stage 2 toddler demonstrates one of the abilities of a child around this development level of creating a block tower.

REFLECTION IN PRACTICE

Helping parents understand developmental milestones

Caregivers are often nervous about their infants and have many questions. Consider how you would respond to each of these questions:

> 'My sister's baby is already walking around the furniture at 9 months of age, but my son is 10 months old and still only crawling.'

> 'My little boy has just started in a new school. He is 6 years old and he has started wetting the bed over the last 3 weeks. He has not wet the bed since he was 4 years old. Should I put him back into a nappy until he settles down?'

Conducting a comprehensive health assessment of an infant requires an evaluation of the degree to which the infant has achieved the developmental tasks of infancy. It is important to remember that although individuals experience similar sequential physical, cognitive, psychosocial and moral changes during the same age periods, there is still a degree of normal variability from one child to another. Developmental tasks that are expected to be achieved during the infancy stage are to:

1. develop a basic, relative sense of trust
2. develop a sense of self as dependent on, but separate from, others, particularly the mother
3. develop and desire affection for and response from others, particularly the mother
4. develop a preverbal communication system, including emotional expression, to communicate needs and desires
5. begin to develop conceptual abilities and a language system
6. begin to learn purposeful fine and gross motor skills, particularly eye–hand coordination and balance (**Figure 2.12**)
7. begin to explore and recognise the immediate environment
8. develop **object permanence**.

Developmental tasks of toddlers (1 to 3 years)

The toddler period is one of steadily increasing growth, fine and gross motor development (**Figure 2.13**), intense activity and discovery, rapid language development, increasingly independent behaviours, and marked personality development. Key gross and fine motor, language and sensory milestones associated with the toddler period can be found in **Table 2.2**.

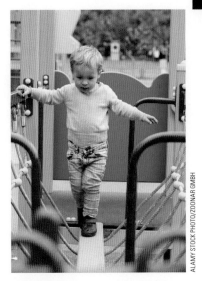

ALAMY STOCK PHOTO/ZOONAR GMBH

FIGURE 2.13 Refinement of skills and a growing sense of independence are most noted in toddlers.

TABLE 2.2 Growth and development during toddlerhood

AGE	GROSS MOTOR	FINE MOTOR	LANGUAGE	SENSORY
12 to 15 months	> Can walk alone well > Walks holding a hand or the rail	> Can feed self with cup and spoon > Puts raisins into a bottle > May hold crayon or pencil and scribble > Builds a tower of two cubes	> Says four to six words > Simple words and incomplete	Binocular vision is developed
18 months	> Runs, falling often > Can jump in place > Can walk up stairs holding on > Plays with push and pull toys	> Can build a tower of three to four cubes > Starting to throw a ball with whole arm	> Says 10 or more words > Points to objects or body parts when asked	Visual acuity 6/6
24 months	> Can walk up and down stairs > Can kick a ball > Can ride a tricycle	> Can draw a circle > Tries to dress self > Can stack six blocks	> Talks a lot > Approximately 150–300-word vocabulary > Use two word combination > Understands commands > Knows first name, refers to self > Verbalises toilet needs	
36 months	> Starting to catch a ball (3 years) > Jumps with both feet > Can stand on one foot for a few seconds	> Can build a tower of eight blocks and create a three-block structure > Can use crayons > Learning to use scissors	> Knows first and last name > Knows the name of one colour > Can sing > Expresses needs > Uses pronouns appropriately > Simple sentences > Can follow simple instructions	

One of the major developmental tasks for toddlers is toilet training. Readiness for toilet training is usually evident in children between the ages of 18 and 36 months. Girls tend to be ready to toilet train earlier than boys, but for independent toileting to occur, the following developmental changes are necessary. Voluntary control of the anal and urethral sphincters must be present including motor skills of sitting, walking and squatting. Fine motor skills needed to remove clothing need to be present along with the cognitive skills of recognising the urge to defecate or urinate, being able to verbalise the urge to do so as well as the willingness and ability to sit on the toilet for 5 to 10 minutes. Parental recognition of the child's level of readiness and willingness to invest the necessary time for toilet training are also essential for the toddler's successful mastery of this task.

REFLECTION IN PRACTICE

Understanding toilet training

Parents often have difficulty with toilet training their child and become frustrated when their first attempts are not successful. What suggestions could you give a mother who has been trying unsuccessfully for the past 2 months with her 2.5-year-old son? The mother says that she had absolutely no problems with her first child, a daughter, at the same age and cannot understand what the problem is this time.

A variety of life events and transitions may produce stress in the toddler. Among the most stressful is personal injury or illness, death of a parent, or loss through separation or divorce.

Children who have been successful in accomplishing the developmental tasks of infancy enter the toddler period with the basic relative trust needed for the achievement of the next tasks. The principal developmental tasks that must be mastered during the toddler stage are to:

1. interact with others less egocentrically
2. acquire socially acceptable behaviours
3. differentiate self from others
4. tolerate separation from key socialising agents (mother or parents)
5. develop increasing verbal communication skills
6. tolerate delayed gratification of wants and desires
7. control bodily functions (toilet training) and begin self-care (feed and dress self almost completely).

REFLECTION IN PRACTICE

Identifying a pre-preps' readiness for school

You are performing a health assessment and physical examination on 5-year-old Jamie for his annual check-up. After the examination, you ask the parents whether they have any questions. Jamie's father expresses concern that the other children in his son's pre-prep class are printing their names, but Jamie appears to have difficulty holding a pencil or crayon. How would you respond to this concern?

HEALTH EDUCATION

The Triple P Parenting Program

A widely recognised parenting and family support resource, available in over 30 countries, is the Triple P Parenting Program (Positive Parenting Program). This program aims to limit severe behavioural, emotional and developmental problems in children, and supports positive parenting techniques to achieve this. The program is based on internationally relevant evidence and can be tailored to individual needs. Further, the Triple P program is evidenced to benefit different cultures and socioeconomic groups. In both Australia and New Zealand, the Triple P program is well established and can be located via online links, child health programs/resources and government-based organisations. The program is a useful resource for healthcare and other professionals who work with children and families.

http://www.triplep.net/

Developmental tasks of preschoolers (3 to 6 years)

During the preschooler period, children are focused on developing initiative and purpose. Play provides the means for physical, mental and social development, and becomes the 'work' of children as they use it to understand, adjust to and work out experiences with their environment (**Figure 2.14**). Preschoolers demonstrate an active imagination and an ability to invent and imitate. They constantly seek to discover the why, what and how of objects and events around them. They are literal in their thinking, are increasingly sociable with other children and adults other than their parents, and are increasingly aware of their places and roles in their families. Key gross and fine motor, language and sensory milestones associated with the preschooler period can be found in **Table 2.3**.

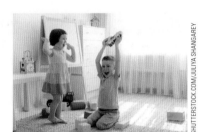

FIGURE 2.14 Play provides these preschoolers with the ability to interact with one another and develop their physical, mental and social skills.

SHUTTERSTOCK.COM/JULIYA SHANGAREY

TABLE 2.3 Growth and development during preschool years

AGE	GROSS MOTOR	FINE MOTOR	LANGUAGE	SENSORY
3 to 6 years	> Can ride a bike with training wheels > Can throw a ball overhand > Skips and hops on one foot > Can climb well > Can skip rope	> Can draw a six-part person > Can use scissors > Can draw circle, square or cross > Likes art projects, likes to paste and string beads > Can button > Learns to tie and buckle shoes > Can brush teeth	> Language skills are well developed, with the child able to understand and speak clearly > Vocabulary grows to over 2000 words > Talks endlessly and asks questions	> Visual acuity is well developed > Focused on learning letters and numbers

The preschooler stage of development is characterised by the refinement of many of the tasks that were achieved during the toddler stage and by the development of the skills and abilities that prepare children for the significant lifestyle change of starting school. Readiness for school is demonstrated by increased attention span and memory, ability to interact cooperatively, ability to tolerate prolonged periods of separation from family, and independence in performing basic self-care activities. Among the principal developmental tasks that must be mastered during the preschooler stage are to:

1. develop a sense of separateness as an individual
2. develop a sense of initiative
3. use language for increasing social interaction
4. interact in socially acceptable ways with others
5. develop a conscience
6. identify gender role and function
7. develop readiness for school.

Developmental tasks of school-age children (6 to 12 years)

With a well-developed sense of trust, autonomy and initiative, school-age children increasingly reduce their dependency on the family as their primary socialising agents and move to the broader world of peers (primarily same-sex peers) in their neighbourhoods and schools, as well as to teachers and adult leaders of social, sports and religious groups. They are increasingly exposed to others' views and seek approval from people outside the home. School-age children become industrious workers as they develop the significant physical, social and intellectual skills needed to operate in the broader and more diverse environment. They strive to be a part of a peer group and to achieve a variety of skills that are approved by others; in so doing, they become competent and confident in their own eyes. Key gross and fine motor, language and sensory milestones associated with this period can be found in **Table 2.4**.

TABLE 2.4 Growth and development during school-age years

AGE	GROSS MOTOR	FINE MOTOR	LANGUAGE	SENSORY
6 to 12 years	> Can ride a skateboard or rip stick > Able to ride two-wheeler bicycle > Plays netball, football	> Can put models together > Likes crafts > Enjoys board games, plays cards	> Vocabulary increases > Language abilities continue to develop	> Reading > Able to concentrate on activities for longer periods

The principal developmental tasks that must be mastered during the school-age stage are to:

1. become a more active, cooperative and responsible family member
2. learn the rules and norms of a widening social, religious and cultural environment
3. increase psychomotor and cognitive skills needed for participation in games and working with others
4. master concepts of time, **conservation** and **reversibility**, as well as oral and written communication skills
5. win approval from peers and adults
6. obtain a place in a peer group
7. build a sense of industry, accomplishment, self-assurance and self-esteem
8. develop a positive self-concept
9. exchange affection with family and friends without seeking an immediate payback
10. adopt moral standards for behaviour.

REFLECTION IN PRACTICE

Friendship in school-age children

Ten-year-old Pahia, who immigrated to Australia from Papua New Guinea 6 months ago, only speaks New Guinea Pidgin. Pahia's English expression has developed quickly, but she still requires support in understanding others and to be understood clearly. Pahia presents to you, the school nurse, with a sore throat. As you are assessing her, she bursts into tears and cries, 'I want to go home [to Papua New Guinea], I don't have any friends.' What is your response to Pahia?

Developmental tasks of adolescents (12 to 18 years)

The adolescent period is one of struggle and sometimes turmoil as the adolescent strives to develop a personal identity and achieve a successful transition from childhood to adulthood. For example, physical and sexual maturity is reached during adolescence, with girls tending to experience both puberty and a growth spurt earlier than boys. In addition, adolescents develop increasingly sophisticated cognitive and interpersonal skills, test out adult roles and behaviours, and begin to explore educational and occupational opportunities that will significantly influence future adult work life and socioeconomic status. Key gross and fine motor, language and sensory milestones associated with this period can be found in **Table 2.5**.

TABLE 2.5 Growth and development during adolescence

AGE	GROSS MOTOR	FINE MOTOR	LANGUAGE	SENSORY
12 to 18 years	> Muscles continue to develop > At times awkward, with lack of coordination	Well-developed skills	Vocabulary is fully developed	Development is complete

REFLECTION IN PRACTICE

Adolescents' reactions to physical changes

As the school nurse, you are presenting sexual education classes to all students in Year 6 at school. While you are explaining sexually transmitted infections, a few of the girls begin to giggle. You overhear one girl saying, 'Ruby doesn't have to worry about getting that, she's got no boobs, so no guy will even look at her.' How would you handle this situation?

Adolescents who have the support and trust of their families as they tackle the developmental tasks of this period are more likely to have a smoother and successful transition from the dependency of childhood to the independence of adulthood. If, however, their parents are too controlling, too permissive or too confrontational during this period, adolescents will experience difficulty in judging the appropriateness of their behaviour and in forming self-identity as competent, worthwhile individuals. If adolescents are able to find sufficient acceptance in a desired peer group or receive more positive than negative responses from the objects of their growing sexual or friendship interests, they will be able to work through feelings of inadequacy and insecurity, and become increasingly self-assured and competent in forming and maintaining adult relationships.

The principal developmental tasks that must be mastered during the adolescent stage are to:

1. develop self-identity and appreciate own achievements and worth
2. form close relationships with peers
3. gradually grow independent from parents
4. evolve own value system and integrate self-concept and values with those of peers and society
5. develop academic and vocational skills and related social, work and civic sensitivities

UNIT 1

6. develop analytic thinking
7. adjust to rapid physical and sexual changes
8. develop a sexual identity and role
9. develop skill in relating to people from different backgrounds
10. consider and possibly choose a career.

Developmental tasks of young adults (18 to 30 years)

Young adulthood is a time of separation from family and commencement of independence of life development, including new commitments, responsibilities, and accountability in social, work and personal relationships (**Figure 2.15**). It is also a period when individuals are exposed to more diverse people, situations and values than ever before. For example, the trend for women, particularly in the Western world but more recently in many Asian countries also, is to choose to extend education and career development over establishing households with children. Another trend is the reduction in focus and choice of young people to establish agricultural and rural lifestyles that support their personal and ongoing family needs. For many countries this may include international immigration, not just migration from rural to metropolitan regions.

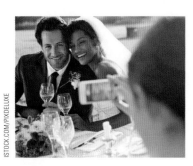

FIGURE 2.15 These young adults look forward to a life together as they celebrate their commitment to one another.

When parents and young adult offspring are able to resolve normal generational differences in philosophy and lifestyles, mastery of the young adult developmental tasks is greatly facilitated. Among the developmental tasks that the young adult must achieve are to:

1. establish friendships and a social group
2. grow independent of parental care and home
3. set up and manage one's own household
4. form an intimate affiliation with another and choose a mate or partner
5. learn to love, cooperate with, and commit to a life partner
6. develop a personal style of living (e.g. shared or single)
7. choose and begin to establish a career or vocation
8. assume social, work and civic responsibility and roles in social, professional, political, religious and civic organisations
9. learn to manage life stresses accompanying change
10. develop a realistic outlook and acceptance of cultural, religious, social and political diversity
11. form a meaningful philosophy of life and implement it in home, employment and community settings
12. begin a parental role for own or life partner's children or for young people in a broader social framework; for example, teaching, health care, volunteer work.

Developmental tasks of early middle adulthood (30 to 50 years)

Middle age, ranging from 30 to 70 years, is the longest stage of the life cycle, and is now often divided into early and late middle adulthood. During early middle adulthood, individuals experience relatively good physical and mental health. They settle into careers, lifestyles, patterns of relationships (married, parental, partnered and single) (**Figure 2.16**), political, civic, social, professional and religious affiliations and activities. During this stage, maximum productivity in work and influence over themselves and their environments is achieved. It is also a period when individuals experience a need to contribute to the next generation (can be referred to as a legacy or personal contribution to life).

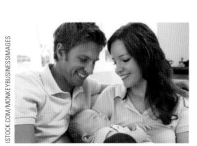

FIGURE 2.16 Young families enjoy their newfound parental roles.

Many who choose to express their generativity through the parental role may, during this period, achieve both the successful launching of their children into responsible adult roles and the associated increase in leisure time and financial resources needed to pursue enjoyable, non-parental goals and activities. Others, following divorce and remarriage/repartnering, may see a merging of offspring into new family groupings and the return to previous parental cycles. An increasing number of others, during or shortly after launching their young adult children into adult roles, may find themselves having to take on the responsibility of chronically ill, ageing parents. Each such life event can generate stress and disruption in individuals' lives with which they must cope. Developing effective coping strategies to manage the stress of life events or role transitions is a developmental task facing individuals in all life stages.

REFLECTION IN PRACTICE

Assessing development of early middle adulthood

During your assessment of adults in this developmental group, you need to consider whether they have achieved the following tasks:

1. attains a desired level of achievement and status in career
2. reviews, evaluates, refines and redirects career goals consistent with one's personal value system
3. continues to learn and refine competencies in areas of personal and career interests
4. manages life stresses accompanying change
5. continues to develop mature relationships with life partner and significant others
6. participates in social, professional, political, religious and community activities
7. copes with an empty nest and possibly a refilled nest
8. adjusts to ageing parents and helps plan support as required
9. continues enjoyable hobbies and leisure activities and begins to develop ones for their post-retirement
10. begins to plan for personal, financial and social aspects of retirement.

Consider the tasks aligned with this age group and apply these to a 35-year-old male who has just been diagnosed with advanced lung cancer. How might this make him feel in relation to achieving these developmental tasks?

Developmental tasks of late middle adulthood (50 to 70 years)

Many individuals during late middle adulthood may be diagnosed for the first time with a chronic health problem, such as arthritis, cardiovascular disease, cancer, diabetes or asthma. In addition, women generally experience a decrease in oestrogen and progesterone production, and undergo **menopause** during their late 40s or early 50s.

Changes also occur during late middle adulthood in work, family, social and community areas. For example, as the family structures change, parents rediscover being a couple and acquire new roles such as becoming grandparents. In addition, the gender developmental differences related to intimacy and autonomy seen in early adulthood begin to converge during late middle adulthood as men and women tend to take on similar life roles (Saxon, Etten & Perkins, 2015).

A variety of development tasks must be achieved by individuals during late middle adulthood. Among these tasks are to:

1. manage life stresses accompanying change
2. maintain interest in current political, cultural and scientific advances, trends and issues

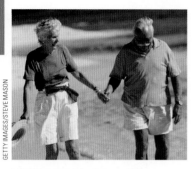

GETTY IMAGES/STEVE MASON

FIGURE 2.17 Adults in late middle adulthood frequently look forward to spending more time with their partner.

3. maintain affiliation with selected social, religious, professional, civic and political organisations
4. adapt to physical and mental changes and health status accompanying ageing
5. continue current activities and develop new interests and leisure activities that can be pursued consistent with changing abilities
6. adjust to more interaction and time spent with life partner without the presence of children (**Figure 2.17**)
7. develop supportive, interdependent relationships with adult children
8. help older parents and relatives cope with lifestyle changes (may include providing a home for them)
9. adjust to possible or actual loss of parents, life partner, older family members, and friends through death or their decreasing abilities to maintain independent living and self-care
10. prepare for and adjust to role changes, changing finances and changing lifestyle resulting from retirement.

Developmental tasks of late adulthood (70 years to death)

How individuals during late adulthood physically and emotionally age and how they confront and adjust to the changes associated with this stage are widely divergent. For those who have achieved the developmental tasks of middle adulthood and are comfortable with the life goals they have achieved, independence from the workplace and time to pursue more leisure activities are welcomed. A loss of work-related status and social outlets, reduced income, a decline in physical and some cognitive capabilities, and decreased resistance to and recovery from illness are often linked to late adulthood. How individuals adapt and cope with these changes is dependent on a number of factors, such as health status, poverty, family relationships, isolation and experiences of abuse or neglect (Saxon, Etten & Perkinsl, 2015).

Among the developmental tasks that must be achieved during late adulthood are to:

1. maintain and develop new activities that help retain functional capacities
2. accept and adjust to changes in mental and physical strength and agility and health status
3. maintain and develop activities that contribute to a continuing sense of usefulness, self-worth and enhanced self-image
4. develop new roles in the family as the oldest member
5. establish affiliation with own age group
6. accept and adjust to changing, possibly restricted, circumstances – social, financial and lifestyle
7. adapt to loss of life partner, family members and friends
8. prepare for the inevitability of own death.

Developmental assessment tools

A variety of developmental assessment tools are available for the nurse to use. Some of the most common tools assess mental, physical, emotional and social functional status of individuals and families. It should be noted that using some of these tools often require specialised training. **Table 2.6** summarises some of the tools that are frequently used.

TABLE 2.6 Examples of developmental assessment tools

TOOL	TARGET POPULATION	ASSESSMENT PARAMETERS	SPECIAL CONSIDERATIONS
Dubowitz Scale of Gestational Age[1]	Newborns	Assessment of gestational age	Useful if no dating or scans available
Denver II[2]	1 month to 6 years old	Personal/social, fine motor/adaptive, language, gross motor skills	Standardised for minority populations
Prechtl's General Movements Assessment (for Cerebral Palsy)[3]	Birth to 5 months corrected age	Assessing for fidgety movements	Fidgety movements are within the normal parameters
HEADSS (Home, Education, Activities, Drugs, Sex, and Suicide) Adolescent Risk Profile[4]	Adolescents	Home, education, activities, drugs, sex, suicide	Identifies high-risk adolescents, and provides a guide for anticipatory guidance
Life Experiences Survey[5]	Young and middle-aged adults	Events that have occurred within the past year, and the type and extent of impact the events have had	Self-administered; identifies respondents at high risk for high stress and in need of stress and coping counselling
Functional Activities Questionnaire (FAQ)[6]	Older adults	Level of independence demonstrated in the performance of activities of daily living	Can be completed by significant other or caregiver
Folstein Mini-Mental State Examination (MMSE)[7]	Older adults	Cognitive function	Can be easily administered in any clinical setting. A telephone version is also available. Assists in determining the need for a more definitive neurological examination
Minimum Data Set (MDS) for Nursing Facility Resident Assessment and Care Screening[8]	Nursing home residents	Cognitive patterns, communication and hearing patterns, vision patterns, physical functioning and structural problems, psychosocial wellbeing, mood and behaviour patterns, activity pursuit patterns, bowel and bladder status, disease diagnoses, health conditions, oral nutritional status, oral and dental status, skin condition, medication use, treatments and procedures, customary activities of daily living routines	Required by federal law for all patients residing in nursing homes
Functional Assessment Screening in the Elderly (FASE)[9]	Older adults	Functional disability	Suggests interventions when abnormal results are present
Beck Depression Inventory (BDI)[10]	Adults	Mood, pessimism, sense of failure, dissatisfaction, guilt, sense of punishment, disappointment in oneself, self-accusations, self-punitive wishes, crying spells, irritability, social withdrawal, indecisiveness, body image, function at work, sleep disturbance, fatigue, appetite disturbance, weight loss, preoccupation with health, loss of libido	Score indicating depression warrants referral to a mental health specialist

[1]Dubowitz, Dubowitz & Golderberg, 1970; [2]Glascoe, Foster, & Wolraich, 1997; [3]Einspieler & Prechtl, 2005; [4]Neinstein, Gordon, Katzman, Rosen & Woods, 2007; [5]Sarason, Johnson & Siegal, 1978; [6]McDowell & Newell, 1996; [7]Folstein, Folstein & McHugh, 1975; [8]Carnevali & Patrick, 1993 + United States of America and InterRAI version 3, 2011; [9]Resnick, 1994; [10]Gallagher, 1986

EXAMINATION **IN BRIEF**

Developmental assessment considerations
Note the consumer's stated chronological age.
> Tailor your questions to the consumer's expected level of ability according to developmental parameters until you can accurately assess the actual developmental level.

> When assessing small children, verify information with the caregiver.
> If a third party is assisting in the interview (for an older person or a consumer with special needs), address all questions to the consumer, not the intermediary.

CHAPTER RESOURCES

REVIEW QUESTIONS

For answers to these questions, see Answer section at the end of the book.

1. During which stage of the consumer interview process does the nurse collect the majority of the consumer's data?
   a. Joining stage
   b. Working stage
   c. Termination stage
   d. Summary stage

2. A consumer at a women's health clinic is telling you about the death of her nephew. She becomes silent and starts to cry. You touch her hand, nod to her, and say 'uh-huh'. You have used the communication technique of:
   a. Making observations
   b. Clarifying
   c. Facilitating
   d. Interpreting

3. The nurse should use listening responses when interviewing a consumer. Which of the following are examples? (Select all that apply.)
   a. Restating
   b. Reflecting
   c. Focusing
   d. Exploring
   e. Interpreting
   f. Encouraging comparisons

4. The nurse tells the consumer, 'Let's look at the environment you are located in when you have an asthma attack and see if we can identify your triggers.' This statement exemplifies the communication technique of:
   a. Confronting
   b. Informing
   c. Collaborating
   d. Presenting reality

5. With which of the following consumers should the nurse use mostly closed questions?
   a. Consumer with impaired hearing
   b. Consumer with impaired vision
   c. Non-English-speaking consumer
   d. Aphasic consumer

6. A patient wants to attach his rosary beads to the IV pole near his bed. What would be the best action for the nurse?
   a. Call the hospital chaplain
   b. Inform the patient that this is not in their job description
   c. Inform the patient that you cannot attach things to the equipment
   d. Tape the beads to the IV pole near his bed.

7. The nurse tells the consumer who was just diagnosed with prostate cancer, 'It's OK to cry. Most people who are given that diagnosis react in a similar fashion.' The nurse used the communication technique of:
   a. Presenting reality
   b. Normalising
   c. Offering false reassurance
   d. Advising

8. A major development task of early middle age is to:
   a. Evolve one's own value system and integrate it with those of family and society
   b. Form a meaningful philosophy of life and implement it in one's own household
   c. Develop a personal style of living and manage one's own household
   d. Work on a life review consistent with one's philosophy

9. One of the principal developmental tasks of adolescents is to:
   a. Manage life stress accompanying change
   b. Be independent of parental care and home
   c. Form an intimate affiliation with another
   d. Develop self-identity and appreciate own achievement and worth

10. When assessing an 18-month-old toddler, the nurse would expect to see:
   a. Building a tower of four blocks, drawing a circle and kicking a ball
   b. Pouring liquids, drawing circles and throwing a ball overhead
   c. Dressing and undressing self, running, jumping, and kicking a ball
   d. Walking up and down stairs, pushing and pulling toys, and skipping rope

FURTHER RESOURCES

> AuslanServices (Interpreters): http://www.auslanservices.com
> Australian Commission on Safety and Quality in Health Care – Australian Charter of Healthcare Rights: https://www.safetyandquality.gov.au/consumers/working-your-healthcare-provider/australian-charter-healthcare-rights
> Australian Commission on Safety and Quality in Health Care: https://www.safetyandquality.gov.au/standards/nsqhs-standards
> Australian Government. Children's health and immunisation: https://www.australia.gov.au/information-and-services/health/childrens-health-and-immunisation

> Australian Human Rights Commission: https://www.humanrights.gov.au/education/face-facts/face-facts-lesbian-gay-bisexual-trans-and-intersex-people
> NZ Human Rights: https://www.hrc.co.nz/
> Interpreting New Zealand: https://interpret.org.nz/
> KidsHealth: https://kidshealth.org.nz/
> Ministry of Health. Child health: https://www.health.govt.nz/our-work/life-stages/child-health
> New South Wales Government, HealthyKids: http://www.healthykids.nsw.gov.au
> Nursing and Midwifery Board of Australia – Code of ethics

for nurses & Code of ethics for midwives: http://www.
nursingmidwiferyboard.gov.au/News/2018-03-01-new-codes-
of-ethics-in-effect.aspx
> Nursing Council of New Zealand – Code of Conduct: https://
www.nursingcouncil.org.nz/Public/Nursing/Code_of_Conduct/
NCNZ/nursing-section/Code_of_Conduct.aspx
> The Paediatric Society of New Zealand: http://www.
paediatrics.org.nz/

> Sign Language Interpreters Association of New Zealand:
http://www.slianz.org.nz
> SMART Recovery Australia: https://smartrecoveryaustralia.
com.au/
> Triple P Positive Parenting Program: https://www.triplep.net/
glo-en/home/
> Child and Family Health Service: https://www.cafhs.sa.gov.au/

REFERENCES

American Academy of Pediatrics. (2020). Newborn and infant nutrition:
a clinical decision support chart. American Academy of Pediatrics.

Australian Bureau of Statistics. (2021). Religious affiliation in Australia.
Exploration of the changes in reported religion in the 2021 Census.
Retrieved 18 April 2022 from https://www.abs.gov.au/articles/
religious-affiliation-australia#:~:text=Religious%20affiliation%20
in%202021,-In%202021%2C%20more&text=In%202021%2C%20the%20
number%20of,No%20religion%20(38.9%25)

Australian Commission on Safety and Quality in Health Care. (2017).
National Safety and Quality Health Service Standards. 2nd ed. Sydney:
ACSQHC.

Australian Government Department of Health. (2022). Australian national
breastfeeding strategy collection. Retrieved 19 May 2022 from https://
www.health.gov.au/resources/collections/australian-national-
breastfeeding-strategy-collection?utm_source=health.gov.au&utm_
medium=callout-auto-custom&utm_campaign=digital_transformation

Australian Institute of Health and Welfare (AIHW). (2020). Australia's
health 2020. Alcohol risk and harm. https://www.aihw.gov.au/reports/
australias-health/alcohol-risk-and-harm

Carnevali, M., & Patrick, M. (Eds.). (1993). Nursing management for the
elderly (3rd ed.). Philadelphia: JB Lippincott.

Commonwealth of Australia. (2019). National Alcohol Strategy 2019–2028.
Canberra: Commonwealth of Australia.

Dubowitz, L. M. S., Dubowitz, V., & Goldberg, C. (1970). Clinical assessment
of gestational age in the newborn infant. Journal of Pediatrics,
77, 1–10.

Einspieler, C., & Prechtl, H. (2005). Prechtl's assessment of general
movements: a diagnostic tool for the functional assessment of the
young nervous system. Mental Retardation and Developmental
Disabilities Research Reviews 11(1), 61–7. doi: 10.1002/mrdd.20051.

Erikson, E. (1974). Dimensions of a new identity. New York: W. W. Norton.

Folstein, M. F., Folstein, S. E., & McHugh, P. R. (1975). 'Mini-mental state'.
A practical method for grading the cognitive state of patients for the
clinician. Journal of Psychiatric Research, 12, 189–98.

Freud, S. (1946). The ego and the mechanism of defense. New York:
International Universities Press.

Gallagher, D. (1986). The Beck Depression Inventory and older adults:
Review of its development and utility. In T. L. Brink (Ed.), Clinical
gerontology: A guide to assessment and intervention (pp. 149–63).
New York: Haworth Press.

Glascoe, F. P., Foster, E. M., & Wolraich, M. L. (1997). An economic analysis
of developmental detection methods. Pediatrics, 99, 830–7.

Hayes, K. (2020). (Ed.). Infant, toddler and child health sourcebook. (1st ed.).
Detroit: Omnigraphics.

Knight, E., & Lappalainen, L. (2017). Clinical Institute Withdrawal Assessment for
Alcohol–Revised might be an unreliable tool in the management of alcohol
withdrawal. Alcohol and Family Physician, 63(9), 691–5.

Kohlberg, L. (1981). The philosophy of moral development: Moral stages
and the idea of justice. New York: Harper & Row.

Kozlowska, K., Scher, S., & Helgeland, H. (2020). Functional somatic
symptoms in children and adolescents: a stress-system approach to
assessment and treatment. (1st ed.). Springer International Publishing.

Lissauer, T., & Carroll, W. (2022). Illustrated textbook of paediatrics.
(6th ed.). Elsevier Limited.

McDowell, I., & Newell, C. (1996). Functional disability and handicap.
Measuring health: A guide to rating scales and questionnaires.
(2nd ed.). New York: Oxford University Press.

Neinstein, L. S., Gordon, C. M., Katzman, D. K., Rosen, D. S., & Woods, E. R.
(Eds.) (2007). Adolescent health care: A practical guide (5th ed.).
New York: Lippincott Williams & Wilkins.

Piaget, J. (1952). The origins of intelligence in children. New York:
International Universities Press.

Quigley, A., Connolly, C., Palmer, B., & Helfgott, S. (2015). A brief guide to
the assessment and treatment of alcohol dependence (2nd ed.). Perth,
Western Australia: Drug and Alcohol Office. Retrieved 15 May 2022
from https://www.mhc.wa.gov.au/media/1171/dependence-brochure-
2014v8web.pdf

Resnick, N. M. (1994). Geriatric medicine and the elderly patient. In L. M.
Tierney, Jr., S. J. McPhee, & M. A. Papadakis (Eds.), Current medical
diagnosis & treatment (33rd ed.), pp. 41–60. Norwalk, CT: Appleton &
Lange.

Sarason, J. G., Johnson, J. H., & Siegal, J. M. (1978). Assessing the impact
of life changes: Development of life experiences survey. Journal of
Consulting Clinical Psychology, 46, 932–46.

Saxon, S. V., Etten, M. J., & Perkins, E. A. (2015). Physical change & aging:
A guide for the helping professions. (6th ed.). New York: Springer
Publishing Company.

Skye, L. M. (2006). Australian Aboriginal Catholic women seek wholeness:
Hearts are still burning. Pacifica 19(3), 283–307.

Statistics New Zealand. (2020). 2018 Census. Retrieved 19 May 2022 from
https://www.stats.govt.nz/2018-census/

Stein-Parbury, J. (2021). Patient & person interpersonal skills in nursing.
(7th ed.). Chatswood: Elsevier Australia.

United States of America and InterRAI. (2011). Minimum Data Sets
MDS 3.0. Retrieved 15 May 2022 from https://www.cms.gov/
Medicare/Quality-Initiatives-Patient-Assessment-Instruments/
NursinHomeQuaityInits/Downloads/Archive-Draft-of-the-MDS-30-
Nursing-Home-Comprehensive-NC-Version-1140.pdf

CHAPTER 3

THE COMPLETE HEALTH HISTORY INCLUDING DOCUMENTATION

LEARNING OUTCOMES

By the end of this chapter you should be able to:

1. identify three different types of health history and the context each type of health history may be used in
2. identify the components of the complete health history
3. describe how to assess the 10 characteristics of a chief complaint when examining present health status and history of the presenting illness
4. demonstrate sensitivity to consumers of different race, religion, cultural background, sexual orientation and socioeconomic status when conducting a health history
5. conduct a complete health history on well and ill consumers, and document appropriately according to context.

BACKGROUND

The health history is usually the first step of consumer assessment. It is the collection of subjective information on the consumer's health status from them and other sources. The health history can provide information on a consumer's health status as well as social, emotional, physical, cultural, developmental and spiritual identities. Consumer strengths and areas of improvement should also be identified. Combined with the physical examination findings, this information should guide the nurse in identifying consumer concerns, which serve as the foundation for their plan of care.

PUTTING IT IN CONTEXT

Problems encountered during history taking

You are taking a health history from Jessica, a 15-year-old female who has presented with abdominal pain. Her mother is not present but waiting outside for you to finish the assessment. You ask Jessica details about her sexual activity and she states, 'That's a bit personal! Why are you asking me this?' You explain that abdominal pain can be caused by many different issues, so you are trying to narrow down the possible area that needs further testing and investigation. Jessica seems to answer your questions fully after this and you feel like you have built rapport with her; she discloses that she had a termination about 6 weeks ago. After you have completed the health history, as Jessica is preparing to leave the room she states, 'You can't tell my mother about the termination I had. I know these sessions are supposed to be confidential.'

Your response will depend on the legal requirements relating to her age, as well as privacy and confidentiality requirements, if the presenting health concern is related to the termination, and if her mother asks for information.

What would the legal requirements be in your environment, if you found yourself presented with this issue?

The health history interview provides the mutual opportunity for the nurse and consumer to become more comfortable with each other and build rapport. The consumer usually feels more at ease with the collection of health history data than with the physical contact necessary for the examination. For this reason, the health history is usually performed prior to the physical examination. Additionally, the health history can help the clinician focus in on specific areas of examination or decide if more comprehensive diagnostic testing may be needed. The health history can be broadly or narrowly focused, depending on the consumer's needs and physical condition. Analysis of the information from the consumer in the health history provides the basis for planning the healthcare education needed by the consumer. The written health history also serves as part of the legal documentation of the consumer's health status. It is a means of communicating information to other healthcare team members, and in this way is an important factor in continuity of care.

Refer to Chapter 2 for communication techniques and strategies for dealing with consumers who have special needs.

TYPES OF HEALTH HISTORY

There are three types of health history: complete, focused and emergency. The choice of which type of health history to use may depend on the healthcare context norms and local requirements, and the clinician's judgement based on the consumer situation and acuity (the care needs of the consumer) (Dalton, Harrison, Malin & Leavey, 2018). The **complete health history**, described in this text, is a comprehensive history of the consumer's past and present health status, and covers many facets of a consumer's life. It is usually gathered during a consumer's initial visit to a healthcare facility on a non-emergency basis and for nursing admission when a consumer is admitted to the hospital.

The **focused history** is shorter and is specific to the consumer's current reason for seeking health care. For example, the consumer who seeks care for a sore throat and fever would have a focused health history taken. This type of history is also used for follow-up care. It documents the consumer's recovery from illness, or progress from a prior visit. However, remember that you may need to switch to a comprehensive or emergency health history if new information surfaces or red flags are evident in the focused health history.

Finally, the **emergency health history** is elicited from the consumer and other sources in an emergency. At times, lifesaving interventions will interrupt the emergency health history as well. Only information that is required immediately to treat the emergent need of the consumer is gathered; once the life-threatening condition is no longer present, the clinician may elicit a more comprehensive history from the consumer.

PREPARING FOR THE HEALTH HISTORY

Taking a complete health history with a consumer may require 30 to 60 minutes. Inform the consumer before the interview starts of the amount of time that will be required. If the health history is not completed within the allotted time, you may need to continue it later to avoid tiring the consumer, depending on their state of health, and willingness to be involved. If the consumer will be spending some time in the healthcare facility, then additional information can be obtained during routine nursing tasks such as bathing or assessing vital signs. Some healthcare agencies request that the literate consumer complete detailed health history forms on admission; in this instance, the nurse can validate the responses during the health history and save valuable time. In addition, information can often be obtained from prior medical records, and then checked and updated during the interview.

Legal documents status

It is essential that health professionals ask the consumer whether he or she has a living will, an advance healthcare directive, and an enduring power of attorney for health care. These documents should be obtained from the consumer at the outset and incorporated into the healthcare record in a prominent place so they can be quickly referred to and immediately seen by other healthcare professionals. Many organisations have policies and processes around the use of advance health directives, which will need to be the basis for how staff interact with and use these documents (Figure 3.1).

For example, consider this for these two consumers:

> A 52-year-old man presenting with shortness of breath tells you he does not want to be 'brought back to life' if his breathing stops. He has had no medical history except major depression. No family members are present.

> An admitted consumer on the ward, a 91-year-old man with multiple life-limiting illnesses, has stated to staff that he does not want resuscitation measures if his cardiac issues escalate. He goes into cardiac arrest the day after being admitted, and family members who are present tell you they want you to 'do everything you can' to resuscitate him.

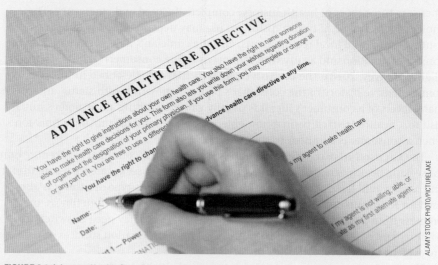

FIGURE 3.1 Advance Health Care Directive paperwork

General approach to the health history

1. Present with a professional appearance and demeanour.
2. Ensure an appropriate environment: for example, good lighting, comfortable temperature, if possible, lack of noise and distractions, and most importantly adequate privacy. Refer to Chapter 2 for additional information.
3. Sit facing the consumer at eye level, with the consumer in a chair or on a bed. Ensure that the consumer is as comfortable as possible because obtaining the health history can be a lengthy process.
4. Ask the consumer whether there are any questions about the interview before it is started.
5. Avoid the use of medical jargon. Use terms the consumer can understand.
6. Reserve asking intimate and personal questions for when rapport is established, and explain why you are collecting this information and how it will be stored.
7. Remain flexible in obtaining the health history. It does not have to be obtained in the exact order it is presented in this chapter or on organisational forms.
8. Remind the consumer that all information will be treated confidentially (keeping in mind the need for mandatory reporting requirements).

IDENTIFYING INFORMATION

The consumer usually completes the identifying information prior to the actual physical examination.

Today's date

Record the date and time that the health history is recorded. If the health history is not written immediately, document the time that the health history was taken and the time when it is recorded. In contexts where documentation is electronic, ensure you clearly identify when the health history was undertaken.

Demographic data

The following demographic data are usually requested for the consumer record:

1. Name
2. Address
3. Phone number
4. Date of birth
5. Birthplace
6. Occupation
7. Work address
8. Work phone number
9. Health insurance/Medicare number/Veteran Affairs/Community Services Card
10. Usual source of health care/Primary healthcare practitioner
11. Source of referral
12. Emergency contact.

THE COMPLETE HEALTH HISTORY ASSESSMENT TOOL

All elements of a complete health history are outlined in the following pages. Figure 3.2 provides an outline of the information needed for a complete health history, which will be explained in more detail in this section.

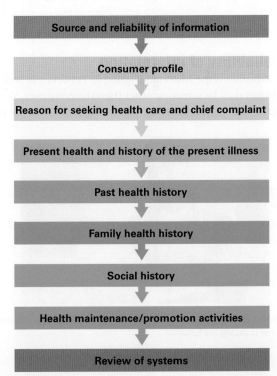

FIGURE 3.2 The complete health history assessment tool

The consumer assessment may be recorded in handwriting. The format of recording may be dictated by your local context rules. In contexts where electronic or digital systems are used to record consumer information, tools or formats may already be embedded to collect this information. An example is the Queensland Health integrated electronic medical record (ieMR), which uses an SBAR (situation, background, assessment, recommendation) format (see **Figure 3.3**). Additionally, in Chapter 11 you can see a free-form medical record entered into an electronic medical record such as Medical Director, which is often found in primary care contexts.

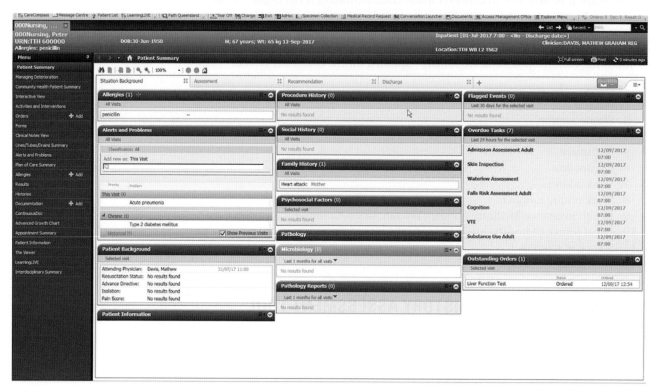

FIGURE 3.3 A digital tool for collecting consumer health assessment information

Source and reliability of information

Usually the adult consumer is the historian (**Figure 3.4**). However, in some instances, such as trauma, the historian may be someone other than the consumer. Note the name of the historian as well as the relationship between the historian and the consumer.

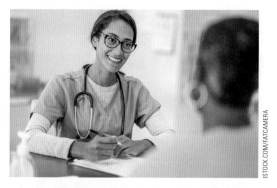

FIGURE 3.4 The nurse needs to note the source of the consumer health history. When working with adult consumers, the consumer is usually the historian.

In addition, assess the reliability of the historian. Consider the mental state of the historian, because emotions and certain medical conditions can influence the retelling of events. For example, the information provided by a consumer with severe Alzheimer's disease may not be accurate. Note if an interpreter is used. (Please ensure you have considered if the consumer requires an interpreter and organise one where required.)

Consumer profile

The **consumer profile** provides demographics that may be linked to health status. Note the consumer's age, gender and **race**, because many diseases are linked to these characteristics. Also note the consumer's marital status, as this may provide clues to support systems. In some organisations national key performance indicators (KPIs) are linked to identifying Indigenous communities. For example, in Queensland (Australia), one KPI is linked to identifying consumers who are Australian Aboriginal, Torres Strait Islander and Pasifika.

Reason for seeking health care and chief complaint

The **reason for seeking health care** is the reason for the consumer's visit and is usually focused on the specific problem. However, the experienced clinician will always assess opportunities for health promotion. Improving a person's ability for self-care should always be a goal the clinician works towards with the consumer. The consumer may present with multiple **chief complaints** for a single visit.

> EXAMPLES OF QUESTIONS TO ELICIT CONSUMER INFORMATION
> > 'What concern(s) bring you here today?' **or** 'What can I help you with today?'
> > 'How long has this condition been concerning you?'

Present health and history of the present illness

The **history of the present illness** is a chronological account of the consumer's primary complaint and the events surrounding it. The chronology can be taken in one of two ways: from the current state of the problem back to its origin (reverse chronology), or from the origin of the symptom leading to the current status (forward chronology). Either approach is acceptable as long as it is consistent with subsequent documentation of chronological events. Usually, the consumer describes one or two signs or symptoms that are abnormal and their progression. Allow the consumer to give the detailed history without interruption where possible, and then ask questions if information is incomplete.

> 'Describe the condition that you are experiencing from the earliest time that it occurred to the present.' (forward chronology)

Ten characteristics of each primary complaint can be ascertained for a complete history:

1. Location
2. Radiation
3. Quality
4. Quantity
5. Associated signs and symptoms
6. Aggravating factors
7. Alleviating factors
8. Setting
9. Timing
10. Impact on quality of life.

Note that some primary complaints may not have all 10 **qualifiers**; hoarseness, for example, may not be characterised by quantity. The primary complaint of abdominal pain will be used to demonstrate the use of these 10 characteristics.

Location

Location refers to the primary area where the symptom occurs or originates. You will want to take note of any changes to this description (if it does change) once you start the physical examination.

EXAMPLES OF QUESTIONS ASSESSING LOCATION

> 'Where does your abdomen hurt? Can you point to the location of the pain?'
> 'Is it in one location or is it spread out (diffuse or localised)?'
> 'Have you ever experienced this type of abdominal pain before? When?'
> 'Does this current pain differ from times you have had it in the past?'

Radiation

Radiation is the spreading of the symptom or other primary complaint from its original location to another part of the body. The areas of radiation can be diagnostic for specific pathologies.

EXAMPLES OF QUESTIONS ASSESSING RADIATION

> 'Does the pain move to another part of your body? If so, where?'
> 'Is the pain presently travelling to any other area?'
> 'Describe how the pain feels in the area to which it radiated.'

Quality

The quality of the primary complaint describes the way it feels to the consumer. Use the consumer's own terms to describe the quality of the primary complaint. For example, if the consumer is having difficulty describing pain, suggest some quality terms such as *gnawing, pounding, burning, stabbing, pinching, aching, throbbing* and *crushing*.

EXAMPLES OF QUESTIONS ASSESSING QUALITY

> 'What does the pain feel like?'
> 'What word would you use to describe it?'
> 'Is the pain deep or closer to the skin/surface?'

Quantity

Quantity depicts the severity, volume, number or extent of the primary complaint. The consumer may refer to the primary complaint with such terms as *minor*, *moderate* or *severe*, and *small*, *medium* or *large*. Although this terminology is important to the history, this information is subjective and is, therefore, difficult to quantify. If the consumer consistently uses the same terms, then a relative scale can be used to assess whether the primary complaint is improving or becoming worse as reported by the consumer.

Another mechanism that can be used to assess the quantity of pain is a numerical scale, known as the **Visual Analog Scale**, which rates pain from 0 (*no pain*) to 10 (*worst pain possible*). Refer to Chapter 6 for additional pain intensity scales.

EXAMPLES OF QUESTIONS ASSESSING QUANTITY OF PAIN

> 'Using a scale of 0 to 10, where 0 is no pain and 10 is the worst pain that you can imagine, rate the pain that you are having now.'
> 'When was the last time that your pain was at this level?'
> 'Has the severity of the pain changed? In what way?'
> 'Has the pain interfered with your normal daily activities? How?'

Associated signs and symptoms

Rarely does a primary complaint occur without affecting other components of the involved system or another body system. **Positive findings** are those associated manifestations that the consumer has experienced along with the primary complaint. Negative findings, also called **pertinent negatives**, are those manifestations expected in the consumer with a suspected pathology but which are denied by the consumer. If the consumer does not mention specific signs or symptoms that might be present with a given illness, ask whether they are present. Document both positive findings and pertinent negatives, because both give clues to the consumer's condition. For example, a consumer with headaches may have nausea, vomiting and diaphoresis as positive **associated manifestations**. Photophobia and phonophobia are pertinent negatives because they might be present in a consumer with headaches but are absent in this consumer at this time; lack of these associated manifestations may lead to a different diagnosis.

EXAMPLES OF QUESTIONS ASSESSING ASSOCIATED SIGNS AND SYMPTOMS
> 'Besides your abdominal pain, are you experiencing any additional symptoms? What are they?'
> 'Have these symptoms occurred before? Do they always occur when you have this type of abdominal pain?'

REFLECTION IN PRACTICE

Variety of alleviating factors
Remember that alleviating factors encompass more than pharmacological interventions. You need to keep in mind the multitude of treatments that consumers implement or seek out to relieve their discomfort. These include, but are not limited to, ice, heat, herbal supplements, exercise, animal-assisted therapy, magnet therapy, meridian therapy, yoga, massage, homeopathy, heat wraps, and other alternative and complementary medicine interventions. It is important to ask about these without judgement or advice when collecting the history. Ensure you collect information and assess the consumer before starting any education interventions, otherwise this may interfere with building rapport and fully exploring the consumer's condition.
> What alleviating factors do you and your friends and family use?
> How effective are they?
> Do you use multiple factors together in certain circumstances to make them more effective?

Aggravating factors
Those factors that worsen the severity of the primary complaint are the **aggravating factors**.

EXAMPLE OF QUESTIONS ASSESSING AGGRAVATING FACTORS
> 'Does anything make your pain worse? How long does this increase in pain last for?'

Alleviating factors
Alleviating factors are events that decrease the severity of the primary complaint.

EXAMPLES OF QUESTIONS ASSESSING ALLEVIATING FACTORS
> 'Does anything decrease the severity of or relieve the pain?'
> 'Has this worked in the past?'
> 'How long did this improvement last for?'

Setting
The setting in which the primary complaint occurs can provide valuable information about the course of the history. The setting can be the actual physical environment in which the consumer is located, the mental state of the consumer, or some activity in which the consumer was involved. The consumer may or may not be aware of any link between the setting and the occurrence of the primary complaint. For instance, the odour of some chemicals can induce headaches in some individuals.

Timing

The timing used to describe a primary complaint has three elements: onset, duration and frequency. Onset refers to the time at which the primary complaint begins and is usually described as *gradual* or *sudden*. Duration depicts the amount of time for which the primary complaint is present. *Continuous* and *intermittent* are terms that can be used to describe the duration of a primary complaint. When possible, the duration of the primary complaint should be stated in specific time increments, such as minutes, hours or days. Frequency describes the number of times the primary complaint occurs and how often it develops (e.g. number of times per day, season of year).

Impact on quality of life

The last two pieces of information needed in the history are the meaning or significance of the primary complaint to the consumer and the impact that the primary complaint has on the consumer. For example, the consumer may be concerned because his or her father started having headaches at his or her age, and subsequently had a stroke.

Secondly, the impact that the primary complaint has on the consumer's lifestyle should be investigated. For example, consider the elderly consumer who complains of minor headache but admits to cancelling routine activities because of the headache. In this case, the condition is presented as mild, but its effects impact significantly on this consumer's life.

Past health history

The **past health history (PHH)** or **past medical history (PMH)** provides information on the consumer's health status from birth to the present. The consumer may think you are ignoring the reason for seeking health care. The following statements can ease the transition.

Medical history

The medical history comprises all medical problems that the consumer has experienced during adulthood and their **sequelae** or aftermath. Chronic illnesses as well as serious episodic illnesses should be included. Forward or reverse chronology can be used to describe the medical history as long as the approach is consistent with the chronological format in the history. If the consumer denies medical illnesses, rephrase your questions. Some consumers may discount 'a little high blood pressure' as being insignificant, or the fact that they take medication for it as no longer affecting them.

EXAMPLES OF QUESTIONS ASSESSING MEDICAL HISTORY

> 'Do you currently receive treatment from a healthcare provider for anything?' **or** 'Have you ever been diagnosed as having an illness? What was it?'
> 'When was the illness diagnosed?'
> 'What is the current treatment for this problem?'
> 'Do you have any difficulty following the prescribed treatment?'
> 'Have you ever been hospitalised for this illness? Where? When? For what period of time? What was the treatment? How did you feel after the treatment?'
> 'Have you ever experienced any complications (sequelae) from this condition? What were they? How were they treated?'

Surgical history

Record a complete account of each surgical procedure, both major and minor, including the year performed, hospital, physician and sequelae, if known.

EXAMPLES OF QUESTIONS ASSESSING SURGICAL HISTORY

> 'Have you ever had surgery? What type?'
> 'Who was your doctor at the time?'
> 'When, where and by whom was the surgery performed?'
> 'Were you hospitalised?'
> 'Were there any complications? How were they treated?'
> 'Are you currently receiving any treatment related to this surgery?'
> 'Have you ever had an adverse effect from anaesthesia?'

CLINICAL **REASONING**

Allergies versus side effects

Many consumers report that they are allergic to specific medications. When questioned further on the specific reaction to a medication, consumers frequently report symptoms such as nausea, headache, diarrhoea and vomiting. While not discounting the consumer's experience with this medication, it is vital to keep in mind that these examples are not drug allergies but adverse reactions to the medication. True drug allergies usually manifest as urticaria, breathing difficulties or anaphylaxis. The sorts of questions you would need to differentiate between what consumers view as side effects or an allergy would include:

> What happened when you took this drug?
> Did you have any breathing difficulties, rashes, swelling in your face or limbs, or a change in blood pressure?
> Did your doctor or treating team change your treatment because of this reaction, or advise you to never have this treatment in the future because of the reaction?

UNIT 1

Allergies

Carefully explore all consumer allergies, which may include medications, topically applied dressings or tapes, or things that touch the skin (e.g. latex in gloves), animals, insect bites, foods and environmental allergens. Allergies are usually written in a conspicuous location in red ink on the consumer's physical chart in order to stand out, or a bright sticker is placed on the chart and other visual triggers are used indicating this consumer has an allergy (e.g. red arm band, medic alert necklace, bracelet or tattoo). For the electronic medical record, once entered this usually is made conspicuous on any subsequent screen related to this consumer.

EXAMPLES OF QUESTIONS ASSESSING ALLERGIES
> 'Are you allergic to any medications? Animals? Foods? Insect bites? Bee stings?'
> 'Are you allergic to anything in the environment?'
> 'Are you allergic to anything that you touch?'
> 'What symptoms do you get when you are exposed to this substance?'
> 'What treatment do you use? Is it effective?'
> 'Have you experienced any complications from the allergies? Which ones?'
> 'Have you ever seen an allergist for this problem? What happened?'
> 'Do you carry an EpiPen with you? Or have you ever needed adrenaline for anything?' (for consumers with life-threatening allergies such as bee stings)

Medications

Past and present consumption of medications, both prescription and over-the-counter (OTC), can affect the consumer's current health status.

CLINICAL **REASONING**

Natural remedies

Natural remedy products are consumed by more of the population than ever before. Whether to improve health or combat illness and pain, this branch of complementary and alternative medicine deserves the nurse's attention. Glucosamine, ginkgo biloba, chondroitin, ephedra, black cohosh and St John's wort are just a few of the many products that consumers ingest. As these products are considered dietary supplements in New Zealand and Australia, they are not held to the same level of scrutiny and accountability as medications. Different brands of the same herbal product can have varying levels of potency and purity. Because many people consider these products to be natural, consumers rarely consider the possibility of herbal products interacting adversely with one another or with prescription medications. For this reason, consumers need to be asked at every encounter which OTC herbal products are being consumed.

Prescription medication

EXAMPLES OF QUESTIONS ASSESSING PRESCRIPTION MEDICATION
> 'What prescription medications are you currently taking? Who prescribed them?'
> 'What prescription medications have you taken in the past? Who prescribed them?'
> 'What is the dose? How often do you take this medication?'
> 'How do you take this medication (e.g. pills, liquid, suppository, drops, inhaler, cream, ointment, patch, injection)?'
> 'For how long have you been taking this medication?'
> 'Have you ever experienced any side effects with this medication?'
> 'Have you ever had an allergic reaction to this medication? What happened?'
> 'Tell me the purpose of this medication.'

CLINICAL **REASONING**

Obtaining an accurate medication history – OTC products
Frequently, consumers discount OTC medications such as aspirin, paracetamol, ibuprofen, vitamins, enemas, cold remedies and antacids. Ask the consumer whether such products are used, because they can adversely interact with prescribed medications and with one another. Also, women frequently overlook birth control pills and men discount medications used for erectile dysfunction; keep this in mind when interviewing.

The outcome of the medication history may point to a need for consumer education. If contact is made with the consumer prior to the healthcare visit, ask the consumer to bring in all medications currently being taken. This will allow you to identify all medications that are in date and if the consumer's account of what they take matches with the prescription on the label. Many consumers keep unused medications past their expiration date. This presents a potential health hazard because some medications lose their potency after a period of time and others become toxic.

Over-the-counter medication

EXAMPLES OF QUESTIONS ASSESSING OVER-THE-COUNTER MEDICATION
> 'Do you currently take any over-the-counter medications? Which ones?'
> 'Why do you take this medication?'
> 'Do you take any other remedies? For what purpose?'
> Repeat all but the first and last questions from the 'Prescription medication' section.
> 'Do you ever take aspirin, paracetamol, ibuprofen, antacids, calcium supplements, nutritional or herbal supplements, vitamins or laxatives? Do you douche? Administer enemas? Do you take allergy pills or cold medications?' (If yes, repeat all but the first and last questions of the previous section.)
> 'Do you consume any probiotics or diet supplements? Which? How much? How often?'

Communicable diseases

Communicable diseases can have a grave impact on the individual as well as on society. Some communicable diseases generate enough of a concern to the community that they are reportable to the public health department. The most talked about communicable disease at present is human immunodeficiency virus (HIV), the virus responsible for acquired immune deficiency syndrome (AIDS). In recent years, there has also been a major focus on hepatitis C and the growing number of consumers diagnosed with it. There is substantial value in asking the consumer about possible exposure to communicable diseases, because pathology may not manifest itself until many years after exposure.

EXAMPLES OF QUESTIONS ASSESSING COMMUNICABLE DISEASES
> 'Have you ever been diagnosed with an infectious or communicable disease (e.g. syphilis, chlamydia, herpes or other sexually transmitted infections), diphtheria, tetanus, pertussis (whooping cough) or tuberculosis? Which one(s)?'
> 'What were your symptoms?'
> 'How were you treated?'
> 'Did you have any complications? What were they? Were there any permanent consequences?'
> 'Have you ever had hepatitis?' (If yes, repeat the second, third and fourth questions.)
> 'Have you ever been told that you are HIV positive or that you have AIDS?' (If yes, repeat the second, third and fourth questions.)
> 'Do you have any tattoos or body piercings? Where were they done?' Tattoos or piercings done in sub-optimal conditions (e.g. many developing countries and unregistered studios/home studios) are more likely to be a cause of concern or higher index of suspicion for exposure to a communicable blood-borne disease.
> 'Have you ever been exposed to someone who had a communicable disease? Which disease(s)?'

Injuries and accidents

A consumer's injury and accident history can reveal a pattern that is amenable to health promotion. For example, a teenager who sustains an injury from falling off his skateboard without a helmet and other protective equipment would be a candidate for health education. Consider the need to use a domestic and family violence screening tool. Please have a look at current tools available from government or specialist support agencies: https://www.justice.qld.gov.au/initiatives/end-domestic-family-violence/our-progress/enhancing-service-responses/dfv-common-risk-safety-framework

EXAMPLES OF QUESTIONS ASSESSING INJURIES AND ACCIDENTS
> 'Have you ever been involved in an accident?' **or** 'Have you ever been injured in any way?'
> 'What occurred? Did you lose consciousness?'
> 'Did you take any precautionary measures? What were they?'
> 'Were you hospitalised? For how long?'
> 'Were there any complications? What were they?'
> 'Were there any long-term effects from this injury/accident?'
> 'Have you ever sustained an injury in a car accident? Describe.'
> 'Have you ever had a broken bone? Stitches? Burns?'
> 'Have you ever been assaulted? Raped? Shot? Stabbed?'
> 'Have you ever been bitten by an animal or insect (e.g. white tail spider, snake, tick)?'

Special needs

The awareness of any cognitive, physical (**Figure 3.5**) or psychosocial disability is essential to providing individualised health care to a consumer. A consumer with Down syndrome, a paraplegic and a consumer with intention to harm themselves all have unique needs. These consumers may receive less than optimal health care if their particular limitations are not identified and considered when planning treatment.

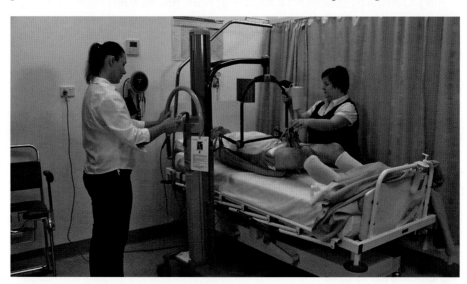

FIGURE 3.5 Consumers with physical special needs, such as a wheelchair or requiring assistance to mobilise, need to have this documented in their health history.

EXAMPLES OF QUESTIONS ASSESSING SPECIAL NEEDS
> 'Do you have any disability, impairment or special need? Can you describe this and how it affects you?'
> 'What type of limitations does this disability/impairment/special need place on you?'
> 'What strategies do you use to limit the effect the disability/impairment/special need has on your lifestyle?'
> 'What support systems help you cope with this disability/impairment/special need?'
> 'Does your disability/impairment/special need place an extra financial burden on you? How do you manage that?'

Blood transfusions

The chance of contracting an infectious disease from a blood transfusion is greatest in consumers who receive many transfusions, such as haemophiliacs, oncology consumers and trauma victims. Blood collection agencies and other organisations are continuously improving their screening tools and history-taking procedures to protect the nation's blood supply. Still, the recipient assumes some risk with every transfusion. Tests are available to screen blood for hepatitis, HIV, and some other viruses. Unfortunately, no approved diagnostic test is available to screen blood for malaria and other infectious diseases. You will need to be mindful of cultural considerations for those who have beliefs that preclude the acceptance of blood transfusions, as even discussing this topic may cause discomfort for some.

EXAMPLES OF QUESTIONS ASSESSING BLOOD TRANSFUSIONS
> 'Have you ever received a blood transfusion (whole blood or any of its components)? When?'
> 'Why did you receive this blood product?'
> 'What quantity did you receive?'
> 'Did you experience any reaction to this blood product? What was it?'

Childhood illnesses

Rarely are adults familiar with a complete history of their childhood illnesses. Ask the consumer about specific childhood diseases by name. Note: although COVID-19 is not considered a childhood illness, ensure that you assess the consumer's history with any communicable disease or virus.

EXAMPLES OF QUESTIONS ASSESSING CHILDHOOD ILLNESSES
> 'Have you ever had any of the following illnesses: varicella (chickenpox), diphtheria, pertussis (whooping cough), measles, mumps, rubella, polio, rheumatic fever or scarlet fever?' (This question is eliminated if previously asked during the communicable diseases section.)
> 'How old were you when the illness occurred?'
> 'Was an actual diagnosis made? By whom?'
> 'Were there any complications? What were they?'

Immunisations

The history of immunisations is closely tied to childhood illnesses. Most immunisations are received in childhood, though some are targeted to adults, pandemics, or when planning to travel. The adult consumer may not recall the exact dates when the immunisations were given, as with childhood illnesses, but should be generally aware that all the regular immunisations were received. Routine immunisations are also associated with different groups. Healthcare workers are frequently given the hepatitis A, B, C, varicella and tuberculosis vaccine, and most recently the COVID-19 vaccines and their mandated boosters. Every April, the adult population and other groups who are considered more susceptible are encouraged to receive the influenza vaccine. Vaccinating in April ensures protection for the peak flu season in the southern hemisphere. Vulnerable groups include children between 6 months and less than 5 years, adults over age 65, Aboriginal and Torres Strait Islander peoples aged 6 months and over, those aged 6 months or over with specific risk (e.g. solid organ transplant recipients, people with HIV or AIDS, people with asplenia), pregnant women and those who are at high risk through occupational exposure (e.g. those who work with the public, healthcare workers, childcare professionals, commercial poultry and pork industry workers etc.) (Australian Government Department of Health and Aged Care, 2022). In addition, travellers to underdeveloped areas of the world receive numerous vaccines prior to visiting specific regions. Immunisation schedules supported by government funding are available across the life span. Review the latest immunisation schedule for further information; this is also discussed in detail in Chapter 20, and websites are provided at the end of this chapter.

Family health history

The family health history records the health status of the consumer, as well as that of immediate blood relatives. At a minimum, the history needs to contain the age and health status of the consumer, spouse, children, siblings and the consumer's parents. Ideally, if possible, the consumer's grandparents, aunts and uncles should be incorporated into the history as well.

The second component of the family health history is the report of occurrences of familial or genetic diseases. Such information is crucial to the consumer and may not have been revealed previously because some familial illnesses do not occur in every generation.

CLINICAL **REASONING**

Practice tip: Family health history and cultural restraints

In some cultures (e.g. Aboriginal and Torres Strait Islander cultures), it is disrespectful to speak of the dead. Thus, the consumer may be reluctant to provide detailed information on the family health history of dead relatives. In these cases, you can ask the consumer whether there is any history of specific diseases in the family, rather than focusing on any specific deceased individual. The consumer may be willing to share in which previous generation and on which side of the family the condition existed. If these approaches are unsuccessful, explain to the consumer the importance of this information because it may provide clues to current health conditions.

EXAMPLES OF QUESTIONS ASSESSING FAMILY HEALTH HISTORY

You may want to preface the family health history questions with the following statement:

> 'Different diseases tend to run in families. I would like to ask you about your family and their health to gain a better understanding of your background.'

You can then continue with questions about the family health history:

> 'Tell me about who makes up your family: spouse, children, siblings and parents.' (Be aware and prepared for consumers who have family issues, and who may become upset talking about their family and those with whom they are no longer in contact.)
> 'Do any of these individuals have any medical illnesses or diseases? What are they?'
> 'Have there been any deaths in your immediate family? What was the cause of death? How old was this person at the time of death?' (Be aware that this may be an inappropriate question for some cultural groups, and for those with recent deaths in the family.)
> 'Has anyone in your family ever had any of the following illnesses? heart disease, sudden cardiac death before age 50, hypertension, stroke, tuberculosis, diabetes mellitus, cancer, kidney disease, blood disorders, sickle cell anaemia, arthritis, epilepsy, migraine headaches, gout, thyroid disease, liver disease, asthma, allergic disorders, obesity, alcoholism, mental illness (schizophrenia, depression), intellectual disability, drug addiction, AIDS, HIV infection'

Social history

The **social history** explores information about the consumer's lifestyle that can affect health. You may have already gleaned some of this information in discussing family in the previous section. If so, aim to add to rather than repeat the same information. Introduce this area of questioning with statements similar to the following.

EXAMPLE OF QUESTIONS ASSESSING SOCIAL HISTORY

> 'Now I would like to ask you some questions about your lifestyle. This information is important because of the effects that different practices can have on your health.'

CLINICAL **REASONING**

Practice tip: Family health history for a consumer who was adopted
Consumers who were adopted have varying degrees of information about their biological parents. Encourage adopted consumers to be frank about their family health history. If the history of the biological parents is unknown, this is documented.

Likewise, the history of adoptive parents can be equally important. Certain environmental factors (such as smoking, drug and alcohol use, and sanitation) may influence the health of the adopted child into their adult years.

Alcohol use

The intermittent and prolonged use of alcohol can interfere with normal metabolism and normal body function.

EXAMPLES OF QUESTIONS ASSESSING ALCOHOL USE
> 'How much alcohol do you drink per week?'
> 'How often do you drink?'
> 'What type of alcohol do you prefer (beer, wine, wine coolers, liquor, spirits)?'
> 'Do you ever consume homemade alcohol or homebrew?'
> 'What quantity do you usually consume at one time?'
> 'Has your drinking pattern changed? In what way?'
> 'When did you first start to drink?'
> 'How long have you been drinking the amount that you are currently consuming?'
> 'At what time of the day do you drink?'
> 'Have you ever lost consciousness or blacked out after drinking?'
> 'Have you ever forgotten what happened when you were drinking?'
> 'Do you drink alone?'
> 'Do you drive after drinking?'
> 'Did you ever drink during pregnancy? How much?' (for women)
> 'Do you think you have a drinking problem?'

CLINICAL **REASONING**

Practice tip: The Alcohol Use Disorders Identification Test (AUDIT)
The Alcohol Use Disorders Identification Test (AUDIT) screening tool is easily administered and can be used to assess a consumer's likelihood of having an alcohol use disorder. This is the internationally developed tool that has translations in 40 languages and significant research supporting the validation of the tool.

There is a shortened version of this tool called the AUDIT-C (a three-question test) that may also be used for a very quick assessment.

Have a look at these two tools at the following links:
> AUDIT: https://auditscreen.org/
> AUDIT-C: https://www.hepatitis.va.gov/alcohol/treatment/audit-c.asp#S1X

Tobacco use

Because of the harmful nature of tobacco products, the consumer's use of tobacco should be ascertained at each visit. If tobacco is used, it is the role of the nurse to encourage the consumer to consider the benefits of quitting. Many resources are available to the nurse to assist the consumer in the smoking cessation process. See websites at end of this chapter.

Some providers quantify tobacco use in the number of packs per day (PPD) for a specified number of years; for example, 2 PPD × 15 years. Additionally, if your consumer uses alcohol and other drugs including tobacco, the Alcohol, Smoking and Substance Involvement Screening Test (ASSIST tool) developed by the World Health Organization may be best to use, and all these elements can be screened for at the one time. Visit the following link to review this tool and support materials published by the World Health Organization: https://www.who.int/publications/i/item/978924159938-2

EXAMPLES OF QUESTIONS ASSESSING TOBACCO USE

> 'Do you use or have you ever used tobacco (cigarettes [filtered or nonfiltered], pipe, cigars)?'
> 'At what age did you start to use tobacco?'
> 'What quantity do you use on a daily basis?'
> 'Has this amount changed? In what way?'
> 'Have you ever tried to quit? How many times? What method(s) did you use? What was the outcome?'
> 'How long ago did you quit?'
> 'Do you think you have a smoking (tobacco) problem?'
> 'Do you live with someone who smokes?'

CLINICAL **REASONING**

Practice tip: Dealing with sensitive topics

How do you ask sensitive questions? Alcohol, drug use and sexual practices are some of the most sensitive areas that are addressed in the health history. Here are some tips for dealing with these sensitive topics:

> Ask these questions in the later stages of the interview after rapport has been established.
> Use direct eye contact (if culturally appropriate); this demonstrates the importance of the topic to the consumer and your lack of embarrassment.
> Pose questions in a matter-of-fact tone.
> Adopt a non-judgemental demeanour. Be aware of your facial expression.
> Use the communication technique of normalising when appropriate (e.g. 'Many high school students drink alcohol or use drugs or engage in sexual relationships on a regular basis. Does this happen at your school? With you?').

Drug use

The questions about use of drugs in this social history section of the complete health history are not to be confused with the medication section under the past health history, which includes the use and abuse of OTC and prescription medications. The questions in this section refer to the use of illegal substances. You may feel uncomfortable asking the consumer whether there has been drug use; remind the consumer that the information will be kept confidential and that the withholding of information may delay necessary treatment.

EXAMPLES OF QUESTIONS ASSESSING DRUG USE

> 'Do you use or have you ever used marijuana, amphetamines, hallucinogens, sedatives, cocaine, crack, heroin, PCP, other inhalants (e.g. petrol or paint), or other recreational or street drugs?'
> 'When did you first start to use drugs?'
> 'What amount and how often do you use?'
> 'Has this changed? In what way?'
> 'In what form do you use the drug (pill, needle, snort, sniff, other)?'
> 'Describe how you inject the drug.'
> 'Do you share needles? Do you clean the needles between uses? How?'
> 'Have you experienced any health problems from the drug use?'
> 'Have you ever overdosed? What happened?'
> 'Have you ever been through a drug rehabilitation program? What was the outcome?'
> 'Do you think you have a drug problem?'

REFLECTION IN PRACTICE

Responding appropriately to sensitive information

Seventeen-year-old Charli is brought to the emergency department by her mother, who explains that she heard a loud noise in the bathroom and ran upstairs to find her daughter unconscious on the floor, with her limbs shaking and jerking. Charli's seizure lasted for approximately 2 minutes. When Charli awoke, she had no memory of the seizure. Charli's mother is concerned as there is no history of epilepsy and she has not had a seizure before. Charli's mother excuses herself to go and provide some information to the administration officer. While she is out of the room, Charli tells you that she takes MDMA occasionally. She then asks, 'Do you think that has anything to do with what happened?'

> How would you respond to Charli's question?
> Do you exhibit any biases when working with people who take street drugs? Do these biases interfere with your nursing care? If so, what actions do you take to control your bias?
> Explore the legal ramifications of working with consumers who take illegal drugs in your city or state. Are there special provisions if the consumer is a minor?

Domestic and intimate partner violence

Domestic and **intimate partner violence (IPV)** is violence that occurs between family members. It can include intimidation, emotional abuse, isolation, minimising, denying and blaming, using children to coerce, threaten or make the partner feel guilty, sexual abuse, rape, male privilege, economic abuse or coercion and threats (Services Australia, 2022). The latest research shows that women are more likely than men to experience family, domestic and sexual violence.

In Australia, 1 in 6 women and 1 in 16 men have experienced physical and/or sexual violence, 1 in 4 women and 1 in 6 men have experienced emotional abuse, and 1 in 5 women and 1 in 20 men have been sexually assaulted or threatened by a current or previous partner (AIHW, 2019). One woman is killed every nine days and one man is killed every 29 days by their partner (AIHW, 2019). Family violence among Australian Aboriginal and Torres Strait Islander communities occurs more frequently than in the general population (AIHW, 2019).

In New Zealand, a survey of women found that intimate partner violence was 1 in 2 for Māori women and 1 in 3 for other women. Those aged 15–29 years were the largest group of people experiencing sexual assault (66%). People who are gay, lesbian or bisexual were more than twice as likely compared to the general population to experience sexual or intimate partner violence. The majority of sexual (94%) or family violence incidents (76%) were not reported to police (New Zealand Ministry of Justice, 2020; New Zealand Ministry of Justice, 2015).

It is vital to be familiar with your country/state's legal statutes regarding mandatory reporting of actual and suspected violence and abuse.

Just as many healthcare providers advocate screening for tobacco and alcohol use for both men and women at each healthcare encounter, some providers recommend routine screening for domestic and intimate partner violence at every healthcare encounter for women. Although men can be the victims of domestic and intimate partner violence, the majority of victims are women. People may not disclose violence unless asked about it and, even then, may initially answer in the negative; however, over 94% of women found it acceptable to be asked about abuse while pregnant (Special Taskforce on Domestic and Family Violence in Queensland, 2015), and the first antenatal visit appears to be the best screening point for pregnant women (Dahlen, Munoz, Schmied & Thornton, 2018; Campo, 2015). In about half of all cases of women murdered, the perpetrator is a current or ex-partner, and approximately 3 in 4 of these women had been assaulted previously by the partner who killed them (Family Violence Death Review Committee, 2017).

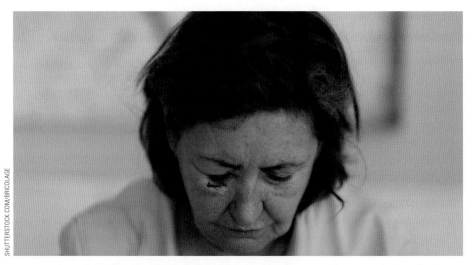

SHUTTERSTOCK.COM/BRICOLAGE

FIGURE 3.6 Seeing a consumer with sutures or other injuries prompts the nurse to inquire about the events that led to the incident, as well as past injuries.

Additionally, significant increases in intimate partner violence were reported during the COVID-19 pandemic, with many victims unable to seek help due to safety concerns (Boxall & Morgan, 2021).

PUTTING IT IN CONTEXT

Assessing for domestic and intimate partner violence

You note that Tasha has come to the ED three times in the past 6 months. Six months ago, she reported falling down the steps and hitting her head. Her old chart documents that she was seen for a mild closed head injury with concussion. Two months ago, Tasha reported falling while roller blading and broke her left arm. Her cast was removed two weeks ago. Today, Tasha presents with multiple facial and mouth lacerations. She tells you that she fell off her bike. You note multiple ecchymoses on the exposed areas of her skin.

You would need to take into consideration her personal safety when questioning her closer. For example, many perpetrators of intimate partner violence will not allow the partner to be alone with a health practitioner when seeking health care. Many health environments have screening tools and processes in place to protect the safety of the consumer and health professionals in these circumstances.

> Investigate your agency's policy on reporting actual and suspected violence or abuse, as this will shape your response and actions.
> Investigate your government's regulations on mandatory reporting of actual and suspected violence or abuse, as this will shape your response and actions.

Some clues that might alert you to the possibility of domestic and intimate partner violence are as follows:
> Frequent injuries, accidents or burns
> Previous injuries for which the individual did not seek health care
> Injury is inconsistent with the consumer's report of how it occurred
> Refusal of the consumer to discuss the injury
> Significant other accompanies the consumer to the ED, answers questions for consumer, and refuses to leave the consumer's side
> Significant other has a history of previous violence or substance abuse
> Vague symptoms such as chronic pain

EXAMPLES OF QUESTIONS ASSESSING DOMESTIC AND INTIMATE PARTNER VIOLENCE

Using the communication technique of normalising, the nurse can screen for potential domestic and intimate partner violence. Some supportive comments might be:

> 'Unfortunately intimate partner violence occurs frequently in lots of families who use our services. Is this what happened to you?'
> 'Domestic and intimate partner violence occurs very frequently in our community. Keeping this in mind, I would like to ask you some questions.'

There are many different ways to screen for IPV. In Australia and New Zealand, the most commonly accepted way for non-domestic-violence health professionals to screen includes asking the following questions:

> 'Within the last year, have you been hit, slapped or hurt in other ways by your partner or ex-partner?'
> 'Has your partner ever physically threatened or hurt you?'
> 'Sometimes partners react strongly in arguments and use physical force. Is this happening to you?'
> 'Does your partner restrict your access to money, social events or friends and family?'
> 'Do you have children? If so are you worried about your children's safety with your partner or ex-partner?'
> 'Are you frightened of your partner or ex-partner?'

If the woman answers 'NO' to these questions, screening is stopped there and you can give her a general information pamphlet then, saying something like: 'Here is some information we give to all women about domestic violence.'

If the woman answers 'YES' to any question, then continue to ask the following questions:

> 'Are you safe to go home when you leave here?'
> 'Would you like some assistance with this?'

A further three questions are also asked if the woman answers 'YES' to any of the above:

> 'Do you have children? (If so) Have they been hurt or witnessed violence?'
> 'With whom are your children now? Where are they?'
> 'Are you worried about their safety?'

(RACGP, 2021; NSW Health, 2022; NSW Health 2020)

Answers that make the health professional concerned for the child/ren's welfare are then required to ensure their actions are in accordance with child protection notifications requirements in their state, territory or area.

Actions taken may then include:

> Giving information about IPV
> Support given and options discussed
> Report to Department of Community and Family Services
> Notify police
> Refer to community or support services.

Screening is generally not completed if the following circumstances apply:

> Presence of a partner where the partner cannot easily be separated from the consumer
> Presence of other family members
> Presence of a child older than three
> Person declines to answer questions.

ADAPTED FROM NSW HEALTH, 2022; NSW HEALTH, 2020.

It is imperative to document physical violence examination findings concisely and accurately. Incorporate drawings of injury locations or use printed anatomical maps on which injuries can be documented. Many EDs have cameras as a resource, so that the staff can photograph injuries to document or include in the consumer's records. This documentation is important, not only for communicating health conditions to other health professionals, but also for use by clinicians who are called to bear witness for police statements and court cases.

Keep in mind that many victims of IPV experience anxiety, depression, substance abuse and posttraumatic stress disorder after their attack and these conditions can last for years. Specific healthcare procedures, such as a gynaecological examination, may invoke memories of the IPV. The nurse needs to be sensitive to the consumer's needs at these times and must try to make the consumer feel as safe as possible in this environment.

Sexual practice

Sexual practice histories focus on healthy sexual practices as well as the transmission of communicable diseases. Various medications can affect sexual function.

Questioning a consumer about sexual practices may be uncomfortable for both consumer and nurse. The consumer may notice your uneasiness with this topic and may feel embarrassed to answer the questions. Examine your personal feelings on sexuality and attain a comfort level that will allow ease in questioning. The health histories in Chapter 17 provide additional information about female and male reproductive health.

EXAMPLES OF QUESTIONS ASSESSING SEXUAL PRACTICE

> 'What term would you use to describe your sexual orientation (heterosexual, homosexual, bisexual, intergender, transgender, other)?'
> 'At what age was your first sexual experience?'
> 'With how many partners are you currently involved? Has this changed?'
> 'What method of birth control do you use? Do you have any questions about it? Would you like additional information on other methods of birth control?'
> 'What measures do you use to prevent exchange of body fluids during sexual activity?'
> 'Do you engage in oral or anal intercourse?'
> 'Have you ever had a sexual partner who had a sexually transmitted infection?'
> 'Do you take any prescription or medications or supplements to help your sexual performance?'

URGENT FINDING

Risk assessment: Dangerous sexual practices

Be alert for individuals who practise potentially lethal sexual practices that involve near-strangulation. In adolescents, this practice is often referred to as auto-eroticism or the 'choking game'. Individuals literally choke one another with their hands, or they can use noose-like materials such as belts, scarves and ropes. Adults usually use more sophisticated techniques to have this auto-erotic experience. The premise of this 'game' is to experience the euphoria that occurs when one is close to unconsciousness or becomes unconscious. In some instances, individuals have died during these activities. If dangerous sexual practices are identified, urgent health education informing the individual of the associated risks needs to be implemented and documented.

CLINICAL **REASONING**

Practice tip: Eliciting the sexual history

Be aware that consumers may refuse to answer questions pertaining to sexual history; try returning to these questions later. Ask the consumer whether a nurse of a different gender would make the consumer more comfortable in discussing sexual practice.

The adolescent consumer may refuse to answer these questions or may provide false answers if the parent or caregiver is in the room. You could ask the caregiver to leave the room at the completion of the health history so that you can ask the consumer whether there is anything else that he or she would like to say.

Be alert for cues that demonstrate the consumer's desire for sexual education, such as questions or requests for written information. Answer the consumer's questions honestly.
> 'Are you satisfied with your sexual performance?'
> 'Do you have any infertility issues? How have you dealt with that?'
> 'Have you ever been sexually abused? What has transpired since? Have you spoken with anybody about this before?'

Travel history

Endemic illnesses may be endogenous to specific regions in the world or to a single country. Consumers sometimes present with symptoms that cannot or may not be attributed to routine illnesses. For these reasons, a complete travel history is warranted when obtaining a health history. As recently seen during the COVID-19 pandemic, the management of communicable diseases may require specific vaccinations pre-travel or impact on where consumers can travel from and to. Checking in with latest border closures, or requirements for travel to and from different destinations, is essential for the traveller who may ask for assistance in interpreting latest advice.

EXAMPLES OF QUESTIONS ASSESSING TRAVEL HISTORY

> 'Where have you travelled either domestically or internationally? Was this a rural or an urban environment? When?'
> 'Did you receive any immunisations before you visited that area?'
> 'Did you need to take any medications prophylactically before or while you were gone?'
> 'Were you ill when you were there?'
> 'Was a diagnosis made? What treatment did you receive? Were there any complications?'
> 'Since returning from this area, have you been ill or not feeling normal?'

Work environment

The work environment can also be hazardous. The nature of employment itself may present health hazards, whether or not safety measures are used. Carpentry, for example, is viewed as a relatively safe employment, although over time carpenters are prone to ischaemia of their fingers from repeated exposure to handheld vibrating tools. Exposure to toxic substances in the work environment, such as asbestos, silica dust and lead, is an additional factor to consider.

EXAMPLES OF QUESTIONS ASSESSING WORK ENVIRONMENT

> 'Describe the work that you do. Is it physically demanding? Is it mentally or emotionally demanding? Do you sit or stand in one place all day/night? Do you undertake repetitive motions in your role?'
> 'How many hours a day do you normally work? For how long have you held this position?'
> 'Do you spend the majority of your work day sitting, standing, walking, running, lifting or biking?'
> 'Do you work with any chemicals? Raw materials?'
> 'Are you exposed to radiation or other pollution? Toxic fumes? Hazardous conditions?'
> 'What safety measures do you practise at work?'
> 'What is the noise level at your place of employment?'
> 'Have you noticed that you are sick on the weekend or on your days off?'
> 'Have you had any work-related accidents or injuries?'
> 'Do you enjoy your work and are you considering changing your profession? Why?'
> 'What other jobs have you held in your lifetime?'

Home environment

When assessing the consumer's home environment, consider both the physical and psychosocial aspects. The physical examination encompasses a broad spectrum of topics: physical condition of the house, safety from toxic substances, and the presence of modern conveniences such as a refrigerator, air conditioner, heater, telephones and electricity. Older houses may have been painted with lead-based paint, which poses a health threat to a young child who chews on wooden items and ingests the paint chips, or have asbestos which can be problematic when renovating or when this material is exposed.

The psychosocial component of the home environment identifies the relative safety of the neighbourhood.

Physical environment

EXAMPLES OF QUESTIONS ASSESSING PHYSICAL ENVIRONMENT
> 'How old are your living quarters (i.e. house or apartment building) and in what condition is the building?
> 'Do you have electricity, heating and air conditioning? What type of heating do you have?'
> 'Do you have running water? Do you have a toilet, bath or shower?'
> 'From what source do you draw your water (e.g. tank, spring, bore, reservoir, town supply)?'
> 'Do you have access to a telephone?'
> 'Do you have smoke detectors? Where? Do you inspect the batteries on a regular basis? Do you have a carbon monoxide detector?'
> 'How many steps separate each floor? Is there a railing?'
> 'Do you have any floor rugs? Are they taped to the floor?'
> 'Do you use a night-light when it is dark?'
> 'Have you adapted your living quarters to fit any special needs?'
> 'What pets do you have? Do they live inside or outside?'
> 'What type of transportation do you use?'
> 'Do you have easy access to a supermarket? Healthcare facility?'
> 'Where do you store your medications, cleaning supplies and other toxic substances? How are they secured?' (if children live in the living quarters)
> 'Are there any problems with pollution near your home?'

Psychosocial environment

EXAMPLE OF QUESTIONS ASSESSING PSYCHOSOCIAL ENVIRONMENT
> 'Do you feel safe in your neighbourhood/home environment?'

Hobbies and leisure activities

Acquiring information on consumers' hobbies and leisure activities is necessary because some activities can pose health risks. For example, repeated exposure to glue used in constructing model cars and planes can lead to respiratory ailments.

EXAMPLES OF QUESTIONS ASSESSING HOBBIES AND LEISURE ACTIVITIES
> 'What hobbies do you have?' **or** 'What do you like to do in your spare time?'
> 'During or after this activity, have you ever felt sick? What happened?'
> 'Have you ever given up some leisure activity because of the effect it had on your health? What happened?'
> 'Have you ever had an injury from your hobby?'
> 'Do you find your hobbies and leisure activities relaxing?'

Stress

Stress is a physiologically defined response to changes that disrupt the resting equilibrium of an individual. Stress can impact on many systems of the body and lead to both negative health outcomes and changes in health behaviours that increase those negative effects (O'Connor, Thayer & Vedhara, 2021). **Distress** is negative stress, or stress that is harmful and unpleasant. **Eustress** is positive stress, stress that challenges the individual, provides motivation and prevents stagnation.

EXAMPLES OF QUESTIONS ASSESSING STRESS
> 'What are the current stressors in your life?'
> 'What do you feel is your greatest stress at the present time?'
> 'Are there recurring themes with the stress that you experience?'
> 'Have you ever progressed from the point of being stressed to panic? What were the circumstances? How did you manage it?'
> 'Are you able to recognise when you become stressed? What does it feel like in your body?'

Education

Elicit information on the consumer's ability to read and write, and tailor your questions and information to this level.

EXAMPLES OF QUESTIONS ASSESSING EDUCATION:
> 'What was the highest schooling level that you completed?'
> 'Describe the type of student that you were.'
> 'What do you do to find out new information?
> 'How do you access new information?'

Military service

Knowledge of overseas tours of duty may provide a vital link to current health status. A consumer may not reveal this information during the travel history because it was work rather than leisure travel. For instance, military personnel who served in the Middle East may have been exposed to many chemical agents. Many of them now have a variety of signs and symptoms collectively called Gulf War syndrome. Some of the troops who were in the Middle East for the Iraq conflict have exhibited various illnesses such as malaria and unknown respiratory pathology. The full extent of the impact on these troops may not be known for some time.

EXAMPLES OF QUESTIONS ASSESSING MILITARY SERVICE
> 'Are you or have you ever been in the military? What was the length of service? Was this active or reserve duty?'
> 'To what regions have you been assigned? For how long were you there? When?'
> 'Have you ever been in combat? Did you have injuries? Do you experience flashbacks?'

Religion

Religion and spirituality can be powerful forces in a consumer's life. You need to be aware of and sensitive to implications that spirituality or religious beliefs may have on the consumer's health status and healthcare practices.

EXAMPLES OF QUESTIONS ASSESSING RELIGION
> 'Are you affiliated with a specific religion?'
> 'Do you currently practise your faith?'
> 'Do your religious beliefs affect your health status? In what way?'
> 'Are there any beliefs that you feel are compromised by seeking health care?'
> 'Are there any religious practices that you may need assistance with?'

Cultural background

Closely associated with health and wellbeing is the consumer's cultural background, which can penetrate all facets of a consumer's life. Integrate familiarity with various cultures into your knowledge base so you will be sensitive to and understand the consumer's cultural heritage.

EXAMPLE OF QUESTIONS ASSESSING CULTURAL BACKGROUND
> 'With what cultural group do you identify yourself?'
> 'What does this mean for different aspects of your life?'
> 'Does this impact on what you eat or how you connect with others in your community?'

Roles and relationships

Family roles, work roles and interpersonal relationships provide clues about possible stressors, areas for health promotion, support systems, and sources of altered psychosocial patterns.

EXAMPLES OF QUESTIONS ASSESSING ROLES AND RELATIONSHIPS
> 'What are your home living arrangements? Do you live with others?'
> 'What type of relationship do you have with these individuals?'
> 'What is your role within your family (e.g. major caregiver, breadwinner, child, student, stay-at-home/housebound caregiver)?'
> 'What responsibilities go along with this role?'
> 'Who gives you support?'
> 'Describe the relationship that you have with your friends and neighbours.'

Characteristic patterns of daily living and functional health assessment

Questions about a consumer's usual lifestyle, or **characteristic patterns of daily living**, reveal information about the consumer's normal daily timetable – meals, work and sleep schedules – and social interactions. If the consumer is disabled or impaired physically or psychologically, you need to perform a functional health assessment (see **Appendix A**). The **functional health assessment** documents a person's ability to perform instrumental activities of daily living and physical self-maintenance activities. This data serves as baseline information upon which the effectiveness of nursing interventions can be evaluated.

EXAMPLES OF QUESTIONS ASSESSING PATTERNS OF DAILY LIVING
> 'Describe a typical day for you, starting from the time you wake up to the time you go to bed.'
> 'Do you need assistance with any activities of daily living? (If yes) Is assistance readily available?'
> 'Do you socialise, meet or talk with people outside your house on a daily basis?'
> 'Does your schedule change on certain days or on the weekend? Describe the change.'

Health maintenance and education activities

Health maintenance activities or **health education activities** are practices a person incorporates into his or her lifestyle to promote healthy living. You can make the transition from the social history to health maintenance or promotion with the following statements:

EXAMPLES OF QUESTIONS AND COMMENTS THAT ASSESS OR INTRODUCE HEALTH MAINTENANCE AND EDUCATION ACTIVITIES
> 'Now I would like to discuss things that you do that improve or maintain your health.'
> 'There are many things you can do to promote healthy living. I would like us to discuss some of those practices.'

Sleep

Many illnesses have sleep pattern disturbances as a characteristic. Increased or decreased hours of sleep or interrupted/changed sleep patterns can both occur. For this reason, you need to learn about the consumer's current and usual sleep habits.

A standardised sleep tool, for example the Epworth Sleepiness Scale developed in Australia (Johns, 2022), can also be used to assess sleep and wakefulness patterns. General questions about sleep include the following:

EXAMPLES OF QUESTIONS ASSESSING SLEEP
> 'At what time do you usually go to bed? At what time do you usually awake?'
> 'How long does it take you to fall asleep? How do you feel when you awaken?'
> 'Is your sleep undisturbed? Do you have difficulty staying asleep? If you wake, is it easy for you to fall back to sleep?'
> 'Do you have any discomfort in your legs when you are in bed trying to sleep?'
> 'Describe the environment in which you sleep (noise level, amount of light, temperature of the room, sleeping arrangement).'

>>

>>

> > 'What strategies (also referred to as sleep hygiene) do you use to fall asleep if you are having difficulty (medication, warm milk, other)? How many times per week do you do this?'
> > 'What is your usual emotional state or mental condition when you go to bed? When you wake?'
> > 'Have you ever been told that you snore loudly or excessively?'
> > 'Do you ever have difficulty staying awake?'
> > 'Does the usual time of your sleep–awake cycle change (working rotating shifts)?'
> > 'Do you take a nap during the day? For how long?'
> > 'Do you have nightmares? How frequent are they?'
> > 'Do you walk in your sleep?'
> > 'Do you experience bedwetting?'
> > 'Do you often wake up with dark circles under your eyes? Puffy eyelids? Bloodshot eyes?'
> > 'Do you ever wake in the night because of pain, shortness of breath (**dyspnoea**), or waking up to pee at night (nocturia)?' (Use non-medical terms wherever possible but document in medical terms.)
> > 'Do you have alcohol, nicotine, high sugar foods or caffeine within 2 hours of bedtime?'
> > 'Do you take any medications or supplements to help you sleep?'

Diet

Refer to Chapter 15 for a more thorough discussion of nutrition and diet history.

EXAMPLES OF QUESTIONS ASSESSING DIET

> 'Are you on any special therapeutic diet (soft foods, low salt, low cholesterol, low fat, etc.)?' (**Figure 3.7**.)
> 'Do you follow any particular diet plan (vegetarian, liquid, commercially available diet food, rice diet, Keto diet, hCG diet, Optifast/Optislim diet, Weight Watchers etc.)?'
> 'How many meals a day do you eat? At what times do you eat? Do you snack? When?'
> 'Has your weight fluctuated in the past year? Can you explain more about this?'

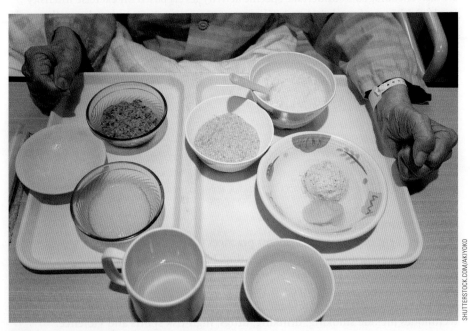

SHUTTERSTOCK.COM/AKIYOKO

FIGURE 3.7 Preventing aspirations: thickening liquids

Exercise

Aerobic exercise appropriate to the consumer's age and physical condition leads to cardiovascular, respiratory and musculoskeletal fitness as well as mental alertness and general mental wellbeing (**Figure 3.8**). Combining aerobic exercise with weightlifting (which increases strength) and calisthenics (which enhances flexibility) establishes a complete physical fitness regimen. Non-aerobic activity also has beneficial effects on the body, even though the target heart rate may not be attained.

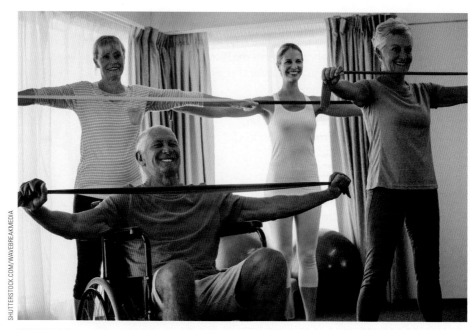

SHUTTERSTOCK.COM/WAVEBREAKMEDIA

FIGURE 3.8 Older adults participating in an exercise class

Australian national guidelines encourage people to be more active and provide specific advice based on age and other parameters. Current advice for adults aged 18–64 includes being active most days, if possible every day, and states hours of activity guidelines based on level of activity (vigorous vs moderate intensity) (Australian Government Department of Health and Aged Care, 2021). New Zealanders are also encouraged to undertake specific activity levels based on exercise intensity levels (2.5 hours of moderate or 1.25 hours of vigorous activity) spread over the week (Ministry of Health, 2021).

EXAMPLES OF QUESTIONS ASSESSING EXERCISE
> 'Do you participate in a formal or informal exercise program? If yes, for how long have you been involved?'
> 'What type of exercise do you do?'
> 'How many times per week do you exercise?'
> 'For how long do you exercise (in minutes)?'
> 'What type of warm-up and cool-down exercises do you do?'
> 'For what period of time do you maintain this elevated heart rate?'
> 'Have you ever experienced any injuries from your exercise regimen? What type?'
> 'Does your health impose any restrictions on your ability to exercise?'

Stress management

The assessment of stress management practices is vital. Some commonly used stress management techniques are exercise, eating, biofeedback, yoga, progressive muscle relaxation, aromatherapy, imagery, massages, verbalisation, praying, humour, pet therapy, music therapy, magnet therapy, reflexology, art work, journaling, storytelling, support groups and meditation. For others, stress management techniques include smoking, drinking, drugs, high-risk sports and violence.

EXAMPLES OF QUESTIONS ASSESSING STRESS MANAGEMENT
> 'When you become stressed, what do you do to help alleviate the stress?'
> 'When do you use this skill? Is it effective for you?'
> 'How do you evaluate the effectiveness of this technique?'
> 'For how long do you need to perform this technique before your stress is reduced?'
> 'How many times per day do you use this technique? Per week?'
> 'Have you tried other stress management skills? How did they work?'

Use of safety devices

The consumer's use or lack of use of safety devices on the job, in the home, during sporting activities and in the environment provides a source for teaching health promotion skills (**Figure 3.9**).

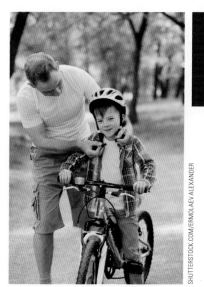

FIGURE 3.9 Wearing safety equipment is essential at all ages.

EXAMPLES OF QUESTIONS ASSESSING SAFETY DEVICES

> 'Do you wear a seatbelt when you are in a car?'
> 'Do you wear a helmet when riding a motorcycle?'
> 'Do your hobbies and leisure activities (e.g. cycling) require the use of safety devices (e.g. helmets)? Do you use them?'
> 'What precautions do you take when using pesticides or fertilisers?'

Health check-ups

Health check-up information demonstrates patterns of healthcare practices by the consumer during illness and health, and provides potential sources of health education.

EXAMPLES OF QUESTIONS ASSESSING HEALTH CHECK-UPS

> 'When was the last time you had the following performed: pulse and blood pressure, complete physical examination, chest X-ray, ECG, urinalysis, blood tests, including blood sugar and cholesterol? What were the results?'
> 'How often do you see a dentist (**Figure 3.10**)? For what reason?'

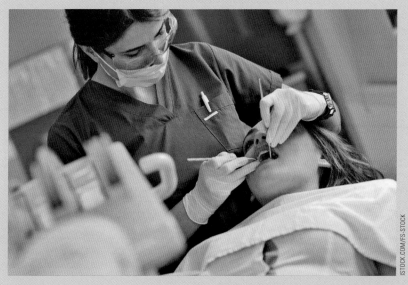

FIGURE 3.10 It is important to ask consumers what other healthcare providers they are seeing, such as the dentist.

> 'How often do you see an eye doctor? For what reason? Have you been checked for glaucoma?'
> 'How often do you have a gynaecological check-up? By whom? What was the date and result of your last Pap smear?' (for women)
> 'Do you know how to perform a breast self-examination? Who taught you? How often do you perform it? Do you have any questions about it?' (for women)
> 'What was the date and the result of your last mammogram?' (for women over 40 or a woman of any age with a strong family history of breast cancer)
> 'Do you know how to perform a testicular self-examination? Who taught you? How often do you perform it? Do you have any questions about it?' (for men)
> 'How often do you have a prostate examination? What was the date and result of your last exam?' (for men)
> 'Do you have any other healthcare providers (psychiatrist, psychologist, podiatrist, occupational or physical therapist, physiotherapist, chiropractor etc.)? For what reason? How often do you see this person?'

Review of systems

The **review of systems (ROS)** is the consumer's subjective response to a series of body system-related questions and serves as a double check that vital information is not overlooked. The ROS covers a broad base of clinical states, but it is by no means exhaustive. The ROS follows a head-to-toe or **cephalocaudal** approach and includes two types of questions: sign- or symptom-related and disease-related. The signs or symptoms and diseases are grouped according to physiological body parts and systems. Some of the diseases may have been discussed earlier in the interview.

Both positive and pertinent negative findings are documented in the ROS. When a response is positive, ask the consumer to describe it as completely as possible. Refer to the 10 characteristics of a chief complaint when gathering more information about positive responses. Table 3.1 lists the symptoms and diseases that can be ascertained during the ROS. Many organisations have pre-printed ROS sheets. These are convenient to use because positive findings can be circled and noted. Negative responses are not circled. As you become more experienced, you can combine the ROS with the physical examination of the consumer. This technique often shortens the interview time with the consumer.

Remember to ask the questions in terms that are understood by the consumer. The following is an appropriate statement to make the transition from the health management or health promotion to the ROS.

EXAMPLES OF QUESTIONS ASSESSING REVIEW OF SYSTEMS (ROS)
> 'Now I would like to ask you if you have experienced a variety of conditions. Most of the questions can be answered with "yes" or "no".'
  Pose the same question for each item in the ROS:
> 'Have you ever had … ?'

TABLE 3.1 Review of systems

General		Consumer's perception of general state of health at the present, difference from usual state, vitality and energy levels, body odours, fever, chills, night sweats
Mental status and neurological system	Neurological	Headache, change in balance, incoordination, loss of movement, change in sensory perception or feeling in an extremity, change in speech, change in smell, syncope, loss of memory, tremors, involuntary movement, loss of consciousness, seizures, weakness, head injury, vertigo, tremor, tic, paralysis, stroke, spasm
	Psychological	Irritability, nervousness, tension, increased stress, difficulty concentrating, mood changes, suicidal thoughts, depression, anxiety, sleep disturbances, eating disorders
Skin		Rashes, itching, changes in skin pigmentation, ecchymoses, change in colour or size of mole, sores, lumps, dry or moist skin, pruritus, change in skin texture, odours, excessive sweating, acne, warts, eczema, psoriasis, amount of time spent in the sun, use of sunscreen, skin cancer
Hair		Alopecia, excessive growth of hair or growth of hair in unusual locations (hirsutism), use of chemicals on hair, dandruff, pediculosis, scalp lesions
Eyes		Blurred vision, visual acuity, glasses, contact lenses, photophobia, excessive tearing, night blindness, diplopia, drainage, bloodshot eyes, pain, blind spots, flashing lights, halos around objects, floaters, **glaucoma**, cataracts, use of sunglasses, use of protective eyewear
Ears		Cleaning method, hearing deficits, hearing aid, pain, phonophobia, discharge, light-headedness (vertigo), ringing in the ears (tinnitus), usual noise level, earaches, infection, piercings, use of ear protection, amount of cerumen, insertion of grommets
Nose and sinuses		Number of colds per year, discharge, itching, hay fever, postnasal drip, stuffiness, sinus pain, sinusitis, polyps, obstruction, epistaxis, change in sense of smell, allergies, snoring
Mouth		Dental habits (brushing, flossing, mouth rinses), toothache, tooth abscess, dentures, bleeding or swollen gums, difficulty chewing, sore tongue, change in taste, lesions, change in salivation, bad breath, caries, teeth extractions, orthodontics
Throat and neck		Hoarseness, change in voice, frequent sore throats, dysphagia, pain or stiffness, enlarged thyroid (goitre), lymphadenopathy, tonsillectomy, adenoidectomy
Lymph nodes		Enlargement, tenderness

>> **TABLE 3.1** *continued*

Musculoskeletal	Joint stiffness, muscle pain, cramps, back pain, limitation of movement, redness, swelling, weakness, bony deformity, broken bones, dislocations, sprains, crepitus, gout, arthritis, osteoporosis, herniated disc
Nails	Change in nails, splitting, breaking, thickened, texture change, onychomycosis, use of chemicals, false nails
Respiratory	Dyspnoea on exertion, shortness of breath, sputum, cough, sneezing, wheezing, haemoptysis, frequent upper respiratory tract infections, pneumonia, emphysema, asthma, tuberculosis, tuberculosis exposure, result of last chest X-ray, Mantoux test
Breasts and axilla	Pain, tenderness, discharge, lumps, change in size, dimpling, rash, benign breast disease, breast cancer, results of recent mammogram
Cardiovascular	Paroxysmal nocturnal dyspnoea, chest pain, cyanosis, heart murmur, **palpitations**, syncope, orthopnoea (state number of pillows used), oedema, cold or discoloured hands or feet, leg cramps, myocardial infarction, hypertension, valvular disease, intermittent claudication, varicose veins, thrombophlebitis, deep vein thrombosis, use of support hose, result of last ECG
Haematological	Easy bruising or bleeding, anaemia, sickle cell anaemia, blood type, exposure to radiation
Gastrointestinal	Change in appetite, nausea, vomiting, diarrhoea, constipation, usual bowel habits, melaena, rectal bleeding, haematemesis, change in stool colour, flatulence, belching, regurgitation, heartburn, dysphagia, abdominal pain, jaundice, ascites, haemorrhoids, hepatitis, peptic ulcers, gallstones, gastro-oesophageal reflux disease, appendicitis, ulcerative colitis, Crohn's disease, diverticulitis, umbilical hernia
Nutrition	Present weight, usual weight, desired weight, food intolerances, food likes and dislikes, where meals are eaten, caffeine intake
Urinary	Change in urine colour, voiding habits, dysuria, hesitancy, urgency, frequency, nocturia, polyuria, dribbling, loss in force of stream, bedwetting, change in urine volume, incontinence, urinary retention, suprapubic pain, flank pain, kidney stones, urinary tract infections
Endocrine	Exophthalmos, fatigue, change in size of head, hands or feet, weight change, heat and cold intolerances, excessive sweating, polydipsia, polyphagia, polyuria, increased hunger, change in body hair distribution, goitre, diabetes mellitus
Female reproductive	Vaginal discharge, change in libido, infertility, sterility, pelvic pain, pain during intercourse, postcoital bleeding; menses: last menstrual period (LMP), menarche, regularity, duration, amount of bleeding, premenstrual symptoms, intermenstrual bleeding, **dysmenorrhoea**, **menorrhagia**, fibroids; menopause: age of onset, duration, symptoms, bleeding; obstetrical: number of pregnancies, number of miscarriages or abortions, number of children, type of delivery, complications; type of birth control, hormone replacement therapy
Male reproductive	Change in libido, infertility, sterility, impotence, pain during intercourse, testicular or penile pain, penile discharge, erections, emissions, hernias, enlarged prostate, type of birth control

CONCLUDING THE HEALTH HISTORY

After completing the ROS, ask the consumer whether there is any additional information to discuss. At the conclusion of the interview, thank the consumer for the time spent in gathering the health history. Inform the consumer what the next step will be (e.g. physical examination, diagnostic tests, treatment) and when to expect it.

Supportive equipment

Some chapters in this text will contain a section on supportive equipment for that particular body system. It is important to assess the supportive equipment as they are healthcare extenders for the consumer. Whether the supportive equipment is supplemental oxygen, a walker or a feeding tube, it needs to be evaluated as you examine the consumer. Correct use of these devices will help the consumer maintain a current level of health, whereas incorrect use can harm the consumer.

DOCUMENTATION

The documentation of the health assessment and physical examination is the legal record of the consumer encounter. It also serves as the medium among health professionals for communicating about the consumer's condition. The consumer record represents a description of the consumer's status and the care delivered to the consumer. The documentation may be read by a multitude of professionals: nurses; doctors; dietitians; physio, speech and occupational therapists; risk managers; utilisation reviewers; quality assurance personnel; accreditation organisations;

lawyers; insurance companies; and, ultimately, the consumer! Because all of these people have access to the consumer's chart, you must document everything in a professional and legally acceptable manner. **Table 3.2** outlines general principles to guide your documentation regardless of whether it is paper-based or electronic documentation. **Table 3.3** provides specific assessment-oriented 'dos' and 'don'ts' for documentation. Each organisation also has its own documentation system. If you perform computerised charting in your workplace, always safeguard your access code to protect yourself.

TABLE 3.2 General documentation guidelines

	IF USING ELECTRONIC MEDICAL RECORDS, PROTECT YOUR ACCESS CODE AND ELECTRONIC SIGNATURE.
1	Ensure that you have the correct consumer record or chart and that the consumer's name and identifying information are on every page of the record.
2	Document as soon as the consumer encounter is concluded to ensure accurate recall of data (follow organisation's guidelines on frequency of charting).
3	Avoid distractions while documenting. This is frequently when errors are made.
4	If interrupted while documenting, reread what you wrote to ensure accuracy.
5	Record date and time of each entry. (This may be a forced function in electronic documentation.)
6	Sign each entry with your full legal name and with your professional credentials, or per your organisation's policy (for paper-based documentation; electronic documentation will bear your access code, so ensure you protect this).
7	Do not sign a note that you did not write (for paper-based documentation; electronic documentation will bear your access code, so ensure you protect this).
8	Do not leave space between entries (for paper-based documentation).
9	Do not insert information between lines (for paper-based documentation).
10	If an error is made while documenting, use a single line to cross out the error, then date, time and sign the correction (check organisational policy); avoid erasing, crossing out, or using correction fluid (for paper-based documentation).
11	Never correct another person's entry, even if it is incorrect (for paper-based documentation).
12	Use quotes to indicate direct consumer responses (e.g. 'I feel lousy').
13	Document in chronological order; if chronological order is not used, state why.
14	Use legible writing (for paper-based documentation).
15	Use a permanent ink pen (for paper-based documentation. Black is usually preferable because of its ability to photocopy well).
16	Document in a complete but concise manner by using phrases and abbreviations as appropriate. Avoid using dangerous abbreviations, acronyms and symbols as specified by your healthcare organisation.
17	When writing numbers less than 1, write a zero to the left of the decimal point; this avoids confusion as to the use of a decimal point.
18	Document telephone calls that relate to the consumer's case.
19	Always reread your notes for accuracy.
20	Record the name of the interpreter if one is used.
21	Avoid using words that have more than one meaning.
22	Remember, from a legal standpoint, if you didn't document it, it wasn't done.

Electronic medical records (EMRs) create a paperless system that can reduce charting/documentation time once the clinician is familiar with the system. EMRs enable the nurse to use voice recognition, narrative writing, and/or check boxes with drop-down menus to record consumers' histories and examination findings. Other advantages of EMRs are their legibility, easy accessibility, ability to be accessed by multiple users simultaneously at different work stations in different areas in real time, and capability of accessing real-time laboratory and diagnostic studies.

TABLE 3.3 Examination-specific documentation guidelines

DO	DON'T
DO record all data that contributes directly to the examination (i.e. positive examination findings and pertinent negatives).	**DON'T** use judgemental language such as 'good', 'poor', 'bad', 'normal', 'abnormal', 'decreased', 'appears to be' and 'seems'.
DO document any parts of the examination that are omitted or refused by the consumer.	**DON'T** use evaluative statements (e.g. 'Consumer is uncooperative,' 'Consumer is lazy'); cite instead specific statements or actions that you observe (e.g. 'consumer said, "I hate this place" and kicked a chair').
DO state time intervals precisely (e.g. 'every 4 hours', 'BD' instead of 'seldom', 'occasionally').	**DON'T** make relative statements about findings (e.g. 'mass the size of an egg'); use specific measurements (e.g. 'mass 3 cm by 5 cm').
DO draw pictures when appropriate (e.g. location of scar, masses, skin lesion, ulcers, deep tendon reflex, etc.).	**DON'T** describe what you did.
DO refer to findings using anatomic landmarks (e.g. left upper quadrant [of abdomen], left lower lobe [of lung], midclavicular line, etc.).	
DO document any change in the consumer's condition during a visit or from previous visits.	
DO describe what you observed.	

Documentation should also reflect information that is relayed verbally, and is the standing record of consumer care (which is based on your assessment of the consumer). Documentation is one of the most important aspects of care as:

> The written patient record survives far into the future and should serve to give a clinical picture of the patient that is accurate, legible, clear and precise. Continuity of care and avoidance of errors depend on this.
>
> Calleja, Aitken & Cooke, 2011, p. 15.

Many health organisations are building structure into all forms of clinical communication, and handover structures are being developed and implemented as a way of improving communication. Calleja et al. (2011) also identify a gap in linking documentation to information that is handed over. To reduce the incidence of this issue, some clinicians are using handover structures to guide any documentation that may usually be unstructured (e.g. nurse's progress notes). One such structure to support this is the SBAR structure (**Figure 3.11**) (Haig, Sutton & Whittington, 2006). Please note there are other similar structures such as ISBAR and ISOBAR. Regardless of the one used in your environment, ensure you understand the structure and what the aim of using it is.

REFLECTION IN PRACTICE

Assessing your documentation
After completing the health history, reflect on the techniques you used to elicit the history. Did you rush the consumer? Did you use too many open-ended or closed questions? Was your documentation concise? What could you have done better?

Many healthcare facilities have pre-printed health history forms that are checklists and require few narrative notes. Other facilities require the nurse to document the health history in its entirety. The health histories that follow throughout the text illustrate how to document the complete health history of an ill consumer and a well consumer.

Chapter 22 gives examples of documentation of a comprehensive and focused health assessment and physical examination.

SBAR Communication

Use the following SBAR steps to communicate issues, problems or opportunities for improvement to coworkers or supervisors. SBAR can be applied to both written and verbal communications.

SITUATION **– State what is happening at the present time that has warranted the SBAR communication.** *Example: Patients and visitors are entering the medical centre through the wrong doors and getting lost trying to find their destination.*

BACKGROUND **– Explain circumstances leading up to this situation. Put the situation into context for the reader/listener.** *Example: The campus has many buildings and is accessible from both E. Washington St. and Eastland Dr. Other entrances are more noticeable than the hospital's main entrance. MD offices do not have good maps to mark and hand to patients when sending them to our campus, and they often misdirect patients.*

ASSESSMENT **– What do you think the problem is?** *Example: People need something that they can carry with them when they are coming to the hospital so they park outside the appropriate entrance.*

RECOMMENDATION **– What would you do to correct the problem?** *Example: Create a campus visitor guide that includes an "aerial" map of the campus as well as a community map and floor by floor maps. Distribute widely, including to physician offices. Make them available to visitors in admission packets and at all entrances.*

FIGURE 3.11 SBAR communication

SOURCE: REPRINTED FROM *THE JOINT COMMISSION JOURNAL ON QUALITY AND PATIENT SAFETY*, VOL 32/ISSUE 3, K HAIG, S SUTTON AND J WHITTINGTON, SBAR: A SHARED MENTAL MODEL FOR IMPROVING COMMUNICATION BETWEEN CLINICIANS, COPYRIGHT 2006, WITH PERMISSION FROM ELSEVIER.

CHAPTER RESOURCES

REVIEW QUESTIONS

For answers to these questions, see Answer section at the end of this book.

1. A consumer at the clinic is complaining of feeling tired for the past few months. What type of health history should the nurse use?
   a. Complete health history
   b. Focused health history
   c. Both a and b
   d. Emergency health history
2. A consumer tells you that she has bloating and increased abdominal sounds, and diarrhoea along with her abdominal pain. What characteristic of a chief complaint do the vomiting and nausea represent?
   a. Location
   b. Radiation
   c. Aggravating factors
   d. Associated manifestations

3. The nurse is conducting a family health history on a consumer who says that he was adopted as a baby. What would be the nurse's next best step?
   a. Ask the consumer to contact the adoption agency to learn his biological parents' health conditions
   b. Continue the health history with the social history
   c. Inquire about medical conditions of his adopted family, as they can affect the consumer's health
   d. Tell the consumer that he has no concerns because he is healthy
4. A consumer reports that he has had increased illicit drug use in the last month. What would be the next appropriate response for the nurse to make?
   a. 'Oh OK, do you like taking drugs?'
   b. 'Well no wonder you have abdominal pain, your liver must be terrible.'
   c. 'Are you quitting any time soon?'
   d. 'How do you view your drug taking? Have you ever considered quitting or reducing your intake?'

5. The nurse documents that the consumer's back pain is 9/10 in the left side of her lower back radiating to the left flank. The consumer reports feeling a stabbing sensation that is accompanied by nausea and vomiting. Which characteristics of a chief complaint are described in this statement? Select all that apply.
    a. Location
    b. Radiation
    c. Quality
    d. Quantity
    e. Setting
    f. Associated manifestations
6. Which of the following statements is true about the review of systems?
    a. It is performed at the beginning of the health history.
    b. It usually follows a cephalocaudal approach.
    c. It is based on a functional assessment.
    d. It is a summary formed by the nurse at the end of the health history.
7. Which of the following chart entries is documented correctly?
    a. The mass is egg-sized.
    b. The mass appears to be smaller than last week.
    c. The mass is located in the left lower quadrant.
    d. The mass does not seem to bother the consumer.
8. Which of the following situations warrants more investigation for possible domestic and intimate partner violence? Select all that apply.
    a. Small oval bruises around the throat of the consumer
    b. A blister on the consumer's lip consistent with a history of cold sores
    c. Frequent urinary tract infections
    d. Consumer refusal to answer questions about past injuries
    e. Vague symptoms such as fatigue, headaches, that have 'caused' clumsiness or small injuries or nonattendance of appointments
    f. A significant other who will not allow the consumer to answer questions
9. Which of the following statements reflect objective documentation? Select all that apply.
    a. Consumer has a poor attitude about losing weight.
    b. Abdominal pain is elicited by palpation in the right upper quadrant.
    c. White nipple discharge is noted bilaterally.
    d. Consumer is uncooperative in taking medications as directed.
    e. Consumer performs five deep breaths every hour.
    f. Swelling of the legs has decreased since yesterday.
10. When undertaking an emergency assessment for the consumer with chest pain, which of the following statements best describes priority of assessment?
    a. Asking the consumer about their lifestyle
    b. Advising the consumer to quit smoking
    c. Assisting the consumer to identify the medications they are on
    d. Asking the consumer questions about their pain, while conducting a physical examination including Airway, Breathing, Circulation and Disability.

CS CLINICAL SKILLS

The following Clinical Skills are relevant to this chapter and can be found in Tollefson & Hillman, *Clinical Psychomotor Skills* 8th edition:
> 25 Clinical handover
> 26 Documentation.

FURTHER RESOURCES

Advance directives
> Advance Care Planning Australia: https://www.advancecareplanning.org.au/
> Advance Directives & Enduring Powers of Attorney: https://www.hdc.org.nz/your-rights/about-the-code/advance-directives-enduring-powers-of-attorney/

Intimate partner violence
> Care directives for clinicians, Australia: https://www.racgp.org.au/clinical-resources/clinical-guidelines/key-racgp-guidelines/view-all-racgp-guidelines/abuse-and-violence/preamble
> New Zealand: http://www.health.govt.nz/our-work/preventative-health-wellness/family-violence

Smoking cessation
> QUITnow: http://www.quitnow.gov.au
> RACGP guidelines for smoking cessation for health professionals: http://www.racgp.org.au/your-practice/guidelines/smoking-cessation
> QUIT New Zealand: http://www.quit.org.nz

Immunisation schedule
> Australia: https://beta.health.gov.au/health-topics/immunisation
> Australian Immunisation Register for health professionals: https://www.humanservices.gov.au/organisations/health-professionals/services/medicare/australian-immunisation-register-health-professionals?utm_id=9
> National Centre for Immunisation Research: http://www.ncirs.edu.au
> New Zealand's Immunisation Schedule: https://www.health.govt.nz/our-work/preventative-health-wellness/immunisation/new-zealand-immunisation-schedule

Travel immunisations
> Australia: Smart Traveller http://smartraveller.gov.au/guide/all-travellers/health/Pages/health-checks-and-vaccinations.aspx
> New Zealand: The Immunisation Advisory Centre http://www.immune.org.nz
> Safetravel: https://www.safetravel.govt.nz/you-go

UNIT 1

Exercise guidelines
> Australia: https://www.health.gov.au/health-topics/physical-activity-and-exercise
> New Zealand: https://www.health.govt.nz/our-work/preventative-health-wellness/physical-activity

Sleep hygiene
http://sleepfoundation.org/ask-the-expert/sleep-hygiene

REFERENCES

Australian Government Department of Health and Aged Care. (2021). Physical activity and exercise guidelines for all Australians. Australian Government: Department of Health and Aged Care. Retrieved from https://www.health.gov.au/health-topics/physical-activity-and-exercise/physical-activity-and-exercise-guidelines-for-all-australians

Australian Government Department of Health and Aged Care. (2022). Australian Immunisation Handbook. Retrieved from https://immunisationhandbook.health.gov.au/contents/vaccine-preventable-diseases/influenza-flu

Australian Institute of Health and Welfare (AIHW). (2019). Family, domestic and sexual violence in Australia, 2019. Cat. No. FDV 3. Canberra: AIHW. https://www.aihw.gov.au/getmedia/b0037b2d-a651-4abf-9f7b-00a85e3de528/aihw-fdv3-FDSV-in-Australia-2019.pdf.aspx?inline=true

Boxall, H., & Morgan, A. (2021). *Intimate partner violence during the COVID-19 pandemic: a survey of women in Australia*. (Research report, 03/2021.) ANROWS. https://www.aic.gov.au/sites/default/files/2022-01/intimate-partner-violence-during-the-covid-19-pandemic.pdf

Calleja, P., Aitken, L. M., & Cooke, M. L. (2011). Information transfer for multi-trauma patients on discharge from the emergency department: mixed-method narrative review. *Journal of Advanced Nursing, 37*(1), 4–18.

Campo, M. (2015). *Domestic and family violence in pregnancy and early parenthood*. Australian Government, Australian Institute of Family Studies. https://aifs.gov.au/resources/policy-and-practice-papers/domestic-and-family-violence-pregnancy-and-early-parenthood

Dahlen, H. G., Munoz, A. M., Schmied, V., & Thornton, C. (2018). The relationship between intimate partner violence reported at the first antenatal booking visit and obstetric and perinatal outcomes in an ethnically diverse group of Australian pregnant women: a population-based study over 10 years. *BMJ Open, e019566*. doi: 10.1136/bmjopen-2017-019566

Dalton, M., Harrison, J., Malin, A., & Leavey, C. (2018). Factors that influence nurses' assessment of patient acuity and response to acute deterioration. *British Journal of Nursing, 27*(4), 212–18. https://www.magonlinelibrary.com/doi/epub/10.12968/bjon.2018.27.4.212

Family Violence Death Review Committee. (2017). Fifth Report Data: January 2009 to December 2015. Family Violence Death Review Committee: Wellington, New Zealand. Retrieved from https://www.hqsc.govt.nz/assets/FVDRC/Publications/FVDRC-FifthReportData-2017.pdf

Haig, K. M., Sutton, S., & Whittington, J. (2006). SBAR: A shared mental model for improving communication between clinicians. *Joint Commission, Journal of Quality and Patient Safety, 32*(3), 167–75.

Johns, M. (2022). About the ESS. The Epworth Sleepiness Scale. https://epworthsleepinessscale.com/about-the-ess/

Ministry of Health. (2021). How much activity is recommended? Retrieved from https://www.health.govt.nz/your-health/healthy-living/food-activity-and-sleep/physical-activity/how-much-activity-recommended

New Zealand Ministry of Justice. (2015). *2014 New Zealand crime and safety survey. Main findings*. https://www.justice.govt.nz/assets/NZCASS-201602-Main-Findings-Report-Updated.pdf

New Zealand Ministry of Justice. (2020). *The New Zealand crime and victims survey. Key findings. Cycle 2, October 2018–September 2019*. https://www.justice.govt.nz/assets/NZCVS-Y2-core-report-v1.1-for-release.pdf

NSW Health. (2020). Prevention and response to violence, abuse and neglect. https://www.health.nsw.gov.au/parvan/Pages/default.aspx

NSW Health. (2022). Policy directive. Domestic Violence – Identifying and responding. https://www1.health.nsw.gov.au/PDS/pages/doc.aspx?dn=PD2006_084

O'Connor, D. B., Thayer, J. F., & Vedhara, K. (2021). Stress and health: a review of psychobiological processes. *Annual Review of Psychology, 72*, 633–88. https://www.annualreviews.org/doi/pdf/10.1146/annurev-psych-062520-122331

Queensland Government Department of Justice and Attorney-General, (n.d.). DFV common risk and safety framework. https://www.justice.qld.gov.au/initiatives/end-domestic-family-violence/our-progress/enhancing-service-responses/dfv-common-risk-safety-framework

RACGP. (2021). Guidelines for preventative activities in general practice (9th ed.). https://www.racgp.org.au/clinical-resources/clinical-guidelines/key-racgp-guidelines/view-all-racgp-guidelines/guidelines-for-preventive-activities-in-general-pr/psychosocial/intimate-partner-violence

Services Australia. (2022). What is family and domestic violence? https://www.servicesaustralia.gov.au/what-family-and-domestic-violence?context=60033#a1

Special Taskforce on Domestic and Family Violence in Queensland. (2015). Not now, not ever report. Retrieved from https://www.publications.qld.gov.au/dataset/not-now-not-ever/resource/533db62b-b2c9-43cc-a5ff-f9e1bc95c7c7

CHAPTER 4

ABORIGINAL AND TORRES STRAIT ISLANDER PEOPLES' HEALTH

LEARNING OUTCOMES

By the end of this chapter you should be able to:

1   describe the identity of Aboriginal and Torres Strait Islander peoples of Australia
2   discuss culturally safe and responsive nursing practice in the context of health assessment and physical examination using the concepts of reflexivity, cultural strengths and intercultural communication
3   reflect on the importance of continually developing self-knowledge, including understanding personal beliefs, privileges, assumptions, values, perceptions, attitudes and expectations, and how these impact on relationships with Aboriginal and Torres Strait Islander peoples
4   discuss the ongoing impacts of colonisation on Aboriginal and Torres Strait Islander peoples in Australian health care, which is evident in forms of racism, internalised racism and resultant systemic barriers to healthcare access for Aboriginal and Torres Strait Islander peoples
5   describe the critical role nurses play in breaking down barriers and enabling equitable and safe access to health care for Aboriginal and Torres Strait Islander peoples
6   improve communication in clinical practice during health assessment and physical examination by engaging with Aboriginal and Torres Strait Islander peoples' ways of 'knowing, being and doing' that can be embedded into health practice as a pathway to building trust and access.

My name is Nicole Hewlett, and I am a proud *palawa* woman from *lutruwita* (Tasmania). I would like to acknowledge that we all stand in footsteps millennia old. May we acknowledge the Traditional Custodians of the lands and waterways we breathe on, whose cultures and customs have nurtured and continue to nurture this land since men and women awoke from the great Dream. We honour the presence of these ancestors who reside in the imagination of this land and whose irrepressible spirituality flows through all creation.

I have been offered the privilege of helping to write this chapter while on Turrbul and Yuggera Country of meeanjin (Brisbane) and would also like to respectfully acknowledge the ancestral spirits that have influenced the Aboriginal wisdom shared with you in this chapter. If you are reading this, then the moment has come for you to learn the lessons that will unfold in these pages. I am not a nurse, so this chapter has been co-authored with nurses to contextualise the learnings to your profession.

>>

>>

> The spirit of this chapter is to take you on a journey in whichever role you take. All peoples in Australia should have equitable access to healthcare knowledge, resources and services, and to thrive with dignity, authority and respect. However, it takes all of us, especially you, as healthcare professionals, to work in solidarity to achieve this reality.
>
> All the authors invite you to take a personal inward journey to the rivers of your mind, which will require your openness and courage to sit with some uncomfortable currents. This journey may produce debris of its own. It is not an easy journey, but one that is powerful, and one which can bring an unimaginable richness to your life. Let us begin to walk together, you have the opportunity to start here and now, *pulingina karati* (welcome, friend).
>
> Nicole Hewlett (2023)

BACKGROUND

In every role a health professional undertakes, whether this is in gathering information to develop care plans and undertaking interventions to help improve the health of consumers, practising in ways that make our consumers feel culturally safe is paramount. If we are unable to provide culturally safe care, the ability of the health professional to gather health and personal information on which care decisions are based, can be reduced, or even completely blocked by the misunderstandings, or inability to uncover the correct information at the right time. Therefore, this journey is vitally important to both your consumers and to you and the healthcare team.

In this chapter, you will encounter many different concepts about health care related to Aboriginal and Torres Strait Islander peoples' cultures when performing health assessment and physical examination: cultural humility, cultural awareness, cultural sensitivity, cultural capability, cultural security, cultural learning and cultural respect. In nursing and midwifery, in other allied health professions, in health education curriculums, and in Australian health policy, these are key concepts when caring for people of a differing culture than your own. In the nursing and midwifery profession, you will see these concepts in the codes of practice, in the professional standards (NMBA, 2016), in curriculums (AGDH, 2014; CATSINaM, 2017a), and in nursing academic literature (Cusack, Kinnear, Ward, Mohamed & Butler, 2018). This section combines the concepts of 'cultural safety' and 'cultural responsiveness'.

Please note that the focus of the chapter is specifically on First Nations people in Australia. Content related to Māori peoples of Aotearoa/New Zealand is referred to throughout the textbook in context of particular health assessments. For further information about Māori peoples in Aotearoa/New Zealand, we recommend that you visit https://www.futureofhealth.govt.nz/maori-health-authority/ as well as https://www.teakawhaiora.nz/, where you will find up-to-date information, policy documents and guidelines for conducting health assessments in a culturally safe context.

INTRODUCTION TO CULTURALLY SAFE AND RESPONSIVE PRACTICE

Cultural safety

Cultural safety uses a broad definition of culture that does not reduce it to ethnicity, but includes age/generation, sexual orientation, socioeconomic status, religious or spiritual belief, ethnic origin, gender and ability. It also recognises that professions and work places have cultures, and cultural safety is as applicable to working with colleagues in providing health care as it is to working with health service users.

CATSINaM (2017a, p. 10)

The concept of *culture* is a component of nursing and midwifery accreditation, standards, and conduct and practice (NMBA, 2016; ANMAC, 2019) in hospital accreditation and registration (ACSQHC, 2017), allied health professions (IAHA, 2019), health policy (AGDH, 2021), and in the national strategy of Closing the Gap (JCCTG, 2020). As you will read later in this chapter, culture and communication are extremely important in clinical practice.

There are many definitions of culture; one is '… a set of meanings, behavioural norms, and values used by members of a particular society, as they construct their unique view of the world' (Alarcon, Foulks & Vakkur, 1998, p. 6). In Australia, racism has its roots in the colonial view of 'an empty land', denying the existence of the original peoples of the land. This racism is evident as late as 50 years ago; evident in the history of the 'White Australia policy' period from 1901–73. This policy informed the development of health professions, including nursing, to see non-white people (especially Aboriginal and Torres Strait Islander peoples) as 'a reservoir of disease that would degenerate and erode the fitness of the white European' (Mayes, 2020, p. 292). However, it is important to recognise that many non-Indigenous peoples have been allies in antiracism and of the human rights of Aboriginal and Torres Strait Islander peoples. Nevertheless, the nursing profession and the healthcare systems need to be further educated and sensitised to create a safe space for Aboriginal and Torres Strait Islander peoples.

Cultural safety describes a state, where people are enabled and feel they can access services that suits their needs, are able to challenge personal or institutional racism levels (when they experience it), establish trust in services and expect effective, quality care.

IAHA (2019, p. 4)

The Australian Health Practitioner Regulation Agency's (Ahpra) definition of 'cultural safety' is:

Cultural safety is determined by Aboriginal and Torres Strait Islander individuals, families and communities. Culturally safe practise [sic] is the ongoing critical reflection of health practitioner knowledge, skills, attitudes, practising behaviours and power differentials in delivering safe, accessible and responsive health care free of racism.

Ahpra (2020)

Cultural safety is central to Aboriginal and Torres Strait Islander peoples' relationships with organisations and service systems: healthy relationships are grounded in trust.

The health care system and the hospitals within it have historically eroded the trust of Aboriginal and Torres Strait Islander people, leading to feelings of being culturally unsafe, which is 'any actions that diminish, demean or disempower the cultural identity and wellbeing of an individual'.

NCNZ (2011, p. 7)

Nurses may have the best of intentions when providing culturally respectful care; however, it is critical to note that experiences of cultural safety can only be determined by Aboriginal and Torres Strait Islander peoples receiving care. Therefore cultural safety does not necessarily require the study of any other cultures. It is largely an inwards journey about landscaping our hearts and attitudes to be open and flexible towards others (see the 'Reflexivity' section below).

The process of seeking cultural safety, like most forms of study and development, is lifelong and it is the receiver of services who determines whether the service is culturally safe or not. Cultural safety is experienced by Aboriginal and Torres Strait Islander people when individual cultural ways of being, preferences and strengths are identified and included in policies, processes, planning, delivery, monitoring and evaluation.

IAHA (2019, p. 4)

Nurses play a vital and important role in creating safe, accessible, person-oriented and informed care for Aboriginal and Torres Strait Islander peoples. Learning to become a culturally competent healthcare professional takes hard work. It is important to acknowledge this, and the authors extend a heartfelt thank you for being here in this moment and taking this journey towards cultural safety as you undertake health assessments and physical examinations.

Cultural responsiveness

Nurses work in teams with other allied health professionals. The Indigenous Allied Health Australia's Cultural Responsiveness Capability Framework (IAHA-CRCF) is a high-quality action-oriented, **First Nations**-focused approach to cultural safety. 'Cultural responsiveness' places particular emphasis on *action*. It is not enough to be motivated or simply understand the need for change; it is about what you *do* to enable safe approaches to care that delivers genuine impact.

Cultural responsiveness is innately transformative and must incorporate knowledge (*knowing*), self-knowledge/behaviour (*being*) and action (*doing*). It is about the approaches we take in engaging with people and how we act to embed what we learn in practice. This requires genuine dialogue to improve practice and health outcomes; it is how we achieve, maintain and govern cultural safety.

Responding *appropriately* is a key part of the 'Registered nurse standards for practice': Standard 1: 1.3; Standard 3: 3.1, 3.5; and Standard 6: 6.1 (NMBA, 2016). The IAHA-CRCF focuses on providing information and support to prepare nurses to engage in this transformation renewal so that, whatever your role, you can learn more about yourself, your capabilities and positively influence the health and wellbeing, quality of life and future aspirations of Aboriginal and Torres Strait Islander peoples, and their families and communities (IAHA, 2019). Part of the challenge in becoming culturally-responsive health professionals is reaching beyond your personal comfort zone so that you can more effectively interact and work with people, families and communities who are both similar and markedly different to you. It is both a personal challenge and an opportunity.

As shown in **Figure 4.1**, there are five key interconnected cultural capabilities in the Nursing and Midwifery Aboriginal and Torres Strait Islander Health Curriculum Framework (NMATSIHCF) (CATSINaM, 2017a). While this chapter will focus on the 'respect for the centrality of cultures' and 'self-awareness' capabilities, it is important to understand that *capabilities* are inherently interconnected and interrelated and that you will naturally build these capabilities at the same time. The NMATSIHCF and IAHA-CRF overlap in terms of cultural respect and central emphasis on culturally safe health care.

A key part of cultural capabilities is developing respectful communication skills. In nursing clinical practice, the *yarning* approach is increasingly adopted as a respectful communication method with interacting with Aboriginal and Torres Strait Islander peoples (see the 'Communication in clinical practice' section for more detail). One aspect of yarning is getting to know some First Nations words (see the 'Further resources' section at the end of the chapter).

Strengths-based communication

There are numerous reports documenting the statistical disadvantage/gaps of Aboriginal and Torres Strait Islander peoples (JCCTG, 2020). The reliance on 'disadvantage statistics' in health policies is known as 'deficit discourse' (Fforde, Bamblett, Lovett, Gorringe & Fogarty, 2013) and while statistics are important for health planning, they do not account for the cultural strengths and resilience of

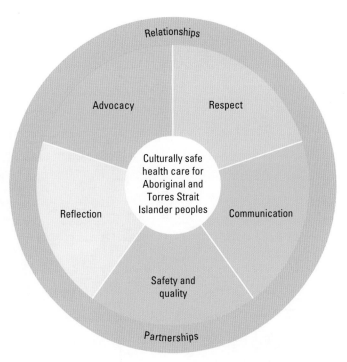

FIGURE 4.1 Graduate Cultural Capability Model: the five key interconnected cultural capabilities required to demonstrate cultural respect

BASED ON COMMONWEALTH OF AUSTRALIA (DEPARTMENT OF HEALTH) MATERIAL

Aboriginal and Torres Strait Islander peoples (Fogarty, Lovell, Langenberg & Heron, 2018). Using 'strengths-based' talk and language is a way to demonstrate respect for cultural identity.

Throughout this chapter, **Aboriginal and Torres Islander peoples** refers to the diverse cultures, languages and nations of the First Peoples of this land we know as Australia (shown in the 'Gambay First Languages Map', https://gambay. com.au). The word *peoples* emphasises this diversity of language groups. There is no single identity among Aboriginal or Torres Strait Islander peoples to describe all nations as a collective, which is often acknowledged in terminology guides that contain examples of 'what not to say' when talking about Aboriginal and Torres Strait Islander peoples (e.g. WIC, 2019). Increasingly, local languages are used to self-identify project names and training programs, because languages are intrinsically connected to Aboriginal and Torres Islander peoples' identities, cultures and Country.

Learning to think about strengths-based talk and language also involves acknowledging the cultural diversity of Aboriginal and Torres Strait Islander peoples. Wherever you train and practise as nurses, seek out local Aboriginal Community Controlled Health Organisations (ACCHOs) that are expert in local cultural protocols and communicating with First Nations communities (see the 'Strength in partnerships' section for more detail).

Diversity and identity

Each coloured patch in **Figure 4.2** attempts to represent a First Nations language, social or nation group. Of the approximate 300 Aboriginal and Torres Strait Islander peoples/groups (AIATSIS, 1996), community varies not only according to geographic location, environment and resources but to each having their own unique cultural practices, histories, languages, beliefs, knowledge and kinship systems. Even within these communities there is significant variability and nuances with the families within the communities and the stories, songlines, values, spiritualities, religion

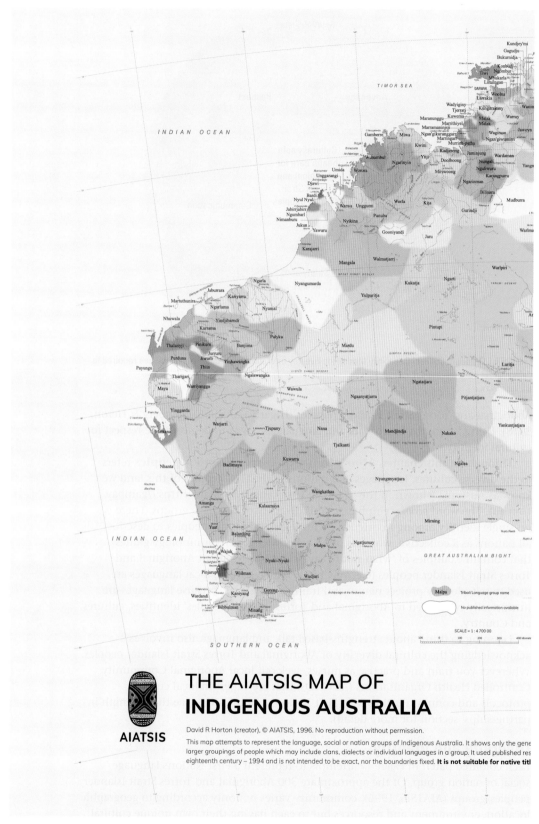

THE AIATSIS MAP OF
INDIGENOUS AUSTRALIA

David R Horton (creator), © AIATSIS, 1996. No reproduction without permission.

This map attempts to represent the language, social or nation groups of Indigenous Australia. It shows only the gene
larger groupings of people which may include clans, dialects or individual languages in a group. It used published res
eighteenth century – 1994 and is not intended to be exact, nor the boundaries fixed. **It is not suitable for native titl**

FIGURE 4.2 AIATSIS map of Aboriginal and Torres Strait Islander peoples of Australia

This map attempts to represent the language, social or nation groups of Aboriginal Australia. It shows only the general locations of larger groupings of people which may include clans, dialects or individual languages in a group. It used published resources from the eighteenth century – 1994 and is not intended to be exact, nor the boundaries fixed. It is not suitable for native title or other land claims. David R Horton (creator), © AIATSIS, 1996. No reproduction without permission. To purchase a print version visit: https://shop.aiatsis.gov.au/

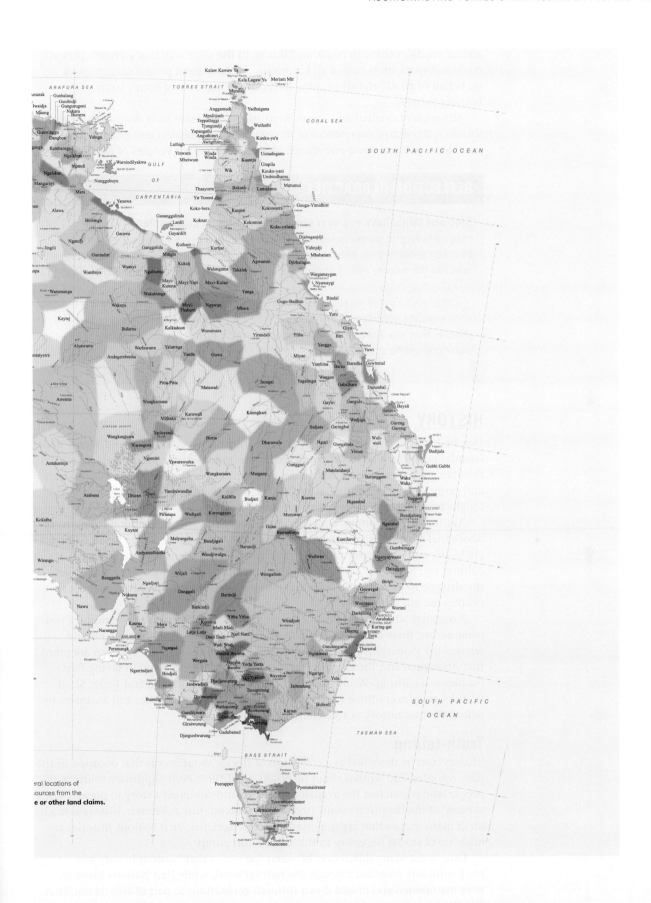

...eral locations of
...ources from the
...e or other land claims.

and/or practices that can be handed down. In the same way that a French person could not speak on behalf of all Europeans, an Aboriginal person cannot speak on behalf of all Aboriginal peoples, let alone Aboriginal *and* Torres Strait Islander peoples.

Although Aboriginal and Torres Strait Islander peoples have distinct cultures and societies, the shared experiences of dispossession, oppression and disadvantage have provided a political bond and shared identity for the First Peoples of Australia.

REFLECTION IN PRACTICE

Stop and think: have you ever struggled with being unaccepted?
Imagine having the people in authority over you automatically assume you are inferior based on something you have no ability to change. What would it feel like to be encouraged to be like the majority culture around you, but then be denied the rights and opportunities to do so?

Indigenous Australians still live with the reality that they are a minority group that is often expected to conform with majority norms, biases and values in regard to culture and lifestyle. They also live with the very real gap in wellbeing that affects their ability to thrive within broader Australian society.

Australians Together (2020)

HISTORY

Despite history being grounded in extreme injustice for Aboriginal and Torres Strait Islander peoples, there has also emerged profound resilience in survival and refusal to adopt the beliefs, tactics and values of colonisation. Despite the massacres, wars and genocide, many Aboriginal and Torres Strait Islander peoples have survived, fought back and maintained their cultures.

At the heart of 'cultural concepts' is the recognition of the cultural strengths of Aboriginal and Torres Strait Islander peoples. Wiradjuri man, Uncle Kevin Gilbert (1933–93, author, activist and artist) described First Nations survival as a great cultural and moral victory because through 'knowing, sharing, caring and respect', the struggle to preserve the knowledge of Aboriginal and Torres Strait Islander peoples remain intact.

No matter which Aboriginal or Torres Strait Islander person or community you come across, these are the children of leaders, of peoples who fought back and resisted the violent invasion of Country and colonisation. These children are proof that Aboriginal and Torres Strait Islander peoples were successful in saving First Peoples and cultures. While there is still much pain, Aboriginal and Torres Strait Islander peoples continue to right injustice, and to honour Elders and ancestors by telling the true history of colonisation.

Truth-telling

'History' can be described as a collection of stories about events that occurred in the past, recorded and written about by observers of these events (primary sources), or people who researched the available resources and compiled a story to present 'their version' of the historical events (secondary sources). Just as Western history is made up of many stories that are important to those societies, First Nations histories are made up of stories necessary to this population group.

One of the many differences between the two is that Western history was predominantly recorded through the written word, while First Nations histories were maintained and passed down through generations as part of an oral tradition. The Western version of history was not successfully challenged by Aboriginal and

Torres Strait Islander peoples until they gained sufficient education and mastery of Western literary traditions, particularly over the last 50 years. Today, this mastery is being achieved by an increasingly significant number of Aboriginal and Torres Strait Islander peoples. This has enabled a different version of history to emerge from the margins. In fact, C. D. Rowley (1970) claimed that Australian history was silent regarding Aboriginal and Torres Strait Islander peoples for almost 150 years.

A significant factor in this silence is that the dominant Western voice that has been historically privileged over First Nations voices has been that of a 'white male historian'. This dominance and bias resulted in a sanitised version of Australian history, one in which the invasion and colonisation of the continent was presented as being peaceful, with no conflicts or battles, when the reality was quite the opposite.

The true history of colonisation is a record of violation and abuse, leaving a legacy of trauma among Aboriginal and Torres Strait Islander peoples. This history can be very shocking to non-Indigenous Australians because many cannot believe that such atrocities could be committed in this country; reactions are often aggressive and focused on denial to escape the uncomfortable emotions that arise.

The contemporary Australian population is composed of peoples from many nations who have chosen Australia as their home. These diverse people who are becoming healthcare professionals will also benefit from understanding the historical legacy of the colonisation of Aboriginal and Torres Strait Islander peoples, so that they are better equipped to provide culturally-responsive care both in urban areas and rural and remote communities.

This history is presented to you, not to make you feel blamed or shamed, but rather for your benefit and that of Aboriginal and Torres Strait Islander peoples. Aboriginal and Torres Strait Islander peoples cannot heal, let alone trust you as a healthcare professional, unless you have an understanding and acceptance in your heart of what has truly happened on this land you call home. Specifically, the truth-telling in this chapter seeks to serve three purposes:

> To address the 'culture of denial', which continues to be perpetuated today and undermines reconciliation and the pathways to healing among Aboriginal and Torres Strait Islander peoples and ultimately all Australians.

> To increase compassion and to reduce the 'blame and shame narrative' that is often placed on Aboriginal and Torres Strait Islander peoples for having complex health, social and emotional wellbeing conditions, and to understand why there is mistrust in using the healthcare system effectively.

> To highlight the 'historical foundations' on which barriers to accessing health care, and the structural inequity of the system, have been built. More specifically and relevantly, this history tells a story of how Aboriginal and Torres Strait Islander peoples' trust continues to be broken by current attitudes, treatment and unsafe environments.

What you read may make you uncomfortable and bring up many emotions for you. Becoming a culturally-responsive health professional is about getting *uncomfortable* to *get comfortable* and thus more effective with interacting and working with those similar or markedly different to you.

It is important to sit with these feelings, lean in and critically reflect (see the 'Bass Model of Holistic Reflection' in **Figure 4.5**), realising that these injustices are our shared injustices and evolve your learning. May this new knowing inspire you to act and genuinely walk alongside Aboriginal and Torres Strait Islander peoples so that you can help to co-create a fairer and more just healthcare environment for all Australians. As nurses you have an important role to play in rebuilding trust with Aboriginal and Torres Strait Islander peoples.

Reflecting on colonisation

Reflecting on colonisation can result in healing, as evidenced in the 2022 apology delivered by the Council of Deans of Nursing and Midwifery (Australia & New Zealand) (CDNM):

> I would like to acknowledge the place of nursing and midwifery education and research, and how this has contributed to culturally unsafe practices and has caused ongoing suffering of Aboriginal and Torres Strait Islander nurses and midwives and their communities through having their cultural practices and contributions to the professions and healthcare ignored, or minimised, through privileging colonial approaches – Professor Karen Strickland.
>
> CDNM (2022)

There are extensive resources available to learn about the history of colonisation. *Colonise* is 'to plant or establish a colony in; form into a colony; settle' (Macquarie Dictionary, 2023b). In summary:

> *Colonisation:* is the impact of the frontier wars (1788–1930s) which were marked by invasion, massacres, genocide, communicable diseases, cultural devastation and a belief in *terra nullius* (land belonging to no-one) (Harris, 2012; Ryan, Debenham, Brown & Pascoe, 2017; Booth, 2021). The trauma from this history is raw and leads to protests about Australia Day/Survival Day and the Change the Date campaign (Ryan, Gilroy & Gibson, 2020).

> *Protection and segregation:* the impact of missions and reserves (1890–1950s) saw Aboriginal and Torres Strait Islander peoples removed from ancestral lands and placed onto missions and reserves, forced into training and education into 'civilised' Western lifestyles and religions, and continued racial discrimination and segregation. After this era it became possible for Aboriginal and Torres Strait Islander women to become nurses and midwives if they trained in a British dominion; but this did not happen in Australia until after 'the end of segregation and introduction of assimilation policies in the 1960s' (Mayes, 2020, p. 298). It was thought that Aboriginal and Torres Strait Islander peoples could not learn the skills and knowledge needed for nursing. It was not until the late 1960s that Aboriginal and Torres Strait Islander peoples could train as nurses and midwives in Australian hospitals (Best, 2018).

> *Breeding out the 'black' to create a 'white Australia': assimilation* (1901–1970s) was 'the process whereby individuals or groups of differing ethnic heritage, as migrant groups, or minority groups, acquire the basic attitudes, habits and mode of life of another all-embracing national culture (distinguished from acculturation)' (Macquarie Dictionary, 2023a). Aboriginal and Torres Strait Islander peoples were forced and coerced to adopt the cultural norms of Western society; in dress, education, work ethic, religion, and in beliefs and behaviours. One aspect of this was the Stolen Generations (which involved nurses and hospitals [Cox, 2007]), where children were removed from their parents, and which resulted in many devastating consequences, such as 'intergenerational trauma' (continued and cumulative effects of discrimination, racism and child removal) that nurses still see in their workplaces today (Power, Lucas, Hayes & Jackson, 2020). The *Bringing them home report* details the practices and consequences of the removal of Aboriginal and Torres Islander children from their families (AHRC, 1997).

> *Self-determination to reconciliation:* this includes an Aboriginal and Torres Strait Islander Voice to Parliament (1973–present). The idea of 'self-determination' is the right of Aboriginal and Torres Strait Islander peoples to 'freely determine their political status and freely pursue their economic, social and cultural development' (UNGA, 2007). The 'reconciliation movement' began in 1999 with the Council for Aboriginal Reconciliation established in response to the 1991 report of the Royal Commission into Aboriginal Deaths in Custody (Johnston, 1991). The Aboriginal and Torres Strait Islander Voice to Parliament movement has a long history rooted in social and political activism for Australian parliaments to create a formal and permanent way for Aboriginal and Torres Strait Islander peoples to influence Australian social policies that relate to them (Arcioni, 2021).

This brief overview of Australian history highlights the role of *power* in determining health outcomes, with the Ahpra definition of cultural safety urging you to consider 'power differentials' and how that contributes to disempowerment (Ahpra, 2020). In the following 'Reflection in practice' box, consider the power of wording about *identity*, which is a contentious issue in Australia (Fforde et al., 2013).

REFLECTION IN PRACTICE

Assumptions of identity

Given this history of colonisation, what do you think the impact of statements such as 'You don't look Aboriginal and/or Torres Strait Islander', or questions such as 'What part/ percentage Aboriginal and/or Torres Strait Islander are you?' have on Aboriginal and Torres Strait Islander peoples?

By asking *everyone* how they identify, you will not offend, but it is important that you ask *everyone*, not just those that you think 'look' Aboriginal and/or Torres Strait Islander, because as this chapter details, history has bred out *some* of the pre-colonial appearance of Aboriginal and Torres Strait Islander peoples.

Nurses and healthcare professionals can overcome assumptions of identity when asking the question: 'Are you an Aboriginal or Torres Strait Islander?' The act of doing so improves the identification of Aboriginal and Torres Strait Islander peoples in health and administrative data collections (Scotney, Guthrie, Lokuge & Kelly, 2010). This allows health planners to shift resources to areas of need, which is a key aspect of improving access to health care.

Barriers to access: health care

> … for Indigenous people to be able to participate in Australian society as equals requires that we be able to live our lives free from assumptions by others about what is best for us. It requires … recognition of our values, cultures and traditions so that they can co-exist with those of mainstream society. It requires respecting our difference and celebrating it within the diversity of the nation – Dr W Jonas, Aboriginal and Torres Strait Islander, Social Justice Commissioner, 1999–2004.
>
> Jonas (2000)

Being subjected to generation after generation of violent conflict, forced relocation from Country, dislocation from ancestral understandings and forced removal from families and communities meant intentional, systematic exclusion and disadvantage for Aboriginal and Torres Strait Islander peoples. These policies and practices have ensured that Aboriginal and Torres Strait Islander peoples have had poor nutrition, inadequate education, lack of employment opportunities and, of course, inadequate health care.

It is important to highlight that this 'history' is recent; in fact, older Aboriginal and Torres Strait Islander peoples were born into a world where they were considered inferior human beings and were not included in the census or allowed to vote. Many spent their youth as domestic servants in Western households doing unpaid work for many years (see the stolen wages link in the 'Further resources' section at the end of the chapter). Horrific acts and policies happened to the Stolen Generations (1910–70s), survivors of the most harmful policy that has ever existed in Australia (see the Healing Foundation website; details under 'Further resources' at the end of the chapter).

The barriers to accessing health care have been established and reinforced by the Western biomedicine world since colonisation and this translates to the reality of *inequity*. While there are many barriers that could be unpacked here, this chapter will focus on the fundamental one that underpins Aboriginal and Torres Strait Islander peoples' barriers to accessing health care and improving health and wellbeing: *racism*.

Racism

'Racism' can be broadly defined as the behaviours, practices, beliefs and prejudices that underlie avoidable and unfair inequalities across groups in society based on race, ethnicity, cultures or religion (Paradies, Chandrakumar & Klocker, 2009). When racist attitudes and behaviours are built into the operations (governance, structures, process and service delivery) of institutions, such as health care, it creates discrimination through prejudice, ignorance, thoughtlessness, racist stereotyping and unsafe physical spaces. For example, a health professional might consider an Aboriginal or Torres Strait Islander person as unsuitable for a kidney transplant, assuming they will be non-compliant with the treatment regime, when, in reality, the patient faces many daily challenges to compliance that the health professional may not consider.

This is known as 'institutionalised *or* systemic racism' and is unrecognised by those involved in it. 'Institutionalised racism' has occurred since colonisation when it was 'lawful' to dispossess and exploit Aboriginal and Torres Strait Islander peoples. It has set up a legacy of discrimination as systems are intrinsically built on non-Indigenous ways of 'knowing, being and doing', which is often at odds with Aboriginal and Torres Strait Islander peoples' ways of 'knowing, being and doing'. Given Australia's history and the lack of education in the general population of Australians about colonisation, there remain entrenched beliefs, assumptions and stereotypes about Aboriginal and Torres Strait Islander peoples. Within healthcare settings, there is no shortage of literature reporting the frequency of racist experiences of Aboriginal and Torres Strait Islander peoples (Paradies et al., 2015). The unequivocal impact of racism is considerable and enduring, with most harm affecting the social and emotional wellbeing of Aboriginal and Torres Strait Islander peoples. It is no surprise that the increased psychological distress, depression and anxiety because of racism is coupled with increased smoking, alcohol and substance misuse (Paradies, Harris & Anderson, 2008).

The impact of these historic and current accumulated experiences is a deep distrust of the health system by Aboriginal and Torres Strait Islander peoples, which, in turn, translates to delays in seeking care, not following recommendations, interruptions in care and avoidance of healthcare services altogether (Cox, 2007). This distrust also influences the number of Aboriginal and Torres Strait Islander peoples who want to work in the healthcare system, which again reduces access to culturally safe health care for Aboriginal and Torres Strait Islander peoples twofold: first, by not having a trusted First Nations healthcare professional who intrinsically understands the client; and second, by decreasing the organic cultural learning opportunities that non-Indigenous practitioners gain by working alongside Aboriginal and Torres Strait Islander peoples.

Internalised racism

Racism and discrimination towards Aboriginal and Torres Strait Islander peoples are realities that are exacerbated by a history of abuse, dispossession and intergenerational trauma occurring and continuing since colonisation. The link between racism and its pervasive impact on Aboriginal and Torres Strait Islander peoples' health is well established and it starts in childhood (Priest, Paradies, Gunthorpe, Cairney & Sayers, 2011). An insidious impact of growing up in a world where you are surrounded by racist stereotypes, beliefs and attitudes towards you and your communities is the 'internalisation of this racism', resulting in many Aboriginal and Torres Strait Islander peoples' feelings of self-doubt, disrespect and disgust towards their own communities.

Many darker-skinned Aboriginal and Torres Strait Islander peoples, particularly those who remain on missions and reserves, carry the shame that has been ingrained since colonisation, and this shame is compounded and confirmed with the everyday racism they experience. For many fair-skinned Aboriginal and Torres Strait Islander peoples, the emotion can often be one of *guilt*; guilt for having fair skin and so being able to access 'white privileges'. (*White privilege* is the unearned and unconscious rights, benefits, entitlements and advantages bestowed on white-skinned people by society simply because they were born white.) Fair-skinned Aboriginal and Torres Strait Islander peoples may also have feelings of shame and betrayal, to appear European on the outside and be treated and assumed as such but feel wholeheartedly different in spirit. This can cause incredible identity distress that is exacerbated by frequent remarks and reminders, such as 'You don't look Aboriginal'. These emotions contribute a reluctance to use the dominant Western health system and/or identify as being of First Nations descent.

The deep intergenerational grief, and unspeakable loss and trauma that is entrenched in the hearts of many Aboriginal and Torres Strait Islander peoples today, has cultivated a deep distrust of the Western healthcare system, and in some cases has created a future of hopelessness. This unfolds in many systemic and layered barriers for Aboriginal and Torres Strait Islander peoples to the effective use of the healthcare system.

You may not be able to change the entire system that you operate in, but you *can* be the change. With reflection and undertaking the uncomfortable journey of educating yourself about Australia's history, you can avoid contributing to the problems in this system and instead be a champion for Aboriginal and Torres Strait Islander peoples. You are capable of critical thinking and profound, transformative growth, but you must truly want this and see the importance of it for not just Aboriginal and Torres Strait Islander peoples, but for yourself as a reflective and caring person, both professionally and personally. See the 'Putting it in context' box following.

PUTTING IT IN CONTEXT

Closing the health gaps

Nurses play an important role in closing the gaps in health outcomes, and leadership in this area is shown by First Nations nurses, and their allies and champions. Nurses *can* help close the gap. See the:

> position statement by the Australian College of Nursing (ACN, 2017)
> Nursing and Midwifery Board of Australia (NMBA) and the Congress of Aboriginal and Torres Strait Islander nurses and midwives (CATSINaM) joint statement on culturally safe care (Cusack et al., 2018)
> nursing research (Stewart, 2018; Power, Lucas, Hayes & Jackson, 2020; Flemington et al., 2022; Power et al., 2022; West et al., 2022)
> leadership from First Nations organisations: Narrunga Kaurna woman and nurse Dr Janine Mohamed as CEO of the Lowitja Institute: Australia's National Institution for Aboriginal and Torres Strait Islander Health Research (Mohamed & West, 2017); and Kalkadunga and Djaku-nde woman and professor Roianne West as the CEO of CATSINaM (Fedele, 2020).

Dr Janine Mohamed said of CATSINaM:

CATSINaM now has the shared responsibility to ensure that cultural safety as an Indigenous nursing philosophy is firstly understood and secondly embedded into systems to ensure that its efficacy is not reliant on individual efforts.

Mohamed & West (2017)

STRENGTH IN PARTNERSHIPS

Partnerships between Aboriginal and Torres Strait Islander peoples and non-Indigenous Australians have always been important for the goal of equitable health care. The NMATSIHCF advocates for a strengths-based approach to facilitating partnerships with First Nations' healthcare professionals, organisations and communities (CATSINaM, 2017a). For registered nurses (RNs), partnerships are important for determining priorities, care planning and person-centred practice (NMBA, 2016). Blignault et al. (2021) state that the development of the Aboriginal Transfer of Care (ATOC) model relied on partnerships between mainstream hospitals and services with First Nations community organisations, First Nations hospital liaison officers, First Nations researchers and First Nations public servants (see **Figure 4.2**). In delivering culturally safe care, *partnerships* mean actively involving Aboriginal and Torres Strait Islander peoples in the decision-making processes. This means working with:

> ACCHOs in health care and social services
> CATSINaM
> IAHA
> National Association of Aboriginal and Torres Strait Islander Health Workers and Practitioners (NAATSIHWP)
> Australian Indigenous Doctors Association (AIDA)
> other organisations that can be found on the Australian Indigenous Health*InfoNet* (https://healthinfonet.ecu.edu.au).

Working in 'partnership' means thinking about concepts of respect, holistic health, relationality and cultural connections, and reflexivity.

Respect

> I love my heritage. I love to celebrate my heritage. It's what connects me to all of you here today. It's what connects me to the land.
>
> Barty in Goodwin (2022)

Respect is at the heart of First Nations' cultures, and it is actively reinforced at all levels (Korff, 2022). In Australia, it is standard protocol when speaking or introducing ourselves to show respect and acknowledge Country, Elders, ancestors and spirits of the place on which we speak. Showing this respect establishes and affirms the identity of the speaker, honours positive connections between peoples and recognises the identity and knowledge of others.

An **Acknowledgment of Country** (different from a Welcome to Country) can be given by non-Indigenous people. It is an opportunity to introduce yourself and show your respect for Country and the waters that you are on, and pay respects to Traditional Custodians of the peoples who have a continuing connection to Country and have done so for over 60 000 years. An Acknowledgment of Country usually takes place at the beginning of an event. An Acknowledgment can also be printed in publications like this book (see an example in the imprint), in the credits of films and television shows, and so on.

A **Welcome to Country** is a ceremony performed by Traditional Custodians to welcome visitors to ancestral land. Unlike an Acknowledgment of Country, this sacred ceremony is conducted by a descendant of the Country that you are on. If no Traditional Custodian is available, an Aboriginal and Torres Strait Islander person from a different clan or a non-Indigenous person can deliver an Acknowledgment of Country.

> [Welcome to Country and Acknowledgement of Country] is a very important way of giving Aboriginal people back their place in society … It's paying respect, in a formal sense, and following traditional custom in a symbolic way – Aunty Joy Murphy Wandin, Aboriginal Elder of the Wurundjeri people.
>
> Keynoteworthy (2019)

Another sign of respect is to consider holistic world views held by Aboriginal and Torres Strait Islander peoples, when you commence a health assessment and physical examination. Standard 4.1 directs the RN to conduct 'assessments that are holistic as well as culturally appropriate' (NMBA, 2016, p. 5).

Holistic health

Aboriginal health does not mean the physical wellbeing of an individual, but refers to the social, emotional, and cultural wellbeing of the whole community. For Aboriginal people this is seen in terms of the whole-life-view. Health care services should strive to achieve the state where every individual is able to achieve their full potential as human beings and must bring about the total wellbeing of their communities.

Gee, Dudgeon, Schultz, Hart & Kelly (2014, p. 56)

In nursing and healthcare literature, the term 'social and emotional wellbeing' (SEWB) is used because it reflects the perspective of Aboriginal and Torres Strait Islander peoples about the interrelatedness of all dimensions of 'being, knowing and doing' (Gee et al., 2014). Western biomedical medicine typically separates the body (physical health), psychology (mental health) and spirituality of the person; the spiritual health of the individual is often not considered at all in the Western treatment and healing process. Medical specialties have been developed around various parts of the body. For example, there are medical practitioners who are experts in specialised areas, such as ophthalmic, cardiovascular, musculoskeletal or neurological. Individuals are seen and treated without reference to their families, communities, kinship systems, connection to Country, lore or culture.

While Western biomedical healthcare constructs of health and wellbeing are typically focused on the individual and the absence of disease, Aboriginal and Torres Strait Islander peoples' view of health can be *holistic*. All social, emotional, physical, cultural and spiritual dimensions of 'being' are inextricably linked and interconnected to Country, cultures and spiritualities (Dudgeon, Bray, Smallwood, Walker & Dalton, 2020). As the Fabric of Aboriginal and Torres Strait Islander Wellbeing Model (see **Figure 4.3**) highlights, for many Aboriginal and Torres Strait Islander peoples, the parts of life that are most important to wellbeing are interwoven through their families, communities and cultures (Garvey et al., 2021).

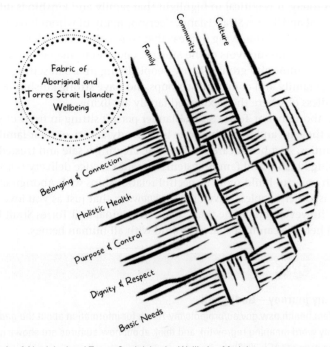

FIGURE 4.3 Fabric of Aboriginal and Torres Strait Islander Wellbeing Model

Note: this model takes inspiration from Aboriginal and Torres Strait Islander peoples' weaving traditions whereby individual strands are twined to 'create fabrics that are both beautiful and strong, the parts of life that are most important to wellbeing for many Aboriginal and Torres Strait Islander people are interwoven through their families, communities and culture.' This model represents the characteristic that the strength of wellbeing is derived from both the strength of the threads and their connections with each other.

GARVEY ET AL. (2021)

UNIT 1

Connection and belonging to family, kinships and communities

Family and kinship systems have always been pivotal to the functioning and wellbeing of ancestral and contemporary First Nations' societies (Gee et al., 2014). In fact, many believe family has been key to how First Nations cultures have survived and continue to survive the effects of colonisation (Walker & Shepherd, 2008). For most Aboriginal and Torres Strait Islander peoples, families play an important role in identity and sense of belonging and connectedness to kinship and culture.

> That extended family take it [family relationships] really seriously and want to be engaged on that life. You will never be an only child. Here's all your other brothers and sisters … You've got all these other mothers and fathers to support and teach you and that's the strength of the system.
>
> Riley (2014)

Kinship establishes where a person fits in their community, and Andrews (2020) states that it helps determine a personal relationship as well as a responsibility towards other people, the universe and Country. Underpinning kinship is the understanding that everything is interrelated and interconnected; that we are all family. Not only are we interconnected to other human beings, but we are all part of creation, including stars, rocks, plants and animals; this connection and belonging to a oneness is 'Dreaming' (Andrews, 2020). Kinship systems are complex and incredibly rich and diverse. They serve to maintain interconnectedness through cultural ties and reciprocal relationships. In turn, a feeling of deep spiritual and cultural belonging is cultivated in the reciprocity of these connections. If you would like to learn more about kinship systems, there are online modules provided by Sydney University; see the 'Further resources' section at the end of the chapter.

While ancestral kinship structures remain important in many First Nations communities today, it is critical to highlight that family and kinship is different for every Aboriginal and Torres Strait Islander person, many of whom have retained kinship connections. Those living in areas that were colonised earlier and most intensively, or who are survivors of the Stolen Generations, may no longer have large family or community groups. Many people living in urban settings still maintain large family and community groups and have strong kinship ties with family, regardless of where their extended family are living.

Only the Aboriginal or Torres Strait Islander person sitting in front of you can tell you who they are and what their role is in the dynamics of their family kinship and communities. As a healthcare professional, creating a safe and trusted space and prioritising kinship and family systems in your practice delivery is a significant way in which you can build more respectful relationships with Aboriginal and Torres Strait Islander peoples. Develop your *knowing*; that just as you love and value your family (however you define that), so do Aboriginal and Torres Strait Islander peoples, and here we can find shared ground with all human beings.

PUTTING IT IN CONTEXT

My rehab, my journey – Gadjigadji

Visit https://aci.health.nsw.gov.au/projects/my-rehab for information about the *gadjigadji* (a Gamilaraay word meaning regrowth), and think about how cultures are shown in every aspect of the project (ACI, 2022):

> What do you observe about the languages and artwork used?

> What do you notice about the consultation process and the implementation resources?

> Do you think these ways of 'knowing, being and doing' would benefit other cultures?

Connection and belonging to Country

We don't own the land, the land owns us. The land is my mother, my mother is the land. Land is the starting point to where it all began. It's like picking up a piece of dirt and saying this is where I started and this is where I'll go. The land is our food, our culture, our spirit and identity.

Knight (1996)

Connection is paramount in Aboriginal and Torres Strait Islander peoples' understanding of the world, and connection to family, kinship, cultures and Country. For millennia, there has been a deep knowing in First Nations cultures that all living connections and ancestral relationships between the natural elements of Country, plants, animals, rivers, stars and people make life possible. Many Aboriginal and Torres Strait Islander peoples do not separate themselves from the lands and waters from which they descend. This connection and belonging to Country define the reciprocal responsibility to care for Country, rather than having ownership or possession of it, and it is considered a privilege to do so (Korff, 2022).

For many Aboriginal and Torres Strait Islander peoples, being on Country is a deep and fundamental spiritual experience. In this environment, ceremonies and rituals can be practised, Dreaming can be shared, and sacred sites can be visited. It is through the performance of ceremonies and storytelling that contact is made with ancestral spirits and guidance and ancient wisdom can be drawn upon (Korff, 2022).

With colonisation, many ancestral groups were forcibly removed from Country so that the British could exploit the wealth and resources of the land. Although many Aboriginal and Torres Strait Islander peoples have been relocated and no longer live on Country, it cannot be emphasised enough that this does not diminish one's cultural and spiritual connections to Country.

One of the initiatives to celebrate cultural diversity is the campaign Know Your Country where nurses can, for example, add an email banner to acknowledge the Country they are working on (Know Your Country, 2022). Although a simple activity, it shows *reflexivity* in thinking about the cultural context of the healthcare service.

Reflexivity

Standard 1.2 of the 'Registered nurse standards for practice' requires nurses to think critically and analyse nursing practice. This involves 'reflection on experiences, knowledge, actions, feelings and beliefs to identify how these shape practice' (NMBA, 2016, p. 3). It is important to clarify what is meant by 'reflection' and to compare this to 'reflexivity' (see **Figure 4.4**). Basic reflection is about developing self-awareness, of identifying and developing an understanding of self-identity in relation to others. Moving into *critical thinking* means deeper exploration of your held beliefs and how they may impact on care provision. Then, analysing your held beliefs and the social context in which they occur can move you into meaningful

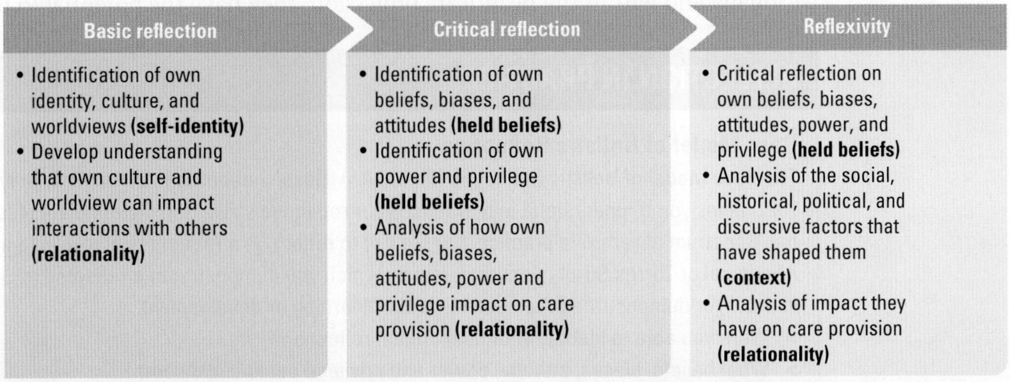

Basic reflection	Critical reflection	Reflexivity
• Identification of own identity, culture, and worldviews **(self-identity)** • Develop understanding that own culture and worldview can impact interactions with others **(relationality)**	• Identification of own beliefs, biases, and attitudes **(held beliefs)** • Identification of own power and privilege **(held beliefs)** • Analysis of how own beliefs, biases, attitudes, power and privilege impact on care provision **(relationality)**	• Critical reflection on own beliefs, biases, attitudes, power, and privilege **(held beliefs)** • Analysis of the social, historical, political, and discursive factors that have shaped them **(context)** • Analysis of impact they have on care provision **(relationality)**

FIGURE 4.4 Spectrum of reflexive practice
DAWSON, LACCOS-BARRETT, HAMMOND & RUMBOLD (2022)

actions for changing your practice with diverse people and those meaningful actions typify reflexivity (see the 'Communication in clinical practice' section).

If unconscious bias and racism can be considered a sickness, then *reflexivity* would be the medicine. Ongoing critical self-reflection and reduction of the power differences are central to being culturally safe and responsive. It is a lifelong journey, as the late Uncle Kevin Gilbert (1988) says, to:

> develop *all* people and encompass them in a code of spiritual being and national conduct, which not only reflects the very essence of life itself and the ultimate continuum for Being, but also will enable us, upon attainment, to project that magnanimity of spirit throughout the world.

As IAHA (2019, p. 4) highlight, 'Cultural safety does not necessarily require the study of any culture other than one's own …' and how you study yourself is a matter of what tool and process best resonates with you. See the 'Reflection in Practice' box following for an example of a tool you might use to take this learning and critical reflection deeper.

While critical reflection will ensure that you unpack the inner workings of your stereotypes, biases, norms, assumptions and belief systems, and question where they came from, being 'reflexive' is about doing activities that transform nursing practice.

Stereotypes

It is important to recognise that we are a product of our environment and that our brains categorise the world based on our experiences. This 'grouping' of information is an efficient way for our brains to process and store vast knowledge and avoid being overloaded. However, this natural tendency for our brain to categorise the world means that we often oversimplify social groups based on visible features (e.g. skin colour, gender, sex and age). These are known as 'stereotypes' and are constructed from direct personal experience, or more commonly, from other people or the media. Although this a natural way that our brains organise themselves, it can be detrimental to the person being stereotyped.

There are still some persistent negative stereotypes about Aboriginal and Torres Strait Islander peoples, which have largely been perpetuated and reinforced by the Australian media. In fact, the *Portrayal of Indigenous health in selected Australian media* study found that 74 per cent of articles about our health focused on negative stories within First Nations communities (Stoneham, Goodman & Daube, 2014). Specifically, the media is often saturated with stories of the poor health of Aboriginal and Torres Strait Islander peoples that focus on alcohol, child abuse, petrol sniffing, violence, crime and deaths in custody. In healthcare practice, these stereotypes become dangerous, as they directly impact on the type of treatments that are provided. For example, Aboriginal and Torres Strait Islander peoples are a third less likely to receive the same care as non-Indigenous people with the same condition (RACP, 2005). If bias and stereotypes go unaddressed and unquestioned, personally and within the healthcare profession, they have the potential to manifest

---

REFLECTION IN PRACTICE

Bass Model of Holistic Reflection
The Bass Model of Holistic Reflection (**Figure 4.5**) (Bass, Sidebotham, Sweet & Creedy, 2022) helps you to understand and practise your reflective skills. Use the template plus the 'Spectrum of reflexive practice' (**Figure 4.4**) to reflect on a recent event involving an Aboriginal or Torres Strait Islander person in which you demonstrated a reflected ability to improve, or demonstrated the need for further learning or development.
> Were you able to identify your own critical reflection?
> What beliefs, biases, attitude, power and privilege could you discern?
> How did it impact on the interaction with the other person?

>>

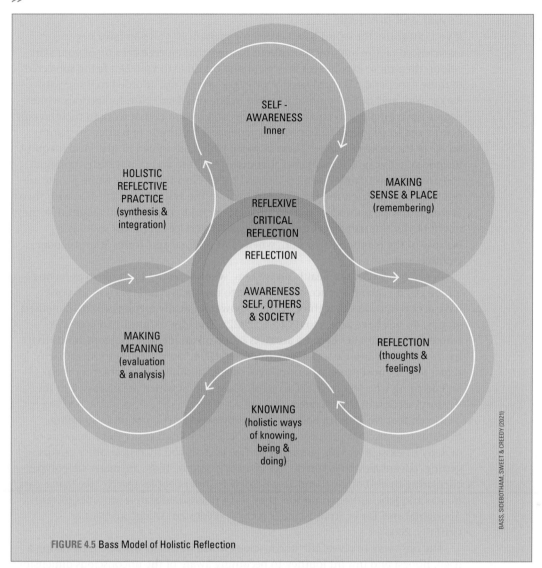

FIGURE 4.5 Bass Model of Holistic Reflection

in maltreatment, miscommunication and racism (both individual and systemic) towards Aboriginal and Torres Strait Islander peoples.

It is important to become aware of our biases and to mitigate the impact that beliefs and attitudes have on our behaviour towards specific groups of people. Many of our stereotypes are unconscious and we may not even be aware of holding them, as demonstrated in the Harvard Project's Implicit Association Test (Project Implicit, 2011) in the following 'Putting it in context' box.

PUTTING IT IN CONTEXT

Implicit Association Test (IAT)

Project Implicit is a non-profit organisation and international collaboration between researchers who are interested in implicit social cognition, thoughts and feelings outside of conscious awareness and control. The goal of the organisation is to educate the public about hidden biases and to provide a 'virtual laboratory' for collecting data on the internet.

The IAT for social attitudes has been developed as a tool for exploring the unconscious roots of thinking and feeling and allows individuals to gain greater awareness about their own unconscious preferences and beliefs.

You can undertake the test at https://implicit.harvard.edu/implicit/.

Power and privilege

If you categorise the world based on your experiences, and you have never experienced racism and the subsequent barriers that emerge because of your skin colour, then these experiences are essentially invisible to you. Not being subjected to these experiences is considered a 'privilege' that is not afforded to those with darker skin, and this is commonly called 'white privilege'. Non-Indigenous white people have privilege in choice, advantages and resources that work in their favour, as opposed to people of colour who experience a multitude of barriers to gaining access to the same resources. These barriers, which are rooted in historical inequity, include systems, policies and laws that disenfranchise and impoverish Aboriginal and Torres Strait Islander peoples (Mayes, 2020). Non-Indigenous white people are not forced to question their behaviours because the system is established with them at the centre, as 'normal' (e.g. non-Indigenous children are seldom taught that they might be discriminated against by police, social services or health systems because of the colour of their skin, whereas Aboriginal and Torres Strait Islander children are).

In the context of the healthcare system, when referring to a person as having 'privilege', it is about the access they have to resources. Those with more power have access to things that those without power, typically members of marginalised groups, do not have access to (PCC4U, 2022). The idea of 'unearned access' is where the inequity lies because access is based on an identity someone holds that has traditionally been associated with power. Here, 'power' refers to the capacity that a person must exercise control over others, deciding what is best for them, and deciding who will have access to resources, all of which are discussed in the 'History' section of this chapter.

Given that we all learn and are shaped by experiences, not understanding that this unconscious privilege and power exists makes it easier to be unaware of or deny its existence. This ignorance can be toxic if you then hear other groups getting 'advantages' that you do not get. For example, there are many stereotypes circulating that Aboriginal and Torres Strait Islander peoples receive free loans, cars, houses and jobs; although untrue, they serve to create negative attitudes towards Aboriginal and Torres Strait Islander peoples (Pedersen, Dudgeon, Watt & Griffiths, 2006).

The only way to reveal the unconscious world in which you live is by taking a deep, honest and inward journey to becoming aware of the unconscious dimensions of yourself. This can be achieved through reflexivity and making changes to your clinical practice.

COMMUNICATION IN CLINICAL PRACTICE FOR HEALTH ASSESSMENT AND PHYSICAL EXAMINATION

'Unsafe cultural practice comprises any action which diminishes, demeans or disempowers the cultural identity and wellbeing of an individual' (NCNZ, 2011, p. 7). The 'Registered nurse standards for practice' contain many aspects of practice that you will be expected to fulfil throughout your nursing career. This includes being responsive to Australia's cultural and linguistic diversity, and to the diverse cultures of Aboriginal and Torres Strait Islander peoples. At universities, nurses are required to learn about First Nations' professional capability: the capacity to work effectively with and for Aboriginal and Torres Strait Islander peoples (Page, Trudgett & Bodkin-Andrews, 2019). In this section are examples of what culturally safe and responsive practice can look like, and some techniques associated with culturally safe communication, such as the RN Standard 2.2 'communicates effectively, and is respectful of a person's dignity, culture, values, beliefs and rights' (NMBA, 2016, p. 5; see Chapter 2).

Shared decision-making

To create equal, two-way sharing of knowledge we must find the space where 'two streams' meet equally. This means we need to remove the underlying belief that you, as the clinician, are the one with all the knowledge and therefore power in the healthcare interaction. In fact, the Aboriginal or Torres Strait Islander person receiving care has incredible cultural knowledge and wisdom to bring to the exchange. In **Figure 4.6**, you will see a patient journey model that was developed with First Nations stakeholders to ensure that whatever health choices Aboriginal and Torres Strait Islander peoples make, they can feel safe and trusted to make informed decisions based on each person's values and beliefs. The different stages of the patient journey, incorporated with *yarning*, ensures shared decision-making, and opening of doors to finding a safe and effective way to health and wellbeing. In turn, this supports the 'purpose and control' weave of the Fabric of Aboriginal and Torres Strait Islander Wellbeing Model (refer to **Figure 4.3**).

What does shared decision-making and a meaningful journey look like? The Daalbirrwirr Gamambigu (Safe Children) Model of care is one way to map out how cultural safety can be embedded in the patient journey through paediatric EDs (Flemington et al., 2022). The aim is for a culturally safe patient journey where First Nations 'families experience respect, dignity and empowerment in their patient journey' (Flemington et al., 2022). Developing a culturally safe patient journey (see **Figure 4.6**) was based on extensive stakeholder yarning, partnerships with a range of service providers, inclusion of Aboriginal people in all aspects of the project, and testing with over 50 Aboriginal and non-Indigenous nurses and health professionals. The patient journey shows the points and pathways where nurses (and other staff) interact with First Nations families.

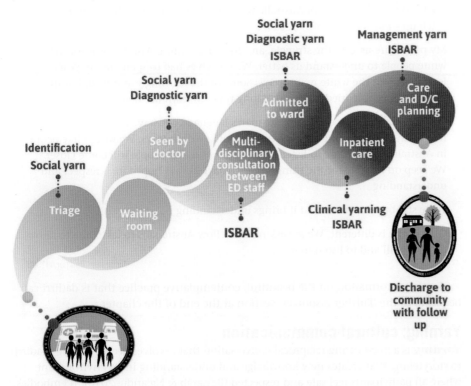

FIGURE 4.6 Culturally safe patient journey

FLEMINGTON ET AL. (2022)

It is at these points and pathways that nurses can be culturally responsive. While you have developed your 'knowing' and your 'being', here we explore how this applies to your 'doing'. What are the ingredients to building connection, trust and respectful two-way relationships with Aboriginal and Torres Strait Islander peoples? It often begins with surrendering your ways of 'knowing, being and doing' and rebuilding yourself in ways of *dadirri*, yarning and shared decision-making; all of which are holistically interconnected.

Dadirri: deep listening

Drawing on her deep respect for Country and a unique and sacred identity with the land, Aboriginal Elder, Dr Miriam-Rose Ungunmerr-Baumann of the Ngangikurungkurr peoples from Daly River (Northern Territory), shares one of the unique and special gifts of her people, 'dadirri' (pronounced *da-did-ee*). Dadirri is a powerful practice of inner, deep listening and quiet, still awareness (Ungunmerr Bauman, 1988). It facilitates deep reflection and contemplation, which brings peace, understanding and increased awareness as you tap into the deep spring that sits inside all of us. In Australia, people from both First Nations and non-Indigenous backgrounds have embraced the ancient practice of dadirri to support healing and wellbeing and reveal pathways to new knowledge.

> In our Aboriginal way, we learnt to listen from our earliest days. We could not live good and useful lives unless we listened. This was the normal way for us to learn – not by asking questions. We learnt by watching and listening, waiting and then acting …

> We cannot hurry the river. We have to move with its current and understand its ways …

> We hope that the people of Australia will wait. Not so much waiting for us – to catch up – but waiting with us, as we find our pace in this world …

> My people are used to the struggle, and the long waiting. We still wait for the white people to understand us better. We ourselves had to spend many years learning about the white man's ways. Some of the learning was forced; but in many cases people tried hard over a long time, to learn the new ways.

> We have learned to speak the white man's language. We have listened to what he had to say. This learning and listening should go both ways. We would like people in Australia to take time to listen to us. We are hoping people will come closer. We keep on longing for the things that we have always hoped for – respect and understanding …

> To be still brings peace – and it brings understanding …

> Our culture is different. We are asking our fellow Australians to take time to know us; to be still and to listen to us …

> Ungunmerr-Baumann (1988)

Further information on the beautiful, contemplative practice that is dadirri can be found in the 'Further resources' section at the end of the chapter.

Yarning: cultural communication

Yarning is a free-flowing reciprocal conversation that involves deep listening (dadirri) to storytelling that creates new knowledge and understanding in an environment where all participants feel safe and respected (Bessarab & Ng'andu, 2010). It embodies and continues First Nations' oral traditions and builds deep reflection and empathy among non-Indigenous participants (Lawrence & Paige, 2016).

> As our ancestors knew, storytelling is a holistic process that engages the heart, body, and spirit along with the mind. Telling our stories is one way of making sense of our own experiences. Listening to others' stories also helps us to understand ourselves as we identify with their experiences. On the other

hand, listening to stories around difference helps to promote empathy and understanding, particularly between people of different cultures. It broadens our knowledge. Storytelling has the power to disrupt stereotypes. It is difficult to judge a person by his or her cultural membership once you have heard his or her story.

Lawrence & Paige (2016, p. 66)

Clinical yarning foregrounds First Nations cultural communication preferences to the important aspects of healthcare conversations (Lin, Green & Bessarab, 2016). It is a way of communicating that is culturally secure and encourages deep listening, and helps to build a trusting relationship.

The 'clinical yarning framework' talks about three types of yarning, which are captured in **Figure 4.7**.

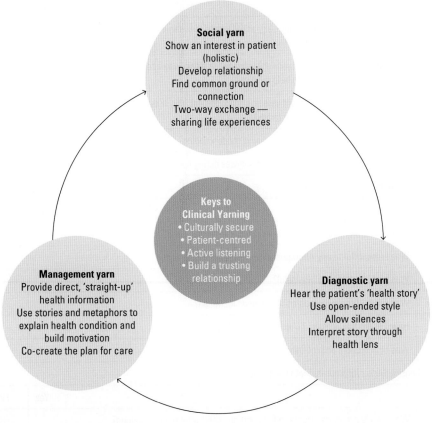

FIGURE 4.7 Keys to clinical yarning

LIN, GREEN & BESSARAB (2016)

To explore and learn how to apply clinical yarning into your practice, there are free online modules available via the Clinical Yarning Project website (see the 'Further resources' section at the end of the chapter). A cultural yarning process informed the ATOC model (Blignault et al., 2021) about strengths-based communication. The ATOC model maps a patient journey for Aboriginal and Torres Strait Islander peoples with chronic disease, and emphasises culturally responsive teamwork, hospital support structures and partnerships with a range of community service providers (Blignault et al., 2021). For shared decision-making, yarning is important for finding a reciprocal way in making decisions with Aboriginal and Torres Strait Islander peoples (ACI, 2021).

Keeping track of culturally safe practice

This chapter has introduced you to new ways of practising nursing. It is important to demonstrate culturally safe practice for nursing accreditation and registration (NMBA, 2016; ANMAC, 2019). One form of evidence is demonstration of cultural safety in patient record-keeping and interprofessional communication. The Daalbirrwirr Gamambigu Project (Flemington et al., 2022) produced a culturally adapted ISBAR (an acronym for 'identify, situation, background, assessment and recommendation') for interprofessional communication, and a cultural safety checklist (see **Figure 4.8**). Your hospital or healthcare organisation can also use tools and checklists to assess organisational-level cultural safety (NSWMoH, 2022). All these forms of evidence are important for your continuing professional development and the accreditation of your healthcare organisation (ACSQHC, 2017).

CULTURAL SAFETY CHECKLIST FOR CLINICIANS			
1 Use of clinical yarning with families			
		Yes	No
i.	Have I engaged in social yarning? e.g. asked where their familly is from, what school the children attend, etc.		
ii.	Have I engaged in diagnostic yarning? (engaged in a two-way information exchange to gather information used to help diagnose)		
iii.	Have I engaged in management yarning? (management plan is clearly explained and formulated in consultation with family)		
iv.	Have I used plain language without being condescending?		
v.	Did I use active listening and allow for silences during conversation?		
2 Incorporation of relationships			
		Yes	No
i.	Was I sincere and authentic when interacting with the family?		
ii.	Was I respectful to any Aboriginal elders present?		
iii.	Was an ALO offered (if available)?		
iv.	Was a family spokesperson/contact person identified?		
v.	Have I asked the question? (Aboriginal identification)		
vi.	Was I transparent and inclusive?		
3 Considerations incorporated into use of ISBAR			
		Yes	No
i.	Were family dynamics, access to transport and carer information included?		
ii.	Was the ALO, social worker and/or community supports included in recommendation section of ISBAR?		
iii.	Were Child & Family Services included in the process?		

FIGURE 4.8 Cultural safety checklist for health professionals
FLEMINGTON ET AL. (2022)

As a nurse, you will spend most of your time with people during hospitalisation or medical treatment, so it is to your advantage to familiarise yourselves with all aspects of their social and emotional wellbeing. It will make your job easier and benefit the person, who will feel that you understand something about their cultures, concerns and issues. When initiating a health assessment and physical examination, you are not expected to be the 'expert' but to have some familiarity with the individual's culture and a willingness to learn about their lives.

There is an increasing number of First Nations' nurses and doctors entering the healthcare arena. While it is not and should not be *their* responsibility to only care for Aboriginal and Torres Strait Islander peoples, or to share their knowledge, you can respectfully ask them for assistance if the issue you are dealing with is culturally related. Choose your questioning moment with care and ensure that you have already built up a relationship of trust and professionalism so they are not going to interpret your questions as bothersome and taking them away from what they should be doing. Remember, there are First Nations healthcare professionals who can assist you (in addition to nurses and doctors, there are interpreters and community health workers). This will in turn impact on the individual's health and rate of healing, and/or their willingness to comply with what you are requesting of them.

'I'm scared of saying or doing the wrong thing' – My letter to you

At the heart of this journey is your ability to genuinely share your time and spirit. In the busy-ness and clinical-ness of the system and its demands, you can see how our two worlds can clash. You may feel awkward doing this at work, perhaps even scared that you are crossing professional boundaries in some way or fearful that you are going to say or do something wrong. Our fear of doing or saying the wrong thing often holds us back. We doubt whether we could really add value or make a difference to the person sitting in front of us.

When we remove the idea that we are there to fix someone's problems and focus instead on the importance of building a trusting relationship (which can still respect professionalism), we often find not only do we have something to offer but that we will gain something beautiful in return.

It is important to emphasise that we need your genuine and meaningful time so that we can read your heart, connect with you our way and this leads to us understanding you. How does anyone trust someone they don't understand? If anything, fear sits there and that is why so many of our people are scared of hospital, health or anything to do with the dominant system. Then, when we have non-Indigenous health professionals coming from that system and mimicking its busy, process-oriented, disconnected and individualistic ways that essentially lack heart, it only further exacerbates our fears. Naturally, we will do everything to avoid anything that makes us feel that way, as any human would.

So, you can see how important each and every one of you is in this dream to create equitable access for our people. You have read this far so clearly you want to be the best nurse you can be, to all people, regardless of cultural background.

When you have the ultimate privilege of connecting with an Aboriginal or Torres Strait Islander person, I encourage you to give the gift of your time and spirit; regardless of whether this environment is clinical, work-related or social. Use the time to share your spirit by offering a bit of your story, not your professional or educational one; strip away that privilege and let us connect with you and better understand your weave in this world. Where did you come from? Who is your family? What makes you, you? Then tell me that you know nothing about my journey, but you are here to listen and learn. And I promise you, every time you speak to an Aboriginal or Torres Strait Islander person, you will learn something deep, something that will move your spirit and change your heart in some special way; but you need to be open to that transformative learning and understand that you don't have to have the answers and we do not expect you to. Just listen and listen deeply so, together, we can walk and dream in solidarity.

Nicole Hewlett (2023)

CHAPTER RESOURCES

REVIEW QUESTIONS

1. What thoughts and assumptions come up for you when you think of Aboriginal and Torres Strait Islander peoples? How has the content in this chapter impacted on those thoughts and assumptions?

2. If a person identifies as having First Nations heritage, why is it important *not* to assume that person is automatically connected to Country, kinship or culture?

3. Why is understanding Australia's history so important to being a culturally-responsive nurse?

4. In your opinion, what are five strengths of First Nations cultures?

5. What are some ways that you can build trust and connection with Aboriginal and Torres Strait Islander peoples and co-workers?

6. Why is your role as a nurse critical to creating access to health care among Aboriginal and Torres Strait Islander peoples?

7. How will you continue your culturally-responsive journey?

FURTHER RESOURCES

Continuing your culturally safe learning journey

> Acquire new knowledge from the IAHA's online cultural safety training modules, which use a cultural responsiveness framework: https://iaha.com.au/iaha-consulting/cultural-responsiveness-training/

> Learn from the CATSINaM cultural safety training e-learning modules: https://anmj.org.au/a-new-cultural-safety-and-cultural-humility-training-program-for-nurses-and-midwives-launched/

> Discover these clinical yarning e-learning modules: https://www.clinicalyarning.org.au/

> Explore Aboriginal and Torres Strait Islander peoples' experiences and learn about local cultures near you: https://www.welcometocountry.com/

> Learn about and practise dadirri: https://www.miriamrosefoundation.org.au/dadirri/

> Visit the Healing Foundation website to learn more about the Stolen Generations and how to educate all age groups: https://healingfoundation.org.au/

> Learn more about Aboriginal kinship systems from Sydney University: https://www.sydney.edu.au/about-us/vision-and-values/our-aboriginal-and-torres-strait-islander-community/kinship-module.html

> Watch this video to understand intergenerational trauma: https://healingfoundation.org.au/intergenerational-trauma/

> Explore more about the history of stolen wages: https://www.creativespirits.info/aboriginalculture/economy/stolen-wages/stolen-wages

> Invest in learning First Nations words: https://www.abc.net.au/radionational/programs/wordup; https://australianaudioguide.com/podcast/word-up/

REFERENCES

Agency for Clinical Innovation (ACI). (2022). *My rehab, my journey Gadjigadji: Improving the experience for Aboriginal people in the rehabilitation environment.* Retrieved from https://aci.health.nsw.gov.au/projects/my-rehab

Alarcon, R. D., Foulks, E. F., & Vakkur, M. (1998). *Personality disorders and culture: Clinical and conceptual interactions.* New York, NY: John Wiley & Sons.

Andrews, M. (2020). *Journey into Dreamtime.* Victoria, Australia: Ultimate World Publishing.

Arcioni, E. (2021). The voice to parliament proposal and 'the people' of the constitution. *Alternative Law Journal, 46*(3), 225–7. https://doi.org/10.1177/1037969X211010827

Australian College of Nursing (ACN). (2017). *Nurses can help close the gap* [Media release]. Retrieved from https://www.acn.edu.au/media-release/nurses-can-help-close-the-gap

Australian Commission on Safety and Quality in Health Care (ACSQHC). (2017). *National safety and quality health service standards* (2nd ed.). Retrieved from http://www.nationalstandards.safetyandquality.gov.au/

Australian Government Department of Health (AGDH). (2014). *Aboriginal and Torres Strait Islander health curriculum framework.* Retrieved from http://www.health.gov.au/internet/main/publishing.nsf/Content/aboriginal-torres-strait-islander-health-curriculum-framework

Australian Government Department of Health (AGDH). (2021). The new *national Aboriginal and Torres Strait Islander health plan 2021–2031.* Retrieved from https://www.health.gov.au/health-topics/aboriginal-and-torres-strait-islander-health/how-we-support-health/health-plan

Australian Health Practitioner Regulation Agency (Ahpra). (2020). *National scheme's Aboriginal and Torres Strait Islander health and cultural safety strategy.* Retrieved from https://www.ahpra.gov.au/About-Ahpra/Aboriginal-and-Torres-Strait-Islander-Health-Strategy/health-and-cultural-safety-strategy.aspx

Australian Human Rights and Equal Opportunity Commission (AHRC). (1997). *Bringing them home: Report of the national inquiry into the separation of Aboriginal and Torres Strait Islander children from their families.* Commonwealth of Australia: AHRC. Retrieved from https://www.humanrights.gov.au/publications/bringing-them-home-report-1997

Australian Institute of Aboriginal and Torres Strait Islander Studies (AIATSIS). (1996). *Map of Indigenous Australia.* Retrieved from https://aiatsis.gov.au/explore/map-indigenous-australia

Australian Nursing and Midwifery Accreditation Council (ANMAC). (2019). *Registered nurse accreditation standards 2019.* Retrieved from https://anmac.org.au/sites/default/files/documents/06920_anmac_reg_nurse_std_ee_2019_updated_fa.pdf

Australians Together. (2020). *A white Australia*. Retrieved from https://australianstogether.org.au/discover-and-learn/our-history/a-white-australia/

Balla, P., Jackson, K., Quayle, A. F., Sonn, C. C., & Price, R. K. (2022). 'Don't let anybody ever put you down culturally … it's not good …': Creating spaces for Blak women's healing. *American Journal of Community 2021 Psychology*, 1–13. https://doi.org/10.1002/ajcp.12607

Bass, J., Sidebotham, M., Sweet, L., & Creedy, D. K. (2022). Development of a tool to measure holistic reflection in midwifery students and midwives. *Women and birth, 35*(5). https://doi.org/10.1016/j.wombi.2021.10.001

Bessarab, D., & Ng'andu, B. (2010). Yarning about yarning as a legitimate method in Indigenous research. *International Journal of Critical Indigenous Studies, 3*(1), 37–50. https://doi.org/10.5204/ijcis.v3i1.57

Best, O. (2018). Training the 'Natives' as Nurses in Australia: So What Went Wrong? In H. Sweet & S. Hawkins (Eds.), *Colonial Caring: A History of Colonial and Post-Colonial Nursing* (104–25). Manchester University Press.

Blignault, I., Norsa, L., Blackburn, R., Bloomfield, G., Beetson, K., Jalaludin, B., & Jones, N. (2021). 'You can't work with my people if you don't know how to': Enhancing transfer of care from hospital to primary care for Aboriginal Australians with chronic disease. *International Journal of Environmental Research and Public Health, 18*(14). https://doi.org/10.3390/ijerph18147233

Booth, A. (2021). *What are the frontier wars?* Retrieved from https://www.sbs.com.au/nitv/what-are-the-frontier-wars/3f2ab8ee-42b1-4c30-b747-fdc3afa35486

Congress of Aboriginal and Torres Strait Islander Nurses and Midwives (CATSINaM). (2017a). The Nursing and Midwifery Aboriginal and Torres Strait Islander Health Curriculum Framework: An adaptation of and complementary document to the 2014 Aboriginal and Torres Strait Islander Health Curriculum Framework. Retrieved from https://catsinam.org.au/2021/01/nursing-and-midwifery-aboriginal-and-torres-strait-islander-health-curriculum-framework/

Congress of Aboriginal and Torres Strait Islander Nurses and Midwives (CATSINaM). (2017b). *A framework for promoting cultural safety in the Australian healthcare system – Partnering for equity: A CATSINaM framework for embedding cultural safety in health services*. Canberra, Australia: Congress of Aboriginal and Torres Strait Islander Nurses and Midwives.

Congress of Aboriginal and Torres Strait Islander Nurses and Midwives (CATSINaM). (2021) *Murra Mullangari: Introduction to cultural safety and cultural humility*. Retrieved from https://catsinam.org.au/murramullangari/

Council of Deans of Nursing and Midwifery (Australia & New Zealand) (CDNM). (2022). *CDNM Apology – delivered at the CATSINaM conference on 19 August 2022*. Retrieved from https://irp.cdn-website.com/1636a90e/files/uploaded/apology_signed.pdf

Cox, L. (2007). Fear, trust and Aborigines: The historical experience of state institutions and current encounters in the health system. *Health and History, 9*(2), 70–92. https://doi.org/10.2307/40111576

Cusack, L., Kinnear, A., Ward, K., Mohamed, J., & Butler, A. (2018). *Joint statement – cultural safety: Nurses and midwives leading the way for safer healthcare*. Retrieved from http://www.nursingmidwiferyboard.gov.au/News/2018-03-23-joint-statement.aspx

Dawson, J., Laccos-Barrett, K., Hammond, C., & Rumbold, A. (2022). Reflexive practice as an approach to improve healthcare delivery for Indigenous peoples: A systematic critical synthesis and exploration of the cultural safety education literature. *International Journal of Environmental Research and Public Health, 19*(11). https://doi.org/10.3390/ijerph19116691

Dudgeon, P., Bray, A., Smallwood, G., Walker, R., & Dalton, T. (2020) *Wellbeing and healing through connection and culture*. Commonwealth of Australia: Lifeline. https://doi:10.6084/m9.figshare.14036774

Fedele, R. (2020). 'It's destiny': Meet new CATSINaM CEO, Professor Roianne West. *Australian Nursing and Midwifery Journal*. Retrieved from https://anmj.org.au/its-destiny-meet-new-catsinam-ceo-professor-roianne-west/

Fforde, C., Bamblett, L., Lovett, R., Gorringe, S., & Fogarty, B. (2013). Discourse, deficit and identity: Aboriginality, the race paradigm and the language of representation in contemporary Australia. *Media International Australia, 149*(1), 162–173. https://doi.org/10.1177/1329878X1314900117

Flemington, T., Fraser, J., Gibbs, C., Shipp, J., Bryant, J., Ryan, A., … Lock Ngiyampaa, M. (2022). The Daalbirrwirr Gamambigu (safe children) model: Embedding cultural safety in child protection responses for Australian Aboriginal children in hospital settings. *International Journal of Environmental Research and Public Health, 19*(9), 5381. https://doi.org/10.3390/ijerph19095381

Fogarty, W., Lovell, M., Lagenberg, J., & Heron, M. J. (2018). *Deficit discourse and strengths-based approaches: Changing the narrative of Aboriginal and Torres Strait Islander health and wellbeing*. The Lowitja Institute & National Centre for Indigenous Studies. Retrieved from https://www.lowitja.org.au/page/services/resources/Cultural-and-social-determinants/racis--/deficit-discourse-strengths-based

Garvey, G., Anderson, K., Gall, A., Butler, T. L., Whop, L. J., Arley, B., … Howard, K. (2021). The Fabric of Aboriginal and Torres Strait Islander Wellbeing: A conceptual model. *International Journal of Environmental Research and Public Health, 18*(15), 7745. https://doi.org/10.3390/ijerph18157745

Gee, G., Dudgeon, P., Schultz, C., Hart, A., & Kelly, K. (2014). Aboriginal and Torres Strait Islander social and emotional wellbeing. In P. Dudgeon, H. Milroy & R. Walker (Eds.), *Aboriginal and Torres Strait Islander Mental Health and Wellbeing Principles and Practice* (Rev. ed., p. 56). Retrieved from https://apo.org.au/node/39689

Gilbert, K. (1988). *Inside black Australia: An anthology of Aboriginal poetry*. Victoria, Australia: Penguin Books Australia.

Goodwin, S. (2022, 18 January). Jelena Dokic breaks down in tears during interview with Ash Barty. *Yahoo Sport Australia*. Retrieved from https://au.sports.yahoo.com/australian-open-2022-jelena-dokic-interview-ash-barty-203259021.html#:~:text=%22I%20love%20my%20heritage%2C%20I,commending%20both%20Dokic%20and%20Barty

Harris, J. (2012). *One blood: 200 years of Aboriginal encounter with Christianity: A story of hope* (3rd ed.). Adelaide, Australia: Concilia Ltd.

Indigenous Allied Health Australia (IAHA). (2019). *Cultural responsiveness in action: An IAHA framework* (3rd ed., version 8). Retrieved from https://iaha.com.au/workforce-support/training-and-development/cultural-responsiveness-in-action-training/

Johnston, E. (1991). *Royal Commission into Aboriginal deaths in custody* [National report, vol. 5]. Canberra, Australia: Australian Government Publishing Service. Retrieved from http://www.austlii.edu.au/au/other/IndigLRes/rciadic/

Joint Council on Closing the Gap (JCCTG). (2020). *National agreement on closing the gap*. Australian Government. Retrieved from https://www.closingthegap.gov.au/national-agreement-closing-gap-glance

Jonas, W. (2000). *Social justice report 2000. Chapter 2: Reconciliation and human rights*. Australian Human Rights Commission. Retrieved from https://humanrights.gov.au/our-work/publications/social-justice-report-2000-chapter-2-reconciliation-and-human-rights

Keynoteworthy. (2019, 2 July). The significance of Welcome to Country: Why every event should have one. *Keynoteworthy*. Retrieved from https://keynoteworthy.com.au/the-significance-of-welcome-to-country-why-every-event-should-have-one/

Knight, S. (1996). *Our land our life* (Timmy Payunka [Payungka] Tjapangati) [Artwork]. Office of Public Affairs, ATSIC Canberra 1996. Retrieved from https://catalogue.nla.gov.au/Record/6102011

Know Your Country. (2022). *We love our Country but how well do we really know it?* Retrieved from https://www.knowyourcountry.com.au/

Korff, J. (2022). *Respect for Elders and culture*. Creative Spirits. Retrieved from https://www.creativespirits.info/aboriginalculture/people/respect-for-elders-and-culture

Lawrence, R. L., & Paige, D. S. (2016). *What our ancestors knew: Teaching and learning through storytelling. New directions for adult and continuing education. New Directions for Adult and Continuing Education, 149,* 63–72. https://doi.org/10.1002/ace.20177

Lin, I., Green, C., & Bessarab, D. (2016). 'Yarn with me': Applying clinical yarning to improve clinician–patient communication in Aboriginal health care. *Australian Journal of Primary Health, 22*(5), 377–82.

Macquarie Dictionary. (2023a). *Assimilation.* Retrieved from https://www.macquariedictionary.com.au/features/word/search/?search_word_type=Dictionary&word=asssimilation&fuzzy=on

Macquarie Dictionary. (2023b). *Colonise.* Retrieved from https://www.macquariedictionary.com.au/features/word/search/?search_word_type=Dictionary&word=colonisation&fuzzy=on

Mayes, C. (2020). White medicine, white ethics: On the historical formation of racism in Australian healthcare. *Journal of Australian Studies 44*(3), 287–302. https://doi.org/10.1080/14443058.2020.1796754

Mohamed, J., & West, R. (2017). *Creating an Indigenous-led movement for cultural safety in Australia.* Retrieved from https://croakey.org/creating-an-indigenous-led-movement-for-cultural-safety-in-australia/

NSW Ministry of Health (NSWMoH). (2022). *NSW health services Aboriginal cultural engagement self-assessment tool.* Sydney, Australia: NSW Government. Retrieved from https://www.health.nsw.gov.au/aboriginal/Pages/cultural-engagement-tool.aspx

Nursing and Midwifery Board Australia (NMBA). (2016). *Registered nurse standards for practice.* Retrieved from https://www.nursingmidwiferyboard.gov.au/codes-guidelines-statements/professional-standards/registered-nurse-standards-for-practice.aspx

Page, S., Trudgett, M., & Bodkin-Andrews, G. (2019). Creating a degree-focused pedagogical framework to guide Indigenous graduate attribute curriculum development [Article]. *Higher Education (00181560), 78*(1), 1–15. https://doi.org/10.1007/s10734-018-0324-4

Palliative Care Curriculum for Undergraduates (PCC4U). (2022). *Topic 2 toolkit: Caring for Australian Indigenous peoples affected by life-limiting illness.* Retrieved from https://pcc4u.org.au/learning/topics/topic2/#:~:text=This%20Focus%20Topic%20Toolkit%3A%20Caring,and%20their%20families%20and%20communities

Paradies, Y., Ben, J., Denson, N., Elias, A., Priest, N., Pieterse, A., Gupta, A., Kelaher, M., & Gee, G. (2015.) Racism as a determinant of health: A systematic review and meta-analysis. *PLoS One, 10*(9). https://doi.org/10.1371/journal.pone.0138511

Paradies, Y., Chandrakumar, L., Klocker, N., Frere, M., Webster, K., Burrell, M., & McLean, P. (2009). *Building on our strengths: A framework to reduce race-based discrimination and support diversity in Victoria* [Full report]. Melbourne, Australia: Victorian Health Promotion Foundation.

Paradies, Y., Harris, R., & Anderson, I. (2008). *The impact of racism on Indigenous health in Australia and Aotearoa: Towards a research agenda.* [Discussion paper no. 4]. Darwin, Australia: Cooperative Research Centre for Aboriginal Health.

Pedersen, A., Dudgeon, P., Watt, S., & Griffiths, B. (2006). Attitudes toward Indigenous Australians: The issue of 'special treatment'. *Australian Psychologist, 41*(2), 85–94. https://doi.org/10.1080/00050060600585502

Power, T., Lucas, C., Hayes, C., & Jackson, D. (2020). 'With my heart and eyes open': Nursing students' reflections on placements in Australian, urban Aboriginal organisations. *Nurse Education in Practice, 49.* https://doi.org/10.1016/j.nepr.2020.102904

Power, T., Wilson, D., Geia, L., West, R., Brockie, T., Clark, T. C., Bearskin, L. B., Lowe, J., Millender, E., Smallwood, R., & Best, O. (2022). Cultural safety and Indigenous authority in nursing and midwifery education and practice. *Contemporary Nurse, 57*(5), 1–6. https://doi.org/10.1080/10376178.2022.2039076

Priest, N. C., Paradies, Y. C., Gunthorpe, W., Cairney, S. J., & Sayers, S. M. (2011). Racism as a determinant of social and emotional wellbeing for Aboriginal Australian youth. *Med Journal of Australia, 194*(10), 546–50. https://doi.org/10.5694/j.1326-5377.2011.tb03099.x

Project Implicit. (2011). *Harvard project's implicit association test.* Retrieved from https://implicit.harvard.edu/implicit/user/demo.australia/au.static/takeatest.htm

Riley, L. (2014). *Aboriginal kinship presentation: Skin names* [Video]. The University of Sydney. Retrieved from https://www.youtube.com/watch?v=ynQEtTfQjQc

Rowley, C. D. (1970). *The destruction of Aboriginal society.* Harmondsworth, United Kingdom: Penguin Books.

Royal Australasian College of Physicians (RACP). (2005). *Inequity and health: A call to action: Addressing health and socioeconomic inequality in Australia.* Retrieved from https://www.racp.edu.au/docs/default-source/advocacy-library/inequity-and-health-policy.pdf

Ryan, L., Debenham, J., Brown, M., & Pascoe, W. (2017). *Colonial frontier massacres in Australia, 1788–1930.* Newcastle, Australia: University of Newcastle. Retrieved from https://c21ch.newcastle.edu.au/colonialmassacres/

Ryan, A., Gibson, C., & Gilroy, J. (2020). #Changethedate: Advocacy as an on-line and decolonising occupation. *Journal of Occupational Science, 27*(3), 405–16. https://doi.org/10.1080/14427591.2020.1759448

Scotney, A., Guthrie, J. A., Lokuge, K., & Kelly, P. M. (2010). 'Just ask!' Identifying as Indigenous in mainstream general practice settings: A consumer perspective. *The Medical Journal of Australia, 192*(10), 609. https://doi.org/10.5694/j.1326-5377.2010.tb03651.x

Stewart, S. (2018). White privilege: What's 'the code' got to do with it? *Australian Midwifery News, 18*(2), 53. https://doi/10.3316/INFORMIT.791987200899592

Stoneham, M. J., Goodman, J., & Daube, M. (2014). The portrayal of Indigenous health in selected Australian media. *The International Indigenous Policy Journal, 5*(1), 1–13.

Te Kaunihera Tapuhi o Aotearoa: Nursing Council of New Zealand (NCNZ). (2011). *Guidelines for cultural safety, the Treaty of Waitangi and Māori health in nursing education and practice.* Retrieved from https://www.nursingcouncil.org.nz/Public/Nursing/Standards_and_guidelines/NCNZ/nursing-section/Standards_and_guidelines_for_nurses.aspx

Ungunmerr, M. R. (1988). *Dadirri: Inner deep listening and quiet still awareness – A reflection by Miriam-Rose Ungunmerr.* Nauiyu (Daly River), Australia: Miriam Rose Foundation. Retrieved from www.miriamrosefoundation.org.au/dadirri/

United Nations General Assembly (UNGA). (2007). *United Nations declaration on the rights of Indigenous peoples.* Retrieved from https://www.un.org/development/desa/indigenouspeoples/wp-content/uploads/sites/19/2018/11/UNDRIP_E_web.pdf

Walker, R., & Shepherd, C. (2008). *Strengthening Aboriginal family functioning: What works and why?* Retrieved from https://aifs.gov.au/resources/policy-and-practice-papers/strengthening-aboriginal-family-functioning-what-works-and-why#:~:text=Aboriginal%20families%20are%20pivotal%20to,belonging%20will%20strengthen%20the%20family

West, R., Saunders, V., West, L., Blackman, R., Del Fabbro, L., Neville, G., Minniss, F. R., Armao, J., van de Mortel, T., Kain, V. J., Corones-Watkins, K., Elder, E., Wardrop, R., Mansah, M., Hilton, C., Penny, J., Hall, K., Sheehy, K., & Rogers, G. D. (2022). Indigenous-led First Peoples health interprofessional and simulation-based learning innovations: Mixed methods study of nursing academics' experience of working in partnership. *Contemporary Nurse, 58*(1), 43–57. https://doi.org/10.1080/10376178.2022.2029518

Woolyungah Indigenous Centre (WIC). (2019). *You can't say that! Hints and tips.* Retrieved from https://documents.uow.edu.au/content/groups/public/@web/@eed/documents/doc/uow272408.pdf

UNIT 2

PHYSICAL EXAMINATION

CHAPTER 5

PHYSICAL EXAMINATION TECHNIQUES

LEARNING OUTCOMES

By the end of this chapter you should be able to:

1   describe how to maintain standard precautions and transmission-based precautions during the physical examination
2   establish an environment suitable for conducting a physical examination
3   describe how to perform inspection, palpation, percussion and auscultation, and identify which areas of the body are assessed with each technique
4   demonstrate inspection, palpation, percussion and auscultation in the clinical setting.

BACKGROUND

Inspection, palpation, percussion and auscultation are the techniques used by the nurse to assess the consumer during a physical examination. This chapter introduces the assessment techniques and equipment used to conduct physical examinations. Before commencing your physical examination, always remember the significance of utilising infection control practices during every encounter involving the consumer. It is important to be aware of the Australian Commission on Safety and Quality in Health Care national priorities that promote, support and encourage the implementation of safety and quality in healthcare provision (ACSQHC, 2019) and the second edition of the National Safety and Quality Health Service Standards (ACSQHC, 2017). Further, in New Zealand, the Health Quality & Safety Commission (2022) works with clinicians, providers and consumers to ensure quality and improvement in health care.

The severe acute respiratory syndrome coronavirus (SARS-CoV-2) that causes coronavirus disease (COVID-19) and the subsequent worldwide pandemic have created significant challenges and changes to many healthcare practices. To date, there have been over 515 million cumulative cases of COVID-19, and over six million cumulative deaths worldwide (World Health Organization (WHO), 2022a). Practice changes to physical examination of persons requiring health care have been considerable. Practice changes include increased use of standard and transmission-based precautions, telehealth, and the use of artificial intelligence to diagnose respiratory sounds. The use of standard precautions and transmission-based precautions will be explored in this chapter and should be applied in the context of the physical examination.

CONSIDERATIONS PRIOR TO COMMENCING PHYSICAL EXAMINATION

Physical examination of a consumer serves many purposes:

1. screening of general wellbeing; the findings will serve as baseline information for future examinations
2. validation of the reason/s that brought the consumer to seek health care
3. monitoring of current health problems
4. identification of health problems/medical diagnoses and treatments.

The need for physical examination depends on factors such as the consumer's health status, contact with healthcare providers, and accessibility to health care. For example, a person with diabetes mellitus, arthritis and glaucoma is likely to access health care more often than a healthy teenager or adult.

Standard precautions

The transmission of hepatitis, human immunodeficiency virus (HIV), severe acute respiratory syndromes (SARS), and other infectious diseases is a primary concern for the nurse and for the consumer. **Standard precautions**, formerly known as 'universal precautions', were developed by the Centers for Disease Control and Prevention (CDC) to protect healthcare professionals and consumers. Australia and New Zealand have developed national guidelines underpinned by the principles of the CDC and WHO guidelines for standard and transmission-based precautions (National Health and Medical Research Council (NHMRC), 2019; Ministry of Health, 2022a). The primary goal of standard precautions is to prevent the exchange of blood and body fluids (**Figure 5.1**). Standard precautions should be practised with every consumer throughout the entire encounter, whether or not the consumer has a known or suspected infectious process.

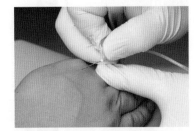

FIGURE 5.1 The nurse is using standard precautions to draw blood.

Standard precautions are the minimum infection control practices that are practised in all healthcare settings (**Figure 5.2**). In Australia the current infection control guidelines are published on a living guideline by the National Health and Medical Research Council (NHMRC, 2019); in New Zealand, the recommendations for standard precautions (Health Quality & Safety Commission, 2022) include:

> hand hygiene
> personal protective equipment (PPE)
> handling and disposing of sharps
> routine management of the physical environment
> reprocessing of reusable instruments and equipment
> respiratory hygiene and cough etiquette.

Hand hygiene

The single most important infection control practice is effective hand hygiene. Hand hygiene includes hand washing with soap and water and alcohol-based hand rub (ABHR). Hand hygiene should be performed according to the five moments of hand hygiene (WHO, 2009). Hand washing with soap and water should occur when hands are visibly dirty, soiled with blood or body fluids or after using the toilet (NHMRC, 2019). In addition, hand washing with soap and water is preferred following exposure to specific microorganisms (e.g. *Clostridium difficile*, norovirus) (NHMRC, 2019). Hand hygiene using ABHR can be used at all other times (WHO, 2009, p. 155).

You must consider the five moments of hand hygiene during every physical examination (see **Figure 5.3**). Some nurses perform hand hygiene in the examination area with the consumer present. It is a nonthreatening way to start the physical assessment, and allows the patient time to ask questions concerning the process. For further information refer to the NHMRC's *Australian guidelines for the prevention and control of infection in healthcare*, 2019, v.11.10 (2021), Living guideline (NHMRC, 2019).

VISITOR RESTRICTIONS MAY BE IN PLACE

STOP

For all staff

Combined contact & droplet precautions*

in addition to standard precautions

Before entering room/care zone

1. Perform hand hygiene
2. Put on gown
3. Put on surgical mask
4. Put on protective eyewear
5. Wear gloves, in accordance with standard precautions

At doorway prior to leaving room/care zone

1. Remove and dispose of gloves if worn
2. Perform hand hygiene
3. Remove and dispose of gown
4. Perform hand hygiene
5. Remove protective eyewear
6. Perform hand hygiene
7. Remove and dispose of mask
8. Leave the room/care zone
9. Perform hand hygiene

What else can you do to stop the spread of infections?
- Always change gloves and perform hand hygiene between different care activities and when gloves become soiled to prevent cross contamination of body sites
- Consider patient placement
- Minimise patient movement

*e.g. Acute respiratory tract infection with unknown aetiology, seasonal seasonal influenza and respiratory syncytial virus (RSV)

For more detail, refer to the Australian Guidelines for the Prevention and Control of Infection in Healthcare and your state and territory guidance.

AUSTRALIAN COMMISSION
ON **SAFETY** AND **QUALITY** IN **HEALTH CARE**

PPE use images reproduced with permission of the NSW Clinical Excellence Commission.

SOURCE: REPRODUCED WITH PERMISSION FROM THE INFECTION PREVENTION AND CONTROL POSTER – COMBINED CONTACT AND DROPLET PRECAUTIONS, DEVELOPED BY THE AUSTRALIAN COMMISSION ON SAFETY AND QUALITY IN HEALTH CARE (ACSQHC). ACSQHC: SYDNEY (2023)

FIGURE 5.2 Standard precautions

VISITOR RESTRICTIONS MAY BE IN PLACE

STOP

For all staff

Combined airborne & contact precautions

in addition to standard precautions

Before entering room/care zone

1. Perform hand hygiene
2. Put on gown
3. Put on a particulate respirator (e.g. P2/N95) and perform fit check
4. Put on protective eyewear
5. Wear gloves in accordance with standard precautions

At doorway prior to leaving room/care zone

1. Remove and dispose of gloves if worn
2. Perform hand hygiene
3. Remove and dispose of gown
4. Leave the room/care zone
5. Perform hand hygiene (in an anteroom/outside the room/care zone)
6. Remove protective eyewear (in an anteroom/outside the room/care zone)
7. Perform hand hygiene (in an anteroom/outside the room/care zone)
8. Remove and dispose of particulate respirator (in an anteroom/outside the room/care zone)
9. Perform hand hygiene

What else can you do to stop the spread of infections?
- Always change gloves and perform hand hygiene between different care activities and when gloves become soiled to prevent cross contamination of body sites
- Consider patient placement
- Minimise patient movement

KEEP DOOR CLOSED AT ALL TIMES

AUSTRALIAN COMMISSION
ON **SAFETY** AND **QUALITY** IN **HEALTH CARE**

PPE use images reproduced with permission of the NSW Clinical Excellence Commission.

SOURCE: REPRODUCED WITH PERMISSION FROM THE INFECTION PREVENTION AND CONTROL POSTER – COMBINED AIRBORNE AND CONTACT PRECAUTIONS, DEVELOPED BY THE AUSTRALIAN COMMISSION ON SAFETY AND QUALITY IN HEALTH CARE (ACSQHC). ACSQHC: SYDNEY (2023)

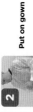

The NHMRC (2019) supports existing WHO (2022b) guidelines that recommend the use of an alcohol-based hand rub (see **Figure 5.4**), as it is more effective against most common infectious agents on hands than hand hygiene using plain or antiseptic soap and water.

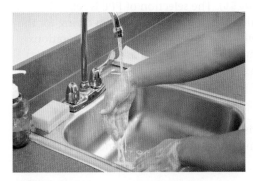

FIGURE 5.3 Hand washing using soap and water

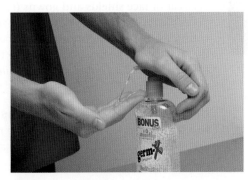

FIGURE 5.4 Hand washing using an alcohol-based hand rub

REFLECTION IN PRACTICE

Five critical moments of hand washing

Can you remember what the five critical moments of hand washing are? You might like to refresh your memory through the Hand Hygiene Australia website: https://www.hha.org.au/hand-hygiene/5-moments-for-hand-hygiene

Figure 5.5 depicts these critical moments. It is based on the 'Your 5 moments for Hand Hygiene', World Health Organization.

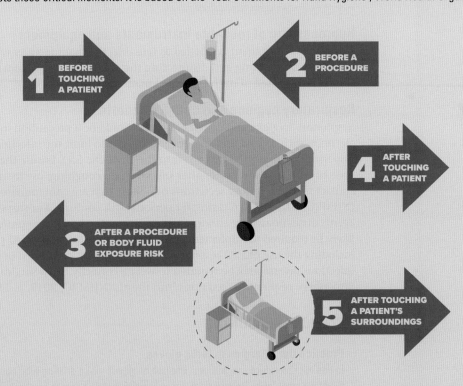

FIGURE 5.5 Five moments for hand hygiene

SOURCE: REPRODUCED WITH PERMISSION FROM 5 MOMENTS FOR HAND HYGIENE POSTER, DEVELOPED BY THE AUSTRALIAN COMMISSION ON SAFETY AND QUALITY IN HEALTH CARE (ACSQHC). ACSQHC: SYDNEY (2021)

In New Zealand, hand hygiene guidelines are also available, and these are based on the same WHO critical moments, and can be accessed via https://www.hqsc.govt.nz/resources/resource-library/hand-hygiene-nz-hand-hygiene-a-guide-for-healthcare-staff/

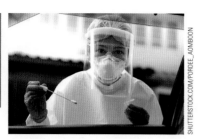

FIGURE 5.6 The nurse must select the appropriate personal protective equipment for every consumer encounter.

Personal protective equipment

Personal protective equipment or PPE refers to equipment that acts as a barrier to protect mucous membranes, airways, skin and clothing from contact with any infectious agent. PPE includes gloves, gowns, masks (surgical/P2 respirator), eyewear or face shields and gowns (**Figure 5.6**). The selection of PPE is related to the potential for exposure to body fluids and infectious processes when caring for the consumer. For further information about the following risks and considerations that relate to PPE you should refer to the NHMRC's *Australian Guidelines for the Prevention and Control of Infection in Healthcare*, 2019, v.11.10 (2021), Living guideline (NHMRC, 2019).

Handling and disposing of sharps

Healthcare workers are exposed to the risk of injury and blood-borne infectious agents such as hepatitis B and C virus and human immunodeficiency virus (HIV) (NHMRC, 2019).

Routine management of the physical environment

Evidence supports that healthcare settings contain infectious agents, although environmental surfaces can be safely decontaminated (NHMRC, 2019). Healthcare facilities should have a specific policy regarding measures for cleaning and disinfecting consumer care areas and the surrounding environment. It is good practice to routinely clean surfaces as follows:

> Clean frequently touched surfaces with detergent solution at least daily, when visibly soiled and after every known contamination.

> Clean general surfaces and fittings when visibly soiled and immediately after spillage.

NHMRC. (2019). AUSTRALIAN GUIDELINES FOR INFECTION PREVENTION, P. 57

Reprocessing of reusable instruments and equipment

If consumer equipment is labelled as reusable, the manufacturer will provide guidelines on cleaning and disinfecting the equipment. If an item is single use, it should be disposed of in the specified manner after it is used.

Respiratory hygiene and cough etiquette

Respiratory hygiene and cough etiquette should be a precaution upheld at all times, such as covering sneezes and coughs to limit the infectious person dispersing respiratory secretions into the air (Table 5.1). Ensure that hands are washed with soap and water after sneezing and coughing; use tissues and watch contact with respiratory secretions or objects that are contaminated by secretions (NHMRC, 2019). When caring for persons with confirmed or suspected infectious agents disseminated by airborne transmission, the healthcare professional may likely be required to implement standard and transmission-based precautions, including the use of a P2 respirator. The person with confirmed or suspected infectious disease may be required to wear a correctly fitted surgical mask to prevent dispersal of respiratory secretions into the air (NHMRC, 2019, p. 112).

CLINICAL **REASONING**

Practice tip: Allergies to latex gloves

In line with standard precautions, the use of gloves when dealing with consumers' bodily fluids is compulsory. Be aware of the possibility that healthcare workers or consumers can have a latex allergy. The reactions range from eczematous contact dermatitis to the extreme of anaphylactic shock. It is important therefore, prior to touching consumers when wearing latex gloves or using other latex products, to check that the consumer does not have any known allergies to latex.

TABLE 5 .1 Steps in respiratory hygiene and cough etiquette

	Anyone with signs and symptoms of a respiratory infection regardless of the cause should follow or be instructed to follow respiratory hygiene and cough etiquette as follows:
STEP 1	Cover the nose/mouth with disposable single-use tissues when coughing, sneezing, wiping and blowing noses.
STEP 2	Use tissues to contain respiratory secretions.
STEP 3	Dispose of tissues in the nearest waste receptacle or bin after use.
STEP 4	If no tissues are available, cough or sneeze into the inner elbow rather than the hand.
STEP 5	Practise hand hygiene after contact with respiratory secretions and contaminated objects/materials.
STEP 6	Keep contaminated hands away from the mucous membranes of the mouth, eyes and nose.
STEP 7	In healthcare facilities, patients with symptoms of respiratory infections should sit as far away from others as possible. If available, healthcare facilities may place these patients in a separate area while waiting for care.

SOURCE: NATIONAL HEALTH AND MEDICAL RESEARCH COUNCIL

Transmission-based precautions

The CDC has developed another level of precautions called **transmission-based precautions**. These precautions are to be used in conjunction with standard precautions. Airborne, droplet and contact transmissions of microorganisms that are known to exist in a consumer, or are suspected in a consumer, are targeted. Contact transmission pathogens, such as impetigo, scabies, *varicella zoster* virus and multidrug-resistant organisms (e.g. MRSA), can be spread directly from person to person. Contact precautions must also be implemented when the consumer has faecal incontinence, excessive wound drainage, or other body secretions, because of the risk of environmental contamination and subsequent transmission. Microorganisms can also be spread indirectly from a contaminated inanimate object to a person. Cohorting of consumers may occur when single rooms are unavailable to allow implementation of contact precautions. Consumer cohorting may be an appropriate infection control strategy during a pandemic (Patterson et al., 2020). Droplet transmission occurs when microorganisms (large-particle droplets >5 microns) are deposited on susceptible body parts via respiratory secretions (sneezing and coughing). Typically, the pathogens in the droplet remain infectious for only a short period of time. Suctioning a consumer can also transmit droplets. *Bacillus pertussis*, *Haemophilus influenzae*, rhinovirus, adenovirus, group A *Streptococcus*, and *Neisseria meningitidis* are examples of pathogens contracted through this mode of transmission. Airborne transmission spreads microorganisms (droplet nuclei or small particles) by air currents and inhalation. These pathogens are infectious over long distances when they are airborne. They can also be passed through ventilation systems. Measles (measles virus), Chickenpox (varicella virus) and tuberculosis (*Mycobacterium tuberculosis*) can spread in this mode. Transmission-based precautions are used in every encounter in every healthcare setting in addition to standard precautions, as some diseases can have more than one mode of transmission (e.g. SARS-CoV). Additional information can be found in the NHMRC (2019) *Australian Guidelines for the Prevention and Control of Infection in Healthcare*, Part 3: Standard and transmission-based precautions. Also, you can view information on the CDC website: http://www.cdc.gov/. Refer to your health institution, or the Australian Government Department of Health: www.health.gov.au within Australia. In New Zealand, refer to *Health and Disability Services (Infection Prevention and Control) Standards* (Standards New Zealand, 2022).

CLINICAL REASONING

Practice tip: PPE for healthcare workers in the context of COVID-19

Caring for consumers in the COVID-19 environment may create a sense of stress or anxiety. Consider the following recommendations, with a flexible approach guided by healthcare facility policy, context, healthcare environment and healthcare professional preferences.

> An assessment of risk of transmission of COVID-19 to healthcare professionals should consider the level of risk (i.e. likely high risk or low risk of SARS-CoV-2 transmission).

> Standard and transmission-based precautions should be following by all healthcare professionals when providing consumer care in the COVID-19 environment. In addition to standard and airborne (transmission) based precautions, the following is recommended when there is likely high-risk SARS-CoV2 transmission:

  • A P2/N95 respirator is preferred when providing care for consumers with confirmed or suspected COVID-19. When a P2/N95 respirator is required, fit testing should occur before the first use, and a seal check should occur prior to each use.

  • Eye protection as described in the guidelines for prevention and control of infection in health care should be worn when providing direct care for consumers with confirmed, suspected or asymptomatic COVID-19.

(ICEG, 2021, June; Ministry of Health, 2022; ACSQHC, 2021)

LEGAL CONSIDERATIONS

In today's litigious society, you must be vigilant when engaging in direct consumer care. Documentation issues have previously been addressed. Equally important is how you execute the health assessment and physical examination. Establishing a trusting and therapeutic relationship that is based on effective communication is a primary element in avoiding legal issues. While performing each step in the physical examination process, you need to inform the consumer of what to expect, where to expect it, and how it will feel. Protests by the consumer need to be addressed prior to continuing the examination. Otherwise, the consumer may claim insufficient informed consent, sexual abuse or physical harassment.

All examinations and procedures, including any injury that may have been caused during the physical examination, must be completely documented. The institutional policy regarding consumer injury in the workplace must be followed.

REFLECTION IN PRACTICE

Consent: Challenging situations

In the following situations think about the strategies you could implement to decrease your legal liability.

> You are preparing to perform a genital exam when the consumer says, 'I've changed my mind. I don't want to do this.' What is your best course of action?

> While performing a breast exam on a consumer, the consumer shrieks, 'What do you think you are doing?' How would you respond to this consumer?

> During deep palpation of the abdomen, your consumer responds, 'Ouch, you hurt me!' How would you respond?

> You are auscultating the lungs of a 42-year-old man. He tells you that he is thinking of suing his previous healthcare provider. The consumer tells you, 'The real problem these days is that no one bothers to listen to the consumer any more.' What would be an appropriate response?

PHYSICAL EXAMINATION TECHNIQUES

Physical examination findings, or objective data, are obtained through the use of four specific diagnostic assessment techniques: inspection, palpation, percussion and auscultation. Usually, these assessment techniques are performed in this order when body systems are assessed. An exception is in the assessment of the abdomen, when auscultation is performed after inspection. Percussion and palpation can alter bowel motility, so they are performed after auscultation. These four techniques validate information provided by a consumer through the health history, or they can verify a suspected physical diagnosis.

Usually, the easiest assessment skills to master are inspection and basic auscultation. Percussion and palpation may take more time and practice to master. With time and practice, the physical examination techniques become second nature, and you will develop your own rhythm and style. You may not perform all examination skills in the order in which they are presented in this text. This practice is acceptable as long as basic guidelines are observed.

Infection control and prevention strategies implemented in response to the COVID-19 pandemic have shifted policy and practice. To safely manage COVID-19 environments, a variety of changes are evident in persons requiring physical examination. Physical examination may require additional infection prevention strategies, time-efficient assessment techniques (Gelfman, 2021), or implementation of telehealth (Monaghesh & Hajizadeh, 2020).

EXAMINATION **IN BRIEF**

Physical assessment techniques

Inspection
> Vision
> Smell

Palpation
> Light palpation
> Deep palpation

Percussion
> Direct percussion
> Indirect percussion

> Recognising percussion sound
> Fist percussion

Auscultation
> Direct auscultation
> Indirect auscultation

Equipment

General approach to physical examination

1. Ensure you are appropriately dressed and act in a professional manner. Ensure your workplace identification is visible.
2. Remove all bracelets, necklaces and earrings that can interfere with the physical examination.
3. Be sure that your fingernails are short and your hands are warm for maximum consumer comfort.
4. Be sure your hair will not fall forwards and obstruct your vision or touch the consumer.
5. Arrange for a well-lit, warm and private room when possible.
6. Ensure all necessary equipment is ready for use and within reach.
7. Introduce yourself to the consumer: for example, 'My name is Sam Annbel. I am the nurse who is caring for you today. I need to assess how your lungs are today.'

8. Clarify with the consumer how he or she wishes to be addressed: Miss Jones, Clara, Dr Casey, Rev. Grimes, and so on.

9. Explain what you plan to do and how long it will take; allow the consumer to ask questions.

10. Instruct the consumer to undress; their underwear can be left on until the end of the examination. Provide a gown and drape for the consumer and explain how to use them.

11. Allow the consumer to undress privately; inform the consumer when you will return to start the examination.

12. Have the consumer void prior to the examination.

13. Wash your hands in front of the consumer to show your concern for cleanliness.

14. Observe standard precautions and transmission-based precautions, as indicated.

15. Ensure that the consumer is accessible from both sides of the examining bed or table.

16. If a bed is used, raise the height so that you do not have to bend over to perform the examination.

17. Position the consumer as dictated by the body system being assessed; **Figure 5.7** illustrates positioning and draping techniques.

18. Enlist the consumer's cooperation by explaining what you are about to do, where it will be done, and how it may feel.

19. Warm all instruments before using them (use your hands or warm water).

20. Examine the unaffected body part or side first if a consumer's complaint is unilateral.

21. Explain to the consumer why you may be spending a long time performing one particular skill: 'Listening to the heart requires concentration and time.'

22. If the consumer complains of fatigue, continue the examination later (if possible).

23. Avoid making crude or negative remarks; be cognisant of your facial expression when dealing with malodorous and dirty consumers, or with disturbing findings (infected wounds, disfigurement, etc.).

24. Conduct the examination in a systematic approach every time. (This decreases the likelihood of forgetting to perform a particular assessment.)

25. Thank the consumer when the physical examination is concluded; inform the consumer what will happen next.

26. Document examination findings in the appropriate section of the consumer health record.

CLINICAL **REASONING**

Practice tip: Key considerations for physical examination

> Stand on the right side of the consumer; establishing a dominant side for examination will decrease your movement around the consumer.
> Perform the examination in a head-to-toe approach.
> Always compare the right and left sides of the body for symmetry.
> Proceed from the least invasive to the most invasive procedures for each body system.
> Always perform the physical examination using a systematic approach. If it is performed the same way each time, you are less likely to forget some part of the examination.

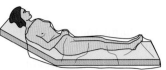

A. Semi-Fowler's 45° angle

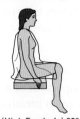

B. Sitting (High Fowler's) 90° angle

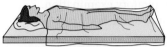

C. Horizontal recumbent (supine)

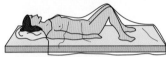

D. Dorsal recumbent

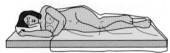

E. Side lying

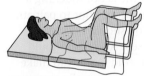

F. Lithotomy

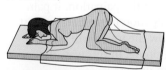

G. Knee-chest

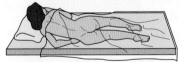

H. Sims'

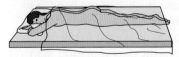

I. Prone

A. SKIN, head and neck; eyes, ears, nose, mouth and throat; thorax and lungs; heart and blood vessels; musculoskeletal; neurological; patients who cannot tolerate sitting up at a 90° angle

B. SKIN, head and neck; eyes, ears, nose, mouth and throat; back; posterior thorax and lungs; anterior thorax and lungs; breasts; axillae; heart and blood vessels; musculoskeletal; neurological

C. BREASTS; heart and blood vessels; abdomen; musculoskeletal

D. FEMALE genitalia; anterior thorax and lungs; breasts; axillae; heart and blood vessels; abdomen; musculoskeletal

E. SKIN; thorax and lungs; bedridden patients who cannot sit up

F. FEMALE genitalia and rectum

G. RECTUM and prostate (in men)

H. RECTUM and female genitalia

I. SKIN; posterior thorax and lungs; hips

FIGURE 5.7 Positioning and draping techniques and areas examined

Inspection

Inspection is usually the first examination technique used during the assessment process. It is an ongoing process that you use throughout the entire physical examination and consumer encounter. **Inspection** is the use of one's senses of vision and smell to consciously observe the consumer. Observing the consumer for even a brief period of time enables you to establish aspects that will help inform your overall consumer assessment, and can be done while you are undertaking other activities with the consumer.

Vision

Use of sight can reveal many facts about a consumer. Visual inspection of a consumer's respiratory status, for example, might reveal a rate of 38 breaths per minute and cyanotic nail beds. In this case, the consumer is tachypnoeic and possibly hypoxic, and would need a more thorough respiratory examination. The process of visual inspection necessitates full exposure of the body part being inspected, adequate overhead lighting and, when necessary, **tangential lighting** (light that is shone at an angle on the consumer to accentuate shadows and highlight subtle findings).

Smell

The nurse's olfactory sense provides vital information about a consumer's health status. The consumer may have a fruity breath odour characteristic of diabetic ketoacidosis. The classic odour emitted by a *Pseudomonas* infection is another well-recognised smell to the experienced nurse.

Palpation

The second examination technique is **palpation**. This is the act of touching a consumer in a therapeutic manner to elicit specific information. Prior to palpating a consumer, some basic principles need to be observed. You should have short fingernails to avoid hurting the consumer as well as yourself. Also, you should warm your hands prior to placing them on the consumer; cold hands can make a consumer's muscles tense, which can distort examination findings. Encourage the consumer to continue to breathe normally throughout the palpation. If pain is experienced during the palpation, discontinue the palpation immediately. Most significantly, inform the consumer where, when and how the touch will occur, especially when the consumer cannot see what you are doing. In this way, the consumer is aware of what to expect in the examination process.

Your hands are the tools used to perform the palpation process. Different sections of the hands are best used for examining certain areas of the body. The dorsum of the hand is most sensitive to temperature changes in the body. Thus, it is more accurate to place the dorsum of the hand on a consumer's forehead to assess the body temperature than it is to use the palmar surface of the hand. The palmar surface of the fingers at the metacarpophalangeal joints, the ball of the hand, and the ulnar surface of the hand best discriminate vibrations, such as a cardiac thrill and fremitus. The finger pads are the portion of the hand used most frequently in palpation. The finger pads are useful in assessing fine tactile discrimination, skin moisture and texture; the presence of masses, pulsations, oedema and crepitation; and the shape, size, position, mobility and consistency of organs (Figure 5.8).

Remember to observe standard precautions when you are performing palpation. Gloves must be worn when examining any open wounds, skin **lesions** or a body part with discharge, as well as internal body parts such as the mouth and rectum.

There are two distinct types of palpation: light and deep palpation. Each of these techniques is briefly described here and covered in greater detail in chapters describing body system examinations in which palpation is specifically used.

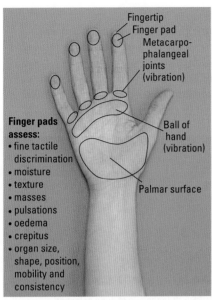

Fingertip
Finger pad
Metacarpo-
phalangeal
joints
(vibration)

**Finger pads
assess:**
• fine tactile
  discrimination
• moisture
• texture
• masses
• pulsations
• oedema
• crepitus
• organ size,
  shape, position,
  mobility and
  consistency

Ball of
hand
(vibration)

Palmar surface

A. Palmar surface

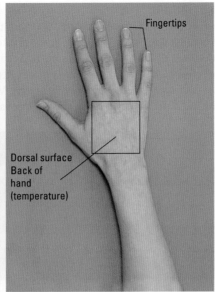

Fingertips

Dorsal surface
Back of
hand
(temperature)

B. Dorsal surface

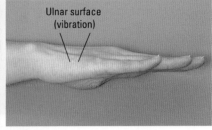

Ulnar surface
(vibration)

C. Ulnar surface

FIGURE 5.8 Parts of the hand used in palpation

CLINICAL REASONING

Practice tip: Sequence of physical examination

When sequencing examination procedures you should progress from the least intrusive to the most intrusive to minimise interference with data. Examinations that may cause discomfort should be performed last whenever possible, in order to prevent consumer anxiety, fear and muscle guarding. For example, palpation of a tender area in the abdomen should be performed last. In the paediatric consumer, the assessment of the ears and throat is usually performed last because these are the most uncomfortable for a child and may cause crying.

Light palpation

Light palpation is performed more frequently than deep palpation and is always done before deep palpation. As the name implies, **light palpation** is superficial, delicate and gentle. In light palpation, the finger pads are used to gain information from the consumer's skin surface to a depth of approximately 1 cm below the surface. Light palpation reveals information on skin texture and moisture; overt, large or superficial masses; and fluid, muscle guarding and superficial tenderness. Perform light palpation by the following steps:

1. Keep the fingers of your dominant hand together, place the finger pads lightly on the skin over the area that is to be palpated. The hand and forearm will be on a plane parallel to the area being assessed.
2. Depress the skin 1 cm in light, gentle, circular motions.
3. Keeping the finger pads on the skin, let the depressed body surface rebound to its natural position.
4. If the consumer is ticklish, lift the hand off the skin before moving it to another area.
5. Using a systematic approach, move the fingers to an adjacent area and repeat the process.
6. Continue to move the finger pads until the entire area being examined has been palpated.
7. If the consumer has complained of tenderness in any area, palpate this area last. **Figure 5.9** shows how light palpation is performed.

Deep palpation

Deep palpation can reveal information about the position of organs and masses, as well as their size, shape, mobility and consistency, and areas of discomfort. Deep palpation uses the hands to explore the body's internal structures to a depth of 4–5 cm or more (**Figure 5.10**). This technique is most often used for examination of the abdomen and the male and female reproductive organs. Variations in this technique are single-handed and bimanual palpation, and are discussed in Chapter 15.

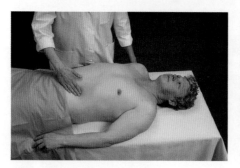

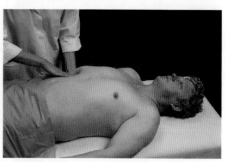

FIGURE 5.9 Technique of light palpation

FIGURE 5.10 Technique of deep palpation

Percussion

Percussion is the technique of striking one object against another to cause vibrations that produce sound. The density of underlying structures produces characteristic sounds. These sounds are diagnostic of normal and abnormal findings. The presence of air, fluid and solids can be confirmed, as can organ size, shape and position. Any part of the body can be percussed, but only limited information can be obtained in specific areas such as the heart. The thorax and abdomen are the most frequently percussed locations.

Percussion sound can be analysed according to its intensity, duration, pitch (frequency), quality and location. **Intensity** refers to the relative loudness or softness of the sound. It is also called the amplitude. **Duration** of percussed sound describes the time period over which a sound is heard when elicited. Frequency describes the concept of **pitch**. Frequency is caused by the sound's vibrations, or the highness or lowness of a sound. Frequency is measured in cycles per second (cps) or hertz (Hz). More rapidly occurring vibrations have a pitch that is higher than that of slower vibrations. The **quality** of a sound is its timbre, or how one perceives it musically. The **location** of a sound refers to the area where the sound is produced and heard.

The process of percussion can produce five distinct sounds in the body: **flatness**, **dullness**, **resonance**, **hyperresonance** and **tympany**. Specific parts of the body elicit distinct sounds when percussed. Therefore, when an unexpected sound is heard in a particular part of the body, the cause must be further investigated.

Table 5.2 illustrates each of the five percussion sounds in relation to its respective intensity, duration, pitch, quality, location and relative density. In addition, examples are provided of normal and abnormal locations of percussed sounds.

TABLE 5.2 Characteristics of percussion sounds

SOUND	INTENSITY	DURATION	PITCH	QUALITY	NORMAL LOCATION	ABNORMAL LOCATION	DENSITY
Flatness	Soft	Short	High	Flat	Muscle (thigh) or bone	Lungs (severe pneumonia)	Most dense
Dullness	Moderate	Moderate	High	Thud	Organs (liver)	Lungs (atelectasis)	
Resonance	Loud	Moderate–long	Low	Hollow	Normal lungs	No abnormal location	
Hyperresonance	Very loud	Long	Very low	Boom	No normal location in adults; normal lungs in children	Lungs (emphysema)	
Tympany	Loud	Long	High	Drum	Gastric air bubble	Lungs (large pneumothorax)	Least dense

Sound waves are better conducted through a solid medium than through an air-filled medium because of the increased concentration of molecules. The basic premises underlying the sounds that are percussed are listed.

1. The more solid a structure, the higher the pitch, the softer the intensity, and the shorter the duration of the sound.
2. The more air-filled a structure, the lower the pitch, the louder the intensity, and the longer the duration of the sound.

There are four types of percussion techniques: direct (immediate), indirect (mediate), **direct fist percussion**, and **indirect fist percussion**. It is important to keep in mind that the sounds produced from percussion are generated from body tissue up to 5 cm below the surface of the skin. If the abdomen is to be percussed, the consumer should have the opportunity to void before the examination.

Direct percussion

Direct percussion or **immediate percussion** is the striking of an area of the body directly. To perform direct percussion:

1. Spread the index or middle finger of the dominant hand slightly apart from the rest of the fingers.
2. Make a light tapping motion with the finger pad of the index finger against the body part being percussed.
3. Note the sound that is produced.

Percussion of the sinuses (**Figure 5.11**) illustrates the use of direct percussion in the physical examination.

Indirect percussion

Indirect percussion is also referred to as **mediate percussion**. This is a skill that takes time and practice to develop and use effectively. Most sounds are produced using indirect percussion. Follow these steps to perform indirect percussion (**Figure 5.12**).

1. Place the nondominant hand lightly on the surface to be percussed.
2. Extend the middle finger of this hand, known as the **pleximeter**, and press its distal phalanx and distal interphalangeal joint firmly on the location where percussion is to begin. The pleximeter will remain stationary while percussion is performed in this location.
3. Spread the other fingers of the nondominant hand apart and raise them slightly off the surface. This prevents interference, and thus dampening, of vibrations during the actual percussion.

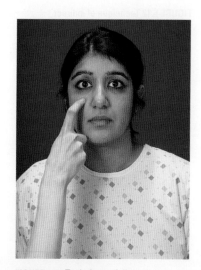

FIGURE 5.11 Technique of direct percussion

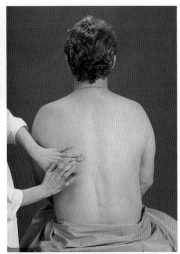

A. Position of hands for posterior thorax percussion

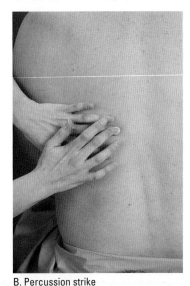

B. Percussion strike

FIGURE 5.12 Technique of indirect percussion

4. Flex the middle finger of the dominant hand, called the **plexor**. The fingernail of the plexor finger should be very short to prevent undue discomfort and injury to the pleximeter. The other fingers on this hand should be fanned.
5. Flex the wrist of the dominant hand and place the hand directly over the pleximeter finger of the nondominant hand.
6. With a sharp, crisp, rapid movement from the wrist of the dominant hand, strike the pleximeter with the plexor. At this point, the plexor should be perpendicular to the pleximeter. The blow to the pleximeter should be between the distal interphalangeal joint and the fingernail. Use the finger pad rather than the fingertip of the plexor to deliver the blow. Concentrate on the movement to create the striking action from the dominant wrist only.
7. As soon as the plexor strikes the pleximeter, withdraw the plexor to avoid dampening the resulting vibrations. Do not move the pleximeter finger.
8. Note the sound produced from the percussion.
9. Repeat the percussion process one or two times in this location to confirm the sound.
10. Move the pleximeter to a second location, preferably the contralateral location from where the previous percussion was performed. Repeat the percussion process in this manner until the entire body surface area being assessed has been percussed.

Recognising percussion sound

When using direct and indirect percussion, the change from resonance to dullness is more easily recognised by the human ear than is the change from dullness to resonance. It is often helpful to close your eyes and concentrate on the sound in order to distinguish whether a change in sounds occurs. This concept has implications for patterns of percussion in areas of the body where known locations have distinct percussible sounds. For example, the techniques of **diaphragmatic excursion** and liver border percussion (advanced practitioner) can proceed in a more defined pattern because percussion can be performed from an area of resonance to an area of dullness. Another helpful hint is to validate the change in sounds by percussing back and forth between the two areas where a change is noted to confirm this change.

As stated earlier, the percussion technique can take considerable time to develop and master. Practising the technique at home or in a teaching environment can be a helpful learning experience; see Clinical reasoning practice tip: Percussion practice.

CLINICAL **REASONING**

Practice tip: Percussion practice
> Percuss two glasses – one filled with water, the other empty. Compare the sounds.
> Percuss the wall of a room and listen for the change in tones when a wall stud is reached.
> Percuss your thigh. Puff your cheeks and percuss them. Compare the sounds.

Fist percussion

Direct and indirect fist percussion are advanced practitioner assessment skills. Note that caution must be exercised when direct or indirect fist percussion is used. Avoid hitting the consumer too hard because this may injure him or her.

Auscultation

Auscultation is the act of active listening to body organs to gather information on a consumer's clinical status. Auscultation includes listening to sounds that are voluntarily and involuntarily produced by the body. The deep inspiration a consumer takes with the lung assessment illustrates a voluntary sound, and heart sounds illustrate involuntary sounds. A quiet environment is necessary for auscultation. Auscultated sounds should be analysed in relation to their relative intensity, pitch, duration, quality and location. There are two types of auscultation: direct and indirect.

Direct auscultation

Direct or **immediate auscultation** is the process of listening with the unaided ear. This can include listening to the consumer from some distance away or placing the ear directly on the consumer's skin surface. An example of direct auscultation is listening to the wheezing that is audible to the unassisted ear in a person having a severe asthmatic attack.

Indirect auscultation

Indirect or **mediate auscultation** describes the process of listening with some amplification or mechanical device. The nurse most often performs indirect auscultation with an acoustic stethoscope, which does not amplify the body sounds, but instead blocks out environmental sounds. Amplification of body sounds can be achieved with the use of a **Doppler** ultrasonic stethoscope. Throughout this text, the use of an acoustic stethoscope is recommended.

Figure 5.13 illustrates the acoustic stethoscope. The earpieces come in various sizes. Choose an earpiece that fits snugly in the ear canal without causing pain. The earpieces block noises from the environment. The earpieces and binaurals should be angled toward the nose. This angle permits the natural direction of the ear canal to be accessed. In this manner, sounds will be directed towards the adult tympanic membrane. The rubber or plastic tubing should be between 30.5 and 40 cm long. Stethoscopes with longer tubing will diminish the body sounds that are auscultated.

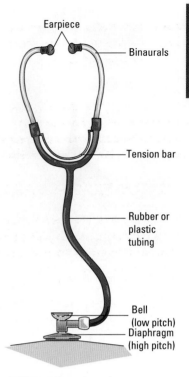

FIGURE 5.13 Acoustic stethoscope

CLINICAL **REASONING**

Practice tip: Headpiece mnemonic
The word 'bellow' can be used to remember the frequency that is transmitted by the headpiece of the stethoscope. The 'bell' transmits 'low' sounds.

The acoustic stethoscope has two listening heads: the bell and the diaphragm. The diaphragm is flat, and the bell is a concave cup. The diaphragm transmits high-pitched sounds, and the bell transmits low-pitched sounds. Breath sounds and normal heart sounds are examples of high-pitched sounds. Bruits and some heart murmurs are examples of low-pitched sounds. Another commonly used stethoscope has a single-sided, dual-frequency listening head. This stethoscope has a single chest piece. The nurse applies different pressures on the chest piece to auscultate high- and low-pitched sounds. In addition, some practitioners are using digital stethoscopes to enhance sound clarity (Figure 5.14). These stethoscopes can amplify natural sounds up to 30 times; they can also function as a traditional acoustic stethoscope with the bell and the diaphragm. The volume can be adjusted on the digital stethoscope, and a mute feature to block the sound of crying children is available.

Another type of stethoscope is the stereophonic stethoscope (Figure 5.15). This type of stethoscope is a two-channel device that augments right- and left-sided auscultatory sounds. Its bell and diaphragm are divided at the diameter of each headpiece.

Prior to auscultating, remove jewellery such as necklaces and bracelets that could move during the examination and cause false noises. Warm the headpieces of the stethoscope in your hands prior to use, because shivering and movement can obscure examination findings. To use the diaphragm, place it firmly against the skin surface to be auscultated. If the consumer has a large quantity of hair in this area, it may be necessary to wet the hair to prevent it from interfering with the sound that

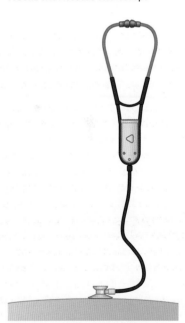

FIGURE 5.14 Digital stethoscope

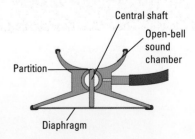

FIGURE 5.15 Stereophonic stethoscope

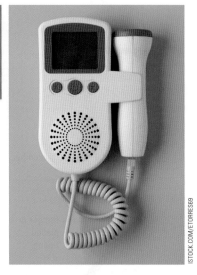

ISTOCK.COM/ETORRES69

FIGURE 5.16 Doppler ultrasonic stethoscope.

is being auscultated. Otherwise, a grating sound may be heard. To use the bell, place it lightly on the skin surface that is to be auscultated. The bell will stretch the skin and act like a diaphragm and transmit high-pitched sounds if it is pressed too firmly on the skin. In both instances, auscultation requires a great deal of concentration. It may be helpful to close your eyes during the auscultation process to help you isolate the sound. Sometimes you can hear more than one sound in a given location. Try to listen to each sound and concentrate on each separately. It is important to clean your stethoscope after each consumer to prevent the transfer of pathogens. Remember, auscultation is a skill that requires practice and patience.

Amplification of body sounds can also be achieved with the use of a Doppler ultrasonic stethoscope (**Figure 5.16**). An electronic stethoscope amplifies body sounds as it filters extraneous sounds. Both high and low frequencies can be auscultated with one headpiece. With the Doppler ultrasonic stethoscope, water-soluble gel is placed on the body part being assessed, and the stethoscope is placed directly on the consumer. The device amplifies the sounds in that region. Fetal heart tones and unpalpable peripheral pulses are frequently assessed via a Doppler ultrasonic stethoscope.

Artificial intelligence (AI) is being used to interpret cough sounds and other audio signals during consumer assessment (Son & Lee, 2022). The COVID-19 pandemic has accelerated investigations using AI diagnostic technology and smartphone-based breathing recordings (Alkhodari & Khandoker, 2022).

Equipment

The physical examination will proceed in an efficient manner if you have gathered all of the necessary equipment beforehand. Ensure your equipment is arranged in order of use and within easy reach. The equipment needed to perform a complete physical examination of the adult consumer includes:

> pen and paper
> marking pen
> tape measure
> ruler
> clean gloves
> penlight or torch
> scales
> thermometer
> sphygmomanometer
> a lamp/good lighting
> tongue depressor
> stethoscope
> otoscope
> nasal speculum
> ophthalmoscope (advanced practice)
> transilluminator
> visual acuity charts
> visual occluder
> tuning fork
> reflex hammer
> sterile needle
> cotton balls
> odours for cranial nerve assessment (coffee, lemon, flowers, etc.)
> small objects for neurological assessment (paper clip, key, cotton ball, pen, etc.)
> water-soluble lubricant
> various sizes of vaginal speculums (advanced practice)
> cervical brush (advanced practice)
> cotton-tip applicator
> cervical spatula (advanced practice)
> slide and fixative

> guaiac material (for testing for faecal material)
> specimen container
> **goniometer**.

The use of these items is discussed in the chapters describing the assessments for which they are used. **Figure 5.17** illustrates some of the equipment used in the physical assessment.

1.	Tuning fork	**15.**	Goniometer
2.	Visual occluder	**16.**	Clean gloves
3.	Ruler	**17.**	Cervical spatula (Ayre spatula)
4.	Visual acuity chart	**18.**	Cervical brush (cytobrush)
5.	Reflex hammer (brush at bottom)	**19.**	Cotton-tip applicator
6.	Reflex hammer	**20.**	Tongue depressor
7.	Pen and marking pen	**21.**	Guaiac material
8.	Penlight (torch)	**22.**	Tape measure
9.	Thermometer	**23.**	Stethoscope
10.	Sphygmomanometer	**24.**	Ophthalmoscope
11.	Slide and fixative	**25.**	Otoscope with speculum
12.	Specimen container	**26.**	Objects for neurological examination (key and cotton ball)
13.	Vaginal speculum		
14.	Lubricant	**27.**	Sterile needle

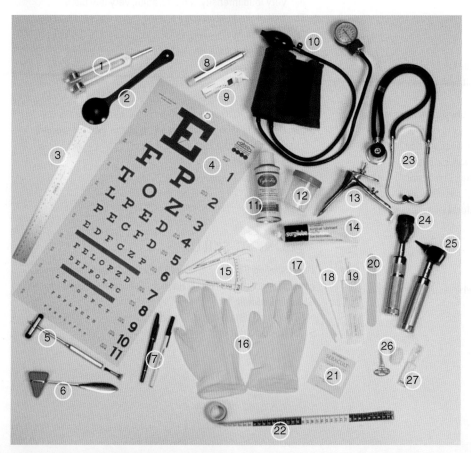

FIGURE 5.17 Equipment used in physical examination

CHAPTER RESOURCES

REVIEW QUESTIONS

For answers to these questions, see Answer section at the end of the book.

1. Which of the following statements accurately reflect standard precautions? Select all that apply.
   a. Recommendations to decrease pathogen transmission in all healthcare settings
   b. Guidelines to maximise precautions to prevent pathogen transmission
   c. Use of a mask when a pregnant woman is given an epidural anaesthetic
   d. The use of alcohol-based hand rub as the primary means of cleaning hands
   e. The disposal of single-use equipment when it is finished being used
   f. The use of EPA-approved disinfectants for use in healthcare settings

2. The nurse palpates the consumer's abdomen, assessing skin texture, moisture and muscle guarding. Which assessment skill is most likely being used?
   a. Light palpation
   b. Direct percussion
   c. Deep palpation
   d. Indirect percussion

Questions 3 and 4 refer to the following situation:
A 53-year-old male is admitted to your unit with a suspected bowel obstruction.

3. In what order would you conduct the physical assessment of the abdomen?
   a. Percussion, inspection, palpation, auscultation
   b. Inspection, auscultation, percussion, palpation
   c. Auscultation, palpation, percussion, inspection
   d. Palpation, percussion, inspection, auscultation

4. What position best facilitates the abdominal assessment?
   a. Sims'
   b. Knee to chest
   c. Horizontal recumbent
   d. High Fowler's

5. The finger pads are used to assess what aspects of a physical examination? Select all that apply.
   a. Oedema
   b. Moisture
   c. Organ size
   d. Temperature
   e. Texture
   f. Vibration

6. Which percussion sound is soft in intensity, short in duration, high in pitch, and has a flat quality?
   a. Flatness
   b. Dullness
   c. Resonance
   d. Tympany

7. Which percussion technique is usually used to assess costovertebral tenderness of a kidney?
   a. Direct percussion
   b. Indirect percussion
   c. Direct fist percussion
   d. Indirect fist percussion

8. Which characteristics best describe hyperresonance?
   a. Soft intensity, short duration, high pitch
   b. Moderate intensity, moderate duration, high pitch
   c. Loud intensity, long duration, high pitch
   d. Very loud intensity, long duration, very low pitch

9. The bell of the stethoscope is used to assess which of the following sounds?
   a. Breath sounds
   b. Bowel sounds
   c. Low sounds
   d. Apical heart rate

10. Which of the following positions is the best to assess the female genitalia and conduct a Pap smear when a woman cannot tolerate the lithotomy position?
    a. Semi-Fowler's
    b. Horizontal recumbent
    c. Sims'
    d. Prone

CS CLINICAL **SKILLS**

The following Clinical Skills are relevant to this chapter and can be found in Tollefson & Hillman, *Clinical Psychomotor Skills,* 8th edition:
> 25 Clinical handover
> 26 Documentation.

FURTHER RESOURCES

> Association for Professionals in Infection Control and Epidemiology (APIC): http://www.apic.org/
> Australasian Society of Clinical Immunology and Allergy: http://www.allergy.org.au
> Australian Commission on Safety and Quality in Health Care: http://www.safetyandquality.gov.au/
> Australian Council on Healthcare Standards: http://www.achs.org.au
> Australian Government Department of Health: http://www.health.gov.au/
> Better Health Channel: http://www.betterhealth.vic.gov.au/
> BloodSafe ELEARNING Australia: https://bloodsafelearning.org.au/course/clinical-transfusion-practice/

> Centers for Disease Control and Prevention: http://www.cdc.gov
> Health Quality & Safety Commission New Zealand: https://www.hqsc.govt.nz/
> Healthdirect Australia: http://www.healthdirect.gov.au/
> Ministry of Health-infection control and prevention: https://www.health.govt.nz/our-work/infection-prevention-and-control#:~:text=Make%20hand%20hygiene%20information%2C%20hand,single%20room%20(if%20available).
> My Stethoscope: The Stethoscope Experts: http://www.mystethoscope.com
> New Zealand Legislation: http://legislation.govt.nz
> New Zealand Ministry of Health: http://www.health.govt.nz/
> Standards New Zealand: https://www.standards.govt.nz/

REFERENCES

Alkhodari, M., & Khandoker, A. H. (2022). Detection of COVID-19 in smartphone-based breathing recordings: A pre-screening deep learning tool. *PloS One, 17*(1), e0262448–e0262448. https://doi.org/10.1371/journal.pone.0262448

Australian Commission on Safety and Quality in Health Care (ACSQHC). (2017). National Safety and Quality Health Service Standards (2nd ed.). Retrieved 18 May 2022 from https://www.safetyandquality.gov.au/sites/default/files/migrated/National-Safety-and-Quality-Health-Service-Standards-second-edition.pdf

Australian Commission on Safety and Quality in Health Care (ACSQHC). (2019). The state of patient safety and quality in Australian hospitals 2019. Retrieved 18 May 2022 https://www.safetyandquality.gov.au/publications-and-resources/state-patient-safety-and-quality-australian-hospitals-2019

Australian Commission on Safety and Quality in Health Care (ACSQHC). (2021). COVID-19: Infection prevention and control risk management. Retrieved 17 May 2022 https://www.safetyandquality.gov.au/publications-and-resources/resource-library/covid-19-infection-prevention-and-control-risk-management-guidance

Gelfman, D. M. (2021). Will the traditional physical examination be another casualty of COVID-19? *The American Journal of Medicine, 134*(3), 299–300. https://doi.org/10.1016/j.amjmed.2020.10.026

Health Quality & Safety Commission New Zealand. (2022). Infection prevention and control. Retrieved 18 May 2022 from https://www.hqsc.govt.nz/our-work/infection-prevention-and-control/ipc-practices/precautions-standard-and-transmission-based

Infection Control Expert Group (ICEG). (2021, June). Guidance on the use of personal protective equipment (PPE) for health care workers in the context of COVID-19. Australian Government. https://www.health.gov.au/committees-and-groups/infection-control-expert-group-iceg

Ministry of Health Manatu Hauora. (2022). Infection prevention and control. New Zealand Government. Retrieved 18 May 2022 https://www.health.govt.nz/our-work/infection-prevention-and-control

Monaghesh, E., & Hajizadeh, A. (2020). The role of telehealth during COVID-19 outbreak: A systematic review based on current evidence. *BMC Public Health, 20*(1), 1193. https://doi.org/10.1186/s12889-020-09301-4

National Health and Medical Research Council (NHMRC). (2019). Australian Guidelines for the Prevention and Control of Infection in Healthcare, (2019), v11.10 31/8/21. Canberra: Commonwealth of Australia. Retrieved 17 May 2022 from https://www.nhmrc.gov.au/about-us/publications/australian-guidelines-prevention-and-control-infection-healthcare-2019

Patterson, B., Marks, M., Martinez-Garcia, G., Bidwell, G., Luintel, A., Ludwig, D., Parks, T., Gothard, P., Thomas, R., Logan, S., Shaw, K., Stone, N., & Brown, M. (2020). A novel cohorting and isolation strategy for suspected COVID-19 cases during a pandemic. *The Journal of Hospital Infection, 105*(4), 632–7. https://doi.org/10.1016/j.jhin.2020.05.035

Son, M.-J., & Lee, S.-P. (2022). COVID-19 diagnosis from crowdsourced cough sound data. *Applied Sciences, 12*(4), 1795. https://doi.org/10.3390/app12041795

Standards New Zealand (2021). Health and disability services standard. https://www.standards.govt.nz/shop/nzs-81342021/

World Health Organization (WHO). (2009). WHO guidelines on hand hygiene in health care. Retrieved 19 May 2022 from: https://www.who.int/publications/i/item/9789241597906

World Health Organization (WHO). (2022a). WHO Coronavirus (COVID-19) dashboard. https://covid19.who.int Retrieved 24 May 2022.

World Health Organization (WHO). (2022b). World hand hygiene day. Retrieved 24 May 2022 https://www.who.int/campaigns/world-hand-hygiene-day

EXAMINATION REQUIREMENTS FOR EVERY CONSUMER

LEARNING OUTCOMES

By the end of this chapter you should be able to:
1 describe the general approach to assessment for all consumers
2 identify factors impacting on assessment for all consumers.

BACKGROUND

A complete physical examination is initiated by performing a general observation of the consumer. This includes a general survey of the physical and psychological status as well as obtaining the consumer's **vital signs** and **pain assessment**. The general survey commences at the time of the initial consumer encounter and provides data about their general health status. Focused observational skills are required to prepare for the physical examination, which centres on the characteristics of illness, demeanour and facial affect or expression, hygiene and grooming, and posture and gait. Vital signs include the consumer's respirations, pulse, temperature, blood pressure (BP) and oxygen saturations. Pain assessment includes the use of an appropriate framework, such as OPQRST and pain intensity scale. These measurements provide information about the consumer's baseline physiological status. In some instances, for example in the emergency department, neurological status should also be assessed by using the AVPU assessment scale (alert, voice, pain, unresponsive), Glasgow Coma Scale (GCS) (Akgun et al., 2018) and/or the Mini Mental Examination (MME). It is important to recognise the normal health-related parameters for the consumer you are assessing, as the nurse must observe for any deviations as potential signs of deterioration. This is because nurses are required to assess and respond to a consumer's acutely deteriorating physiological or mental status in an appropriate and timely way (ACSQHC, 2022).

Refer to Chapter 1 for guidance on a systematic approach for examination requirements.

URGENT FINDING

Recognition of physiological deterioration
Nurses must be alert for any red flags that can identify a consumer's physiological deterioration and understand their responsibility in being vigilant, take into consideration the following:

\>>

Vital signs
> Frequency of assessment should suit clinical acuity.
> Regular monitoring as part of a systematic physical assessment includes:
  - respiratory rate
  - oxygen saturation
  - heart rate
  - blood pressure
  - temperature
  - level of consciousness and pain assessment.
> Monitor and document observations in a chart that provides visual graphical information, displaying trends that can be tracked over time.
> The response or action required when deviations from normal are detected and timely interventions for the safety of the consumer maintained.

Other physiological observations and assessment
> Depending on the clinical situation, to support timely recognition of deterioration, other assessment data and observations should also be monitored and taken into consideration. These include fluid balance, occurrence of seizures, chest pain, respiratory distress, pallor, capillary refill, pupil size and reactivity, sweating, nausea and vomiting, as well as additional biochemical and haematological analyses.

Note: It is each healthcare professional's responsibility to be aware of the protocol in their facility regarding escalation of care, as an essential requirement for responding appropriately to clinical deterioration. Protocols are safety nets that set out an organisation's process required to respond to deterioration (including response to abnormal vital signs and deviations from normal physiological observations and assessments).

For more information on standards and protocols related to the deteriorating consumer visit ACSQHC – National Consensus Statement: Essential elements for recognising and responding to acute physiological deterioration (3rd edn.), https://www.safetyandquality.gov. au/publications-and-resources/resource-library/national-consensus-statement-essential-elements-recognising-and-responding-acute-physiological-deterioration-third-edition

PLANNING FOR PHYSICAL EXAMINATION

The planning phase refers to evaluating subjective data to narrow the focus of the physical examination, determining what objective data needs to be gathered, as well as considering the environment and equipment that will be required.

Objective data is:
> collected during the physical examination of the consumer
> usually collected after subjective data
> information that is measured or observed by the clinician as opposed to being reported by the consumer
> vital to the overall health assessment, to enable you to make clinical decisions that are representative of the whole consumer picture.

Environment

General survey, vital signs, level of consciousness and pain assessment can be undertaken in most physical environments in healthcare settings. Adequate privacy and lighting is required as for any health assessment, as well as minimal noise for accurate auscultation and data collection.

Equipment
> Stethoscope
> Watch with a second hand

> Thermometer (gloves and lubricant if using a rectal thermometer)
> Sphygmomanometer
> Pulse oximeter
> Pen light (torch)
> Relevant documentation

CLINICAL REASONING

Practice tip: Additional observational cues
When observing the consumer, take a moment to look more broadly for clues about their health status. For example, in the immediate environment you may notice an inhaler, a nasal spray, a hearing aid, orthotic inserts in shoes or used tissues. These clues provide additional information about the individual's health status.

IMPLEMENTATION: CONDUCTING THE GENERAL SURVEY

Initial observations include collecting information about the consumer's physical status, psychological status, and signs and symptoms of distress.

EXAMINATION IN BRIEF

General survey, vital signs, pain, neurological status

Examination of physical status
> Stated age versus apparent age
> General appearance
> Body fat
> Body conformation and posture
> Motor activity
> Body and breath odours

Examination of psychological status
> Mental status and cognitive function
> Facial expressions

> Dress, grooming and personal hygiene
> Mood and manner
> Speech and communication
> Distress

Examination of vital signs
> Respiration
> Pulse
> Temperature
> Blood pressure
> Oxygen saturation
> Pain assessment

Examination of physical status

Observe the consumer's:

E
1. stated age versus apparent age
2. general appearance
3. body fat
4. body conformation and posture
5. motor activity
6. body and breath odours.

Stated age versus apparent age

N The consumer's stated chronological age should be congruent with the apparent age.

A It is significant for a consumer to appear older or younger than the stated chronological age.

P > Endocrine deficiencies of growth hormone associated with dwarfism can manifest in a younger-than-chronological-age appearance in younger life and premature ageing later in life.

E Examination   **N** Normal findings   **A** Abnormal findings   **P** Pathophysiology

> > Genetic syndromes (e.g. Turner) manifest in an 'old-person' facial appearance.
> > Chronic disease, severe illness (such as cancer and AIDS), and prolonged sun exposure that causes facial wrinkling can all lead to a consumer looking older than his or her chronological age.

General appearance

E Observe body symmetry, any obvious anomaly, and the consumer's apparent level of wellness (**Figure 6.1**). In addition, note any gross observation such as use of a walker, assistance from a caregiver, or distinctive markings (e.g. multiple piercings, tattoos).

N The consumer should exhibit body symmetry, no obvious deformity, and a well appearance. The level of gross normal observations is varied.

A Asymmetry is seen when a paired body part does not look the same on the contralateral side.

P The unilateral facial drooping of Bell's palsy, a limb appearing at an abnormal angle, and unilateral paralysis are examples of body asymmetry.

A A missing limb, cleft lip, and burned facial skin are examples of obvious anomalies.

P The pathophysiology of each of these is varied and needs to be investigated further via history and physical assessments.

A The consumer who shows signs of being ill, such as pain, respiratory distress, pallor, sweating, nausea and vomiting is an abnormal finding.

P A consumer who appears ill needs to be carefully assessed via the history and physical examination, to quickly identify if there are signs of acute physiological or mental health deterioration, and immediate action taken.

E Observe for skin colouration (see Chapter 8 for detailed information).

N Normally, the skin is a uniform whitish-pink or brown colour, depending on the consumer's race.

A The appearance of cyanosis (dusky blue), jaundice (yellow-green to orange cast or colouration) or pallor of skin, sclera or mucous membranes is abnormal in both light- and dark-skinned individuals.

P The pathophysiology of each of these is varied and needs to be investigated further via health history and physical examination.

Body fat

N Body fat should be evenly distributed. Research has indicated that it is body fat content, not body weight that is most closely linked to pathology. For example, a person can be within normal limits on height and weight charts but have a high proportion of body fat to lean body mass.

A **Obesity** occurs when there are large amounts of body fat. This poses a serious health risk to the consumer and warrants a comprehensive nutritional assessment (see Chapter 15).

P Excess caloric intake and decreased energy expenditure are the most common causes of obesity.

P Some disease processes such as hypothyroidism, which slows the basic metabolic rate, may result in obesity.

A Cushing syndrome manifests in a rounded, moonlike face, truncal obesity, fat pads on the neck, and relatively thin limbs.

P Excessive production of cortisol resulting from an anterior pituitary tumour or large doses of prolonged steroid therapy produces Cushing syndrome.

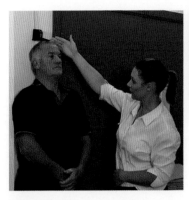

FIGURE 6.1 The nurse can make observations about the consumer's general appearance while talking with them and preparing for the physical examination.

E Examination **N** Normal findings **A** Abnormal findings **P** Pathophysiology

A A thin or frail appearance occurs when there are limited body fat stores. Severely limited fat stores can be a life-threatening condition.

P Energy expenditures that exceed caloric intake will result in decreased fat stores. This may be caused by several conditions, including:

> anorexia nervosa, which results in inadequate intake of calories from food and over-expenditure of energy by means of exercise

> hyperkinetic states, in which the body's metabolic needs are greater than the ability to ingest calories. Adolescent growth spurts result in tall, thin teens because the increased metabolic demands for growing tissue exceed the calories teens can consume

> chronic disease processes that may be due to hyperkinetic states or a result of malabsorption diseases.

Body conformation and posture

N Limbs and trunk should appear proportional to body height; posture should be erect (see **Figure 6.2**). A person's arm span (fingertip to fingertip) should be approximately equal to their height, and body length (crown to pubis) should be about equal to the length from the pubis to the feet.

A A slumped or humpbacked appearance is abnormal.

P **Osteoporosis**, especially in postmenopausal women, may cause a slumped or humpbacked appearance.

P Consumers experiencing depression may also present with a slumped posture.

A Long limbs relative to trunk length are abnormal.

P Marfan syndrome, an inherited disease, can result in the development of long limbs; long, thin fingers; a tall, thin appearance; and poorly developed muscles due to a defect in the elastic fibres of connective tissues. The consumer's arm span is greater than their height.

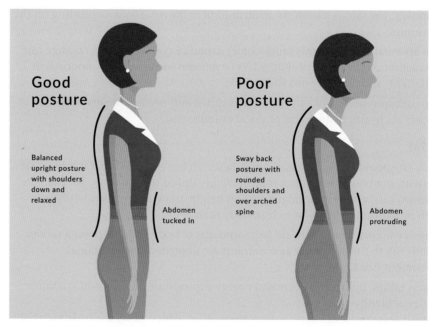

FIGURE 6.2 Example of good and poor posture
GETTY IMAGES/WETCAKE

Motor activity

N Gait as well as other body movements should be smooth and effortless. All body parts should have controlled, purposeful movement.

E Examination   **N** Normal findings   **A** Abnormal findings   **P** Pathophysiology

A An unsteady gait or movements that are slow, absent or require great effort are abnormal. Tremors or movements that seem uncontrollable by the consumer are also abnormal.

P Arthritis can result in slow and difficult movement because joint movement is painful. See Chapter 16 for additional information.

P Neurological disturbances can result in tics, paralysis or ataxia, and can cause difficulty with the smoothness of movement. See Chapter 7 for additional information.

REFLECTION IN PRACTICE

Assessing the consumer with severe odours
You are examining a young person and about to take their oral temperature. At this time, you note they have severe halitosis. Consider how you would progress with this observation, and the approach you would take, including the questions you would pose to discover the cause of the odour. In these situations it is imperative to maintain respect for the consumer's dignity.

Body and breath odours

N Normally, there is no apparent odour from consumers. It is normal for some people to have bad breath related to the types of foods ingested or due to individual digestive processes and reflux.

A Severe body or breath odour is abnormal.

P Poor hygiene can cause body odours due to perspiration and bacteria left on the skin.

P An alcohol smell on the breath can result from alcohol ingestion or from ketoacidosis in a diabetic consumer.

P Bad breath can result from poor oral hygiene, allergic rhinitis, or from infections such as tonsillitis, rhinosinusitis or pneumonia.

P Severe vaginal infections can result in an offensive body odour.

Examination of psychological status

Observe the consumer's:

E 1. mental status and cognitive function (level of consciousness)
  2. facial expressions
  3. dress, grooming and personal hygiene
  4. mood and manner
  5. speech and communication
  6. distress.

Mental status and cognitive function

N The consumer should appear awake and alert, and be generally oriented to person, place and date/time. When using assessment tools such as AVPU or Glasgow Coma Scale (GCS), normal function is 'A' in AVPU or a score of 15 for GCS (see **Figure 6.3**). Mini Mental State Examination (see **Figure 6.4**) also should show normal function for attention, memory, judgement, insight, spatial perception, calculation, abstraction, thought processes and thought content. The consumer with normal function has no plans to harm self or others.

A Altered level of consciousness.

P Confusion, lethargy, stupor, permanent vegetative state, locked-in syndrome, coma or brain death (see Chapter 7 for detailed information) can alter a person's level of consciousness.

E Examination   **N** Normal findings   **A** Abnormal findings   **P** Pathophysiology

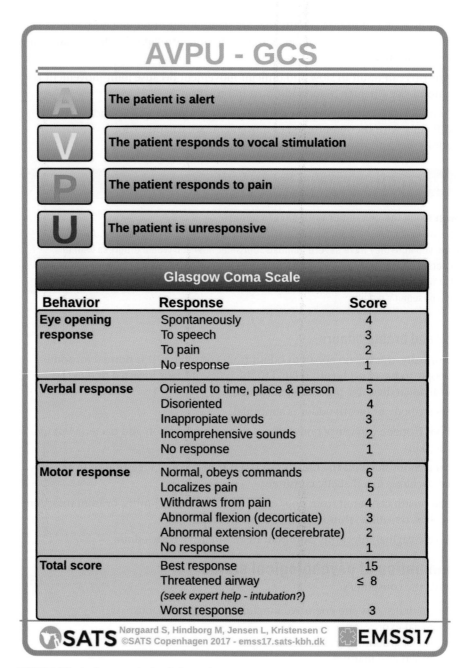

AVPU - GCS

A	The patient is alert
V	The patient responds to vocal stimulation
P	The patient responds to pain
U	The patient is unresponsive

Glasgow Coma Scale

Behavior	Response	Score
Eye opening response	Spontaneously	4
	To speech	3
	To pain	2
	No response	1
Verbal response	Oriented to time, place & person	5
	Disoriented	4
	Inappropiate words	3
	Incomprehensive sounds	2
	No response	1
Motor response	Normal, obeys commands	6
	Localizes pain	5
	Withdraws from pain	4
	Abnormal flexion (decorticate)	3
	Abnormal extension (decerebrate)	2
	No response	1
Total score	Best response	15
	Threatened airway	≤ 8
	(seek expert help - intubation?)	
	Worst response	3

SATS Nørgaard S, Hindborg M, Jensen L, Kristensen C
©SATS Copenhagen 2017 - emss17.sats-kbh.dk **EMSS17**

FIGURE 6.3 Scales for assessing level of consciousness

SATS: Danish Student Society of Anesthesiology and Traumatology

A Altered attention, memory, judgement, insight, spatial perception, calculation, abstraction, thought processes and thought content.

P Dementia, delirium, neurological injury, infection or disease, intellectual disability, effect of drugs and alcohol, psychosis, bipolar affective disorders, schizophrenia, endogenous anxiety states or depressed states, brain lesions or growths can cause altered cognitive function.

A Expresses plans or intention to harm self or others.

P Suicidal or homicidal ideation can occur when mental disorders, particularly depression, substance abuse and schizophrenia, are present and active.

E Examination **N** Normal findings **A** Abnormal findings **P** Pathophysiology

Mini-Mental State Examination (MMSE)

Patient's Name: _____   Date: _____

Instructions: Ask the questions in the order listed.
Score one point for each correct response within each question or activity.

Maximum Score	Patient's Score	Questions
5		"What is the year? Season? Date? Day of the week? Month?"
5		"Where are we now: State? County? Town/city? Hospital? Floor?"
3		The examiner names three unrelated objects clearly and slowly, then asks the patient to name all three of them. The patient's response is used for scoring. The examiner repeats them until patient learns all of them, if possible. Number of trials: _____
5		"I would like you to count backward from 100 by sevens." (93, 86, 79, 72, 65, …) Stop after five answers. Alternative: "Spell WORLD backwards." (D-L-R-O-W)
3		"Earlier I told you the names of three things. Can you tell me what those were?"
2		Show the patient two simple objects, such as a wristwatch and a pencil, and ask the patient to name them.
1		"Repeat the phrase: 'No ifs, ands, or buts.'"
3		"Take the paper in your right hand, fold it in half, and put it on the floor." (The examiner gives the patient a piece of blank paper.)
1		"Please read this and do what it says." (Written instruction is "Close your eyes.")
1		"Make up and write a sentence about anything." (This sentence must contain a noun and a verb.)
1		"Please copy this picture." (The examiner gives the patient a blank piece of paper and asks him/her to draw the symbol below. All 10 angles must be present and two must intersect.) 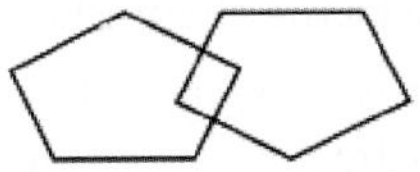
30		**TOTAL**

FIGURE 6.4 Mini Mental State Examination

Facial expressions

N Facial expressions should be appropriate for what is happening in the environment and should change naturally.

A Unchanging or flat facial expression/affect, inappropriate facial expression, tremors or tics are abnormal.

P Apathy or depression may cause lack of facial expression due to feelings of lethargy or sadness.

P Dementia may cause inappropriate facial expressions because the consumer's perception of reality is distorted.

P Cranial nerve (CN) dysfunction or impingement of CN VII may show asymmetry in muscle control in the face, which includes abnormal facial movements. Bell's palsy, a condition resulting in paralysis of the muscles in the face, may cause the mouth to droop and the affected side of the face to appear flaccid, with the inability to completely close the eye on the affected side.

E Examination   **N** Normal findings   **A** Abnormal findings   **P** Pathophysiology

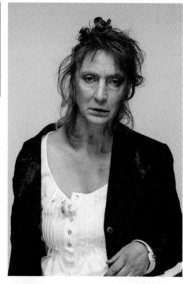

FIGURE 6.5 Assessing a consumer's psychological presence, specifically dress, grooming and personal hygiene. A dishevelled appearance is an abnormal finding.

ALAMY STOCK PHOTO/SCOTT RYLANDER

Dress, grooming and personal hygiene

N Normally, consumers should appear clean and neatly dressed. Clothing choice should be appropriate for the weather. Norms and standards for dress and cleanliness may vary among cultures.

A A dishevelled, unkempt appearance or clothing that is inappropriate for the weather (such as a wool coat in hot weather) is abnormal.

P Psychological or psychiatric disorders such as depression (characterised in part by lethargy, mood swings, anhedonia [or lack of pleasure in activities], fatigue), psychotic disorders (characterised by a distortion in thinking) and dementia (processes that alter perceptions of reality) may be reflected in inappropriate appearance (hair, make-up) or through inappropriate clothing selection.

P Poor self-esteem or a homeless lifestyle may be reflected by general neglect of personal hygiene, grooming and dress.

P An unshaven, unclean appearance may reflect abuse or neglect of the consumer by the consumer's caregiver.

Mood and manner

N Generally, a consumer should be cooperative and pleasant.

A An uncooperative, hostile or tearful adult or an adult who seems unusually elated or who has a flat affect needs further assessment.

P Psychiatric conditions such as depression, manic disorders, paranoid disorders and psychotic disorders produce a distortion in reality (distorted thinking and perceptions), resulting in abnormal behaviours. Dementia or confusion in the elderly can also result in disturbances of mood and manner. See Chapter 7 for a more complete discussion.

Speech and communication

N The consumer should respond to questions and commands easily. Speech should be clear and understandable. Pitch, rate, content and volume should be appropriate to the circumstances.

A Speech that is slow, slurred, mumbled, very loud or rapid needs to be assessed further.

P Hyperthyroidism can cause rapid speech because of hormones that are stimulatory in nature and result in hypermetabolism and hyperactivity.

P Alcohol ingestion can cause slow, mumbled or slurred speech because alcohol affects the central nervous system, causing transient brain dysfunction.

P Hearing difficulties may be associated with loud speech because individuals with decreased ability to hear may not be able to hear themselves at normal conversational decibels.

P Strokes or brain injury can result in aphasia if the speech centre in the brain is affected, or language dysfunction such as dysphasia. Lesions in the brain can impact on communication with other dysfunctions such as dysphonia, aphonia, dysarthria, apraxia, agraphia and alexia.

P Damage to CN XII, the hypoglossal nerve, can cause inability to speak or changed lingual sounds; speech changes may include lisps.

Distress

Observe the consumer for:

E 1. laboured breathing, wheezing or cough, or laboured speech
2. painful facial expression, sweating, or physical protection of painful area
3. serious or life-threatening occurrences such as **seizure** activity, active and severe bleeding, gaping wounds and open fractures.

E Examination   **N** Normal findings   **A** Abnormal findings   **P** Pathophysiology

4. signs of emotional distress or anxiety that may include, but are not limited to, tearfulness, nervous tics or laughter, avoidance of eye contact, cold clammy hands, excessive nail biting, inability to pay attention, autonomic responses such as diaphoresis, or changes in breathing patterns.

N Breathing should be effortless, without cough or wheezing. Speech should not leave a consumer breathless. The face should be relaxed, and the individual should be willing to move all body parts freely. There should be no serious or life-threatening conditions. The consumer should not perspire excessively or show signs of emotional distress such as nail biting or avoidance of eye contact (**Figure 6.6**).

A The presence of shortness of breath with laboured speech, wheezing or cough is abnormal.

P Pulmonary disease may be present. See Chapter 13 for additional information.

A Pain, as evidenced by facial grimacing, crying, moaning, sweating or protection of a body part, is an abnormal finding.

P Tissue damage results in pain, and further investigation is needed into the character, location, intensity and occurrence of the pain, as well as factors associated with increased and decreased pain.

A Excessive nail biting, avoidance of eye contact, nervous laughter, tearfulness or lack of interest may be indicators of emotional distress or emotional pain.

P Nervous habits are often displayed when a person is in an uncomfortable or new situation. A tearful or sad affect can result from emotional pain related to situations the consumer may be experiencing or has experienced. Often, there is an attempt made to disguise emotional distress.

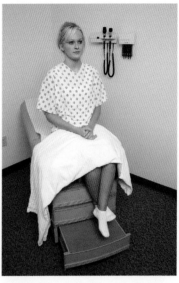

FIGURE 6.6 The general survey includes assessing every consumer for signs of distress.

URGENT FINDING ⚠

Recognition of deterioration in a person's mental state

Mental state deterioration can be due to internal factors, including exacerbation of mental illness, psychological distress, physical conditions such as delirium, atypical responses to prescribed treatments, or intoxication with licit or illicit substances. Deterioration in mental state can also be attributed to factors arising from an individual's social context or their response to the environment. It is important to note that individuals experience and express deterioration in mental state in different ways (ACSQHC, 2017).

Acute deterioration in a consumer's mental state can occur in any healthcare setting, and this in itself is an adverse outcome. However, this acute change can also be associated with further adverse outcomes including attempted suicide, increased aggression and the traumatic use of restrictive practices, if not managed in a timely manner.

The key for a nurse to identify deterioration in a person's mental state is observing any changes in current or usual behaviours, cognitive function, perception or emotional state by using relevant screening processes at presentation, during physical examination and health history taking.

Common signs of deterioration in mental state can include the following.

> Reported by the consumer/family:

- mood disturbance (elevated or irritable mood; depression)
- psychotic symptoms (paranoid ideas; hallucinations; delusions)
- situational crisis
- attempted self-harm
- risk of harm to others
- verbal commands to do harm to self or others
- suicidal ideation

>>

>>

> > Observed behaviours:
>   - ambivalence about treatment
>   - restlessness
>   - confusion
>   - agitation
>   - physical/verbal aggression
>   - bizarre/disoriented behaviour
>   - withdrawn/uncommunicative

(Adapted from ACSQHC, 2017)

When a consumer's mental state is observed to have changed, the nurse must determine the immediate actions needed to prevent further deterioration by following the escalation protocol in place in their healthcare facility.

For more information on standards and protocols related to the deteriorating mental state of the consumer, visit ACSQHC (2017) – National Consensus Statement: Essential elements for recognising and responding to deterioration in a person's mental state, https://www.safetyandquality.gov.au/publications-and-resources/resource-library/national-consensus-statement-essential-elements-recognising-and-responding-deterioration-persons-mental-state.

EXAMINATION OF VITAL SIGNS

Vital sign measurements include respiration, pulse, temperature, blood pressure and oxygen saturations (if indicated). Note that the vital sign measurements adopted in this textbook are based on the current evidence-based literature. You may note slight variations to these parameters published in other literature sources. It is important that you check your health service for guidelines on what the 'normal ranges' are to ensure you respond and act as appropriate in your work environment.

General approach to vital signs assessment

1. Gather equipment.
2. Explain the procedure to the consumer.
3. Select equipment according to the consumer's age, size and developmental level, and the site selected for assessment. Specific decision-making criteria are discussed under each section.
4. Warm the stethoscope headpiece before touching the consumer with it.
5. Assess vital signs and record findings.

CLINICAL REASONING

Practice tip: Frequency of assessing vital signs

Vital signs should be assessed as often as prescribed (as per the clinical pathway/policy/protocol in the health service area) or as often as the consumer's condition requires. Within active plans of care, vital sign frequency is often ordered by a medical officer or nurse practitioner (e.g. every 6 hours); however, this should be considered the minimum frequency for vital signs to be taken. If the consumer's condition changes, nurses can increase frequency of vital signs as often as required by the change in their condition. For example, for a consumer who has a drop in blood pressure, the nurse may re-evaluate the person's vital signs every half-hour. This may also trigger an escalation protocol, which should be documented and revisited often.

Respiration

Respiration is the act of breathing. Breathing supplies oxygen to the body and occurs in response to changes in the concentration of oxygen (O_2), carbon dioxide (CO_2) and hydrogen (H^+) in the arterial blood. Inhalation, or inspiration, occurs when air is taken into the lungs. Exhalation, or expiration, refers to the airflow out of the lungs.

Inspiration occurs when the diaphragm and the intercostal muscles contract. This can be observed by the movement of the abdomen outwards and the movement of the chest upwards and outwards, resulting in the lungs filling with air. Expiration occurs when the external intercostal muscles and the diaphragm relax. The abdomen and the chest return to a resting position.

Respiratory rate is measured in breaths per minute. One respiratory cycle consists of one inhalation and one expiration. A complete discussion of respiratory assessment is found in Chapter 13.

To assess respiratory rate:

E 1. Stand in front of or to the side of the consumer.
2. Discreetly observe the consumer's breathing (rise and fall of the chest). These observations are best done with the consumer unaware of what you are doing. If the consumer is aware that you are counting respirations, the breathing pattern may be altered.
3. Count the number of respiratory cycles that occur in 1 minute.

N Table 6.1 lists the normal respiratory rates for different ages. Respiratory rates decrease with age and may vary with excitement, anxiety, fever, exercise, medications and altitude.

TABLE 6.1 Respiratory rate

AGE	RESTING RESPIRATORY RATE (BREATHS PER MINUTE)	AVERAGE
Newborn	30–50	40
1 year	20–40	30
3 years	20–30	25
6 years	16–22	19
10 years	16–20	18
14 years	14–20	17
Adult	12–20	18

A **Tachypnoea** is a respiratory rate greater than 20 breaths per minute in an adult.

P Hypoxaemia and metabolic acidosis are common causes of tachypnoea. The increased respiratory rate is a compensatory mechanism to provide the body with more oxygen and eliminate excess hydrogen ions when the body's metabolism is increased.

P Stress and anxiety cause the release of catecholamines, which can elevate the respiratory rate.

A **Bradypnoea** is a respiratory rate less than 12 breaths per minute in an adult at rest.

P Head injury resulting in increased intracranial pressure in the respiratory centre of the brain can cause bradypnoea.

P Medications or chemicals such as narcotics, barbiturates and alcohol depress the respiratory centre of the brain and can cause bradypnoea.

P A lower metabolic rate that occurs during normal sleep can result in bradypnoea.

A **Apnoea** is the absence of spontaneous breathing for 10 or more seconds.

P Many causes of apnoea are unknown.

P **Traumatic brain injury** may lead to apnoea from injury of the brain stem. Death ensues in the absence of respirations and pulse.

E Examination **N** Normal findings **A** Abnormal findings **P** Pathophysiology

CLINICAL **REASONING**

Practice tip: Assessing respiration
Respirations are the most sensitive vital signs for detecting deterioration. To assist collection of accurate counts, respirations can be measured when assessing the radial or apical pulse. Observe and count the consumer's chest movements when they are unaware, as this provides an accurate assessment of their respirations. Alternatively, if respirations are shallow and difficult to observe, put the individual's arm across the chest while taking a radial pulse and feel the chest rise while observing respirations.

Pulse

As the heart contracts, blood is ejected from the left ventricle (stroke volume) into the aorta. A pressure wave is created as the blood is carried to the peripheral vasculature. This palpable pressure is the **pulse**. Pulse assessment can determine heart rate and rhythm, and the estimated volume (strength) of blood being pumped by the heart.

Rate

Pulse rate is the number of pulse beats counted in 1 minute. Several factors influence heart rate or pulse rate. These include:

> the S-A (sinoatrial) node, which fires automatically at a rate of 60 to 100 times per minute and is the primary controller of pulse rate and heart rate
> parasympathetic or vagal stimulation of the autonomic nervous system, which can result in decreased heart rate
> sympathetic stimulation of the autonomic nervous system, which results in increased heart rate
> baroreceptor sensors, which can detect changes in blood pressure and influence heart rate. Elevated blood pressure can decrease heart rate, whereas decreased blood pressure can increase heart rate.
Other factors influencing heart rate include:
> age. The heart rate generally decreases with age.
> sex. The average heart rate for females is higher than the average heart rate for males.
> activity. The heart rate increases with activity. Athletes will have a lower resting heart rate than the average person because of their increased cardiac strength and efficiency.
> emotional status. Heart rate increases with anxiety.
> pain. Heart rate increases with pain.
> environmental factors. Temperature and noise level can alter the heart rate.
> stimulants. Caffeinated beverages and tobacco elevate the heart rate.
> medications. Drugs such as digoxin decrease the heart rate; drugs such as amphetamines increase the heart rate.
> disease state. Abnormal clinical conditions can affect the heart rate (e.g. increased heart rate in hyperthyroidism, fever and haemorrhage).

Rhythm

Pulse rhythm refers to the pattern of pulses and the intervals between pulses. Pulses can be regular or irregular. A regular pulse occurs at regular intervals with even intervals between each beat. Normal sinus rhythm is an example of a regular pulse.

An irregular pulse can be regularly irregular or irregularly irregular. A regular irregular rhythm is one in which an abnormal conduction occurs in the heart, but at regular intervals. Ventricular bigeminy is an example of a regularly irregular rhythm. In ventricular bigeminy, the irregular conduction, called a premature ventricular complex (PVC), occurs prior to the expected QRS complex. This PVC occurs at a regular rhythm (every other beat).

An irregularly irregular rhythm has no predictable pattern. Atrial fibrillation is an example of an irregularly irregular rhythm.

Volume

Pulse volume (also called pulse strength or amplitude) reflects the stroke volume and the **systemic vascular resistance (SVR)**. It can range from absent to bounding. Table 6.2 displays the most commonly used 4-point scale; however, your clinical area may have other guidelines so it is important to refer to these. When reporting pulse volume, 2+/4+ indicates a normal pulse (2+) on a 4-point scale. Refer to the Clinical reasoning practice tip: Peripheral pulse documentation, for schematic representations. If a pulse is not palpable, then attempt to ascertain its presence with a Doppler ultrasonic stethoscope. The letter 'D' in a pulse chart or stick figure represents the pulse that was detected by using this mechanical device.

CLINICAL **REASONING**

Practice tip: Peripheral pulse documentation

You can document the pulse volume (strength) of a consumer's pulses by drawing a small stick figure and labelling the pulses accordingly (Figure 6.7A) or by recording the pulses in tabular format (Figure 6.7B).

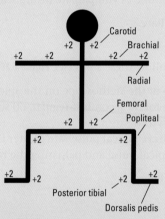

Scale = 4+

A. Stick figure peripheral pulse documentation

	CAROTID	BRACHIAL	RADIAL	FEMORAL	POPLITEAL	PT	DP
R	2+	2+	2+	1+	1+	D	D
L	2+	2+	2+	2+	1+	1+	1+

Scale = 4+
D = Doppler ultrasonic stethoscope

B. Tabular peripheral pulse documentation

FIGURE 6.7 Methods for charting peripheral pulses

TABLE 6.2 The 4-point scale for measuring pulse volume (strength)

SCALE	DESCRIPTION OF PULSE
0	Absent
1+	Thready/weak
2+	Normal
3+	Increased
4+	Bounding

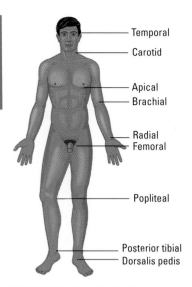

- Temporal
- Carotid
- Apical
- Brachial
- Radial
- Femoral
- Popliteal
- Posterior tibial
- Dorsalis pedis

FIGURE 6.8 Peripheral pulse sites

Site

Peripheral pulses can be palpated where the large arteries are close to the skin surface. There are nine common sites for assessment of pulse, as indicated in **Figure 6.8**. When routine vital signs are assessed, the pulse is generally measured at one of two sites: radial or apical.

Measuring the apical pulse is indicated for consumers with an irregular pulse or known cardiac or pulmonary disease. The assessment of apical pulse can be accomplished through palpation but is most commonly accomplished through auscultation.

Radial pulse

To palpate the radial pulse, follow these steps.

E 1. Place the pad of your first, second and/or third finger on the site of the radial pulse, along the radial bone on the thumb side of the inner wrist (see **Figure 6.9**).
2. Press your fingers gently against the artery with enough pressure so that you can feel the pulse. Pressing too hard will obliterate the pulse.
3. Count the pulse rate using the second hand of your watch. If the pulse is regular, count for 30 seconds and multiply by 2 to obtain the pulse rate per minute. If the pulse is irregular, count for 60 seconds.
4. Identify the pulse rhythm as you palpate (regular or irregular).
5. Identify the pulse volume as you palpate (using scales from **Table 6.2**).

N A P Refer to section on Rate.

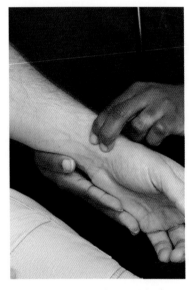

FIGURE 6.9 Palpation of the radial pulse

Apical pulse

To assess the apical pulse, follow these steps (see **Figure 6.10**).

E 1. Place the diaphragm of the stethoscope on the apical pulse site.
2. Count the pulse rate for 30 seconds if regular, 60 seconds if irregular.
3. Identify the pulse rhythm.
4. Identify a **pulse deficit** (apical pulse rate greater than the radial pulse rate) by listening to the apical pulse and palpating the radial pulse simultaneously.

N A P Refer to section on Rate.

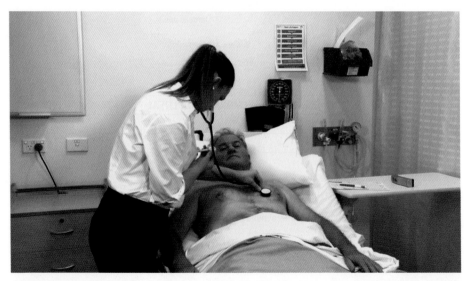

FIGURE 6.10 Auscultation of the apical pulse

Rate

N Normal pulse rates vary with age. Table 6.3 depicts ranges for normal pulse rates by age. The heart rate normally increases during periods of exertion. Athletes commonly have resting heart rates below 60 beats per minute because of the increased strength and efficiency of the cardiac muscle.

TABLE 6.3 Pulse rate: Normal range according to age

AGE	RESTING PULSE RATE (BEATS PER MINUTE)	AVERAGE
Newborn	100–170	140
1 year	80–160	120
3 years	80–120	110
6 years	70–115	100
10 years	70–110	90
14 years	60–110	85–90
Adult	60–100	72

A **Tachycardia** refers to a pulse rate faster than 100 beats per minute in an adult.

P Psychophysiological stressors such as trauma, blood volume losses, anaemia, infection, fear, fever, pain, hyperthyroidism, shock and anxiety can increase pulse rate because of increased metabolic demands placed on the body.

P Some tachycardia may not have clinical significance; however, in consumers with myocardial disease, tachycardia can be a sign of decreased cardiac output, congestive heart failure, myocardial ischaemia or dysrhythmias.

A **Bradycardia** refers to slow pulse rates. Pulse rates that fall below 60 beats per minute in adults are considered to be bradycardic.

P Medications such as cardiotonics (digoxin) and beta blockers decrease the heart rate.

P Bradycardia usually occurs with excessive vagal stimulation or decreased sympathetic tone. Conditions that may cause bradycardia are eye surgery, increased intracranial pressure, myocardial infarction, hypothyroidism and prolonged vomiting.

A **Asystole** refers to the absence of a pulse. Palpate or auscultate for a pulse for 10–15 seconds to establish asystole.

P Cardiac arrest resulting from biological or clinical death results in asystole.

P Pulseless electrical activity (electromechanical dissociation) caused by, for example, hypovolaemia, pneumothorax, cardiac tamponade or acidosis results in the absence of a pulse despite the presence of electrical activity in the heart muscle.

A A pulse deficit occurs when the apical pulse rate is greater than the radial pulse rate.

P Dysrhythmias (such as atrial fibrillation, premature ventricular contractions, second-degree heart block, third-degree heart block) and heart failure can cause pulse deficits because some heart contractions are too weak to produce a pulse pressure to the peripheral site. Severe vascular disease can also cause pulse deficits.

Rhythm

N Normal pulse rhythm is regular, with equal intervals between each beat.

A **Dysrhythmias**, or **arrhythmias**, refer to pulse rhythms that are not regular. They may consist of irregular beats that are random, or irregular beats that present in a regular pattern.

P Cardiac dysrhythmias that are atrial and ventricular in origin cause abnormal rhythms, such as atrial flutter and ventricular fibrillation.

E Examination N Normal findings A Abnormal findings P Pathophysiology

Volume

N The pulse volume is normally the same with each beat. A normal pulse volume can be felt with a moderate amount of pressure of the fingers and obliterated with greater pressure.

A Small, weak pulses are referred to as weak or thready pulses or as pulses easily obliterated with light pressure.

P Decreased cardiac stroke volume caused by heart failure, hypovolaemic shock or cardiogenic shock can result in weak pulses.

P A low pulse amplitude occurs in states of increased peripheral vascular resistance, such as in aortic stenosis and constrictive pericarditis.

P Weak pulses occur in conditions in which ventricular filling time is decreased, such as in dysrhythmias.

A Bounding pulses are full, forceful pulses that are difficult to obliterate with pressure.

P Hyperkinetic states such as exercise, fever, anaemia, anxiety and hyperthyroidism can cause bounding pulses.

P Early stages of septic shock are characterised by bounding pulses because of decreased peripheral vascular resistance.

Temperature

Scales, variables, routes, and measurement methods for assessing temperature are outlined.

Temperature scales

In Australia and New Zealand, degree Celsius is the most commonly used measurement scale for **temperature**, which reflects the degree of core body heat. Figure 6.11 summarises and correlates both Celsius and Fahrenheit scales and gives the conversion formulas.

Variables affecting body temperature

Core body temperature is established by the temperature of blood perfusing the area of the hypothalamus (the body's temperature control centre), which triggers the body's physiological response to temperature. An ideal thermometer would accurately measure central brain stem temperature at the hypothalamus. Invasive procedures that provide temperatures of the arterial blood, oesophagus or bladder are reliable indicators of core temperature, but are impractical. More practical methods for measurement of body temperature are less reliable and can result in variations in body temperature readings. In addition, there are physiological variables that affect body temperature. These include:

> **circadian rhythm** patterns. Normal body temperature (as well as pulse and blood pressure) fluctuates with a consumer's activity level and the time of day. Core body temperature is lower during sleep than during waking activities, being lowest in the early morning just before awakening from sleep, and highest in the afternoon or early evening. A 0.5°C to 1.0°C fluctuation in body temperature throughout the day is considered within the normal range.

> hormones. In women, increased production of progesterone at the time of ovulation raises the basal body temperature about 0.35°C.

> age. Infants and young children are affected by the environmental temperature to a much greater extent than adults because their thermoregulation mechanisms are not fully developed. The elderly are more sensitive to extremes of environmental temperature due to a decrease in thermoregulatory controls.

> exercise. Body temperature rises due to increased metabolic activity.

> stress. Stimulation of the sympathetic nervous system increases the production of adrenaline, resulting in increased metabolic activity and higher body temperature.

Celsius	Fahrenheit
42	107.6
41	105.8
40	104.0
39	102.2
38	100.4
37	98.6
36	96.8
35	95.0
34	93.2

To convert:

(9/5 × temperature in Celsius) + 32°
= temperature in Fahrenheit

5/9 × (temperature in Fahrenheit − 32°)
= temperature in Celsius

FIGURE 6.11 Correlation between Celsius and Fahrenheit scales

 E Examination N Normal findings 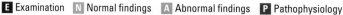 A Abnormal findings P Pathophysiology

> environmental extremes of hot or cold.
> health status. Temperature deviations can occur in illnesses such as infections. as well as in hypothalamus dysfunction.

Measurement routes

There are four basic routes by which temperature can be measured: oral, rectal, axillary and tympanic. Each method has advantages and disadvantages. The advantages and disadvantages of each route are summarised in Table 6.4.

TABLE 6.4 Advantages and disadvantages of four routes for body temperature measurement

ROUTE	NORMAL RANGE	ADVANTAGES	DISADVANTAGES
Oral			
Average 37.0°C	35.5–37.5°C	Convenient; accessible	**Safety:** Consumers need to be alert and cooperative, and cognitively capable of following instructions for safe use. **Physical abilities:** Consumers need to be able to breathe through the nose and be without oral pathology or recent oral surgery; route not applicable for comatose or confused consumers. **Accuracy:** Oxygen therapy by mask, as well as ingestion of hot or cold drinks immediately before oral temperature measurement, affects accuracy of the reading.
Rectal			
Average 0.4°C higher than oral	36.6–38.0°C	Considered most accurate	**Safety:** Contraindicated following rectal surgery. Risk of rectal perforation in children less than 2 years of age. Risk of stimulating Valsalva manoeuvre in cardiac consumers. **Physical aspects:** Invasive, uncomfortable, and possibly embarrassing.
Axillary			
Average 0.6°C lower than oral	35.5–37.5°C	Safe; non-invasive	**Time frame:** Glass thermometer must be left in place for 5 minutes to obtain accurate measurement. Glass and mercury thermometers are no longer used in healthcare facilities. Placement and position of thermometer tip affect reading.
Tympanic			
Calibrated to oral or rectal scales	35.8–38.0°C	Convenient, fast, safe, non-invasive; does not require contact with any mucous membrane	**Accuracy:** Research is inconclusive as to accuracy of readings and correlations with other body temperature measurements. Technique affects reading. Tympanic membrane is thought to reflect the core body temperature.

Oral method

E 1. Place the thermometer (Figure 6.12) at the base of the tongue and to the right or left of the frenulum, and instruct the individual to close the lips and to avoid biting the thermometer. Ensure that it has been at least 15 minutes since the individual consumed a hot or cold beverage or food.
2. Leave the thermometer in the mouth until the device has signalled that the maximum body temperature has been reached.
3. Remove the thermometer from the person's mouth.

Rectal method

E 1. Position individual with the buttocks exposed. Adults may be more comfortable lying on the side (with knees slightly flexed), facing away from you, or prone.
2. Put on nonsterile gloves.
3. Lubricate the tip of the thermometer with a water-soluble lubricant.
4. Ask the individual to take a deep breath; insert the thermometer into the anus 1.5 to 2.5 cm, depending on the person's age.
5. Do not force the insertion of the thermometer or insert into faeces.

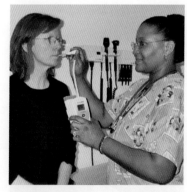

FIGURE 6.12 Taking a consumer's oral temperature with an electronic thermometer

E Examination **N** Normal findings **A** Abnormal findings **P** Pathophysiology

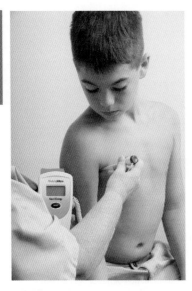

FIGURE 6.13 Taking a consumer's axillary temperature

E 6. Leave the thermometer in the rectum until the device has signalled that the maximum body temperature has been reached.

7. Remove the thermometer from the individual's rectum.

Axillary method

E 1. Place the thermometer into the middle of the axilla (Figure 6.13) and fold the individual's arm across the chest to keep the thermometer in place.

2. Leave the thermometer in the axilla until the device has signalled that the maximum body temperature has been reached.

3. Remove the thermometer from the individual's axilla.

Electronic thermometer

E 1. Remove the electronic thermometer from the charging unit (Figure 6.14).

2. Attach a disposable cover to the probe.

3. Using one of the methods described (oral, rectal or axillary), measure the temperature.

4. Listen for the sound or look for the symbol that indicates maximum body temperature has been reached.

5. Observe and record the reading.

6. Remove and discard the probe cover.

7. Return the electronic thermometer to the charging unit.

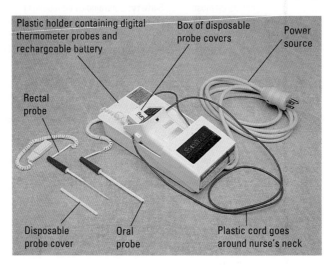

FIGURE 6.14 A battery-operated thermometer

Tympanic thermometer

E 1. Attach the probe cover to the nose of the thermometer (Figure 6.15).

2. Gently place the probe of the thermometer over the entrance to the ear canal. If the individual is under 3 years old, pull the **pinna** down, aiming the probe towards the opposite eye. If the individual is over 3 years old, grasp the pinna and pull gently up and back, aiming the probe towards the opposite ear (Figure 6.16). Make sure there is a tight seal.

3. Press the start button on the thermometer handle.

4. Wait for the beep, remove the probe from the ear, and read the temperature.

5. Discard the probe cover.

6. Return the tympanic thermometer to the charger unit.

N Normal body temperatures are described in Table 6.4.

A **Hyperthermia**, pyrexia or fever are conditions in which body temperatures exceed 38.5°C. Clinical signs of hyperthermia include increased respiratory rate and pulse, shivering, **pallor** and thirst.

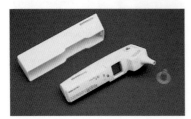

FIGURE 6.15 A tympanic thermometer

E Examination   **N** Normal findings   **A** Abnormal findings   **P** Pathophysiology

P There can be many causes of hyperthermia (including infection), which results from an increased basal metabolic rate.

A **Hypothermia** occurs when the body temperature is below 34°C. Clinical signs of hypothermia include decreased body temperature and initial shivering that ceases as drowsiness and coma ensue. **Hypotension**, decreased urinary output, lack of muscle coordination, and disorientation also occur as hypothermia progresses.

P Hypothermia can be caused by prolonged exposure to cold, such as immersion in cold water or administration of large volumes of unwarmed blood products.

P Hypothermia can be induced to decrease the tissues' need for oxygen, such as during cardiac surgery.

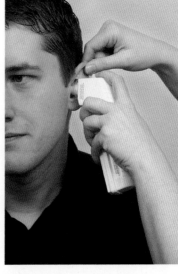

FIGURE 6.16 Taking a consumer's temperature with a tympanic thermometer

---

URGENT FINDING ⚠

Hypothermia – importance of assessment

Hypothermia can cause bradycardia and cardiac arrest. The focus of care for those with hypothermia is on comprehensive and multiple methods of rewarming, with close cardiac monitoring. As the person's temperature increases, arrythmias can develop. It is important to identify the consumer's full history and assessment to ensure correct treatment. Resuscitation efforts do not stop until the person is at a normal body temperature and all other interventions have been exhausted.

Blood pressure

Blood pressure measures (in millimetres of mercury [mmHg]) the force exerted by the flow of blood pumped into the large arteries. Arterial blood pressure is determined by blood flow and the resistance to blood flow as indicated in the following formula:

$$MAP = CO \times TPR$$
$$\text{mean arterial pressure (MAP)} = \text{cardiac output (CO)} \times \text{total peripheral resistance (TPR)}$$

Changes in blood pressure can be used to monitor changes in cardiac output. Ineffective pumping, decreased circulating volume, as well as changes in the characteristics of the blood vessels, can affect blood pressure. There is a diurnal variation in blood pressure, as characterised by a high point in the early evening and a low point during the early deep stage of sleep.

Korotkoff sounds

Korotkoff sounds are generated when the flow of blood through the artery is altered by inflating the blood pressure cuff that is wrapped around the extremity. Korotkoff sounds may be heard by listening over a pulse site that is distal to the blood pressure cuff. As the air is released from the bladder of the cuff, the pressure on the artery changes from that which completely occludes blood flow to that which allows free flow. As the pressure against the artery wall decreases, five distinct sounds occur.

> **Phase I:** The first audible sound heard as the cuff pressure is released. Sounds like clear tapping and correlates to systolic pressure (the force needed to pump the blood out of the heart).

> **Phase II:** Sounds like swishing or a murmur. Created as the blood flows through blood vessels narrowed by the inflation of the blood pressure cuff.

> **Phase III:** Sounds like clear, intense tapping. Created as blood flows through the artery, but cuff pressure is still great enough to occlude flow during diastole.

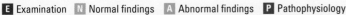

E Examination   **N** Normal findings   **A** Abnormal findings   **P** Pathophysiology

> **Phase IV:** Sounds are muffled and are heard when cuff pressure is low enough to allow some blood flow during diastole. The change from the tap of Phase III to the muffled sound of Phase IV is referred to as the first diastolic reading.
> **Phase V:** No sounds are heard. Occurs when cuff pressure is released enough to allow normal blood flow. This is referred to as the second diastolic reading.

Measuring blood pressure

Systolic pressure represents the pressure exerted on the arterial wall during **systole**, when the ventricles are contracting. Diastolic pressure represents the pressure in the arteries when the ventricles are relaxed and filling. Blood pressure is recorded as a fraction, with the top number representing the systole and the bottom number(s) representing the **diastole**. If the first and second diastolic sounds are recorded, the first diastolic sound is written over the second. For example, 120/90/80 indicates that 120 mmHg is the systolic pressure, 90 mmHg is the first diastolic sound, and 80 mmHg is the second diastolic sound. **Pulse pressure** is the difference between the diastolic and systolic blood pressures.

Measurement sites

There are several potential sites for blood pressure measurement. The preferred site is the brachial pulse site, where the brachial artery runs across the antecubital fossa. The posterior thigh, where the popliteal artery runs behind the knee joint, can also be used. A site should not be used if there is pain or injury around or near the site; for instance, a postmastectomy consumer should have blood pressure assessed on the unaffected side. Surgical incisions; intravenous, central venous or arterial lines; or areas with poor perfusion should be avoided for blood pressure measurement. Consumers with arteriovenous (AV) fistulas or AV shunts should not have blood pressure measured in those extremities.

Equipment

Blood pressure is measured indirectly with a Doppler or a stethoscope and a **sphygmomanometer**, which consists of the blood pressure cuff, connecting tubes and air pump, and manometer. Blood pressure cuffs come in several sizes (**Figure 6.17**). The size of the cuff bladder should be 80% of the circumference of the limb being assessed (JNC, 2003). The cuff should completely encircle the limb.

A manometer is attached to the cuff via a second tube. The **aneroid manometer** is a calibrated dial with a needle that points to numbers representing the air pressure within the cuff (**Figure 6.18**).

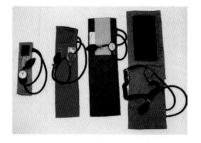

FIGURE 6.17 Blood pressure cuffs come in various sizes.

HEALTH EDUCATION

Home blood pressure monitoring devices

Many consumers take their blood pressure at home for numerous reasons, for example to monitor antihypertensive medication treatment. Periodically, consumers should be instructed to bring their home devices to their healthcare provider appointment. The consumer should be observed taking their blood pressure to assess their technique. Reinforcing correct technique can positively influence an individual's compliance with their medical treatment.

It is also appropriate to compare the blood pressure reading on the home device with that obtained in the healthcare provider's office. The measurements should correlate within 5 mmHg of each other. This assists to determine if the readings from home are accurate and reflect the consumer's actual blood pressure.

FIGURE 6.18 An aneroid manometer dial

Blood pressure assessment

A Doppler ultrasonic stethoscope can also be used to obtain blood pressure. It is especially useful when blood pressure sounds are difficult to hear, such as with infants or very obese consumers.

E

1. Ensure that the consumer has not had any caffeine or tobacco products in the past 30 minutes. Allow the consumer to rest for 5 minutes before you take the blood pressure.
2. Select an appropriate size cuff.
3. Position the consumer. The consumer may be sitting, standing or supine. At the first encounter, all three positions are recommended.
4. Position the arm or leg to be used so that the extremity is at a level equal to the heart to prevent a false reading (**Figure 6.19**). At subsequent encounters, the sitting position is usually the position of choice. Ensure that the consumer's feet are firmly on the floor in this position.
5. Apply the deflated blood pressure (BP) cuff:
    a. Upper arm: Wrap the BP cuff snugly around the bare upper arm. The bottom of the BP cuff should be 3 to 5 cm above the antecubital fossa. The centre of the bladder should be directly above the brachial artery.
    b. Leg: Wrap the BP cuff around the bare thigh, with the bottom of the BP cuff slightly above the knee. The popliteal artery below the cuff is used for BP measurement. This is usually easier if the consumer is in the prone position.
6. Establish a baseline systolic blood pressure (palpating the blood pressure), if needed:
    a. Palpate the brachial or radial artery with the finger pads of your nondominant hand distal to the BP cuff.
    b. Inflate the BP cuff, and note when the artery pulsation is no longer palpable.
    c. Release the air from the BP cuff, and wait 1 to 2 minutes.
7. Palpate the pulse distal to the BP cuff.
8. Place the bell of the stethoscope over the blood pressure site (the diaphragm may be used if sounds are hard to hear):
    a. If a Doppler ultrasonic stethoscope is to be used, apply conducting gel to the site where the pulse was palpated.
    b. Place the Doppler transducer over the site.
9. Inflate the BP cuff to approximately 20 mmHg above the established baseline blood pressure or 20 mmHg above where the Korotkoff sounds disappear.
10. Slowly open the valve and release the pressure at a rate of 2 to 3 mmHg per second.
11. Listen for the Korotkoff sounds:
    a. Onset of Korotkoff sounds correlates to systolic pressure.
    b. Muffling or disappearance of sounds correlates to diastolic pressures.
12. Deflate the BP cuff completely.
13. Record the blood pressure reading(s). The extremity used and position of the consumer are important data to record along with the blood pressure reading. Refer to Clinical reasoning practice tip: Accurate documentation of blood pressure.

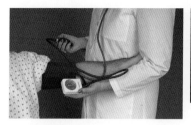

A. When taking a blood pressure measurement, the nurse can manually elevate the arm to the level of the consumer's heart.

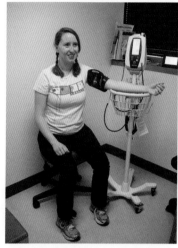

B. The nurse can also rest a consumer's elevated arm at the level of the heart using equipment. Note that this seated consumer has her feet resting on the floor.

FIGURE 6.19 Measuring a consumer's blood pressure

E Examination   **N** Normal findings   **A** Abnormal findings   **P** Pathophysiology

TABLE 6.5 Normal blood pressure range according to age and sex*

AGE (FEMALE)	SYSTOLIC (MMHG)	DIASTOLIC (MMHG)
1	97–103	52–56
5	103–109	66–70
10	112–118	73–76
15	120–127	78–81
≥ 18	< 120	< 80
AGE (MALE)	**SYSTOLIC (MMHG)**	**DIASTOLIC (MMHG)**
1	94–103	49–54
5	104–112	65–70
10	111–119	73–78
15	122–131	76–81
≥ 18	< 120	< 80

*The measurements listed for paediatric consumers are included; however blood pressure is not taken routinely for children unless they are in ICU or in a critical condition.

TABLE 6.6 Errors in blood pressure measurement

IF READING SHOWS	SUSPECT
inaccurately high blood pressure	Blood pressure cuff is too short or too narrow (e.g. using a regular blood pressure cuff on an obese arm), or the brachial artery may be positioned below the heart. The consumer may also be stressed, be in an emotional state, or have just completed physical activity.
high diastolic blood pressure	Unrecognised **auscultatory gap** (a silent interval between systolic and diastolic pressures that may occur in hypertensive consumers or because you deflated the blood pressure cuff too rapidly); immediate reinflation of the blood pressure cuff for multiple blood pressure readings (resultant venous congestion makes the Korotkoff sounds less audible). If the consumer supports his or her own arm, then sustained muscular contraction can raise the diastolic blood pressure by 10%.
inaccurately low blood pressure	Blood pressure cuff is too long or too wide; the brachial artery is above the heart.
low systolic blood pressure	Unrecognised auscultatory gap (a rapid deflation of the cuff or immediate reinflation of the cuff for multiple readings can result in venous congestion, thus making the Korotkoff sounds less audible and the pressure appear lower).

CLINICAL REASONING

Practice tip: Accurate documentation of blood pressure

It is important to record the position of the consumer during the blood pressure measurement, as there can be differences (e.g. sitting and standing can have a marked difference), and identify postural hypotension. Document consumer position as follows:

> supine
> sitting or standing

Also, record where the blood pressure was taken. Use the following abbreviations:

> RA = (right arm)   LA = (left arm)
> RL = (right leg)   LL = (left leg)

Examples of blood pressure readings are:

> 160/122 mmHg LL (supine)
> 98/52 mmHg RA (sitting)
> 118/85 mmHg LA (standing)

CLINICAL REASONING

Practice tip: Palpating the blood pressure

If you are unable to hear a consumer's blood pressure and there is no electronic monitor or amplification device available, you can use the palpation method. Conduct the blood pressure measurement as described in steps 1–6 using the brachial artery. When releasing air from the cuff, note when the brachial artery is palpable. This correlates with the systolic pressure. This blood pressure is then documented as a number over palpated (e.g. 115/palpated). It should also be noted that an audible BP reading was unable to be obtained.

TABLE 6.7 Classification of blood pressure in adults

DIAGNOSTIC CATEGORY[a]	SYSTOLIC (MMHG)		DIASTOLIC (MMHG)
Optimal	<120	and	<80
Normal	120–129	and/or	80–84
High-normal	130–139	and/or	85–89
Grade 1 (mild) hypertension	140–159	and/or	90–99
Grade 2 (moderate) hypertension	160–17	and/or	100–109
Grade 3 (severe) hypertension	≥180	and/or	≥110
Isolated systolic hypertension	>140	and	<90

[a] When a consumer's systolic and diastolic BP levels fall into different categories, the higher diagnostic category and recommended action/s apply.

SOURCE: NATIONAL HEART FOUNDATION OF AUSTRALIA. GUIDELINE FOR THE DIAGNOSIS AND MANAGEMENT OF HYPERTENSION IN ADULTS – 2016. MELBOURNE: NATIONAL HEART FOUNDATION OF AUSTRALIA, 2016.

N Normal blood pressure varies with age. As a person ages, blood pressure generally increases. **Table 6.5** presents general ranges for normal blood pressure at different ages. Normally, baroreceptors help a consumer to maintain normal blood pressure when changing from a supine to a sitting or a standing position. (Baroreceptors are the receptors located in the walls of most of the great arteries that sense hypotension and initiate reflex vasoconstriction and tachycardia to bring the blood pressure back to normal.) Processes that increase cardiac output, such as exercise, will normally increase blood pressure. Pulse pressure is normally 30 to 40 mmHg. **Table 6.6** lists errors in blood pressure measurement.

P **Hypertension**, or high blood pressure, is usually confirmed when an adult consumer has blood pressure readings remaining consistently above 120 mmHg systolic and 80 mmHg diastolic on two consecutive visits after an initial screening. See **Table 6.7** for the classification of hypertension.

P The cause of hypertension in 90% of consumers who have it is unknown. It is thought that the mechanisms that maintain the therapeutic fluid volume in the body (e.g. the heart, kidneys, nervous system, renin–angiotensin–aldosterone system) may be abnormal. The other 10% of the population with high blood pressure have secondary hypertension. All of the following pathophysiologies of hypertension are secondary in nature.

P Arteriosclerosis reduces arterial compliance. Elastic and muscular tissues of arteries are replaced with fibrous tissue as part of the normal ageing process, making the vessels less able to contract and relax in response to systolic and diastolic pressures. When the systolic pressure alone is elevated in the elderly, it is called isolated systolic hypertension.

P Processes decreasing the size of the arterial lumen cause hypertension. Hypercholesterolaemia results in deposits of plaque along the inner walls of the vessels, reducing the size of the arterial lumen and increasing blood pressure.

E Examination   **N** Normal findings   **A** Abnormal findings   **P** Pathophysiology

P Processes that increase the viscosity of the blood, such as sickle cell crisis, cause greater friction between molecules of the blood and, thus, higher blood pressure.

P Chronic steroid use, Cushing syndrome, thyroid disease and parathyroid dysfunction can all cause hypertension.

P High blood pressure may result from diseases affecting other regulatory blood pressure processes. For example, kidney disease, which affects the production of antidiuretic hormone, a hormone that helps control body fluid balance, can cause hypertension. An adrenal gland tumour, or phaeochromocytoma, can increase blood pressure because of adrenaline and noradrenaline secretion.

P Overload of fluids from poor renal function or indiscriminate intravenous fluid administration (particularly in children) can result in hypertension.

P Stress can increase blood pressure. Stimulation of the sympathetic nervous system increases cardiac output and vasoconstriction, thus increasing blood pressure.

P A consumer's stress level can increase when in the presence of a healthcare provider. Consumers who have elevated blood pressure in an office or hospital environment only are said to have 'white coat syndrome'. When these individuals have their blood pressure taken in the community, it is frequently within an acceptable range.

A Blood pressure falling below normal range is considered to be hypotension, or low blood pressure, which results in inadequate tissue perfusion and oxygenation. If the standing systolic blood pressure is more than 30 mmHg below the supine systolic pressure, it may indicate that the person has orthostatic hypotension. (See Chapter 14.) Slow response by baroreceptors when an individual transitions from a lying to a standing position can result in transitory orthostatic hypotension. When this occurs, the individual may feel dizzy and is at risk for falls.

P Processes drastically reducing circulatory blood volume, such as hypovolaemic shock, cause hypotension.

P Medications such as nitroglycerine (glyceryl trinitrate) and antihypertensives lower blood pressure.

P Anaphylactic shock, resulting from massive histamine release, and circulatory collapse cause severe hypotension.

A A difference of greater than 10 to 15 mmHg between the blood pressure in each arm is abnormal.

P This difference in blood pressure between arms can be caused by coarctation of the aorta, aortic aneurysm, atherosclerotic obstruction, and subclavian steal syndrome. These conditions all result in an increased pressure proximal to the narrowing and a decreased pressure distal to the narrowing of the aorta or whatever is causing the obstruction.

A A systolic blood pressure that is greater in the arms than in the legs is abnormal.

P This blood pressure difference between the arms and the legs is caused by constriction or obstruction of the aorta, which can result from an increase in stroke volume ejection velocity, increased cardiac output, peripheral vasodilation, and decreased distensibility of the aorta or major arteries.

A A decreased pulse pressure is abnormal.

P A decreased pulse pressure can result from a decreased stroke volume (cardiac tamponade, shock and tachycardia) or increased peripheral resistance (aortic stenosis, coarctation of the aorta, mitral stenosis or mitral regurgitation, and cardiac tamponade).

A An increased pulse pressure is abnormal.

P An increased pulse pressure can result from increased stroke volume (aortic regurgitation) or increased peripheral vasodilation (fever, anaemia, heat, exercise, hyperthyroidism and arteriovenous fistula).

E Examination **N** Normal findings **A** Abnormal findings **P** Pathophysiology

CLINICAL **REASONING**

Practice tip: Automatic blood pressure cuffs – decreasing complications

If your consumer is receiving a drug such as heparin, aspirin or other thrombolytic therapy, this makes them susceptible to bleeding complications (**Figure 6.20**). If you are using an automatic blood pressure cuff on a consumer who is having thrombolytic therapy, take the following precautions to prevent any bleeding complications that may occur in the arm that is being used for non-invasive blood pressure monitoring:

> Adjust the maximal inflation pressure on the automatic blood pressure machine to the individuals' last systolic blood pressure. Otherwise, the blood pressure cuff could inflate as high as a systolic blood pressure of 200 mmHg.

> Once your consumer's blood pressure is stable, increase the intervals between measurements. If you do not, the blood pressure cuff could inflate as often as every minute. Also, you can switch the mode from automatic to manual, so that you avoid unnecessary inflations of the blood pressure cuff.

> Place the blood pressure cuff on the arm opposite any intravenous infusions. If this is not possible, then try the thigh as a site for blood pressure measurement.

> Whenever permissible, rotate the cuff site and remember to remove it at least every shift to assess the consumer's skin.

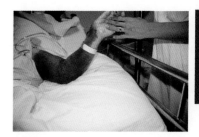

FIGURE 6.20 Proper placement and monitoring of an automatic blood pressure cuff will reduce the risk of injury or trauma to the consumer. This Caucasian consumer had an automatic blood pressure cuff placed on the left arm while also receiving a heparin infusion in that arm.

Oxygen saturation (SpO$_2$)

Haemoglobin is responsible for transporting oxygen from the lungs to other parts of the body, where the oxygen can be used by other cells. Oxyhaemoglobin (HbO$_2$) is the bright red haemoglobin that is a combination of haemoglobin and oxygen from the lungs. One haemoglobin molecule can carry a maximum of four oxygen molecules. One hundred haemoglobin molecules together carry a maximum of 400 (100 × 4) oxygen molecules. If these 100 haemoglobin molecules were carrying 380 oxygen molecules they would be carrying (380/400) × 100 = 95% of the maximum number of oxygen molecules. Thus, this would be 95% saturation. When arterial oxyhaemoglobin saturation is measured non-invasively by a pulse oximetry device, the symbol is charted as SpO$_2$ (Berman, Snyder, Frandsen, Kozier & Kozier, 2020).

Reasons for assessing a consumer's oxygen saturation

There are multiple reasons for low oxygen saturation, including cardiovascular disease, chronic obstructive pulmonary disease, pneumonia, cardiomyopathy and dehydration. When the bloodstream does not receive enough oxygen from either the lungs or the heart, or a disease or illness is depleting the oxygen from the bloodstream, the organs and the brain suffer. Injury and blood loss will also cause low oxygen saturation.

Central cyanosis, the traditional clinical sign of **hypoxaemia**, is an insensitive marker, occurring only at 75–80% saturation. Consequently, pulse oximetry has a wide range of applications including:

> individual pulse oximetry readings that can be invaluable in clinical situations where hypoxaemia may be a factor; for example, in a confused elderly person

> continuous recording that can be used during **anaesthesia** or sedation, or to assess hypoxaemia during sleep studies to diagnose obstructive sleep apnoea

> pulse oximetry that can replace blood gas analysis in many clinical situations unless PaCO$_2$ or acid–base state is needed

> pulse oximetry that assists with determining the effectiveness of O$_2$ supplementation usage

> neonatal care – the safety limits for oxygen saturation are higher and narrower (95–97%) than those of adults.

Measuring oxygen saturation (pulse oximetry)

Pulse oximeters give a non-invasive estimate of the arterial haemoglobin oxygen saturation. A probe with LEDs (light-emitting diodes) is used to generate red and infrared light through a translucent part of the body. The probe is connected by a cable to an oximeter device and the light waves emitted by the LED are absorbed and then reflected back. The arteriolar bed normally pulsates and absorbs variable amounts of light during systole and diastole, as blood volume increases and decreases. The ratio of light absorbed at systole and diastole is translated into an oxygen saturation measurement. Oxygen saturation should always be above 95%, although in those with longstanding respiratory disease this may be lower corresponding to disease severity.

CLINICAL REASONING

Practice tip: Reasons for low oxygen levels
When assessing a consumer who has presented with respiratory symptoms, the following can indicate low oxygen levels:
> shortness of breath/difficulty breathing/dyspnoea
> extreme fatigue
> chest tightness
> tingling fingers
> water retention (especially feet and ankles)
> chronic cough
> mental confusion.

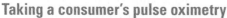

Taking a consumer's pulse oximetry

The oximeter probe can be applied to the earlobe, the toe, or the bridge of the nose; however, it is most commonly sited on a finger digit (Figure 6.21). These areas are highly vascular and this is a requirement of the oximeter device to detect the degree of change in the light transmitted.

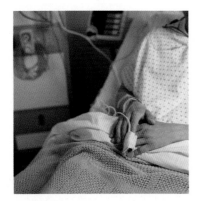

FIGURE 6.21 A consumer with a pulse oximeter probe attached to a finger digit
GETTY IMAGES/SEAN JUSTICE

1. Select the probe with particular attention to correct sizing and where it is to go. The digit should be clean (remove nail varnish).
2. Position the probe on the chosen site, avoiding excess force.
3. If a finger probe is used, the hand should be rested on the chest rather than held in the air, in order to minimise motion artefact.
4. Allow several seconds for the pulse oximeter to detect the pulse and calculate the oxygen saturation.
5. Look for a displayed waveform. Without this, any reading is meaningless.
6. Read off the displayed oxygen saturation and pulse rate.
   Be cautious interpreting figures where there has been an instantaneous change in saturation; for example, 99% falling suddenly to 85%. This is physiologically not possible.
7. If in doubt, rely on your clinical judgement, rather than the value given by the machine.
8. Record the pulse oximetry reading accurately.

URGENT FINDING

False SpO$_2$ when carbon monoxide poisoning is suspected
Consumers with suspected smoke inhalation or carbon monoxide poisoning will have an inaccurate pulse oximetry reading. This is because carbon monoxide attaches itself to haemoglobin molecules, preventing the uptake of oxygen molecules. The oximeter does not differentiate between oxyhaemoglobin or the haemoglobin molecules with carbon monoxide molecules attached. In this situation the oximeter will give a normal reading when this is not the case. This is a dangerous scenario so, for this reason, pulse oximetry should not be used on individuals who may have inhaled smoke (e.g. in a house fire). In these cases, urgent specialised blood tests (arterial blood gases) will need to be taken to identify accurate oxygenation levels.

Variables affecting pulse oximetry

The function of a pulse oximeter is affected by many variables.

> Poor positioning of the probe can cause inaccurate readings due to various problems. This can be a particular problem with very small fingers and very large ones. Make sure the probe is well on the finger.

> In the case of a consumer with cold hands and feet, and/or a very weak pulse, a pulse oximeter may display a reading that may not be accurate.

> An irregular heartbeat, or the consumer moving, shivering or fitting can cause inaccurate recordings of pulse oximetry readings.

> It should be noted that pulse oximetry does not give an indication of a consumer's ventilation, only their oxygenation status; therefore, it can give a false sense of security if supplemental oxygen is being given. In addition, there may be a delay between the occurrence of a potentially hypoxaemic event such as respiratory obstruction and a pulse oximeter detecting low oxygen saturation.

> It is important to remember that pulse oximetry is only one way of monitoring breathing. It is also necessary, as a minimum, to record respiratory rate and, if pulse oximetry is used, the amount of oxygen they are receiving *must* be recorded.

> A single one-off reading often is not much use; trends over a period of time give more information.

> As with all clinical assessments the 'whole picture' must be looked at.

(Adapted from Berman et al., 2020)

REFLECTION IN PRACTICE

Using clinical judgement when taking vital signs

Mr Godfrey is a 75-year-old man hospitalised for pneumonia. He has a history of confusion and combative behaviour, particularly at night. His IV had to be replaced last night because, in his confusion and agitation, he pulled it out. You are working the night shift, and it is 2:00 a.m.

Mr Godfrey is in a sound sleep, and appears comfortable. He has vital signs ordered to be taken every 4 hours. His vital signs were last taken at 10:00 p.m. and were as follows:

> Respirations: 14 per minute
> Pulse: 90 beats per minute
> Blood pressure: 132/88 mmHg LA (supine)
> Temperature: 37.1°C (aural)
> SpO_2 98%, on a Hudson mask at 8 L/min.
> What are the major issues related to completing Mr Godfrey's vital signs at this present time?
> What are the possible actions you could take, and what are the potential consequences of each?

CLINICAL **REASONING**

Providing end-of-life care

The majority of Australians over 65 die in healthcare facilities, with 50% dying in the acute care setting, 36% in residential aged care facilities, and 14% dying elsewhere (AIHW, 2021). Providing care to people who are near the end of life includes quality-of-life considerations, and care that focuses on assessing the physical, psychosocial and spiritual needs of the individual and their families.

Identifying that a person is in the last days or weeks of life can be challenging, and the withdrawing of treatment can be a complex process. However, there are guidelines and polices available to aid healthcare professionals to provide the best care for the dying person (CareSearch, 2021). Care of an individual who is imminently dying involves both

>>

clinical and ethical considerations, and care based on the needs of the person and their specific clinical context. The individual's needs will vary depending on age, disease status, and social and cultural context. The Australian Commission on Safety and Quality in Health Care (2021) has developed guidelines on delivering comprehensive end-of-life care for different settings, to ensure appropriate person- and family-centred care.

Assessing and planning care for the dying person is based on the fundamental principles of recognising dying, communication and decision-making, and encompasses reviewing the individual's:

> medical condition and care
> need for interventions
> personal care needs, such as bathing and feeding.

It also involves:

> communicating with the dying person, family/carer(s), including explanation of the plan of care
> documentation completed as per local health service documentation policies.

The key concerns for a person at the end of life relate to:

> pain and symptom management
> preparation for the end of life
> relationships between the consumer, family members and healthcare providers
> achieving a sense of completion (Steinhauser et al., 2000).

Assessing and managing a person at end of life does not necessarily imply use of equipment or invasive tests. However, assessing changes in signs and symptoms can be gathered from talking with, observing and examining the individual. Symptom management is specific to the person who is dying and their response to care interventions. Assessment is based on signs and symptoms of:

> pain
> restlessness and agitation
> skin integrity
> fever
> nausea and/or vomiting
> respiratory secretions
> breathlessness
> emotional or psychological distress.

Examples of signs and symptoms that are suggestive that a person is in the final stage of end of life include agitation, Cheyne–Stokes breathing, deterioration in level of consciousness, mottled skin, and noisy respiratory secretion.

Further information can be obtained from the following:

> AIHW (Australian Institute of Health and Welfare). (2021). Interfaces between the aged care and health systems in Australia – where do older Australians die? (June). Retrieved from https://www.aihw.gov.au/getmedia/56c1f616-8b2c-493e-8e1c-2db5083ad59d/aihw-age-106.pdf.aspx?inline=true
> Australian Commission on Safety and Quality in Health Care. (2021). Delivering and supporting comprehensive end-of-life care: a user guide. Sydney: ACSQHC. Retrieved from https://www.safetyandquality.gov.au/our-work/end-life-care
> CareSearch. (2021). Care of the dying person – clinical evidence – finding evidence – evidence. Retrieved from https://www.caresearch.com.au/tabid/6220/Default.aspx
> Palliative Care Australia. (2018). National Palliative Care Standards (5th ed). Retrieved from https://palliativecare.org.au/wp-content/uploads/dlm_uploads/2018/02/PalliativeCare-National-Standards-2018_web-3.pdf

PAIN

Pain is 'an unpleasant sensory and emotional experience associated with, or resembling that associated with, actual or potential tissue damage' (IASP, 2020). It is a complex sensory experience that has received significant clinical attention over the last 40 years. Pain has become the focus of many clinical research projects as a single clinical phenomenon, not just as a symptom of clinical pathology.

Perception of pain

Pain is a unique, subjective, personal experience that most people experience some time in their lives. There is a small percentage of people who do not feel pain due to a genetic condition (Hellier, 2016). Pain affects a person's physical, psychological and social being. It is vital to remember that not every person experiences the same level of pain in response to similar stimuli. Sometimes the source of the pain cannot be identified, and this may be due to the result of multi-layered brain systems.

A person's response to pain can be influenced by their previous pain experience, their mood, beliefs about pain, culture and their ability to cope. Pain is what an individual perceives it to be; so it is important to remember that a consumer's report is the most reliable indicator of their pain status.

Source of pain

The source of the pain refers to its origin in the body. Pain can be grouped by its origin as well as its duration. Cutaneous, somatic, visceral and referred pain are the types of pain grouped by origin. Cutaneous pain arises from the stimulation of cutaneous nerves. This pain usually has a burning quality. Somatic pain originates from bone, tendons, ligaments, muscles and nerves, and is frequently caused by musculoskeletal injury. Visceral pain arises from the organs. Diseased organs can change size, usually resulting in stretching of the organ, leading to pain. Acute appendicitis is an example of visceral pain. Referred pain is perceived in a location other than where the pathology is occurring. The location of the referred pain is in the dermatome of the spinal cord that is innervating the affected viscera and where the organ was located in its embryonic stage. An example of referred pain is the pain of pancreatitis felt on the left shoulder.

Pain pathophysiology comprises two categories: nociceptive and neuropathic. It is important to identify which category of pain a consumer is experiencing as treatment is different for each.

Nociceptive pain

Nociceptive pain arises from somatic or visceral stimulation. **Nociception**, or pain perception, is a multistep process that involves the nervous system as well as other body systems **(Figure 6.22)**. A noxious stimulus occurs, which stimulates the **nociceptors** (receptive neurones of pain sensation that are located in the skin and various viscera). The noxious stimulus can be many things (e.g. trauma, burn, chemical exposure, internal body inflammation, internal body growth of tissue). Transduction of the noxious stimulus travels to the spinal cord via the nociceptors. This transduction causes the conversion of one energy (travelling stimulus) from another (noxious stimulus). Cell damage from the noxious stimulus causes the release of certain chemicals or sensitising nociceptors. Prostaglandins (PG), bradykinins (BK), serotonin (5 HT), substance P (SP), hydrogen (H^+), potassium (K^+), histamine (H) and leukotrienes are all sensitising substances. Substance P is unique because it is released only when pain fibres are stimulated.

Activating the sensitising substances leads to an action potential in which the pain sensation is moved via afferent nerves to the spinal cord. Two types of nerve fibres participate in the action potential: A-delta fibres, myelinated neurones that transmit acute, sharp, shooting and localised pain; and C fibres, nonmyelinated

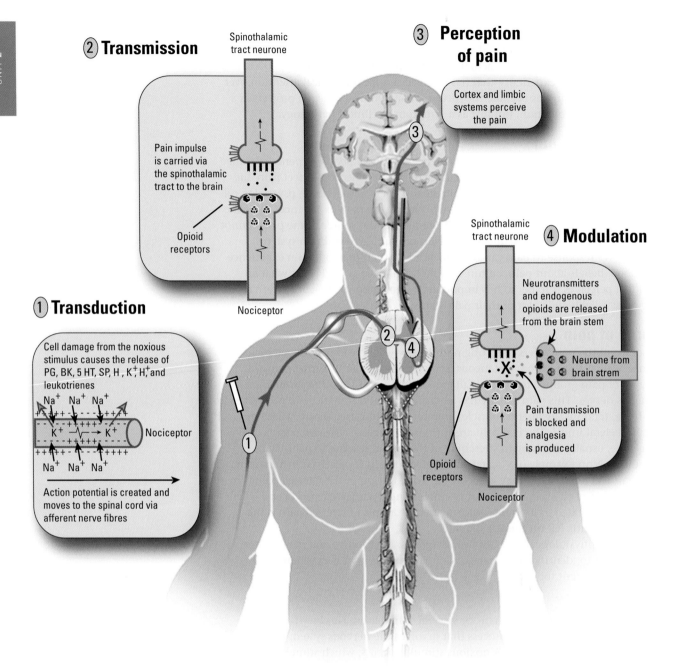

② **Transmission**

Spinothalamic
tract neurone

Pain impulse
is carried via
the spinothalamic
tract to the brain

Opioid
receptors

Nociceptor

③ **Perception
of pain**

Cortex and limbic
systems perceive
the pain

③

① **Transduction**

Cell damage from the noxious
stimulus causes the release of
PG, BK, 5 HT, SP, H , K^+,H^+,and
leukotrienes

Na^+ Na^+ Na^+

K^+ $\longrightarrow$ K^+ Nociceptor

Na^+ Na^+ Na^+

Action potential is created and
moves to the spinal cord via
afferent nerve fibres

② ④

①

④ **Modulation**

Spinothalamic
tract neurone

Neurotransmitters
and endogenous
opioids are released
from the brain stem

Neurone from
brain strem

X

Pain transmission
is blocked and
analgesia
is produced

Opioid
receptors

Nociceptor

FIGURE 6.22 Nociception

neurones that transmit dull, throbbing, and poorly localised pain. These nerve
fibres carry the pain impulse from the spinal cord via the spinothalamic tract to the
brain stem and thalamus. The thalamus relays information to the cortex (which
is capable of identifying past pain memories) and to the limbic system (where the
emotional component of pain is formed). It is in these areas of the brain that pain is
consciously perceived.

The last step of nociception is modulation. Modulation is the inhibition of
nociceptor impulses. Neurones from the brain stem release neurotransmitters
(e.g. serotonin, norepinephrine [NE], gamma-aminobutyric acid [GABA], 5 HT,
and endogenous opioids [e.g. enkephalins, dynorphins and β-endorphins]) as the
pain message descends from the brain stem to the spinal cord. Collectively, these
substances block the transmission of pain and produce analgesia.

Neuropathic pain

Neuropathic pain can result from injury or lesions in the central nervous system (CNS) or the peripheral nervous system (PNS). This can cause **paraesthesia**, such as numbness, tingling, electrical or burning sensations, for example that experienced with lower back pain or herpes zoster. Neuropathic pain may be difficult to treat clinically; however, with careful diagnosis and use of combination treatments, there is an excellent chance of improving the pain and the consumer returning to normal function.

Types of pain

Acute, cancer and chronic (persistent) pain is pain that is grouped by duration. Acute pain has a sudden onset, a duration of 3–6 months and has a likely limited duration. It ranges in intensity from mild to severe. It usually has an identifiable cause, such as surgery or trauma. Cancer pain is pain of more than 6 months duration. This persistent pain can be due to a tumour, inflammation, blocked ducts, pressure on other body parts, treatment and necrosis. Chronic (persistent) pain also lasts more than 6 months. It can occur with and without an identifiable cause. The pain can remain even after an initial injury is healed. Back pain and fibromyalgia are examples of chronic (persistent) pain.

Variables affecting pain

A consumer's past response to pain, as well as successful pain reduction measures, greatly influence future pain management. Indeed a consumer's age, sex, previous experience with pain, and cultural expectations can affect their response to pain.

Age

Studies indicate that pain is perceived by our youngest members of society – neonates. As children grow, they learn how to respond to pain by modelling others' behaviours, and pain management can be learned via direct and indirect observation. Children can learn how to communicate their pain (crying/verbalising), when to seek help, and whom they should seek out for care. As they reach adolescence, children may become more stoic about pain.

Older adults, especially those who have chronic pain, may also not complain about their pain until it becomes debilitating. This failure to seek treatment for pain is frequently due to the perception that the pain means something is seriously wrong, or the consumer may not have the resources to seek treatment. Older adults also have a lifetime of experiences with different types of pain, and that greatly influences how they choose to deal with new pain. Conditions such as hearing loss, loss of speech, and aphasia can all hamper communication of needs regarding pain. Further, older individuals with cognitive impairment may not have the capacity to give a reliable report during assessment. To conduct a comprehensive assessment, include the consumer's self-report and the caregiver's report, and observe the person using pain assessment tools during your assessment. Behaviours that suggest that pain is present are changes in facial expressions, vocalisations, changes in activity patterns and interpersonal interactions.

Sex

Studies have shown that females have a lower pain tolerance or threshold than males and report pain more frequently. Females tend to dwell on the psychological aspects of pain, whereas males emphasise its physiological aspects (Keogh, 2014; Keogh & Arendt-Nielsen, 2004). In many cultures, men stoically endure pain without seeking medical help, whereas women express pain more openly and verbally.

Culture

A cultural group's norms, expectations and acceptance of pain as a normal part of life can influence how a person experiences pain. This can be further shaped by their individual experiences and learnings. It is important to approach each consumer in a culturally safe way. Refer to Chapter 4 for more detailed information on cultural safety.

Healthcare professionals

A healthcare professional's knowledge of pain management may affect how the person in pain is treated. Studies have shown that there is a deficiency of adequate education regarding pain management for healthcare professionals (Watt-Watson et al., 2002). Gender differences between healthcare professionals and the person in pain may also determine differences in treatments (Safdar et al., 2009). Poorer management for their pain may be provided to females, ethnic and racial populations (Burgess et al., 2014). Collaboration between the consumer in pain and the healthcare professional can lead to improved care.

Effects of pain on the body

Pain affects everyone in different ways. Acute pain usually manifests itself differently from chronic (persistent) pain, although there are some common elements. Physiological responses to pain occur during the acute stage of pain. These include tachycardia, tachypnoea, hypertension, diaphoresis, dilated pupils and an altered immune response. Additional responses to pain include complaints of pain, crying, moaning, frowning, anger, fear, anxiety, depression, suicidal ideation, decreased appetite, sleep deprivation, altered concentration, pacing, rubbing the affected body part, and protecting or splinting the affected body part. These responses to pain are by no means all-inclusive. Pain can affect every system in the human body, and unrelieved pain can take its toll on the health of the consumer over time. Just as pain is a unique experience for the person in pain, so is the consumer's response to pain.

Pain assessment

A comprehensive pain assessment should be conducted on each consumer in a healthcare setting. Further, a consumer should be referred for a pain assessment as determined by their health status and the availability of care. Pain is to be measured in terms of intensity and quality appropriate to the consumer's age and then documented in their records. Pain is a critical vital sign of a consumer's wellbeing, thus assessment of pain is mandatory.

Many consumers present to the healthcare system with a principal complaint of pain. Assessing pain comprehensively is commonly guided by a framework such as the mnemonic OPQRST: Onset, Position/Palliates, Quality, Radiates, Severity, Time + Treatment. This is a useful tool for people who can self-report pain (ensure you consider age, verbal and cognitive ability).

The approach using OPQRST as an assessment tool

> *Onset* – did anything provoke the pain: 'What were you doing when the pain started (exercise, activity, resting)?' 'Was it a sudden or gradual onset, or an ongoing chronic issue?'
> *Position or Palliates* – the site of the pain: 'Where is the pain?' 'What makes the pain better or worse?'
> *Quality* – a description of the pain: 'What does the pain feel like?' 'What words would you use to describe the pain (sharp/ dull/crushing)?'
> *Radiates* – does the pain radiate: 'Point to where it hurts the most. Where does your pain go from there?' 'Does the pain move anywhere else?'
> *Severity* – it is important to remember that pain is subjective and relative to each individual consumer. 'On a scale of 1 to 10, 1 being minimal pain and 10 the worst pain imaginable, how would you rate your pain?'
> *Time* – this is a reference to when the pain started or how long ago it started: 'When did the pain start?' 'How long did it last for?'
> *Treatment* – self-treatment: 'Have you attempted to relieve the pain?' 'Have you taken any medication for it?'

(Adapted from Ahmadi et al., 2016; and Hui & Bruera, 2014)

Many healthcare institutions have their own pain assessment flow sheet that incorporates these main pain assessment features.

Pain intensity rating scales are available to assess the severity of a consumer's pain experience (**Figure 6.23**). The Visual Analog Scale (VAS) is perhaps the easiest to use in any setting because it requires no additional resources. The VAS contains a 10 cm line; one end is labelled 'no pain' and the other end is labelled 'most severe pain imaginable'. The consumer indicates where on the spectrum their pain currently lies. This is noted and used as a reference for current and future pain assessment to trend the consumer's verbal reports of pain.

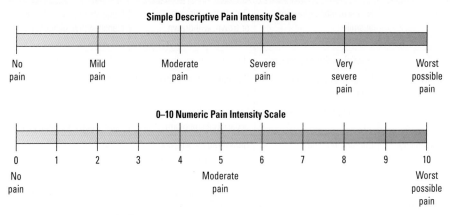

FIGURE 6.23 Pain Intensity Scale

SOURCE: *ACUTE PAIN MANAGEMENT: OPERATIVE OR MEDICAL PROCEDURES AND TRAUMA*. QUICK REFERENCE GUIDE NO. 1A. CLINICAL PRACTICE GUIDELINE (AHCPR PUBLICATION NO. 92-0032), BY THE ACUTE PAIN MANAGEMENT GUIDELINE PANEL, 1992, ROCKVILLE, MD: AGENCY FOR HEALTH CARE POLICY AND RESEARCH [NOW AGENCY FOR HEALTHCARE RESEARCH AND QUALITY].

Categorical pain intensity scales include:

> the Pain Intensity Scale (Acute Pain Management Guideline Panel, 1992) (**Figure 6.23**), a quick and easy tool to implement

> the Faces, Legs, Activity, Cry and Consolability (FLACC) pain scale, used for children 6 months to 5 years who cannot verbalise (**Table 6.8**). This scale, initially used to assess post-operative pain levels in children, is also accurate and reliable in all children with pain (Kochman et al., 2017).

> the Wong–Baker FACES Pain Rating Scale (**Figure 6.24**), is recommended for children over the age of 3 years. It is important that the nurse explains this scale to the child at each assessment encounter.

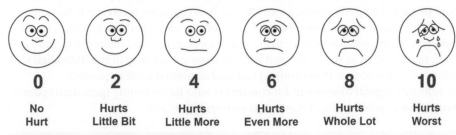

FIGURE 6.24 Wong–Baker FACES Pain Rating Scale

* Please note you may also see a FACES pain scale that is endorsed by the International Association for the Study of Pain (IASP) at http://www.iasp-pain.org/Education/Content.aspx?ItemNumber=1519

SOURCE: © 1983 WONG-BAKER FACES FOUNDATION. WWW.WONGBAKERFACES.ORG. USED WITH PERMISSION. ORIGINALLY PUBLISHED IN *WHALEY & WONG'S NURSING CARE OF INFANTS AND CHILDREN*. © ELSEVIER INC.

With each scale, the consumer has control over each of his or her own pain assessment encounters. These reports can provide information on whether the individual's pain is alleviating or worsening. This information also allows the nurse to evaluate the effectiveness of the consumer's pain regimen.

Assessing pain in consumers who are unable to communicate poses a challenge for nurses (Hockenberry & Wilson, 2018). Many pain tools have been developed and tested to assist in these situations. For example, the FLACC tool, which assesses behaviour (Table 6.8) is useful. Another example is the Abbey Pain Scale, which measures pain in consumers with dementia who cannot verbalise (Abbey et al., 2004). These tools have been found to be valid and reliable pain measurement scales.

TABLE 6.8 FLACC Behavioural Scale

CATEGORIES	SCORING		
	0	1	2
Face	No particular expression or smile	Occasional grimace or frown; withdrawn, disinterested	Frequent to constant frown, clenched jaw, quivering chin
Legs	Normal position or relaxed	Uneasy, restless, tense	Kicking or legs drawn up
Activity	Lying quietly, normal position, moves easily	Squirming, shifting back and forth, tense	Arched, rigid or jerking
Cry	No cry (awake or asleep)	Moans or whimpers, occasional complaint	Crying steadily, screams or sobs; frequent complaints
Consolability	Content, relaxed	Reassured by occasional touching, hugging, or being talked to; distractible	Difficult to console or comfort

Note: Each of the five categories Face, Legs, Activity, Cry and Consolability is scored from 0 to 2, which results in a total score between 0 and 10.
SOURCE: COPYRIGHT © 2002, THE REGENTS OF THE UNIVERSITY OF MICHIGAN. ALL RIGHTS RESERVED.

Pain management

One of the most difficult and challenging clinical practice areas is pain management. Acute pain can often be treated with various interventions and is relatively short lived. This is not the case with chronic pain from any aetiology. Ideally, cancer pain and chronic (persistent) pain should be managed in an interdisciplinary team environment that includes the consumer and their family. The goal is to have the individual's pain managed with pharmacological and non-pharmacological treatments, to allow them to achieve the highest level of functioning possible.

Treatment approaches to pain (acute and chronic) can include pharmacological measures that are appropriate for the type of pain; for example, analgesics, anti-epileptics, nonsteroidal anti-inflammatories and opioids, just to name a few. Non-pharmacological interventions include physical therapy, application of hot/ cold therapy, and psychological measures such as cognitive behavioural therapy.

The goal cannot always be to alleviate all of the consumer's pain. Some chronic pain conditions, such as osteoarthritis and diabetic peripheral neuropathy, have no cure. In cases such as these, the goal is to decrease the severity of the individual's pain symptoms so that the consumer can lead as normal a life as possible. Conducting regular assessment for consumers who have chronic (persistent) pain is imperative to achieve this, because it is an ongoing process.

REFLECTION IN PRACTICE

Communicating appropriately in difficult situations
You are working in the community health clinic, taking a health history from a new female consumer. She states that she has had acute lower back pain for the past 2 years. She tells you 'I want a really strong medication because my pain is really bad. Do not tell me to use hot packs. I know how stingy you people can be giving the good stuff.'
> What questions would you ask her?
> How would you proceed?

CHAPTER RESOURCES

REVIEW QUESTIONS

For answers to these questions, see Answer section at the end of the book.

1. You are assessing a consumer's physical status and note that the consumer looks thin and frail. What condition might this consumer have?
   a. Cushing syndrome
   b. Hypokinetic state
   c. Malabsorption disease
   d. Hypothyroidism

2. Smelling an alcohol odour on a consumer may indicate which of the following conditions?
   a. Vaginal infection
   b. Allergic rhinitis
   c. Tonsillitis
   d. Ketoacidosis

3. Which of the following is true about the pulse rate?
   a. Parasympathetic stimulation causes an increase in pulse rate.
   b. Medications such as digoxin can increase the pulse rate.
   c. Caffeine and tobacco decrease the pulse rate.
   d. The sinoatrial node is the primary controller of pulse rate.

4. You are assessing a consumer who has just presented to the emergency room after being knocked off his bike. You have just completed taking his vital signs and record his temperature as T 36.2°C (tympanic). What conclusion do you make about the consumer's temperature?
   a. The consumer's temperature is within normal limits.
   b. The rectal route is the best method to use in a trauma consumer to determine temperature.
   c. Tympanic thermometers are inaccurate if the consumer has lost a lot of blood.
   d. The Celsius scale is the most accurate scale to use when documenting temperature.

5. The nurse counts 10 respirations in 1 minute while the consumer is asleep. What assessment does the nurse make about this consumer?
   a. The consumer has obstructive sleep apnoea.
   b. The consumer has bradypnoea.
   c. The consumer is hypoxic.
   d. The consumer is stressed.

6. Your consumer is connected to a heart monitor and you recognise their electrical rhythm as atrial fibrillation. You also palpate the consumer's carotid pulse. Which of the following describes the rhythm of the heart rate and pulse?
   a. Regular
   b. Regularly regular
   c. Regularly irregular
   d. Irregularly irregular

7. A consumer's pulse volume is documented as 1+/4+. This means the consumer's pulse is:
   a. Absent
   b. Thready
   c. Normal
   d. Bounding

8. The nurse takes a consumer's blood pressure at the clinic. The blood pressure is 84/55. The consumer states that this is very low for him. The nurse suspects that an error has occurred during the blood pressure measurement. Which of the following can cause an inaccurately low blood pressure?
   a. The blood pressure cuff is too large.
   b. The consumer smoked a cigarette five minutes before the measurement was taken.
   c. The blood pressure cuff is too small.
   d. The brachial artery was positioned below the heart.

9. The nurse obtains a blood pressure of 138/92 mmHg on a consumer's right arm while he is in the sitting position. What blood pressure classification characterises this reading?
   a. Normal
   b. Prehypertension
   c. Stage 1 hypertension
   d. Stage 2 hypertension

10. Neuropathic pain is characterised by which of the following?
    a. A change in organ size, such as in acute appendicitis
    b. Left shoulder pain that is felt during pancreatitis
    c. A sudden onset that is life-limiting after surgery
    d. A burning or tingling, such as with herpes zoster

11. Which of these statements is not a misconception regarding pain?
    a. Medication is the only treatment to be used for pain.
    b. Consumers will always tell the nurse when they are in pain.
    c. The consumer should expect to have pain while in hospital.
    d. Pain is whatever the experiencing person reports.

12. Considerations during an assessment of pain in older people are that they:
    a. Have a decreased pain threshold
    b. Have a reduction in their sensory perception
    c. Have an alteration in their mental function
    d. Are expected to experience chronic pain

CS CLINICAL SKILLS

The following Clinical Skills are relevant to this chapter and can be found in Tollefson & Hillman, *Clinical Psychomotor Skills,* 8th edition:
> 10 Temperature, pulse and respiration measurement
> 11 Blood pressure measurement
> 12 Monitoring pulse oximetry
> 13 Pain assessment
> 19 Focused respiratory health history assessment and physical assessment
> 23 Height, weight (BMI) and waist circumference measurement
> Part 8: Pain management
> 75 Non-pharmacological pain management interventions – therapeutic massage
> 76 Non-pharmacological pain management interventions – conventional transcutaneous electrical nerve stimulation.

FURTHER RESOURCES

> Australian Pain Management Association: http://www.painmanagement.org.au/
> Heart Foundation (Australia) – Information for Professionals: http://www.heartfoundation.org.au/Information-for-professionals/pages/information-professionals.aspx
> Heart Foundation (New Zealand): http://www.heartfoundation.org.nz/

> International Association for the Study of Pain: http://www.iasp-pain.org
> New Zealand Pain Society: http://www.nzps.org.nz/
> World Health Organization Palliative WHO's Cancer Pain Ladder: http://www.who.int/cancer/palliative/painladder/en/

REFERENCES

Abbey, J., Piller, N., De Bellis, A., Esterman, A., Parker, D., Giles, L., & Lowcary B. (2004).The Abbey Pain Scale: A 1 minute numerical indicator for people with end stage dementia. *Palliative Nursing, 10,* 6–13.

Ahmadi, A., Bazargan-Hejazi, S., Zadie, A. H., Euasobhon, P., Ketumarn, R., & Mohammadi, R. (2016). Pain management in trauma: a review study. *Journal of Injury and Violence Research, 8*(2), 89–98. doi: 10.5249/jivr.v8i2.707

Akgun, F. S., Ertan, C., & Yucel, N. (2018). The prognastic efficiencies of modified early warning score and main emergency evaluation score for emergency department consumers. *Nigerian Journal of Clinical Practice, 21*(12), 1590–5. https://doi.org/10.4103/njcp.njcp_58_18

Australian Commission on Safety and Quality in Health Care (ACSQHC). (2017). National Consensus Statement: Essential elements for recognising and responding to deterioration in a person's mental state. Retrieved 22 May 2022 from https://www.safetyandquality.gov.au/publications-and-resources/resource-library/national-consensus-statement-essential-elements-recognising-and-responding-deterioration-persons-mental-state

Australian Commission on Safety and Quality in Health Care (ACSQHC). (2021). Delivering and supporting comprehensive end-of-life care: a user guide. Retrieved from https://www.safetyandquality.gov.au/our-work/end-life-care

Australian Commission on Safety and Quality in Health Care (ACSQHC). (2022). National Consensus Statement: Essential elements for recognising and responding to acute physiological deterioration (3rd ed.). Retrieved 22 May 2022 from https://www.safetyandquality.gov.au/publications-and-resources/resource-library/national-consensus-statement-essential-elements-recognising-and-responding-acute-physiological-deterioration-third-edition

Australian Institute of Health and Welfare (AIHW). (2021). Interfaces between the aged care and health systems in Australia – where do older Australians die? (June). Retrieved from https://www.aihw.gov.au/getmedia/56c1f616-8b2c-493e-8e1c-2db5083ad59d/aihw-age-106.pdf.aspx?inline=true May 8TH 2021

Berman, A., Snyder, S., Frandsen, G., Kozier, A., & Kozier, B. (2020). *Kozier and Erb's fundamentals of nursing: Concepts, process and practice* (5th Australian ed., 5th adaptation ed.). Frenchs Forest, NSW: Pearson Education Australia.

Burgess, D. J., Phelan, S., Workman, M., Hagel, E., Nelson, D. B., Fu, S. S., Widome, R., & van Ryn, M. (2014). The effect of cognitive load and patient race on physicians' decisions to prescribe opioids for chronic low back pain: A randomised trial. *Pain Medicine, 15*(6), 965–74. doi: https://doi.org/10.1111/pme.12378

CareSearch. (2021). Care of the dying person – clinical evidence – finding evidence – evidence. Retrieved 20 May 2022 from https://www.caresearch.com.au/tabid/6220/Default.aspx May 8th 2021

Hellier, J. L. (2016). *The five senses and beyond: The encyclopedia of perceptio*n. ABC-CLIO. pp. 118–19. ISBN 1440834172.

Hockenberry, M., & Wilson, D. (2018). *Wong's nursing care of infants and children* (11th ed.). St Louis, Missouri: Elsevier.

Hui, D., & Bruera, E. (2014). A personalized approach to assessing and managing pain in patients with cancer. *Journal of Clinical Oncology, 32*(16), 1640–6. http://doi.org/10.1200/JCO.2013.52.2508

International Association for the study of Pain (IASP). (2020). ISAP announces revised definition of pain. Retrieved 29 March 2023 from https://www.iasp-pain.org/publications/iasp-news/iasp-announces-revised-definition-of-pain/

Joint National Committee on Prevention, Detection, Evaluation, and Treatment of High Blood Pressure and the National High Blood Pressure Education Program Coordinating Committee (JNC). (2003). The seventh report of the Joint National Committee on Prevention, Detection, Evaluation, and Treatment of High Blood Pressure (NIH Publication No. 03-5233). *Archives of Internal Medicine, 157.*

Keogh, E. (2014). Gender differences in the nonverbal communication of pain: A new direction for sex, gender, and pain research? *Pain, 155*(10), 1927–31.

Keogh, E., & Arendt-Nielsen, L. (2004). Sex differences in pain. *European Journal of Pain, 8*(5), 395–6.

Kochman, A., Howell, J., Sheridan, M., Kou, M., Shelton Ryan, E. E., Lee, S., Zettersten, W., & Yoder, L. (2017). Reliability of the Faces, Legs, Activity, Cry, and Consolability Scale in assessing acute pain in the pediatric emergency department. *Pediatric Emergency Care, 33*(1), 14–17. doi: 10.1097/PEC.0000000000000995

Merkel, S. I., Voepel-Lewis, T., Shayevitz, J. R., & Malviya, S. (1997). The FLACC: A behavioral scale for scoring postoperative pain in young children. *Pediatric Nursing, 23*(3), 293–7.

National Heart Foundation of Australia. (2016). Guideline for the diagnosis and management of hypertension in adults – 2016. Retrieved 26 May 2022 from https://www.heartfoundation.org.au/images/uploads/publications/PRO-167_Hypertension-guideline-2016_WEB.pdf.

Palliative Care Australia. (2018). National Palliative Care Standards (5th ed) Retrieved 20 May 2022 from https://palliativecare.org.au/wp-content/uploads/dlm_uploads/2018/02/PalliativeCare-National-Standards-2018_web-3.pdf

Safdar, B., Heins, A., Homel, P., Miner, J., Neighbor, M., DeSandre, P., & Todd, K.H. (2009). Impact of physician and patient gender on pain management in the emergency department – A multicenter study. *Pain Medicine, 10*(2), 364–72. https://doi.org/10.1111/j.1526-4637.2008.00524.x

Watt-Watson, J., Stevens, B., Garfinkel, P., Streiner, D., & Gallop, R. (2002). Relationship between nurses' pain knowledge and pain management outcomes for their postoperative cardiac patients. *Journal of Advanced Nursing, 36*(4), 535–45. https://doi.org/10.1046/j.1365-2648.2001.02006.x

CHAPTER 7

MENTAL STATUS AND NEUROLOGICAL TECHNIQUES

LEARNING OUTCOMES

By the end of this chapter you should be able to:

1 describe the divisions of the nervous system and their functions
2 identify the characteristics of the most common mental health and neurological complaints
3 perform a mental status assessment and document the results
4 examine the neurological system in a systematic manner and document the results
5 explain the pathophysiology of any abnormal results obtained
6 discuss the clinical reasoning in evaluating outcomes of health assessment and physical examination including documentation requirements for recording information, health education given and referral to other health practitioners as appropriate.

BACKGROUND

Hundreds of thousands of people across Australia and New Zealand receive a diagnosis related to mental health and neurological issues each year. The following is a snapshot of incidence for some selected neurological and mental health disorders.

Alzheimer's disease, the most common form of dementia, is estimated to have affected around 70 000 New Zealanders in 2022 and is expected to increase to approximately 170 000 by 2050 (Alzheimers New Zealand, 2022). In Australia, it is estimated that there were more than 400 000 Australians living with dementia in 2023 (Dementia Australia, 2023), nearly two-thirds of whom are women (AIHW, 2022a). This represents a significant rise from 2009 figures, when approximately 245 000 Australians had dementia. In 2023, there were more than 28 000 people with younger-onset dementia (Dementia Australia, 2023). The impact on health and burden on life is very high for people as dementia progresses, but as yet the disease cannot be prevented, cured or slowed.

Parkinson's disease is a progressive and degenerative neurological condition that impairs the control of movement due to insufficient quantities of dopamine. Parkinson's disease affects approximately 100 000 people in Australia, with an average of 38 new diagnoses of the disease every day (Shake It Up Australia Foundation, n.d.). Twenty per cent of people with Parkinson's are under 50 years of age, and 10% are diagnosed before age 40 (Shake It Up Foundation Australia, n.d.). In New Zealand approximately 11 000 people have Parkinson's disease, and a recent study has predicted this to double by 2040 (New Zealand Brain Institute, n.d.). Prevalence of Parkinson's differs by ethnic group; a New Zealand study found that people of European ancestry had the highest incidence of the disease in that country (Pitcher et al., 2018).

Motor neurone disease (MND) begins with a weakness of the muscles in the hands or feet and eventually leads to generalised paralysis, including the inability to speak or swallow, usually leading to death within approximately three years (Dharmadasa et al., 2017). Motor neurone disease affects more than 2000 people in Australia, and an average of two people are diagnosed each day (Brain Foundation, 2022). Deaths are also rising from MND each year. In 2020, 741 people died from MND, significantly more than the 457 people who died from MND in 2000 (Motor Neurone Disease Australia, 2020). In New Zealand, the number of people living with MND is around 1 in 15 000, meaning there are currently over 400 people living with the disease, 35% of whom are under 65 (Motor Neurone Disease New Zealand, 2020).

Stroke is a sudden-onset injury to brain cells that causes cell injury and death. Symptoms appear in the location of the body controlled by the injured part of the brain. **Stroke** occurs due to a disruption of blood supply to the brain cells, as a result of arteries that either become blocked (ischaemic stroke) or burst (haemorrhagic stroke) in the brain (Stroke Foundation, 2018). More people are surviving stroke. By the year 2050, the number of new strokes each year in Australia is expected to top 50 000; in 2020, the figure was 27 428 (Stroke Foundation, 2020). In Australia, nearly 450 000 people are living with the effects of stroke (Stroke Foundation, 2022). Prevalence of stroke in Aboriginal and Torres Strait Islander peoples is higher than for other populations, and in all populations it is 17% higher in regional locations than most metropolitan locations (Stroke Foundation, 2022). In New Zealand, stroke is the second biggest killer and the leading cause of serious disability in adults (Stroke Foundation New Zealand, n.d.). Over 9500 people experience stroke every year in New Zealand, and that number is predicted to rise by 40% by 2028 (Stroke Foundation New Zealand, n.d.). Over 75% of strokes are preventable.

Traumatic brain injury (TBI) is an injury to the brain caused by a direct physical force to the head or body (trauma) that results in impairments for the person (Brain Injury Australia, n.d.). Causes of blunt TBI include road trauma, falls, and being struck by an object or person (O'Reilly et al., 2022). Prevalence and incidence are difficult to determine because of the number of gradations in TBI severity, but it is estimated that around 200 000 Australians suffer from a TBI, with 20 000 of them hospitalised every year (Connectivity, n.d.). In Australia, males are more than twice as likely to sustain a TBI than females, and Indigenous people are twice as likely as non-Indigenous people to present to emergency departments with a TBI (Esterman et al., 2018). In New Zealand, incidence of TBI is significantly higher in rural areas than in cities, with higher prevalence in males aged 0–34 and Māori people, than in those of European descent (Bentley, Singhal, Christey & Amey, 2022).

HEALTH EDUCATION

Preventing traumatic neurological injuries

Teach your consumers the importance of reducing the risk for traumatic injury:

> Always wear a helmet when riding a motorcycle or bicycle, rollerblading, skateboarding, horseback riding, skiing and snowboarding.

> Buckle your seat belt whenever you are in a car, even if it is fitted with airbags. Avoid placing children in car seats in the front passenger seat of the car if airbags are installed.

> When diving into water, look for signs indicating water depth and obey 'No Diving' signs. Enter the water in a safer way (walk in) to identify how deep the water is to avoid other injuries (e.g. fractured lower limbs, pelvis or spinal injuries).

Mental health disorders or mental illness are common in Australia and New Zealand. Each year, around one in five people experience mental illness, and/or medium to high levels of mental distress (Mindframe, 2022; HPA, 2020), some experiencing more than one mental illness at a time. Here are some important considerations for health professionals:

> Over 2 in 5 (44%) of Australians experience a mental disorder in their lifetimes. Anxiety disorders were the most prevalent (17%), followed by affective disorders (8%) and substance use disorders (3%) (AIHW, 2022b). Women are more likely to be diagnosed with depression, and men with substance abuse. Males 16–24 years old were the most likely to have experienced symptoms of a mental health disorder in the previous 12 months (AIHW, 2022a).

> Mental health disorders are a leading cause of disability burden in Australia and New Zealand, accounting for 13% of Australia's disease burden in 2018 (the fourth highest) (AIHW, 2022b) and an estimated cost of $12 billion in New Zealand (New Zealand Government, 2018). Major depression accounts for more days lost to illness than almost any other physical or mental health disorder.

> Māori and Pasifika people have a higher prevalence of mental health disorders than the general population in New Zealand, and much of this can be accounted for by socio-demographic disparity (New Zealand Government, 2018). For Pasifika people, time spent in the New Zealand environment is positively correlated with higher levels of mental health disorders. There is a substantial difference in the mental health disease burden on Aboriginal and Torres Strait Islander people compared with non-Indigenous Australians, with the years of healthy life lost to mental and substance use disorders in First Nations people found to be 2.4 times higher (AIHW, 2022b).

The nervous system controls all body functions and thought processes and, therefore, will be discussed first. The complex interrelationships among the various divisions of the nervous system permit the body to maintain homeostasis; to receive, interpret and react to stimuli; and to control voluntary and involuntary processes, including cognition.

ANATOMY AND PHYSIOLOGY

The structure and function of the central nervous system and the peripheral nervous system are discussed.

Macrostructure

The scalp and skull are two protective layers covering the brain. The scalp performs a unique function in that it moves freely, helping to protect and cushion the head from traumatic injury. The skull is a rigid, bony cavity that has a fixed volume of approximately 1500 mL.

Meninges

There are three layers of meninges (protective membranes), known as the dura mater, arachnoid mater and pia mater, located between the brain and the skull (Figure 7.1). The dura mater is the thick, tough outermost layer. Below the dura mater is a small serous space known as the subdural space.

The arachnoid mater lies between the dura mater and the pia mater. Below the arachnoid mater is the subarachnoid space, where **cerebrospinal fluid (CSF)** is circulated. Portions of the arachnoid mater, called arachnoid villi, project into the subarachnoid space (Figure 7.1). These serve to absorb CSF.

The pia mater is thin and vascular. It is the innermost layer of the meninges. The pia mater helps form the choroid plexuses, which are vascular structures located in the ventricles of the brain that produce CSF.

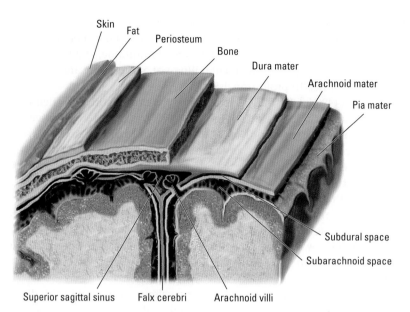

Skin
Fat
Periosteum
Bone
Dura mater
Arachnoid mater
Pia mater
Subdural space
Subarachnoid space
Superior sagittal sinus
Falx cerebri
Arachnoid villi

FIGURE 7.1 Location and structure of the meninges

Central nervous system

The brain and the spinal cord make up the central nervous system (CNS). The brain is divided into four main components: the cerebrum, the diencephalon, the cerebellum and the brain stem. Each of these areas is subdivided into various anatomic areas.

Cerebrum

The cerebrum is the largest portion of the brain. It is incompletely divided into right and left hemispheres by the longitudinal **fissure**. The two hemispheres are connected by the corpus callosum, which serves as a communication link between the left and right hemispheres.

The cerebral cortex, or the outermost layer of the cerebrum, contains grey matter. Higher cognitive functioning is dependent on the cerebral cortex and its interaction with other parts of the nervous system. The cerebral cortex is involved in memory storage and recall, and conscious understanding of sensation, vision, hearing and motor function. The basal ganglia are located deep within the cerebral hemispheres and function intricately with the cerebral cortex and the cerebellum in regulating motor activity.

Each cerebral hemisphere is divided into four lobes: the frontal, parietal, temporal and occipital lobes. The locations and functions of each of the cerebral lobes are illustrated in **Figure 7.2**. A fifth lobe called the limbic lobe is anatomically part of the temporal lobe and is involved in emotional behaviour and self-preservation.

Diencephalon

The diencephalon, a relay centre for the brain, is composed of the thalamic structures: the thalamus, the epithalamus and the hypothalamus. The hypothalamus is important in body temperature regulation, pituitary hormone control and autonomic nervous system responses. It also plays a role in behaviour via its connections with the limbic system.

Cerebellum

The cerebellum lies inferior to the occipital lobe and behind the brain stem. It is divided into two lateral lobes and a medial part called the vermis. The vermis is concerned primarily with maintenance of posture and equilibrium. Each cerebellar hemisphere is responsible for coordination of movement of the ipsilateral (same) side of the body.

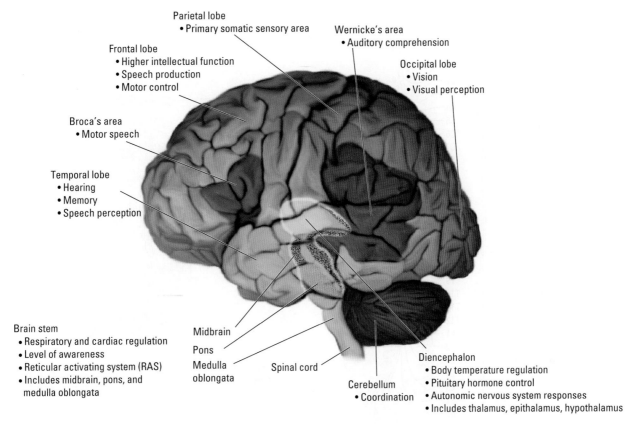

Parietal lobe
• Primary somatic sensory area

Frontal lobe
• Higher intellectual function
• Speech production
• Motor control

Wernicke's area
• Auditory comprehension

Occipital lobe
• Vision
• Visual perception

Broca's area
• Motor speech

Temporal lobe
• Hearing
• Memory
• Speech perception

Brain stem
• Respiratory and cardiac regulation
• Level of awareness
• Reticular activating system (RAS)
• Includes midbrain, pons, and medulla oblongata

Midbrain
Pons
Medulla oblongata
Spinal cord

Cerebellum
• Coordination

Diencephalon
• Body temperature regulation
• Pituitary hormone control
• Autonomic nervous system responses
• Includes thalamus, epithalamus, hypothalamus

FIGURE 7.2 The locations and functions of the cerebral lobes, diencephalon, cerebellum and brain stem

Brain stem

The brain stem is located immediately below the diencephalon and is divided into the midbrain, the pons and the medulla oblongata. The reticular formation, a complex network of sensory fibres in the brain stem, contains centres that control respiratory, cardiovascular and vegetative functions. The ascending reticular activating system (RAS) is located in the brain stem and extends to the cerebral cortex. The RAS is mostly excitatory and is essential for arousal from sleep, maintaining attention, and perception of sensory input.

The midbrain contains the nuclei of cranial nerves III (oculomotor) and IV (trochlear), which are associated with control of eye movements. The pons is located between the midbrain and the medulla oblongata. Sensory and motor nuclei of cranial nerves V (trigeminal), VI (abducens), VII (facial) and VIII (acoustic) are located in the pons. The medulla oblongata is located between the pons and the spinal cord. It contains the nuclei of cranial nerves IX (glossopharyngeal), X (vagus), XI (spinal accessory) and XII (hypoglossal). Also located in the medulla oblongata are the centres for reflexes such as sneezing, swallowing, coughing and vomiting, as well as the centres regulating the respiratory and cardiovascular systems.

Spinal cord

The spinal cord is a continuation of the medulla oblongata. It exits the skull at the foramen magnum and begins at the upper border of the atlas (C1), continuing downwards to the conus medullaris, a tapered ending of the cord at about the level of the first or second lumbar vertebrae (see **Figure 7.3A**). From the conus medullaris, a connective tissue filament called the 'filum terminale' continues down to its attachment at the coccyx (see **Figure 7.3B**).

A cross-section of the spinal cord will show that the central part of the cord is grey matter. The grey matter is in the shape of an H. White matter surrounds the grey matter.

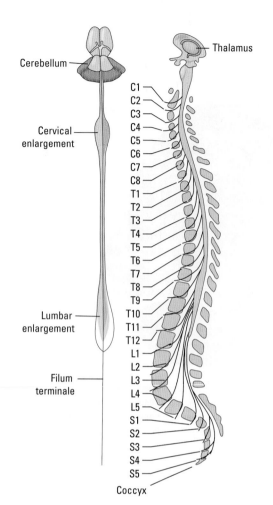

A. The spinal cord and spinal nerves

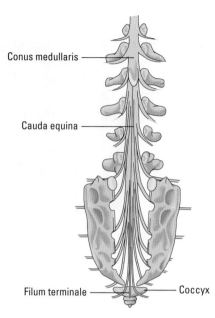

B. Close-up of the caudal region of the spinal nerves

FIGURE 7.3 The spinal cord

The grey matter is made up of nerve cell bodies and short segments of unmyelinated fibres. The posterior portion of the H is called the dorsal horn, and the anterior portion is the ventral horn. The dorsal horn contains cell bodies of sensory (afferent) neurones, which receive and transmit sensory messages from the afferent fibres in the spinal nerve. The ventral horn contains cell bodies of motor (efferent) neurones, which send axons into the spinal nerves and innervate skeletal muscles, carrying signals from the brain and the spinal cord.

Motor pathways of the CNS

There are three motor pathways in the CNS: the corticospinal or pyramidal tract, the extrapyramidal tract and the cerebellum.

Pyramidal tract

The corticospinal pathway descends from the motor area of the cerebral cortex, through the midbrain, the pons and the medulla. At the level of the medulla, 90% of the fibres of the corticospinal tract decussate (cross) to travel down the opposite side of the spinal cord, becoming the lateral corticospinal tract. The remaining fibres travel down the spinal cord in a tract known as the anterior corticospinal tract. Fibres of the lateral corticospinal tract synapse in the anterior horn (grey matter) at all levels of the cord just before they leave the cord (**Figure 7.4**). The motor neurones above this synapse in the anterior horn are known as upper motor neurones. Upper motor neurones connect the cerebral cortex with the anterior horn and are entirely contained within the CNS. Lower motor neurone cell bodies are located in

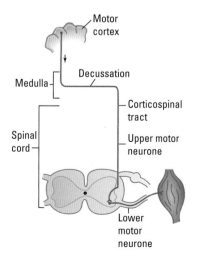

FIGURE 7.4 Motor pathways of the CNS

the anterior horn, where they connect with the corticospinal tract. Lower motor neurones innervate skeletal muscle at the myoneural junction. They are responsible for purposeful, voluntary movement.

Extrapyramidal tract

This pathway includes all motor neurones in the motor cortex, basal ganglia, brain stem and spinal cord that are outside the corticospinal, or pyramidal, tract (henceforth referred to as extrapyramidal). The extrapyramidal tract is responsible for controlling body movement, particularly gross automatic movements (e.g. walking), and for controlling muscle tone.

Sensory pathways of the CNS

The sensory portion of the peripheral nervous system consists of afferent neurones divided into somatic afferent and visceral afferent neurones. Somatic afferent fibres originate in skeletal muscles, joints, tendons and skin. Visceral fibres originate in the viscera. Both types of afferent fibres carry impulses from both the external and the internal environments to the CNS.

Afferent fibres containing impulses, or messages, enter the spinal cord through the dorsal roots. From the spinal cord the message travels via the spinothalamic tracts or the posterior column to the thalamus and sensory cortex. The thalamus receives the message and interprets a general sensation. The impulse synapses with another sensory neurone to the sensory cortex, where the message is fully interpreted (**Figure 7.5**).

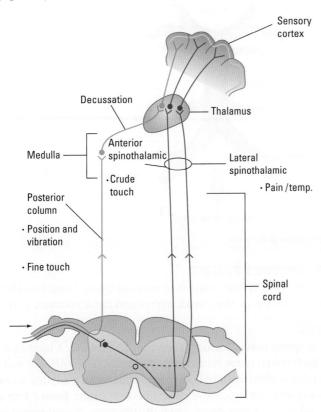

FIGURE 7.5 Sensory pathways of the CNS

Spinothalamic tracts

In the spinal cord, the spinothalamic tracts synapse with a second sensory neurone and then decussate to the opposite side. The message is then carried up the tract. The lateral spinothalamic tract carries pain and temperature sensations, and the anterior spinothalamic tract carries the sensations of crude or light touch.

Posterior column

The posterior column carries position, vibration and fine-touch sensations. The nerve impulse enters the spinal cord and travels upwards to the medulla, where a synapse with a second sensory neurone occurs. The neurone decussates to the opposite side of the medulla and continues on to the thalamus and sensory cortex.

Blood supply

Blood is supplied to the brain by two pairs of arteries: the internal carotid arteries (anterior circulation) and the vertebral arteries (posterior circulation). At the base of the brain lies the circle of Willis, an arterial anastomosis that links the anterior and posterior blood supplies (**Figure 7.6**).

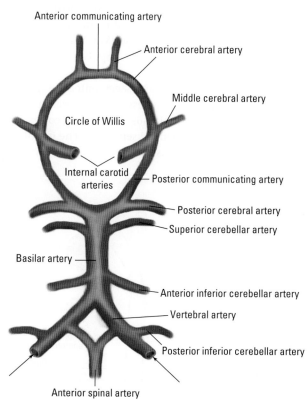

FIGURE 7.6 Major arteries of the brain

Peripheral nervous system

The peripheral nervous system consists of nervous tissue found outside the CNS, including the spinal nerves, the cranial nerves and the autonomic nervous system.

Spinal nerves

The 31 pairs of spinal nerves include 8 cervical, 12 thoracic, 5 lumbar, 5 sacral and 1 coccygeal. Each spinal nerve is made up of a dorsal (afferent) root and a ventral (efferent) root. Each afferent spinal nerve root innervates a specific area of the skin, called a **dermatome**, for superficial cutaneous sensations. **Figure 7.7** illustrates both the anterior and the posterior dermatomal distributions. Spinal nerves leaving the right side of the cord supply the right side of the body, and those leaving the left side supply the left side.

Each of the eight cervical nerves exits above its corresponding vertebra. Each of the spinal nerves below the cervical portion exits below its corresponding vertebra. The spinal cord is not as long as the vertebral column, so the lumbar and sacral nerves are comparatively long. These longer roots are called the cauda equina, meaning 'horse's tail' (see **Figure 7.3B**).

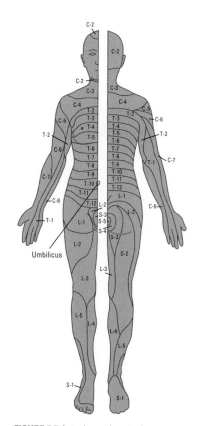

FIGURE 7.7 Anterior and posterior dermatomal distributions

Cranial nerves

There are 12 pairs of cranial nerves. They are designated with Roman numerals I to XII in order of their position. Some cranial nerves have purely motor functions and some have only sensory functions. Others have mixed sensory and motor functions. Table 7.1 summarises the functions of the cranial nerves, and Table 7.2 gives a mnemonic to remember them.

TABLE 7.1 The 12 cranial nerves and their functions

NAME AND NUMBER	FUNCTION
Olfactory (I)	Smell
Optic (II)	Visual acuity, visual fields, fundoscopic examination
Oculomotor (III)	Cardinal fields of gaze (EOM movement), eyelid elevation, pupil reaction, doll's eyes phenomenon
Trochlear (IV)	EOM movement
Trigeminal (V)	Motor: strength of temporalis and masseter muscles
	Sensory: light touch, superficial pain and temperature to face, corneal reflex
Abducens (VI)	EOM movement
Facial (VII)	Motor: facial movements
	Sensory: taste anterior two-thirds of tongue
	Parasympathetic: tears and saliva secretion*
Acoustic (VIII)	Cochlear: gross hearing, Weber and Rinne tests
	Vestibular: vertigo, equilibrium, nystagmus
Glossopharyngeal (IX)	Motor: soft palate and uvula movement, gag reflex, swallowing, guttural and palatal sounds
	Sensory: taste posterior one-third of tongue
	Parasympathetic: carotid reflex, chemoreceptors*
Vagus (X)	Motor and sensory: same as CN IX
	Parasympathetic: carotid reflex, stomach and intestinal secretions, peristalsis, involuntary control of bronchi, heart innervation*
Spinal accessory (XI)	Sternocleidomastoid and trapezius muscle movements
Hypoglossal (XII)	Tongue movement, lingual sounds

*Cannot be directly assessed.

EOM = extraocular muscle; CN = cranial nerve.

REFLECTION IN PRACTICE

Cranial nerve mnemonics

How do you remember this type of detailed information? Mnemonics can assist you in remembering the name of each cranial nerve and whether each nerve has a sensory function, a motor function, or both (see Table 7.2).

TABLE 7.2 Mnemonics to remember cranial nerves

FIRST LETTER OF CRANIAL NERVE	NUMBER OF CRANIAL NERVE	FUNCTION OF CRANIAL NERVE
On (Olfactory)	I	Some
Old (Optic)	II	Say
Olympus's (Oculomotor)	III	Marry
Towering (Trochlear)	IV	Money
Tops (Trigeminal)	V	But
A (Abducens)	VI	My
Finn (Facial)	VII	Brother
And (Acoustic)	VIII	Says
German (Glossopharyngeal)	IX	Bad
Viewed (Vagus)	X	Business
Some (Spinal accessory)	XI	Marry
Hops (Hypoglossal)	XII	Money

For cranial nerve function, S = sensory nerve, M = motor nerve, B = both sensory and motor nerves.

Autonomic nervous system

The autonomic nervous system (ANS) is divided into two functionally different subdivisions: the sympathetic and the parasympathetic nervous systems. The ANS functions without voluntary control to maintain the body in a state of homeostasis. Most organs that are under the influence of the ANS have dual innervation of both sympathetic and parasympathetic systems.

The sympathetic nervous system, sometimes called the thoracolumbar system, controls 'fight or flight' actions. The parasympathetic nervous system (craniosacral) is responsible for 'general housekeeping' of the body. See **Table 7.3** for specific system responses to autonomic stimulation.

TABLE 7.3 Sympathetic versus parasympathetic response

SYSTEM	SYMPATHETIC RESPONSE	PARASYMPATHETIC RESPONSE
Neurological	Pupils dilated Heightened awareness	Pupils normal size
Cardiovascular	Increased heart rate Increased myocardial contractility Increased blood pressure	Decreased heart rate Decreased myocardial contractility
Respiratory	Increased respiratory rate Increased respiratory depth Bronchial dilatation	Bronchial constriction
Gastrointestinal	Decreased gastric motility Decreased gastric secretions Sphincter contraction Increased glycogenolysis Decreased insulin production	Increased gastric motility Increased gastric secretions Sphincter dilatation
Genitourinary	Decreased urine output Decreased renal blood flow	Normal urine output

Reflexes

A reflex action is a specific response to an adequate stimulus and occurs without conscious control. The stimulus can occur in a joint, a muscle or the skin, and is transmitted to the CNS by one or more sensory neurones. The impulse enters the spinal cord through the dorsal root of a spinal nerve, where it synapses. Following synapse in the cord, the anterior motor neurones send an impulse via motor neurones to the endplates of the skeletal muscle, causing the effector muscle to react (Figure 7.8).

A monosynaptic reflex, such as the patellar reflex, involves two neurones: one sensory and one motor. Polysynaptic reflexes involve many neurones in addition to the sensory and motor limbs of the reflex arc. Reflexes are classified into three main categories: muscle stretch, or deep tendon reflexes (DTR); superficial reflexes; and pathological reflexes.

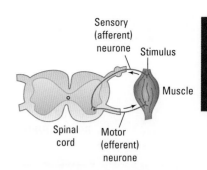

FIGURE 7.8 Monosynaptic reflex arc

ASSESSMENT: TAKING THE CONSUMER'S HEALTH HISTORY

Assessment is the first phase of the nursing process, and involves collecting subjective information about the consumer's health status in order to identify consumer problem areas to focus on.

Subjective data is most frequently collected during a health history and serves as the starting point for the health professional to base the depth of their assessment on.

The sections for the health history include:

> **Consumer profile**

> **Chief complaint** (explained systematically using variations of location, quality, quantity, associated manifestations, aggravating factors, alleviating factors, setting and timing. This is a variation on the OPQRST assessment mnemonic you may use for other conditions such as pain assessment)

> **Past health history** (including medical history, surgical history, allergies, medications, injuries and accidents, special needs and childhood illnesses)

> **Family health history**

> **Social history** (including alcohol, tobacco and drug use, sexual practice, work and home environment, hobbies and leisure activities, stress and culture).

HEALTH HISTORY		
CONSUMER PROFILE	The mental status and neurological health history provides insight into the link between a consumer's life and lifestyle, mental status and neurological information and pathology. Diseases that are age-, sex- and race-specific for the neurological system are listed.	
	AGE	**Mental status disorders:** > Delirium (any) > Dementia (usually aged 60 and over) > Depression (any) > Acute confusion (any) > Other psychiatric disorders such as schizophrenia, psychosis, anorexia nervosa, bulimia **Neurological:** > Multiple sclerosis (MS) (20–40) > Myasthenia gravis (20–30) > Fibromyalgia (25–50) > Syringomyelia (30) > Huntington's disease (30–40) > Parkinson's disease (>50) > Alzheimer's disease (middle age–old age)

HEALTH HISTORY

	SEX	**FEMALE**	Alzheimer's disease, myasthenia gravis, MS, meningiomas, pseudotumor cerebri, migraine headaches, fibromyalgia
		MALE	Cervical spine injuries, cluster headache, dyslexia (boys)
	CULTURAL BACKGROUND	**CAUCASIAN**	Parkinson's disease, Alzheimer's disease, multiple sclerosis
		ASIAN OR PASIFIKA	Intracranial haemorrhage
CHIEF COMPLAINT	Common chief complaints for mental status and the neurological system are defined, and information on the characteristics of each sign or symptom is provided.		
	1. HEADACHE	See Chapter 9	
	2. SEIZURE	A transient disturbance of cerebral function caused by an excessive discharge of neurones	
		LOCATION	Body parts involved
		QUALITY	General or localised
		QUANTITY	Number of minutes or seconds, weekly, monthly, every few months
		ASSOCIATED MANIFESTATIONS	Incontinence, injury (tongue, cheeks, limbs), memory loss, cyanosis, respiratory arrest, postictal headache, somnolence, confusion
		AGGRAVATING FACTORS	Television viewing, bright lights, sleep deprivation, stress, flashing lights, hyperventilation, fever in children or infants, alcohol (use or withdrawal), **hyperglycaemia, hypoglycaemia**
		ALLEVIATING FACTORS	Medications
		SETTING	Sequence of events: warning (aura) such as headache, abdominal discomfort, euphoria or depression, visual hallucination Types and phase: Generalised tonic-clonic or generalised motor seizures, absence or generalised non-motor seizures, focal seizures, febrile convulsions, post-ictal phase
		TIMING	First occurrence, age at onset of seizures, associated trauma or presumed cause, sleeping hours, first awakening, menses
	3. SYNCOPE	Abrupt loss of consciousness of brief duration due to decreased oxygen or glucose supply to the brain	
		QUALITY	Total versus partial loss of consciousness
		QUANTITY	Duration of seconds, minutes or hours; daily, monthly
		ASSOCIATED MANIFESTATIONS	Nausea, diaphoresis, dimmed vision, increased salivation, gastrointestinal bleeding, dyspnoea, chest pain, palpitations, hemiparesis, transient focal deficits, seizures, migraine headache, associated illness (myocardial infarction, diabetes mellitus type 1)
		AGGRAVATING FACTORS	Injury, intense emotion, carotid occlusion, cardiovascular disorders, exertion, anaemia, hypoglycaemia, insulin peak, crowded space, decreased atmospheric oxygen
		ALLEVIATING FACTORS	Cool air, change in position, oxygen, glucose, medication, volume infusions
		SETTING	Hot, stuffy room; standing still for long periods of time

>>

HEALTH HISTORY

4. TREMOR	Repetitive, often regular, oscillatory movements of a body part caused by contraction of opposing muscle groups; usually involuntary	
	LOCATION	Voice, face, arms, hands, trunk
	QUALITY	Postural, intention/essential, rest
	AGGRAVATING FACTORS	Fatigue, anxiety, caffeine, movement; hyperthyroidism, cerebellar disease, MS, Parkinson's disease; lithium, tricyclic antidepressants
	ALLEVIATING FACTORS	Rest, propranolol, benzodiazepines, L-dopa, primidone, alcohol intake
	SETTING	Head or hands outstretched against gravity; with tasks requiring precision or fine motor grasp
	TIMING	Age of onset; intermittent, constant
5. PAIN	A sensation of discomfort, distress or suffering	
	LOCATION	Anatomic location (e.g. lower back, head)
	QUALITY	Aching, stabbing, throbbing, cramping
	ASSOCIATED MANIFESTATIONS	Crying, hysteria, muscular tenseness, depression, shortness of breath, diaphoresis, splinting or protective behaviours, focal deficits, limited range of motion, sleep disturbance
	AGGRAVATING FACTORS	Stress, excessive exercise, lifting, coughing or sneezing, posture changes, trauma, illness, extreme temperatures, humidity
	ALLEVIATING FACTORS	Medications, heat, cold, distraction, physical therapy
	TIMING	Minutes to constant; early morning, late day; daily, monthly
6. PARAESTHESIA	Abnormal sensations such as numbness, pricking, tingling	
	LOCATION	Anatomic location (e.g. arms, hands, legs, feet)
	QUALITY	Aching, stabbing, pins and needles, numbness
	ASSOCIATED MANIFESTATIONS	Pain, stiffness, changes in gait, pulseless extremities, pallor, injury, ulcers, muscle wasting, traumatic injury
	AGGRAVATING FACTORS	Activity, extreme cold, diabetes mellitus
	ALLEVIATING FACTORS	Medication, warmth, position changes
7. DISTURBANCES IN GAIT	Abnormal way of moving on foot, walking or running	
	QUALITY	Ataxic, spastic hemiplegia, hemiplegic, scissors, festinating, steppage, antalgic, apraxic, Trendelenburg
	ASSOCIATED MANIFESTATIONS	Vertigo, visual impairments, blackouts, stroke, focal weakness, muscle wasting, abnormal movements or posture, spasticity, falling
	AGGRAVATING FACTORS	Fatigue, alcohol ingestion, vitamin D deficiency
	ALLEVIATING FACTORS	Rest, supportive equipment
	SETTING	Level ground versus uneven terrain, stroke, neuromuscular pathology

>>

UNIT 2

HEALTH HISTORY

8. VISUAL CHANGES	Changes in visual acuity, visual fields, colour perception, depth perception	
	QUALITY	Blindness in particular field of vision; scotoma; perception of flashing, bright lights; blurriness
	ASSOCIATED MANIFESTATIONS	Vertigo, dizziness, nausea, weakness, headache
	AGGRAVATING FACTORS	Darkness, fatigue, bright lights, reading, alcohol ingestion, medication
	ALLEVIATING FACTORS	Rest, medication, glasses
	TIMING	Abrupt, gradual, constant, intermittent, morning, evening
9. VERTIGO	The sensation of moving in space or objects moving around the person; also may be referred to as dizziness, light-headedness	
	QUALITY	Spinning sensations, dizziness or light-headedness
	ASSOCIATED MANIFESTATIONS	Nausea, vomiting, headache, tinnitus, deafness, discharge from ear, cranial nerve palsies, hemiparesis, seizure, loss of consciousness, chest pain, palpitations, falling
	AGGRAVATING FACTORS	Motion, movement of head, changes in atmospheric pressure (weather), heights, amusement rides, anxiety, alcohol ingestion, pain, medications
	ALLEVIATING FACTORS	Medications, lying down, maintaining a still posture
	SETTING	Amusement rides, glassed-in elevators, rising from a seated or supine position
	TIMING	Sudden, gradual; seconds, minutes, days, months; constant, intermittent
10. MEMORY DISORDERS	Change in ability to remember events or facts	
	QUALITY	Recent or remote (long-term) memory loss
	ASSOCIATED MANIFESTATIONS	Irritability, anxiety, agitation, confabulation, associated trauma, depression, fearfulness
	AGGRAVATING FACTORS	Distraction, anxiety, medications, alcohol ingestion, drug abuse, unfamiliar environment, sleep deprivation, anaesthesia, hypoxia, electrolyte imbalance, high altitude
	ALLEVIATING FACTORS	Visual or auditory cues, familiarity with environment, oxygen, electrolyte replacement, narcotic reversal, detoxification
	SETTING	Unfamiliar environment
	TIMING	Night-time, upon awakening
11. DIFFICULTY WITH SWALLOWING OR SPEECH	Inability to swallow food or drink, choking, or aspiration; changes in enunciation of words, speed and volume of speech, content of speech, or comprehension of written or verbal language, word salad, making up of new words	
	ASSOCIATED MANIFESTATIONS	Excessive drooling and saliva, paresis, dysarthria, weight loss, dehydration, irritability, depression, disease or damage to the CNS such as stroke or cerebral palsy, confusion
	AGGRAVATING FACTORS	Fatigue, position, prolonged tracheal intubation, alcohol intake, stress levels

>>

HEALTH HISTORY			
		ALLEVIATING FACTORS	Rest, quiet environment, thickened liquids, soft foods, varied communication tools
		SETTING	Loud, chaotic environment; after a prolonged intubation, at times of crisis or high stress
	12. SUICIDAL IDEATION	Describes thoughts of life not being worth living. May range from fleeting thoughts to concrete plans engaging in behaviour intended to end one's life. May have preoccupation with distressing thoughts to end one's life, may feel like they are a burden to others. May report feelings of helplessness and hopelessness, negative outlook on life, may feel like they are a burden to others and that life is not worth living and expressing regret about being alive or ever having been born	
		ASSOCIATED MANIFESTATIONS	Previous or failed suicide attempts, excessive risky behaviour (e.g. increase in alcohol or drug use, careless driving), self-imposed social isolation, purchasing or acquiring firearms, stockpiling medications or drugs, getting affairs in order or giving away possessions, saying or writing final 'goodbyes' to others, change in mood (depression, anxiety), reports feeling helpless or hopeless, talks about taking revenge or overwhelming feelings of shame, physical agitation or depression, significant decline in day-to-day activities, may also exhibit no associated manifestations
		AGGRAVATING FACTORS	Alcohol/drug intake, social isolation, bullying, situational crisis, crisis of identity, sexuality, gender or personality, family history of suicide, recent suicide in family members or friends, victim of abuse, violence or neglect, fatigue, sleep deprivation, other mental health disorders, breakdown of social or family support systems, owning a firearm, military service, gambling, financial debt, deterioration in physical health, witness to family violence
		ALLEVIATING FACTORS	Psychosocial support, crisis support referrals, counselling, medication, further psychiatric assessment to rule out other mental health disorders
		SETTING	Any
	13. MOOD ALTERATION	Two types of presentations: depression related or mania related. Some conditions will have manifestations of both (e.g. those with bipolar disorder or borderline personality disorder). Depressive-related signs and symptoms: Extreme tiredness and lack of energy, persistent lethargy, crying often or for long periods of time, indifference to others or for normal interests/activities, increased sleep, difficulty waking in the morning, increased or decreased appetite, weight gain or loss, feelings of worthlessness or guilt, inability to concentrate, indecisive, anxiety, irritability, suicidal thoughts, decreased libido, headaches, body aches, pains, cramps or digestive problems. Mania-related signs and symptoms: Elevated mood – feeling extremely energised, creative, feels 'interesting'; rapid thinking and speech, physical agitation, weight loss, decreased sleep, recklessness – risk-taking behaviours not usually exhibited; increased sexual desire, irritability, grandiose plans and beliefs, lack of insight, inability to concentrate.	
		ASSOCIATED MANIFESTATIONS	Relationship breakdown, loss of job/ability to work, decreased ability in managing self and relationships, financial stress (e.g. mania can cause people to spend all their savings in short period of time, whereas those who are depressed have reduced ability to earn money). In some cases of severe depression, presence of psychotic symptoms can be identified such as hallucinations (seeing, hearing, smelling, tasting or sensing things that are not apparent to others) or delusions (false beliefs that are firmly held, despite evidence opposite to the belief).

>>

HEALTH HISTORY

		AGGRAVATING FACTORS	This is dependent on cause. Situational crisis, change in sleep patterns, season (winter or summer), alcohol or drug use, genetic predisposition, hormone changes (in line with menstrual cycle, menopause and andropause, thyroid disorders), illness, onset of other disorders such as dementia, schizophrenia and attention deficit hyperactivity disorder. Borderline personality disorder more common in women, onset early 20s and intensity may lessen with age.
		ALLEVIATING FACTORS	This is dependent on cause. For example, if seasonally related, then a change in season or exposure to light. If related to changes in hormone levels or other diagnosed disorders, adherence to medication regimen.
		SETTING	Seasonal Affective Disorder (SAD) is related to season and length of days. Winter and autumn onset, more common in locations with significantly shortened days. Summer onset, more common in locations that have long hot days.
PAST HEALTH HISTORY	The various components of the past health history are linked to neurological pathology and neurology-related information.		
	MEDICAL HISTORY	**NEUROLOGIC SPECIFIC**	Amyotrophic lateral sclerosis (ALS), MS, tumours, Guillain-Barré syndrome, cerebral aneurysm, arteriovenous malformations (AVM), stroke, migraines, Alzheimer's disease, myasthenia gravis, congenital defects, metabolic disorders, childhood seizures, TBI, neuropathies, peripheral vascular disease, Parkinson's disease
		NON-NEUROLOGIC SPECIFIC	Hypertension, heart disease, cardiac surgery, invasive procedures, diabetes mellitus, leukaemia, hypoglycaemia
	SURGICAL HISTORY	Craniotomy, laminectomy, carotid endarterectomy, transsphenoidal hypophysectomy, cordotomy, aneurysm repair (surgical or radiological)	
	MEDICATIONS	Antidepressants, antiseizure medications, narcotics, antianxiety medications, antipsychotic medications	
	COMMUNICABLE DISEASES	Encephalitis, meningitis or poliomyelitis, AIDS, botulism, syphilis, cat scratch fever (*Bartonella henselae*), rickettsial infections, toxoplasmosis	
	INJURIES AND ACCIDENTS	Closed head injury, chronic subdural haematoma, spinal cord injury, peripheral nerve damage	
FAMILY HEALTH HISTORY	Congenital defects such as neural tube defects, hydrocephalus, AVM, headaches, epilepsy, Alzheimer's disease, Huntington's chorea, muscular dystrophies, lipid storage diseases, Gaucher's disease, Niemann-Pick disease. Neurological diseases that are familial are listed.		
SOCIAL HISTORY	The components of the social history are linked to neurological factors and pathology.		
	ALCOHOL USE	Consumers suffering from chronic alcoholism may exhibit the following abnormal findings: Korsakoff's psychosis, polyneuropathy, Wernicke's encephalopathy, tremor	
	TOBACCO USE	Increased risk of stroke	
	DRUG USE	Neurological signs of drug use are listed in **Table 7.4**	
	SEXUAL PRACTICE	Neurosyphilis; impotence secondary to neuropathies, MS or lower motor neurone lesions	
	TRAVEL HISTORY	Arthropod-borne encephalitis (Japanese B, Murray Valley), malaria	
	WORK ENVIRONMENT	Exposure to continuous loud noise, performing repetitive-motion tasks, toxic chemical exposure (carbon dioxide, insecticides)	
	HOME ENVIRONMENT	Exposure to toxic chemicals (carbon dioxide, insecticides), lead paint	
	HOBBIES AND LEISURE ACTIVITIES	Use of protective equipment; participation in contact sports or high-risk activities such as football, soccer, hockey, boxing, race car driving, motorcycling; hobbies involving repetitive motion (needlework)	
	STRESS	Headaches; migraine headaches, fibromyalgia flares, or MS can be exacerbated by stress	

TABLE 7.4 Neurological signs of drug ingestion

ASSESSMENT PARAMETER	DRUG				
	HALLUCINOGENS (E.G., PCP, LSD)	CANNABIS (MARIJUANA) (NOTE THIS HAS HALLUCINOGENIC PROPERTIES TOO)	NARCOTICS (E.G., HEROIN, MORPHINE, CODEINE)	SEDATIVE – HYPNOTICS (E.G., ALCOHOL, BENZODIAZEPINES, BARBITUATES, KETAMINE)	CNS STIMULANTS (COCAINE, MDMC, AMPHETAMINES)
Pupils	Dilated	Normal	Pinpoint	Normal	Dilated
	React to light		Fixed		React to light
Deep tendon reflexes	Hyperactive	Normal	Normal	Hypoactive	Hyperactive
Speech	Normal	Often normal	Normal or dulled	Slurred	N/A
Coordination	Normal	Normal	Normal or unsteady	Ataxia	N/A
Sensorium	Often clear	Usually clear	Dulled	Confusion	May be confused
Sensory perception	Distorted	Distorted	Dulled	Dulled	Heightened
Memory	Unchanged	Transient loss	Unchanged	Impaired	Unchanged
Hallucinations	Any type	Rare	Rare	N/A	N/A
Delusions	Variable	Paranoid	N/A	N/A	Paranoid

PERSON-CENTRED HEALTH EDUCATION

When conducting a health assessment, opportunities for the provision of person-centred health education will arise. This is a significant consideration in relation to the assessment process for examination of the person's mental health and neurological status due to the stigma associated with mental illness, and the associated quality of life limitations that mental illness and neurological disorders have on the person and their families. These occasions are identified as individualised education and may generate further data that can be added to the assessment. All education given should be documented so that in future, health professionals can assess the impact of previous information provided to the consumer. (Refer to Chapter 1 for initiating Health education.) Refer to the following examples.

INDIVIDUALISED HEALTH EDUCATION INTERVENTIONS	
This information provides a bridge between the health maintenance activities and neurological function.	
Sleep	Narcolepsy, insomnia, mindfulness for stress reduction to improve sleep quality
Diet	Beriberi (vitamin B$_1$), pellagra (niacin), maintaining medication adherence
Exercise	Increased muscle strength, increased coordination, provides stress relief, and linked to improved sleep and overall wellbeing
Use of safety devices	Helmet, seat belt, eye shields and other protective equipment
Health check-ups	Developmental milestones review, post TBI or mental health diagnosis may need to have relationship support/referral

PLANNING FOR PHYSICAL EXAMINATION

The planning phase refers to evaluating subjective data to narrow the focus on physical examination, determining what objective data needs to be gathered, as well as considering the environment and equipment that will be required.

> **Objective data** is:
> > collected during the physical examination of the consumer
> > usually collected after subjective data
> > information that is measured or observed by the clinician as opposed to being reported by the consumer
> > vital to the overall health assessment, to enable you to make clinical decisions that are representative of the whole consumer picture.

Evaluating subjective data to focus physical examination

Before commencing the physical examination of the person's mental health and neurological status, consider what information the health history has provided. Critical consideration, linked to knowledge of anatomy and physiology, should focus the physical assessment so your examination will be more effective and efficient.

Environment

Assessment of the consumer's mental health and neurological status needs to be done in a suitable environment. This means controlling the level of light, and somewhere for the consumer to feel secure that confidentiality can be maintained, as well as a safe environment for staff if the person is agitated, restless or experiencing changes in mood. Staff should position themselves where they are able to clearly exit and obtain assistance with consumers who may be unpredictable or unstable. As you are likely to require several different pieces of equipment for this assessment, enough bench space for you to lay out your equipment will allow you to work methodically through the assessment.

Equipment

> Cotton wisp
> Cotton-tipped applicators
> Penlight (torch)
> Tongue blade
> Vials containing odorous materials (coffee, orange extract, vinegar)
> Vials with solutions for tasting: quinine (bitter), glucose solution (sweet), lemon or vinegar (sour), saline (salty)
> Snellen chart or Rosenbaum pocket screener

IMPLEMENTATION: CONDUCTING THE PHYSICAL EXAMINATION

Implementation of the physical examination requires you to consider your scope of practice as well. In this section, depending on your context, you may be performing a foundation examination with aspects of advanced examination if you are practising in a specialised area.

EXAMINATION **IN BRIEF: MENTAL STATUS AND NEUROLOGICAL ASSESSMENT**

Examination of mental status

Level of consciousness (LOC)

Physical appearance and behaviour
> Posture and movements
> Facial expression
> Dress, self-care, grooming and personal hygiene
> Mood and affect

Speech and communication

Cognitive abilities and mentation
> Attention
> Memory
> Judgement
> Insight
> Spatial perception

>>

> Calculation
> Abstract reasoning
> Thought process and content
> Suicidal ideation

Mental health

Sensory examination

Exteroceptive sensation

> Light touch

Proprioceptive sensation

> Motion and position

Examination of cranial nerves

Olfactory nerve (CN I)

Optic nerve (CN II)

> Visual acuity
> Visual fields
> Fundoscopic examination

Oculomotor nerve (CN III)

> Cardinal fields of gaze
> Eyelid elevation
> Pupil reactions

Trochlear nerve (CN IV)

> Cardinal fields of gaze

Trigeminal nerve (CN V)

> Motor component
> Sensory component

Abducens nerve (CN VI)

> Cardinal fields of gaze

Facial nerve (CN VII)

> Motor component
> Sensory component

Acoustic nerve (CN VIII)

> Cochlear division
> Vestibular division

Glossopharyngeal and vagus nerves (CN IX and CN X)

Spinal accessory nerve (CN XI)

Hypoglossal nerve (CN XII)

Examination of motor system

Pronator drift

Examination of cerebellar function

Coordination

Gait

General approach to neurological assessment

1. Greet the consumer and explain the assessment techniques you will be using.
2. Maintain a quiet, unhurried, self-confident demeanour to help relieve any feelings of anxiety or discomfort, and to help the consumer relax during the assessment.
3. Provide a warm, quiet and well-lit environment.
4. After the mental status examination (if required), ask the consumer to remove all street clothes, and provide an examination gown for the consumer to put on.
5. Begin the assessment with the consumer in a comfortable (where appropriate), upright sitting position or, for the consumer on bed rest, position the consumer comfortably, preferably with the head of the bed elevated, or flat, whichever is tolerated best or is within activity orders for the consumer.

HEALTH EDUCATION

Risk factors for stroke

Consider the following risk factors for stroke and where appropriate provide individualised education to increase awareness.

Significant risk factors for stroke include:

> hypertension
> physical inactivity (increases risks of hypertension, type 2 diabetes mellitus and obesity)
> diabetes mellitus
> cocaine and methamphetamine use
> marijuana use
> cigarette smoking

>>

>>

> hyperlipidaemia
> migraines
> atrial fibrillation and flutter
> history of cerebral aneurysm
> sickle cell disease
> alcohol abuse
> kidney dysfunction
> obesity
> oral contraceptive use, especially in women over age 35 who smoke and have hypertension
> environmental factors (such as lead exposure, pollution, temperature).

Sources include Healthdirect (2022), Parekh, Pemmasani & Desi (2020); Madsen et al. (2018); Stark et al. (2021).

A complete examination includes an assessment of mental status, sensation, cranial nerves, motor function, cerebellar function and reflexes. For consumers with minor or intermittent symptoms, a rapid screening examination may be used, as outlined in **Table 7.5**.

TABLE 7.5 Neurological screening assessment

ASSESSMENT PARAMETER	ASSESSMENT SKILL	COMMENTS
Mental status	Perform Glasgow Coma Scale (GCS) with motor assessment component and pupil assessment.	If GCS < 15, perform full assessment of mental status and consciousness. If motor assessment is abnormal or asymmetrical, perform complete motor and sensory assessment. URGENT FINDING: if GCS score drops by 2 or more, activate a medical emergency response.
	Note general appearance, personal hygiene and dress (level of self-care and appropriate to season), affect (facial expression), speech content, memory, logic, mood, and manner, judgement and speech patterns during the history.	If any abnormalities or inconsistencies are evident, perform full mental status assessment.
Sensation	Assess pain and vibration in the hands and feet, light touch on the limbs.	If deficits are identified, perform a complete sensory assessment.
Cranial nerves	Assess CN II, III, IV, VI: visual acuity, gross visual fields, fundoscopic examination, pupillary reactions and extraocular movements.	If any abnormalities exist, perform complete assessment of all 12 cranial nerves.
	Assess CN VII, VIII, IX, X, XII: facial expression, gross hearing, voice, and tongue.	If any abnormalities exist, perform complete assessment of all 12 cranial nerves.
Motor system	Muscle tone, strength and posture Abnormal movements Hand grasp	If deficits are noted, perform a complete motor system assessment.
Cerebellar function	Observe the consumer's: 1 gait on arrival 2 ability to: • walk heel-to-toe • walk on toes • walk on heels • hop in place • perform shallow knee bends. Check 3 Romberg's test 4 Finger-to-nose test 5 Fine repetitive movements with hands	If any abnormalities exist, perform complete cerebellar assessment.
Reflexes	Assess the deep tendon reflexes and the plantar reflex.	If an abnormal response is elicited, perform a complete reflex assessment.

Examination of mental status

Much of the mental status assessment should be done during the interview, with the consumer comfortably positioned facing you. Mental status may also continue to be assessed throughout the neurological assessment. Assess level of consciousness, physical appearance and behaviour, speech and communication, cognitive abilities and mentation while conversing with the consumer. Assess suicidal ideation and mood by asking specific questions.

Note: Mental status and neurological examination may also be performed independently of each other, but they are usually undertaken together to ensure a comprehensive initial assessment. If a consumer is displaying signs of irritability and paranoia or aggression, aspects of the neurological examination may be delayed or be more appropriately undertaken at another time when a more focused mental status and neurological examination is undertaken.

CLINICAL **REASONING**

Practice tip: Commence mental status assessment when you first meet the consumer

1. Begin your assessment as the consumer approaches you. Observe gait, posture, mode of dress, involuntary movements, speech, and other features that will help guide and refine your assessment priorities.
2. The history should be holistic because neurological disorders can affect all body systems.
3. The history should be age-sensitive:
   • Utilise other family members when appropriate.
   • Acknowledge adolescents' ability to speak for themselves.
   • Do not make assumptions regarding elderly or young consumers' ability to describe their own health histories.
4. Allow the consumer to remain clothed during the history and mental status assessment.
5. Consider language and cultural norms when obtaining the history and performing the mental status assessment.

Level of consciousness (LOC)

Consciousness is the level of awareness of the self and the environment. Conscious behaviour requires arousal, or wakefulness, and awareness, or cognition and affect. Arousal is controlled by the reticular activating system (RAS). The RAS activates the cortex after receiving stimuli from the somatic and special sensory pathways. Awareness is a higher-level function of the cerebral cortex, which interprets incoming sensory stimuli. Aspects of awareness at a higher level include judgement and thinking, which are generally assessed as part of the cognitive assessment. Orientation is awareness of self and environment.

E 1. Observe the consumer's eyes when you enter the room (environmental stimuli). Note whether the consumer's eyes are open or whether they open when you enter the room (prior to any verbalisation). Note the consumer's response to any general environmental stimuli, such as noises or lights.
2. If the consumer's eyes are closed, introduce yourself (verbal stimuli). Observe whether the consumer's eyes open, whether he or she responds verbally and appropriately, and whether he or she follows verbal commands.
3. If the consumer does not respond to verbal stimuli, lightly touch or squeeze the consumer's hand or gently shake the consumer awake.
4. If the consumer is not responding to environmental or verbal stimuli, proceed to the application of a painful stimulus.
   a. Apply pressure with a pen to the nail bed of each extremity, or
   b. Firmly pinch the trapezius muscle, or
   c. Apply pressure to the supraorbital ridge or the manubrium.

E Examination **N** Normal findings **A** Abnormal findings **P** Pathophysiology

E 5. Observe the consumer's reaction to the painful stimulus. Note whether the consumer's eyes open.

6. Observe whether the consumer can localise the painful stimulus by reaching for the area being stimulated. Strength of the consumer's extremities can be assessed by the strength and distance of movement during his or her attempt to reach the painful stimulus. Note any abnormal motor responses.

7. Compare the motor responses and strength of the responses of right versus left sides of the consumer.

8. Note whether the consumer responds verbally to the painful stimulus.

9. Assess orientation by asking questions related to person, place and time:
   a. Person: name of the consumer, name of spouse or significant other
   b. Place: where the consumer is now (what town, what state), where the consumer lives
   c. Time: the time of day, month, year, season.

10. Determine the **Glasgow Coma Scale (GCS)** (see **Figure 7.9**) score, an international method for grading neurological responses of the injured or severely ill consumer. It is monitored in consumers who have the potential for rapid deterioration in level of consciousness. The GCS assesses three parameters of consciousness: eye opening, verbal response and motor response.

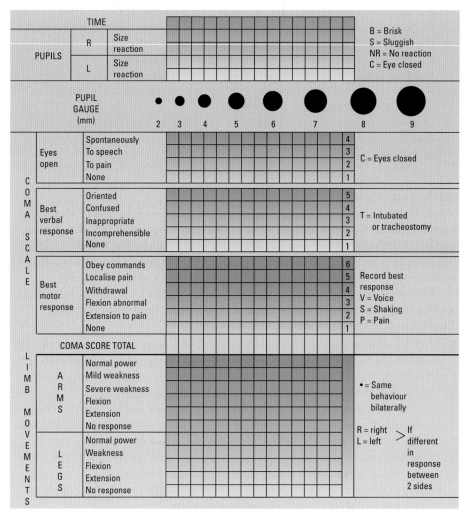

FIGURE 7.9 Neurological flow sheet, including Glasgow Coma Scale

CLINICAL REASONING

Glasgow Coma Scale
Most often, the GCS is included in neurological assessment documentation. This includes:
> vital signs
> motor movement and strength
> pupillary size and reactions.
    This provides a more in-depth evaluation of the neurological status of the consumer.
However, using the GCS *does not replace* undertaking a full mental status assessment.

N The consumer's best response to each of these categories is what is recorded.
The sum of the three categories is the total GCS score. The highest score of
responsiveness is 15 and the lowest is 3. A score of 15 would indicate a fully
alert, oriented individual.

A P See Table 7.6.

TABLE 7.6 Levels of consciousness: Abnormalities and pathophysiology

LOC	GCS	RESPONSE TO STIMULI	PUPIL RESPONSE	PATHOPHYSIOLOGY	PROGNOSIS
Confusion	14	Spontaneous but may be inappropriate Memory faulty Reflexes intact	Normal	Metabolic derangements Diffuse brain dysfunction	Good chance of recovery Must treat primary cause
Lethargy	13–14	Requires stimulus to respond (verbal, touch) Reflexes intact	Normal to unequal	Metabolic derangements Medications Increased ICP	Good chance of recovery Must treat primary cause
Stupor	12–13	Requires vigorous, continuous stimuli to respond Reflexes intact	Normal, unequal, or sluggish	Metabolic derangements Medications Increased ICP	Good chance of recovery Must treat primary cause
Unresponsive wakefulness syndrome OR Unaware and unresponsive state	8–10	Responds to pain No cognitive response Reflexes abnormal	Normal	Anoxic ischaemic insults	Irreversible
Locked-in syndrome	6	Awake and aware	Normal	Lesion in ventral pons All four extremities and lower cranial nerves paralysed Myasthenia gravis Acute polyneuritis	Poor prognosis
Coma	3–6	Abnormal Varied response to pain Reflexes abnormal or absent	Abnormal Dilated or pinpoint	Anoxia Traumatic injury Space-occupying lesion Cerebral oedema	Prognosis dependent on length of time in coma
Brain death	3	No response Reflexes abnormal or absent	Abnormal Dilated or pinpoint	Anoxia Structural damage	Irreversible

LOC – level of consciousness; GCS – Glasgow Coma Scale; ICP – intracranial pressure

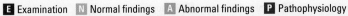
E Examination N Normal findings A Abnormal findings P Pathophysiology

CLINICAL REASONING

Practice tip: Application of painful stimuli
1. Application of painful stimuli is extremely upsetting to significant others and therefore should not be performed without a comprehensive explanation.
2. Apply only the amount of pressure needed to elicit a response.
3. Alternate sites when possible.
4. Pain applied centrally (e.g. trapezius muscle squeeze) that results in a response always indicates involvement of the cerebrum. Pain applied to an extremity (e.g. pen pressure on a nail bed) may elicit a reflex response or cerebral response, or both.

Great care is needed when interpreting the significance of response to pain with consumers in profound coma.

Note: Care needs to be taken in choosing when and where painful stimuli should be applied. If always applied to the same soft tissue, injury and tissue breakdown will occur and may need treatment for pressure injury.

Physical appearance and behaviour

Posture and movements

E
1. Observe the person's ability to wait patiently (dependent also on environmental factors).
2. Note if consumer's posture is relaxed, slumped or stiff.
3. Observe the consumer's movements for control and symmetry.
4. Observe the consumer's gait (see Chapter 16).

N The consumer should appear relaxed with the appropriate amount of concern for the examination. The consumer should exhibit erect posture, a smooth gait, and symmetrical body movements.

A Restlessness, tenseness and pacing can be abnormal.

P These may be signs of anxiety or metabolic disorders, which should alert you to further investigate these problems.

Note: At times you may need to just undertake a mental status assessment or an abbreviated neurological assessment separately due to the consumer's condition. The neurological assessment described in this text is comprehensive rather than focused or abbreviated.

A Slumped posture, slow gait, poor eye contact and slow responses can be abnormal findings. (However, consider that lack of eye contact may be a cultural difference – see Chapter 4.)

P These may be signs of depression.

A Stooped, flexed or rigid posture; drooping neck; deformities of the spine; and tics are abnormal findings.

P Consumers with kyphosis, scoliosis, Parkinson's disease, cerebral palsy, osteoporosis, schizophrenia, muscular atrophy, myasthenia gravis or stroke may exhibit these signs.

REFLECTION IN PRACTICE

Influences on dress, self-care, grooming and personal hygiene
Dress and self-care are influenced by the consumer's economic status, age, home situation and ethnic background. Information obtained during the health history will assist you in determining appropriate dress and grooming for each consumer. It is helpful to directly ask the consumer about self-care routines and clothing choices when there is a question as to appropriateness.

How would you phrase this type of questioning so that it does not sound judgemental? Practise with your colleagues, friends or family members.

 Examination Normal findings Abnormal findings 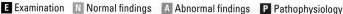 Pathophysiology

Facial expression

E Observe for appropriateness of, variations in, and symmetry of facial expressions.

N Facial expressions should be appropriate to the content of the conversation and should be symmetrical.

A Extreme, inappropriate or unchanging facial expressions, or asymmetrical facial movements, are abnormal.

P Abnormal facial expressions demonstrate anxiety, depression, or the unchanging facial expression of a consumer with Parkinson's disease. They may also indicate a lesion in the facial nerve (CN VII).

Dress, self-care, grooming and personal hygiene

E 1. Note the appearance of the consumer's clothing, specifically:
- cleanliness
- condition
- age appropriateness
- weather appropriateness
- appropriateness for the consumer's socioeconomic group or cultural affiliations.
2. Observe the consumer's personal grooming (hair, skin, nails, teeth) for:
- adequacy
- symmetry
- odour.

N The consumer should be clean and should wear appropriate clothing for age, weather and socioeconomic status.

A Poor personal hygiene such as uncombed hair, body odour or unkempt clothing is usually abnormal.

P These signs may be indications of depression, schizophrenia or dementia.

A Excessive, meticulous care and attention to clothing and grooming are abnormal behaviours.

P These signs may indicate obsessive-compulsive behaviour.

A Obvious one-sided differences in grooming and dressing or the use of only one side of the body is abnormal.

P Stroke in the parietal lobe may cause the consumer to be aware of only one side of the body, which is termed 'one-sided neglect'.

Mood and affect

E 1. Observe the consumer's interaction with you and others where possible (e.g. in waiting room or with other staff), paying particular attention to both verbal and nonverbal behaviours.
2. Note if the consumer's affect appears labile, blunted or flat. Note if their choice of words also denotes mood.
3. Note the variations in the consumer's affect with a variety of topics.
4. Note any extreme emotional responses during the interview.

N The appropriateness and degree of affect should vary with the topics and the consumer's cultural norms, and be reasonable, or eurhythmic (normal).

A Blunted affect, manifested by the consumer shuffling into the examination room, slumping into a chair, moving slowly and not making eye contact, is abnormal.

P A blunted affect may indicate psychotic disorders. It may also indicate frontal lobe dysfunction associated with traumatic brain injury or brain tumour.

A Unresponsive, inappropriate affect is abnormal.

P A flat, unresponsive affect may indicate depression or schizophrenia.

E Examination **N** Normal findings **A** Abnormal findings **P** Pathophysiology

A Anger, hostility and paranoia are abnormal responses in most clinical situations.

P These may be the responses of an individual experiencing paranoia.

A Euphoric, dramatic, disruptive, irrational or elated behaviours are abnormal in most clinical situations. Significant changes in mood, not necessarily related to context, are abnormal.

P A consumer with bipolar disorder might display these responses during the manic phase, or experience significant changes in mood.

Speech and communication

Speech and communication skills should be assessed throughout the entire interview and physical assessment.

E 1. Note voice quality, which includes voice volume and pitch.
2. Assess articulation, fluency and rate of speech by engaging the consumer in normal conversation. Ask the consumer to repeat words and sentences after you, or to name objects you point out.
3. Assess for quantity of information in conversation. In conversation, is the consumer able to answer the questions asked in a coherent manner. Observe for pressured, loud, slurred, mumbled, poverty of speech, or word salad.
      Word salad is a confused or unintelligible mixture of seemingly random words and phrases. A person may attempt to communicate an idea, but words and phrases may appear to be random and unrelated and come out in an incoherent sequence. This can be present in people with schizophrenia or dementia.
4. Note the consumer's ability to carry out requests during the assessment, such as pointing to objects within the room as requested. Ask questions that require 'yes' or 'no' responses.
5. Write simple commands for the consumer to read and perform: for example, 'point to your nose' or 'tap your right foot'. Reading ability may be influenced by the consumer's educational level or visual impairment.
6. Ask the consumer to write his or her name, birthday, a sentence the consumer composes, or a sentence that you dictate. Note the consumer's spelling, grammatical accuracy and logical thought process (be aware that the consumer's level of schooling may affect this as well).

N The consumer should be able to produce spontaneous, coherent speech. The speech should have an effortless flow with normal inflections, volume, pitch, articulation, rate and rhythm. Content of the message should make sense. Comprehension of language should be intact. The consumer's ability to read and write should match the consumer's educational level. Non-native speakers may exhibit some hesitancy or inaccuracy in written and spoken language.

A **Aphasia** is an impairment (often complete absence) of language functioning.

P Aphasias are classified by involved anatomy, behavioural speech manifestations, fluency of speech (fluent: rhythm, grammar and articulation are normal; nonfluent: speech production is limited and speech is poorly articulated), and comprehension (receptive) versus expression (expressive) deficits. Other categories include amnesic (the inability to recall specific types of words) and central (a deficit in the coordination among the speech areas). **Table 7.7** has a summary of the characteristics and pathophysiology of specific aphasias. Most consumers with an aphasia will have some components of several aphasia classifications (e.g. a consumer with transcortical motor aphasia will usually have some degree of transcortical sensory aphasia).

URGENT FINDING

The confused consumer – missed diagnosis

The confused consumer should be thoroughly assessed for aphasia, especially after a fall or a brain injury. A missed diagnosis because of 'confusion' can be fatal if aphasia is present and due to a subdural haematoma (SDH). Check for other signs associated with an SDH, including headache, slow cerebration (functioning of the brain), decreasing level of consciousness, and ipsilateral pupil dilatation with a sluggish response to light. An SDH can have an acute onset (within hours to days after moderate to severe injury) or chronic (days to weeks after minor injury). Any person with this history should be referred to a medical officer or emergency department for urgent brain imaging.

A **Dysphasia**, an impairment of language functioning, which may be complete or partial, is abnormal. May include loss or impairment to understand language, speak, read or write.

P Causes include stroke or TBI to left side (usually) of brain, causing damage on this side of the brain.

URGENT FINDING

Acting on signs of stroke

According to the Stroke Foundation (2018), the most common signs of stroke are facial weakness, arm weakness and difficulty with speech.

Other signs include:

> weakness, numbness or paralysis of the face, arm or leg on either or both sides of the body
> difficulty speaking or understanding
> dizziness, loss of balance or an unexplained fall
> loss of vision, sudden blurring or decreased vision in one or both eyes
> headache, usually severe and abrupt onset or unexplained change in the pattern of headaches
> difficulty swallowing.

In Australia, the following poster is used to raise awareness of seeking help as soon as possible. New Zealand uses the same acronym, but 111 is the emergency number to call.

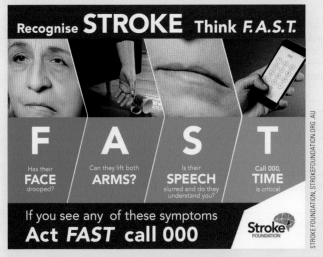

FIGURE 7.10 Stroke symptoms recognition

A stroke is a medical emergency and just like a 'heart attack' where time means more heart cell death, a stroke is a 'brain attack' and time is related to more brain cell injury/death. Any person who experiences these symptoms should be assisted to seek emergency care urgently.

E Examination **N** Normal findings **A** Abnormal findings **P** Pathophysiology

UNIT 2

A **Dysarthria**, a disturbance in muscular control of speech, is abnormal.

P Dysarthria is due to ischaemia affecting motor nuclei of CN X and CN XII, defects in the premotor or motor cortex that provide motor input for the face throat and mouth, or cerebellar disease.

A **Dysphonia**, difficulty making laryngeal sounds, is abnormal and can progress to **aphonia** (total loss of voice).

P Dysphonia is usually caused by lesions of CN X or swelling and inflammation of the larynx.

URGENT FINDING

The consumer with dysphonia

Consumers with signs of dysphonia (impaired laryngeal speech) are at high risk for dysphagia (difficulty with swallowing) and therefore aspiration. A thorough assessment of swallowing is warranted before the consumer may eat unassisted, otherwise this consumer may not be able to protect their airways. Depending on your resources and scope, you may need to refer to a speech therapist to have swallowing comprehensively assessed.

A **Apraxia**, the inability to convert the intended speech into the motor act of speech, is abnormal.

P Apraxia is due to dysfunction in the precentral gyrus of the frontal lobe.

A **Agraphia**, the loss of the ability to write, is abnormal.

P Agraphia is caused by lesions of Broca's and Wernicke's areas in the dominant side of the brain.

A **Alexia**, the inability to grasp the meaning of written words and sentences (word blindness), is abnormal.

P Alexia is usually due to a lesion of the angular gyrus and the occipital lobe.

TABLE 7.7 Classification of aphasias

APHASIA	PATHOPHYSIOLOGY	CHARACTERISTICS
Broca's aphasia	Motor cortex lesion, Broca's area	Speech slow and hesitant, the consumer has difficulty in selecting and organising words. Naming, word and phrase repetition, and writing impaired. Subtle defects in comprehension.
Wernicke's aphasia	Left hemisphere lesion in Wernicke's area	Auditory comprehension impaired, as is content of speech. Consumer unaware of deficits. Naming severely impaired.
Anomic aphasia	Left hemisphere lesion in Wernicke's area	Consumer unable to name objects or places. Comprehension and repetition of words and phrases intact.
Conduction aphasia	Lesion in the arcuate fasciculus, which connects and transports messages between Broca's and Wernicke's areas	Consumer has difficulty repeating words, substitutes incorrect sound for another sound (e.g. *dork* for *fork*).
Global aphasia	Lesions in the frontal-temporal area	Both oral and written comprehension severely impaired; naming, repetition of words and phrases, ability to write impaired.
Transcortical sensory aphasia	Lesion in the periphery of Broca's and Wernicke's areas (watershed zone)	Impairment in comprehension, naming and writing. Word and phrase repetition intact.
Transcortical motor aphasia	Lesion anterior, superior or lateral to Broca's area	Comprehension intact. Naming and ability to write impaired. Word and phrase repetition intact.

Cognitive abilities and mentation

Assessment of cognitive function includes testing for attention, memory, judgement, insight, spatial perception, calculation, abstraction, thought processes and thought content.

E Examination   **N** Normal findings   **A** Abnormal findings   **P** Pathophysiology

Attention

E 1. Pronounce a list of numbers slowly (approximately 1 second apart), starting with a list of two numbers and progressing to a series of five or six numbers. For example: 2, 5; 3, 7, 8; 1, 9, 4, 3; 1, 5, 4, 9, 0.

2. Ask the consumer to repeat the numbers in correct order, both forwards and backwards.

3. Give the consumer a different series of the same number of digits, if the consumer is unable to repeat the first series correctly. Stop after two misses of any length series.

4. Serial 7s is another way of assessing attention and concentration. Instruct the consumer to begin with the number 100 and to count backwards by subtracting 7 each time: 100, 93, 86, 79, 72, 65, etc.

5. The consumer may also try serial 3s (counting backwards from 100 by 3s) if unable to perform serial 7s.

N The consumer should be able to correctly repeat the series of numbers up to a series of five numbers. The consumer should be able to recite serial 7s or serial 3s accurately to at least the 40s or 50s from 100 within 1 minute. (Be aware this test will not be appropriate for people who have issues with numeracy.)

A If the consumer has a short attention span, the consumer will not be able to repeat the numbers in sequence or perform serial 7s or 3s.

P Dementia, neurological injury or disease, and intellectual disability may impair attention.

CLINICAL REASONING

Preparing for cognitive mental status screening

The Mini Mental State Exam (MMSE) is a widely used tool for assessing cognitive mental status, detecting impairment following the course of an illness, and monitoring response to treatment; however, this needs to be contextually appropriate. The MMSE is most useful in screening for the cognitive deficits seen in syndromes of dementia and delirium. The MMSE has been adapted to many contexts; some are available online or through your healthcare organisation.

A mental status examination usually assesses appearance, behaviour, affect, mood, cognition, speech and thought form, thought content, perception, history obtained from family/carers, orientation, concentration, short-term and long-term memory, and cortical function.

Assessment of cognitive function

You should have on hand:

> pre-printed lists of objects, phrases and numbers for consumer recall and explanation

> answers to long-term memory questions to accurately assess recall

> alternative tests prepared for consumers with language barriers, aphasia, deafness, blindness, etc.

> paper and pencils for consumer to use to respond.

One version is accessible via https://oxfordmedicaleducation.com/geriatrics/mini-mental-state-examination-mmse/

Content specific for children can be found at https://www.rch.org.au/clinicalguide/guideline_index/Mental_state_examination/

Cultural differences will need to be considered. Some examples include:

- A medical practitioner's example of working in Australian Aboriginal communities: http://www.aams.org.au/mark_sheldon/ch8/ch8_mental_state_exam.htm

- Transcultural mental health centre: https://www.dhi.health.nsw.gov.au/transcultural-mental-health-centre-tmhc/health-professionals/cross-cultural-mental-health-care-a-resource-kit-for-gps-and-health-professionals/cross-cultural-mental-health-assessment

- The Centre of Best Practice in Aboriginal & Torres Strait Islander Suicide Prevention: https://cbpatsisp.com.au/clearing-house/best-practice-screening-assessment/

E Examination   **N** Normal findings   **A** Abnormal findings   **P** Pathophysiology

Memory

E 1. Assess immediate recall in conjunction with attention span as discussed previously.

2. Give a list of three items that the consumer is to remember and repeat in 5 minutes. Have the consumer repeat the items to check initial understanding. During the 5 minutes, carry on conversation as usual. Ask the consumer to repeat the items again after the 5-minute time frame.

3. If the consumer is unable to remember one or more of the objects, show a list containing the objects along with others, and check recognition.

4. Record the number of objects remembered over the number of objects given.

5. Long-term memory is memory that is retained for at least 24 hours. Commonly asked questions for testing long-term memory include name of spouse, spouse's birthday, mother's maiden name, name of the Prime Minister and the consumer's birthday.

N The consumer should be able to correctly respond to questions and to identify all the objects as requested.

A Memory loss is abnormal.

P Memory loss may be caused by pathologies such as nervous system infection, trauma, stroke, tumours, Alzheimer's disease, seizure disorders, alcohol and drug toxicity. Memory is located in the temporal lobe and the hippocampus. Damage to these areas, in the form of haemorrhage, ischaemia, compression or herniation, will cause memory impairment. See Table 7.4 for neurological signs of drug ingestion.

Judgement

E 1. During the interview, assess whether the consumer is responding appropriately to social, family and work situations that are discussed.

2. Note whether the consumer's decisions are based on sound reasoning and decision making.

3. Present hypothetical situations and ask the consumer to make decisions as to what his or her responses would be. For example: 'What would you do if you were driving and noticed a police car with flashing lights behind you?' or 'What would you do if you saw smoke in your house?'

4. Interview the consumer's family or directly observe the consumer to assess judgement more carefully.

N The consumer should be able to evaluate and act appropriately in situations requiring judgement.

A Impaired judgement, the inability to act appropriately in situations, is abnormal.

P Frontal lobe damage, dementia, psychotic states and an intellectual disability may cause the consumer to exhibit lack of appropriate judgement.

Insight

Insight is the ability to realistically understand oneself.

E 1. Ask the consumer to describe personal health status, reason for seeking health care, symptoms, current life situation and general coping behaviours.

2. If the consumer describes symptoms, ask what life was like prior to the appearance of the symptoms, what life changes the illness has introduced, and whether the consumer feels a need for help.

N The consumer should demonstrate a realistic awareness and understanding of self.

A Unrealistic perceptions of self are abnormal.

P Lack of insight may occur in the euphoric stages of bipolar affective disorders, endogenous anxiety states or depressed states.

E Examination **N** Normal findings **A** Abnormal findings **P** Pathophysiology

Spatial perception
(May be considered advanced practice depending on context)
Spatial perception is the ability to recognise the relationships of objects in space.

E 1. Ask the consumer to copy figures that you have previously drawn, such as a circle, triangle, square, cross, and a three-dimensional cube.
2. Ask the consumer to draw the face of a clock, including the numbers around the dial.
3. Ask the consumer to identify a familiar sound while keeping their eyes closed; for example, a closing door, running water or a finger **snap**.
4. Have the consumer identify right from left body parts.

N The consumer should be able to draw the objects without difficulty and as closely as possible to the original drawing, and to identify familiar sounds and left and right body parts.

A **Agnosia**, the inability to recognise the form and nature of objects or persons, is abnormal. It may be visual, auditory or somatosensory. For example, the consumer may be unable to name or recognise objects, faces or familiar objects by touch, or to identify the meaning of nonverbal sounds.

P Lesions in the nondominant parietal lobe impair the consumer's ability to appreciate self in relation to the environment and to conceive three-dimensional objects. Lesions in the occipital lobe will cause visual agnosia, and temporal lesions will cause auditory agnosia.

A Apraxia, the inability to perform purposeful movements despite the preservation of motor ability and sensation, is abnormal. **Constructional apraxia** is the inability to reproduce figures on paper (**Figure 7.11**).

P Apraxia is usually associated with lesions of the precentral gyrus of the frontal lobe.

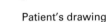
Diamond   Patient's drawing

FIGURE 7.11 Constructional apraxia

Calculation
The consumer's ability to perform serial 7s was discussed in the section on attention and is also an assessment of calculation (note: be aware of consumer's abilities in numeracy).

E 1. Ask the consumer to add 3 to 100, then 3 to that number, until numbers greater than 150 are reached.
2. Note the amount of time and difficulty associated with the calculations.

N The consumer should be able to calculate the correct numbers upon subtraction or addition within educational abilities and with fewer than four errors in less than 1½ minutes.

A **Dyscalculia**, the inability to perform calculations, is abnormal (unless low level of schooling or issues are identified with numeracy).

P Dyscalculia may be caused by depression or anxiety, dementia or an intellectual disability. The most common cause of dyscalculia is focal lesions in the dominant parietal lobe; however, calculation deficits have also been ascribed to focal lesions in the frontal, temporal and occipital lobes.

Abstract reasoning
E 1. Ask the consumer to describe the meaning of a familiar fable, proverb or metaphor. Use examples that are meaningful within the context of the consumer's culture and language. Some examples from Australian and New Zealand culture are:
   - A storm in a tea cup
   - Opening a can of worms
   - Don't let the cat out of the bag
   - You shouldn't look a gift horse in the mouth
   - It's raining cats and dogs
2. Note the degree of concreteness versus abstraction in the answers.

E Examination **N** Normal findings **A** Abnormal findings **P** Pathophysiology

N Consumers should be able to give the abstract meanings of proverbs, fables or metaphors within their cultural understanding.

A Conceptual concreteness, the inability to describe in abstractions, to generalise from specifics, and to apply general principles, is abnormal.

P Alterations of cognitive processes causing concreteness in thought may occur in consumers with dementia, frontal tumours or schizophrenia. Concreteness in thought processes may also indicate low intelligence.

Thought process and content

E 1. Observe the consumer's pattern of thought for relevance, consistency, coherence, logic and organisation.
2. Listen throughout the interview for flaws in content of conversation.

N Thought processes should be logical, coherent and goal-oriented. Thought content should be based on reality.

A Unrealistic, illogical thought processes and interruptions of the thinking processes, such as blocking, are abnormal. Blocking is demonstrated when an extended pause occurs during a sentence due to a repressed or painful subject matter. Sometimes, the thoughts following are unrelated to what the consumer was discussing.

P Abnormal thought processes are often due to psychotic symptoms.

A Flight of ideas, demonstrated when the consumer changes from subject to subject within a sentence, is abnormal. This is frequently due to distractions or word associations with a resultant lack of sense of purpose of the conversation.

P Consumers suffering from manic episodes of bipolar affective disorder often demonstrate flight of ideas.

A **Confabulation**, the making up of answers unrelated to facts, is abnormal.

P Confabulation is often related to ageing, memory loss, disorientation, Korsakoff's psychosis or psychopathic disorders.

A **Echolalia**, the involuntary repetition of a word or sentence that was uttered by another person, is abnormal.

P Consumers suffering from dementia or schizophrenia often demonstrate echolalia.

A **Neologism**, a word coined by the consumer that is meaningful only to the consumer, is an abnormal finding.

P Consumers with delirium or schizophrenia may exhibit neologism.

A Delusions of persecution, grandiose delusions, hallucinations, illusions, obsessive-compulsiveness and paranoia are examples of abnormal thoughts.

P Abnormal thought content is demonstrated in consumers suffering from schizophrenia or dementia and in people who may be affected by substances.

Suicidal ideation

If the consumer has expressed feelings of sadness, hopelessness, despair, worthlessness or grief, explore his or her feelings further with more specific questions such as:

E 1. Have you ever felt so bad that you wanted to hurt yourself?
2. Do you ever feel that life isn't worth living?
3. Do you feel like hurting yourself now?

N The consumer should provide a negative response and be able to verbalise his or her self-worth.

A An affirmative response is abnormal and requires probing such as:
> Do you have a plan to hurt yourself?
> What would happen if you were dead?
> Continued affirmative responses and expressions of worthlessness and hopelessness should be interpreted as suicidal ideation, a psychiatric emergency that requires immediate referral to a specialist.

E Examination   **N** Normal findings   **A** Abnormal findings   **P** Pathophysiology

P Suicidal ideation is associated with mental disorders, particularly depression, substance abuse and personality disorders.

CLINICAL REASONING

Suicide risk factors and clinical decision making

Suicide was the fifteenth leading cause of all deaths in Australia in 2020. In the 15–44-year-old age group it was the leading cause of death. In 2020, there were 3139 deaths from suicide in Australia (Australian Bureau of Statistics, 2021). As in most states in Australia, in Queensland males remain overrepresented for death rates by suicide and there were higher percentages of deaths by suicide related to remoteness (Leske, Adam, Catakovic, Weir & Kolves, 2022).

Consider the following risk factors for suicide when undertaking a health history and deciding where to focus attention:

> Living with a mental illness diagnosis
> Female (more non-fatal suicide behaviour)
> Male (more fatal suicide behaviour)
> Prior non-fatal suicide behaviour
> Family member with suicide behaviour (both fatal and non-fatal) history
> Substance use and overuse
> Unwillingness to seek help because of stigma
> Barriers to accessing mental health treatment
> Stressful life events or loss
> Easy access to lethal methods such as guns and poisons
> Is thinking about suicide, with or without a plan
> Have a history of living with post-traumatic stress disorder

Risk factors identified should prompt the health practitioner to explicitly explore any self-harm plans, means and opportunity, and refer to emergency mental health services as outlined in your mental health legislation if a positive plan and risk are identified.

Be aware of your language around suicide when assessing consumers. As a health professional you need to be sure that your language does not present suicide as a desired outcome (e.g. 'successful suicide' or 'unsuccessful suicide'; try 'died by suicide' or 'took their own life') or add to the stigma, such as associating suicide with a crime or a sin (e.g. saying 'commit/ed suicide'; try 'took their own life', or 'suicide death' instead) (Everymind, 2022).

Table 7.8 compares and contrasts the various clinical parameters that distinguish dementia, depression, delirium and acute confusion.

TABLE 7.8 Distinguishing dementia, depression, delirium and acute confusion

PARAMETER	DEMENTIA	DEPRESSION	DELIRIUM	ACUTE CONFUSION
Definition	Deterioration of all cognitive function with little or no disturbance of consciousness or perception	An abnormal emotional state characterised by feelings of sadness, despair and discouragement	A disorder of perception with heightened awareness, hallucinations, vivid dreams and intense emotional disturbances	An inability to think with customary speed, clarity and coherence
Onset	Gradual	Variable	Sudden	Variable
Pathophysiology	> Alzheimer's disease > Metabolic disorders > Stroke > Head injury	> Inherited: neurochemical abnormalities > Situational: acute loss of significant person > Stroke > Parkinson's disease > Alzheimer's disease > Medications (e.g. steroids)	> Withdrawal from alcohol and other drugs > Drug intoxication > Encephalitis > Traumatic injury > Febrile states > Hypoxia > Fluid and electrolyte imbalance	> Metabolic disorders > Drug intoxication > Traumatic injury > Febrile states

>>

E Examination   **N** Normal findings   **A** Abnormal findings   **P** Pathophysiology

UNIT 2

>> **TABLE 7.8** *continued*

PARAMETER	DEMENTIA	DEPRESSION	DELIRIUM	ACUTE CONFUSION
Attention	Impaired	Intact	Impaired: heightened or dulled	Impaired: dulled
Memory	> Short-term: impaired first > Long-term: intact for a while	Intact	> Short-term: impaired > Long-term: intact	> Short-term: impaired > Long-term: may be intact
Judgement	Impaired	Intact	> Grossly impaired > Impulsive > Volatile	Impaired
Insight	Impaired	May be intact	Impaired	Impaired
Spatial perception	Impaired	Intact	Intact	May be impaired
Calculation	Impaired	May be intact	May be intact	Impaired
Abstract reasoning	Impaired	Intact	Impaired	Impaired
Thought process and content	Impaired	Intact	Impaired, hallucinations present	Impaired, incoherent

CLINICAL REASONING

Practice tip: Depression acronym

An easy way to remember the symptoms of clinical depression is to use the acronyms CAPS or SIG-E-CAPS

C	Concentration impaired or decreased
A	Appetite changes
P	Psychomotor function decreased
S	Suicidal ideations and sleep disturbances

SOURCED FROM HTTPS://WWW.NURSEBUFF.COM/NURSING-ASSESSMENT-MNEMONICS/

S	Sleep changes – increased during day or decreased at night
I	Interest loss in activities that used to interest them
G	Guilt or worthlessness – depressed elderly tend to devalue themselves
E	Energy reduction/lack of – fatigue is a common presenting symptom
C	Cognition/Concentration – reduced cognition and/or difficulty concentrating
A	Appetite change – loss (common) or gain of weight (sometimes)
P	Psychomotor – agitation, anxiety or lethargy
S	Suicide – suicidal thoughts or preoccupation with death (elderly consumers with higher risk factors for this include living alone, male, alcoholism, comorbid physical illness)

ADAPTED FROM HTTP://WEBMEDIA.UNMC.EDU/INTMED/GERIATRICS/REYNOLDS/PEARLCARDS/DEPRESSION/SIGECAPS.HTM

CLINICAL REASONING

Mental state examination

An easy way to remember the categories of a mental state examination is to use the acronym 'I AM A STAR':

> I: Introduce yourself. For example: Hello my name is …
> A: Appearance and behaviour
> M: Movement and gait
> A: Affect and mood
> S: Speech
> T: Thought pattern
> A: Attention and concentration
> R: Respond and record

ADAPTED FROM GIBSON, H. (2009). USING MNEMONICS TO INCREASE KNOWLEDGE OF AN ORGANIZING CURRICULUM FRAMEWORK. *TEACHING AND LEARNING IN NURSING*, 4(2), 56–62.

Mental health

Findings during the cognitive functioning examination may indicate the need for further mental health screening. **Table 7.9** summarises findings common to mental illness that may lead the practitioner to refer the consumer for further diagnostic study.

TABLE 7.9 Mental illnesses

DISORDER	DEFINING CHARACTERISTICS	POPULATION CHARACTERISTICS
Anxiety disorders > Panic > Phobias > Generalised anxiety disorder > Obsessive-compulsive disorder > Trauma and stressor-related disorders	A group of conditions that share extreme or pathological anxiety as the principal disturbance of mood or emotional tone	> Common across cultures > Early age onset > Relapsing or recurrent episodes > Periods of disability > Significant overlap with mood and substance abuse disorders
Panic disorder > Panic attack > Panic disorder	The consumer has experienced recurrent unexpected panic attacks and develops persistent concern over having recurring attacks or changes behaviour to avoid or minimise such attacks Panic attacks are abrupt surges of intense fear or intense discomfort that reach a peak within minutes accompanied by physical and or cognitive symptoms	> Twice as common in women as men > Onset most common between adolescence and mid-adult life > Significant overlap with mood, substance abuse, psychotic disorders > Panic attacks can be used as a descriptive specifier for any anxiety disorder
Phobias > Agoraphobia > Social phobia > Specific phobias	Marked fear of specific objects or situations Fear and anxiety to the specific phobias must be intense and severe The amount of fear experienced may vary with proximity to the feared object and may occur in anticipation of or in the actual presence of the object or situation	> Experienced by approximately 8% of the population > Typically begin in childhood > There is a second peak in the middle 20s of adulthood > Animal, natural environment and situational-specific phobias are predominantly experienced by females, whereas blood injection-injury phobia is experienced by both sexes
Generalised anxiety disorder	Protracted period of anxiety and worry accompanied by multiple associated physical and cognitive symptoms Persistent and excessive worry about various domains that the individual finds difficult to control	> Twice as common in women as men > Half of cases begin in childhood or adolescence > Symptoms increase with life stress or difficulties
Obsessive-compulsive disorder	Obsessions are recurrent; intrusive thoughts, impulses or images that are perceived as inappropriate, grotesque or forbidden Compulsions are repetitive behaviours or mental acts that reduce the anxiety that accompanies an obsession	> Equally common among the sexes > Begins in adolescence to young adult life in males > Males have an earlier onset than females > Female onset typically is young adult life > Familial pattern > Strongly associated with Tourette disorder > Significant overlap with other anxiety disorders and major depressive disorder

>> **TABLE 7.9** continued

DISORDER	DEFINING CHARACTERISTICS	POPULATION CHARACTERISTICS
Acute and post-traumatic stress disorders	Acute: the anxiety and behavioural disturbances that develop within the first month after exposure to an extreme trauma If the symptoms persist for more than 1 month and are associated with functional impairment, the diagnosis is changed to post-traumatic stress disorder	> Twice as prevalent in females as males > Develop in approximately 9% of those exposed to extreme trauma > Rape > Physical assault > Near-death experience > Witnessing murder and combat

Mood disorders
> Major depressive disorder
> Persistent depressive disorder – dysthymia
> Bipolar disorder
> Cyclothymia
	A cluster of mental disorders best recognised by depression or mania
	Common feature of depressive disorders is the presence of sad, empty or irritable mood accompanied by somatic and cognitive changes that significantly affect the individual's capacity to function
		> Rank among the top 10 causes of worldwide disability
		> More prevalent in women
		> Leading cause of absenteeism and diminished productivity at work
		> Common comorbidities include anxiety disorder, personality disorders, and chronic medical conditions
		> May be caused by:
		  • Dominant hemispheric strokes
		  • Hyperthyroidism
		  • Antihypertensives
		  • Cushing disease
		  • Oral contraceptives
		  • Pancreatic cancer
		  • Alcohol withdrawal

Major depressive disorder	Five or more of the following symptoms have been present for the same 2-week period and represent a change from previous functioning; at least one symptom is either depressed mood or loss of interest or pleasure: > Depressed mood > Loss of interest or pleasure > Significant weight loss when not dieting > Insomnia or hypersomnia > Psychomotor agitation or retardation > Fatigue or loss of energy > Feeling of worthlessness > Diminished ability to think or concentrate; indecisiveness > Recurrent thoughts of death or suicidal ideation	> More common among females > Most severe depressions more common among the elderly > At least 50% will recur
Dysthymia – persistent depressive disorder	A chronic form of depression; symptoms are constant for a 2-year period (1 year for children)	> Twice as many females as males are diagnosed > Early onset (childhood, adolescence or early adult life) > Affects about 2% of adults each year > If onset in childhood before 21 years old, associated strongly with subsequent substance abuse and comorbid personality disorders > Susceptible to major depression episode superimposed on dysthymia
Bipolar disorder > Type I (manic episode may have been preceded by hypomanic or major depressive episodes) > Type II (hypomanic episodes only)	Recurrent mood disorder featuring one or more episodes of mania or mixed episodes of mania/hypomania and depression	> Equally common in males and females > Affects about 2% of adult population > Lifetime risk of suicide in individuals with bipolar disorder is estimated to be at least 15 times that of the general population. A past history of suicide behaviour and days spent depressed in the past years are associated with greater risk of suicide behaviour
Cyclothymic disorder	Chronic fluctuating mood disturbance involving numerous periods of hypomanic symptoms and periods of depressive symptoms that are distinct from each other Manic and depressive states of insufficient intensity or duration to merit a diagnosis of bipolar disorder or major depressive disorder	> 33% higher risk than general population to develop bipolar disorder I or II > Cyclothymic disorder onset is usually adolescence or early adult life

>> **TABLE 7.9** *continued*

DISORDER	DEFINING CHARACTERISTICS	POPULATION CHARACTERISTICS
Schizophrenia	Profound disruption in cognition and emotion. Two or more of the following symptoms persist for a significant portion of time during a 1-month period: > Delusions > Hallucinations > Disorganised speech > Grossly disorganised or catatonic behaviour > Negative symptoms: affective flattening, **alogia** (inability to express oneself through speech) or **avolition** (lack of motivation for work or other goal-directed activity)	> Onset during young adulthood > Women experience later onset than men > One-year prevalence in adults is estimated to be 1.3% > Associated with significantly higher mortality rate than the general population > Suicide > Comorbid medical illness: visual and dental problems, hypertension, diabetes, hyperlipidaemia and sexually transmitted diseases

SOURCE: INFORMATION CONDENSED FROM HARRISON, C., CHARLES, J. & BRITT, H. (2015). COMORBIDITIES AND RISK FACTORS AMONG PATIENTS WITH SCHIZOPHRENIA. *AUSTRALIAN FAMILY PHYSICIAN, 44*(11), 2015 PAGES 781–3.

CLINICAL **REASONING**

The elderly depressed consumer

It is often difficult to differentiate between depression and early dementia in the elderly. The clinical presentation of apathy, difficulty concentrating, memory loss, and general inability to keep up with the demands of everyday life is common to both depression and early dementia. It is imperative to also remember that the elderly may have other aetiologies that may account for their behaviour, such as thyroid disease, altered glucose metabolism, electrolyte imbalance and polypharmacy. A complete health history and physical examination are warranted, and referral if abnormal findings are present.

Sensory examination

Sensation should be tested early in the neurological assessment because of the detail involved and because the cooperation of the consumer is required. The conclusions of the assessment may be unreliable if the consumer becomes fatigued.

The sensory examination is divided into three sections. First, the exteroceptive sensations (superficial sensations that originate in the sensory receptors in the skin and mucous membranes) are tested. These are the sensations of light touch, superficial pain and temperature.

Next, the proprioceptive sensations (deep sensations, with sensory receptors in the muscles, joints, tendons and ligaments) are assessed. **Proprioception** is tested with the modalities of motion and position, and vibration sense.

Finally, the cortical sensations (those that require cerebral integrative and discriminative abilities) are assessed. **Stereognosis**, **graphaesthesia**, two-point discrimination, and extinction are tested.

Exteroceptive sensation

1. Explain the procedure to the consumer before starting the examination.
2. The sensory examination is carried out with the consumer's eyes closed.
3. For a thorough sensory examination, the consumer should be in a supine position.
4. The consumer should be cooperative and reliable, although the pain examination may be performed on comatose consumers.
5. Note the consumer's ability to perceive the sensation.
6. Much of the sensory component of the neurological examination is subjective; observe the reactions of the consumer by watching their face for grimacing, or for withdrawal of the stimulated extremity.
7. Compare the consumer's sensation on the corresponding areas bilaterally.
8. Note whether any sensory deficits follow a dermatome distribution.
9. The borders of any area exhibiting changes in sensation should be mapped by dermatomes (see **Figure 7.7**).

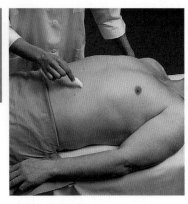

FIGURE 7.12 Assessment of light touch

Light touch

E 1. Use a wisp of cotton and apply the stimulus with very light strokes (**Figure 7.12**). If the skin is calloused, or for thicker skin on the hands and soles, the stimulus may need to be intensified, although care must be taken not to stimulate subcutaneous tissues.
  2. Begin with distal areas of the consumer's limbs and move proximally.
  3. Test the hand, lower arm, abdomen, foot and leg. Examination of sensation of the face is discussed in the cranial nerves section.
  4. To prevent the consumer from being able to predict the next touch, alter the rate and rhythm of stimulation. Also, vary the sites of stimulation, keeping in mind that the right and left sides must be compared.
  5. Instruct the consumer to respond by saying 'now' or 'yes' when the stimulus is felt, and to identify the area that was stimulated either verbally or by pointing to it.

Proprioceptive sensation

Motion and position

E 1. Grasp the consumer's index finger with your thumb and index finger. Hold the finger at the sides (parallel to the plane of movement) in order not to exert upwards or downwards pressure with your fingers and thus give the consumer any clues as to which direction the finger is moving. The consumer's fingers should be relaxed.
  2. Have the consumer shut their eyes, and show the consumer what 'up' and 'down' feel like by moving the finger in those directions.
  3. Use gentle, slow and deliberate movements. Begin with larger movements that become smaller and less perceptible.
  4. Instruct the consumer to respond 'up,' 'down,' or 'I can't tell' after each time you raise or lower the finger.
  5. Repeat this several times. Vary the motion in order not to establish a predictable pattern.
  6. Repeat steps 2–5 with the finger of the consumer's opposite hand, and then with the great toes.
  7. If there appears to be a deficit in motion sense, proceed to the proximal joints such as wrists or ankles, and repeat the test.

N The consumer should be able to correctly identify the changes of position of the body.

A Inability to perceive direction of movement is abnormal.

P Peripheral neuropathies will interfere with position sense. A lesion of the posterior column will cause an ipsilateral loss of position sense. Lesions of the sensory cortex, the thalamus, or the connections between them (thalamocortical connections) may also disrupt position sense.

More detailed assessment such as vibration sense, cortical sensation (such as stereognosis, graphaesthesia, two-point discrimination and extinction) is usually undertaken in advanced assessment and can be found in the online content.

Examination of cranial nerves

A complete examination of the 12 cranial nerves is necessary when a baseline assessment is desired, if a tumour of a specific cranial nerve is suspected, or if periodic assessment is needed after surgery or radiation treatments. An abbreviated cranial nerve examination is an integral part of a neurological screening examination. The screening examination would include cranial nerves II, III, IV and VI: visual acuity and gross visual fields, fundoscopic examination, pupillary reactions, and extraocular movements; cranial nerves VII, VIII, IX, X and XII: facial musculature and expression, gross hearing, voice and inspection of the tongue.

E Examination **N** Normal findings **A** Abnormal findings **P** Pathophysiology

Olfactory nerve (CN I)

E 1. Ask the consumer to close their eyes.
2. Test each side separately by asking the consumer to occlude one nostril by pressing against it with a finger. Determine whether the nasal passages are patent by asking the consumer to breathe through first one nostril and then through the other while occluding the opposing nostril by pressing against it with a finger. Assessment of the olfactory nerve may be delayed if the consumer has a severe cold, allergic rhinitis, nasal packing, had recent oral surgery, or if nasal steroids have been used for a prolonged period.
3. Ask the consumer to hold the test vial close to the nostril and inhale deeply in order to cause the odour to surround the mucous membranes and adequately stimulate the olfactory nerve (**Figure 7.13**).
4. Ask the consumer to identify the contents of each vial.
5. Present one odour at a time and alternate them from nostril to nostril. Keep aromatic substances such as cloves, coffee, orange, peanut butter or chocolate in closed glass vials until they are presented to the consumer. Avoid using noxious odours such as alcohol, camphor, ammonia, acetic acid or formaldehyde, which may stimulate the trigeminal nerve endings in the nasal mucosa.
6. Allow enough time to pass between presentation of vials to prevent confusion of the olfactory system.
7. Record the number of substances tested and the number of times the consumer was able to correctly identify the contents.
8. Note whether a difference between the right and the left sides was apparent.

N The consumer should be able to distinguish and identify the odours with each nostril.

A **Anosmia**, the loss of the sense of smell, is abnormal.

P Total loss of the sense of smell may be caused by trauma to the cribriform plate, sinusitis, colds or heavy smoking. Unilateral anosmia may be the result of an intracranial neoplasm, such as a meningioma of the sphenoid ridge compressing the olfactory tract or bulb.

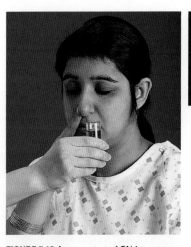

FIGURE 7.13 Assessment of CN I

Optic nerve (CN II)

Visual acuity
E **N** **A** **P** See Chapter 10.

Visual fields
E **N** **A** **P** See Chapter 10.

Fundoscopic examination
E **N** **A** **P** See Chapter 10.

Oculomotor nerve (CN III)

Cardinal fields of gaze
E **N** **A** **P** See Chapter 10.

Eyelid elevation
E **N** **A** **P** See Chapter 10.

Pupil reactions (direct, consensual, accommodation)
E **N** **A** **P** See Chapter 10.

Trochlear nerve (CN IV)

Cardinal fields of gaze
E **N** **A** **P** See Chapter 10.

E Examination   **N** Normal findings   **A** Abnormal findings   **P** Pathophysiology

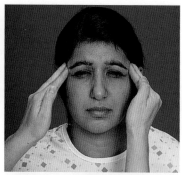

A. Temporalis muscles

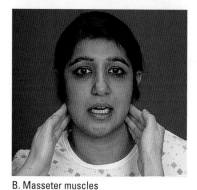

B. Masseter muscles

FIGURE 7.14 Assessment of the motor component of CN V

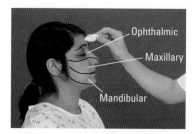

Ophthalmic

Maxillary

Mandibular

FIGURE 7.15 Assessment of the sensory component of CN V: Light touch

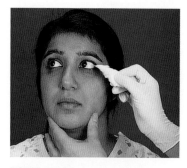

FIGURE 7.16 Assessment of the sensory component of CN V and motor component of CN VII: Corneal reflex

Trigeminal nerve (CN V)

Motor component

E 1. Instruct the consumer to clench the jaw.
2. Palpate the contraction of the temporalis (**Figure 7.14A**) and masseter (**Figure 7.14B**) muscles on each side of the face by feeling for contraction of the muscles with the finger pads of the first three fingers.
3. Ask the consumer to move the jaw from side to side against resistance from your hand. Feel for weakness on one side or the other as the consumer pushes against resistance.
4. Test the muscles of mastication by having the consumer bite down with the molars on each side of a tongue blade and comparing the depth of the impressions made by the teeth. If you can pull the tongue blade out while the consumer is biting on it, there is weakness of the muscles of mastication.
5. Observe for fasciculation and note the bulk, contour and tone of the muscles of mastication.

Sensory component

E 1. Instruct the consumer to close their eyes.
2. Test light touch by using a cotton wisp to lightly stroke the consumer's face in each area of the sensory distribution of the trigeminal nerve (**Figure 7.15**).
3. Instruct the consumer to respond by saying 'now' each time the touch of the cotton wisp is felt.
4. Test and compare both sides of the face.
5. To assess superficial pain sensation, use a sterile needle. Before testing, show the consumer how the sharpness of the needle feels compared to the dullness of the opposite, blunt end. Testing with the blunt end will give some reliability to the assessment.
   a. Instruct the consumer to respond by saying 'sharp' or 'dull' when each sensation is felt.
   b. Irregularly alternate the sharp and dull ends, and again test each distribution area of the trigeminal nerve on both sides of the face.
6. Test temperature sensation if other abnormalities have been detected. Use vials of hot and cold water.
   a. Touch the vials to each dermatomal distribution area, alternating hot and cold.
   b. The consumer should respond by saying 'hot' or 'cold'.
7. Because sensation to the cornea is supplied by the trigeminal nerve, test the corneal reflex (the motor component is CN VII). The corneal reflex should not be routinely assessed in conscious consumers, unless there is a clinical suspicion of trauma to CN V or CN VII.
   a. Ask the consumer to open their eyes and look away from you.
   b. Approach the consumer out of the line of vision to eliminate the blink reflex. You can stabilise the consumer's chin with your hand if it is moving.
   c. Lightly stroke the cornea with a slightly moistened cotton wisp (to avoid irritating the cornea) (**Figure 7.16**). Avoid stroking just the sclera or the lashes of the eye. An alternative technique is to instil normal saline eye drops instead of a light stroke of a cotton wisp.
   d. Observe for bilateral blinking of the eyes.
   e. Repeat on the opposite eye.

E Examination **N** Normal findings **A** Abnormal findings **P** Pathophysiology

N The temporalis and masseter muscles should be equally strong on palpation. The jaw should not deviate and should be equally strong during side-to-side movement against resistance. The volume and bulk of the muscles should be bilaterally equal. Sensation to light touch, superficial pain and temperature should be present on the sensory distribution areas of the trigeminal nerve. The corneal reflex should cause bilateral blinking of eyes.

A Lesions of the trigeminal nerve may give rise to either reduced sensory perception or to facial pain, both of which are abnormal.

P Aneurysms of the internal carotid artery next to the cavernous sinus may give rise to severe pain in the ophthalmic or mandibular distribution of the trigeminal nerve due to the pressure of the aneurysm on the nerve. Neoplasms that compress the gasserian ganglion or root, such as meningiomas, pituitary adenomas and malignant tumours of the nasopharynx, may cause facial pain and impairment of sensation. Head injuries, especially basilar skull fractures, may give rise to facial anaesthesia and paralysis of the muscles of mastication.

A Trigeminal neuralgia (tic douloureux), characterised by brief, paroxysmal, unilateral facial pain along the distribution of the trigeminal nerve, is abnormal. The pain can be provoked by touch or movement of the face, such as in tooth brushing, yawning, chewing or talking. There is no associated motor weakness.

P Trigeminal neuralgia may occur in consumers with multiple sclerosis due to demyelination of the root of CN V. The consumer with a posterior fossa tumour may have trigeminal neuralgia. In most cases, there is no aetiology found.

A Postherpetic neuralgia is found most often in the elderly. The pain is continuous and is described as a constant, burning ache with occasional stabbing pains. The stabbing pain may begin spontaneously or may be provoked by touch. The pain is unilateral and tends to follow the distribution of the ophthalmic distribution of the trigeminal nerve. It is abnormal.

P *Herpes zoster* involvement of the trigeminal nerve causes postherpetic neuralgia. Inflammatory lesions are found throughout the trigeminal pathways.

A Tetanus is characterised by tonic spasms interfering with the muscles that open the jaw (trismus). **Dysphagia** and spasms of the pharyngeal muscles are also observed in tetanus. Tetanus is abnormal.

P Motor root involvement of the trigeminal nerve causes the spasm of the masseter muscles.

Abducens nerve (CN VI)

Cardinal fields of gaze
E N A P See Chapter 10.

Facial nerve (CN VII)

Motor component
E 1. Observe the consumer's facial expressions for symmetry and mobility throughout the examination.
2. Note any asymmetry of the face, such as wrinkles or lack of wrinkles on one side of the face or one-sided blinking.
3. Test muscle contraction by asking the consumer to:
   a. frown
   b. raise their eyebrows
   c. wrinkle their forehead while looking up
   d. close their eyes lightly and then keep them closed against your resistance (Figure 7.17)
   e. smile, show teeth, purse lips, and whistle
   f. puff out the cheeks against the resistance of your hands.

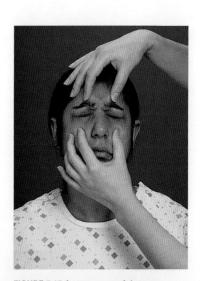

FIGURE 7.17 Assessment of the motor component of CN VII: Opening the consumer's eyes against resistance

E Examination N Normal findings A Abnormal findings P Pathophysiology

E 4. Observe for symmetry of facial muscles and for weakness during the above manoeuvres.

5. Note any abnormal movements such as tremors, tics, grimaces or immobility.

N Normal findings of the motor portion of the facial nerve include symmetry between the right and the left sides of the face as well as between the upper and lower portions of the face at rest and while executing facial movements. There should be an absence of abnormal muscle movement.

A **Bell's palsy** (idiopathic facial palsy), characterised by complete flaccid paralysis of the facial muscles on the involved side, is abnormal. The affected side of the face is smooth, the eye cannot close, the eyebrow droops, the labiofacial fold is gone, and the mouth may droop. Loss of the sensation of taste in the anterior two-thirds of the tongue may occur.

P Bell's palsy is caused by damage to the facial nerve. It is a lower motor neurone paralysis because the damage occurs along the facial nerve from its origin to its periphery.

A Supranuclear facial palsy is characterised by paralysis in the lower one-third to two-thirds of the face; the upper portion of the face is spared. The nasolabial fold is flat, and the eye on the affected side can close, although may be weaker. The consumer may be unable to keep the eye closed against resistance applied by the nurse. The muscles of the upper portion of the face remain intact. Supranuclear facial palsy is abnormal.

P Supranuclear facial palsy is due to an upper motor neurone lesion of the facial nerve.

Sensory component

E 1. Sensory examination of the facial nerve is limited to testing taste. The portions of the tongue that are tested are:
   a. the tip of the tongue for sweet and salty tastes
   b. along the borders and at the tip for sour taste
   c. the back of the tongue and the soft palate for bitter taste.

2. Test both sides of the tongue with each solution.

3. The consumer's tongue should protrude during the entire assessment of taste, and talking is not allowed. In order for the consumer to identify the substance, the words sweet, salty, bitter and sour should be written on a card so that the consumer can point to what is tasted. Be sure the consumer does not see which solution is being tested.

4. Cotton swabs may be used as applicators, using a different one for each solution.

5. Dip the cotton swab into the solution being tested and place it on the appropriate part of the tongue.

6. Instruct the consumer to point to the word that best describes the taste perception.

7. Instruct the consumer to rinse the mouth with water before the next solution is tested.

8. Repeat steps 5–7 until each solution has been tested on both sides of the tongue.

N Normal sensation would be accurate perceptions of sweet, sour, salty and bitter tastes.

A **Ageusia** (loss of taste) and **hypogeusia** (diminution of taste) are abnormal.

P Age, excessive smoking, extreme dryness of the oral mucosa, colds, medications, lesions of the medulla oblongata and lesions of the parietal lobe may cause alterations in the sense of taste.

E Examination   **N** Normal findings   **A** Abnormal findings   **P** Pathophysiology

Acoustic nerve (CN VIII)

Cochlear division

Hearing
E N A P   See Chapter 11.

Weber and Rinne tests
E N A P   See Chapter 11.

Vestibular division
The vestibular division of CN VIII assesses for **vertigo**.

E   1. During the history, ask the consumer if vertigo is experienced.
   2. Note any evidence of equilibrium disturbances. Refer to the section on cerebellar examination.
   3. Note the presence of nystagmus.

N   Vertigo is not normally present.

A   Vertigo describes an uncomfortable sensation of movement of the environment or the movement of self within a stationary environment; it is often accompanied by nausea, vomiting and nystagmus.

P   Vertigo is caused by a disorder of the labyrinth or the vestibular nerve. Causative factors may include migraine headache, which causes a disruption in the supply of the internal auditory artery. Tumours of the cerebellopontine angle may cause vertigo by compressing the vestibular nerve. Head injuries that involve the labyrinth may cause vertigo. Blockage of the Eustachian tube during ascent in an aeroplane may lead to vertigo.

A   Ménière's disease, characterised by vertigo that lasts for minutes or hours, low-pitched roaring tinnitus, progressive hearing loss, nausea and vomiting, is abnormal. The consumer also experiences pressure in the ear.

P   The main pathological finding is distension of the endolymphatic system, with degenerative changes in the organ of Corti.

Glossopharyngeal and vagus nerves (CN IX and CN X)
The glossopharyngeal and vagus nerves are tested together because of their overlap in function.

E   1. Examine soft palate and uvula movement and gag reflex as described in Chapter 11.
   2. Assess the consumer's quality of speech for a nasal quality or hoarseness. Ask the consumer to produce guttural and palatal sounds, such as *k*, *q*, *ch*, *b* and *d*.
   3. Assess the consumer's ability to swallow a small amount of water. Observe for regurgitation of fluids through the nose. If the consumer is unable to swallow, observe how oral secretions are handled.
   4. The sensory examination of the glossopharyngeal and vagus nerves is limited to taste on the posterior one-third of the tongue. This examination was previously discussed in the section on CN VII.

N   Refer to Chapter 11 for normal soft palate and uvula movement and gag reflex findings. The speech is clear, without hoarseness or a nasal quality. The consumer is able to swallow water or oral secretions easily. Taste (sweet, salty, sour and bitter) is intact in the posterior one-third of the tongue.

A   Unilateral lowering and flattening of the palatine arch; weakness of the soft palate; deviation of the uvula to the normal side; mild dysphagia, regurgitation of fluids, and nasal quality of the voice; loss of taste in the posterior one-third of the tongue; and hemianaesthesia of the palate and pharynx, are abnormal.

P   Unilateral glossopharyngeal and vagal paralysis, such as with trauma or skull fractures at the base of the skull, will cause these symptoms.

E Examination   **N** Normal findings   **A** Abnormal findings   **P** Pathophysiology

🄰 Marked nasal quality of the voice, difficulty with guttural and palatal sounds, severe dysphagia with liquids, and inability of the palate to elevate on phonation, are abnormal.

🄿 Bilateral vagus nerve paralysis will cause these more marked symptoms, and often occurs simultaneously with signs and symptoms of other lower brain stem cranial nerve dysfunctions, such as in progressive bulbar palsy in amyotrophic lateral sclerosis (ALS).

Spinal accessory nerve (CN XI)

🄴 1. Place the consumer in a seated or a supine position. Inspect the sternocleidomastoid muscles for contour, volume and fasciculation.
2. Place your right hand on the left side of the consumer's face. Instruct the consumer to turn the head sideways against the resistance of your hand (Figure 7.18A).
3. Use the other hand to palpate the sternocleidomastoid muscle for strength of contraction. Inspect the muscle for contraction.
4. Repeat steps 2 and 3 in the opposite direction. Compare the strength of the two sides.
5. To assess the function of the trapezius muscle, stand behind the consumer and inspect the shoulders and scapula for symmetry of contour. Note any atrophy or fasciculation.
6. Place your hands on top of the consumer's shoulders and instruct the consumer to raise the shoulders against the downwards resistance of your hands (Figure 7.18B). This can be performed in front of or behind the consumer.
7. Observe the movements and palpate the contraction of the trapezius muscles. Compare the strength of the two sides.

🄽 The consumer should be able to turn their head against resistance with a smooth, strong and symmetrical motion. The consumer should also demonstrate the ability to shrug the shoulders against resistance with strong, symmetrical movement of the trapezius muscles.

🄰 Inability to turn the head towards the paralysed side, and a flat, noncontracting muscle on that side are abnormal findings. The contralateral sternocleidomastoid muscle may be contracted.

🄿 These findings are the result of unilateral paralysis of the sternocleidomastoid muscle due to trauma, tumours, or infection affecting the spinal accessory nerve.

🄰 The inability of the consumer to elevate one shoulder, asymmetrical drooping of the shoulder and scapula, and a depressed outline of the neck are abnormal findings. The involved shoulder may also show atrophy and fasciculation of the muscles.

🄿 Unilateral paralysis of the trapezius muscle may be suspected, usually due to trauma, tumours or infection.

🄰🄿 For information on torticollis, see Chapter 9.

Hypoglossal nerve (CN XII)

🄴 1. See Chapter 11 for assessment of tongue movement.
2. Assess lingual sounds by asking the consumer to say 'la la la'.

🄽 See Chapter 11 for normal tongue movements. Lingual speech is clear.

🄰 Inability or difficulty in producing lingual sounds is abnormal. The speech sounds lispy and clumsy.

🄿 Lesions of the hypoglossal nerve will cause difficulty in pronunciation of lingual sounds.

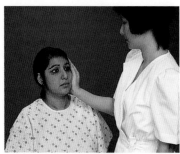

A. Strength of sternocleidomastoid muscle

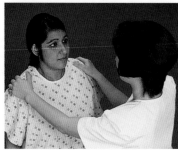

B. Strength of trapezius muscle

FIGURE 7.18 Assessment of CN XI

Examination of motor system

For **E N A P** on muscle size, tone, strength and involuntary movements see Chapter 16. See the following for additional abnormal findings and pathophysiology.

A Extrapyramidal rigidity is evident when resistance is present during passive movement of the muscles in all directions and lasts throughout the entire range of motion. It may involve both flexor and extensor muscles and is abnormal.

P Extrapyramidal rigidity is due to lesions located in the basal ganglia.

A **Decerebrate rigidity** (decerebration) is characterised by rigidity and sustained contraction of the extensor muscles and is abnormal. The arms are adducted, extended and hyperpronated. The legs are stiffly extended and the feet are plantar flexed (**Figure 7.19A**). The back and neck may be arched and the teeth clenched (opisthotonos).

P Decerebration may be found in unconscious consumers with deep, bilateral diencephalic injury that progresses to midbrain dysfunction. Decerebrate rigidity may also occur due to midbrain and pontine damage, which occurs with compression of these structures due to expanding cerebellar or posterior fossa lesions. Severe metabolic disorders that depress diencephalic and forebrain function may also cause decerebration.

A **Decorticate rigidity** (decortication) is characterised by hyperflexion of the arms (flexion of the arm, wrist and fingers, adduction of the arms), hyperextension and internal rotation of the legs, and plantar flexion (**Figure 7.19B**). It is abnormal.

P Decorticate rigidity is found in unconscious consumers with cerebral hemisphere lesions that interfere with the corticospinal tract.

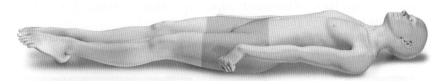

A. Decerebrate rigidity (abnormal extension)

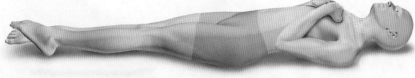

B. Decorticate rigidity (abnormal flexion)

FIGURE 7.19 Motor system dysfunction

Pronator drift

E 1. Have the consumer extend the arms out in front with palms up for 20 seconds.
2. Observe for downwards drifting of an arm.

N There should be no downwards drifting of an arm.

A Downwards drifting of an arm is abnormal.

P Downwards drifting of an arm may indicate hemiparesis, such as in stroke.

Examination of cerebellar function (coordination and gait)

Motor coordination refers to smooth, precise and harmonious muscular activity. Movement requires the coordination of many muscle groups. Coordination is an integrated process involving complicated neural integration of the motor and premotor cortex, basal ganglia, cerebellum, vestibular system, posterior columns and peripheral nerves.

E Examination   **N** Normal findings   **A** Abnormal findings   **P** Pathophysiology

Equilibratory coordination refers to maintenance of an upright stance and depends on the vestibular, cerebellar and proprioceptive systems. Nonequilibratory coordination refers to smaller movements of the extremities and involves the cerebellar and proprioceptive mechanisms.

Incoordination is categorised into three different types of syndromes: cerebellar, vestibular and posterior column syndromes. Incoordination is not considered to be secondary to involuntary movements, paresis or alterations of muscle tone.

Gait refers to the consumer's manner of walking.

Coordination

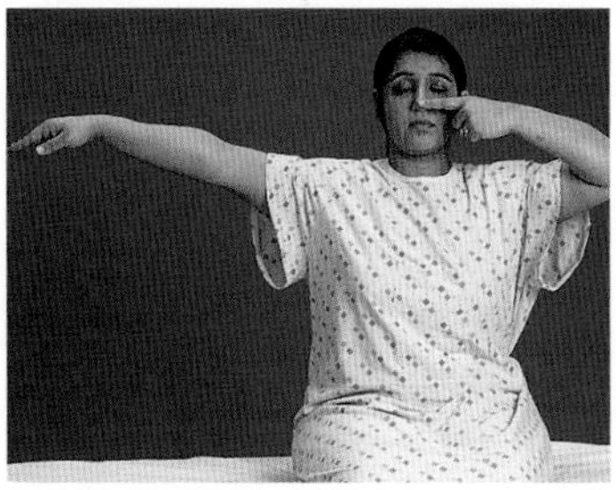

FIGURE 7.20 Assessment of coordination: Fingertip-to-nose touch

E
1. Instruct the consumer to sit comfortably facing you, with eyes open and arms outstretched. Ensure that consumers who wear corrective lenses (glasses or contacts) are wearing them prior to assessing their coordination.
2. Ask the consumer to first touch the index finger to the nose, then to alternate rapidly with the index finger of the opposite hand.
3. With their eyes closed, have the consumer continue to rapidly touch the nose with alternate index fingers (Figure 7.20).
4. With their eyes open, ask the consumer to again touch finger to nose. Next, ask the consumer to touch your index finger, which is held about 45 cm away from the consumer.
5. Change the position of your finger as the consumer rapidly repeats the manoeuvre with one finger.
6. Repeat steps 4 and 5 with the other hand.
7. Observe for intention tremor or overshoot or undershoot of the consumer's finger.
8. To assess rapid alternating movements, ask the consumer to rapidly alternate patting their knees, first with the palms and then alternating palms with the backs of the hands (rapid supinating [see Figure 7.21A] and pronating [see Figure 7.21B] of the hands).
9. Ask the consumer to repeatedly touch the thumb to each of the fingers of the hand in rapid succession from index to the fifth finger, and back.

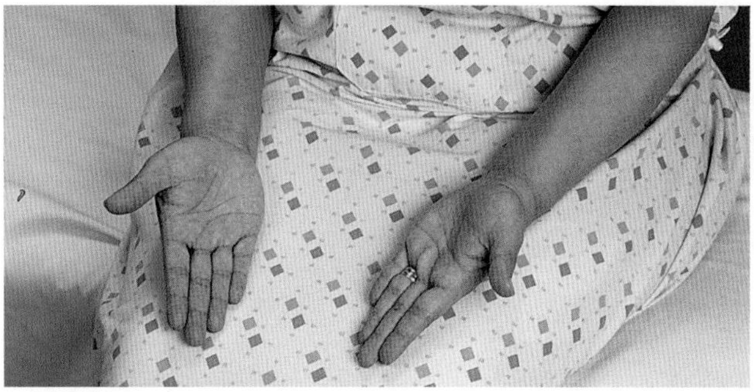

A. Supination

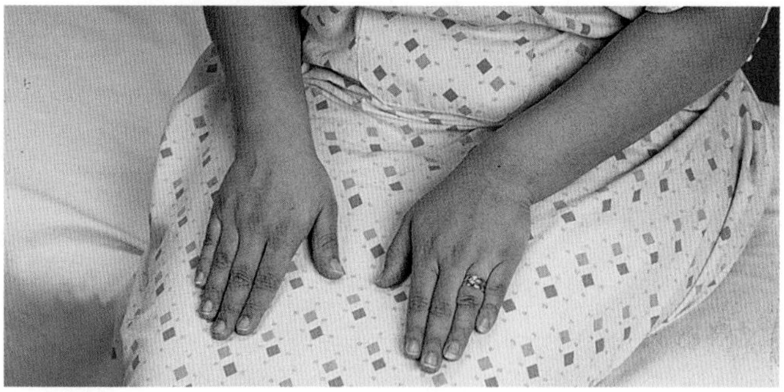

B. Pronation

FIGURE 7.21 Assessment of coordination: Rapid alternating hand movements

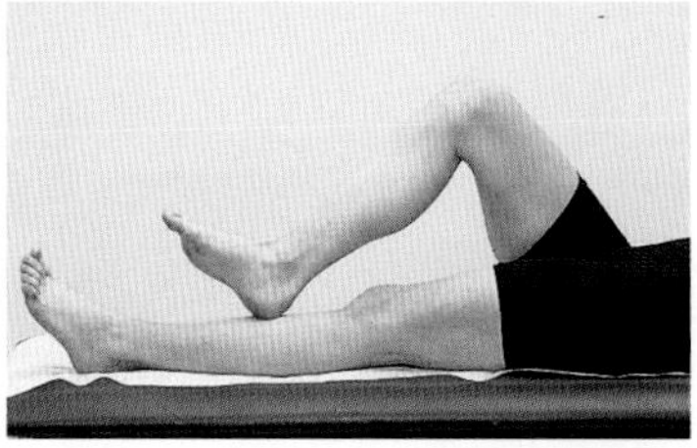

FIGURE 7.22 Assessment of coordination: Heel slide

E
10. Repeat step 9 with the other hand.
11. Observe coordination and the ability of the consumer to perform these in rapid sequence.
12. With the consumer in a seated or supine position, ask the consumer to place the heel just below the knee on the shin of the opposite leg and to slide it down to the foot (Figure 7.22).
13. Repeat with the opposite foot.
14. Observe coordination of the two legs.

E Examination N Normal findings A Abnormal findings P Pathophysiology

E 15. Ask the consumer to draw a circle or a figure 8 with a foot either on the ground or in the air (**Figure 7.23**).
16. Repeat with the other foot.
17. Observe for coordination and regularity of the figure.
18. Test the lower extremities for rapid alternating movement by asking the consumer to rapidly extend the ankle ('tap your foot') or to rapidly flex and extend the toes of one foot.
19. Repeat with the opposite foot.
20. Note rate, rhythm, smoothness and accuracy of the movements.

N The consumer is able to rapidly alternate touching finger to nose and moving finger from nose to your finger in a coordinated fashion. The consumer is able to perform alternating movements in a purposeful, rapid, coordinated manner. The consumer demonstrates the ability to purposefully and smoothly run heel down shin with equal coordination in both feet and to draw a figure 8 or circles with the foot.

A **Dyssynergy**, the lack of coordinated action of the muscle groups, is abnormal. The consumer is unable to carry out smooth, coordinated movements. The consumer's movements appear jerky, irregular and uncoordinated. **Dysmetria**, impaired judgement of distance, range, speed and force of movement, is abnormal. The consumer misjudges distance and overshoots.

P **Dysdiadochokinesia**, the inability to perform rapid alternating movements, is abnormal. The consumer is unable to abruptly stop one movement and begin another opposite movement.
Cerebellar disease causes all of these abnormal findings.

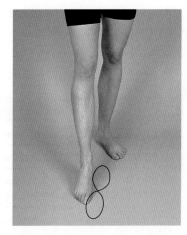

FIGURE 7.23 Assessment of coordination: Figure 8

Gait
E N A P See Chapter 16 for assessment of gait.

EVALUATION OF HEALTH ASSESSMENT AND PHYSICAL EXAMINATION FINDINGS

In the evaluation phase of a health assessment, the focus is on ensuring the data gathered is complete, accurate and documented appropriately. (See case study as an example of the focused assessment, and Chapter 22 for a comprehensive health assessment.) In evaluating the data you should:
> draw on your critical thinking and problem-solving skills to make sound clinical decisions
> act on abnormal data (include communicating findings to other health professionals)
> ensure documentation reflects the outcomes of the clinical decisions/actions taken. (Refer to Chapter 3, which discusses in detail why documentation is so important and how this may be undertaken in different health settings.)
The case study that follows steps you through this process.

UNIT 2

CASE STUDY 1

THE CONSUMER WITH DELIRIUM

This case study illustrates the application and objective documentation of the mental health status and neurological assessment.

Mrs Nina Tabone is a 91-year-old lady who resides at home and presents with symptoms of delirium.

HEALTH HISTORY		
CONSUMER PROFILE	91-year-old, widowed, lives home alone	
CHIEF COMPLAINT	Periods of confusion, distress and sleep disturbance	
HISTORY OF THE PRESENT ILLNESS	Consumer has been confused for short periods during the afternoon and evening, and spent a disturbed night, waking every 2 hours (approximately) and calling out in distress.	
PAST HEALTH HISTORY	**MEDICAL HISTORY**	Hypertension (idiopathic) for last 35 years Osteoarthritis with reduced mobility in left hip (ambulates with walker) since a fall 8 months ago resulted in a fractured left neck of femur. Arthritis in hands with considerable deformity. Still lives home alone, but recently has had daughter staying with her since she had COVID-19 a month ago. Has been treated twice over past 6 months for chest infection. Has had productive cough for past two days, sputum now green and yellow.
	SURGICAL HISTORY	Appendectomy at age 16 Left hip replacement 8 months ago (following a fall)
	ALLERGIES	Penicillin – rash
	MEDICATIONS	Ibuprofen prn for headache Lisinopril 10 mg mane for hypertension Lasix 40 mg mane for fluid Caltrate with vitamin D 600 mg once daily for osteoarthritis
	COMMUNICABLE DISEASES	Denies
	INJURIES AND ACCIDENTS	Fractured left neck of femur 8 months ago
	SPECIAL NEEDS	Self-ambulates with walker. Food preparation ability is now minimal; had been using Meals on Wheels, but since daughter has come to stay has not been able to manage as well as she used to before having had COVID-19
	BLOOD TRANSFUSIONS	Denies
	CHILDHOOD ILLNESSES	Chickenpox, measles, mumps as child. No sequelae
	IMMUNISATIONS	Up to date
FAMILY HEALTH HISTORY	Nil known	
SOCIAL HISTORY	**ALCOHOL USE**	Nil
	TOBACCO USE	Nil
	DRUG USE	Nil
	DOMESTIC AND INTIMATE PARTNER VIOLENCE	Widowed, usually lives alone, daughter staying with her since she had COVID-19 one month ago
	SEXUAL PRACTICE	No longer sexually active
	TRAVEL HISTORY	Immigrated to Melbourne with husband in 1950s

>>

>>

HEALTH HISTORY

	WORK ENVIRONMENT	Retired
	HOME ENVIRONMENT	Lives at Bundaberg now in a lowset unit at the beach.
	HOBBIES AND LEISURE ACTIVITIES	Watching television and listening to speaking books
	STRESS	Becomes frustrated with deformed hands and decreasing ambulatory ability
	EDUCATION	Went to Grade 6
	ECONOMIC STATUS	Middle class
	RELIGION	Roman Catholic
	CULTURAL BACKGROUND	Sicilian
	ROLES AND RELATIONSHIPS	Mother, grandmother, great grandmother
	CHARACTERISTIC PATTERNS OF DAILY LIVING	Goes to respite twice a week, otherwise wakes early and has coffee and bread with butter. Has early lunch and dinner, and bed by 8 p.m. Days that she goes to respite, leaves the house at 10 a.m. and returns at 4.30 p.m.
HEALTH MAINTENANCE ACTIVITIES	**SLEEP**	6 hours/night, usually restful; no sleep aids used
	DIET	Low salt
	EXERCISE	Ambulates with difficulty with walker
	STRESS MANAGEMENT	Listening to music and speaking books
	USE OF SAFETY DEVICES	Seat belt in care
	HEALTH CHECK-UPS	GP visit when ill, does not like to go to the doctor

PHYSICAL EXAMINATION

MENTAL STATUS

1 Physical appearance and behaviour:
   a Posture and movements: lying on ambulance stretcher, curled up in left lateral position
   b Dress, grooming and personal hygiene: has been incontinent of urine (which is unusual), dressing gown wadded up to waist, bed clothes twisted
   c Facial expression: grimacing
   d Affect: distressed
2 Communication: mumbling
3 Level of consciousness: awake, alert and disorientated; GCS = 14 oriented to person, not place, part of day (morning, afternoon or evening), month or year
4 Cognitive abilities and mentation:
   a Attention: unfocused, easily wanders, appears to be responding to things/people the nurse is unable to see
   b Memory: intact long-term, short-term confused about where she is and why she is here
   c Judgement: unable to focus consumer to answer
   d Insight: unable to assess – consumer not able to focus
   e Spatial perception: unable to assess – consumer not able to focus
   f Calculation: unable to assess – consumer not able to focus
   g Abstract reasoning: unable to assess – consumer not able to focus
   h Thought process and content: confused, distressed about not recognising room and people, talking to people who are not present (particularly husband who is deceased)
   i Suicidal ideation: unable to assess – consumer not able to focus

>>

>>

PHYSICAL EXAMINATION

SENSORY	1 Exteroceptive sensation:
	  a Light touch: equal and intact bilaterally
	  b Superficial pain: did not assess, consumer too distressed
	  c Temperature: did not assess, consumer too distressed
	2 Proprioceptive sensation:
	  a Motion and position: did not assess, consumer too distressed
	  b Vibration sense: did not assess, consumer too distressed
	3 Cortical sensation:
	  a Stereognosis, graphaesthesia, two-point discrimination, extinction: did not assess, consumer
	    too distressed

CRANIAL NERVES	I: Smells – did not assess, consumer too distressed and confused II: Visual acuity with glasses; visual fields intact as focuses on nurse until leaves visual field, unable to assess further. When responding to things the nurse cannot see, states she is calling the cat in the corner of the room to come and eat. There is no cat in the room. III, IV, and VI: EOM intact, pupils equal, round, react to light, accommodation (PERRLA) V: Did not assess, consumer too distressed VII: Intact; no facial palsy, ptosis or asymmetry; taste deferred VIII: Gross hearing intact; did not assess further, consumer too distressed IX and X: Intact gag reflex, uvula midline; taste deferred XI: Did not assess, consumer too distressed XII: Tongue midline, speech mumbling
MOTOR	1 Size: equal bilaterally 2 Tone: did not assess, consumer too distressed 3 Strength: did not assess, consumer too distressed, but gripping sides of bed with equal strength bilaterally 4 Involuntary movements: none 5 Pronator drift: did not assess, consumer too distressed
CEREBELLAR FUNCTION	1 Coordination: unable to assess 2 Gait: unable to assess
DIAGNOSTIC DATA	Sputum collected

EVALUATION AND CLINICAL REASONING FOR CASE STUDY

Considerations for making clinical decisions for this consumer need to take into account the scope of practice of the nurse assessing the consumer. Nurses in advanced practice positions, such as nurse practitioners and, depending on the role, remote area nurses with endorsement for advanced practice, may be able to make diagnostic decisions and prescribe medications without referring to a medical officer. The majority of nurses, however, work within a scope of practice in which nurses will collect the above information, consider all the data, refer to a medical officer and carry out the prescribed interventions, with some autonomy on assessing the consumer's level of education required for providing additional advice. Nurses are often required to monitor the consumer's response to these interventions, and to decide on what symptoms or developments are significant to report to the medical officer. Being able to appropriately decide when this should occur relies on the nurse applying a good understanding of underlying pathophysiology, consumer symptoms, baseline data and critical thinking to consider all this information in a meaningful way for directing consumer care. This is the process that is referred to as clinical reasoning. The phases presented in the clinical reasoning

cycle are stepped out below, drawing on information presented and collected during the health history and physical assessment. We then work through the cycle components that are relevant to this case study (cycle components are bolded).

Nurses have a positive impact on **consumer outcomes** and the use of systematic clinical reasoning skills in this situation is critical to supporting the consumer.

For Mrs Tabone, the 91-year-old woman who presents with confusion, sleep disturbance and distress, the following significant data needs to be considered.

Collecting cues/information

Recall and Review: In the first instance you will need to reflect on what you know about delirium, confusion, and why and how this manifests in the elderly population.

Chief complaint and history of present illness

> Periods of confusion, distress and sleep disturbance over past 18 hours.
> Consumer has been confused for short periods during the afternoon and evening, and spent an unrestful night, waking every 2 hours (approximately) and calling out in distress.

Processing information

Interpret: These symptoms and details of history outline the scope of the issue for this consumer, and we would need to ensure that this is not their usual behaviour. For this we need to rely on the daughter's knowledge of this consumer's usual condition. Usually Mrs Tabone is alert and lucid and has not displayed these symptoms before.

Medical history

> Hypertension (idiopathic) for last 35 years.
> Osteoarthritis with reduced mobility in left hip (ambulates with walker usually) since a fall 8 months ago resulted in a fractured left neck of femur. Arthritis in hands with considerable deformity.
> Still lives home alone, but recently has had daughter staying with her since she had COVID-19 a month ago. Has been treated twice over past 6 months for chest infection. Has had productive cough for past two days, sputum now green and yellow.

Interpret, Match and Infer: Mrs Tabone's medical history is important to note as this tells us that she is vulnerable to recurring chest infections, especially as she has likely become frailer since her operation and her increasing immobility. Also her recent infection with COVID-19 may make her more open to other infections.

Allergies

> Penicillin: rash

Medications

> Ibuprofen prn for headache
> Lisinopril 10 mg mane for hypertension
> Lasix 40 mg mane for fluid
> Caltrate with vitamin D 600 mg once daily for osteoarthritis

Infer and Relate: Both use of medications and past allergies need to be accurate and considered as it will be likely that Mrs Tabone may need to have further medications prescribed, but we also need to see if any of the medications she has been on are new or could cause these types of symptoms.

Mental status

1 Physical appearance and behaviour:
  a Posture and movements: lying in bed, curled up in left lateral position
  b Dress, grooming and personal hygiene: has been incontinent of urine (which is unusual), dressing gown wadded up to waist, bed clothes twisted
  c Facial expression: grimacing
  d Affect: distressed
2 Communication: mumbling
3 Level of consciousness: awake, alert and disorientated; GCS = 14 orientated to person, not place, part of day (morning, afternoon or evening), month or year

4 Cognitive abilities and mentation:
  a Attention: unfocused, easily wanders, appears to be responding to things/people the nurse is unable to see
  b Memory: intact long-term, short-term confused about where she is and why she is here
  c Thought process and content: confused, distressed about not recognising room and people, talking to people who are not present (particularly husband who is deceased)

Interpret: Mrs Tabone shows marked changes in mental status, is easily distracted by stimuli not apparent to the nurse, shows signs of confusion and is not oriented to the location she is in. Although Mrs Tabone is not usually orientated to date, she is usually orientated to her location, month and year. She has been incontinent of urine, unusual for this lady as she usually is able to ambulate in time to reach the toilet. Unable to focus Mrs Tabone without distressing her to undertake detailed mental status such as calculation etc.

Cranial nerves

> II: Visual acuity with glasses; visual fields intact as focuses on nurse until leaves visual field, unable to assess further. When responding to things the nurse cannot see, states she is calling the cat in the corner of the room to come and eat. There is no cat in the room.
> III, IV and VI: EOM intact, PERRLA
> VII: Intact; no facial palsy, ptosis or asymmetry; taste deferred
> VIII: Gross hearing intact; did not assess further, consumer too distressed
> IX and X: Intact gag reflex, uvula midline; taste deferred
> XII: Tongue midline, speech mumbling
> Motor – strength: did not assess, consumer too distressed, but gripping sides of bed with equal strength bilaterally
> Involuntary movements: none

Distinguish and Infer: Assessment of some of Mrs Tabone's cranial nerves show no signs of other neurological issues or symptoms of stroke or transient ischaemic attack. This allows us to rule out mechanical neurological issues and surmise that delirium caused by chemical imbalance or delirium caused by sepsis may be responsible for her change in mental status.

The above supposition of infection causing delirium would need to be further substantiated by undertaking respiratory assessment, and to also look for symptoms of sepsis such as pyrexia.

Match and Infer: Since Mrs Tabone has had recurring chest infections, has reduced mobility, has had a recent COVID-19 infection, has symptoms of a productive cough, the other symptoms (rapid onset of confusion, sleep disturbance, distress and visual hallucinations) AND lack of further neurological findings (such as facial palsy, slurred speech) point to delirium as a probable cause of Mrs Tabone's change in condition.

Putting it all together – synthesise information

The nurse in this case would document all of these abnormalities, and refer to the medical officer. As it is likely antibiotics will be prescribed, the nurse will need to check that medication prescribed is not of the penicillin family (as consumer has allergy to this) or has contraindications or adverse interactions with Mrs Tabone's antihypertensive drugs.

Actions based on assessment findings

The nurse should also provide additional education for interventions that do not require a doctor's order, such as:

1 inhaling steam to help loosen secretions
2 continue use of ibuprofen for analgesia and comfort measures
3 rest and sleep as much as possible until symptoms improve; this will aid the body's immune response
4 orientate consumer regularly without distressing consumer
5 monitor consumer closely since confusion can increase risk of falls, or higher risk for injury via hot drinks etc.

The final step in the process is accurate documentation. The nurse must document findings, referrals, interventions, advice and education given. The consumer would continue to have ongoing long-term management and follow-up by specialist medical staff in collaboration with general practitioner.

THE CONSUMER WITH EARLY ONSET DEMENTIA

This case study illustrates the application and objective documentation of the mental health status and neurological assessment.

HEALTH HISTORY

CONSUMER PROFILE	Mrs Margie Thomms is a 53-year-old who lives at home with her husband.	
CHIEF COMPLAINT	Confusion and behavioural change, especially inappropriateness, angry outbursts and impulsivity with hyperactivity, particularly pacing.	
HISTORY OF THE PRESENT ILLNESS	Husband describes gradual deterioration in cognitive function including memory loss, and lack of tact in social interactions over last six months to one year.	
PAST HEALTH HISTORY	**MEDICAL HISTORY**	History of anxiety and previous addiction to diazepam and alcohol treated successfully after rehabilitation 10 years ago
	SURGICAL HISTORY	Previous caesarean section 20 years ago
	ALLERGIES	Nil
	MEDICATIONS	Fish oil
	COMMUNICABLE DISEASES	Nil
	INJURIES AND ACCIDENTS	Recent fall without injury
	SPECIAL NEEDS	Independent with mobility
	BLOOD TRANSFUSIONS	Nil
	CHILDHOOD ILLNESSES	Chickenpox as a child
	IMMUNISATIONS	All immunisations up to date
FAMILY HEALTH HISTORY	Nil known	
SOCIAL HISTORY	**ALCOHOL USE**	Nil (previous dependence as noted in medical history)
	TOBACCO USE	Nil
	DRUG USE	Nil (previous dependence as noted above)
	DOMESTIC AND INTIMATE PARTNER VIOLENCE	Nil

>>

HEALTH HISTORY

	SEXUAL PRACTICE	Previously sexually active in stable relationship; now difficulty connecting emotionally and physically
	TRAVEL HISTORY	Immigrated from the United Kingdom to Australia 20 years ago
	WORK ENVIRONMENT	Former school teacher; currently on sick leave
	HOME ENVIRONMENT	Two-storey house with level external access
	HOBBIES AND LEISURE ACTIVITIES	Previously played piano, however no longer showing interest. Enjoyed family gatherings but now has difficulty with social situations – ranging from quiet and withdrawn to inappropriate and tactless in conversation
	STRESS	Angry outbursts usually related to frustration or misunderstanding situation
	EDUCATION	University education
	ECONOMIC STATUS	Middle class
	RELIGION	Anglican
	CULTURAL BACKGROUND	Anglo-Scottish
	ROLES AND RELATIONSHIPS	Wife, mother, grandmother
	CHARACTERISTIC PATTERNS OF DAILY LIVING	Previously managed household duties (cooking, laundry, shopping) but now unable to organise self to carry out these duties Difficulty with initiating social gatherings with family
HEALTH MAINTENANCE ACTIVITIES	SLEEP	7 hours/night on 'good night'; sometimes up several times at night
	DIET	Previously had healthy diet, now periods of binge eating
	EXERCISE	Walking was main exercise but now not motivated
	STRESS MANAGEMENT	Listening to music. Previously enjoyed reading, however now unable to focus
	USE OF SAFETY DEVICES	Nil
	HEALTH CHECK-UPS	Regular GP who has known her over 20 years

PHYSICAL EXAMINATION

MENTAL STATUS

1 Physical appearance and behaviour:
  a Posture and movements: sitting in chair with stooped posture
  b Dress, grooming and personal hygiene: unkempt appearance – hair uncombed, obvious body odour; food stains on shirt; still maintaining continence as per family
  c Facial expression: puzzled expression
  d Affect: flattened
2 Communication: some word-finding difficulties; some preservation
3 Level of consciousness: awake, alert and disorientated; GCS = 14 orientated to person, not place, part of day (morning, afternoon or evening), month or year
4 Cognitive abilities and mentation:
  a Attention: difficult to keep on track in conversation; tangential conversation
  b Memory: intact long-term, short-term confused about where she is and why she is here
  c Judgement: does not demonstrate insight. Family expresses concern about her ability to manage her finances and recently had to take away her credit cards as she was not able to manage her spending
  d Insight: as above – lacking insight and empathy for others
  e Spatial perception: normal, no neglect
  f Calculation: unable to carry out serial 7s
  g Abstract reasoning: not able to explain proverb 'people in glass houses shouldn't throw stones'
  h Thought process and content: confused
  i Suicidal ideation: no suicidal ideation

>>

PHYSICAL EXAMINATION

SENSORY	1 Exteroceptive sensation:
	  a Light touch: equal and intact bilaterally
	  b Superficial pain: normal
	  c Temperature: normal
	2 Proprioceptive sensation: normal
	3 Cortical sensation: unable to understand commands

CRANIAL NERVES	Intact except for smell, which was impaired
MOTOR	1 Size: no obvious wasting of muscle groups 2 Strength: upper and lower limb 5/5 bilaterally 3 Tone: normal 4 Involuntary movements: none 5 Pronator drift: no drift
CEREBELLAR FUNCTION	1 Coordination: intact finger-to-nose test and heel-to-shin 2 Gait: no ataxia

DIAGNOSTIC DATA

MRI	Report: significant right hemisphere atrophy in the frontal and anterior temporal region
VITAL SIGNS & LABORATORY DATA	All within normal limits

EVALUATION AND CLINICAL REASONING FOR CASE STUDY

Considerations for making clinical decisions for this consumer need to take into account the scope of practice of the nurse assessing the consumer. Nurses in advanced practice positions, such as nurse practitioners and, depending on the role, remote area nurses with endorsement for advanced practice, may be able to make diagnostic decisions and prescribe medications without referring to a medical officer. The majority of nurses, however, work within a scope of practice in which nurses will collect the above information, consider all the data, refer to a medical officer and carry out the prescribed interventions, with some autonomy on assessing the consumer's level of education required for providing additional advice. Nurses are often required to monitor the consumer's response to these interventions, and to decide on what symptoms or developments are significant to report to the medical officer. Being able to appropriately decide when this should occur relies on the nurse applying a good understanding of underlying pathophysiology, consumer symptoms, baseline data and critical thinking to consider all this information in a meaningful way for directing consumer care. This is the process that is referred to as clinical reasoning. The phases presented in the clinical reasoning cycle are stepped out below, drawing on information presented and collected during the health history and physical assessment. We then work through the cycle components that are relevant to this case study (cycle components are bolded).

For Mrs Margie Thomms, the 53-year-old woman who presents with confusion and behavioural change, the following significant data needs to be considered.

Collecting cues/information

Recall and Review: Reflect on what you know about dementia, focusing on frontal temporal dementia including presentation, age of onset and pattern of illness.

Chief complaint and history of present illness

> Behavioural and cognitive changes in previously healthy woman

Processing information

Interpret: The family is often a major source of information when the consumer presents with dementia. Although in the first instance the questions are addressed to the consumer, it is important to use family members as a resource when collecting data and interpreting assessment findings.

Medical history

Although this consumer had a past history of both anxiety and problems with drug and alcohol addiction, she successfully recovered and there is no history of dependence currently. Mrs Thomms' only medication is fish oil. There is no medication history that would suggest a cause for her behavioural changes. Vital signs and laboratory data are within normal limits.

Putting it all together – synthesise information

Mrs Thomms presents with a decline in her cognitive and behavioural function while maintaining her motor and sensory function. She is able to ambulate independently and manage most activities of daily living and is continent. Mrs Thomms is not able to carry out her normal roles both at home and in her professional role as a teacher. Because she has lost the ability to be empathetic towards others, this also affects her social role both within her family and within her social circle.

Actions based on assessment findings

The priorities for this consumer are as follows.

In hospital:

1 Assess falls risk.
2 Assess level of agitation and risk to consumer, family and staff members.
3 Provide a single room if possible and limit visitors to two each time.
4 Manage periods of agitation; may need one-on-one nursing if at risk of leaving the hospital. Avoid mechanical restraint as it may lead to escalation of agitation.
5 Discuss with team the pros and cons of medication to manage behaviour if indicated.
6 Document findings in progress notes and develop a behavioural management program for staff members caring for Mrs Thomms.

On discharge home:

1 Address safety and environmental concerns: safety of home appliances, securing food to prevent bingeing, supervision when crossing roads given impulsiveness, driving restrictions and anger-management strategies for Mrs Thomms and her family members.
2 Managing finances: may require referral to social worker to assist.
3 Managing challenging behaviours: educate family carers on how to manage challenging behaviours as well as provide written information.
  a Speak calmly.
  b Use simple one-step commands.
  c Positively reinforce appropriate behaviour.
  d Provide a restful environment at mealtime (quiet music, soft lighting).
  e Educate family to not engage in lengthy explanations or try to rationalise with Mrs Thomms.
  f Combat restlessness by engaging in walking program.
  g Consider community resources for a walking program and other programs, and make appropriate referrals.
  h Document in the progress notes the education provided to family on discharge.

THE CONSUMER WITH DEPRESSION AND ANXIETY

CASE STUDY 3

This case study illustrates the application and objective documentation of the mental health status and neurological assessment.

HEALTH HISTORY

CONSUMER PROFILE	Mr Joseph Shaw, a 25-year-old single male, currently living with parents	
CHIEF COMPLAINT	Reports low mood for 12 months, distress, sleep disturbance, panic attacks	
HISTORY OF THE PRESENT ILLNESS	Consumer has reported suicidal thoughts over the past 2 months, has been unable to go out in public places over the past 6 months, experiencing increase in panic attacks, reports lowered mood for 12 months.	
PAST HEALTH HISTORY	**MEDICAL HISTORY**	Nil
	SURGICAL HISTORY	Nil
	ALLERGIES	Nil
	MEDICATIONS	Cipramil 20 mg mane
	COMMUNICABLE DISEASES	Denies
	INJURIES AND ACCIDENTS	Sporting injuries as teenager; no surgery required
	SPECIAL NEEDS	Nil
	BLOOD TRANSFUSIONS	Denies
	CHILDHOOD ILLNESSES	Chickenpox as child
	IMMUNISATIONS	All immunisations as per requirement
FAMILY HEALTH HISTORY	Mother: type 2 diabetes, father: hypertension	

HEALTH HISTORY

SOCIAL HISTORY	ALCOHOL USE	6 standard drinks daily
	TOBACCO USE	20 cigarettes daily
	DRUG USE	Cannabis use, reports using 1 gram weekly
	DOMESTIC AND INTIMATE PARTNER VIOLENCE	Nil
	SEXUAL PRACTICE	Sexually active, currently not in a relationship
	TRAVEL HISTORY	Nil
	WORK ENVIRONMENT	Currently unemployed
	HOME ENVIRONMENT	Lives with parents in family home, youngest child – not close to siblings; they are significantly older than him
	HOBBIES AND LEISURE ACTIVITIES	Listening to music, watching television, art
	STRESS	Worried about future plans of studying and employment
	EDUCATION	Completed Year 12, was enrolled in Bachelor of Education, completed 2 years and has recently deferred university
	ECONOMIC STATUS	Middle class background, both parents work full-time, only child still living at home
	RELIGION	Anglican
	CULTURAL BACKGROUND	English
	ROLES AND RELATIONSHIPS	Son, sibling
	CHARACTERISTIC PATTERNS OF DAILY LIVING	Prefers to spend the day in his bedroom, will have dinner with his parents; contact with friends is through social media
HEALTH MAINTENANCE ACTIVITIES	SLEEP	Disturbed sleep overnight, prefers to spend the day sleeping
	DIET	Poor appetite, reports that he has lost 6 kg in the past 3 months
	EXERCISE	No exercise currently
	STRESS MANAGEMENT	Listening to music, drawing, using THC and alcohol to help relax
	USE OF SAFETY DEVICES	Nil
	HEALTH CHECK-UPS	Linked in with his local GP and sees her fortnightly

PHYSICAL EXAMINATION

MENTAL STATUS	1 Physical appearance and behaviour: young male, thin-built, tanned complexion, unshaven, wearing glasses, stains on clothing, staring at the floor during conversation, poor eye contact, responsive to questions asked. Accompanied by parents to interview
	2 Mood: reports low mood over the past 12 months, rates mood 3/10
	3 Affect: flat
	4 Speech: softly spoken, normal rate, volume, tone
	5 Thought form: logical and coherent in conversation
	6 Thought content: reports feeling helpless and hopeless about future plans, suicidal thoughts for the past 2 months; worried about his future and whether he will be better again. Reports panic attacks in public places and has been avoiding going out
	7 Perception: denies perceptual disturbances

>>

PHYSICAL EXAMINATION

8 Insight/Judgement: he is aware of the reasons for attending the appointment and displays intact judgement

9 Cognition: attention focused, is able to respond to questions asked, pausing at times between questions due to feeling overwhelmed

10 Level of consciousness: alert and orientated to time, place, person

11 Memory: intact

DIAGNOSTIC DATA

Further psychiatric assessment required, physical observations taken

EVALUATION AND CLINICAL REASONING FOR CASE STUDY

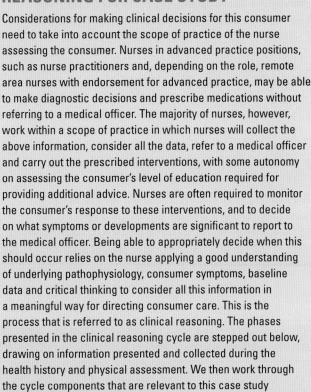

Considerations for making clinical decisions for this consumer need to take into account the scope of practice of the nurse assessing the consumer. Nurses in advanced practice positions, such as nurse practitioners and, depending on the role, remote area nurses with endorsement for advanced practice, may be able to make diagnostic decisions and prescribe medications without referring to a medical officer. The majority of nurses, however, work within a scope of practice in which nurses will collect the above information, consider all the data, refer to a medical officer and carry out the prescribed interventions, with some autonomy on assessing the consumer's level of education required for providing additional advice. Nurses are often required to monitor the consumer's response to these interventions, and to decide on what symptoms or developments are significant to report to the medical officer. Being able to appropriately decide when this should occur relies on the nurse applying a good understanding of underlying pathophysiology, consumer symptoms, baseline data and critical thinking to consider all this information in a meaningful way for directing consumer care. This is the process that is referred to as clinical reasoning. The phases presented in the clinical reasoning cycle are stepped out below, drawing on information presented and collected during the health history and physical assessment. We then work through the cycle components that are relevant to this case study (cycle components are bolded).

For Mr Shaw, the 25-year-old single male who presents with low mood, suicidal thoughts and panic attacks, the following significant data needs to be considered.

Collecting cues/information

Recall and Review: In the first instance, you will need to reflect on what you know about anxiety, depression and substance use, and why and how this manifests in the young adult population.

Chief complaint and history of present illness

> Low mood for the past 12 months
> Suicidal thoughts over the past 2 months
> Panic attacks, sleep disturbance
> Decline in functioning for the past 12 months
> Substance use to help cope with symptoms

Processing information

Interpret: These symptoms and details of history outline the scope of the issue for this consumer and we would need to conduct further assessments to assist with providing further information to clarify diagnosis and formulate a plan of care. For this we need to further assess Mr Shaw.

Medical history

> Mr Shaw's medical history is not the reason for his presentation, so it is not relevant in the current assessment. He is reporting physical symptoms of chest tightness and shortness of breath, but this is related to him reporting panic attacks.

Medications

> Cipramil 20 mg mane
> Mr Shaw was prescribed Cipramil by his GP 7 months ago. He does report that he felt an improvement in his mood for 3 months after commencing Cipramil, but since then he has experienced further decline in his mood. He reports that he takes his medications daily. He will require review of his antidepressant medication due to reporting further decline in his depressive symptoms.

Mental status

1 Physical appearance and behaviour: young male, thin-built, tanned appearance, unshaven, wearing glasses, stains on clothing, staring at the floor during conversation, poor eye contact, responsive to questions asked. Accompanied by parents to interview

2 Mood: reports low mood for the past 12 months, rates mood 3/10

3 Affect: flat

4 Speech: softly spoken, normal rate, volume, tone

5 Thought form: logical and coherent in conversation

6 Thought content: reports feeling helpless and hopeless about future plans, suicidal thoughts for the past 2 months, worried about his future and whether he will be better again. Reports panic attacks in public places and has been avoiding going out.

7 Perception: denies perceptual disturbances

8 Insight/Judgement: is aware of the reasons for attending the appointment and displays intact judgement

9 Cognition: attention focused, is able to respond to questions asked, pausing at times between questions due to feeling overwhelmed

10 Level of consciousness: alert and orientated to time, place, person

11 Memory: intact

Interpret: Mr Shaw shows marked changes in his mood. He presents with poor eye contact, helpless and hopeless themes, feeling no pleasure in activities, increased worry about his future plans, thoughts of suicide to end his life. He displays understanding about his symptoms and is willing to seek help for his mental health. He has been financially reliant on his parents since deferring university and resigning from his casual position, which Mr Shaw reports has been a significant stressor. He reports that he noticed a decline in his mood due to increased stress from university studies and death of a close friend.

Substance use

Mr Shaw reports using cannabis, alcohol and smoking cigarettes daily to help him feel relaxed. He states that he is unsure about whether he is dependent on substances.

Suicidal thoughts

Mr Shaw reports that he has had plans of hanging himself previously, stated that he is comfortable approaching his family for support if required, although he is not close to his siblings. Currently he denies any active plans, but states that he does not see the point of living due to his current mental state.

Family history

Parents are very supportive and Mr Shaw reports having a close relationship with his parents. Nil known history of mental illness in his family.

Mr Shaw reports decline in his mood for the past 12 months, with panic attacks and suicidal ideation, sleep disturbance, and substance use. There is lack of evidence about perceptual disturbances. He denies psychotic symptoms and his family is in agreeance that Mr Shaw does experience depression and anxiety. His presenting symptoms point to a diagnosis of major depression with anxiety features.

Putting it all together – synthesise information

The nurse in this case would document all these findings and refer this to the medical officer. The likely outcome would be that Mr Shaw would be further referred to a psychiatrist for review of his medications and further treatment.

Actions based on assessment findings

The nurse should also provide additional education for interventions that do not require a doctor's order such as:

1. Using deep-breathing techniques when feeling highly anxious.
2. Use of mindfulness, relaxation techniques to help manage anxiety.
3. Establishing a daily routine at home to assist with structuring.
4. Education about the impact of substance use on his mood and anxiety.
5. Monitor consumer closely due to suicidal thoughts; establish therapeutic relationship to ensure that consumer feels comfortable to discuss his concerns.
6. Referral to social worker for assistance with financial support, linking in with assistance at university.

The final step in the process is accurate documentation. The nurse must document findings, referrals, interventions, advice and education given. The consumer would continue to have ongoing management and follow-up by specialist medical staff in collaboration with general practitioner.

CHAPTER RESOURCES

REVIEW QUESTIONS

For answers to these questions, see Answer section at the end of this book.

1. You are assessing a consumer who has reported feeling 'low' for suicide risk factors. Which of the following increases the risk for suicide attempts? Select all that apply.
   a. Suicidal thoughts without a specific plan
   b. Verbal expression of increasing self-worth
   c. Male sex
   d. Previous non-fatal suicide behaviours
   e. Does not take illicit substances
   f. Increased alcohol use
   g. Renewed interest in school or work
2. When assessing your consumer's mental status, you note that she is alert but talks with a monotone and little expression. This indicates:

a. Flat affect
b. Aphasia
c. Altered level of consciousness
d. Acute confusion

3. Janet, a 40-year-old female, has presented with severe depression and suicidal ideation. She reports that she is not responding to antidepressant medication prescribed by her GP. What are the common symptoms of depression? Select all that apply.
   a. Perceptual disturbance
   b. Low mood
   c. Sleep disturbance
   d. Anhedonia
   e. Thought disorder
   f. Weight changes

4. What is the objective assessment for emotion in a mental status examination?
   a. Mood
   b. Thought form
   c. Affect
   d. Thought content

5. Your consumer presents for a check-up reporting a sudden collapse that lasted 15 seconds. The consumer is now awake but feels nauseas and has a headache. He has a history of diabetes mellitus type 1, and his current blood glucose level is 2.9 mmol/L. You suspect he has which condition?
   a. Syncope
   b. Concussion
   c. Vertigo
   d. Seizure

6. Which of the following conditions are risk factors for stroke? Select all that apply.
   a. Atrial fibrillation
   b. Physical inactivity
   c. Liver disease
   d. Hypertension
   e. Use of codeine
   f. Obesity

7. The son of your 80-year-old female consumer expresses concern about his mother's cognitive mental status. You tell the consumer a list of three items and have the consumer repeat them to check initial understanding. By having the consumer recall the three items 5 minutes later, you are assessing what cognitive function?
   a. Judgement
   b. Attention
   c. Memory
   d. Abstract reasoning

8. Consumers with delirium may show which of the following symptoms?
   a. Perception is mostly affected and has a sudden onset, hallucinations, emotional disturbance, and may be volatile and impulsive
   b. All cognitive processes are affected, onset is gradual, and may have intact long-term memory
   c. Emotional state is mostly affected, could have gradual or sudden onset, may be in response to a situation or inherited neurochemical abnormalities. Attention, memory and judgement are all intact
   d. Show signs of slowed speech, lack of mental clarity and coherence, with variable onset, short-term and long-term memory may be impaired, spatial perception is impaired and may be incoherent

9. You are assessing a consumer who has arrived to the emergency department with a headache and difficulty speaking. The treating team are suspecting a stroke may

be the cause. A student nurse asks you what the term is for the impaired laryngeal speech you are witnessing with the consumer. This is an example of:
   a. Hyperaesthesia
   b. Hypophonia
   c. Dysphonia
   d. Dysaesthesia

10. The consumer you are seeing has a shingles outbreak on the C4–C5 dermatomes. Where would you observe an erythematous, vesicular rash? Select all that apply.
    a. Chin
    b. Clavicular area
    c. Neck
    d. Trapezius muscle area
    e. Biceps muscle area
    f. Scalp

11. With your consumer sitting relaxed and facing you, have them perform the following sequence of activities: With arms outstretched, alternately bring in each hand and touch the tip of each index finger to his nose. Next, have the consumer rapidly alternate patting his knees with the palmar, then the dorsal, aspects of his hands. Finally, have the consumer rapidly extend and tap his foot. Which component of the neurological exam are you assessing?
    a. Sensory function
    b. Cerebellar function
    c. Cranial nerves
    d. Mental status

12. A 25-year-old female reports a history of anxiety and nervousness. She comes in due to recent panic attacks. You know the 'fight or flight' response is controlled by the sympathetic nervous system. What characteristic symptoms might this consumer experience with acute anxiety or panic? Select all that apply.
    a. Heightened awareness
    b. Increased gastric secretions
    c. Decreased gastric motility
    d. Bronchial constriction
    e. Increased heart rate
    f. Increased urine output

CS CLINICAL SKILLS

The following Clinical Skills are relevant to this chapter and can be found in Tollefson & Hillman, *Clinical Psychomotor Skills*, 8th edition:
> 16 Mental status assessment
> 20 Focused neurological health history and physical assessment
> 27 Healthcare teaching
> 73 Seclusion management
> 74 Electroconvulsive therapy care.

FURTHER RESOURCES

> Alzheimer's New Zealand: http://www.alzheimers.org.nz/
> Brain Injury Australia: https://www.braininjuryaustralia.org.au/
> Brain Injury New Zealand: http://www.brain-injury.org.nz/
> Community and Public Health New Zealand: https://www.cph.co.nz/your-health/youth-mental-health/
> Dementia Australia: https://www.dementia.org.au/
> Headspace National Youth Mental Health Foundation (Australia): https://headspace.org.au/
> Mental Health Australia: https://mhaustralia.org/
> Mental Health Foundation of New Zealand: https://www.mentalhealth.org.nz/

> MS Australia: http://www.msaustralia.org.au/
> MS Society of New Zealand: http://www.msnz.org.nz/
> Neurological Foundation of New Zealand: http://www.neurological.org.nz/
> Royal Australian and New Zealand College of Psychiatrists: http://www.ranzcp.org/
> Stroke Foundation (Australia): https://strokefoundation.org.au/
> Stroke Foundation of New Zealand: http://www.stroke.org.nz/

REFERENCES

Alzheimers New Zealand. (2022). Facts and figures. Retrieved 05 December 2022 from: https://alzheimers.org.nz/explore/facts-and-figures/

Australian Bureau of Statistics. (2021). Causes of death, Australia. ABS. https://www.abs.gov.au/statistics/health/causes-death/causes-death-australia/latest-release.

Australian Institute of Health and Welfare (AIHW). (2022a). Dementia in Australia. Retrieved 5 December 2022 from: https://www.aihw.gov.au/reports/dementia/dementia-in-aus/contents/summary

Australian Institute of Health and Welfare (AIHW). (2022b). Mental health: prevalence and impact. Retrieved 5 December 2022 from: https://www.aihw.gov.au/reports/mental-health-services/mental-health

Bentley, M., Singhal, P., Christey, G., & Amey, J. (2022). Characteristics of patients hospitalised with traumatic brain injuries. *Medical Journal of New Zealand, 135*(1550). Retrieved 5 December 2022 from: https://journal.nzma.org.nz/journal-articles/characteristics-of-patients-hospitalised-with-traumatic-brain-injuries-open-access

Brain Foundation. (2022). Motor neurone disease. Retrieved 5 December 2022 from: https://brainfoundation.org.au/disorders/motor-neurone-disease/

Brain Injury Australia. (n.d.). What is TBI? Retrieved 5 December 2022 from: http://braininjury-au.info/Severe_TBI/Brain_Injury_3A_TBI.htm

Connectivity: Traumatic Brain Injury Australia. (n.d.). Have you suffered a traumatic brain injury? Retrieved 5 December 2022 from: https://www.connectivity.org.au

Dementia Australia. (2023). Key facts and statistics. Retrieved 05 December 2022 from: https://www.dementia.org.au/statistics

Dharmadasa, T., Henderson, R. D., Talman, P. S., Macdonell, R. A. L., Mathers, S., Schultz, D. W., … Kiernan, M. C. (2017). Motor neurone disease: progress and challenges. *Medical Journal of Australia, 206*(8), 357–62. doi: 10.5694/mja16.01063

Esterman, A., Thomson, F., Fitts, M., Gilroy J., Fleming J., Maruff P., … Bohanna I. (2018). Incidence of emergency department presentations for traumatic brain injury in Indigenous and non-Indigenous residents aged 15–64 over the 9-year period 2007–2015 in North Queensland, Australia. *Injury Epidemiology, 12*(5):40. doi: 10.1186/s40621-018-0172-9

Everymind. (2022). Midframe. Suicide: communicating about suicide. An Everymind product, funded by the Australian government under the National Suicide Prevention Leadership and Support Program. Retrieved 31 October 2022 from https://mindframe.org.au/suicide/communicating-about-suicide/language

Healthdirect. (2022). Stroke. Australian Government Retrieved 31 October 2022 https://www.healthdirect.gov.au/stroke#prevention

Health Promotion Agency (HPA). (2020). Mental Health in Aotearoa. Retrieved 5 December 2022 from: https://www.hpa.org.nz/sites/default/files/Mental_Health_Aotearoa_Insight_2020.pdf

Leske, S., Adam, G., Catakovic, A., Weir, B., & Kolves, K. (2022). *Suicide in Queensland: annual report 2022*. Australian Institute for Suicide Research and Prevention, World Health Organization collaborating centre for research and training in Suicide Prevention, School of Applied Psychology, Griffith University, Brisbane, Queensland, Australia.

Madsen, T. E., Howard, V. J., Jimenez, M., Rexrode, K. M., Acelajado, M. C., Kleindorfer, D., & Chaturvendi, S. (2018). Impact of convention stroke risk factors in women. An update. *Stroke, 49*, 536–42. doi: 10.1161/STROKEAHA.117.018418

Mindframe. (2022). Mental ill-health – Data and statistics. Retrieved 5 December 2022 from: https://mindframe.org.au/mental-health/data-statistics

Motor Neurone Disease (MND) Australia. (2020). MND research statistics. Retrieved 5 December 2022 from: https://www.mndaustralia.org.au/research/for-researchers/mnd-research-statistics

Motor Neurone Disease New Zealand. (2020). Basic facts about MND. Retrieved 5 December 2022 from: https://mnd.org.nz/about-mnd/what-is-mnd/basic-facts-about-mnd/

New Zealand Brain Institute. (n.d.). Prevalence and incidence of Parkinson's in New Zealand. Retrieved 5 December 2022 from: https://www.nzbri.org/Labs/parkinsons/Epidemiology/

New Zealand Government. (2018). Mental Health and Addiction Inquiry, 1.4.1 Mental health and addiction in New Zealand. Retrieved 5 December 2022 from: https://mentalhealth.inquiry.govt.nz/inquiry-report/he-ara-oranga/chapter-1-the-inquiry/1-4-context/

O'Reilly, G., Curtis, K., Kim, Y., Mitra, B., Hunter, K., Ryder, C., … Fitzgerald, M. C. (2022). The Australian Traumatic Brain Injury National Data (ATBIND) project: a mixed methods study protocol. *Medical Journal of Australia, 217*(7): 361–5. doi: 10.5694/mja2.51674. Retrieved 5 December 2022 from: https://www.nzbri.org/Labs/parkinsons/Epidemiology/

Parekh, T., Pemmasani, S., & Desai, R. (2020). Marijuana use among young adults (18-44 years of age) and risk of stroke. A behavioural risk factor surveillance system survey analysis. *Stroke, 51*, 308–10. doi: 10.1161/STROKEAHA.119.027828

Pitcher, T. L., Myall, D. J., Pearson, J. F., Lacey, C. J., Dalrymple-Alford, J. C., Anderson, T. J., & MacAskill, M. R. (2018). Parkinson's disease across ethnicities: A nationwide study in New Zealand. *Movement Disorders*. doi: 10.1002/mds.27389

Shake It Up Australia Foundation. (n.d.) About Parkinson's. Retrieved 5 December 2022 from: https://shakeitup.org.au/understanding-parkinsons/

Stark, B. A., Roth, G. A., Adebayo, O. M., Akbarpour, S., Aljunid, S. M., Alvis-Guzman, N., … Castañeda-Orjuela, C. A. (2021). Global, regional, and national burden of stroke and its risk factors, 1990–2019: a systematic analysis for the Global Burden of Disease Study 2019. *Lancet Neurology, 20*(10), 795–820. https://doi.org/10.1016/S1474-4422(21)00252-0

Stroke Foundation. (2018). About Stroke. Retrieved 29 August 2018 from https://strokefoundation.org.au/About-Stroke

Stroke Foundation. (2020). Top 10 facts about stroke. Retrieved 5 December 2022 from: https://strokefoundation.org.au/about-stroke/learn/facts-and-figures

Stroke Foundation. (2022). Learn about stroke. Retrieved 5 December 2022 from: https://strokefoundation.org.au

Stroke Foundation New Zealand. (n.d.). Facts and FAQs. Retrieved 5 December 2022 from: https://www.stroke.org.nz/facts-and-faqs

CHAPTER **8**

INTEGUMENTARY

LEARNING OUTCOMES

By the end of this chapter you should be able to:
1 describe the anatomy and physiology of the integumentary system
2 demonstrate a physical assessment of the skin, hair and nails
3 identify pathophysiological changes to hair and nails, and explain possible aetiologies
4 explain the warning signs of carcinoma in pigmented lesions
5 identify health education opportunities for clients in regard to specific conditions
6 discuss the clinical reasoning to evaluate outcomes of health assessment and physical examination including documentation requirements for recording information, health education given and relevant health referral.

BACKGROUND

In Australia and New Zealand, hair, skin and nail conditions experienced by people are largely affected by location, socioeconomic status and physical environment (more specifically the work environment). Examples of common skin conditions are outlined according to these three factors.

> **Location:** Australia and New Zealand have the highest and second-highest rates of melanoma in the world, likely due to mostly fair-skinned populations and high ultraviolet (UV) radiation (Verma et al., 2022). Tropical diseases and infections are a significant health concern in northern Australia, particularly bacterial and fungal infections resulting from the humid environment or contact with vegetation, infected soils, coral reefs and fish (Australian Government Department of Health, 2018). Skin conditions such as eczema are aggravated by, and thus more prominent in, the colder mountainous regions of southern Australia and New Zealand. Poor access to timely health care is also associated with living in a rural or remote area (AIHW, 2022).

> **Socioeconomic status:** Aboriginal and Torres Strait Islander peoples in remote and coastal communities in Australia struggle to control outbreaks of pediculosis (head lice), impetigo (school sores) and scabies, all of which have significant complications (Davidson, Knight & Bowen, 2020). Although these conditions regularly occur and are picked up in school environments (Mullane et al., 2019), they are not only found in school environments, and the potential for epidemic outbreaks is prevalent in both Australia and New Zealand. Poor socioeconomic status and the barriers facing Indigenous peoples of Australia and New Zealand in accessing health care contribute to poor knowledge about self-care practices in hygiene and nutrition. Such outcomes are usually apparent in assessment findings for hair, skin and nails.

> **Physical environment:** Hot sun and high UV levels can cause issues such as sunburn and skin cancer. Environmental factors, paired with individual factors,

contribute to Australia and New Zealand having the highest incidence in the world for melanoma skin cancers (Melanoma Institute Australia, 2022). Melanoma is the third most common cancer in New Zealand and accounts for close to 80% of skin cancer deaths (Melanoma New Zealand, 2022). In Australia, new melanoma diagnoses account for 11% of all cancers (Cancer Australia, 2022), and approximately 17 000 Australians are diagnosed with invasive melanoma each year (Melanoma Institute Australia, 2022). Men are more likely to develop and die from a melanoma (Cancer Australia, 2022). Melanoma was the 10th most common cause of cancer death in Australia in 2020 (Cancer Australia, 2022). However, more common than melanoma are basal cell carcinomas (one of the non-melanoma skin cancers), which affect a large proportion of Australians and New Zealanders. Skin cancers kill more people in New Zealand than road traffic crashes (Health Promotion Agency, New Zealand, 2018). Snow and ice conditions in New Zealand and parts of the southern Australian Great Dividing Range can cause health problems such as frostbite and xeroderma, which affect the person's integumentary system.

This chapter provides a review of the skin and its appendages: hair and nails. Techniques for examination of the integumentary system are addressed, as is an approach to evaluating skin lesions.

ANATOMY AND PHYSIOLOGY

The skin, also known as the **integumentary system** or cutaneous tissue, is the largest organ system of the body. It shelters most of the other organ systems and, if assessed carefully, can provide a noninvasive window through which to observe the body's level of functioning.

The skin, hair and nails, along with their functions, are discussed.

Skin

The surface area of the skin covers approximately 6 square metres in the average adult, with a thickness varying from 0.2 to 1.5 mm, depending on the region of the body and the person's age. Morphologically speaking, the skin is composed of three main layers: the epidermis, the dermis and the subcutaneous tissue, or hypodermis (**Figure 8.1**).

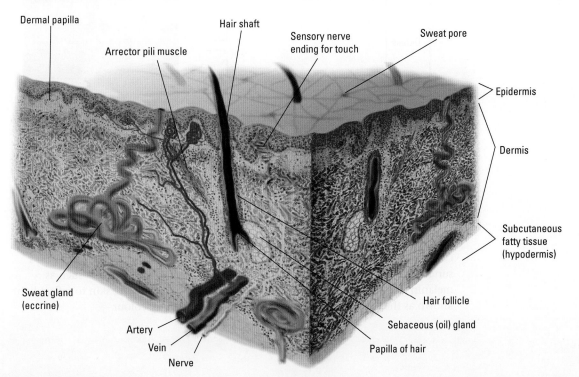

FIGURE 8.1 Structures of the skin

Epidermis

The **epidermis** is a multilayered outer covering consisting of four layers throughout the body, except for the palms of the hands and soles of the feet, where there are five layers (see **Figure 8.2**). The top layer, called the **stratum corneum**, is in a continual state of **desquamation** (shedding), as new skin cells are pushed up from the lower layers; a complete turnover of cells occurs every 3 to 4 weeks.

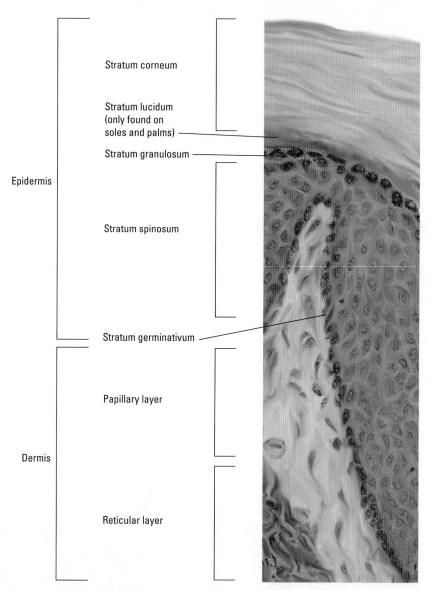

Stratum corneum

Stratum lucidum (only found on soles and palms)

Stratum granulosum

Epidermis

Stratum spinosum

Stratum germinativum

Papillary layer

Dermis

Reticular layer

FIGURE 8.2 Part of the epidermal and dermal layers of the skin

The epidermis, with the exception of the palmar and plantar surfaces, is normally smooth. All epidermal surfaces are devoid of blood vessels. Despite the absence of vessels, blood pigments, such as oxyhaemoglobin and reduced haemoglobin in the corium or dermis, are responsible for the vascular colour transmitted to the skin's surface. Other factors that affect the skin's colour are various pigments such as melanin and carotene. Epidermal thickness and the ability of the skin to reflect light, known as the Tyndall effect, also influence integumentary colour.

Dermis

The **dermis**, or corium, is the second layer of the skin. It is approximately 20 times thicker than the epidermis in certain areas of the body and can be divided into two layers: the papillary layer and the reticular layer (see **Figure 8.2**). The **papillary layer**, or upper layer, is composed primarily of loose connective tissue, small elastic fibres, and an extensive network of capillaries that serve to nourish the epidermis. The **reticular layer**, the lower layer of the dermis, is formed by a dense bed of vascular connective tissue that also includes nerves and lymphatic tissue. This layer also provides structural support for the skin. Intermeshed with the connective tissue are hair follicles, sweat glands, sebaceous glands and adipose tissue.

The fibrous connective tissue in the dermis gives the skin its strength and elasticity. The fibrous tissues provide structural support for the epidermis and form dermal 'ridges' to which the epidermis conforms and anchors, creating 'epidermal ridges' known as fingerprints. These ridges develop during the first trimester of fetal development and, although they enlarge with growth, their pattern remains the same throughout life and enhances with age. In general, the dermis is thicker over the dorsal and lateral surfaces such as the palmar and plantar surfaces. It is much thinner over the ventral and medial surfaces, and is especially thin in areas such as the eyelids, scrotum and penis.

Subcutaneous tissue

Beneath the dermis is the **subcutaneous tissue**, or superficial fascia. It is composed of either loose areola connective tissue or adipose tissue, depending on its location in the body. The subcutaneous layers attach the skin to the underlying bones. These layers act as a temperature insulator and help regulate body heat; they also encompass fat stores for energy use and contain an extensive venous plexus layer, which acts as a reservoir for the blood that warms the surface of the skin.

Distributed around the dermal blood vessels and the subcutaneous tissue are the skin's mast cells. These cells number from 7000 to 20 000 per cubic centimetre of skin. **Mast cells** are the body's major source of tissue histamine and they trigger the body's reaction to allergens.

Glands of the skin

There are two main groups of glands in the skin: the sebaceous glands and the sweat glands.

Sebaceous glands

The **sebaceous glands** are sebum-producing glands that are found almost everywhere in the dermis except for the palmar and plantar surfaces. They are also part of the apparatus that contains the hair follicle and the **arrector pili muscle**, which causes contraction of the skin and hair, resulting in 'goose bumps'. The ducts of the sebaceous glands open into the upper part of the hair follicle and are responsible for producing **sebum**, an oily secretion that is thought to retard evaporation and water loss from the epidermal cells. Sebaceous glands are most prevalent in the scalp, forehead, nose and chin.

Sweat glands

The two main types of **sweat glands** are **apocrine glands**, which are associated with hair follicles, and **eccrine glands**, which are not associated with hair follicles. The secretory apparatus of both types of sweat glands is located in the subcutaneous tissue. Eccrine glands open directly onto the skin's surface and are widely distributed throughout the body. Apocrine glands are found primarily in the axillae, genital and rectal areas, nipples and navel. These glands become functional during puberty, and secretion occurs during emotional stress or sexual stimulation. After puberty, apocrine glands are responsible for the characteristic body odour when sweat mixes with the natural bacterial flora normally present on the skin surface.

Hair

With few exceptions (the palmar and plantar surfaces, lips, nipples and the glans penis), hair is distributed over the entire body surface. Exceptions to 'normal' hair distribution or too much hair or loss of hair are considered conditions that may respond to treatment. Causes of these conditions may be linked as a side effect to certain drugs, a genetic predisposition, high levels of physical or emotional stress, endocrine abnormalities or as markers of other disease processes. The abundance and texture of hair are dependent on an individual's age, sex, race and heredity. **Vellus hair**, or fine, faint hair, covers most of the body. In general, **terminal hair** is the coarser, darker hair of the scalp, eyebrows and eyelashes. In the axillary and pubic areas, terminal hair becomes increasingly evident in both males and females with the onset of puberty. Males also tend to develop coarser, thicker chest and facial hair.

Most hair shafts are composed of three layers: the cuticle, or outer layer; the cortex, or middle layer; and the medulla, or innermost layer. Hair colour is determined by the **melanocytes** produced in the cells at the base of each follicle; an abundance of pigment produces darker hair colour, and smaller amounts produce a lighter colour.

Nails

Like hair, nails are composed of modified keratin and are layers of cells that arise from undifferentiated epithelial tissue called the **matrix**. The **nail plate**, tissue that covers the distal portion of the digits and provides protection, is approximately 0.5 to 0.75 mm thick. The nail consists of the **nail root**, which lies posteriorly to the cuticle and is attached to the matrix; the **nail bed**, which is the vascular bed located beneath the nail plate; and the **periungual tissues**, which surround the nail plate and the free edge of the nail (**Figure 8.3**). At the proximal end of each nail is a white, crescent-shaped area known as the **lunula**. This structure is obscured by the cuticle in some individuals.

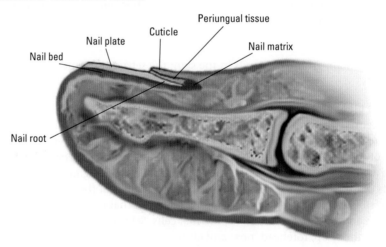

FIGURE 8.3 Structures of the nail

The normally translucent nail plate is given a pinkish cast by the underlying vascular bed in light-skinned individuals and a brownish cast in dark-skinned individuals. In many disease processes, the colour of the nail bed may vary. For instance, a decrease in oxygen content of the blood will cause the nail beds to appear **cyanotic**, or variations of colour from blue (in a fair-skinned person) to grey or dark brown (in darker-skinned people). The nail plate is formed continuously as the plate is pushed forwards by new growth from the germinative layer of the matrix. Fingernails take about five months to grow and cover from base to tip, and toenails can take up to 10 months to grow; however, growth varies with age, season, nutrition, climate, health status and activity.

Function of skin

The skin has many functions, but perhaps the most important one is its ability to serve as a protective barrier against invasion from environmental hazards and pathogens. It provides boundaries against materials that might enter the body, such as toxic chemicals, and provides boundaries for fluids and mobile tissues, such as blood, within the body. An intact integument is also responsible for the protection of underlying organs, which would otherwise be vulnerable to injury because of exposure.

Temperature regulation is carried out by the skin through the production of perspiration. During states of increased body temperature, large quantities of sweat are produced by the eccrine glands. As perspiration reaches the skin's surface, rapid evaporation takes place, and the body's temperature begins to decrease. The skin's vascular system also plays a role in heat control. When vasodilation occurs, much of the heat can be lost through radiation and conduction. Conversely, vasoconstriction helps to maintain body heat.

The skin contains receptors for pain, touch, pressure and temperature. These receptors originate in the dermis and terminate as either free nerve endings throughout the skin's surface or as special touch receptors that are encapsulated and found predominantly in the fingertips and lips. Each hair found on the body also contains a basal nerve fibre that acts as a tactile receptor. Sensory signals that help determine precise locations on the skin are transmitted along rapid sensory pathways, and less distinct signals such as pressure or poorly localised touch are sent via slower sensory pathways.

The skin acts as an organ of excretion for substances such as water, salts and nitrogenous wastes. The skin produces cells for wound repair and is the site for the production of vitamin D. The skin is also an indicator of nonverbal language and emotions via blushing and facial expressions. The skin may further be used for the purpose of identification via fingerprints and birthmarks. Skin colour is one of the most visible variations between people across our diverse populations. Skin colour can impact on melanin production, risks associated with sun or UV damage, and can be a focus of health promotion, a barometer of health and wellness and plays a large part in people's self-identity and self-image.

Function of hair

Hair provides warmth, protection and sensation to the underlying systems. Terminal hair of the scalp and face provides warmth, shields against UV light, and filters dust and particulate matter. Vellus hair enhances tactile sensation and sensory perception. In some cultures, hair is a status symbol of beauty and wealth. Even though physiological functions of hair have modified with changes to lifestyle and evolution, psychologically and socially, hair serves a very important function especially for self-image. Unwanted changes to hair location, quality and presence can impact greatly on the individual's sense of wellness and self.

Function of nails

Nails provide protection to the distal surface of the digits and can be used for self-protection. In some cultures, nail length in both men and women is a qualifier of social and economic status and self-image.

ASSESSMENT: TAKING THE CONSUMER'S HEALTH HISTORY

Assessment is the first phase of the nursing process. It involves collecting subjective information about the consumer's health status in order to identify consumer problem areas to focus on.

Subjective data is most frequently collected during a health history and serves as the starting point for the health professional to base the depth of their assessment on. The sections for the health history include:

> **Consumer profile**
> **Chief complaint** (explained systematically using variations of location, quality, quantity, associated manifestations, aggravating factors, alleviating factors, setting and timing. This is a variation on the OPQRST assessment mnemonic you may use for other conditions such as pain assessment)
> **Past health history** (including medical history, surgical history, allergies, medications, injuries and accidents, special needs and childhood illnesses)
> **Family health history**
> **Social history** (including alcohol, tobacco and drug use, sexual practice, work and home environment, hobbies and leisure activities, stress and culture).

HEALTH HISTORY

CONSUMER PROFILE	The skin, hair and nails health history provides insight into the link between a consumer's life/lifestyle and skin, hair and nails information and pathology. Diseases that are age-, sex- and race-specific for the skin, hair and nails are listed.		
	AGE	**SKIN**	> Fungal infections, diseases of sebaceous glands, such as acne vulgaris (13–26 years) > Lupus erythematosus, psoriasis, hyperpigmented macular lesions, skin tags (acrochordon), dermatophyte infections (25–60 years) > Basal cell carcinoma (BCC) (older adults) > Melanoma (all ages)
		HAIR	> Male pattern alopecia (adolescence to young adulthood) > Thinning, greying, loss of hair in axillary and pubic areas, excessive facial hair (middle to old age)
	SEX	**SKIN**	Skin pathology is consistently more prevalent among males than females; dermatophyte infections, skin tumours, fungal infections, and increased incidence of tumours related to occupational hazards and hygiene; Kaposi's sarcoma associated with immunodeficiency conditions
		HAIR	> Female: female pattern alopecia, increased facial hair with ageing > Male: alopecia, increased coarse nose and ear hair with ageing
	CULTURAL BACKGROUND	**DARK-SKINNED**	Keloid formation, dermatosis papulosa nigra, hyperpigmentation and hypopigmentation, traumatic marginal alopecia, seborrhoeic dermatitis, pseudofolliculitis barbae, acne keloidalis, granuloma inguinale, Mongolian spots, albinism, hypopigmented sarcoidosis, granulomatosis skin lesions
		LIGHT-SKINNED	Squamous and basal cell carcinoma, actinic keratosis, psoriasis

>>

>>

HEALTH HISTORY			
CHIEF COMPLAINT	Common chief complaints for the skin, hair and nails are defined, and information on the characteristics of each sign and symptom is provided.		
	1. PRURITUS	Cutaneous itching that may have a multitude of aetiologies	
		LOCATION	Generalised or localised
		QUALITY	Superficial or deep sensation of itching, intensity of itching, interference with sleep habits
		ASSOCIATED MANIFESTATIONS	Rashes, lesions, oedema, angioedema, anaphylaxis, excoriation or ulcers as the result of scratching, lichenification (thickening of the skin), systemic disease
		AGGRAVATING FACTORS	Exposure to chemicals, sunlight, plants, food, animals, stress, climate, parasites, xerosis (dry skin), drug reaction, systemic disease processes, contact dermatitis, types of clothing (frequently wool)
		ALLEVIATING FACTORS	Dietary changes, medications, antihistamines, biofeedback, cool baths, types of clothing (frequently cotton), increased skin hydration, ultraviolet-band light therapy
		SETTING	Work, home, school or recreational environment
		TIMING	Preprandial or postprandial, nocturnal, seasonal, during periods of stress, associated with menstrual cycle
	2. RASH	A cutaneous eruption that may be localised or generalised	
	3. LESION	A circumscribed pathological change in the tissues	
		LOCATION	Location of where it started and spread, distribution over the body, percentage of body involved, following dermatomes
		QUANTITY	Grouping or arrangement: discrete, grouped, confluent, linear, annular, polycyclic, generalised, zosteriform
		QUALITY	Morphology: macule, patch, papule, plaque, nodule, cyst, wheal, vesicle, pustule, bulla, tumour, lichenification, crust, erosion, fissure, ulcer, atrophy
		ASSOCIATED MANIFESTATIONS	Oedema, angioedema, anaphylaxis, excoriation or ulcers as the result of scratching, lichenification, systemic disease, allergies, fever, induration
		AGGRAVATING FACTORS	Exposure to chemicals, sunlight, plants, food, animals, stress, climate, parasites, xerosis, drug reaction, systemic disease processes, contact dermatitis, radiation, types of clothing (frequently wool)
		ALLEVIATING FACTORS	Dietary changes, medications, antihistamines, biofeedback, cool baths, types of clothing (frequently cotton), increased skin hydration, ultraviolet-band light therapy, surgery
		SETTING	Work, home, school or recreational environment
		TIMING	When it started, preprandial or postprandial, nocturnal, seasonal, during periods of stress, associated with menstrual cycle

>>

UNIT 2

HEALTH HISTORY

PAST HEALTH HISTORY	The various components of the past health history are linked to skin, hair and nails pathology and skin-, hair- and nails-related information.		
	MEDICAL HISTORY	**SKIN-SPECIFIC**	Allergies, eczema, atopic dermatitis, melanoma, albinism, vitiligo, psoriasis, skin cancer, athlete's foot, birthmarks, body piercing, tattoos, urticaria
		NON-SKIN-SPECIFIC	Renal disease, diabetes mellitus, lupus erythematosus, peripheral vascular disease, idiopathic thrombocytopaenia purpura (ITP), Rocky Mountain spotted fever, liver disease, hepatitis, collagen diseases, cardiac dysfunction, sexually transmitted infections, Lyme disease, arthritis, lymphoma, thyroid disease, pregnancy, Addison's disease, pernicious anaemia, HIV, cytomegalovirus, Epstein-Barr virus, measles, mumps, rubella, coxsackievirus, adenovirus, drug hypersensitivities, varicella, herpes zoster, herpes simplex, Kawasaki disease, toxic shock syndrome, carcinoma, tuberculosis, viral syndromes
		HAIR-SPECIFIC	Allergies, alopecia, lice, bacterial or fungal infections of the scalp, brittle hair, rapid hair loss, trichotillomania, trauma, congenital anomalies
		NON-HAIR-SPECIFIC	Renal disease, diabetes mellitus, cardiac dysfunction, peripheral vascular disease, thyroid disease, pregnancy, Addison's disease, HIV, anaemia, malnutrition, stress, chemotherapy, radiation therapy
		NAIL-SPECIFIC	Allergies, psoriasis, bacterial or fungal infections, trauma, brittle nails, nail biting, congenital anomalies
		NON-NAIL-SPECIFIC	Iron-deficiency anaemia, chronic infection, malnutrition, Raynaud's disease, hypoxia, acute infections, syphilis
	SURGICAL HISTORY	Keloid and scar formation, plastic surgery for birthmarks, skin grafts, reconstructive surgery, excision biopsy	
	ALLERGIES	Medication, insect stings, foods, soaps, laundry detergent, chemicals, fibres (wool), metals (nickel), animal dander, pollens, grasses, cosmetics, signs/symptoms of first manifestation of allergic reaction	
	MEDICATIONS	Reaction manifested in skin changes after use of prescription or over-the-counter drugs	
	COMMUNICABLE DISEASES	Varicella, roseola, measles, scabies, bacterial or fungal infections, HIV Sexually transmitted infections: syphilis, gonorrhoea, chancroid, genital warts (see Chapter 17 for further information)	
	INJURIES AND ACCIDENTS	Chemical inhalation, trauma, burns, toxin contamination	
	SPECIAL NEEDS	Poor eyesight can lead to poor hygiene; frequent skin trauma prevents early detection and treatment of skin diseases; bedridden or wheelchair bound with possibility of pressure injury and compromise of skin integrity	
	BLOOD TRANSFUSIONS	Skin eruptions, pruritus	
	CHILDHOOD ILLNESSES	Refer to section on communicable diseases in Chapter 3	

>>

HEALTH HISTORY		
FAMILY HEALTH HISTORY	Skin, hair and nail diseases that are familial in nature are listed.	
	SKIN-SPECIFIC	Allergies, eczema, melanoma, albinism, vitiligo, psoriasis, non-melanoma skin cancer
	HAIR-SPECIFIC	Allergies, alopecia, brittle hair, hair loss
	NAIL-SPECIFIC	Brittle nails
SOCIAL HISTORY	The components of the social history are linked to skin, hair and nail factors/pathology.	
	ALCOHOL USE	Hepatotoxicity and subsequent skin manifestations that accompany liver failure, such as jaundice and pruritus; skin bruising and trauma from falls and ataxia; telangiectasia of the nose, neck and upper chest
	TOBACCO USE	Yellow discolouration of fingertips on smoking hand, leathery facial appearance
	DRUG USE	Skin manifestations from intravenous drug use, such as injection sites or tracks; these are especially prevalent in the forearms, behind the knees, toe webs, finger webs, and under the nails
	SEXUAL PRACTICE	Various sexually transmitted infections may manifest in the genital region; these are discussed in Chapters17
	TRAVEL HISTORY	> Tropical regions: fungal infections, contact dermatitis, tropical eczema, leishmaniasis > Insect bites and stings: insects indigenous to certain climates, such as fire ants, bees, spiders, wasps > High-altitude areas: light-sensitive eruptions and winter eczema
	WORK ENVIRONMENT	> Chemical: contact dermatitis, burns > Sunlight: skin eruptions, increased incidence of basal or squamous cell carcinoma (SCC), burns, wrinkles, senile freckles, lightened hair, excessive exposure to ultraviolet radiation > Excessive exposure to water: drying and cracking of skin, pruritus, soft nails, damaged hair shafts > Insect bites: rashes, urticaria, oedema, angioedema, pruritus > Operating heavy or sharp equipment: trauma, laceration > Excessive exposure to wind and cold temperatures: ageing, drying and cracking of skin > Pollution: contact dermatitis > Tar and pitch: act as both photosensitiser and carcinogen
	HOME ENVIRONMENT	Chemicals used in cleaning can cause contact dermatitis; excessive exposure to water can cause dry, cracked skin, soft nails and damaged hair shafts; excessive heat in the home can dry skin and cause pruritus; infected kittens and puppies may lead to tinea capitis
	HOBBIES AND LEISURE ACTIVITIES	Gardening with exposure to chemicals, sunlight, contact dermatitis (e.g. chrysanthemums, primula, tomato plants, grevillea, English ivy, occasionally rhus trees; lantana or vegetables such as parsnip or celery may cause photo-contact dermatitis) and insect bites; outdoor summer sports or activities increase sun and insect-bite exposure; outdoor winter activities increase frostbite and exposure; excessive exposure to chlorine and salt water damages hair; the climate in northern Australia particularly as well as excessive use of tanning salons may lead to skin carcinoma
	STRESS	Skin eruptions such as eczema, urticaria, acne and psoriasis may have a psychological component in some cases; body image disorder as a result of skin disease and hair loss
	ECONOMIC STATUS	People of lower socioeconomic status may develop skin eruptions associated with poor hygiene because of insufficient resources, infestations associated with overcrowding, and infections associated with malnutrition Scabies and impetigo are common in conditions where housing is crowded and nutrition and socioeconomic status is poor – therefore common in Aboriginal and Torres Strait Islander communities

CLINICAL **REASONING**

Practice tip: Focusing health history – self-care behaviours and risk
Before undertaking the physical examination, the following specific questions will assist you to identify self-behaviours and potential risk factors that may enable you to opportunistically provide person-centred health education.

> Skin care habits:
  • Do you use lotions, perfumes, cologne, cosmetics, soaps, oils, shaving cream, after-shave lotion, electric or standard razor?
  • What type of home remedies do you use for skin lesions and rashes?
  • How often do you bathe or shower?
  • Do you use a tanning bed or salon?
  • What type of sun protection do you use?
  • Have you ever had a reaction to jewellery that you wore?
  • Do you wear hats, visors, gloves, long sleeves or pants, sunscreen when in the sun?
  • How much time do you spend in the sun?
> Hair care habits:
  • Do you use shampoo, conditioner, hair spray, setting products (e.g. mousse or gel)?
  • Do you colour, dye or bleach your hair?
  • What products do you use?
  • Do you wear a wig or hairpiece?
  • Do you have greying hair or hair loss?
  • Do you use a hair dryer, heated curlers, hair straightener or curling iron?
  • Do you tightly braid your hair?
> Nail care habits:
  • Do you get manicures or pedicures?
  • What type of nail care do you practise (trimming, clipping, use of polish, nail tips, acrylics)?
  • Do you bite your nails?
  • Do you suffer from nail splitting or discolouration?

PERSON-CENTRED HEALTH EDUCATION

When conducting a health assessment, opportunities for the provision of person-centred health education will arise. This is a significant consideration in relation to the assessment process for examination of the skin, hair and nails, due to their associated personal identity aspects and lifestyle choices for preventative care. These occasions are identified as individualised education and may generate further data that can be added to the assessment. All education given should be documented so that in the future, health professionals can assess the impact of previous information provided to the consumer. (Refer to Chapter 1 for initiating health education.)

INDIVIDUALISED HEALTH EDUCATION INTERVENTIONS	
Assessing the person for the following health-related activities can assist in identifying the need for education about these factors. This information provides a bridge between health maintenance activities and the function of skin, hair and nails.	
Sleep	Sleep disturbances caused by symptoms such as itching or burning
Diet	Allergies to food can cause skin eruptions such as urticaria; diets high in fat and cholesterol may be connected to the development of xanthelasmatous lesions; vitamin deficiencies result in skin, hair and nail changes; see Chapter 15 for further information
Exercise	Increased risk for cutaneous trauma associated with contact sports and sun exposure with outdoor sports and activities
Use of safety devices	Sunblock/sunscreen with appropriate sun protection factor (SPF) to prevent UV exposure; lotions and creams to prevent drying and cracking of skin; protective gloves when handling harsh, irritating chemicals; use of protective clothing for environmental conditions

PLANNING FOR PHYSICAL EXAMINATION

The planning phase refers to evaluating subjective data to narrow the focus on physical examination, determining what objective data needs to be gathered, and considering the environment and equipment that will be required.

Objective data is collected during the physical examination of the consumer. It is:

> usually collected after subjective data

> information that is measured or observed by the clinician as opposed to being reported by the consumer

> vital to the overall health assessment, to enable you to make clinical decisions that are representative of the whole consumer subjective data to focus physical examination.

Before commencing the physical examination of the consumer's integumentary system (e.g. skin, hair, nails), consider what information the health history has provided. Critical consideration, linked to knowledge of anatomy and physiology, should focus the physical assessment so your examination will be more effective and efficient.

Environment

Assessment of the hair, skin and nails needs to be done in a suitable environment that can provide privacy and a comfortable temperature, as you will need to be able to completely undress the person to access all of his or her skin.

Equipment

> Magnifying glass
> Good source of natural light
> Penlight
> Nonsterile gloves
> Small centimetre ruler

HEALTH EDUCATION

Reducing exposure to integumentary irritants

Workplace-related skin disease is a common and expensive issue in Australia and New Zealand. It can impact people at any time of life, even if there is no history of allergies and which could mostly be prevented (Skin Health Institute, 2022).

Allergic contact dermatitis is the leading workplace-related skin disease in Australia and New Zealand, and hands are the most commonly affected body part. Many workplaces will provide support for workers to help them reduce their exposure to these irritants with products, procedures and guidelines. The following professions are most commonly affected:

> Hairdresser
> Food handler (bakers, caterers, cooks and confectioners)
> Health workers (especially nurses)
> Construction and industry workers
> Leather and shoe manufacturers
> Florists
> Gardeners
> Metal workers
  To reduce exposure, follow these guidelines:
> In the workplace, always follow Occupational Safety and Health Administration and employer's safety guidelines.
> Follow the directions on the labels of all products; pay special attention to warning labels.
> If using a personal care product for the first time, perform a patch test to evaluate for sensitivity.
> Use rubber gloves when handling toxins or caustic substances.
> Contact a poison control centre for treatment guidelines if exposed to toxic or caustic substances.
> Notify HAZMAT (hazardous materials) officials if a dangerous chemical or toxin exposure occurs.

IMPLEMENTATION: CONDUCTING THE PHYSICAL EXAMINATION

Implementation of the physical examination requires you to consider your scope of practice as well. In this section, depending on your context, you may be performing foundation assessment with aspects of advanced assessment if you are practising in a specialised area.

EXAMINATION IN BRIEF: SKIN, HAIR AND NAILS

Examination of the skin

Inspection
> Colour
> Bleeding, ecchymosis and vascularity
> Lesions

Palpation
> Moisture
> Temperature
> Tenderness
> Texture
> Turgor
> Oedema

Examination of the hair

Inspection
> Colour
> Distribution
> Lesions

Palpation
> Texture

Examination of the nails

Inspection
> Colour
> Shape and configuration

Palpation
> Texture

General approach to examination of the skin

1. Ensure that the room is well lit. Daylight is the best source of light, especially when determining skin colour. However, if daylight is unavailable, overhead fluorescent lights should be added.
2. Use a handheld magnifying glass to aid in inspection when simple visual inspection is not adequate.
3. Explain to the consumer each step of the examination process prior to initiating the assessment.
4. Ensure consumer privacy by providing drapes.
5. Ensure the comfort of the consumer by keeping the room at an appropriate temperature.
6. Warm hands by washing them in warm water prior to the examination.
7. Gather equipment on a table prior to initiating the examination.
8. Ask the person to undress completely and put on a gown, leaving the back untied.
9. Perform the examination in a cephalocaudal fashion.
10. For episodic illness, the skin examination is incorporated into the regional physical examination.

Examination of the skin

In each area, observe for colour, bleeding, ecchymosis, vascularity, lesions, moisture, temperature, texture, turgor and oedema.

Inspection

E 1. Facing the consumer, inspect the colour of the skin of the face, eyelids, ears, nose, lips and mucous membranes.
2. Inspect the anterior and lateral aspects of the neck, then behind the ears.

E Examination **N** Normal findings **A** Abnormal findings **P** Pathophysiology

E 3. Inspect arms and dorsal and palmar surfaces of the hands. Pay special attention to the webs between the fingers.

4. Have the consumer move to a supine position with arms placed over the head.

5. Lower gown to uncover chest and breasts.

6. Inspect intramammary folds and ridges. Pendulous breasts may need to be raised to complete this inspection.

7. Assess axillae, and then cover chest and breasts with gown.

8. Raise gown to uncover abdomen and anterior aspect of the lower extremities; place a sheet over the genital area.

9. Inspect abdomen, anterior aspect of the lower extremities, dorsal and plantar surfaces of the feet, and toe webs.

10. Don gloves and uncover genital area.

11. Inspect inguinal folds and genitalia.

12. Remove and discard gloves.

13. Have the consumer turn to a side-lying position on the examination table so their back is facing you.

14. Inspect back and posterior neck and scalp. Specifically look for **naevi** or other lesions.

15. Inspect posterior aspect of the lower extremities.

16. Don nonsterile gloves and raise the gluteal cleft and inspect the gluteal folds and perianal area; then remove and discard the gloves.

17. Cover the person and assist them back to a sitting position.

18. Wash hands.

CLINICAL **REASONING**

Practice tip: Tattoos and body piercings

It is important to inspect the skin and note the presence and location of tattoos and body piercings (**Figure 8.4**). Some consumers react to the ink in the tattoo and develop various skin disorders. Body piercing sites should be assessed for signs of infection (e.g. erythema, purulent discharge, increased skin temperature). Remember to assess all body areas. The ears, umbilicus, eyebrows, lips, nares, tongue, vagina and scrotum are often pierced. Ask the patient if they change or remove piercings, or have any concerns with their piercings. Document the location of all tattoos and body piercings in relation to anatomical location.

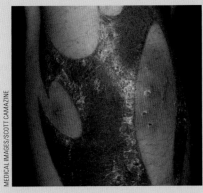 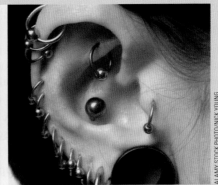

FIGURE 8.4 Tattoos and body piercings

E Examination   **N** Normal findings   **A** Abnormal findings   **P** Pathophysiology

Colour

E Assess for colouration.

N Normally, the skin is a uniform whitish-pink or brown colour, depending on the person's race. Exposure to sunlight results in increased pigmentation of sun-exposed areas. Dark-skinned persons may normally have a freckling of the gums, tongue borders, and lining of the cheeks; the gingiva may appear blue or variegated in colour.

A The appearance of cyanotic (dusky blue) fingers, lips or mucous membranes is abnormal in both light- and dark-skinned individuals. In light-skinned individuals, the skin has a bluish tint. The earlobes, lower eyelids, lips, oral mucosa, nail beds, and palmar and plantar surfaces may be especially cyanotic. Dark-skinned individuals have an ashen-grey to pale tint, and the lips and tongue are good indicators of **cyanosis**.

P Cyanosis occurs when there is greater than 0.05 g/mL of deoxygenated haemoglobin in the blood. In order for cyanosis to be an accurate indicator of arterial oxygen (PaO$_2$), two conditions must be met: the consumer must have normal haemoglobin and **haematocrit** as well as normal perfusion. For example, a consumer with **polycythaemia** (elevated number of red blood cells) can be cyanotic but have adequate oxygenation. The problem lies in the fact that the consumer has too many red blood cells rather than too little oxygen. Conversely, a consumer with **anaemia** (reduced number of red blood cells) can be hypoxaemic but not cyanotic. In this case, the consumer has too little haemoglobin. Central cyanosis is secondary to marked heart and lung disease; peripheral cyanosis can be secondary to systemic disease, or vasoconstriction stimulated by cold temperatures or anxiety.

A The appearance of **jaundice** (yellow-green to orange cast or colouration) of skin, sclera, mucous membranes, fingernails, and palmar or plantar surfaces in the light-skinned individual is abnormal (**Figure 8.5A**). Jaundice in dark-skinned individuals may appear as yellow staining in the sclera, hard palate, and palmar or plantar surfaces.

P Jaundice is caused by an increased serum bilirubin level of greater than 0.02 mg/mL associated with liver disease or haemolytic disease. Severe burns and sepsis also can produce jaundice.

A A yellow discolouration of the palmar and digital creases is abnormal.

P Xanthoma striata palmaris is caused by hyperlipidaemia.

A A greyish cast to the skin is abnormal.

P A greyish cast is seen in consumers with renal concerns and is associated with chronic anaemia along with retained urochrome pigments. Slight jaundice may also be found in the consumer with renal disease.

A Sustained bright red or pink colouration in light-skinned individuals is abnormal. Dark-skinned individuals may have no underlying change in colouration. Palpation may be used to ascertain signs of warmth, swelling or induration.

P Hyperaemia occurs because of dilated superficial blood vessels, increased blood flow, febrile states, local inflammatory condition or excessive alcohol intake.

A A bright red to ruddy, sustained appearance that is evident on the integument, mucous membranes and palmar or plantar surfaces is abnormal in both light- and dark-skinned individuals.

P Polycythaemia, as noted earlier, is an increased number of red blood cells and results in this ruddy appearance.

A A dusky rubor of the extremities when in a dependent position, which can be associated with tissue necrosis, is abnormal.

E Examination **N** Normal findings **A** Abnormal findings **P** Pathophysiology

P Venous stasis results from venule engorgement and diminished blood flow, which occurs in congestive heart failure and **atherosclerosis**.

A A pale cast to the skin that may be most evident in the face, mucous membranes, lips and nail beds is abnormal in light-skinned individuals. A yellow-brown to ashen-grey cast to the skin along with pale or grey lips, mucous membranes and nail beds is abnormal in dark-skinned individuals.

P Pallor is due to decreased visibility of the normal oxyhaemoglobin. This can occur when the person has decreased blood flow in the superficial vessels, as in shock or **syncope**, or when there is a decreased amount of serum oxyhaemoglobin, as in anaemia. Localised pallor may be secondary to arterial **insufficiency**.

A A brown cast to parts of the skin can be generalised or discrete.

P A brown colouration occurs when there is a deposition of melanin, which can be caused by genetic predisposition, pregnancy, Addison's disease (deficiency in cortisol leading to enhanced melanin production), café au lait spots (**Figure 8.5B**) and sunlight.

P Acanthosis nigricans is a condition in which the skin becomes brownish and thicker, almost leathery in appearance (**Figure 8.5C**). This usually occurs in the axillae, on the flexoral surfaces of the groin and neck, and around the umbilicus. Acanthosis nigricans occurs in obesity, diabetes mellitus, and with medications such as steroids.

A A white cast to the skin as evidenced by generalised whiteness, including of the hair and eyebrows, is abnormal (see **Figure 8.5D**).

P This lack of colouration is caused by **albinism**, a congenital inability to form melanin.

P **Vitiligo** is a condition marked by patchy, symmetrical areas of white on the skin and is abnormal (see **Figure 8.5E**).

P This condition can be caused by an acquired loss of melanin. Trauma can also lead to hypopigmentation, especially in dark-skinned individuals.

A An erythematous, confluent eruption in a butterfly-like distribution over the face is abnormal.

P Systemic lupus erythematosus, a connective tissue disorder, is the most likely aetiology.

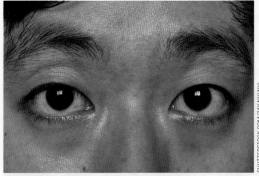

A. Jaundice. Note the yellowing of the skin as well as the eyes (in fair-skinned people). In some darker-skinned people, often this may only be apparent in the conjunctiva of the eyes

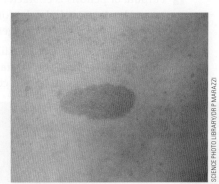

B. Café au lait spots

FIGURE 8.5 Skin colour abnormalities

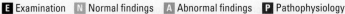

E Examination **N** Normal findings **A** Abnormal findings **P** Pathophysiology

URGENT FINDING

Signs of abuse when assessing integumentary system

Areas of ecchymosis are often signs of trauma that could be the result of physical abuse, but are often presented as resulting from an injury or 'clumsiness' from the consumer. Ecchymotic areas at the base of the skull or on the face, buttocks, breasts or abdomen should warrant a high index of suspicion for abuse, especially if found in children or pregnant women, as should burns (e.g. cigarettes, iron) and belt buckle or bite marks. In addition, lacerations, scars, haematomas and puncture wounds should carry a high index of suspicion. Patterned injuries, such as those caused by ropes or chains, need to be investigated further.

Signs of physical abuse can also be present in the hair. Hair that is singed or unusually kinked may have been exposed to fire. Alopecia can be caused by repeated pulling. Describe injuries in relation to type, age (old/new) and anatomical location.

Any signs of abuse should be investigated further and referred as necessary. Check your responsibilities for mandatory reporting with your state/territory or federal law. Further information relating to investigating possible abuse can be found in Chapter 3.

Bleeding, ecchymosis and vascularity

E Inspect the skin for evidence of bleeding, ecchymosis or increased vascularity.

N Normally, there are no areas of increased vascularity, ecchymosis or bleeding.

A Bleeding from the mucous membranes, previous venipuncture sites or lesions should be considered abnormal.

P Spontaneous bleeding can be indicative of clotting disorders, trauma or use of antithrombolytic agents such as warfarin or heparin.

A **Petechiae** are violaceous (red-purple) discolourations of less than 0.5 cm in diameter (see **Figure 8.6A**). Petechiae do not blanch. In dark-skinned individuals, evaluate for petechiae in the mucous membranes and axillae.

P Petechiae can indicate an increased bleeding tendency or embolism; causes include intravascular defects or infections.

A **Purpura** is a condition characterised by the presence of confluent petechiae or confluent ecchymosis over any part of the body (see **Figure 8.6B**).

P Purpura or peliosis is characterised by haemorrhage into the skin and can be caused by decreased platelet formation. Lesions vary, depending on the type of purpura; pigmentation changes may become permanent.

A **Ecchymosis** is a violaceous discolouration of varying size, also called a black-and-blue mark (see **Figure 8.6C**). In dark-skinned consumers, these discolourations are deeper in colour.

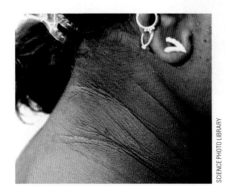
C. Acanthosis nigricans

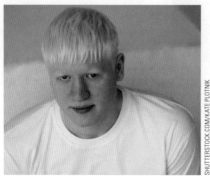
D. Albinism. Note the lack of colouration.

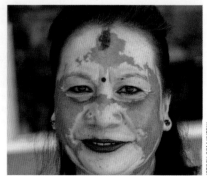
E. Vitiligo

FIGURE 8.5 *continued* Skin colour abnormalities

E Examination **N** Normal findings **A** Abnormal findings **P** Pathophysiology

P Ecchymosis is caused by extravasation of blood into the skin as a result of trauma; it can also occur with heparin or warfarin use or liver dysfunction.

A An erythematous dilation of small blood vessels is abnormal (see **Figure 8.6D**).

P This erythematous dilation describes a telangiectasia. Erythematous dilations tend to appear on the face and thighs; they occur more frequently in women.

A **Spider angiomas** are bright red and star-shaped (see **Figure 8.6E**). There is often a central pulsation noted with pressure, and this pressure results in blanching in the extensions. Most often, these lesions are noted on the face, neck and chest. They are a type of telangiectasia.

P Causes of spider angiomas include pregnancy, liver disease and hormone therapy. They are normal in a small percentage of the population and are more prevalent in women.

A **Venous stars** are linear or irregularly shaped, blue vascular patterns that do not blanch with pressure (**Figure 8.6F**). These are often noted on the legs near veins or on the anterior chest.

P Venous stars are caused by increased venous pressure in the superficial veins.

A **Cherry angiomas** are bright red, circumscribed areas that may darken with age (see **Figure 8.6G**). They can be flat or raised and may show partial blanching with pressure. Most often, they are found on the trunk.

P These vascularities are of unknown aetiology and are pathologically insignificant except for cosmetic appearance.

A A bright red, raised area that has well-defined borders and does not blanch with pressure is abnormal (see **Figure 8.6H**).

P Strawberry haemangiomas, or strawberry marks, are congenital malformations of closely packed, immature capillaries. This condition is also known as naevus vascularis. They regress as the child grows and are usually gone in a few years.

A A burgundy, red or violaceous macular/vascular patch that is located along the course of a peripheral nerve is abnormal (**Figure 8.6I**).

P This macular/vascular patch is a port-wine stain, or naevus flammeus. The port-wine stain is composed of mature, but thin-walled, capillaries. The lesion is usually present at birth and is frequently located on the face. A port-wine stain can be indicative of underlying disorders, such as Sturge-Weber syndrome.

A In light-skinned individuals, a purple to black discolouration is abnormal (**Figure 8.6J**). In dark-skinned individuals, very dark to black discolouration is abnormal.

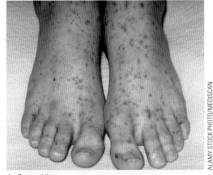

A. Petechiae

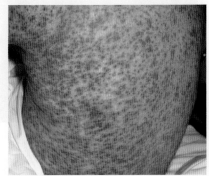

B. Purpura

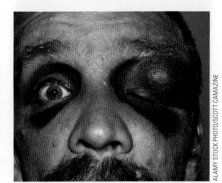

C. Ecchymosis

FIGURE 8.6 Bleeding, ecchymosis and vascular abnormalities of the skin

E Examination **N** Normal findings **A** Abnormal findings **P** Pathophysiology

P These findings can indicate different stages of necrosis, or tissue death. Conditions that starve the affected body part of oxygen, whether in acute or chronic situations, can cause necrosis. Diabetes mellitus, disseminated intravascular coagulation, acute hypovolaemia, and severe electric charge are some of the conditions that can cause necrosis.

A Dark brown or blackened areas of skin that are oedematous and painful are abnormal (see **Figure 8.6K**). These areas may drain a thin liquid that has a sweet, foul odour. Crepitus may be palpated in the affected areas.

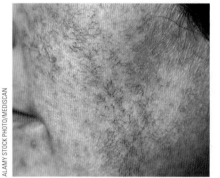
D. Telangiectasia usually occurs in women and on the face.

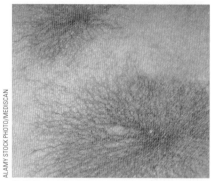
E. Spider angioma

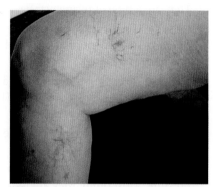
F. Venous star

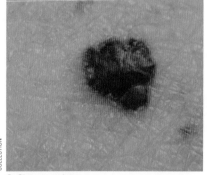
G. Cherry angioma

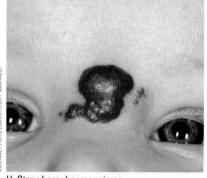
H. Strawberry haemangioma

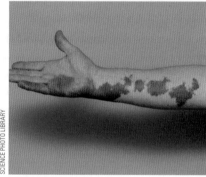
I. Naevus flammeus

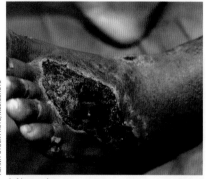
J. Necrosis

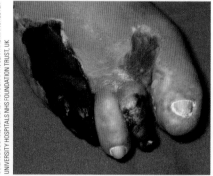
K. Gas gangrene

FIGURE 8.6 continued Bleeding, ecchymosis and vascular abnormalities of the skin

E Examination **N** Normal findings **A** Abnormal findings **P** Pathophysiology

P Gas gangrene, or clostridial myonecrosis, is a Gram-positive infection that affects skeletal muscles that have decreased oxygenation. The clostridia organisms are endogenous to the gastrointestinal tract and are also found in the soil. Consumers who experience circulatory compromise, such as in diabetes mellitus, arterial insufficiency, trauma and constricting casts, are at risk for developing gas gangrene. Consumers who have contaminated wounds and decreased vascularity to the affected area are also at risk for developing gas gangrene.

HEALTH EDUCATION

Evaluating skin lesions

A simple approach to teaching people how to decide to seek medical review for skin lesions is an essential tool for nurses. The following ABCDE mnemonic for evaluating skin lesions is easy to remember.

> A (**A**symmetrical): Is the lesion asymmetrical?
> B (**B**orders): Are the borders of the lesion irregular?
> C (**C**olour): Is the colour of the lesion uneven, irregular or multicoloured?
> D (**D**iameter): Has the lesion's diameter changed recently?
> E (**E**levation): Has the lesion become elevated?

If the answer is 'yes' to any of the questions in this evaluation, consumers should be referred to or advised to go to their medical officer or skin lesion/cancer clinic for further assessment.

Lesions

E 1. Inspect the skin for lesions, noting the anatomic location. Lesions can be localised, regionalised or generalised. They can involve exposed areas or skin folds (see **Table 8.1**).
2. Note the grouping or arrangement of the lesions: discrete, grouped, confluent, linear, annular, polycyclic, generalised or zosteriform (see **Figure 8.7**).
3. Inspect the lesions for elevation (flat or raised).
4. Using a ruler, measure the lesions.
5. Describe the colour of the lesions.
6. Note any exudate for colour or odour.
7. Note the morphology of the skin lesions. Skin lesions can be primary, originating from previously normal skin, or secondary, originating from primary lesions. For specific descriptions of primary lesion morphology, see **Figure 8.8**. For specific descriptions of secondary lesion morphology, refer to **Figure 8.9**.

TABLE 8.1 Anatomic locations of various skin lesions

LESION	LOCATION
Basal cell carcinoma	Medial and lateral canthi, nasolabial fold
Rosacea	Face
Acne vulgaris	Face, back, shoulders, chest
Furuncle	Nose, neck, face, axillae, buttocks
Lesions resulting from light exposure (squamous cell carcinoma, solar lentigo, solar keratosis)	Forehead, cheeks, tops of the ears, neck, dorsal surface of hands and forearms, lateral arms
Seborrhoeic keratosis, spider angioma	Face, trunk, upper extremities
Impetigo, verruca vulgaris (warts)	Arms, legs, buttocks, face, hands, fingers, knees

>>

E Examination N Normal findings A Abnormal findings P Pathophysiology

>> **TABLE 8.1** *continued*

LESION	LOCATION
Herpes zoster	Along the cutaneous spinal nerve tracks, almost always unilateral
Kaposi's sarcoma	Widespread: trunk, head, tip of nose, periorbital, penis, legs, palms, soles
Erythema nodosum	Lower legs
Stasis dermatitis	Sock area
Cutaneous moniliasis	Moist folds behind the ears, under the breasts, in the axilla, umbilicus, along the inguinal and pudendal regions, in the gluteal and perineal areas
Adult atopic eczema	Mainly flexor surfaces of the body
Psoriasis	Mainly scalp, elbows, extensor surfaces of the body (rarely on the face and skin folds)
Contact dermatitis	Affects surfaces in contact with irritating agents
Pediculosis pubis	Pubic and axillary areas

CLINICAL **REASONING**

Practice tip: Wound evaluation

If a wound is present, the following assessment process should be undertaken (Benbow, 2016). Assess:

1. the person (examine all areas of the skin for signs of scarring, dermatological disorders, skin changes, condition of skin, nails and hair of the extremities, skin colour temperature, pulse, capillary refill and oedema)
2. the region around the wound
3. the current dressing (type, condition, time since last changed)
4. exudate (colour, amount, odour)
5. wound base and edge (measure the borders of the wound with a centimetre ruler)
6. periwound skin
7. management of the wound to date, knowledge levels and related problems.

Draw a picture in your notes to depict necrotic areas, drains and other features.
Describe location in relation to anatomical landmarks.

Wound assessment should take a holistic, person-centred view. A useful framework to undertake this is the 9 Cs of wound care (Baranoski, Ayello & Langemo, 2008):

> Cause of the wound
> Clear picture of what the wound looks like
> Comprehensive picture of the consumer
> Contributing factors
> Communication with other healthcare practitioners
> Continuity of care
> Centralised location for wound care information
> Components of the wound care plan
> Complications of the wound.

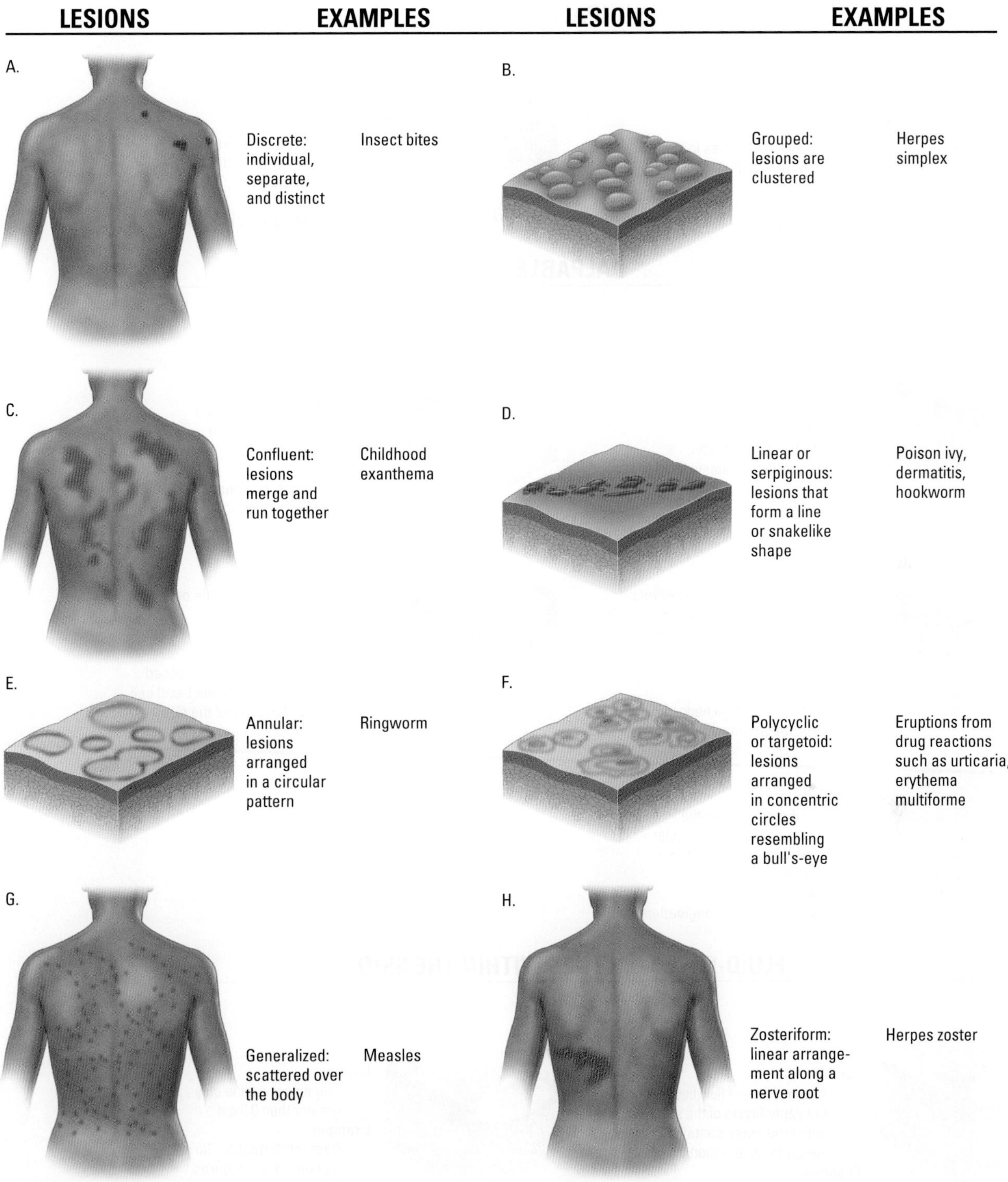

LESIONS	EXAMPLES	LESIONS	EXAMPLES

A.

Discrete: individual, separate, and distinct

Insect bites

B.

Grouped: lesions are clustered

Herpes simplex

C.

Confluent: lesions merge and run together

Childhood exanthema

D.

Linear or serpiginous: lesions that form a line or snakelike shape

Poison ivy, dermatitis, hookworm

E.

Annular: lesions arranged in a circular pattern

Ringworm

F.

Polycyclic or targetoid: lesions arranged in concentric circles resembling a bull's-eye

Eruptions from drug reactions such as urticaria, erythema multiforme

G.

Generalized: scattered over the body

Measles

H.

Zosteriform: linear arrangement along a nerve root

Herpes zoster

FIGURE 8.7 Arrangement of lesions

NONPALPABLE

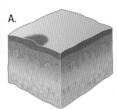

A.

Macule:
Localized changes in skin
color of less than 1 cm
in diameter
Example:
Freckle

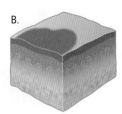

B.

Patch:
Localized changes in skin
color of greater than 1 cm
in diameter
Example:
Vitiligo, stage 1 of pressure
ulcer

PALPABLE

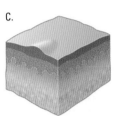

C.

Papule:
Solid, elevated lesion less
than 0.5 cm in diameter
Example:
Warts, elevated nevi,
seborrheic keratosis

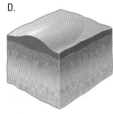

D.

Plaque:
Solid, elevated lesion
greater than 0.5 cm
in diameter
Example:
Psoriasis, eczema,
pityriasis rosea

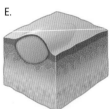

E.

Nodules:
Solid and elevated; however,
they extend deeper than
papules into the dermis or
subcutaneous tissues,
0.5-2.0 cm
Example:
Lipoma, erythema nodosum,
cyst, melanoma, hemangioma

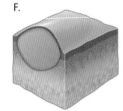

F.

Tumor:
The same as a nodule only
greater than 2 cm

Example:
Carcinoma (such as advanced
breast carcinoma); **not** basal cell
or squamous cell of the skin

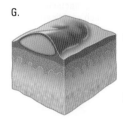

G.

Wheal:
Localized edema in the
epidermis causing irregular
elevation that may be red
or pale
Example:
Insect bite, hive, angioedema

FLUID-FILLED CAVITIES WITHIN THE SKIN

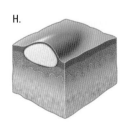

H.

Vesicle:
Accumulation of fluid between
the upper layers of the skin;
elevated mass containing
serous fluid; less than 0.5 cm
Example:
Herpes simplex, herpes
zoster, chickenpox, scabies

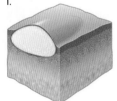

I.

Bullae:
Same as a vesicle only
greater than 0.5 cm
Example:
Contact dermatitis, large
second-degree burns,
bullous impetigo, pemphigus

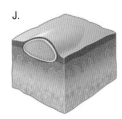

J.

Pustule:
Vesicles or bullae that
become filled with pus,
usually described as less
than 0.5 cm in diameter
Example:
Acne, impetigo, furuncles,
carbuncles, folliculitis

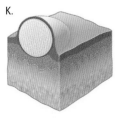

K.

Cyst:
Encapsulated fluid-filled or
a semi-solid mass in the
subcutaneous tissue or
dermis
Example:
Sebaceous cyst, epidermoid
cyst

FIGURE 8.8 Morphology of primary lesions

ABOVE THE SKIN SURFACE

A.
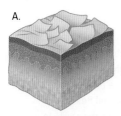
Scales:
Flaking of the skin's surface
Example:
Dandruff, psoriasis, xerosis

B.
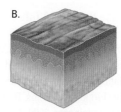
Lichenification:
Layers of skin become thickened and rough as a result of rubbing over a prolonged period of time
Example:
Chronic contact dermatitis

C.
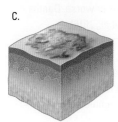
Crust:
Dried serum, blood, or pus on the surface of the skin
Example:
Impetigo, acute eczematous inflammation

D.
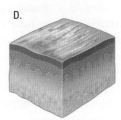
Atrophy:
Thinning of the skin surface and loss of markings
Example:
Striae, aged skin

BELOW THE SKIN SURFACE

E.
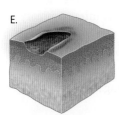
Erosion:
Loss of epidermis
Example:
Ruptured chickenpox vesicle

F.
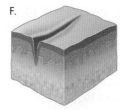
Fissure:
Linear crack in the epidermis that can extend into the dermis
Example:
Chapped hands or lips, athlete's foot

G.
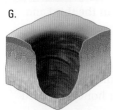
Ulcer:
A depressed lesion of the epidermis and upper papillary layer of the dermis
Example:
Stage 2 pressure ulcer

H.
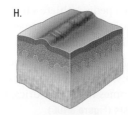
Scar:
Fibrous tissue that replaces dermal tissue after injury
Example:
Surgical incision

I.
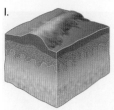
Keloid:
Enlarging of a scar past wound edges due to excess collagen formation (more prevalent in dark-skinned persons)
Example:
Burn scar

J.
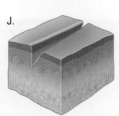
Excoriation:
Loss of epidermal layers exposing the dermis
Example:
Abrasion

FIGURE 8.9 Morphology of secondary lesions

N No skin lesions should be present except for freckles, birthmarks or moles (naevi), which may be flat or elevated.

A A non-palpable lesion that is less than 2 cm in size, light brown in colour, and appearing on the face, arms or hands is abnormal (**Figure 8.10A**).

P This non-palpable lesion describes a **lentigo**. It is a hyperpigmented disorder that occurs in body areas that are exposed to the sun. They can increase in size as the person ages.

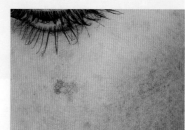

COURTESY OF ROBERT A. SILVERMAN, M.D., CLINICAL ASSOCIATE PROFESSOR, DEPARTMENT OF PEDIATRICS, GEORGETOWN UNIVERSITY.

A. A lentigo occurs in sun-exposed areas of the body

FIGURE 8.10 Common skin lesions

E Examination   **N** Normal findings   **A** Abnormal findings   **P** Pathophysiology

CLINICAL **REASONING**

Practice tip: MRSA infections

The incidence of skin and soft tissue infections caused by methicillin-resistant *Staphylococcus aureus* (MRSA) has significantly increased in the outpatient population (called Community-Associated MRSA). MRSA is carried by approximately 30% of the population (either on their skin or in their nose or mouth), and is often not a problem for healthy people (Turnidge, Coombs, Daley, Nimmo & Australian Group of Antimicrobial Resistance (AGAR) participants, 2000–14, 2016). However, in some circumstances, it has the ability to cause outbreaks of infection that can cause serious poor health outcomes or worse. Deaths due to MRSA infections have occurred in young and old alike (Turnidge et al., 2016).

Risk factors are close living quarters (e.g. childcare centres, sporting groups, military barracks, dormitories, prisons and other institutions) and poor hygiene (e.g. sharing towels, bedsheets, sports equipment, handling soiled clothes and other personal items, and skin contact).

All suspect lesions or wounds need to be cultured for MRSA. MRSA is a notifiable condition required to be reported by doctors, hospitals and laboratory technicians. Reporting is confidential.

A Intertriginous exudative patches that are beefy red in colour, well demarcated, pruritic and erythematous are abnormal.

P Moniliasis, also known as candidiasis, is a yeast infection that may invade numerous areas of the body but normally occurs in the axillae, inframammary areas, groin, and gluteal regions (**Figure 8.10B**).

A A pink to red papulosquamous annular lesion with raised borders that expands peripherally and has a clearing centre is abnormal.

P Tinea corporis is caused by *Trichophyton*, a dermatophyte (fungal) infection (**Figure 8.10C**).

A Toe web lesions that are macerated and have scaling borders are abnormal.

P Tinea pedis (athlete's foot) is very common and often erupts in the third and fourth interdigital spaces; with time, the lesions will spread over the plantar surface. Tinea pedis is caused by *Trichophyton mentagrophytes* (**Figure 8.10D**).

A Vesicles or bullae that measure 1 to 2 cm and become pustular and rupture easily, discharging straw-coloured fluid, are abnormal. The purulent drainage becomes thick as it dries, producing light brown or golden or honey-coloured crusts (**Figure 8.10E**).

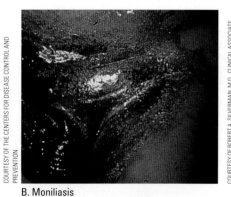

COURTESY OF THE CENTERS FOR DISEASE CONTROL AND PREVENTION

B. Moniliasis

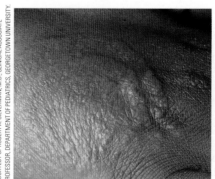

COURTESY OF ROBERT A. SILVERMAN, M.D., CLINICAL ASSOCIATE PROFESSOR, DEPARTMENT OF PEDIATRICS, GEORGETOWN UNIVERSITY.

C. Tinea corporis

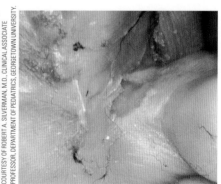

COURTESY OF ROBERT A. SILVERMAN, M.D., CLINICAL ASSOCIATE PROFESSOR, DEPARTMENT OF PEDIATRICS, GEORGETOWN UNIVERSITY.

D. Tinea pedis

FIGURE 8.10 *continued* Common skin lesions

E Examination **N** Normal findings **A** Abnormal findings **P** Pathophysiology

P Impetigo is usually caused by group A streptococcus or *Staphylococcus aureus* and is highly contagious. It is typically found in children in summer, and can be associated with poor hygiene, crowding, contact sports and minor skin trauma that is untreated.

A A diffuse red area that is warm, oedematous, painful and indurated is abnormal (**Figure 8.10F**).

P These findings suggest cellulitis, an acute bacterial infection (usually staphylococcal or streptococcal) of the skin and subcutaneous tissues. Cellulitis can result from trauma to the skin, foreign bodies in the skin and underlying infection.

P A lesion that starts as a tender, deep red **papule** and develops into a well-defined, **erythematous** and painful mass with purulent material is abnormal. This describes a furuncle, commonly called a boil. It can be a firm or fluctuant lesion. Furuncles are usually caused by staphylococci.

A A flat or raised lesion with a black interior is abnormal.

P A comedo, or blackhead, is usually seen on the face, chest, shoulders or back. Comedones are due to increased keratinisation in the hair follicle from an unknown aetiology. They are associated with acne.

A Comedones accompanied by pustules (with yellow or white centres), red papules (**Figure 8.10G**), nodules and cysts are abnormal.

P Acne vulgaris usually occurs in the middle to late teen years and is caused by an inflammation of the sebaceous follicles. Acne vulgaris is associated with hormonal changes. It can be located on the face, chest, shoulders and back. Lesions that appear punched out may be present from scarring of previously active acne lesions.

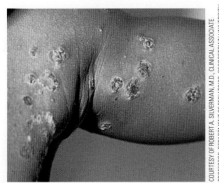

E. Impetigo

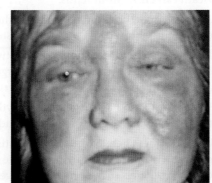

F. Cellulitis

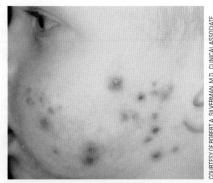

G. Acne papules and nodules visible on a child's face

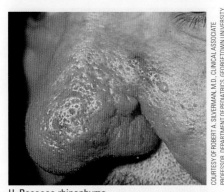

H. Rosacea rhinophyma

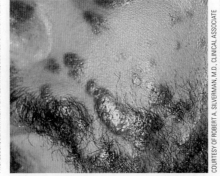

I. Kaposi's sarcoma

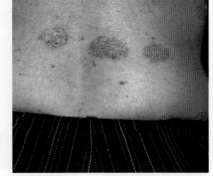

J. Psoriasis

FIGURE 8.10 *continued* Common skin lesions

E Examination **N** Normal findings **A** Abnormal findings **P** Pathophysiology

A Rosacea that is red or purple on the lower nose and is accompanied by thickening of the affected skin and enlargement of the follicular orifices is abnormal (**Figure 8.10H**).

P This condition is rosacea rhinophyma. The cause is unknown, although it is aggravated by alcohol, spicy foods, hot liquids, sunlight, extremes in temperature, exercise and stress.

A Reddish salmon-coloured macular lesions are abnormal.

A Elevated purple to brown lesions (in light-skinned consumers) and bluish lesions (in dark-skinned consumers) that are spongy, painful and pruritic are abnormal (**Figure 8.10I**).

P Both of these abnormal findings are typical lesions of Kaposi's sarcoma. The reddish-salmon lesions are early findings, and the purplish or bluish lesions are more advanced lesions. Kaposi's sarcoma is a neoplastic disorder that is thought to have a genetic, hormonal and viral aetiology. It is frequently found in consumers infected with the AIDS virus, immunocompromised consumers and older adults.

A Pruritic, silvery scales of the epidermis that have clearly demarcated borders and underlying erythema are abnormal. These lesions are circular and are found primarily on the elbows, knees and behind the ears, but can be found in other areas as well (see **Figure 8.10J**).

P The aetiology of psoriasis is unknown, but it has a genetic component and may be aggravated by cold weather, trauma and infection.

On rare occasions, psoriasis can progress to pustular psoriasis (see **Figure 8.10K**). Erythema develops throughout the body, especially in flexural areas. Pustules develop over the erythema and can easily rupture. The consumer is often febrile. Death can ensue from sepsis.

A A chronic superficial inflammation of the face, scalp, buttocks or extremities that evolves into pruritic, red, weeping, crusted lesions is abnormal (see **Figure 8.10L**).

P Eczema, also known as atopic dermatitis, is a multifaceted disease process that is often associated with asthma and allergic rhinitis. The aetiology is unknown, and a family history of related disorders is usually noted.

A It is abnormal to have oedema and erythema along with red, pruritic vesicles that may discharge an exudate that leads to crusting (see **Figure 8.10M**).

P This describes allergic contact dermatitis. The consumer must come in direct contact with the irritant to develop the dermatitis. Contact dermatitis is also caused by metals such as nickel, detergents, cosmetics, rubber, topical medications, food, shampoo, hair dye and clothing.

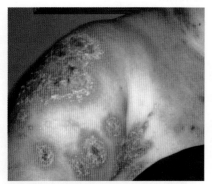

K. Pustular psoriasis

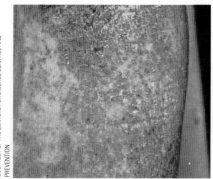

COURTESY OF THE CENTERS FOR DISEASE CONTROL AND PREVENTION.

L. Eczema

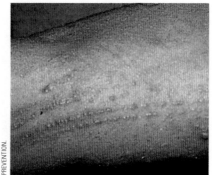

COURTESY OF THE CENTERS FOR DISEASE CONTROL AND PREVENTION.

M. Allergic contact dermatitis

FIGURE 8.10 *continued* Common skin lesions

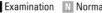
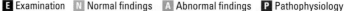

E Examination   **N** Normal findings   **A** Abnormal findings   **P** Pathophysiology

CHAPTER 8

A Red, pruritic papules or vesicles with S-shaped or straight-line burrows are abnormal (**Figure 8.10N**). These lesions can be intensely pruritic.

P Scabies is caused by the parasitic *Sarcoptes scabiei* mite, and may be visible as a small, dark area within the vesicle. It is highly contagious and can sometimes be spread through infected clothing or bedding. It is endemic in many resource-poor communities where there is poor sanitation, overcrowding and social disruption.

A Red papules, vesicles, open sores, and crusting on the face, in the mouth, or on the genitalia are abnormal (**Figure 8.10O**).

P Herpes simplex virus I is usually responsible for these lesions, which are more common on the face and in the mouth. After the initial exposure, the consumer can often predict an outbreak because of the presence of numbness, burning, itching or soreness at the eruption site.

A Red macular and papular lesions that are intensely pruritic are abnormal (see **Figure 8.10P**).

P Varicella, or chickenpox, usually starts on the trunk and proceeds to the extremities. Papules progress to thin-walled vesicles, pustules and crusts. The consumer may exhibit all of the different lesions simultaneously. Varicella is caused by the varicella -zoster virus, which is highly contagious, especially in children.

A Red, extremely painful vesicles with paraesthesia that are closely grouped in a dermatomal pattern are abnormal (see **Figure 8.10Q**).

P Herpes zoster, or shingles, is caused by a reactivation of the varicella zoster virus. The virus remains dormant after the initial varicella inoculation. It frequently occurs in elderly individuals. The lesions are similar to those of varicella, but they tend to develop more slowly.

P Herpes zoster that involves the ophthalmic branch of the fifth cranial nerve is called herpes zoster ophthalmicus. Anterior uveitis, keratitis, optic neuritis and retinal necrosis are possible complications of this condition. These consumers need to be evaluated by an ophthalmologist within 24 hours.

A Flat, purpuric macules or atypical target lesions that are widespread and/or located on the thorax and progress to blistering are abnormal (**Figure 8.10R**).

P These lesions are characteristic of Stevens-Johnson syndrome. Medications such as phenytoin, sulfonamides and penicillin are frequently the causative agent. Serious complications can occur with this condition if not diagnosed and treated early.

A An excessive enlarging of a scar past wound edges is abnormal.

P Keloids are formed from excess collagen formation.

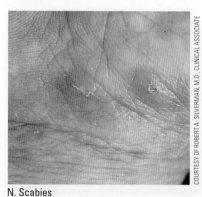
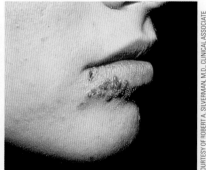
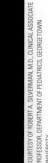
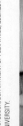
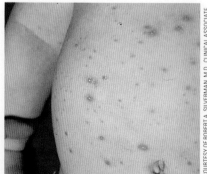
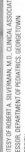

COURTESY OF ROBERT A. SILVERMAN, M.D., CLINICAL ASSOCIATE PROFESSOR, DEPARTMENT OF PEDIATRICS, GEORGETOWN UNIVERSITY.

N. Scabies

O. Herpes simplex virus I

P. Varicella

FIGURE 8.10 *continued* Common skin lesions

E Examination **N** Normal findings **A** Abnormal findings **P** Pathophysiology

A A maculopapular **rash** that is brownish pink and starts around the ears, face and neck and then progresses over the trunk and limbs is abnormal (see **Figure 8.10S**).

P Rubeola (measles) is a viral infection that is highly contagious, and is characterised by high fever, cough, rash, and Koplik's spots (whitish-blue spots with a red halo) on the buccal or labial mucosa.

A Rubella (German measles) displays a fine, pinkish, macular rash that becomes confluent and pinpoint after the second day (see **Figure 8.10T**).

P Rubella is an RNA virus in nature and spreads from the face and neck to the trunk.

A Flesh-coloured, hyperkeratotic papules that have black dots on them are abnormal.

P Common warts, or verruca vulgaris, are viral in origin. The black dots represent thrombosed blood vessels. Warts that occur on the feet are called plantar warts (**Figure 8.10U**).

A Discrete, flesh-coloured, dome-shaped papules that are slightly umbilicated in the centre (**Figure 8.10V**) are abnormal.

P This describes molluscum contagiosum, a self-limiting viral infection. The papules may be found anywhere on the body except the palmar and plantar surfaces. When found on the genitalia of children, sexual abuse must be considered.

A A flesh-coloured or brown pedunculated nodule is abnormal.

P Skin tags, or achrochordon, are benign nodules (**Figure 8.10W**). They are frequently removed if they are in an area that receives repeated movement such as a bra line, or if they are annoying to the consumer.

A Small, pinkish-brown papules that are slightly raised and retract beneath the skin when compressed are abnormal.

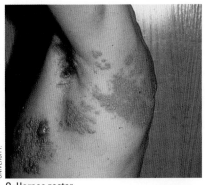

COURTESY OF ROBERT A. SILVERMAN, M.D., CLINICAL ASSOCIATE PROFESSOR, DEPARTMENT OF PEDIATRICS, GEORGETOWN UNIVERSITY.

Q. Herpes zoster

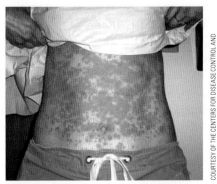

R. Stevens-Johnson syndrome

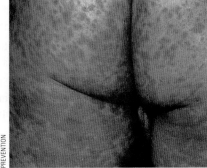

COURTESY OF THE CENTERS FOR DISEASE CONTROL AND PREVENTION

S. Rubeola

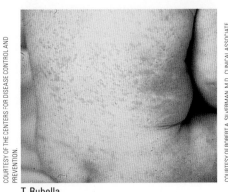

COURTESY OF THE CENTERS FOR DISEASE CONTROL AND PREVENTION.

T. Rubella

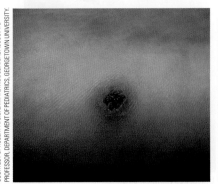

COURTESY OF ROBERT A. SILVERMAN, M.D., CLINICAL ASSOCIATE PROFESSOR, DEPARTMENT OF PEDIATRICS, GEORGETOWN UNIVERSITY.

U. Plantar wart

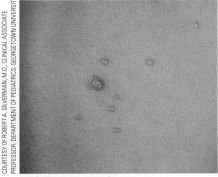

COURTESY OF ROBERT A. SILVERMAN, M.D., CLINICAL ASSOCIATE PROFESSOR, DEPARTMENT OF PEDIATRICS, GEORGETOWN UNIVERSITY.

V. Molluscum contagiosum

FIGURE 8.10 *continued* Common skin lesions

E Examination **N** Normal findings **A** Abnormal findings **P** Pathophysiology

P These are dermatofibromas, or benign papules. Occasionally, they may also be scaly in appearance.

A Pruritic, red wheals (urticarial rash) that vary in size from very small to large and are sometimes accompanied by maculopapular eruptions, vesicles and bullae are abnormal (**Figure 8.10X**).

P Urticaria can be acute or chronic in nature. This itchy skin lesion is linked to histamine release within the body (**Figure 8.10Y**). Exposure to food, drugs, infections, chemicals and physical stimuli (pressure, sun, cold weather or water, exercise) are among the causes of urticaria.

A Lesions that are brownish-tan, red, white, blue, pink, purple or grey and that have irregular borders and notching are abnormal. These lesions can be flat or elevated.

P Malignant melanoma (**Figure 8.10Z**) is a cancerous lesion that is associated with repeated sun exposure. Those individuals with light skin and blue eyes are particularly at risk for malignant melanoma. These neoplastic lesions can also be related to precancerous lesions such as naevi.

A Basal cell carcinomas (**Figure 8.11A**) and squamous cell carcinomas (**Figure 8.11B**) are abnormal. They may appear as scaly sores, ulcers, or pearly/waxy skin that do not heal or change back to 'normal' looking skin, to a raised nodule or papule on the skin varying in colour from reddish tan, pale or bright pink, or many other colours all the way through to dark brown or black lesions (Mayo Clinic, 2021a; Mayo Clinic, 2021b).

P Basal cell carcinomas and squamous cell carcinomas are both malignant carcinomas of the epidermal layers of the skin. They most often only infiltrate locally; however, if not treated may metastasise to other areas of the body. They are most often linked to disfigurement from surgery related to removal of the carcinoma (AIHW, 2016). Both of these types of cancers are easily treated when small.

A Perifollicular papules are abnormal.

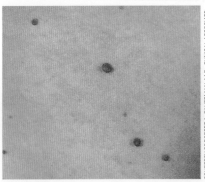

W. Skin tags

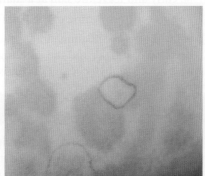

X. Urticaria

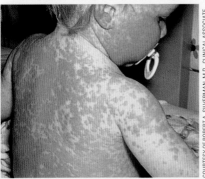

Y. Exanthematous drug eruption

Z. Malignant melanoma

FIGURE 8.10 *continued* Common skin lesions

E Examination **N** Normal findings **A** Abnormal findings **P** Pathophysiology

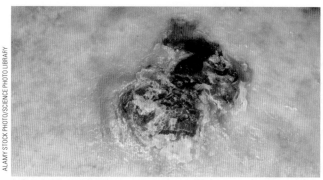

A. Basal cell carcinoma

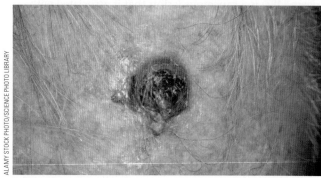

B. Squamous cell carcinoma

FIGURE 8.11 Basal cell and squamous cell carcinomas

P Pseudofolliculitis barbae, or ingrown hair, is caused by hair tips that penetrate into the skin rather than exiting through the follicular orifice. It usually occurs in the beard area, particularly in African American men, because their hair may be curly and leave the skin at a sharp angle.

A Pustules at the opening of the hair follicle are abnormal.

P Folliculitis is an inflammation of the hair follicle. Infecting agents may be bacterial or fungal, and the resulting inflammation is named for the causative agent (e.g. staphylococcal folliculitis, tinea barbae).

HEALTH EDUCATION

Skin self-assessment and warning signs

Teach the consumer to check moles and other lesions in front of a mirror once a month for the warning signs. If the mole or lesion is on a posterior surface, the consumer should ask a partner to check it on a monthly basis. A photo can be taken for future comparisons. Consumers with a personal or family history of skin cancer should have a skin examination every 6–12 months by a qualified professional.

Danger signs in potentially cancerous lesions

1. Rapid change in size
2. Change in colouration
3. Irregular border or butterfly-shaped border
4. Elevation in a previously flat mole
5. Multiple colourations in a lesion
6. Change in surface characteristics, such as oozing
7. Change in sensation, such as pain, itching or tenderness
8. Change in surrounding skin, such as inflammation or induration
9. Bleeding or ulcerative appearance in a mole
   Consumer referral is required for any of the above-mentioned abnormal findings because of the risk of carcinoma.

E Examination   **N** Normal findings   **A** Abnormal findings   **P** Pathophysiology

CLINICAL REASONING

Wound healing

Wound healing for normal wounds goes through four phases (see Figure 8.12). This includes **re-epithelialisation** in the proliferative phase, which is the migration of epithelial cells inwards from the wound edges and from any surrounding hair follicles or eccrine glands. Scab formation may prohibit re-epithelialisation because of diminished moisture. **Granulation tissue** is a combination of inflammatory cells, new vessels and white blood cells that forms a matrix at the base of the wound. The granulation tissue provides a foundation on which re-epithelialisation occurs.

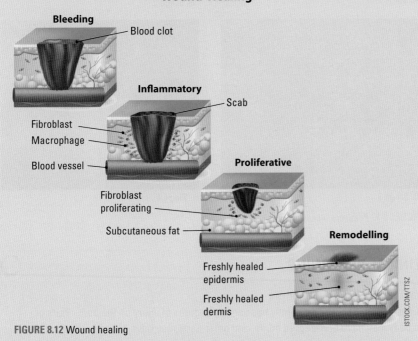

FIGURE 8.12 Wound healing

Scar formation may take several months. New scars are thick, darkened and vascular in appearance. Over time, the scar tissue flattens and becomes less vascular; however, old scars remain slightly darker or discoloured compared with the surrounding tissue.

Try to view as many wounds as possible (even by looking at wounds on the internet and in your textbooks) and identify the tissue you can see and describe this in practice progress notes.

CLINICAL REASONING

Practice tip: Stages of pressure ulcers

Uniform standards for staging pressure ulcers are used for consumers with pressure areas on any portion of the body. Ensuring you use the correct staging to refer to the wound is essential in ensuring accurate communication and management of the wound across multiple health practitioners.

> Stage 1 In light-skinned consumers, the area is reddened, but the skin is not broken; in dark-skinned consumers, the pigmentation is enhanced (Figure 8.13A).
> Stage 2 Epidermal and dermal layers have sustained injury (Figure 8.13B).
> Stage 3 Subcutaneous tissues have sustained injury (Figure 8.13C).
> Stage 4 Muscle tissue and perhaps bone have sustained injury (Figure 8.13D).

>>

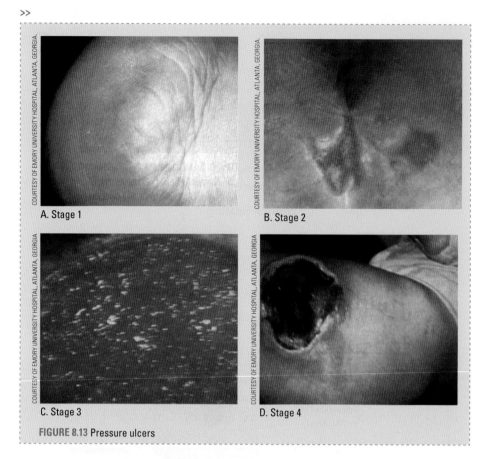

A. Stage 1

B. Stage 2

C. Stage 3

D. Stage 4

COURTESY OF EMORY UNIVERSITY HOSPITAL, ATLANTA, GEORGIA.

FIGURE 8.13 Pressure ulcers

CLINICAL REASONING

Practice tip: Identifying burns

A consumer with burns frequently has varying degrees of injury on the body. Parts of the body may have first-degree burns, and other parts may have second-, third- or fourth-degree burns.

Once burns have been identified, estimation tools should be used to calculate the total body surface area (TBSA%) affected, and this is used to make decisions of clinical management and resuscitation volumes of fluid given in the first 24 hours post-burn. This is an essential component of physical assessment. Different burns estimation tools are available for use, and will vary depending on local practice, age and BMI (body mass index) of the consumer, and whether the burns are small and scattered or large and grouped together. Care must be taken to be as accurate as possible with these calculations as they can significantly impact on the resuscitation and outcomes of the consumer in recovery.

For example, the following suggestions are made to use the best placed tool to assess the following burns in a consumer:

For large burns use Rule of 9s (if BMI of consumer is <30, and patient is an adult), modified Lund-Browder (if BMI is 30–39.9, may be used for both adults and paediatrics) (Figure 14A and B) or Rule of 7s (if BMI is >40) [not widely used in Australia].

For small scattered burns use the palmar method (total hand surface of consumer is approximately 1% of consumer's body surface) (Figure 14C).

(Victorian Adult Burns Service, 2022; Pham, Collier & Gillenwater, 2018)

>>

>>

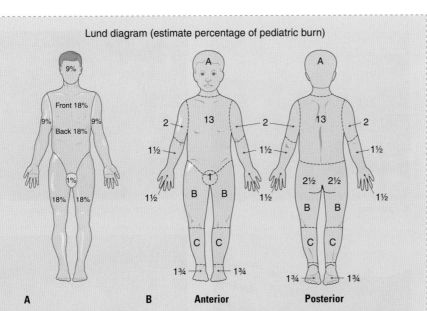

Lund diagram (estimate percentage of pediatric burn)

A. Rule of 9s (for adults) and B. Lund-Browder chart (for children)

Relative percentage of body surface area (% BSA) affected by growth

Body part	Age				
	0 yr	1 yr	5 yr	10 yr	15 yr
a = ½ of head	9 ½	8 ½	6 ½	5 ½	4 ½
b = ½ of 1 thigh	2 ¾	3 ¼	4	4 ¼	4 ½
c = ½ of 1 lower leg	2 ½	2 ½	2 ¾	3	3 ¼

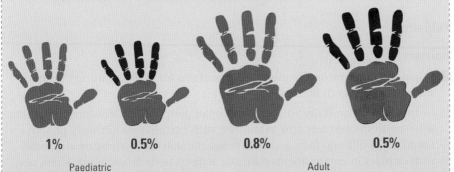

1%   0.5%   0.8%   0.5%

Paediatric   Adult

C. Palmar method

FIGURE 8.14 Tools for estimating extent of burns

The following descriptions and photographs will assist you in identifying burn injuries:
> Epidermal (Figure 8.15A): the epidermis is injured or destroyed; there may be some damage to the dermis; hair follicles and sweat glands are intact; the skin is red and dry; painful, no blisters.
> Partial thickness (superficial dermal or mid dermal) (Figure 8.15B): the epidermis and upper layers of the dermis are destroyed; the deeper dermis is injured; hair follicles, sweat glands and nerve endings are intact; the skin is red and blistery with exudate; painful. Blisters are present.
> Deep dermal partial thickness (Figure 8.15C): the epidermis and dermis are destroyed; subcutaneous tissue may be injured; hair follicles, sweat glands and nerve endings are destroyed; the skin is white, red, black, tan or brown with a leathery-looking appearance; painless because nerve endings are destroyed.
> Full thickness (Figure 8.15D): the epidermis and dermis are destroyed; subcutaneous tissue, muscle and bone may be injured; hair follicles, sweat glands and nerve endings are destroyed; the skin is white, red, black, tan or brown with exposed and damaged subcutaneous tissue, muscle or bone; painless.

>>

>>

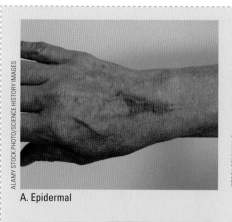
A. Epidermal

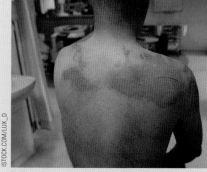
B. Superficial dermal partial thickness

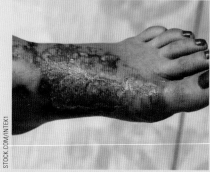
C. Deep dermal partial thickness

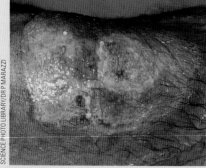
D. Full thickness

FIGURE 8.15 Types of burns

Palpation

Moisture

E Palpate all non-mucous membrane skin surfaces for moisture using the dorsal surfaces of the hands and fingers.

N Normally, the skin is dry with a minimum of perspiration. Moisture on the skin will vary from one body area to another, with perspiration normally present on the hands, axilla and face, and in between the skin folds. Moisture also varies with changes in environment, muscular activity, body temperature, stress, and activity levels. Body temperature is regulated by the skin's production of perspiration, which evaporates to cool the body.

A Excessive dryness of the skin, **xerosis**, as evidenced by flaking of the stratum corneum and associated **pruritus**, is abnormal.

P Hypothyroidism and exposure to extreme cold and dry climates can lead to xerosis.

A Very dry, large scales that are light coloured or brown are abnormal (**Figure 8.16**).

P Ichthyosis vulgaris is a skin abnormality originating from a keratin disorder. It can be associated with atopic dermatitis.

A Diaphoresis is the profuse production of perspiration.

P Causes include hyperthyroidism, increased metabolic rate, sepsis, anxiety and pain.

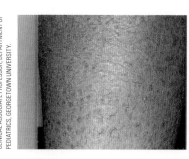
FIGURE 8.16 Ichthyosis vulgaris

E Examination   **N** Normal findings   **A** Abnormal findings   **P** Pathophysiology

Temperature

E Palpate all non-mucosal skin surfaces for temperature using the dorsal surfaces of the hands and fingers.

N Skin surface temperature should be warm and equal bilaterally. Hands and feet may be slightly cooler than the rest of the body.

A Hypothermia is a cooling of the skin, and may be generalised or localised.

P Generalised hypothermia is indicative of shock or some other type of central circulatory dysfunction. Localised hypothermia is indicative of arterial insufficiency in the affected area.

A Generalised hyperthermia is the excessive warming of the skin and may be generalised or localised.

P Generalised hyperthermia may be indicative of a febrile state, hyperthyroidism, or increased metabolic function caused by exercise. Localised hyperthermia may be caused by infection, trauma, sunburn or windburn.

Tenderness

E Palpate skin surfaces for tenderness using the dorsal surfaces of the hands and fingers.

N Skin surfaces should be nontender.

A Tenderness over the skin structures can be discrete and localised or generalised.

P Discrete tenderness may indicate a localised infection such as cellulitis, and generalised tenderness can indicate systemic illness such as lymphoma or allergic reaction.

Texture

E 1. Evaluate the texture of the skin using the finger pads.
   2. Evaluate surfaces such as the abdomen and medial surfaces of the arms first.
   3. Compare these areas to areas that are covered with hair.

N Skin should normally feel smooth, even and firm, except where there is significant hair growth. A certain amount of roughness can be normal.

A Roughness can occur on exposed areas such as the elbows, the soles of the feet and the palms of the hands.

P Roughness can be due to wool clothing, cold weather, occupational exposures, or the use of soap. In addition, generalised roughness can be associated with systemic diseases such as scleroderma, hypothyroidism and amyloidosis. Localised thickening and roughness can be a result of chronic pruritus (**lichenification**) due to scratching, which causes a thickening of the epidermis.

A Areas of hyperkeratosis and increased roughness that are found in the lower extremities are abnormal.

P This type of texture change may be indicative of peripheral vascular disease, which causes abated circulation and diminished nourishment of cutaneous layers.

A The skin can feel very soft and silk-like.

P Generalised softness can result from hyperthyroidism secondary to elevated metabolism.

E Examination   **N** Normal findings   **A** Abnormal findings   **P** Pathophysiology

UNIT 2

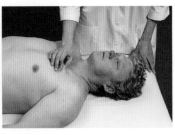

FIGURE 8.17 Assessment of skin turgor

Turgor

E Palpate the skin **turgor**, or elasticity, which reflects the skin's state of hydration.
1. Pinch a small section of the consumer's skin between your thumb and forefinger. The anterior chest, under the clavicle, and the abdomen are optimal areas to assess.
2. Slowly release the skin.
3. Observe the speed with which the skin returns to its original contour when released (**Figure 8.17**).

N When the skin is released, it should return to its original contour rapidly.

A Decreased skin turgor is present when the skin is released and it remains pinched, and only slowly returns to its original contour.

P **Dehydration**, or lack of fluid in the tissues, is the main cause of decreased skin turgor. The ageing process and scleroderma can also decrease the turgor of the skin.

A Increased turgor or tension causes the skin to return to its original contour too quickly.

P Increased turgor can be indicative of connective tissue disease caused by an increase of granulation tissue.

Oedema

E Palpate the skin for **oedema**, or accumulation of fluid in the intercellular spaces.
1. Firmly imprint your thumb against a dependent portion of the body, such as the arms, hands, legs, feet, ankles or sacrum.
2. Release the pressure.
3. Observe for an indentation on the skin.
4. Rate the degree of oedema. Pitting oedema is rated on a 4-point scale (**Figure 8.18**).
5. Check for symmetry and measure circumference of affected extremities.

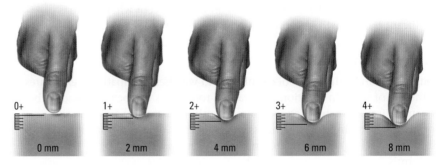

0+ No pitting oedema
1+ Mild pitting oedema. 2 mm depression that disappears rapidly.
2+ Moderate pitting oedema. 4 mm depression that disappears in 10–15 seconds.
3+ Moderately severe pitting oedema. 6 mm depression that may last more than 1 minute.
4+ Severe pitting oedema. 8 mm depression that can last more than 2 minutes.

FIGURE 8.18 Pitting oedema grading scale

N Oedema is not normally present.

A Oedema is present if the skin feels puffy and tight. It can be localised in one area (**Figure 8.19**) or generalised throughout the body. There are many different types of oedema (**Table 8.2**).

P Localised oedema may be due to dependency; however, generalised or bilateral oedema is caused by increased hydrostatic pressure, decreased capillary osmotic pressure, increased capillary permeability or obstruction to lymph flow. This occurs in congestive heart failure or kidney failure.

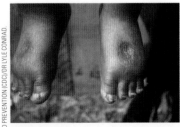

FIGURE 8.19 Assessment of pitting oedema

E Examination **N** Normal findings **A** Abnormal findings **P** Pathophysiology

TABLE 8.2 Types of oedema

TYPE	DESCRIPTION
Pitting	Oedema that is present when an indentation remains on the skin after applying pressure
Non-pitting	Oedema that is firm with discolouration or thickening of the skin; results when serum proteins coagulate in tissue spaces
Angioedema	Recurring episodes of noninflammatory swelling of skin, brain, viscera and mucous membranes (**Figure 8.20**); onset may be rapid, with resolution requiring hours to days
Dependent	Localised increase of extracellular fluid volume in a dependent limb or area
Inflammatory	Swelling due to an extracellular fluid effusion into the tissue surrounding an area of inflammation
Noninflammatory	Swelling or effusion due to mechanical or other causes not related to congestion or inflammation
Lymphoedema	Oedema due to the obstruction of a lymphatic vessel

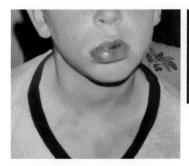

FIGURE 8.20 Angioedema of the lips

PUTTING IT IN CONTEXT

Evaluation of oedema

Mrs Johnstone is a 68-year-old woman with a history of asthma and diabetes. She has not had any issues with wounds or skin concerns before. She presents to the clinic to have her many moles assessed, and you notice her feet and ankles are significantly swollen. Upon asking, Mrs Johnstone says her ankles have been swollen for the last 2 days, but are not painful. On assessment you note her left ankle oedema is 2+ and her right is 3+. She states she has never had this before. As a healthcare professional you will need to decide what to do next.

If the oedema is severe enough, it can prohibit the evaluation of pathological conditions that are manifested by colouration changes. Two plus (2+) oedema warrants referral if it is newly onset. Significant, severe oedema (3+ to 4+) warrants immediate evaluation. In Mrs Johnstone's case, she would qualify for a priority referral to have this investigated. Oedema can cause local issues with skin and limbs, but may also be a marker for cardiac concerns as well.

Examination of the hair

Inspection

Colour

 Inspect scalp hair, eyebrows, eyelashes and body hair for colour.

Hair varies from dark black to pale blond depending on the amount of melanin present. As melanin production diminishes, hair turns grey. Hair colour may also be chemically changed.

Patches of grey hair that are isolated or occur in conjunction with a scar are abnormal.

Patches of grey hair not associated with ageing can be indicative of nerve damage.

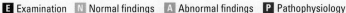

E Examination **N** Normal findings **A** Abnormal findings **P** Pathophysiology

Distribution

E Evaluate the distribution of hair on the body, eyebrows, face and scalp.

N The body is covered in vellus hair. Terminal hair is found in the eyebrows, eyelashes and scalp, and in the axilla and pubic areas after puberty. Males may experience a certain degree of normal balding and may also develop terminal facial and chest hair. Native Americans, Asians and those from the Pacific Rim may have a light distribution of hair.

A The absence of pubic hair, unless purposefully removed, is abnormal in the adult.

P Diminished or absent pubic hair may be indicative of endocrine disorders, such as anterior pituitary adenomas, or chemotherapy.

A Male or female pattern baldness (**alopecia**) may be abnormal in some individuals if associated with pathology. Alopecia areata is a circumscribed bald area (see **Figure 8.21A**).

P Androgenetic alopecia is a common, progressive hair loss that is caused by a combination of genetic predisposition and androgenetic effects on the hair follicle; however, alopecia may be secondary to chemotherapy and radiation, infection, stress, drug reactions, lupus and traction. A pathological aetiology of alopecia should be ruled out.

A Total scalp baldness, or alopecia totalis, is abnormal.

P Autoimmune diseases, emotional crisis, stress or heredity can cause alopecia totalis.

A Hair loss in linear formations is abnormal (see **Figure 8.21B**).

P Linear alopecia can be caused by frequent pressure on hair follicles leading to their inability to produce new hair. In addition, traction alopecia can be caused by the use of curlers and wearing the hair in a tightly pulled ponytail, whereby traction is continually applied. This is common among individuals who wear cornrows.

A Excess facial and body hair is abnormal (see **Figure 8.21C**).

P **Hirsutism** is manifested by excessive body hair. It is indicative of endocrine disorders such as hypersecretion of adrenocortical androgens and polycystic ovary syndrome. In women, this disorder is manifested as excess facial and chest hair.

P Hirsutism can also result as a side effect of medications such as cyclosporin.

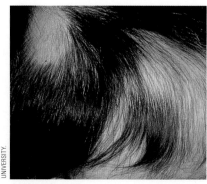

COURTESY OF ROBERT A. SILVERMAN, M.D., CLINICAL ASSOCIATE PROFESSOR, DEPARTMENT OF PEDIATRICS, GEORGETOWN UNIVERSITY.

A. Alopecia areata

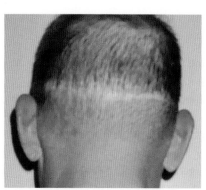

B. Linear alopecia developed in this man from daily wearing of his military uniform cap.

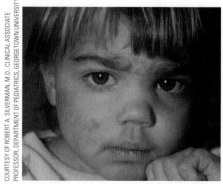

COURTESY OF ROBERT A. SILVERMAN, M.D., CLINICAL ASSOCIATE PROFESSOR, DEPARTMENT OF PEDIATRICS, GEORGETOWN UNIVERSITY.

C. Hirsutism caused by the drug cyclosporin

FIGURE 8.21 Abnormalities of the head and scalp

E Examination   **N** Normal findings   **A** Abnormal findings   **P** Pathophysiology

A Areas of broken-off hairs in irregular patterns with scaliness, but no infection, are abnormal (see **Figure 8.21D**).

P Trichotillomania is the manipulation of the hair by twisting and pulling, leading to reduced hair mass. This can be an unconscious action or a sign of psychiatric illness.

A Broken-off hairs with scaliness and follicular inflammation are abnormal (see **Figure 8.21E**). The area may be painful and purulent with boggy nodules.

P Tinea capitis (ringworm) is a fungal infection, frequently caused by dermatophytic trichomycosis.

A The scalp is covered with yellow-brown scales and crusts. The scalp may be oily. Oedema may be present (see **Figure 8.21F**).

P Seborrhoeic dermatitis is caused by increased production of sebum by the scalp.

Lesions

E 1. Don gloves and lift the scalp hair by segments.
   2. Evaluate the scalp for lesions or signs of infestation.

N The scalp should be pale white to pink in light-skinned individuals and light brown in dark-skinned individuals. There should be no signs of infestation or lesions. Seborrhoea, commonly known as dandruff, may be present.

A Abnormal manifestations include head lice.

P Head lice (pediculosis capitis) may be distinguished from dandruff in that dandruff can be easily removed from the scalp or hair, whereas nits (see **Figure 8.21G**), which are the lice larvae, are attached to the hair shaft and are difficult to remove. Both seborrhoea and head lice may cause itching.

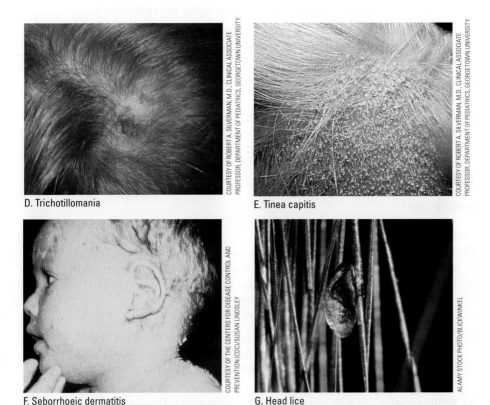

D. Trichotillomania

E. Tinea capitis

F. Seborrhoeic dermatitis

G. Head lice

COURTESY OF ROBERT A. SILVERMAN, M.D., CLINICAL ASSOCIATE PROFESSOR, DEPARTMENT OF PEDIATRICS, GEORGETOWN UNIVERSITY.

COURTESY OF ROBERT A. SILVERMAN, M.D., CLINICAL ASSOCIATE PROFESSOR, DEPARTMENT OF PEDIATRICS, GEORGETOWN UNIVERSITY.

COURTESY OF THE CENTERS FOR DISEASE CONTROL AND PREVENTION (CDC)/SUSAN LINDSLEY

ALAMY STOCK PHOTO/BLICKWINKEL

FIGURE 8.21 *continued* Abnormalities of the head and scalp

E Examination   **N** Normal findings   **A** Abnormal findings   **P** Pathophysiology

PUTTING IT IN CONTEXT

Dealing with impetigo in school-based populations (school sores)

As the school nurse in a primary school, you are asked to assess the skin of each first-grade student after a parent notifies the school that their child has been diagnosed with school sores. You discover that seven children have blister-like sores, some of which appear to be filled with pus, others have extensive scab formation. As you are aware this condition is extremely contagious, you call the affected children's parents to pick up their children and seek treatment. Many parents are at a loss as how to manage this issue, particularly if their child has good hygiene practices. You know treatment is to kill the bacteria that cause the infection, which is usually treated with topical or oral antibiotics.

> What information do you need to give to parents in this situation? (Consider prevention-related information for children who have not yet been infected, as well as treatment and isolation requirements based on local guidelines.)

> What are your responsibilities for the wellbeing of the entire school? Children at many schools have segregated lunch and play areas. (Consider your responsibility here in relation to this being a communicable condition, and one that also has stigma associated with it.)

> What are local methods of managing an impetigo outbreak in your schools and childcare centres?

Palpation

Texture

E 1. Palpate the hair between your fingertips.
2. Note the condition of the hair from the scalp to the end of the hair.

N Hair may feel thin, straight, coarse, thick or curly. It should be shiny and resilient when traction is applied and should not come out in clumps in your hands.

A Brittle hair that easily breaks off when pulled or hair that is listless and dull is abnormal.

P Brittle, dull hair or hair that is broken off can be indicative of malnutrition, hyperthyroidism, use of chemicals such as permanents, or infections secondary to damage of the hair follicle.

Examination of the nails

Inspection

Colour

E 1. Inspect the fingernails and toenails, noting the colour of the nails.
2. Check capillary refill by depressing the nail until blanching occurs.
3. Release the nail and evaluate the time required for the nail to return to its previous colour.
4. Perform a capillary refill check on all four extremities.

N Normally, the nails have a pink cast in light-skinned individuals and are brown in dark-skinned individuals. Capillary refill is an indicator of peripheral circulation. Normal capillary refill may vary with age, but colour should return to normal within 2–3 seconds.

A White striations or dots in the nail bed are abnormal (**Figure 8.22A**).

P Leukonychia (Mees bands) may result from trauma, infections, vascular diseases, psoriasis and arsenic poisoning.

E Examination   **N** Normal findings   **A** Abnormal findings   **P** Pathophysiology

A An entire nail plate that is white is abnormal.

P Leukonychia totalis may result from hypocalcaemia, hypochromic anaemia, leprosy, hepatic cirrhosis and arsenic poisoning.

A A brown colour in the nail plate is abnormal.

P Melanonychia may result from Addison's disease and malaria.

A Bluish nails are abnormal.

P Bluish nails may result from cyanosis, venous stasis, and sulfuric acid poisoning.

A Red or brown linear streaks in the nail bed are abnormal (**Figure 8.22B**).

P Splinter haemorrhages can result from subacute bacterial endocarditis, mitral stenosis, trichinosis, cirrhosis and nonspecific causes.

A It is abnormal for the proximal end of the nail bed to be white and the distal portion to be pink.

P Lindsey's nails (half-and-half nails) can result from chronic renal failure and hypoalbuminaemia.

A A yellow or white hue in a hyperkeratotic nail bed is abnormal (**Figure 8.22C**).

P Onychomycosis is a fungal infection of the nail.

Shape and configuration

E 1. Assess the fingernails and toenails for shape, configuration and consistency.
2. View the profile of the middle finger and evaluate the angle of the nail base (**Figure 8.23**).
3. Have the consumer bring the distal phalanges together, as illustrated in **Figure 8.24**. Note the position of the nail beds in relation to each other.

N The nail surface should be smooth and slightly rounded or flat. Curved nails are a normal variant. Nail thickness should be uniform throughout, with no splintering or brittle edges. The angle of the nail base should be approximately 160°. Longitudinal ridging is a normal variant. There is a diamond-shaped opening at the base of the nail beds in nails that are normal when assessed, as in **Figure 8.24**.

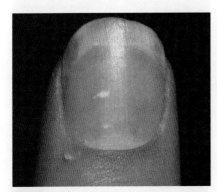

A. Leukonychia

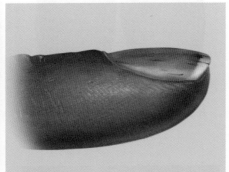

B. Splinter haemorrhages

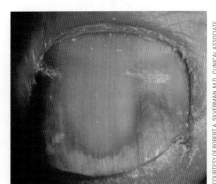

C. Onychomycosis

FIGURE 8.22 Abnormal colour changes of the nail bed

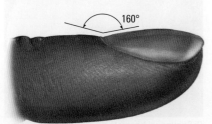

A. Normal nail angle

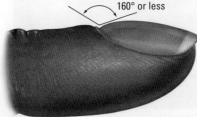

B. Curved nail variant of normal

FIGURE 8.23 Evaluate the angle of the nail base

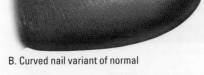

Diamond-shaped opening

FIGURE 8.24 Assess the configuration of the nail beds

E Examination   **N** Normal findings   **A** Abnormal findings   **P** Pathophysiology

A An angle of the nail base greater than 160°, along with sponginess of the nail bed, is abnormal.

A Nail beds that do not meet medially and do not have a diamond-shaped opening at their base are abnormal (**Figure 8.25**).

P Clubbing can result from longstanding hypoxia and lung cancer.

A Thin nail plates with cuplike depressions and concave, or spoon-shaped, nails are abnormal (see **Figure 8.26A**).

P Koilonychia can result from iron deficiency anaemia, chronic infections, malnutrition or Raynaud's disease.

A Separation of the nail from the nail bed is abnormal.

P Onycholysis can result from hypo- and hyperthyroidism, repeated trauma, Raynaud's disease, syphilis, eczema and acrocyanosis.

A Painful, red swelling of the nail fold is abnormal (**Figure 8.26B**).

P Paronychia can be caused by *Candida albicans*, bacteria, and repeated exposure of the nails to moisture.

A Purpura or ecchymosis under the nail plate is abnormal (**Figure 8.26C**).

P Subungual haematoma is caused by trauma to the digit and nail, leading to haemorrhage into the matrix and nail bed.

A The distal portion of the nail plate may become embedded in periungual tissues (**Figure 8.26D**). The periungual tissues may become inflamed and have purulent discharge.

P Onychocryptosis (ingrown nail) is caused by growth of the distal nail plate into periungual tissues, secondary to increased lateral nail pressure, resulting in trauma to the tissues.

A Nails that become white, thin and curved under the free edge are abnormal.

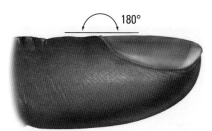

A. Early clubbing

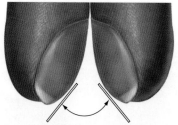

B. Clubbing seen from a lateral view

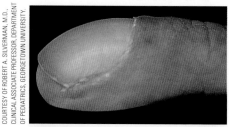

COURTESY OF ROBERT A. SILVERMAN, M.D., CLINICAL ASSOCIATE PROFESSOR, DEPARTMENT OF PEDIATRICS, GEORGETOWN UNIVERSITY.

C. Established clubbing

FIGURE 8.25 Clubbing

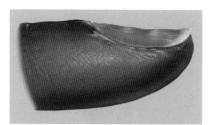

A. Koilonychia

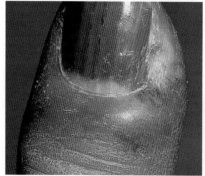

B. Paronychia

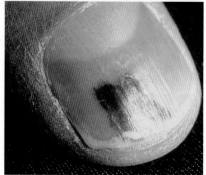

C. Subungual haematoma

FIGURE 8.26 Examples of abnormalities of the shape and configuration of the nail

E Examination   N Normal findings   A Abnormal findings   P Pathophysiology

P Eggshell nails may be caused by systemic diseases, medications, dietary deficiencies, nervous disorders or sleeping with the hand fisted.

A Nails that atrophy, shrink and fall off are abnormal (Figure 8.26E).

P Onychatrophia may result from injury to the nail matrix and from systemic diseases.

A Nails that **hypertrophy** (become abnormally thick and overgrown) are abnormal.

P Onychauxis is caused by systemic infection, electrolyte imbalance and hereditary predisposition.

A A nail that is split or brittle with lengthwise ridges is abnormal (Figure 8.26F).

P Onychorrhexis may result from trauma to the nail, toxic exposure to solvents or harsh nail filing.

Palpation

Texture

E 1. Palpate the nail base between your thumb and index finger.
2. Note the consistency.

N The nail base should be firm on palpation.

A A spongy nail base is an early indication of clubbing.

P Clubbing is the result of impaired tissue oxygenation over a prolonged period of time, as in chronic bronchitis, emphysema and heart disease. See Chapters 13 and 14 for further information.

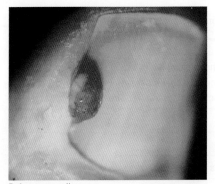 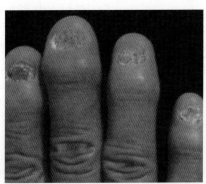 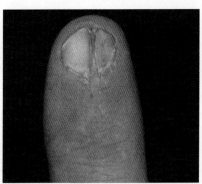

D. Ingrown nail | E. Onychatrophia | F. Onychorrhexis

COURTESY OF ROBERT A. SILVERMAN, M.D., CLINICAL ASSOCIATE PROFESSOR, DEPARTMENT OF PEDIATRICS, GEORGETOWN UNIVERSITY.

FIGURE 8.26 continued Examples of abnormalities of the shape and configuration of the nail

EVALUATION OF HEALTH ASSESSMENT AND PHYSICAL EXAMINATION FINDINGS

In the evaluation phase of a health assessment, the focus is on ensuring the data gathered is complete, accurate and documented appropriately (see case study as an example of the focused assessment; see Chapter 22 for a comprehensive health assessment). In evaluating the data you should:
> draw on your critical thinking and problem-solving skills to make sound clinical decisions
> act on abnormal data (include communicating findings to other health professionals)
> ensure documentation reflects the outcomes of the clinical decisions/actions taken. (Refer to Chapter 3, which discusses in detail why documentation is so important and how this may be undertaken in different health settings.)
The case study that follows steps you through this process.

E Examination **N** Normal findings **A** Abnormal findings **P** Pathophysiology

THE CONSUMER WITH HERPES ZOSTER

This case study illustrates the application and objective documentation of the skin, hair and nails assessment.

Mrs Amrita Singh presents with an abdominal rash.

HEALTH HISTORY

CONSUMER PROFILE	62-year-old married female of Indian descent (identifies as Hindi)	
CHIEF COMPLAINT	'I have this painful rash on my lower belly.'	
HISTORY OF THE PRESENT ILLNESS	Four days ago, Mrs Singh reported burning right lower quadrant (RLQ) pain, malaise, and a 37.5°C temperature. The pain started as a 1–2/10 and progressed over the next 24 hours to 8/10. She denied radiation of pain, or nausea, vomiting, diarrhoea, constipation. She denies history of Crohn's disease, ulcerative colitis, and diverticulitis; and still has appendix. Ibuprofen did not help the pain. Nothing made the pain worse. Consumer was concerned and went to the local ED, fearful of appendicitis. She had blood work and an abdominal CT scan, which were negative. Consumer was sent home with instructions to follow up with her GP. Last night, Mrs Singh noted a rash on her lower abdomen and presents today for evaluation.	
PAST HEALTH HISTORY	MEDICAL HISTORY	Hypothyroidism, age 52 Malaria, age 35 and multiple times since Eczema since age 12
	SURGICAL HISTORY	Nil
	ALLERGIES	Denies medication, bee sting/insect, food and environmental
	MEDICATIONS	Levothyroxine 100 mcg orally in the morning Hydrocortisone valerate 0.2% cream BD prn to affected areas Ca^{++} 500 mg orally BD prn Ibuprofen 200–600 mg orally prn 6 hourly
	COMMUNICABLE DISEASES	Denies
	INJURIES AND ACCIDENTS	Wrist fracture age 12 when she fell jumping over a ditch, grew up in remote area of India, little access to health care; mother 'made' up a splint for her; never had medical care for the fracture
	SPECIAL NEEDS	Denies
	BLOOD TRANSFUSIONS	Denies
	CHILDHOOD ILLNESSES	Not sure – had a few illnesses with rashes and fever
	IMMUNISATIONS	No immunisations as a child due to economic status; believes she was fully immunised at age 26 when she immigrated to Australia with her husband.
SOCIAL HISTORY	ALCOHOL USE	Denies
	TOBACCO USE	Denies
	DRUG USE	Denies
	DOMESTIC AND INTIMATE PARTNER VIOLENCE	States she was 'hit with a stick' or fist (demonstrates closed fist) by her father growing up; he would frequently 'discipline' her and her siblings, and became angry easily with all his children and his wife; denies sexual abuse
	SEXUAL PRACTICE	Husband of 40 years only partner
	TRAVEL HISTORY	Mrs Singh has often visited poorer parts of India during her adult life, and grew up in very poor area with few amenities.

>>

>>

HEALTH HISTORY

	WORK ENVIRONMENT	She lived in India until her mid-20s, working with her father's animals and farming, then with her husband's family in the food markets in Delhi. Often, she was miles from public transportation and medical care. Once she immigrated to Australia, she cared for home and children, but visited India often to care for older relatives and assist her husband's family business importing foods to Australia and New Zealand.
	HOME ENVIRONMENT	Currently resides in an older 1-level house with all modern appliances; has lived in various houses throughout her life, ranging from mud-hut houses, to wooden houses with no running water or any appliances
	HOBBIES AND LEISURE ACTIVITIES	Enjoys cooking for family, watching television and reading
	STRESS	Has extended family who want to immigrate to Australia to live with her and her husband and family, but is concerned about being able to cope with the extra people and expense, even though she feels obliged to assist. 'I am required to help them, all our family, my husband has promised.'
	EDUCATION	Primary school year 5 equivalent, but undertook some night classes in Australia once immigrated for language, numeracy and literacy
	ECONOMIC STATUS	'We are comfortable and have everything we need, but I am not sure we can support all our family if they move to Australia.'
	MILITARY SERVICE	Denies
	RELIGION	Hindi
	CULTURAL BACKGROUND	Indian (Kutch region)
	ROLES AND RELATIONSHIPS	Married for 40 years to husband. 'He is a wonderful husband. I am very lucky; other girls in my village did not have such a good match. Now we live here in Australia and my children have many opportunities we did not have in my village.' Enjoys relationships with 4 daughters and one son and her 3 grandchildren, who live within 10 km of her house. Her youngest daughter still resides at home – this causes some issues with her and her husband as this daughter does not want to marry or study, but wishes to travel around the world, doing work that allows her to come and go as she pleases.
	CHARACTERISTIC PATTERNS OF DAILY LIVING	States her schedule changes daily. The most important times of her day are the time she spends caring for her family.
HEALTH MAINTENANCE ACTIVITIES	SLEEP	Has difficulty falling asleep and staying asleep; never tried any sleep aid
	DIET	Mostly Indian food, some meat but prefers vegetables and rice, curries and savouries
	EXERCISE	Walks 30–60 minutes daily, weather permitting
	STRESS MANAGEMENT	'I pray.'
	USE OF SAFETY DEVICES	Wears seat belt
	HEALTH CHECK-UPS	'In the past, I always had medical checks when we came home from India; now, I just seek medical care when I am sick ... really sick.'

>>

>>

PHYSICAL EXAMINATION				
EXAMINATION OF THE SKIN	**INSPECTION**	COLOUR	Uniformly brown	
		BLEEDING, ECCHYMOSIS AND VASCULARITY	No bleeding, ecchymosis or increased vascularity	
		LESIONS	20–30 vesicles of varying sizes over lower abdomen, dermatomal level T 9–10 with extended base of erythema; mild oedema of area, no crusting of vesicles	
	PALPATION	MOISTURE	Mild xerosis	
		TEMPERATURE	Hands/feet/trunk all warm and equal	
		TENDERNESS	Nontender except for hyperaesthesia in regions inferior and superior to the lesions	
		TEXTURE	Smooth	
		TURGOR	Skin returns to original contour immediately	
		OEDEMA	No oedema except as noted above	
EXAMINATION OF THE HAIR	**INSPECTION**	COLOUR	Black with grey roots, shiny	
		DISTRIBUTION	No hirsutism or alopecia	
		LESIONS	No infestations	
	PALPATION	TEXTURE	Mildly coarse, brittle	
EXAMINATION OF THE NAILS	**INSPECTION**	COLOUR	Light brown with brisk cap refill	
		SHAPE AND CONFIGURATION	Smooth and flat; no splintering or brittle edges; nail edge less than 160°	
	PALPATION	TEXTURE	Firm	

EVALUATION AND CLINICAL REASONING FOR CASE STUDY

The assessment and clinical decisions you make should reflect your scope of practice. For example, advanced practice health professionals, such as nurse practitioners and remote nurses with endorsement, may be able to make diagnostic decisions and prescribe medications without referring to a medical officer.

Fundamentally, all health professionals collect, evaluate and act on person-focused health information, which will at times include referral to, or collaboration with, other healthcare team members. Nurses assess consumer responses to interventions and determine when to escalate key changes in a consumer's condition. The clinical reasoning cycle provides health professionals with a framework to consider all this information in a meaningful way for planning consumer care. These phases are stepped out below, and draw on information presented and collected during the health history and physical examination. We then work through the cycle components that are relevant to this case study (cycle components are bolded).

For Mrs Amrita Singh, the 62-year-old woman who presents with a painful rash over her lower abdomen, the significant data that needs to be considered includes the following.

Collecting cues/information

Recall and Review: In the first instance you will need to reflect on what you know about rashes and their connections to disease processes, infection, allergies and lifestyle aspects such as nutrition.

Chief complaint and history of present illness
> Painful rash on lower abdomen.
> Four days ago, consumer reported burning RLQ pain, malaise, and a 37.5°C temperature.
> Pain started as a 1–2/10 and progressed over the next 24 hours to 8/10. Consumer denied radiation of pain, or nausea, vomiting, diarrhoea, constipation. Ibuprofen did not help the pain. Nothing made the pain worse.
> Denies history of Crohn's disease, ulcerative colitis and diverticulitis; still has appendix.
> Consumer had blood work and an abdominal CT, which were negative, and was sent home with instructions to follow up with her GP.
> Last night, consumer noted a rash on her lower abdomen and presents today for evaluation.

Processing information

Interpret, Discriminate and Infer: These symptoms and details of history outline the scope of the issue for this consumer. The absence of specific disease (Crohn's disease, ulcerative colitis etc.) is significant, as it rules out other reasons for the symptoms and narrows the field of causes for the symptoms.

Match and Predict: Pain at this level that is not relieved by simple analgesia will need to be managed in another way, as it is too painful to remain untreated — otherwise consumers will continue to re-present regardless of other management.

Medical history

> Not sure about childhood diseases; had some illnesses with rashes and fever
> Had little medical attention as young person, no immunisation until mid-20s
> History of malaria, eczema and hypothyroidism

Infer: Amrita's medical history, while not pinpointing a specific childhood illness, shows she has experienced rashes and fever as a child, and little medical attention makes it likely she would have received tribal/home remedies only.

Relate and Infer: Her medical history of malaria and hypothyroidism puts her at risk of becoming run down and immunologically compromised. Eczema is present and shows she is likely to be affected by stress-related skin disorders as well.

Social history and health maintenance activities

> Work history and travel history to poor parts of India, living and working in conditions that are likely to be dirty, and exposure to many people in low socioeconomic conditions
> Stressed about possibility of family immigrating to Australia and ability to support them here
> Has travelled often to India to assist in family business or care for older relatives as is her 'requirement to do so'
> Grown-up children, good relationships, still has one daughter living at home, this daughter does not conform to family expectations, but is supported living at home
> Has difficulty falling asleep and staying asleep; never tried any sleep aid

Relate, Infer and Predict: Amrita's social information supports her medical history of likely being exposed to many viruses in poor conditions, with little access to medical assistance. There are also her feelings of obligation to her family, the stress caused by the possibility of their immigration and the extra work this will bring for her. Alongside this, Amrita has been dealing with stress on a longer-term basis around her daughter's life choices and the conflict this is causing in her family. Amrita is not sleeping well, so this will be affecting her ability to deal with stress and to allow her body to recuperate.

Physical assessment

> 20–30 vesicles of varying sizes over lower abdomen, dermatomal level T 9–10 with extended base of erythema; mild oedema of area, no crusting of vesicles, mild xerosis
> Nontender except for hyperaesthesia in regions inferior and superior to the lesions

Interpret, Discriminate and Infer: This information shows the extent of the vesicles' area, the physical location and the patterns that correspond to dermatomes or nerve tracts, all of which are important cues to consider. The type of vesicle, extent of erythema, oedema and pain and tenderness in surrounding regions are also important in considering the cause of the vesicles. Also important are whether they are infected, weeping or may be infectious. This will affect how to contain the infectious risk to others as well.

Putting it all together – synthesise information

Considering all the cues above, it is likely that the vesicles are caused by the herpes zoster virus. As Amrita is unsure what childhood illnesses she may have had, it is probable that she has had chickenpox (varicella virus). Once a person has had chickenpox there is a risk of experiencing an outbreak of herpes zoster after the initial infection, perhaps many years later, and usually it is triggered by stress and the body becoming run-down. This condition is also known as shingles and fits with the other symptoms of an initial localised pain without radiation, malaise, low-grade fever then, within 48 hours, appearance of vesicles (often fluid-filled) and increasing pain not affected by other variables.

The nurse in this case would document all these abnormalities, and refer to the medical officer, as the consumer may have the duration of the symptoms shortened with antiviral medications, analgesia and anti-inflammatories. As it is likely these medications will be prescribed (non-steroidal anti-inflammatory drugs such as ibuprofen usually do not require prescription), the nurse will need to check again that the consumer has no drug allergies and that the medications prescribed will have no contraindications or adverse interactions with Amrita's current medications.

Actions based on assessment findings

The nurse should also provide additional education for interventions that do not require a doctor's order, such as:
1 Apply cool cloths or cloth-wrapped ice packs over the lesions or take a cool bath twice a day.
2 Avoid exposure to warm and hot water because this could lead to further itching and irritation.
3 Cover lesions with a clean cloth or loose-fitting gauze after cleansing because they are contagious to people who have not had chickenpox before.
4 Trim fingernails to reduce the chance of bacterial infection from scratching.
5 Avoid wearing tight clothing over the rash because this could irritate the rash further.

The final step in the process is accurate documentation. The nurse must document findings, referrals, interventions, advice and education given. The consumer would continue to have ongoing long-term management and follow-up by specialist medical staff in collaboration with general practitioner.

CHAPTER RESOURCES

REVIEW QUESTIONS

For answers to these questions, see Answer section at the end of the book.

1. Which of the following are functions of the skin? Select all that apply.
   a. Serves as a protective barrier to pathogens
   b. Filters dust and particulate matter
   c. Excretes water, salts and nitrogenous wastes
   d. Regulates temperature
   e. Produces vitamin E
   f. Permits sensory perception

2. The consumer mentions to the nurse that there are a lot of skin problems in his family. Which of the following does the nurse recognise as familial skin conditions? Select all that apply.
   a. Squamous cell cancer
   b. Melanoma
   c. Eczema
   d. Psoriasis
   e. Shingles
   f. Tinea pedis

3. While inspecting the skin of a consumer, you note circular lesions that are pruritic, and have a silvery scale appearance with clearly demarcated borders on the elbows and knees. What medical condition might you suspect this consumer has?
   a. Psoriasis
   b. Second-degree burns
   c. Ichthyosis vulgaris
   d. Diabetes mellitus

4. A consumer complains of pruritus over the trunk and upper limbs. You note a raised red, itchy rash. What is a possible aetiology of this rash?
   a. Ringworm
   b. Herpes zoster
   c. Drug reaction
   d. Dermatitis

5. The nurse teaches her consumer about skin cancer prevention measures. Which of the following should be included in the discussion? Select all that apply.
   a. Using sunscreen when the anticipated time of outdoor activity is more than two hours
   b. Using a tanning bed no more than once a month
   c. Avoiding the sun between 10:00 a.m. and 4:00 p.m.
   d. Reapplying sunscreen every four hours while swimming
   e. Applying a lip balm with an SPF of 30 or higher
   f. Using sunscreen even on cloudy days

6. Which of the following might the nurse expect to see in a consumer who had an insect bite or a reaction to an allergy shot?
   a. A macule
   b. A vesicle
   c. A wheal
   d. A cyst

7. A chronic superficial inflammation of the face and extremities that evolves into pruritic, red, weeping, crusted lesions is usually associated with which of the following conditions?
   a. Contaminated clothing and bedding
   b. Contact with harsh detergent
   c. Cold weather and trauma
   d. Asthma and allergic rhinitis

8. The skin lesions that occur in impetigo are best described by which of the following findings?
   a. A maculopapular rash with erythemic borders that appears first on the wrists
   b. A blotchy maculopapular rash that appears first on the cheeks
   c. Vesicles that measure 2 cm, are pustular and rupture easily, and have straw-coloured discharge
   d. Flesh-coloured, hyperkeratotic papules that are slightly umbilicated

9. A consumer shows you the area on her arm where she burned herself with an iron. The skin is red and painful but has no blistering. What type of burn do you suspect the consumer incurred?
   a. Epidermal
   b. Partial thickness
   c. Deep dermal partial thickness
   d. Full thickness

10. The consumer tells you that when she was a child her finger was caught in a piece of machinery that damaged her fingernail. What type of nail condition might the consumer have?
    a. Onychorrhexis
    b. Clubbing
    c. Onychophagy
    d. Eggshell nails

CS CLINICAL SKILLS

The following Clinical Skills are relevant to this chapter and can be found in Tollefson & Hillman, *Clinical Psychomotor Skills,* 8th edition:
> 5 Hand hygiene
> 6 Personal protective equipment
> 7 Aseptic non touch technique
> 27 Healthcare teaching
> 59 Pressure area care – preventing pressure injuries
> Part 13: Wound management
> 67 Dry dressing technique
> 68 Complex wounds – drain, suture or clip removal
> 69 Complex wounds – wound irrigation
> 70 Complex wounds – packing a wound.

FURTHER RESOURCES

> Australia and New Zealand Burn Association: http://www.anzba.org.au/
> Australian Dermatology Nurses Association: http://www.adna.org.au/
> Cancer Council Australia: http://www.cancer.org.au/home.htm
> Cancer Society of New Zealand: http://www.cancernz.org.nz/
> International Society for Burn Injuries: http://www.worldburn.org
> New Zealand Dermatology Nurses Society Incorporated (NZDNS): https://www.nzdermatologynurses.nz/

REFERENCES

Australian Government Department of Health. (2018). Communicable diseases information. Retrieved 2 September 2018 from http://www.health.gov.au/internet/main/publishing.nsf/content/ohp-communic-1

Australian Institute of Health and Welfare (AIHW). (2016). Skin cancer in Australia. Cat. no. CAN 96. Canberra: AIHW. https://www.aihw.gov.au/getmedia/0368fb8b-10ef-4631-aa14-cb6d55043e4b/18197.pdf.aspx?inline=true

Australian Institute of Health and Welfare (AIHW). (2022). Rural and remote health. Retrieved 5 December 2022 from https://www.aihw.gov.au/reports/rural-remote-australians/rural-and-remote-health

Baranoski, S., Ayello, E. A., & Langemo, D. K. (2008). Wound assessment. In S. Baranoski and E. A. Ayello (Eds.), *Wound care essentials: practice principles* (2nd ed.). Ambler PA: Lippincott, Williams and Wilkins.

Benbow, M. (2016). Best practice in wound assessment. *Nursing Standard, 30*(27), 40–7. Retrieved 2 September 2018 from https://rcni.com/sites/rcn_nspace/files/ns.30.27.40.s45.pdf

Cancer Australia. (2022). Melanoma of the skin. Retrieved 5 December 2022 from https://www.canceraustralia.gov.au/cancer-types/melanoma/statistics

Davidson, L., Knight, J., & Bowen, A. (2020). Skin infections in Australian Aboriginal children: a narrative review. *Medical Journal of Australia, 212*(5): 231–7. doi:10.5694/mja2.50361

Health Promotion Agency, New Zealand, Nov 2018, SS102, Skin Cancer in New Zealand. Retrieved 5 December 2022, from: https://www.hpa.org.nz/sites/default/files/4.3%20SS102%20Skin%20Cancer%20Facts%20Infographic.pdf

Mayo Clinic. (2021a). Basal cell carcinoma. Mayo Clinic website. https://www.mayoclinic.org/diseases-conditions/basal-cell-carcinoma/symptoms-causes/syc-20354187. Updated 1 October 2021. Accessed 18 July 2022.

Mayo Clinic. (2021b). Squamous Cell Carcinoma. Mayo Clinic website. https://www.mayoclinic.org/diseases-conditions/squamous-cell-carcinoma/symptoms-causes/syc-20352480. Updated 13 May 2021. Accessed 18 July 2022.

Melanoma Institute Australia. (2022). A report into melanoma – a national health priority. Retrieved 5 December 2022 from: https://melanoma.org.au/wp-content/uploads/2022/03/MIA-and-MPA_SoN-Report_Final-Report_28-March-2022.pdf

Melanoma New Zealand. (2022). Melanoma facts and risk factors. Retrieved 5 December 2022, from: https://www.melanoma.org.nz/facts-risk-factors

Mullane, M., Barnett, T., Cannon, J., Carapetis, J. R., Christophers, R., Coffin, J., … Bowen, A. C. (2019). SToP (See, Treat, Prevent) skin sores and scabies trial: study protocol for a cluster randomised, stepped-wedge trial for skin disease control in remote Western Australia. *British Medical Journal* 9: e030635. doi:10.1136/bmjopen-2019-030635

Pham, C. H., Collier, Z. J., & Gillenwater, J. (2018). Changing the way we think about burn size estimation. *Journal of Burn Care & Research, 39*(suppl_1), S39–S40. https://doi.org/10.1093/jbcr/iry006.073

Skin Health Institute. (2022). Occupational Contact Dermatitis. https://www.skinhealthinstitute.org.au/page/96/occupational-dermatitis . Accessed 18 July 2022.

Turnidge, J., Coombs, G., Daley, D., Nimmo, G., & Australian Group on Antimicrobial Resistance (AGAR) participants 2000–14. (2016). *MRSA: A tale of three types: 15 years of survey data from AGAR.* Sydney, Australia: Australian Commission of Safety and Quality in Health Care. Retrieved 2 September 2018 from https://www.safetyandquality.gov.au/wp-content/uploads/2016/11/MRSA-A-Tale-of-Three-Types.pdf

Verma, C., Lehane, J., Neale, R., & Janda, M. (2022). Review of sun exposure guidance documents in Australia and New Zealand. Public Health Research and Practice *32*(1):e3212202.

Victorian Adult Burns Service. (2022). Burn % TBSA. Burns Management Guidelines. https://www.vicburns.org.au/burn-assessment-overview/burn-tbsa/. Accessed 18 July 2022.

CHAPTER 9

HEAD, NECK AND REGIONAL LYMPH NODES

LEARNING OUTCOMES

By the end of this chapter you should be able to:

1 identify the anatomic structures of the head and neck
2 identify the lymph nodes of the head and neck
3 describe the health history for the head, neck and regional lymph nodes
4 demonstrate the physical examination of the head, neck and regional lymph nodes
5 explain normal findings, common abnormalities and pathophysiology of these abnormalities in the physical examination of the head, neck and regional lymph nodes
6 discuss the clinical reasoning in evaluating outcomes of health assessment and physical examination, including documentation, health education provision and relevant health referral.

BACKGROUND

The most common head, neck and regional lymph node disorders are head and neck cancers (of which there is a higher incidence in males) (Cancer Australia, 2022a), malignant neoplasms of lymphoid and other tissue, headache and thyroid cancer (AIHW, 2022a).

Headache is one of the most common health problems experienced by Australians and New Zealanders. As no major studies have been undertaken in either country, statistics related to prevalence and cost are based on overseas research findings (Headache Australia, 2023). Individuals aged between 20 and 50 years are more likely than others to encounter headaches (Headache Australia, 2023). Cancer of the thyroid gland is a significant health problem, with a marked increase in annual incidence in Australia from 2.7 to 14 cases per 100 000 people between 1982 and 2022 (Cancer Australia, 2022b). There is no single explanation for this increase, which is evident across all adult age groups and socioeconomic bands; however, research points to a link between obesity and thyroid cancer (Laaksonen et al., 2021). In New Zealand, thyroid cancer disproportionately affects women and prevalence is higher among Pasifika people (Health Navigator New Zealand, 2021). Also of note is the low mortality rate for thyroid cancer: 0.4 deaths per 100 000 people (Cancer Australia, 2022b).

The most common oral health problems are tooth decay and gum disease (AIHW, 2020). Oral health is a significant issue for Aboriginal and Torres Strait Islander peoples, with hospitalisation rates for dental conditions in 2019–20 reported to be 1.8 times higher than for non-First Nations people (AIHW, 2022b). Gingivitis, the most common type of periodontal disease, is seen more commonly in First Nations children, especially those living in remote areas, and is almost twice as prevalent as the rate in the broader community (AIHW, 2022c) . Thirty-four per cent of First Nations Australian children aged between 4 and 14 years (in 2014–15) self-reported a tooth or gum problem (Australian Indigenous HealthInfoNet, 2017).

Major causes of periodontal disease among First Nations people in Australia include poor oral hygiene and lack of access to appropriate diet and dental services (AIHW, 2022c) as well as the high prevalence of smoking (37% in 2018–19 of those aged 15 years and over; almost three times the rate of the general population) (Australian Government Department of Health and Aged Care, 2020). Systemic disadvantage and intergenerational trauma in Aboriginal and Torres Strait Islander communities, in addition to inaccessibility of appropriate services, contribute to a range of health issues, including oral health.

Māori and Pasifika people also experience poorer oral health and attend the dentist less frequently than the broader population of New Zealand. Children are 1.5 times more likely to have had a tooth extracted due to decay (Ministry of Health, 2018). Lack of access to services is a significant risk factor for periodontal disease; it is important that you are aware of the services available for consumers close to where they live.

Assessment of the head and neck provides a wide range of critical clues about the functions of various body systems. As you assess the head and neck, you will learn about the skin, endocrine function, musculoskeletal integrity and neurological function. You should refer to the relevant chapters in this textbook to assist in your understanding of these health assessment areas.

ANATOMY AND PHYSIOLOGY

The skull, face, neck, thyroid, lymph nodes and blood supply are discussed in the following sections.

Skull

The skull is a complex bony structure that rests on the superior end of the vertebral column (Figure 9.1). The skull protects the brain from direct injury, and provides a surface for the attachment of the muscles that assist with mastication and the production of facial expressions.

The cranial bones of the skull are connected by immovable joints called **sutures**. The most prominent sutures are the coronal suture, the sagittal suture and the lambdoidal suture. The junction of the coronal and sagittal sutures is called the **bregma**.

Face

The face of every individual has its own unique characteristics, which are influenced by factors such as ethnicity, state of health, emotions and environment. Facial structures are symmetrical, so that the eyes, eyebrows, nose, mouth, nasolabial folds and palpebral fissures look the same on both sides.

Neck

The neck is made up of seven flexible cervical vertebrae that support the head while allowing it maximum mobility. The first cervical vertebra, the **atlas**, articulates with the occipital condyles to support and balance the head. The second vertebra, the **axis**, has an odontoid process that extends into the ring of the atlas, allowing it to pivot as the head is turned from side to side. The seventh cervical vertebra has a long spinous process called the **vertebra prominens**, which serves as a useful landmark during physical assessment of the neck, back and thorax.

The major muscles of the neck are the sternocleidomastoids and the trapezii (Figure 9.2). The sternocleidomastoid muscles extend from the upper portion of the sternum and the clavicle to the mastoid process and allow the head to bend laterally, rotate, flex and extend. They also divide each side of the neck into two triangles: the anterior cervical and the posterior cervical, which serve as assessment landmarks. The **anterior triangle** is formed by the mandible, the trachea and the sternocleidomastoid muscle, and contains the anterior cervical lymph nodes, the trachea and the thyroid gland. The **posterior triangle**, the area between

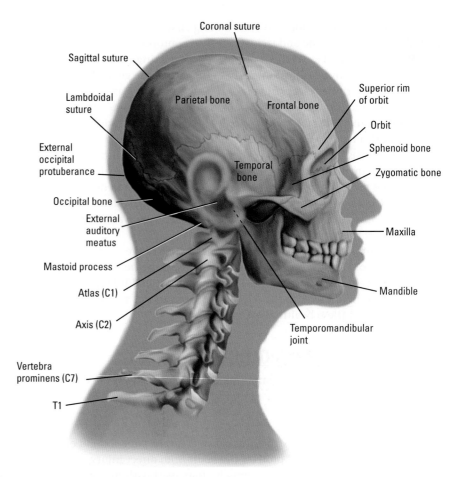

FIGURE 9.1 Bones of the face and skull (lateral view)

the sternocleidomastoid and the trapezius muscles with the clavicle at the base, contains the posterior cervical lymph nodes (**Figure 9.3**).

The trapezii extend from the occipital bone down the neck to insert at the outer third of the clavicles, at the acromion process of the scapula, and along the spinal column to the level of T12. They allow the shoulders and scapula to move up and down, and rotate the scapula medially.

Thyroid

The thyroid gland, the largest endocrine gland in the body, secretes thyroxine (T_4) and triiodothyronine (T_3), which regulate the rate of cellular metabolism.

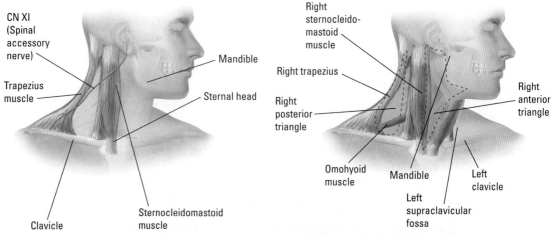

FIGURE 9.2 Major cervical muscles

FIGURE 9.3 Anterior and posterior cervical triangles

The gland, a flattened, butterfly-shaped structure with two lateral lobes connected by the **isthmus**, weighs about 25 to 30 g and is slightly larger in females (**Figure 9.4**). The isthmus rests on top of the trachea, inferior to the cricoid cartilage.

Lymph nodes

An extensive system of lymphatic vessels drains the head and neck and is an important part of the immune system (**Figure 9.5**). Lymphatic tissue in the nodes is responsible for the filtering and sequestration of pathogens and other harmful substances. Lymph nodes are usually less than 1 cm, round or ovoid in shape, and smooth in consistency. When nodes are enlarged or tender, it is important to assess for infection or malignancy. Note the direction in which each node drains (**Figure 9.5**). If a tender or enlarged lymph node is found on clinical examination, assess the entire lymph node area, as well as the area that the involved node drains. For example, if a consumer's posterior cervical node is enlarged, examine the posterior scalp, the ear (both externally and internally) and the skin of the posterior neck for pathology.

Blood supply

The blood supply to the head and neck is quite extensive, with arterial and venous patterns. Major arteries that carry blood to the head and neck include the common carotids (which bifurcate into the internal and external carotid arteries), the brachiocephalic artery (the right common carotid artery branches from this), the subclavian arteries, and the temporal arteries. Deoxygenated blood from the head and neck is returned to the heart via the internal and external jugular veins, the brachiocephalic vein, and the subclavian veins (**Figure 9.6**).

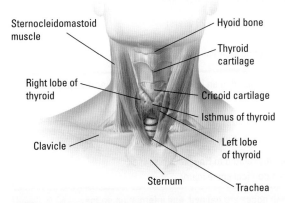

FIGURE 9.4 Structures of the thyroid gland

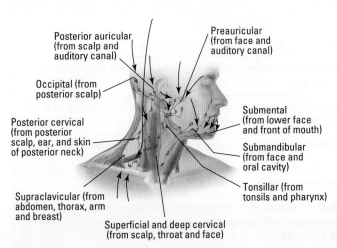

FIGURE 9.5 Lymph nodes of the head and neck and drainage patterns

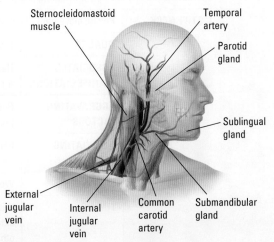

FIGURE 9.6 Major veins and arteries of the neck

ASSESSMENT: TAKING THE CONSUMER'S HEALTH HISTORY

Assessment is the first phase of the nursing process, and involves collecting subjective information about the consumer's health status in order to identify consumer problem areas to focus on.

Subjective data is most frequently collected during a health history, and serves as the starting point for the health professional to base the depth of their assessment on.

The sections for the health history include:

> **Consumer profile**
> **Chief complaint** (explained systematically using variations of location, quality, quantity, associated manifestations, aggravating factors, alleviating factors, setting and timing. This is a variation on the OPQRST assessment mnemonic you may use for other conditions such as pain assessment)
> **Past health history** (including medical history, surgical history, allergies, medications, injuries and accidents, special needs and childhood illnesses)
> **Family health history**
> **Social history** (including alcohol, tobacco and drug use, sexual practice, work and home environment, hobbies and leisure activities, stress and culture).

HEALTH HISTORY

CONSUMER PROFILE	The head and neck and regional lymph nodes health history provides insight into the link between a consumer's life/lifestyle and head, neck and regional lymph nodes information and pathology. Diseases that are age- and sex-specific for the head, neck and regional lymph nodes are listed.		
	AGE	> Lymphadenopathies related to Hodgkin's disease (11–29 years) > Cervical spine trauma (young adults) > Hyperthyroidism (reproductive years in young women) > Temporal arteritis (older adults) > Decreased mobility of the cervical spine related to an inflammatory or degenerative process (older adults)	
	SEX	FEMALE	> Hypothyroidism or hyperthyroidism, thyroid cancer, migraines > Degenerative cervical bone disease
		MALE	> Lymphadenopathy related to Hodgkin's disease > Trauma-related cervical spine injury
CHIEF COMPLAINT	Common chief complaints for the head, neck and regional lymph nodes are defined, and information on the characteristics of each sign or symptom is provided.		
	1. STIFF NECK	Painful movement of the neck that restricts range of motion	
		QUALITY	Limited range of motion, either passive or active
		ASSOCIATED MANIFESTATIONS	Headache, neck tenderness, swelling, fever, numbness and tingling in arms or hands
		AGGRAVATING FACTORS	Position (sitting, standing, lying down), immobilisation of position for a prolonged period, mobility, stress, weather
		ALLEVIATING FACTORS	Immobility or rest, certain positions, analgesics, muscle relaxants, heat
		SETTING	Work, driving, stress
		TIMING	With all movements, with rotating movements only, with flexion and extension only, with weather changes, after falls, motor vehicle or other accidents

>>

2. NECK MASS		Discrete area of swelling found in the neck
	QUALITY	Mobile, nonmobile, smooth, irregular, tender, nontender
	ASSOCIATED MANIFESTATIONS	Shortness of breath, hoarseness, weight loss, fever and chills, dysphagia, ear pain, prior radiation therapy to head/neck
	AGGRAVATING FACTORS	Eating, talking, movement, tight clothing around the neck, swallowing
	ALLEVIATING FACTORS	Avoidance of tight clothing, analgesic medications, decreased dietary intake
	TIMING	Longstanding, recent
3. HEADACHE		Pain felt within the head, behind the eyes, or at the nape of the neck (Table 9.1)
	LOCATION	Temporal, frontal, occipital, orbital, hemicranial/bilateral, neck, facial pain, behind the eyes, and upper shoulders
	QUALITY	Neck pain: aching, sore, dull, sharp Head pain: throbbing, sharp, dull, aching
	ASSOCIATED MANIFESTATIONS	Neck pain: fever, headache, swelling, tenderness Head pain: nausea and vomiting, aura (visual, olfactory, auditory, tactile), diplopia, blurred vision, irritability, sneezing, rhinorrhoea, weakness, dizziness, photophobia, phonophobia, hypertension, nosebleed, cough
	AGGRAVATING FACTORS	Neck pain: stress, trauma, ageing, position, mobility, weather changes Head pain: stress, fatigue, foods, noxious odours, caffeine intake, coughing, alcohol intake, smoke, hunger, season, menstruation, chemicals, toxins
	ALLEVIATING FACTORS	Medications such as analgesics, anti-inflammatory agents, ergotamine, caffeine or caffeinated medications, antidepressants, triptan medications; position change; rest; sleep; shaking head; food intake
	SETTING	Work, outdoors, relationship to biologic events, stressful environment, change in weather, head trauma
	TIMING	Acute and sudden onset, at rest with weather changes Head pain: constant intermittent, in the morning, at the end of the day, premenstrual, seasonal Neck pain: with movement
4. HEAD INJURY		
	QUALITY	Open, closed
	ASSOCIATED MANIFESTATIONS	Light-headedness, photophobia, phonophobia, poor attention and concentration, sleep disturbances, depression, neck pain, nausea, vomiting, projectile vomiting, dizziness or vertigo, headache, seizure activity, loss of consciousness, amnesia, visual disturbances, gait disturbances, speech disturbances, confusion, drowsiness, abnormal behaviour, abnormal movement of extremities, change in respiratory pattern, discharge from nose or ear, head or neck lacerations/abrasions/ecchymoses
	ALLEVIATING FACTORS	Ice, analgesics, rest, surgical intervention
	SETTING	Mechanism of injury, use of helmet or protective headgear, use of seat belt, violent activity, fall, sports injury, motor vehicle collision, alcohol or drug use, concurrent history of seizure disorder, heart disease or diabetes mellitus

>>

>>

PAST HEALTH HISTORY			
	MEDICAL HISTORY	**HEAD, NECK AND REGIONAL LYMPH NODES SPECIFIC**	Hypo or hyperthyroidism, hypo or hyperparathyroidism, sinus infections, migraine headache, cancer, head injury, skull fracture, Bell's palsy, Cushing syndrome, lymphadenopathy, recent lumbar puncture
		NON–HEAD, NECK AND REGIONAL LYMPH NODES SPECIFIC	Phaeochromocytoma
	SURGICAL HISTORY		Thyroidectomy, parathyroidectomy, facial reconstruction, cosmetic surgery, neurosurgery, other surgery related to the head or neck
	MEDICATIONS		Antibiotics, steroids, anticonvulsants, chemotherapy, thyroxine, propranolol, analgesics, oral contraceptives, radioiodine (I^{131}), propylthiouracil, methimazole
	COMMUNICABLE DISEASES		Meningitis, encephalitis
	INJURIES AND ACCIDENTS		Obstruction caused by foreign bodies, trauma to the head or neck, chemical splashes to the face, noxious fumes, sports injuries, motor vehicle accidents
	SPECIAL NEEDS		Tracheostomy, paralysis
FAMILY HEALTH HISTORY	Head and neck diseases that are familial are listed. Thyroid disease, migraines		
SOCIAL HISTORY	The components of the social history are linked to head and neck factors or pathology.		
	ALCOHOL USE		Predisposes to accidents and head injury
	TOBACCO USE		Cigarette smoking is a primary risk for cancer of the lips, oral cavity and pharynx
	WORK ENVIRONMENT		Risk of head injury, exposure to toxins or chemicals, carbon monoxide
	HOME ENVIRONMENT		Risk of falls and head injury due to loose rugs or absence of handrails, carbon monoxide exposure

TABLE 9.1 Classification of headaches

Vascular aetiologies	> Migraine headaches > Cluster headaches > Subarachnoid haemorrhage > Subdural haematoma > Infarction > Cerebral aneurysm > Temporal arteritis > Vasculitis
Muscle contraction	> Tension headache
Intracranial aetiologies	> Brain tumours > Increased intracranial pressure from hydrocephalus, pseudotumor cerebri > Intracranial infection (e.g. meningitis, encephalitis, abscess) > Ischaemic cerebrovascular disease
Systemic aetiologies	> Infection > Post-lumbar puncture > Hypertension > Exertion from coitus, cough, exercise > Postictal > Phaeochromocytoma > Premenstrual syndrome

>>

>> **TABLE 9.1** *continued*

Food-related aetiologies	> Nitrites (e.g. hot dogs, bacon, processed meats) > Tyramine (e.g. cheese, chocolate) > Monosodium glutamate (MSG) (e.g. Chinese food) > Alcohol > Some artificial sweeteners > Food allergy
Facial or cervical aetiologies	> Sinusitis > Temporomandibular joint dysfunction > Dental lesions > Trigeminal neuralgia > Cervical spine radiculopathy
Ocular-related aetiologies	> Narrow angle glaucoma > Uveitis > Extraocular muscle paralysis > Eye strain
Metabolic aetiologies	> Hypoxia > Hypercapnia > Hypoglycaemia
Drug aetiologies	> Alcohol and alcohol withdrawal > Caffeine and also caffeine withdrawal > Nitrates > Oral contraceptives > Oestrogen > Nicotine
Environmental aetiologies	> Change in barometric pressure (from weather or altitude) > Carbon monoxide poisoning > Tobacco smoke > Glaring or flickering lights > Odours
Miscellaneous aetiologies	> Fever > Influenza > Head trauma > Otitis media > Parotitis > Pregnancy > Fatigue and decreased sleep > Psychogenic disorders > Stress It is worth noting that a way to categorise headaches is provided by the International Headache Society (IHS). In 2018 the IHS published the third edition of the *International Classification of Headache Disorders* (ICHD-3). This edition contains the most current guidelines. Headaches are classified into three parts. Part 1: primary headaches; Part 2: secondary headaches; and Part 3: neuropathies and facial pains and other headaches (IHS, 2018).

PERSON-CENTRED HEALTH EDUCATION

When conducting a health assessment, opportunities for the provision of person-centred health education will arise. This is a significant consideration in relation to the assessment process for examination of the head, neck and regional lymph nodes. These occasions are identified as individualised education, and may generate further data that can be added to the assessment. All education given should be documented so that in future, health professionals can assess the impact of previous information provided to the consumer. (Refer to Chapter 1 for initiating health education.) Refer to the following examples.

INDIVIDUALISED HEALTH EDUCATION INTERVENTIONS	
Assessing the consumer for the following health-related activities can assist in identifying the need for education about these factors. This information provides a bridge between the health maintenance activities and head and neck function.	
Sleep	May be increased due to head injury
Diet	Recent weight gain or loss
Stress	Demands of employment, home, school

HEALTH EDUCATION

Risk factors for migraine headache
The following are risk factors for people who are susceptible to developing migraine headaches. These risks should be considered when gathering health assessment data for a person who has verbalised experiencing headaches.
> Adolescence to age 40
> Female
> Family history of migraines
> Allergies
> Increased stress
> Caffeine intake
> Oral contraceptive and hormone use
> Tyramine, monosodium glutamate, sulfites, or nitrite consumption
> Sleep disorders

Non-pharmacological headache intervention
Consumers should be informed of alternative strategies that may reduce or alleviate a headache. Some suggestions include relaxation techniques, a quiet environment, a dark room, lying down, walking, music, muscle stretching, warm or cool compresses to the head, herbal tea, and a neck or temple massage. Encourage the consumer to experiment with these techniques to determine what is effective, and to use the effective method when headaches occur.

PUTTING IT IN CONTEXT

The consumer experiencing migraines
You are a community nurse visiting a 55-year-old female who had surgery 4 days ago.
As you are performing a dressing change, the woman tells you that she has had migraine headaches all her life and she 'can't take them anymore'. She confides to you that all her past healthcare providers dismissed her headaches as 'nothing'. She also tells you that a lot of her family members suffer from migraines.
> How would you respond to this consumer?
> What questions would you ask her?
> What non-pharmacological strategies could you suggest she use?

PLANNING FOR PHYSICAL EXAMINATION

The planning phase refers to evaluating subjective data to narrow the focus on physical examination, determining what objective data needs to be gathered, as well as considering the environment and equipment that will be required.

At this time, you will identify which of the four diagnostic techniques you will need to implement the physical examination, and how you will sequence these. For the physical examination of the head, neck and regional lymph nodes, you will include inspection, palpation and auscultation.

Objective data is:

> collected during the physical examination of the consumer
> usually collected after subjective data
> information that is measured or observed by the clinician as opposed to being reported by the consumer
> vital to the overall health assessment, to enable you to make clinical decisions that are representative of the whole consumer picture.

Evaluating subjective data to focus physical assessment

Before commencing the physical examination of the consumer's head, neck and regional lymph nodes, consider what information the health history has provided. Critical consideration, linked to knowledge of anatomy and physiology, should focus the physical assessment so your examination will be more effective and efficient.

Environment

Assessing the head, neck and regional lymph nodes requires a physical environment in the healthcare setting that has:

> a flat table/surface for the consumer to lie on
> minimal noise for accurate auscultation of specific sounds
> adequate lighting
> adequate privacy for the consumer.

Equipment

Assemble items before placing the consumer on the examination table. Materials should be arranged in order of use and within easy reach.

> Stethoscope
> Glass of water
> Flat table/surface.

IMPLEMENTATION: CONDUCTING THE PHYSICAL EXAMINATION

Implementation of the physical examination requires you to consider your scope of practice. In this section, depending on your context, you may be performing a foundation assessment or the addition of advanced assessment techniques if you are practising in a specialised area.

EXAMINATION IN BRIEF: HEAD, NECK AND REGIONAL LYMPH NODES

Examination of the head

Inspection
> Shape of the head

Palpation

Examination of the scalp

Inspection and palpation

Examination of the face

Inspection
> Symmetry
> Shape and features

Examination of the mandible

Palpation and auscultation

Examination of the neck

Inspection
Palpation

Examination of regional lymphatics: the thyroid gland

Inspection
Palpation
> Anterior approach
> Posterior approach

Auscultation

Examination of regional lymphatics: the lymph nodes

Inspection
Palpation

General approach to examination of head, neck and regional lymph nodes

Physical examination of the head, neck and regional lymph nodes has two major components:

1. assessment of the head and neck
2. assessment of the lymph nodes.

Prior to the assessment:

1. Meet the consumer and explain the examination techniques that you will be using.
2. Ensure that the environment is at a warm, comfortable room temperature to provide the consumer comfort.
3. Use a quiet room that will be free from interruptions.
4. Ensure that the light in the room provides sufficient brightness to allow adequate observation of the consumer.
5. Place the consumer in an upright sitting position on the examination table, or gain access to the head of the supine, bedbound consumer by removing nonessential equipment or bedding (for consumers who cannot tolerate the sitting position).
6. If the consumer is wearing a wig or headpiece, ask the consumer to remove it.
7. Visualise the underlying anatomic structures during the examination process to permit an accurate description of the location of any pathology.
8. Always compare the right and left sides of the head, neck and face.
9. Use the same systematic approach every time the examination is performed.

Examination of the head

Inspection

Shape of the head

E 1. Have the consumer sit in a comfortable position.
2. Face the consumer, with your head at the same level as their head.
3. Inspect the head for shape and symmetry.

N The head should be normocephalic and symmetrical.

A **Hydrocephalus** is an enlargement of the head without enlargement of the facial structures (see **Figure 9.7A**).

P Hydrocephalus is caused by an abnormal accumulation of cerebrospinal fluid within the skull.

A **Acromegaly** is an abnormal enlargement of the skull and bony facial structures.

P Acromegaly is caused by excessive secretion of growth hormone from the pituitary gland (see **Figure 9.7B**).

A **Craniosynostosis** is characterised by abnormal shape of the skull or bone growth at right angles to suture lines, exophthalmos, and drooping eyelids.

P Craniosynostosis is caused by the premature closure of one or more sutures of the skull before brain growth is complete.

Palpation

E 1. Place the finger pads on the scalp and palpate all of its surface, beginning in the frontal area and continuing over the parietal, temporal and occipital areas.
2. Assess for contour, masses, depressions and tenderness.
3. Palpate the temporal artery, which is located anterior to the tragus of the ear.

E Examination **N** Normal findings **A** Abnormal findings **P** Pathophysiology

N The normal skull is smooth, nontender, and without masses or depressions. The temporal artery is usually a weaker peripheral pulse (1+/4+ or 1+/3+) than the other peripheral pulses of the body (see **Table 6.2** in Chapter 6: pulse is explained, including the flow quality of the pulse). The artery is nontender, smooth and readily compressible.

A Masses in the cranial bones that feel hard or soft are abnormal.

P These types of masses may be carcinomatous metastasis from other regions of the body or may result from lymphomas, multiple myeloma or leukaemia.

A Palpation elicits localised oedema over the bony frontal portion of the skull.

P Osteomyelitis of the skull may develop following acute or chronic sinusitis if the infection extends out from the sinuses into the surrounding bone.

A Firm palpation reveals a softening of the outer bone layer.

P **Craniotabes** is a softening of the skull caused by hydrocephalus or demineralisation of the bone due to rickets, osteogenesis imperfecta or syphilis.

A A temporal artery that is hard in consistency and tender is abnormal.

P This can indicate temporal arteritis. In temporal arteritis, the temporal arteries may also be more tortuous.

Examination of the scalp
Inspection and palpation

E 1. Part the hair repeatedly all over the scalp and inspect the scalp for lesions or masses.
   2. Place the finger pads on the scalp and palpate for lesions or masses.

N The scalp should be shiny, intact, and without lesions or masses.

A A laceration or a laceration with bleeding is abnormal.

P Direct trauma can cause lacerations to the scalp.

A A gaping laceration with profuse bleeding is abnormal.

P If the laceration on the scalp is gaping, it indicates a deep wound that may further indicate a compound skull fracture as a result of some type of trauma.

A Palpation reveals a localised, easily movable accumulation of blood in the subcutaneous tissue.

P Haematomas can result from direct trauma to the skull.

A Palpation may reveal either single or multiple masses that are easily movable. They are round, firm, nontender, and arise from either the skin or the subcutaneous tissue.

P These are sebaceous cysts that form as a result of retention of secretions from sebaceous glands.

A Nonmobile, fatty masses with smooth, circular edges may be palpated deeper in the scalp.

P These masses are benign fatty tumours known as **lipomas**.

Examination of the face
Inspection
Symmetry

E 1. Have the consumer sit in a comfortable position facing you.
   2. Observe the consumer's face for expression, shape, and symmetry of the following structures: eyebrows, eyes, nose, mouth, ears.

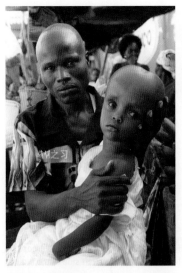

A. Hydrocephalus

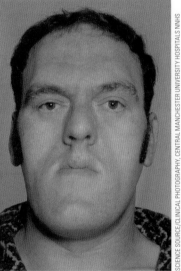

B. Acromegaly

FIGURE 9.7 Abnormal head shapes

ALAMY STOCK PHOTO/BOAZ ROTTEM

SCIENCE SOURCE/CLINICAL PHOTOGRAPHY, CENTRAL MANCHESTER UNIVERSITY HOSPITALS NNHS FOUNDATION TRUST, UK

E Examination **N** Normal findings **A** Abnormal findings **P** Pathophysiology

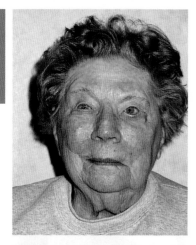

FIGURE 9.8 Bell's palsy. Note the drooping left lower eyelid and left side of the mouth.
SOURCE: COURTESY OF MARY A. HITCHO

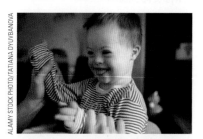

ALAMY STOCK PHOTO/TATIANA DYUVBANOVA

FIGURE 9.9 Down syndrome

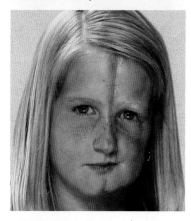

FIGURE 9.10 Scleroderma
SOURCE: COURTESY OF THE SCLERODERMA FOUNDATION, WWW.SCLERODERMA.ORG

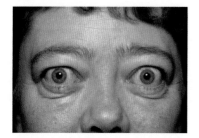

FIGURE 9.11 Exophthalmos of Graves' disease
SCIENCE PHOTO LIBRARY/CLINICAL PHOTOGRAPHY

N The facial features should be symmetrical. Both palpebral fissures should be equal and the nasolabial fold should present bilaterally. It is important to remember that slight variations in symmetry are common. Slanted eyes with inner epicanthal folds are normal findings in consumers of Asian descent.

A Structures are absent or deformed. There is a definite asymmetry of facial expression, palpebral fissures, nasolabial folds and the corners of the mouth.

P Asymmetry of the palpebral fissures, nasolabial folds, the mouth and facial expression may indicate damage to the nerves innervating facial muscles (cranial nerve VII), as in stroke or Bell's palsy (**Figure 9.8**).

PUTTING IT IN CONTEXT

Sensitivity to consumers with facial disfigurement

Scarring can have a significant impact on a person's self-esteem, especially when visible on the face. You are working in the plastics surgical ward and you are admitting a consumer who has multiple partial thickness burns to her face and upper extremities. She has been admitted for skin grafts. As you meet her for the first time, she says, 'I look horrible. I know people don't like to look at me and I am very self-conscious of this.'

> How would you respond verbally and nonverbally to her comment and her disfigurement?

Shape and features

E 1. Face the consumer.
2. Observe the shape of the consumer's face.
3. Note any swelling, abnormal features, or unusual movement.

N The shape of the face can be oval, round or slightly square. There should be no oedema, disproportionate structures, or involuntary movements.

A Inspection of the face may reveal slanted eyes with inner epicanthal folds; a short, flat nose; and a thick, protruding tongue.

P These findings are likely to indicate the presence of **Down syndrome**, or Trisomy 21, a chromosomal aberration (**Figure 9.9**).

A An abnormally wide distance between the eyes is **hypertelorism**.

P Hypertelorism is a congenital anomaly.

A Facial skin is shiny, contracted and hard. The face appears to have furrows around the mouth (**Figure 9.10**).

P Scleroderma is a collagen disease of unknown cause. Sclerosis of the skin, as well as visceral organs (oesophagus, lungs, heart, muscles, kidneys), occurs.

A The face is thin with sharply defined features and prominent eyes (**exophthalmos**) in Graves' disease (**Figure 9.11**).

P Graves' disease is an autoimmune disorder associated with increased circulating levels of T_3 and T_4.

A The consumer's face is round and swollen with characteristic periorbital oedema and dry, dull skin (**Figure 9.12**).

P This condition is known as myxoedema and is associated with hypothyroidism.

E Examination **N** Normal findings **A** Abnormal findings **P** Pathophysiology

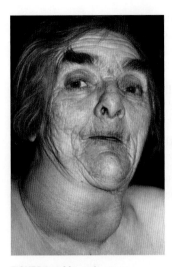

FIGURE 9.12 Myxoedema
SCIENCE PHOTO LIBRARY /DR P. MARAZZI

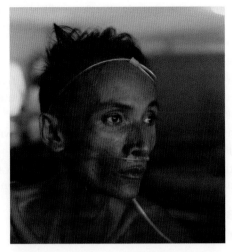

FIGURE 9.13 This shows a cachectic face in a 40-year-old man with tuberculosis. Also note his cachectic torso.
GETTY IMAGES/ROBERT NICKELSBERG

CLINICAL **REASONING**

Body art piercing

Over the last decade there has been a surge in people receiving body art such as piercing and tattoos. Although this has become a more common and accepted practice, it is not without risks. Bloodborne infections can occur and include hepatitis B and C, HIV, STIs and staphylococcal infections. Australia and New Zealand have guidelines in place for safe piercing and tattooing (refer to relevant legislation in Australia, for example Queensland Government, 2016, 2017; NSW Health, 2022; and HealthEd Ministry of Health New Zealand, 2019).

A case to consider

Your consumer has a history of acne, chronic sinusitis and allergies. She informs you that she plans to get her eyebrows and nares pierced.

> How would you respond to her?
> How would you encourage this consumer to have her body piercing done safely?

As piercing is a common practice, it is important to check the body artist practices, according to the relevant legislative requirements. Ensure use of sterile equipment and appropriate and relevant post care. Penetrating the surface of the skin means there is a risk of infection for the individual. Post care includes information about healing times (an eyebrow usually takes about 6–8 weeks and a nose about 8–12 weeks), and the appropriate cleansing procedure to utilise (to keep the site clean to reduce the risk of infection).

A The eyes are sunken and the cheeks are hollow in cachexia (see **Figure 9.13**).

P **Cachexia** is a profound state of wasting of the vital tissues that is associated with cancer, malnutrition and severe chronic illnesses.

A The consumer's face is immobile and expressionless with a staring gaze and raised eyebrows in Parkinson's disease.

P Parkinson's disease is the degeneration of basal ganglia, resulting from a deficiency of the neurotransmitter dopamine.

A The faces of some Caucasians show a dusky blue discolouration beneath the eyes ('allergic shiners') along with creases below the lower eyelids (Dennie's lines) and open mouth due to mouth breathing.

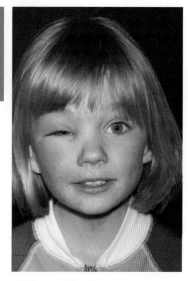

FIGURE 9.14 Allergic facies
SCIENCE PHOTO LIBRARY /DR P. MARAZZI

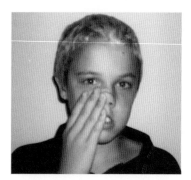

FIGURE 9.15 This young boy has a characteristic nasal crease from the repeated action of the 'nasal salute' caused by allergies.

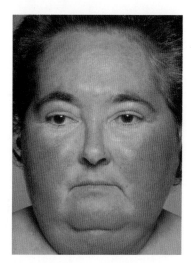

FIGURE 9.16 Cushing syndrome
SCIENCE SOURCE/CLINICAL PHOTOGRAPHY, CENTRAL MANCHESTER UNIVERSITY HOSPITALS NHS FOUNDATION TRUST, UK

P The consumer with chronic allergies or allergic rhinitis develops this characteristic of allergic facies or allergic gape. This can occur in seasonal or perennial allergic rhinitis (**Figure 9.14**).

A A transverse crease is noted across the nose.

P This is a characteristic finding in consumers with allergies and allergic rhinitis who frequently are observed to do the 'nasal salute' or upwards wiping of the nose (**Figure 9.15**).

A The consumer has a rounded 'moon face' along with red cheeks and excess hair on the jaw and upper lip (**Figure 9.16**).

P This is the facies of Cushing syndrome, which is caused by increased production of adrenocorticotropic hormone (ACTH) or prolonged steroid ingestion.

Examination of the mandible
Palpation and auscultation

E 1. Use the fingertips of both index and middle fingers to locate the temporomandibular joint anterior to the tragus of the ear on both sides.
2. Hold the fingertips firmly in place over the joints and ask the consumer to open and close the mouth.
3. As the consumer opens and closes the mouth, observe the relative smoothness of the movement and whether or not the consumer notices any discomfort.
4. Remove the hands.
5. Hold the bell of the stethoscope over the joint.
6. Listen for any sound while the consumer opens and closes the mouth.

N The consumer should experience no discomfort with movement. The temporomandibular joint should articulate smoothly and without clicking or crepitus.

A The consumer complains of tenderness when the mouth is opened and closed. Palpation or auscultation reveals clicking or crepitus.

P Tenderness in the joint may be from the inflammation of migratory arthritis.

A Crepitus is present from the articulation of irregular bone surfaces found in osteoarthritis.

P Clicking may follow a 'snapping' sound if there is displaced cartilage.

A The mouth remains in an open and fixed position.

P Following a wide yawn or trauma to the chin, the temporomandibular joint is dislocated and will not function. This condition requires reduction.

Examination of the neck
Inspection

E 1. Have the consumer sit facing you, with the head held in a central position.
2. Inspect for symmetry of the sternocleidomastoid muscles anteriorly, and the trapezii posteriorly.
E 3. Have the consumer touch the chin to the chest, to each side, and to each shoulder.
4. Assess for limitation of motion.
5. Note the presence of a stoma or tracheostomy.

N The muscles of the neck are symmetrical with the head in a central position. The consumer is able to move the head through a full range of motion without complaint of discomfort or noticeable limitation. The consumer may be breathing through a stoma or tracheostomy.

E Examination **N** Normal findings **A** Abnormal findings **P** Pathophysiology

Ⓐ Asymmetry of the neck is abnormal (see **Figure 9.17**).

Ⓟ Asymmetrical masses can be benign or malignant, but they all must be evaluated further.

Ⓐ The consumer complains of pain with flexion or rotation of the head.

Ⓟ Pain with flexion can be associated with the pain and muscle spasm caused by meningeal irritation of meningitis (see Chapter 7). Generalised discomfort may be related to trauma, spasm, inflammation of muscles or diseases of the vertebrae.

Ⓐ There is a slight or prominent lateral deviation of the consumer's neck. The sternocleidomastoid muscles, and to a lesser extent the trapezii and scalene muscles, may also be prominent on the affected side. The muscles frequently hypertrophy as a result of powerful contractions.

Ⓟ This condition is called **torticollis** (**Figure 9.18**). Causes can be:
1. congenital: resulting from a haematoma or partial rupture at birth of the sternocleidomastoid, causing a shortening of the muscle
2. ocular: a head posture assumed to correct for ocular muscle palsy and resulting diplopia
3. acute spasm: commonly associated with the inflammation of viral myositis or trauma such as sleeping with the head in an unusual position
4. other: phenothiazine therapy and Parkinson's disease, as the result of increased cholinergic activity in the brain.

Ⓐ Range of motion of the neck is reduced.

Ⓟ Degenerative changes of osteoarthritis may result in decreased ability for full range of motion. This condition is usually painless unless nerve root irritation has occurred. Crepitus, or a crunching sound on hyperextension of the neck, may also be observed.

Palpation

Ⓔ 1. Stand in front of the consumer.
2. With the finger pads, palpate the sternocleidomastoid muscles.
3. Note the presence of masses or tenderness.
4. Stand behind the consumer.
5. With the finger pads, palpate the trapezius.
6. Note the presence of masses or tenderness.

Ⓝ The muscles should be symmetrical without palpable masses or spasm.

Ⓐ A mass is palpated in the musculature.

Ⓟ A mass may be a tumour, either primary or metastatic.

Ⓐ A spasm may be felt in the muscles.

Ⓟ Muscle spasm may be due to varied causes such as infections, trauma, chronic inflammatory processes or neoplasms.

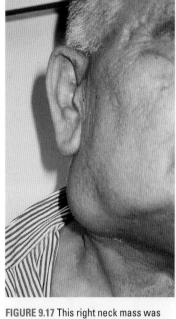

FIGURE 9.17 This right neck mass was identified as squamous cell carcinoma.
COURTESY OF DR. DANIEL D. ROONEY

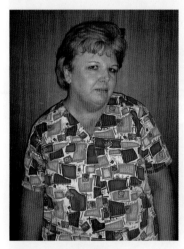

FIGURE 9.18 Torticollis

URGENT FINDING ⚠

Immobilisation of potential neck injury

If a neck injury is suspected, the cervical spine is the most vulnerable as over half of all spinal injuries occur in the cervical area. Careful handling of the victim, minimising spinal alignment and calling for emergency assistance are key precautions. Watch for the following assessment cues that reflect the signs of spinal injury: the head or neck is in an abnormal position, breathing difficulties, loss of function in limbs (ANZCOR, 2016).

Ⓔ Examination   Normal findings Ⓐ Abnormal findings Ⓟ Pathophysiology

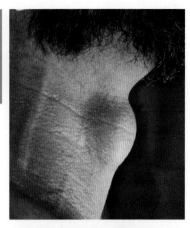

FIGURE 9.19 Solitary thyroid nodule
COURTESY OF DR ANDREW B. SILVA, PEDIATRICOTOLARYNGOLOGY

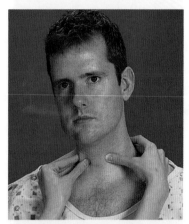

A. Anterior approach

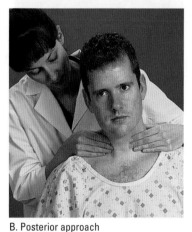

B. Posterior approach

FIGURE 9.20 Examination of the thyroid gland

Examination of regional lymphatics: the thyroid gland
Inspection

E 1. Secure tangential lighting, and shine it at an oblique angle on the consumer's anterior neck.
2. Face the consumer.
3. Ask the consumer to look straight ahead with the head slightly extended.
4. Have the consumer drink a sip of water and swallow twice.
5. As the consumer swallows, observe the front of the neck in the area of the thyroid and the isthmus for masses and symmetrical movement.

N Thyroid tissue moves up with swallowing, but often the movement is so small that it is not visible on inspection. In males, the thyroid cartilage, or Adam's apple, is more prominent than in females.

A A mass or enlargement of the thyroid that moves upwards with swallowing is not normal.

P Many **goitres** (enlarged thyroid glands) or thyroid nodules are visible and may indicate a variety of thyroid diseases (**Figure 9.19**).

Palpation

Palpation of the thyroid gland may be done using both anterior and posterior approaches (**Figure 9.20**).

Anterior approach

P 1. Stand in front of the consumer.
2. Ask the consumer to flex the head slightly forwards.
3. Place the right thumb on the thyroid cartilage and displace the cartilage to the consumer's right.
4. Grasp the elevated and displaced right lobe of the thyroid gland with the thumb and index and middle fingers of the left hand.
5. Palpate the surface of the gland for consistency, nodularity and tenderness.
6. Have the consumer swallow, and then palpate the surface again.
7. Repeat the procedure on the opposite side.

N No enlargement, masses or tenderness should be noted on palpation.

A Palpation reveals the gland to be smooth, soft and slightly enlarged but less than twice the size of a normal thyroid gland.

P This is referred to as physiological hyperplasia and can be seen premenstrually, during pregnancy, or from puberty to young adulthood in females. Symmetrical enlargement may also be noted in consumers who live in areas of iodine deficiency. These are referred to as nontoxic diffuse goitres or endemic goitres.

A Palpation reveals the gland to be two to three times larger than normal size.

P This is diffuse toxic hyperplasia of the thyroid, or Graves' disease, an autoimmune disorder that is the most common type of hyperthyroidism. Table 9.2 distinguishes between the signs and symptoms of thyroid disorders. In addition, Table 9.3 identifies signs and symptoms of parathyroid disease. Because the parathyroid glands can be affected with thyroid manipulation, it is imperative that the examiner has the clinical knowledge of pathology of the parathyroid glands.

E Examination **N** Normal findings **A** Abnormal findings **P** Pathophysiology

A Asymmetrical enlargement of the thyroid and the presence of two or more nodules are found.

P These are thyroid adenomas (benign epithelial tumours) that usually occur after the age of 30. A nontoxic, diffuse goitre may become nodular as the consumer ages.

A Palpation reveals a solitary nodule in the thyroid tissue.
A solitary nodule is suggestive of carcinoma (**Figure 9.19**).

A Lateral deviation of the trachea is noted on palpation, but you are unable to identify a specific goitre.

P This may be a retrosternal goitre. This type of goitre sometimes occurs in a consumer with a short neck, or it may be a goitre with many adenomatous nodules.

TABLE 9.2 Signs and symptoms of thyroid disease

Hypothyroidism and hyperthyroidism are diseases that can occur from birth until later years of life. They can be congenital or acquired. The primary laboratory tests that are used to screen for these conditions are the thyroid stimulating hormone (TSH), T_3 and T_4.

SYSTEM	HYPOTHYROIDISM	HYPERTHYROIDISM
General	Tired, weak	Fatigue, weak
Skin	Dry, cold, coarse	Sweaty, warm
Hair	Alopecia	Thin hair
Head and neck	Hoarseness, puffy face	Lid lag, exophthalmos, goitre
Ears and mouth	Impaired hearing, macroglossia	None
Respiratory	Dyspnoea	Tachypnoea
Cardiovascular	Bradycardia, cool extremities, peripheral oedema	Tachycardia, palpitations
Gastrointestinal	Constipation	Diarrhoea
Musculoskeletal	Carpal tunnel syndrome	Muscle weakness
Neurological	Difficulty concentrating, decreased memory, paraesthesia, decreased deep tendon reflexes	Hyperactivity, irritability, tremor, insomnia
Reproductive	Amenorrhoea	Oligomenorrhoea, gynaecomastia in men, decreased libido, decreased fertility
Endocrine	Cold intolerance	Heat intolerance
Weight	Weight gain with decreased appetite	Weight loss with increased appetite

A Tenderness of the thyroid is found on palpation.

P Tenderness of an enlarged, firm thyroid suggests thyroiditis.

E Examination   **N** Normal findings   **A** Abnormal findings   **P** Pathophysiology

TABLE 9.3 Signs and symptoms of parathyroid disease

Hypoparathyroidism and hyperparathyroidism are diseases that can occur congenitally or be acquired. Both are primarily conditions of calcium imbalance. In hypoparathyroidism, the consumer is in a state of hypocalcaemia; in hyperparathyroidism, the consumer is hypercalcaemic. The body has four parathyroid glands, located posterior to the thyroid. Occasionally, they are accidentally removed when a consumer undergoes thyroid surgery. The parathyroid glands are not accessible to direct physical examination, but parathyroid conditions can be detected by astute history taking and physical assessment data synthesis.

HYPOPARATHYROIDISM	HYPERPARATHYROIDISM
Muscle spasms	Recurrent nephrolithiasis
Facial grimacing	Peptic/duodenal ulcers
Laryngeal spasm	Mental status changes
Seizures	Proximal muscle weakness
Mental status changes	Fatigue
Tetany	Muscle atrophy
Chvostek sign (see Chapter 16)	Osteitis fibrosa cystica
Trousseau sign (see Chapter 16)	

Posterior approach

E 1. Have the consumer sit comfortably. Stand behind the consumer.
2. Have the consumer lower the chin slightly in order to relax the neck muscles.
3. Place the thumbs on the back of the consumer's neck and bring the other fingers around the neck anteriorly with their tips resting on the lower portion of the neck over the trachea.
4. Move the finger pads over the tracheal rings.
5. Instruct the consumer to swallow. Palpate the isthmus for nodules or enlargement.
6. Have the consumer incline the head slightly forwards.
7. Press the fingers of the left hand against the left side of the thyroid cartilage to stabilise it while placing the fingers of the right hand gently against the right side.
8. Instruct the consumer to swallow sips of water.
9. Note consistency, nodularity and tenderness as the gland moves upwards.

N A P Refer to Anterior approach.

Auscultation

If the thyroid is enlarged, auscultation should be performed.

E 1. Stand in front of the consumer.
2. Place the bell of the stethoscope over the right thyroid lobe.
3. Auscultate for bruits.
4. Repeat on the left thyroid lobe.

N Auscultation should not reveal bruits.

A Auscultation reveals the presence of a bruit over an enlarged thyroid gland.

P Bruits occur with increased turbulence in blood vessels and are due to the increased vascularisation of a thyroid gland that is enlarged due to diffuse toxic goitre.

REFLECTION IN PRACTICE

Pregnant woman with neck asymmetry

It is widely recognised that thyroid disease can affect the pregnant woman and the development of the fetus. In the presence of iodine deficiency, enhanced thyroid stimulation during pregnancy can lead to goitre formation in the mother and fetus.

You are assessing a pregnant 22-year-old woman who has recently moved to New Zealand from Samoa. She has received limited medical care her entire life and no prenatal care for this pregnancy. She presents with a unilateral bulge on the left side of her neck. How would you proceed with gaining a health history and physical examination? What might be the aetiology of this neck asymmetry?

For further information refer to your organisation's clinical guidelines or the Australian Government, Pregnancy Care Guidelines: https://www.health.gov.au/resources/pregnancy-care-guidelines

HEALTH EDUCATION

Risk factors for thyroid cancer

When assessing a consumer's neck for possible thyroid abnormalities, identify risk factors for thyroid cancer. Keep in mind the following considerations.

> Age (females 40–50 years; male 60–70 years)
> Female sex
> Diet low in iodine
> History of head or neck radiation, especially in childhood
> Exposure to nuclear weapons (Hiroshima)
> Genetics (e.g. familial medullary thyroid carcinoma)

If the consumer is identified as having any of these risks, discuss the need for further investigation and the need for a health referral.

Examination of regional lymphatics: the lymph nodes

Inspection

E 1. Stand in front of the consumer.
   2. Expose the area of the head and neck to be assessed.
   3. Inspect the nodal areas of the head and neck for any enlargement or inflammation.

N Lymph nodes should not be visible or inflamed.

A Enlargement and inflammation is present in specific nodes.

P Lymph nodes can be enlarged and inflamed when there is a localised or generalised infection in the body. This attempt to prevent the spread of infection occurs as a part of the body's immune response to infection.

Palpation

E 1. Have the consumer sit comfortably.
   2. Face the consumer and conduct the assessment of both sides of the neck simultaneously.
   3. Move the pads and tips of the middle three fingers in small circles of palpation using gentle pressure.

E Examination   **N** Normal findings   **A** Abnormal findings   **P** Pathophysiology

E 4. Follow a systematic, routine sequence beginning with the preauricular, postauricular, occipital, submental, submandibular and tonsillar nodes. Move down to the neck and evaluate the anterior cervical chain, the posterior cervical chain, and the supraclavicular nodes (see Figure 9.21).

5. Note size, shape, delimitation (discrete or matted together), mobility, consistency and tenderness.

N Lymph nodes should not be palpable in the healthy adult consumer; however, small, discrete, movable nodes are sometimes present but are of no significance.

A Palpable lymph nodes are abnormal.

P Palpable lymph nodes are frequently seen in acute bacterial infections such as streptococcal pharyngitis. The anterior cervical nodes are usually affected and may be warm, firm, tender and mobile. A lymph node that is larger than 1 cm in size should be evaluated in greater depth.

P An enlarged postauricular node is sometimes found in consumers with ear infections.

P Enlarged, hard, tender nodes are seen in lymphadenitis (inflammation of the lymph nodes). The affected node is the site of the inflammation.

P Enlarged nodes, particularly of the anterior and posterior cervical chains, may be found in infectious mononucleosis. These nodes are usually tender.

P An enlarged node in the left supraclavicular area (Virchow's node) may point to malignancy in the abdominal or thoracic regions.

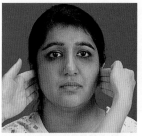
A. Preauricular

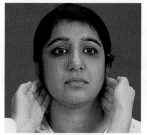
B. Postauricular

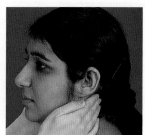
C. Occipital

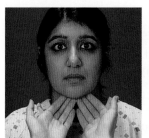
D. Submental

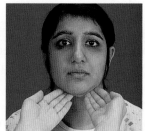
E. Submandibular

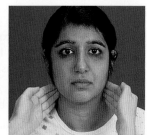
F. Tonsillar

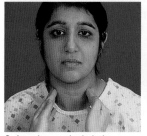
G. Anterior cervical chain

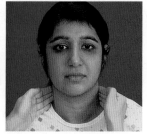
H. Posterior cervical chain

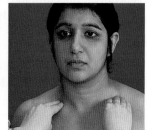
I. Supraclavicular

FIGURE 9.21 Palpation of lymph nodes

E Examination   **N** Normal findings   **A** Abnormal findings   **P** Pathophysiology

P Nontender, firm or hard nodes that are nonmobile may indicate a malignancy in the head and neck area, or metastasis from the region that the lymph node drains.

P Consumers with malignant lymphomas may also present with nodes that are firm, hard or rubbery; nontender; and fixed. In Hodgkin's disease, the cervical nodes are frequently the first to be palpable.

P Palpable lymph nodes can result from a variety of other pathological processes, including blood dyscrasias, AIDS, tuberculosis, surgical procedures that traumatise the nodes, blood transfusions or chronic illness.

EVALUATION OF HEALTH ASSESSMENT AND PHYSICAL EXAMINATION FINDINGS

In the evaluation phase of a health assessment, the focus is on ensuring the data gathered is complete, accurate and documented appropriately (see case study as an example of the focused assessment; see Chapter 22 for a comprehensive health assessment). In evaluating the data you should:

> draw on your critical thinking and problem-solving skills to make sound clinical decisions

> act on abnormal data (include communicating findings to other health professionals)

> ensure documentation reflects the outcomes of the clinical decisions/actions taken (refer to Chapter 3, which discusses in detail why documentation is so important and how this may be undertaken in different health settings).

The case study that follows steps you through this process.

By using the following case study, you will be able to follow this process.

THE CONSUMER WITH HYPERTHYROIDISM, GRAVES' DISEASE

This case study illustrates the application and objective documentation of the head, neck and regional lymph node assessment.

Samuel Norris is a 54-year-old man who has not been feeling well the past few months.

HEALTH HISTORY

CONSUMER PROFILE	54-year-old male
CHIEF COMPLAINT	'I just haven't felt right for the past couple of months.'
HISTORY OF THE PRESENT ILLNESS	Consumer reports that he was doing well until 9 months ago, when he saw his general practitioner for his 6-month check-up for hypertension and hyperlipidaemia. At that time, he was noted to have tonsillar enlargement and was referred to an ENT specialist. Subsequently, he was diagnosed with squamous cell carcinoma of the tonsils. His tonsils were removed and he received a 6-week course of external beam radiation to the tonsillar region. He had an uneventful postoperative period and resumed work. About 2 months ago, Samuel developed signs of myalgias and complained of general weakness. He denies experiencing dysphagia, hoarseness, any fever, shortness of breath, palpitations, diarrhoea, tremor, heat intolerance. He has lost 4 kg since his surgery. Samuel is concerned about the effects of his current health status because he has no more sick leave this year due to his earlier surgery and radiation therapy treatments.

>>

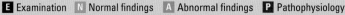

E Examination **N** Normal findings **A** Abnormal findings **P** Pathophysiology

>>

HEALTH HISTORY			
PAST HEALTH HISTORY	**MEDICAL HISTORY**		Hypertension for 10 years, controlled with medications. Takes BP at home every two days and records the results
	SURGICAL HISTORY		Appendectomy 1975 ACL repair 1996 Tonsillectomy, 3.5 months ago
	ALLERGIES		Allergic to penicillin, breaks out in hives
	MEDICATIONS		Metoprolol 50 mg oral daily Ezetimibe 10 mg oral daily Aspirin 100 mg oral daily
	COMMUNICABLE DISEASES		Chickenpox, age 3
	INJURIES AND ACCIDENTS		1993 playing AFL and tore ACL, repaired early 1996
	SPECIAL NEEDS		Nil reported
	BLOOD TRANSFUSIONS		Nil reported
	CHILDHOOD ILLNESSES		Mumps, age 4
	IMMUNISATIONS		Had latest influenza vaccination and his tetanus is up to date
FAMILY HEALTH HISTORY	Denies family history of thyroid disease		
SOCIAL HISTORY	**ALCOHOL USE**		2 beers each night at home and after work on Friday. Goes out for a few beers with work friends sometimes
	TOBACCO USE		8–10 cigarettes a day for the past 6 months; prior to this he smoked 40 cigarettes/day for 30 years and an occasional cigar on the weekend
	DRUG USE		Marijuana in high school; continued use on irregular basis until age 30
	DOMESTIC AND INTIMATE PARTNER VIOLENCE		States no issues
	SEXUAL PRACTICE		Good relationship with wife of 30 years
	TRAVEL HISTORY		Travels interstate to follow touring car championships
	WORK ENVIRONMENT		Manager of a busy Australia Post service vehicle maintenance unit. Has a few staff and been there for 20 years. Work space is crowded; he has a dirty office from exhaust fumes from cars all day
	HOME ENVIRONMENT		Lives in low-set brick home with wife and 23-year-old son. No major environmental risks noted
	HOBBIES AND LEISURE ACTIVITIES		Poker once a month, watching touring car and rally car races in New Zealand on TV, attending Australian touring car races when able
	STRESS		'My health and bills, bills, bills and work, work, work.'
	EDUCATION		'I finished high school, and that was enough for me.'
	ECONOMIC STATUS		'We aren't starving.'
	MILITARY SERVICE		None
	RELIGION		Uniting Church
	CULTURAL BACKGROUND		Caucasian
	ROLES AND RELATIONSHIPS		Samuel and his wife get along 'OK'. 'I get on well with my son. He lives at home and we love watching the car racing and car rallies together.' 'Bit of stress with the big boss at work, but nothing I can't handle.'

>>

>>

HEALTH HISTORY

	CHARACTERISTIC PATTERNS OF DAILY LIVING	Wakes at 5:30 a.m., showers, has coffee and cereal; arrives at work at 7 a.m.; smokes a cigarette; black coffee throughout the day; fast-food for lunch, but lately has been trying to cut down on fried food; leaves work at 4 p.m., comes home and has 2 beers; eats dinner with wife and son, if he is at home, and then watches TV; in bed by 10 p.m.
HEALTH MAINTENANCE ACTIVITIES	**SLEEP**	7½ hours per night; usually feels rested
	DIET	'I grab something when I can at work. It should be low-fat, low-cholesterol with lots of fish; I am trying to be better about my diet.'
	EXERCISE	'Oh not much, but I want to do more.'
	STRESS MANAGEMENT	'A good beer helps me relax.'
	USE OF SAFETY DEVICES	'At work we are very regulated. That's a big part of my role, to ensure the safety of vehicles and drivers.'
	HEALTH CHECK-UPS	'Usually 6 monthly for my BP and general health; I have had more visits lately with the tonsil cancer.'

PHYSICAL EXAMINATION

EXAMINATION OF THE HEAD	**INSPECTION**	**SHAPE OF THE HEAD**	Normocephalic and symmetrical
	PALPATION	Skull smooth, no tenderness, masses or depressions; temporal artery 1+/4+ with mild tenderness, mildly stiff vessel	
EXAMINATION OF THE SCALP	**INSPECTION AND PALPATION**	Scalp smooth and intact, no lesions or masses	
EXAMINATION OF THE FACE	**INSPECTION**	**SYMMETRY**	Symmetrical, no involuntary movements or swelling
		SHAPE AND FEATURES	Round, no oedema or involuntary movements; no exophthalmos
EXAMINATION OF THE MANDIBLE	**PALPATION AND AUSCULTATION**	Temporomandibular joint articulates smoothly, no clicking or crepitus	
EXAMINATION OF THE NECK	**INSPECTION**	Muscles symmetrical, full range of movement	
	PALPATION	No palpable masses or spasms reported	
EXAMINATION OF THE REGIONAL LYMPHATICS: THE THYROID GLAND	**INSPECTION**	Moves with swallowing	
	PALPATION	**ANTERIOR APPROACH**	No enlargement
		POSTERIOR APPROACH	No discrete nodules, nontender
	AUSCULTATION	Bruits noted	
EXAMINATION OF THE REGIONAL LYMPHATICS: THE LYMPH NODES	**INSPECTION**	Enlargement noted	
	PALPATION	Adenopathy (enlargement noted)	

DIAGNOSTIC DATA

	Complete metabolic panel – Within normal ranges	
	CONSUMER'S VALUES	**NORMAL RANGE**
TSH	<0.30 mIU/L	0.30–5.00 mIU/L
FREE T$_4$	>23 pmol/L	11–23 pmol/L

>>

>>

HEALTH HISTORY		
FREE T₃	>6.7 pmol/L	3.5–6.7 pmol/L
CRP	80 mg/L	<12 mg/L
	Nuclear medicine scan of thyroid gland with uptake: Multiple pinhole images of the thyroid show a mild diffuse goitre. The thyroid is mildly enlarged. The lobes are biconvex in configuration with homogeneous uptake of the radionuclide throughout the parenchyma of both lobes. No discrete nodules are identified. 6- and 24-hour radioactive uptake measurements are mildly elevated at 28.7% and 42.6%.	
	Impression: Mild diffuse toxic goitre	

EVALUATION AND CLINICAL REASONING FOR CASE STUDY

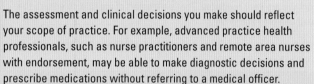

The assessment and clinical decisions you make should reflect your scope of practice. For example, advanced practice health professionals, such as nurse practitioners and remote area nurses with endorsement, may be able to make diagnostic decisions and prescribe medications without referring to a medical officer.

Fundamentally, all health professionals collect, evaluate and act on consumer-focused health information, which will at times include referral to, or collaboration with, other healthcare team members. Nurses assess consumer responses to interventions and determine when to escalate key changes in a consumer's condition. The clinical reasoning cycle provides health professionals with a framework to consider all this information in a meaningful way for planning consumer care. These phases are stepped out below, and draw on information presented and collected during the health history and physical examination. We then work through the cycle components that are relevant to this case study (cycle components are bolded).

For Samuel Norris, the significant data that needs to be considered includes the following.

Collecting cues/information

Recall and Review: In the first instance you will need to reflect on what you know about hyperthyroidism. This is characterised by hyperactivity and enlargement of the thyroid gland. There are a number of causes of hyperthyroidism, and the most common is Graves' disease. In this case scenario, Samuel Norris has been diagnosed with Graves' disease. This is an autoimmune disease of unknown aetiology in which the body's own immune system causes the thyroid gland to produce excess thyroid hormone. Antibodies to the thyroid stimulating hormone (TSH) receptor sites develop in individuals, causing the thyroid gland to release either T₃ or T₄ or both of these. Clinical signs develop as a result of the excessive release of thyroid hormones, in which remissions and exacerbations are common patterns even when the person is treated.

Chief complaint and history of present illness (subjective data)

> States 'I just haven't felt right for the past couple of months'.
> 9 months previously, noted tonsillar enlargement, subsequently diagnosed with squamous cell carcinoma of the tonsils. Treated with surgical removal and 6-week course of radiation therapy

> Over the last 2 months, has experienced myalgia and generalised weakness
> Weight loss 4 kg since surgery
> Verbalised concern about present health status and the lack of sick leave remaining if illness continues

Processing information

Interpret: These symptoms and details of history outline the scope of the issue for this consumer and how it affects their wellbeing and ability to self-manage.

Health maintenance activities

> Diet is poor (fast-foods, fried food, regular coffee), on the run, but wants to do better with diet
> Limited exercise but aware more is desirable
> Other issues: Smoker (8–10 cigarettes/day, occasional cigar), alcohol each night (2 beers)

Physical assessment

> Enlarged lymph nodes noted
> Thyroid functioning tests elevated
> Elevated CRP (indicates inflammation)
> Bruits detected in the thyroid gland
> Nuclear scan findings indicate mild diffuse goitre
> Elevated BP (for past 10 years, medication controlled)
> Smoker
> Respiration rate 30/minute

Interpret, Discriminate, Infer and Predict: The significance of these findings indicate that Samuel Norris has Graves' disease, which requires medical and long-term follow-up and management. He also has a high cardiovascular risk factor profile, which will necessitate long-term education and behavioural lifestyle management changes.

Putting it all together – synthesise information

The role of the nurse in this case is to work with the medical practitioners to ensure Samuel fully understands the nature and extent of his current health problem and the lifelong management required. The medical officer will review and prescribe initial medication treatment for Samuel. Samuel will be referred to a specialist endocrinologist for further consideration of his medical management. Diagnosis was confirmed through review of thyroid functioning tests (decreased TSH levels, all other thyroid function tests increased) and radioactive iodine uptake investigation (greater uptake of radioactive iodine noted).

Care options centre on specialist medical staff deciding the most appropriate treatment pathway for Samuel – there is no single treatment option for Samuel. This may include medication management to reduce the production of thyroxine (preferred option, pending situation); radiation, using radioactive iodine therapy; or surgical intervention involving partial or full removal of the thyroid gland.

Actions based on assessment findings

Other areas that need to be considered for Samuel include:

1 Cardiovascular risk factor modification: given Samuel's high risk-factor profile it is critical that the nurse provides education, referral and support on how to approach risk-factor reduction. Samuel will need to target smoking – smoking cessation; diet – encourage a balanced healthy diet; exercise – undertaking some form of physical exercise at least 5 times per week.

2 Anxiety and concern about limited sick leave time available at work: Due to the ongoing sick role and lengthy time off work, the nurse should give Samuel the opportunity to express his feelings about this and provide information about contacting his employer regarding present illness in the view to working out a return-to-work plan. Provide support options through pastoral care, counselling and other social support structures.

3 Broader education about living with thyroid disease, how to manage this, with particular emphasis on compliance with medication and modifications to present lifestyle, will be important.

The final step in the process is accurate documentation. The nurse must document findings, referrals, interventions, advice and education given. The consumer would continue to have ongoing long-term management and follow-up by specialist medical staff in collaboration with Samuel's general practitioner.

CHAPTER RESOURCES

REVIEW QUESTIONS

For answers to these questions, see Answer section at the end of the book.

1. The nurse is conducting an admission health history of a consumer and asks about family health history. The nurse recognises which of the following pathologies to be familial conditions of the head and neck? Select all that apply.
   a. Hyperthyroidism
   b. Sinusitis
   c. Migraines
   d. Torticollis
   e. Bell's palsy

2. The posterior triangle of the neck is formed by the:
   a. Mandible, trachea and sternocleidomastoid muscle
   b. Omohyoid muscle, trachea and trapezius muscle
   c. Sternum, sternocleidomastoid muscle and mandible
   d. Sternocleidomastoid muscle, trapezius muscle and the base of the clavicle

3. Adam, a 23-year-old male, presents to the emergency department with a long history of allergic rhinitis. What physical examination findings might Adam exhibit? Select all that apply.
   a. Dry, dull facial skin
   b. Round and swollen face
   c. Immobile and expressionless face
   d. Excess hair on the jaw and upper lip
   e. Darkened areas beneath the eyes
   f. Transverse nasal crease

4. While inspecting a consumer's face, you note their slanted eyes with inner epicanthal folds; a short, flat nose; and a thick, protruding tongue. What condition do these findings suggest?
   a. Hydrocephalus
   b. Craniosynostosis
   c. Bell's palsy
   d. Down syndrome

5. Amelie reports feeling intermittent muscle spasms and facial grimacing. Which of these conditions is she most likely experiencing?
   a. Hypothyroidism
   b. Hyperthyroidism
   c. Hypoparathyroidism
   d. Hyperparathyroidism

6. Which of the following assessment findings describes the consumer with Cushing syndrome?
   a. Red cheeks, increase in hair on the upper lip, large cheeks
   b. An abnormally wide distance between the eyes
   c. Facial skin that is shiny, contracted and hard
   d. Sunken eyes and hollow cheeks

7. Risk factors for thyroid cancer include:
   a. Thyroid adenoma, male sex, diet high in sodium
   b. Exposure to nuclear fallout, female sex, diet high in phosphates
   c. History of thyroid radiation, male sex, diet low in potassium
   d. Genetics, female sex, diet low in iodine

8. While inspecting a consumer, you note that the consumer's neck deviates sharply to the left. The consumer also has a prominent left sternocleidomastoid muscle. What may be causing this consumer's condition?
   a. Osteoarthritis
   b. Acute spasm
   c. Trigeminal neuralgia
   d. Thyroid cancer

9. Which of the following is a normal finding of lymph
   node assessment?
   a. Small, discrete, movable nodes
   b. Enlarged node in the left supraclavicular area
   c. Nontender, fixed, hard node
   d. Nonmobile, rubbery, erythematous node
10. The consumer with a sore throat is most likely to have tender
    and enlarged lymph nodes in which area?
    a. Preauricular
    b. Tonsillar

c. Supraclavicular
d. Postauricular

CS CLINICAL SKILLS

The following Clinical Skill is relevant to this chapter and can
be found in Tollefson & Hillman, *Clinical Psychomotor Skills*,
8th edition:
> 27 Healthcare teaching.

FURTHER RESOURCES

> ABC Health and Wellbeing: http://www.abc.net.au/health/library/stories/2005/06/16/1831822.htm
> Australian Government Department of Health and Aged Care – Aboriginal and Torres Strait Islander health: https://www.health.gov.au/health-topics/aboriginal-and-torres-strait-islander-health?utm_source=health.gov.au&utm_medium=callout-auto-custom&utm_campaign=digital_transformation
> Australian Thyroid Foundation: https://www.thyroidfoundation.org.au/
> Better Health Channel: http://www.betterhealth.vic.gov.au/
> Cancer Council: http://www.cancer.org.au/

> Endocrine Society of Australia: http://www.endocrinesociety.org.au/
> healthdirect Australia: http://www.healthdirect.gov.au/
> Health Navigator New Zealand: https://www.healthnavigator.org.nz/health-a-z/o/overactive-thyroid/
> International Headache Society (IHS): https://ihs-headache.org/en/resources/guidelines/
> Lymphoma Australia: http://www.lymphoma.org.au/
> Mayo Clinic: http://www.mayoclinic.com
> Migraine & Headache Australia: http://headacheaustralia.org.au/
> New Zealand Ministry of Health: http://www.health.govt.nz/

REFERENCES

Australian Government Department of Health and Aged Care. (2020). Smoking and tobacco and Aboriginal and Torres Strait Islander peoples. Retrieved 27 October 2022 from https://www.health.gov.au/topics/smoking-and-tobacco/smoking-and-tobacco-throughout-life/smoking-and-tobacco-and-aboriginal-and-torres-strait-islander-peoples

Australian Indigenous HealthInfoNet. (2017). National Aboriginal and Torres Strait Islander social survey 2014–15 released. Retrieved 27 October 2022 from https://healthinfonet.ecu.edu.au/about/news/4088/

Australian Institute of Health and Welfare (AIHW). (2020). 1.11 Oral Health. Aboriginal and Torres Strait Islander Health Performance Framework. Retrieved 8 December 2022 from: https://www.indigenoushpf.gov.au/measures/1-11-oral-health

Australian Institute of Health and Welfare (AIHW). (2022a). Cancer data in Australia. Retrieved 6 December 2022 from: https://www.aihw.gov.au/getmedia/43903b67-3130-4384-8648-39c69bb684b5/Cancer-data-in-Australia.pdf.aspx?inline=true

Australian Institute of Health and Welfare (AIHW). (2022b). Oral and dental care in Australia. Retrieved 8 December 2022 from: https://www.aihw.gov.au/reports/dental-oral-health/oral-health-and-dental-care-in-australia/contents/hospitalisations

Australian Institute of Health and Welfare (AIHW). (2022c). Indigenous health and wellbeing. Retrieved 8 December 2022 from: https://www.aihw.gov.au/reports/australias-health/indigenous-health-and-wellbeing#Hearing%20health,%20eye%20health%20and%20oral%20health

Australian Resuscitation Council and New Zealand Resuscitation Council (ANZCOR). (2016). ANZCOR Guideline 9.1.6 – Management of suspected spinal injury. Retrieved 21 October 2022 from https://resus.org.au/guidelines/

Cancer Australia. (2022a). Head and neck cancer. Retrieved 6 December 2022 from: https://www.canceraustralia.gov.au/cancer-types/head-and-neck-cancer/statistics

Cancer Australia. (2022b). Thyroid cancer. Retrieved 6 December 2022 from: https://www.canceraustralia.gov.au/cancer-types/thyroid-cancer/statistics

Headache Australia. (2023). Prevalence and cost of headache. Retrieved 25 May 2023 from http://headacheaustralia.org.au/what-is-headache/prevalence-and-cost-of-headache/

Health Navigator New Zealand. (2021). Thyroid cancer. Retrieved 6 December 2022 from: https://www.healthnavigator.org.nz/health-a-z/t/thyroid-cancer/

HealthED Ministry of Health New Zealand. (2019). Body-piercing and tattooing: Protecting your health. Retrieved 19 October 2022 from https://www.healthed.govt.nz/resource/body-piercing-and-tattooing-protecting-your-health

International Headache Society (IHS). (2018). The International Classification of Headache Disorders, 3rd edition. Retrieved 19 October 2022 from https://ichd-3.org/

Laaksonen, M., MacInnis, R., Canfell, K., Shaw, J. E., Magliano, D. J., Banks, E., … Vajdic, C. M. (2021). Thyroid cancers potentially preventable by reducing overweight and obesity in Australia: A pooled cohort study. *International Journal of Cancer 150*(8), 1281–90. https://doi.org/10.1002/ijc.33889

Ministry of Health. (2018). Oral health. Māori health. Retrieved 8 December 2022 from: https://www.health.govt.nz/our-work/populations/maori-health/tatau-kahukura-maori-health-statistics/nga-mana-hauora-tutohu-health-status-indicators/oral-health

NSW Health. (2022). Body art and tattooing businesses. Retrieved 19 October from https://www.health.nsw.gov.au/environment/factsheets/Pages/tattooing.aspx

Queensland Government. (2017). Body piercing – so you are thinking of getting a piercing. Retrieved 19 October 2022 from http://conditions.health.qld.gov.au/HealthCondition/condition/20/40/17/body-piercing-so-you-are-thinking-of-gettin

Queensland Government, Queensland Health (2016). Personal appearance services. Retrieved 27 October 2022 from https://www.health.qld.gov.au/public-health/industry-environment/personal-appearance/services/legislation

CHAPTER 10

EYES

LEARNING OUTCOMES

By the end of this chapter you should be able to:

1 identify the structures of the eyes
2 discuss the system-specific history for the eyes
3 describe normal findings in the physical examination of the eyes
4 describe common abnormalities found in the physical examination of the eyes
5 perform a foundation level physical examination of the eyes
6 identify health education opportunities for consumers in regard to specific eye conditions
7 discuss the clinical reasoning in evaluating outcomes of health assessment and physical examination including documentation requirements for recording information, health education given and relevant health referral.

BACKGROUND

Health assessment and physical examination of the eyes provides information about the consumer's nutritional, endocrine, cardiovascular, gastrointestinal and neurological systems. This chapter provides a comprehensive guide to examining the eye, and the factors that affect it. How comprehensive your assessment is may also depend on your role and scope of practice. For example, most nurses in general areas do not undertake examination of the retina or conduct field tests; however, nurses in specialised areas or advanced practice roles may do so. Nevertheless, eye-related health problems occur in over 55% of the Australian population (more commonly in females than males) (AIHW, 2021a), which makes eye-related health issues one of the most common health problems in Australia.

Common conditions that will be discussed include:

> refractive error issues such as myopia, presbyopia and hyperopia
> **cataracts**
> glaucoma
> age-related macular degeneration
> diabetic retinopathy
> eye injuries/trauma such as corneal ulceration and foreign bodies.

Eye conditions are very common, with an estimated 13 million Australians having one or more chronic (long-term) eye conditions, including 131 000 with complete or partial blindness (AIHW, 2021a). Vision impairment is not, however, equally distributed across the Australian population. Aboriginal and Torres Strait Islander people are three times as likely as non-First Nations Australians to be blind or have low vision (AIHW, 2021b), and despite these higher rates of vision loss, research shows that Aboriginal and Torres Strait Islander people use eye health services at lower rates than non-First Nations Australians. Barriers to accessing eye care include a lack of specialist services in rural and remote areas, the complexity of the patient journey, a lack of coordination within and between services, and uncertainty about service providers and the cost of treatment (Razavi, Burrow & Trzesinski, 2018). The main causes of vision impairment in Australia are refractive error and cataracts (AIHW, 2021a).

In New Zealand, it is estimated that there are 180 000 New Zealanders with moderate to severe functional vision loss. The most common eye conditions underlying blindness and low vision are age-related macular degeneration (AMD), diabetic retinopathy, glaucoma and cataracts (Blind Low Vision NZ, 2022). The Māori people have a higher prevalence of diabetic retinopathy and keratoconus, develop cataracts 10 years younger than non-Māori people, and have decreased access to strabismus surgery (Chilibeck, Mathan, Ng & McKelvie, 2020).

LEADING EYE HEALTH RELATED CONCERNS

> Globally, at least 2.2 billion people have a near or distance vision impairment. In 50% of these cases, vision impairment could have been prevented or has yet to be addressed. These 1 billion people include those with moderate or severe distance vision impairment or blindness due to unaddressed refractive error (88.4 million), cataract (94 million), age-related macular degeneration (8 million), glaucoma (7.7 million) and diabetic retinopathy (3.9 million), as well as near vision impairment caused by unaddressed presbyopia (826 million) (World Health Organization, 2022). Recent modelling by Vision 2020 Australia suggests that around 840 000 Australians are currently living with vision loss, and that by 2030 this could exceed 1.04 million (Vision 2020, 2021).

> Glaucoma is the leading cause of irreversible visual impairment internationally with **primary open angle glaucoma** (POAG) being the predominant subtype of glaucoma (Zhang, Wang, Li & Jiang, 2021). Currently, about 80 million people worldwide have glaucoma and numbers are increasing due in part to the rapidly ageing population (Glaucoma Research Foundation, 2022). In Australia, over 300 000 people have glaucoma and one in 50 will develop glaucoma in their lifetime. It is estimated that about half of the cases of glaucoma remain undetected (Glaucoma Australia, 2022). Primary open angle glaucoma is a condition in which increased intraocular pressure causes damage to the optic nerve (Glaucoma Australia, 2022). The rise in pressure is often due to impaired drainage of fluid out of the eye. There is no pain or other related symptoms to warn of its presence. While anyone may develop glaucoma, some people are at a higher risk, including those with a family history of the disease and anyone over the age of 50. There is a 10-fold chance of immediate relatives of an affected person contracting POAG (CERA, 2022).

> **Age-related macular degeneration (ARMD)** is the leading cause of blindness in both Australia and New Zealand (Macular Disease Foundation Australia, n.d.(a); Macular Degeneration New Zealand, 2020; Vision Australia, 2022). As its name suggests, ARMD affects the macular region of the retina. Early detection is the best chance of halting progression in cases of wet ARMD where sudden loss of vision occurs. Dry ARMD results in a gradual loss of central vision (Macular Degeneration New Zealand, 2020). One in seven people over 50 will develop ARMD (Macular Degeneration New Zealand, 2020).

> Other conditions and injuries also impact vision, such as diabetes mellitus (people with diabetes mellitus are at risk of developing diabetic-related retinopathy) (AIHW, 2021a; Macular Disease Foundation Australia, n.d.(b)). Eye injuries (falls, assaults, sport and work-related accidents) are also a significant proportion of reasons for visual impairment, responsible for 10–27% of operating department, 38–65% of emergency department and 5–16% of all eye

hospital patient admissions. The majority of people hospitalised for eye injuries are male (Hoskin, 2020).

Diseases, disorders and injuries affecting vision can have enormous effects on the individual's ability to care for self and others, and therefore makes assessment of the eyes extremely important. Among older people, vision-related issues become more pronounced, significantly reducing their quality of life and contributing to depression (Sturrock, 2018). Risk factors for eye-related problems can be useful to consider when preparing to assess a consumer (see **Table 10.1**).

TABLE 10.1 Risk factors for eye problems

AGE AND SEX	Increased prevalence of problems as age increases Women are more likely than men to suffer vision impairment Diet High intake of protein, vitamins A, B and riboflavin protects against some forms of cataract High dietary fat is a risk for macular degeneration High fish consumption may protect against macular degeneration
GENETICS	People who have a family member with macular degeneration are three times more likely to develop it. Aboriginal Australians have lower levels of refractive error and better visual acuity, which is likely to be genetic.
OTHER FACTORS	Smoking and excessive alcohol consumption can increase the risk of some types of cataracts as well as macular degeneration. Excessive sun exposure also may pre-dispose to eye-related problems. Population groups: Specific population groups can be at higher risk of avoidable vision loss and include Aboriginal and Torres Strait Islanders, the elderly, people with a family history of eye disease, those with diabetes mellitus, and societal groups that are marginalised or disadvantaged.
FOR DIABETIC PEOPLE	15–30% will also have diabetic retinopathy Accounts for significantly worse vision than those without diabetes Are at a higher risk for glaucoma and cataracts

ADAPTED FROM KAMIŃSKA, PINKAS, WRZEŚNIEWSKA-WAL, OSTROWSKI & JANKOWSKI, M. (2023); AUSTRALIAN DEPARTMENT OF HEALTH AND AGED CARE (2023)

ANATOMY AND PHYSIOLOGY

External structures

The external structures of the eye comprise the eyelids or palpebra, the conjunctiva, the lacrimal glands, and the extraocular muscles. The eyelids consist of smooth muscle covered with a very thin layer of skin; they admit light to the eye while protecting and maintaining lubrication of the eye. The interior surface of the lid muscle is covered with a pink mucous membrane called the **palpebral conjunctiva**. Alongside the palpebral conjunctiva is the **bulbar conjunctiva**. The bulbar conjunctiva folds back over the anterior surface of the eyeball and merges with the cornea at the **limbus**, the junction of the sclera and the cornea (**Figure 10.1**). The conjunctiva contains blood vessels and pain receptors that respond quickly to outside insult. Eyelashes are evenly spaced along lid margins and curve outwards to protect the eye by filtering particles of dirt and dust from the external environment. Eyebrows are symmetrical and evenly distributed above the eyelids.

The opening between the eyelids is called the **palpebral fissure**. Upper and lower eyelids meet at the inner **canthus** on the nasal side and at the outer canthus on the temporal side. Embedded just beneath the lid margins are the meibomian glands, which secrete a lubricating substance onto the surface of the eye. The **tarsal plates** are connective tissue that gives shape to the upper lids.

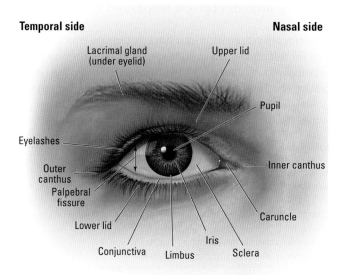

Temporal side

Nasal side

Lacrimal gland
(under eyelid)

Upper lid

Pupil

Eyelashes

Outer
canthus

Inner canthus

Palpebral
fissure

Caruncle

Lower lid

Iris

Conjunctiva   Limbus   Sclera

FIGURE 10.1 External view of the right eye

Lacrimal apparatus

The **lacrimal apparatus** is made up of the lacrimal gland and ducts. The lacrimal glands, located above and on the temporal side of each eye, are responsible for the production of tears, which lubricate the eye. Tears drain through the inferior and superior **puncta** at the inner canthus, through the nasolacrimal duct and the lacrimal sac to the inferior turbinate in the nose. The **caruncle**, which contains sebaceous glands, is the round, red structure in the inner canthus.

Extraocular muscles

Six extraocular muscles extend from the scleral surface of each eye and attach to the bony orbit. These voluntary muscles work in concert to move the eyes with great precision in several directions to provide a single image to the brain. These muscles are the superior, inferior, medial and lateral recti, and the superior and inferior obliques.

Internal structures

The globes of the eyes are spherical structures that are encased in the protective bony orbits of the face, along with the lacrimal gland and extrinsic muscles of the eye. Only a small portion of the anterior surface of the eye is exposed. The eye itself is approximately 2.5 cm in diameter and has three layers: a tough, outer fibrous tunic (sclera); a middle, vascular tunic; and the innermost layer, which contains the retina (**Figure 10.2**).

Outer layer

The outer tunic consists of the transparent cornea on the outer portion, which is continuous with the **sclera**, an opaque material that in most people appears white and covers the structures inside the eye. The **cornea** is a nonvascular, transparent surface that covers the iris and is continuous with the conjunctival epithelium. The sclera protects the eye and is a surface for the attachment of the extraocular muscles. The posterior portion of the sclera contains an opening for the entrance of the optic nerve and various blood vessels.

Middle layer

The pigmented, middle vascular tunic, or uveal layer, is composed of the **choroid**, the ciliary body, and the iris. The choroid is a vascular tissue that lines the inner surface of the eye just beneath the retina. It provides nutrition to the retinal pigment epithelium and helps absorb excess light.

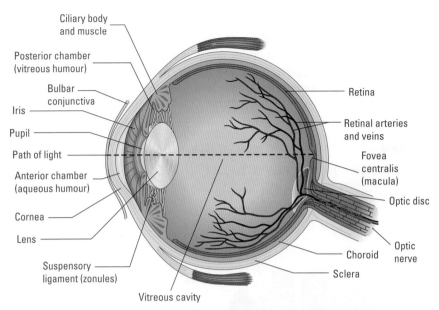

Ciliary body
and muscle

Posterior chamber
(vitreous humour)

Bulbar
conjunctiva

Iris

Pupil

Path of light

Anterior chamber
(aqueous humour)

Cornea

Lens

Suspensory
ligament (zonules)

Vitreous cavity

Retina

Retinal arteries
and veins

Fovea
centralis
(macula)

Optic disc

Optic
nerve

Choroid

Sclera

FIGURE 10.2 Lateral cross section of the interior eye

The **ciliary body** is an anterior extension of the uveal tract; it siphons serum from the systemic blood flow to produce the aqueous humour needed to nourish the corneal endothelium. Zonules are small strands of tissue extending from the ciliary body to the crystalline **lens**. Zonules hold the lens in place and allow it to change shape in order to refract light from various focusing distances. The **iris**, the most anterior portion of the uveal tract, provides a distinctive colour for the eye that is genetically determined. It is comprised of smooth muscle that regulates the entrance of light. The **pupil**, an opening in the centre of the iris, regulates the amount of light entering the eye. The pupil reacts to light and the closeness of objects by stimulation of the sympathetic nervous system, which dilates it, and the parasympathetic nervous system, which constricts it.

The central cavity of the eye posterior to the lens is filled with a clear, gelatinous material called **vitreous humour**, which helps maintain the shape of the eye and the position of the internal structures.

Visual images pass through the structures and aqueous humour of the **anterior chamber**, the space anterior to the pupil and iris, and the vitreous humour of the **posterior chamber**, the space immediately posterior to the iris, to the fundus of the eye, where the retina is located.

Inner layer

The innermost layer of the eyeball, the **retina**, is an extension of the optic nerve, which lines the inside of the globe and receives light impulses to be transmitted to the occipital lobe of the brain. Paired retinal arteries and veins branch from the optic disc towards the periphery, growing smaller as they extend outwards. Generally, retinal arteries are smaller and a lighter red than veins and often have a silver-looking 'arterial light reflex'.

The **optic disc** is a round or oval area with distinct margins located on the nasal side of the retina. Retinal fibres join at the optic disc to form the optic nerve. Nerve fibres from the temporal visual fields cross at the optic chiasm.

The **physiologic cup** is a pale, central area in the optic disc occupying one-third to one-fourth of the disc. In the temporal area of the retina, the tiny, darker **macula**, with the **fovea centralis** at its centre, contains a high concentration of the **cones** necessary for colour vision, reading ability, and other tasks requiring fine visual discrimination. The fovea is the area of sharpest vision. Other portions of the retina contain a high concentration of **rods**, which provide dark and light discrimination and peripheral vision.

Visual pathway

Objects in the field of vision reflect light, which is received by sensory neurones in the retina; these images are received upside down and reversed. From there they pass along nerve fibres through the optic disc and the optic nerve. Fibres from the left half of each eye pass through the optic chiasm to the right side of the brain, and fibres from the right side of each eye pass to the left side of the visual cortex of the occipital lobe of the brain (see **Figure 10.3**).

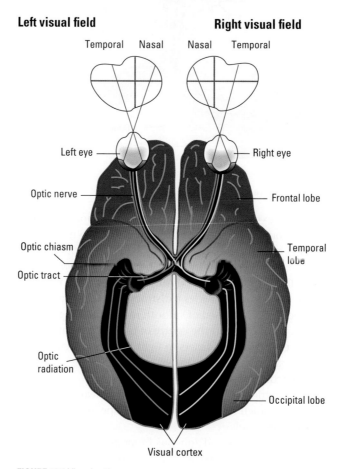

FIGURE 10.3 Visual pathway

ASSESSMENT: TAKING THE CONSUMER'S HEALTH HISTORY

Assessment is the first phase of the nursing process, and involves collecting subjective information about the consumer's health status in order to identify consumer problem areas to focus on.

Subjective data is most frequently collected during a health history and serves as the starting point for the health professional to base the depth of their assessment on. The sections for the health history include:

> **Consumer profile**

> **Chief complaint** (explained systematically using variations of location, quality, quantity, associated manifestations, aggravating factors, alleviating factors, setting and timing. This is a variation on the OPQRST assessment mnemonic you may use for other conditions such as pain assessment)

>>

> > **Past health history** (including medical history, surgical history, allergies, medications, injuries and accidents, special needs and childhood illnesses)
> > **Family health history**
> > **Social history** (including alcohol, tobacco and drug use, sexual practice, work and home environment, hobbies and leisure activities, stress and culture).

We have included a guide for foundation eye assessment below. Eye examination scope of practice may differ depending on where you are located, so the foundation assessment outline included here is relevant.

Many readers will find that some information included in this chapter is at an advanced level. Please note the headings identified and adjust your reading accordingly.

HEALTH HISTORY			
CONSUMER PROFILE	The eye health history provides insight into the link between a consumer's life/lifestyle and eye information and pathology. Diseases that are age-, sex- and race-specific for the eyes are listed.		
	AGE	> Cataract (congenital, elderly) > Presbyopia (middle age) > Hypertensive retinopathy (middle age to elderly) > Glaucoma (middle age to elderly) > Age-related macular degeneration (elderly) > Entropion, ectropion (elderly) > Dry eyes (elderly)	
	SEX	**FEMALE**	Dry eyes, thyroid-related ophthalmopathy
	CULTURAL BACKGROUND	Cataract, diabetic retinopathy, trachoma (Aboriginal and Torres Strait Islander peoples) (Australia is the only developed country to still have trachoma), diabetic retinopathy (Māori and Pasifika), age-related macular degeneration, and melanoma of the eye (Caucasians)	
CHIEF COMPLAINT	Common chief complaints for the eyes are defined, and information on the characteristics of each sign or symptom is provided.		
	1. CHANGES IN VISUAL ACUITY	Change in ability to see clearly	
		LOCATION	One eye or both eyes
		QUALITY	Dimming of vision, blurred vision, diplopia, visual field loss, legal blindness, fading of colour vision
		ASSOCIATED MANIFESTATIONS	Headache, rhinorrhoea, sneezing, vertigo, 'floaters' (spots of different sizes that float across the visual field and are caused by changes in the vitreous humour), flashes of light, aura, nausea and vomiting, generalised muscle weakness, eye pain or pressure, infection (herpes simplex/herpes zoster or cytomegalovirus)
		AGGRAVATING FACTORS	Allergens, stress, lack of sleep, decreased lighting, darkness (night), refractive changes, systemic diseases
		ALLEVIATING FACTORS	Improved lighting, medication, corrective glasses, rest or sleep, adequate hydration
		SETTING	Work environment, increased reading, computer work, night driving
		TIMING	With ageing, at night, after trauma, with or after a headache, seasonal, sudden onset, gradual onset

>>

>>

2. PAIN	Discomfort in the eye	
	QUALITY	Aching, sharp, throbbing, burning
	ASSOCIATED MANIFESTATIONS	Drainage, conjunctival injection, decreased vision, herpes simplex/herpes zoster, increased tearing, headache
	AGGRAVATING FACTORS	Foreign body in the eye, sunlight or very bright light, contact lenses, trauma, allergens
	ALLEVIATING FACTORS	Closing of eye or eyes, removal of contacts, medications, sunglasses, avoiding allergens
	SETTING	Work environment (increased reading or computer work), recreational area, outdoors
	TIMING	Sudden onset, gradual onset, with reading
3. DRAINAGE	Discharge of liquid from the eye	
	QUALITY	Type, colour
	ASSOCIATED MANIFESTATIONS	Crusting on the lids, pain, itching, redness of the eye or the lids, headache
	AGGRAVATING FACTORS	Allergens, eye make-up, chlorine, poor hygiene, upper respiratory infection
	ALLEVIATING FACTORS	Medications, hypoallergenic or no eye make-up, avoiding allergens, good hand washing
	SETTING	Outdoors, swimming pool
	TIMING	In the morning, continuous, intermittent, seasonal
4. ITCHING	Irritation that causes the consumer to scratch or rub	
	QUALITY	Mild, severe
	ASSOCIATED MANIFESTATIONS	Rhinitis, sneezing, drainage, burning sensation in the eye, gritty sensation in the eye, conjunctivitis, headache
	AGGRAVATING FACTORS	Allergens, contact lenses, eye make-up
	ALLEVIATING FACTORS	Medications, cold compresses to the eyes, removal of contacts, avoiding allergens and eye make-up
	SETTING	Indoors, outdoors
	TIMING	Seasonal, intermittent, continuous
5. DRYNESS	Reduced amount of lubricating secretions in the eye	
	ASSOCIATED MANIFESTATIONS	With systemic disease, redness of the eye, reduced tearing, itching
	AGGRAVATING FACTORS	Decreased humidity, wind, reading
	ALLEVIATING FACTORS	Artificial tears, humidified air
	SETTING	Outdoors, indoors with decreased humidity
	TIMING	With ageing, during the winter (decreased humidity), post-menopause

>>

PAST HEALTH HISTORY	The various components of the past health history are linked to eye pathology and eye-related information.		
	MEDICAL HISTORY	EYE-SPECIFIC	Myopia, hyperopia, strabismus, diplopia, astigmatism, glaucoma, cataracts, conjunctivitis, hordeolum, pterygium, blepharitis, chalazion, trachoma, age-related macular degeneration, prosthesis
		NON-EYE-SPECIFIC	Diabetes mellitus, renal disease, atherosclerotic disease, hypertension, thyroid disease, inflammatory processes, infections (viral or bacterial), immunosuppressive disease, nutritional disturbances, collagen vascular diseases, multiple sclerosis, myasthenia gravis, stroke, pituitary tumours
	SURGICAL HISTORY	Cataract extraction, lens implant, LASIK (laser-assisted in situ-keratomileusis; laser vision correction), repair of detached retina, neurosurgery, enucleation of eye, optic nerve decompression, prosthesis insertion	
	ALLERGIES	> Pollen: watery or itchy eyes > Insect stings: swelling around the eyes > Animal dander: watery or itchy eyes	
	MEDICATIONS	Carbonic anhydrase inhibitors, nonselective β-blockers, mast cell stabilisers, antibiotics, antihistamines, decongestants, corticosteroids, artificial tears, mydriatics, myotics	
	INJURIES AND ACCIDENTS	Foreign bodies; trauma to the eyes or surrounding structures of the eyes	
	SPECIAL NEEDS	Legal blindness, glasses/contacts for driving/reading	
	CHILDHOOD ILLNESSES	Rubella and visual sequelae (blindness), congenital syphilis, strabismus	
FAMILY HEALTH HISTORY	Eye diseases that are familial are listed.		
	Myopia, hyperopia, strabismus, colour blindness, cataracts, glaucoma, age-related macular degeneration, retinitis pigmentosa, retinoblastoma, neonatal blindness secondary to cataracts from mother contracting rubella in pregnancy.		
SOCIAL HISTORY	The components of the social history are linked to eye factors and pathology.		
	TOBACCO USE	Smoking is associated with macular degeneration and cataracts	
	TRAVEL HISTORY	Prolonged facial exposure to sun; facial exposure to contaminated waste	
	WORK ENVIRONMENT	Exposure to toxins/chemicals, infections, allergens, eye strain from long hours reading/computer use	
	STRESS	Can be linked with decreased vision	

PERSON-CENTRED HEALTH EDUCATION

When conducting a health assessment, opportunities for the provision of person-centred health education will arise. This is a significant consideration in relation to the assessment process for examination of the eyes due to conditions that are impacted by lifestyle choices or related to genetic risk. These occasions are identified as individualised education and may generate further data that can be added to the assessment. All education given should be documented so that in future, health professionals can assess the impact of previous information provided to the consumer. (Refer to Chapter 1 for initiating health education.) Refer to the following examples.

INDIVIDUALISED HEALTH EDUCATION INTERVENTIONS	
Assessing the consumer for the following health-related activities can assist in identifying the need for education about these factors. This information provides a bridge between the health maintenance activities and eye functions.	
Diet	Vitamin deficiencies may affect vision; uncontrolled glucose levels in consumers with diabetes can increase risk of diabetic neuropathy
Use of safety devices	Safety glasses, goggles or face shields for sports, job, or home projects; sunglasses in bright ultraviolet light
Health check-ups	Eye examination, intraocular pressure check, knowing family history to enable close monitoring of early signs and symptoms of family-related risk
Tobacco use	Smoking is associated with age-related macular degeneration

PLANNING FOR PHYSICAL EXAMINATION

The planning phase refers to evaluating subjective data to narrow the focus on physical examination, determining what objective data needs to be gathered, as well as considering the environment and equipment that will be required.

At this time, you will identify which of the four diagnostic techniques you will need to implement the physical examination, and how you will sequence these. For the physical examination of the eyes you will include inspection and palpation.

Objective data is:

> collected during the physical examination of the consumer

> usually collected after subjective data

> information that is measured or observed by the clinician as opposed to being reported by the consumer

> vital to the overall health assessment, to enable you to make clinical decisions that are representative of the whole.

Environment

Assessment of the eyes needs to be done in a suitable environment that can provide control of light levels, and often somewhere for the consumer to sit to increase his or her ability to be still during the examination.

Equipment

> Penlight
> Nonsterile gloves
> Snellen chart
> Snellen E chart
> Rosenbaum near vision pocket screening card
> Vision occluder
> Cotton-tipped applicator.

IMPLEMENTATION: CONDUCTING THE PHYSICAL EXAMINATION

Implementation of the physical examination requires you to consider your scope of practice as well. In this section, depending on your context, you may be performing foundation assessment with aspects of advanced assessment if you are practising in a specialised area.

Assessment of the eyes should be carried out in an orderly fashion, moving from the extraocular structures to the intraocular structures. The eye assessment usually includes testing of associated cranial nerves and can be performed in the following order:

1. Determination of visual acuity
2. Determination of visual fields
3. Assessment of the external eye and lacrimal apparatus
4. Evaluation of extraocular muscle function

EXAMINATION IN BRIEF: EYES

Examination of visual acuity

Inspection
> Distance vision
> Near vision
> Colour vision

Examination of visual fields

Examination of external eye and lacrimal apparatus

Inspection
> Eyelids, eyebrows and eyelashes
> Lacrimal apparatus

Palpation
> Lacrimal apparatus

Examination of extraocular muscle function

Inspection
> Corneal light reflex
> Cover/uncover test
> Cardinal fields of gaze

Examination of anterior segment structures

Inspection
> Conjunctiva
> Sclera
> Cornea
> Anterior chamber
> Iris
> Pupil
> Lens

General approach to examination of the eyes

1. Greet the consumer and explain the techniques that you will be using.
2. Use a quiet room that will be free from interruptions.
3. Ensure that the light in the room provides sufficient brightness to allow adequate observation of the consumer.
4. Place the consumer in an upright sitting position on the examination table.
5. Visualise the underlying structures during the assessment process to allow adequate description of findings.
6. Always compare the two eyes.
7. Use a systematic approach that is followed consistently each time the assessment is performed.

Examination of visual acuity

The examination of visual acuity (cranial nerve II) is a simple, non-invasive procedure that is carried out with the use of a Snellen chart and an occluder to cover the consumer's eye. The **Snellen chart** contains letters of various sizes with standardised visual acuity numbers at the end of each line of letters (**Figure 10.4A**). The numbers indicate the degree of visual acuity when the consumer is able to read that line of letters at a distance of 6 metres. For instance, a consumer who has a visual acuity of 6/24 can read at 6 metres what a consumer with 6/6 vision is able to read at 24 metres.

It is sometimes difficult to have a space of 6 metres available for the placement of the chart, but the distance can be simulated with the use of mirrors if necessary. For all vision screening, the chart should be illuminated with a diffuse light source to prevent spotlighting or glare. Otherwise 3-metre Snellen charts are also available. Please note that for the purposes of this examination you are testing for concerns and changes, not whether the person needs vision correction, as is done in ophthalmology clinics.

Advanced Assessment

70 ft – 21 m

G

60 ft – 18 m

WV

50 ft – 15 m

GSBE

40 ft – 12 m

NOIHW

30 ft – 9 m

JHERLC

20 ft – 6 m

NOSZLEPH

15 ft – 4.5 m

ULYTHBXPGO

10 ft – 3 m

SWMBWGCPTT

7 ft – 2.1 m

OHDCWNYZWAV

4 ft – 1.2 m

HNUOCI CRTWWDQMVBF

A. Snellen vision chart

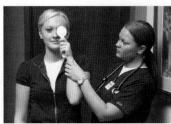

B. Assist the patient in occluding the eye

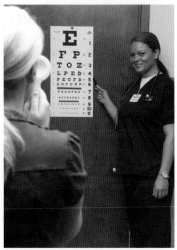

C. Assessing distance vision

FIGURE 10.4 Visual acuity testing

Inspection

Distance vision

E 1. Ask the consumer to stand or sit facing the Snellen chart at a distance of 6 metres.
2. If the consumer normally wears glasses, ask that they be removed. Contact lenses may be left in the eyes, but you must note that vision is corrected when documenting the results of the vision test. If possible, also note the strength of the contact lenses that the consumer is wearing.
3. Instruct the consumer to cover the left eye with the occluder (**Figure 10.4B**) and to read as many lines on the chart as possible.
4. Note the number at the end of the last line the consumer was able to read (**Figure 10.4C**).
5. If the consumer is unable to read the letters at the top of the chart, move the consumer closer to the chart. Note the distance at which the consumer is able to read the top line.
6. Repeat the test, occluding the right eye.
7. Repeat the test for the right eye with the left eye occluded.
8. If the consumer normally wears glasses, the test should be repeated with the consumer wearing the glasses, and this should be so noted (corrected or uncorrected).

N The consumer who has a visual acuity of 6/6 is considered to have normal visual acuity. This means that the consumer is able to read the line indicated at 6 metres in both eyes.

A The consumer is unable to read the chart with an uncorrected visual acuity of 6/9 in one eye, vision in the two eyes is different by two lines or more, or acuity is absent.

E Examination   **N** Normal findings   **A** Abnormal findings   **P** Pathophysiology

P The consumer may have a refractive error related to a difference in the refractive power of the cornea. **Figure 10.5A** illustrates how light rays focus on the retina in a normal eye. In **myopia** (near-sightedness), the axial length of the globe is longer than normal, resulting in the image not being focused directly on the retina; this condition can be changed with corrective lenses (see **Figure 10.5B**). If the consumer is amblyopic, no corrective lenses will improve vision. **Amblyopia** is the permanent loss of visual acuity resulting from strabismus that was not corrected in early childhood, or certain medical conditions (alcoholism, uraemia, diabetes mellitus).

P The consumer may have corneal opacities that are congenital, due to lesions that have scarred the cornea (e.g. herpes simplex), from trauma, or from degeneration and dystrophies.

P Visual acuity can be decreased because of opacities of the lens caused by senile or traumatic cataracts.

P Systemic autoimmune diseases such as inflammatory bowel disease, arthritis or other collagen vascular diseases can be associated with inflammation of the iris (iritis), which will affect visual acuity. Iritis can also be idiopathic.

P Inflammation of the retina caused by toxoplasmosis or by the presence of blood in the vitreous humour following haemorrhage can be responsible for decreased visual acuity.

P Systemic diseases, such as hypertension or diabetes mellitus, and trauma may damage the choroid and retina, causing decreased visual acuity.

P Visual acuity can be impaired by pathology affecting the optic nerve, such as multiple sclerosis, tumours or abscesses of the nerve itself, optic atrophy, papilloedema resulting from increased intracranial pressure, optic neuritis, or neovascularisation of the optic nerve.

E Examination   **N** Normal findings   **A** Abnormal findings   **P** Pathophysiology

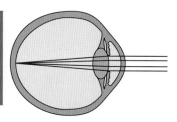

A. Normal eye
Light rays focus on the retina.

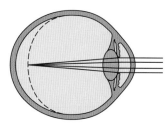

B. Myopia (nearsightedness)
Light rays focus in front
of the retina.

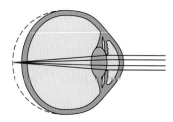

C. Hyperopia (farsightedness)
Light rays focus behind
the retina.

FIGURE 10.5 Eye refraction

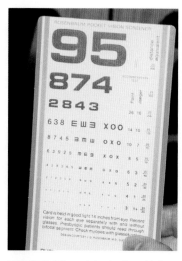

FIGURE 10.6 Near vision testing with the Rosenbaum pocket vision screener

Near vision

E 1. Use a pocket Snellen chart, Rosenbaum card (see **Figure 10.6**), or any printed material written at an appropriate reading level.
2. If the pocket vision card is available, have the consumer sit comfortably and hold the card 35 cm from the face without moving it.
3. Ask the consumer to read the smallest line possible (if other printed material is used, you will only be able to gain a general understanding of the consumer's near vision).

N Until the consumer is in their late 30s to late 40s, reading is generally possible at a distance of 35 cm.

A A consumer in this age range who cannot read at 35 cm is considered **presbyopic**. Younger persons may have difficulty seeing up close because they have **hyperopia**, or farsightedness (**Figure 10.5C**).

P The normal ageing process causes the lens to harden (nuclear sclerosis), decreasing its ability to change shape and therefore focus on near objects.

Colour vision

E Colour vision is usually tested in young children. If there is suspicion that the consumer has a colour vision deficit, have the consumer identify the primary colours on the Snellen chart or colours in the examining room. More specific testing is conducted by optometrists and ophthalmologists.

N The consumer should be able to identify colours correctly.

A The colour vision defect is designated as red/green, blue/yellow, or complete when the consumer sees only shades of grey.

P Defects in colour vision can result from diseases of the optic nerve, macular degeneration, pathology of the fovea centralis, nutritional deficiency, or may be hereditary.

Examination of visual fields

The confrontation technique is used to test visual fields of each eye (CN II). The visual field of each eye is divided into quadrants, and a stimulus is presented in each quadrant.

E 1. Sit or stand approximately 60–90 cm away from and opposite the consumer, with your eyes at the same level as the consumer's (see **Figure 10.7A**).
2. Have the consumer cover their right eye with the right hand or an occluder.
3. Cover your left eye in the same manner.
4. Have the consumer look at your uncovered eye with his or her uncovered eye.
5. Hold your free hand at arm's length equidistant from you and the consumer and move it or a held object, such as a pen, into your and the consumer's field of vision from nasal, temporal, superior, inferior and oblique angles.
6. Ask the consumer to say 'now' when your hand is seen moving into the field of vision. Use your own visual fields as the control for comparison to the consumer's.
7. Repeat the procedure for the other eye.

N The consumer is able to see the stimulus at about 90° temporally, 60° nasally, 50° superiorly and 70° inferiorly (**Figure 10.7B**).

A If the consumer is unable to identify movement that you perceive, a defect in the visual field is presumed. The portion of the visual field loss should be noted and the consumer referred to an optometrist or ophthalmologist.

P Defects in the consumer's visual field can be associated with tumours, strokes or neurological diseases such as glaucoma or retinal detachment.

E Examination **N** Normal findings **A** Abnormal findings **P** Pathophysiology Advanced Assessment

Examination of external eye and lacrimal apparatus

The assessment of the external eye includes the eyelids and the lacrimal apparatus. Pathology of the eyelids is among the most common eye complaints of consumers seeing a healthcare provider.

Inspection

Eyelids, eyebrows and eyelashes

E 1. Ask the consumer to sit facing you.
2. Observe the consumer's eyelids for drooping, infection, tumours or other abnormalities.
3. Note the distribution and symmetry of the eyelashes and eyebrows and any lesions.
4. Instruct the consumer to focus on an object or a finger held about 25–30 cm away and slightly above eye level.
5. Move the object or finger slowly downwards and observe for a white space of sclera between the upper lid and the limbus.
6. Observe the blinking of the eyes.
7. Ask the consumer to open the eyelids as wide as possible without touching them with their fingers.

N The eyelids should appear symmetrical with no drooping, infections or tumours of the lids. Eyelids of Asians normally slant upwards. When the eyes are focused in a normal frontal gaze, the lids should cover the upper portion of the iris. The consumer can raise both eyelids symmetrically (CN III). Slight **ptosis**, or drooping of the lid, can be normal. When the eye is closed, no portion of the cornea should be exposed. Normal lid margins are smooth, with the lashes evenly distributed and sweeping upwards from the upper lids and downwards from the lower lids. Eyebrows are present bilaterally and are symmetrical and without lesions or scaling.

A The consumer has either unilateral or bilateral, constant or intermittent ptosis of the lid (**Figure 10.8**). If part of the pupil is occluded, there may be wrinkling of the forehead above the affected eye in an attempt to compensate by using the frontalis muscle to lift the lid.

P Ptosis can be either congenital or acquired. In congenital ptosis, there is failure of the levator muscle to develop. This condition may be associated with pathology of the superior rectus muscle as well. If the ptosis is acquired, it is related to one of three factors:

1. Mechanical: heavy lids from lesions, adipose tissue, swelling or oedema
2. Myogenic: muscular diseases such as myasthenia gravis or multiple sclerosis
3. Neurogenic: paralysis from damage or interruption of the neural pathways such as cranial nerve III palsy

A An area of white sclera appears between the upper lid and the limbus, widening as the object is moved downwards.

P This condition is called lid lag and may indicate the presence of thyrotoxicosis or increased circulating levels of free thyroxine or triiodothyronine.

A The consumer is unable to bring about complete lid closure. This is generally a unilateral condition.

P This condition is referred to as **lagophthalmos** and can be associated with Bell's palsy, stroke, trauma or **ectropion** (everted right eyelid) (**Figure 10.9**).

A The turning inwards, or inversion, of the lower lid is referred to as **entropion** and can cause severe discomfort to the consumer as the eyelashes abrade the cornea (trichiasis) (**Figure 10.10**). If left untreated, it can cause inflammation, corneal scarring and eventual ulceration.

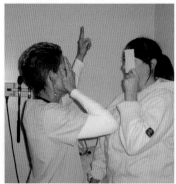

A. The nurse and patient should be approximately at an eye-to-eye level

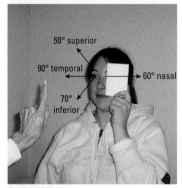

50° superior

90° temporal

60° nasal

70° inferior

B. Visual fields range

FIGURE 10.7 Testing visual fields by confrontation

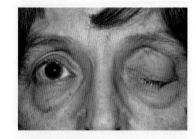

FIGURE 10.8 Ptosis
SCIENCE PHOTO LIBRARY/DR P MARAZZI

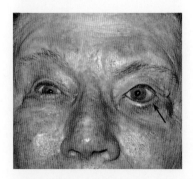

FIGURE 10.9 Ectropion right lower eyelid
COURTESY OF MARY A. HITCHO

E Examination   **N** Normal findings   **A** Abnormal findings   **P** Pathophysiology

UNIT 2

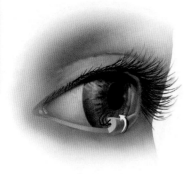

FIGURE 10.10 Entropion

P Entropion is caused by spasms or advancing age (senile). In senile entropion, there is a loss of muscle tone, which causes the lid to fold inwards.

A The turning outwards, or eversion, of the lower lid is referred to as ectropion and may be unilateral or bilateral. With ectropion, the lower lids appear to be sagging outwards.

P The normal ageing process can cause the muscles to lose their tone and relax, or they may be affected by Bell's palsy.

A The consumer exhibits excessive blinking that may or may not be accompanied by increased tearing and pain.

P The causes of excessive blinking can be voluntary or involuntary:

1. Voluntary: irritation to the cornea or the conjunctiva, or stress and anxiety (usually disappears when stimulus is removed)
2. Involuntary: tonic spasms of the orbicularis oculi muscle called blepharospasm; often seen in elderly individuals as well as in consumers with CN VII lesions, irritation of the eye, fatigue and stress

A The lids are black and blue, bluish, yellow or red, depending on race and skin colour.

P Colour changes in the lids can result from the following:

1. Redness: generalised redness is nonspecific; however, redness in the nasal half of the lid may indicate frontal sinusitis. Redness adjacent to the lower lid can indicate disease of the lacrimal sac or nasolacrimal duct, such as dacryocystitis; and redness in the temporal portion of the lid can result from **dacryoadenitis**, an inflammation of the lacrimal gland.
2. Bluish: cyanosis can result from orbital vein thrombosis, orbital tumours, or aneurysms in the orbit.
3. Black and blue: ecchymosis is caused by bleeding into the surrounding tissues following trauma (black eye).

A Swelling or oedema is noted in the eyelid.

P Swelling or oedema may be noted in nonocular conditions such as inflammation associated with allergies, herpes simplex virus, systemic diseases, medications that contribute to swelling from fluid overload, trichinosis, early myxoedema, thyrotoxicosis and contact dermatitis.

A There is an acute localised inflammation, tenderness and redness, with the consumer complaining of pain in the infected area. This is called a **hordeolum**.

P *Staphylococcus* is generally the infecting organism that causes a hordeolum.

There are two types of hordeolum:

1. Internal: affects the meibomian glands, is usually large, may point to the skin or conjunctival side of the lid
2. External: often called a 'stye', an infection of a sebaceous gland, usually points to the skin side of the lid, extending to the lid margin

Infections of the glands of the eyelid can be caused by improper removal of make-up, dry eyes or seborrhoea. There may be some connection between a hordeolum and increased handling of the lids in activities such as inserting and removing contact lenses.

A There is a chronic inflammation of the meibomian gland in either the upper or the lower lid. It generally forms over several weeks and, in many cases, points towards the conjunctival side of the lid, usually not on the lid margin. There is no redness or tenderness.

P This inflammation is referred to as a **chalazion** and its cause is unknown.

E Examination **N** Normal findings **A** Abnormal findings **P** Pathophysiology

A The lids are inflamed bilaterally and are red-rimmed, with scales clinging to both the upper and the lower lids. The consumer complains of itching and burning along the lid margins. There may also be some loss of the eyelashes.

P This is **blepharitis**, which may be either staphylococcal or seborrhoeic. Often a consumer has both types simultaneously. If the consumer has seborrhoeic infections elsewhere (scalp or eyebrows), it is more likely that the blepharitis is of the seborrhoeic type.

A Raised, yellow, nonpainful plaques are present on upper and lower lids near the inner canthus.

P These lesions are **xanthelasma**, a form of xanthoma frequently associated with hypercholesterolaemia.

A The eyebrows have scaling areas.

P This is caused by seborrhoea.

Lacrimal apparatus

E 1. Have the consumer sit facing you.
2. Identify the area of the lacrimal gland. Note any swelling or enlargement of the gland or elevation of the eyelid. Note any enlargement, swelling, redness, increased tearing or exudate in the area of the lacrimal sac at the inner canthus.
3. Compare to the other eye in order to determine whether there is unilateral or bilateral involvement.

N There should be no enlargement, swelling or redness; no large amount of exudate; and minimal tearing.

A There is inflammation and painful swelling beside the nose and near the inner canthus and possibly extending to the eyelid.

P **Dacryocystitis** is caused by inflammatory or neoplastic obstruction of the lacrimal duct.

Palpation

Lacrimal apparatus

E 1. To assess the lacrimal sac for obstruction, don gloves.
2. Gently press the index finger near the inner canthus, just inside the rim of the bony orbit of the eye.
3. Note any discharge from the punctum.

N There should not be excessive tearing or discharge from the punctum.

A Mucopurulent discharge is noted.

P Obstruction anywhere along the system from the lacrimal sac to the point at which the ducts empty below the inferior nasal turbinate can cause mucopurulent discharge.

A There is an overflowing of tears from the eye.

P This condition is epiphora, which is caused by obstruction of the lacrimal duct.

Examination of extraocular muscle function

Six extraocular muscles control the movement of each eye in relation to three axes: vertical, horizontal and oblique (see **Figure 10.11**). Assessing extraocular function is carried out by observing corneal light reflex or alignment, using the cover/uncover test, and by testing the six cardinal fields of gaze (cranial nerves III, IV and VI).

E Examination **N** Normal findings **A** Abnormal findings **P** Pathophysiology   Advanced Assessment

UNIT 2

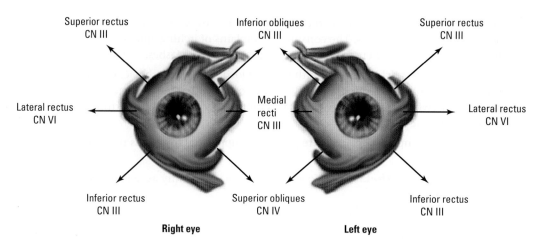

Superior rectus
CN III

Inferior obliques
CN III

Superior rectus
CN III

Lateral rectus
CN VI

Medial
recti
CN III

Lateral rectus
CN VI

Inferior rectus
CN III

Superior obliques
CN IV

Inferior rectus
CN III

Right eye

Left eye

FIGURE 10.11 Direction of movement of extraocular muscles

Inspection

Corneal light reflex (Hirschberg test)

E 1. Instruct the consumer to look straight ahead.
2. Focus a penlight on the corneas approximately 30 cm away from the consumer at the midline.
3. Observe the location of reflected light on the cornea.

N The reflected light (light reflex) should be seen symmetrically in the centre of each cornea.

A There is a discrepancy in the placement of one of the light reflections.

P Asymmetrical corneal light reflexes indicate an extraocular muscle imbalance that may be related to a variety of causes, depending on the consumer's age and medical condition: neurological, such as myasthenia gravis, multiple sclerosis, stroke, neuropathies of diabetes mellitus; uncorrected childhood strabismus (misalignment); trauma; or hypertension. The condition of one eye constantly being deviated is called **strabismus**, or tropia: **esotropia** is an inward turning of the eye; **exotropia** is an outward turning of the eye (**Figure 10.12**).

Cover/uncover test

E 1. Ask the consumer to look straight ahead and to focus on an object in the distance.
2. Place an occluder over the left eye for several seconds and observe for movement in the uncovered right eye.
3. As the occluder is removed, observe the covered eye for movement.
4. Repeat the procedure with the same eye, having the consumer focus on an object held close to the eye.
5. Repeat on the other side.

N If the eyes are in alignment, there will be no movement of either eye.

A If the uncovered eye shifts position as the other eye is covered, or if the covered eye shifts position as it is uncovered, a phoria, or latent misalignment of an eye, exists.

P This condition is a mild weakness elicited by the cover/uncover test and has two forms: **esophoria**, nasal or inwards drift, and **exophoria**, a temporal or outwards drift (see **Figure 10.13**).

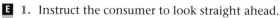

A. Right esotropia

B. Right exotropia

FIGURE 10.12 Strabismus

E Examination   **N** Normal findings   **A** Abnormal findings   **P** Pathophysiology   Advanced Assessment

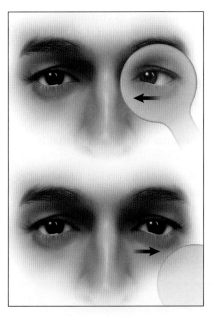

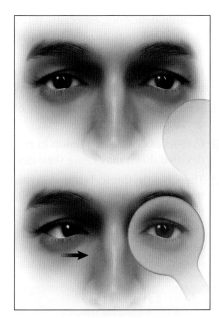

Left covered eye is weaker.
(Left exophoria)

Right uncovered eye is weaker.
(Right esophoria)

FIGURE 10.13 Cover/uncover test

Cardinal fields of gaze (extraocular muscle movements)

E
1. Place the consumer in a sitting position facing you.
2. Place your nondominant hand just under the consumer's chin or on top of the consumer's head as a reminder to hold the head still.
3. Ask the consumer to follow an object (finger, pencil or penlight) with the eyes.
4. Move the object through the six fields of gaze (**Figure 10.14**) in a smooth and steady manner, pausing at each extreme position to detect any **nystagmus**, or involuntary movement, and returning to the centre after each field is tested.
5. Note the consumer's ability to move the eyes in each direction.
6. Move the object forward to about 12 cm in front of the consumer's nose at the midline.
7. Observe for convergence of gaze.

N Both eyes should move smoothly and symmetrically in each of the six fields of gaze and converge on the held object as it moves towards the nose. A few beats of nystagmus with extreme lateral gaze can be normal. A number of abnormalities cause changes in a person's ability to demonstrate all cardinal fields. The most common findings are presented in the text.

A There is a lack of symmetrical eye movement in a particular direction.

P Inability to move the eye in a given direction indicates a weakness in the muscle responsible for moving the eye in that direction.

A Abnormal eye movements consist of failure of an eye to move outwards (CN VI), inability of an eye to move downwards when deviated inwards (CN IV), or other defects in movement (CN III).

P Traumatic ophthalmoplegia may be caused by fracture of the orbit near the foramen magnum, causing damage to the extraocular muscles or CN II, III, IV and VI. Basilar skull fractures that involve the cavernous sinus may also cause extraocular muscle palsy.

E Examination **N** Normal findings **A** Abnormal findings **P** Pathophysiology

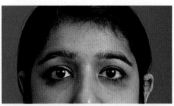

A. Eyes midline

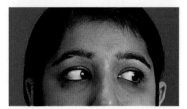

B. Left lateral gaze

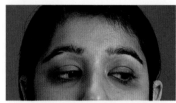

C. Left lateral inferior gaze

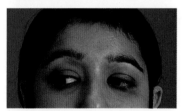

D. Right lateral inferior gaze

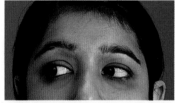

E. Right lateral gaze

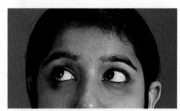

F. Right lateral superior gaze

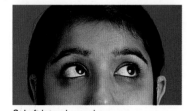

G. Left lateral superior gaze

FIGURE 10.14 Cardinal fields of gaze

P Vitamin deficiency, especially thiamine (which may occur in chronic alcoholism), may cause extraocular muscle palsy and nystagmus. Usually CN VI is affected.

P Herpes zoster, syphilis, scarlet fever, whooping cough and botulism are infections that may affect CN III, IV and VI, causing extraocular muscle palsy.

A If one eye deviates down and the other eye deviates up, it is called skew deviation.

P Cerebellar disease or a lesion in the pons on the same side as the eye that is deviated down may cause skew deviation.

A There is a rhythmic, beating, involuntary oscillation of the eyes as the object is held at points away from the midline. Movement is usually lateral, vertical or rotary. Nystagmus can be jerky, with fast and slow components, or rhythmic, similar to the pendulum of a clock.

P Nystagmus may be caused by a lesion in the brain stem, cerebellum, vestibular system, or along the visual pathways in the cerebral hemispheres.

HEALTH EDUCATION

Eye hygiene – assessment and education
If a consumer wears contact lenses, inquire what type is worn. Ask the consumer what the disinfecting criteria are for that type of lens, the frequency of lens replacement, and the daily duration of wear time. Determine whether the consumer is adhering to these protocols. Failure to comply with contact lens cleaning procedures, wear time, and recommended replacement schedule can lead to corneal abrasions and ocular infections.

Persons who use eye make-up should be sure to replace such items as old mascara and eyeliner frequently to avoid the possibility of bacterial colonisation. In the event of an episode of conjunctivitis, all items should be discarded to prevent reinfection from make-up that could be contaminated.

Examination of anterior segment structures
Inspection

Conjunctiva
To assess the bulbar conjunctiva:

E 1. Separate the lid margins with the fingers.
2. Have the consumer look up, down, and to the right and left.
3. Inspect the surface of the bulbar conjunctiva for colour, redness, swelling, exudate or foreign bodies. Note whether there is **injection** or redness around the cornea or towards the periphery.
4. With the thumb, gently pull the lower lid towards the cheek and inspect the surface of the bulbar conjunctiva for colour, inflammation, oedema, lesions or foreign bodies.

N The bulbar conjunctiva is transparent, with small blood vessels visible in it. It should appear white except for a few small blood vessels, which are normal. No swelling, injection, exudate, foreign bodies, or lesions are noted.

A P The palpebral conjunctiva is examined only when there is a concern about its condition. Examining the palpebral conjunctiva is advanced practice, and is usually not undertaken by most nurses.

A A yellow nodule is noted on the nasal side of the bulbar conjunctiva adjacent to the cornea. It may be on the temporal side as well. This lesion is painless unless it becomes inflamed.

E Examination **N** Normal findings **A** Abnormal findings **P** Pathophysiology

P This lesion is called a **pinguecula**. It is a nodular degeneration of the conjunctiva and is thought to be a result of increased exposure to ultraviolet light.

A A unilateral or bilateral triangle-shaped encroachment onto the conjunctiva is abnormal (**Figure 10.15**). This lesion always occurs nasally and remains painless unless it becomes ulcerated. If the lesion covers the cornea, loss of vision may occur.

P This lesion is called a **pterygium** and is caused by excessive ultraviolet light exposure.

A The consumer exhibits a sudden onset of a painless, bright red appearance on the bulbar conjunctiva.

P This is a subconjunctival haemorrhage and may result from the pressure exerted during coughing, sneezing, or a Valsalva manoeuvre. It can also be attributed to anticoagulant medications or uncontrolled hypertension.

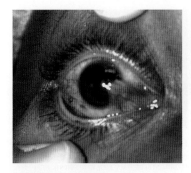

FIGURE 10.15 Pterygium

COURTESY OF SALIM I. BUTRUS, M.D., SENIOR ATTENDING, DEPARTMENT OF OPHTHALMOLOGY, WASHINGTON HOSPITAL CENTER, WASHINGTON, DC, & ASSOCIATE CLINICAL PROFESSOR, GEORGETOWN UNIVERSITY MEDICAL CENTER, WASHINGTON, DC.

Sclera

E While assessing the conjunctiva, inspect the sclera for colour, exudate, lesions and foreign bodies.

N In light-skinned individuals, the sclera should be white with some small, superficial vessels and without exudate, lesions or foreign bodies. In dark-skinned individuals, the sclera may have tiny brown patches of melanin, or a greyish-blue or 'muddy' colour.

A The colour of the sclera is uniformly yellow.

P This condition is known as jaundice or scleral icterus and is due to colouring of the sclera with bilirubin, which infiltrates all tissues of the body. This is an early manifestation of systemic conditions such as hepatitis, sickle cell disease, gallstones and physiological jaundice of the newborn.

A The sclera is blue.

P This finding is a distinctive feature of osteogenesis imperfecta and is due to the thinning of the sclera, which allows the choroid to show through.

REFLECTION IN PRACTICE

Corneal abrasion
You are examining a 55-year-old male with severe eye pain, photophobia and tearing. This is his fourth visit in the past 6 months. His previous three visits were for confirmed corneal abrasions caused by not wearing protective eye wear while servicing machinery (particularly while lying underneath the machinery looking up). While you are examining the consumer, he tells you that he hates wearing protective glasses because they fog up and he can't see what he is doing. What type of physical examination would you perform? List some strategies you could use to promote eye health in this consumer.

Cornea

E 1. Stand in front of the consumer.
2. Shine a penlight directly on the cornea.
3. Move the light laterally and view the cornea from that angle, noting colour, discharge and lesions.

N The corneal surface should be moist and shiny, with no discharge, cloudiness, opacities or irregularities.

A A greyish, well-circumscribed ulcerated area on the cornea is abnormal (**Figure 10.16**).

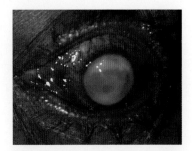

FIGURE 10.16 Corneal ulceration. Note the injection and hypopyon (purulent material in the anterior chamber), which frequently occur with corneal ulceration.

COURTESY OF SALIM I. BUTRUS, M.D., SENIOR ATTENDING, DEPARTMENT OF OPHTHALMOLOGY, WASHINGTON HOSPITAL CENTER, WASHINGTON, DC, & ASSOCIATE CLINICAL PROFESSOR, GEORGETOWN UNIVERSITY MEDICAL CENTER, WASHINGTON, DC.

E Examination   **N** Normal findings   **A** Abnormal findings   **P** Pathophysiology

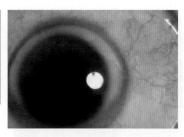

FIGURE 10.17 Arcus senilis

COURTESY OF SALIM I. BUTRUS, M.D., SENIOR ATTENDING, DEPARTMENT OF OPHTHALMOLOGY, WASHINGTON HOSPITAL CENTER, WASHINGTON, DC, & ASSOCIATE CLINICAL PROFESSOR, GEORGETOWN UNIVERSITY MEDICAL CENTER, WASHINGTON, DC.

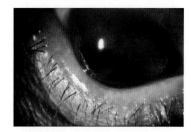

FIGURE 10.18 Keratoconus

COURTESY OF SALIM I. BUTRUS, M.D., SENIOR ATTENDING, DEPARTMENT OF OPHTHALMOLOGY, WASHINGTON HOSPITAL CENTER, WASHINGTON, DC, & ASSOCIATE CLINICAL PROFESSOR, GEORGETOWN UNIVERSITY MEDICAL CENTER, WASHINGTON, DC.

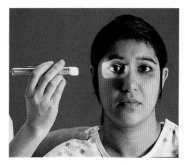

FIGURE 10.19 Examining the anterior chamber

P The most common cause of this condition is a corneal ulceration resulting from a bacterial infection.

A A tree-like configuration on the corneal surface is identified. The consumer complains of mild discomfort, photophobia and, in some cases, blurred vision (depending on the location of the lesions).

P This type of ulceration is caused by the herpes simplex virus. The consumer usually has a history of having had a cold sore somewhere on the face.

A There is a hazy grey ring about 2 mm in width just inside the limbus (**Figure 10.17**).

P This common finding is **arcus senilis**, a bilateral, benign degeneration of the peripheral cornea. It can be found at any age but is most common in older individuals. If found in a young person, may be associated with hypercholesterolaemia.

A A steamy or cloudy cornea is abnormal. The consumer also has ocular pain.

P Glaucoma is caused by increased intraocular pressure. Refer to anterior chamber assessment.

A Any irregularities in the appearance of the cornea are abnormal.

P Keratoconus (**Figure 10.18**) is the conical protrusion of the centre of the cornea. It is a noninflammatory condition in which the cornea thins, sometimes leading to the need for corneal transplant surgery.

P A corneal scar forms at the site of past injury or inflammation.

P Corneal laceration can occur secondary to trauma.

Anterior chamber

The anterior chamber is that compartment of the eye found between the cornea and the iris. The space between the flat plane of the iris and the periphery of the cornea must be adequate to allow drainage of aqueous fluid out of the eye. If this angle is too narrow, drainage is inadequate, the pressure of the aqueous fluid in the anterior chamber increases, and glaucoma develops. If intraocular fluid pressure remains high, optic nerve damage and visual field loss occur.

To differentiate a normal from a narrowed angle:

E 1. Face the consumer and shine a light obliquely through the anterior chamber from the lateral side towards the nasal side (see **Figure 10.19**).
2. Observe the distribution of light in the anterior chamber (see **Figure 10.20**).
3. Repeat the procedure with the other eye.

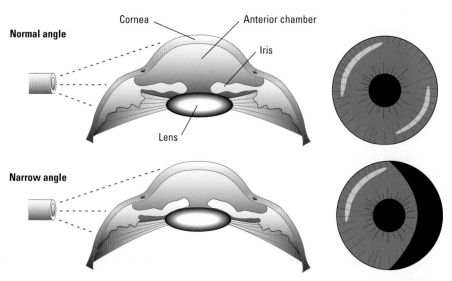

FIGURE 10.20 Evaluating the angle of the anterior chamber

E Examination   **N** Normal findings   **A** Abnormal findings   **P** Pathophysiology   Advanced Assessment

CHAPTER 10

N In a normal eye, the entire iris will be illuminated.

A The eye has a narrow angle, with the decreased space between the iris and the cornea appearing as a crescent-shaped shadow on the far portion of the iris.

P The narrow angle is an anatomic variant that can predispose an individual to the development of angle-closure glaucoma. As ageing progresses, the lens thickens, which may cause even further narrowing of the angle.

Iris

E With the penlight, inspect the iris for colour, nodules and vascularity.

N Normally, the colour is evenly distributed over the iris, although there can be a mosaic variant. It is normally smooth and without apparent vascularity.

A There is a heavily pigmented, slightly elevated area visible in the iris.

P This lesion can be a benign iris naevus or a malignant melanoma. An iris naevus is much more common than melanoma.

A The inferior portion of the iris is obscured by blood.

P This is a **hyphaema** and is caused by bleeding from vessels in the iris as a result of direct trauma to the globe. It can also occur as a result of eye surgery.

A An absent wedge portion of the iris is abnormal.

P The shape of the iris changes after surgical removal of a cataract; the pupil may also have an irregular shape.

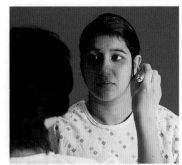

A. Starting position with penlight to side of pupil

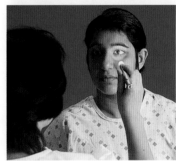

B. Move the penlight directly in front of the pupil

FIGURE 10.21 Pupil assessment

Pupil

E 1. Stand in front of the consumer in a darkened room.
2. Note the shape and size of the pupils in millimetres.
3. Move a penlight from the side to the front of one eye without allowing the light to shine on the other eye (see **Figure 10.21**).
4. Observe the pupillary reaction in that eye. This is the direct light reflex. Note the size of the pupil receiving light stimulus and the speed of pupillary response to light.
5. Repeat in the other eye.
6. Move the penlight in front of one eye, and observe the other eye for pupillary constriction. This is the consensual light reflex.
7. Repeat the procedure on the other eye.
8. Instruct the consumer to shift the gaze to a distant object for 30 seconds.
9. Instruct the consumer to then look at your finger or an object held in your hand about 10 cm from the consumer.
10. Note the reaction and size of the pupils. **Accommodation** occurs when pupils constrict and converge to focus on objects at close range.

N The pupils should be deep black, round, and of equal diameter, ranging from 2 to 6 mm. Pupils should constrict briskly to direct and consensual light and to accommodation (CN III). Small differences in pupil size (**anisocoria**) may be normal in some people.

A The pupil that constricts to less than 2 mm in diameter is termed miotic. The pupil that dilates to more than 6 mm in diameter is termed mydriatic.

P Abnormal pupillary size can be caused by medications such as sympathomimetics or parasympathomimetics, iritis, or disorders such as CN III paralysis, which can occur as a result of a carotid artery aneurysm. These abnormalities may also be due to nerve damage or trauma (see for further pathologies).

A The pupil has an irregular shape.

P This is a common finding associated with the surgical removal of cataracts and iridectomy.

E Examination   N Normal findings   A Abnormal findings   P Pathophysiology   Advanced Assessment

A When the direct light reflex is defective, the pupil dilates in response to light, but consensual reaction is appropriate. This is called a Marcus Gunn pupil.

P Optic nerve damage in the optic chiasm, such as in trauma, results in destruction of the afferent pathways of the pupillary light reflex (deafferented pupil).

A The hippus phenomenon occurs after the pupil has been stimulated by direct light. Light causes the pupil to constrict, but then the pupil appears to rhythmically vacillate in size from a larger to a smaller diameter.

P Hippus may be caused by a lesion in the midbrain.

A The presence of midposition, round, regular and fixed (5–6 mm) pupils that may show hippus is abnormal.

P These signs usually indicate midbrain damage that interrupts the light reflex but may leave accommodation intact.

Lens

E 1. Stand in front of the consumer.
2. Shine a penlight directly on the pupil. The lens is behind the pupil.
3. Note the colour.

N The lens is transparent in colour.

A One or more of the pupils are not deep black.

P In an adult, a pearly grey appearance of one or both pupils may indicate an opacity (cloudiness) in the lens (cataract) (see **Figure 10.22**).

P A senile cataract is the most common type. Progressively blurred distance vision is the main symptom, although near vision may be improved because of greater convexity of the lens.

P A unilateral cataract may occur soon after eye injury caused by a foreign body. Along with the lens opacity, there may be intraocular haemorrhage or aqueous or vitreous humour leaking from the globe. The consumer reports an immediate blurring of vision.

P Bilateral cataracts found in infants or young children are congenital cataracts. These cataracts are probably genetically determined, although maternal rubella in the first trimester can also be responsible.

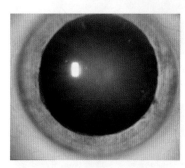

FIGURE 10.22 Cataract

COURTESY OF SALIM I. BUTRUS, M.D., SENIOR ATTENDING, DEPARTMENT OF OPHTHALMOLOGY, WASHINGTON HOSPITAL CENTER, WASHINGTON, DC, & ASSOCIATE CLINICAL PROFESSOR, GEORGETOWN UNIVERSITY MEDICAL CENTER, WASHINGTON, DC.

TABLE 10.2 Pupil abnormalities

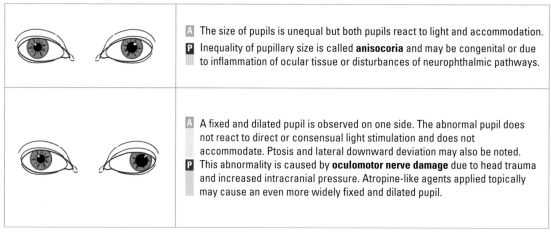

	A The size of pupils is unequal but both pupils react to light and accommodation. **P** Inequality of pupillary size is called **anisocoria** and may be congenital or due to inflammation of ocular tissue or disturbances of neurophthalmic pathways.
	A A fixed and dilated pupil is observed on one side. The abnormal pupil does not react to direct or consensual light stimulation and does not accommodate. Ptosis and lateral downward deviation may also be noted. **P** This abnormality is caused by **oculomotor nerve damage** due to head trauma and increased intracranial pressure. Atropine-like agents applied topically may cause an even more widely fixed and dilated pupil.

>>

E Examination   **N** Normal findings   **A** Abnormal findings   **P** Pathophysiology   ▓ Advanced Assessment

>> **TABLE 10.2** *continued*

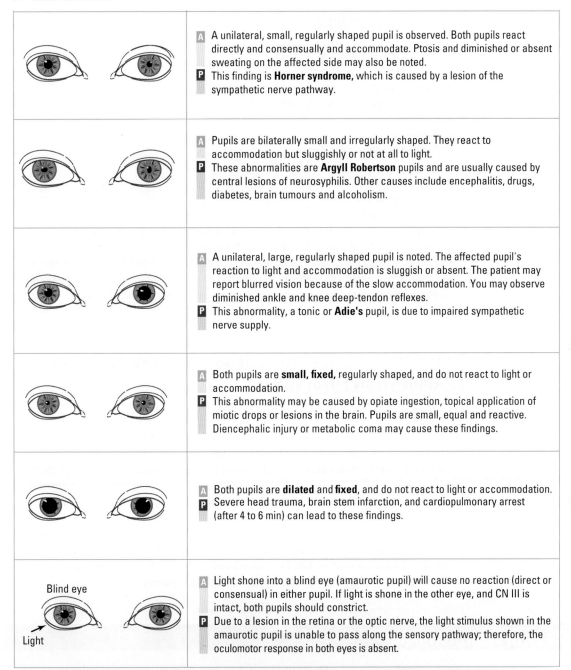

	A A unilateral, small, regularly shaped pupil is observed. Both pupils react directly and consensually and accommodate. Ptosis and diminished or absent sweating on the affected side may also be noted.
	P This finding is **Horner syndrome,** which is caused by a lesion of the sympathetic nerve pathway.
	A Pupils are bilaterally small and irregularly shaped. They react to accommodation but sluggishly or not at all to light.
	P These abnormalities are **Argyll Robertson** pupils and are usually caused by central lesions of neurosyphilis. Other causes include encephalitis, drugs, diabetes, brain tumours and alcoholism.
	A A unilateral, large, regularly shaped pupil is noted. The affected pupil's reaction to light and accommodation is sluggish or absent. The patient may report blurred vision because of the slow accommodation. You may observe diminished ankle and knee deep-tendon reflexes.
	P This abnormality, a tonic or **Adie's** pupil, is due to impaired sympathetic nerve supply.
	A Both pupils are **small, fixed,** regularly shaped, and do not react to light or accommodation.
	P This abnormality may be caused by opiate ingestion, topical application of miotic drops or lesions in the brain. Pupils are small, equal and reactive. Diencephalic injury or metabolic coma may cause these findings.
	A Both pupils are **dilated** and **fixed**, and do not react to light or accommodation.
	P Severe head trauma, brain stem infarction, and cardiopulmonary arrest (after 4 to 6 min) can lead to these findings.
Blind eye Light	**A** Light shone into a blind eye (amaurotic pupil) will cause no reaction (direct or consensual) in either pupil. If light is shone in the other eye, and CN III is intact, both pupils should constrict.
	P Due to a lesion in the retina or the optic nerve, the light stimulus shown in the amaurotic pupil is unable to pass along the sensory pathway; therefore, the oculomotor response in both eyes is absent.

REFLECTION IN PRACTICE

Consumer with potential multiple eye pathologies

Sally is a 82-year-old woman with a history of severe asthma and hypertension. Sally lives with her son Max who is a smoker. Sally has taken oral corticosteroids for 5 years to help control her asthma. Today, she presents with seeing halos around lights, scratchy dry eyes and on review Sally is found to be within the morbidly obese weight range with a BMI of 41. What questions would you pose to this consumer? Knowing Sally's history, describe some possible findings on the physical examination of her eyes.

E Examination   **N** Normal findings   **A** Abnormal findings   **P** Pathophysiology

CLINICAL REASONING

Practice tip: Cataract risk factors

Consider the following when assessing consumers:

> Increasing age
> Ultraviolet light exposure (sun exposure)
> Hypertension
> Obesity
> Previous eye injuries or surgery
> Smoking
> Diabetes
> Steroid use (prolonged)
> Excessive alcohol use

Since cataract correction is one of the most common eye-related reasons people seek health care (second only to refractive error correction), understanding the risk factors for people when undertaking assessment for other health reasons can lead to early detection. Applying these risk factors to consumers who do not have cataracts yet can also provide you with an opportunity for health education to help people prevent their development or at least seek help early.

(MAYO CLINIC, 2021)

EVALUATION OF HEALTH ASSESSMENT AND PHYSICAL EXAMINATION FINDINGS

In the evaluation phase of a health assessment, the focus is on ensuring the data gathered is complete, accurate and documented appropriately (see case study as an example of the focused assessment; see Chapter 22 for a comprehensive health assessment). In evaluating the data you should:

> draw on your critical thinking and problem-solving skills to make sound clinical decisions
> act on abnormal data (includes communicating findings to other health professionals)
> ensure documentation reflects the outcomes of the clinical decisions/actions taken (refer to Chapter 3, which discusses in detail why documentation is so important and how this may be undertaken in different health settings).

The case study that follows steps you through this process.

CASE STUDY

THE CONSUMER WITH SENILE CATARACT

This case study illustrates the application and the objective documentation of the eye assessment.

Mr Teroma Kunle, a 59-year-old man, presents complaining of gradually decreasing vision in both eyes.

HEALTH HISTORY

CONSUMER PROFILE	59-year-old male of Nigerian descent
CHIEF COMPLAINT	'Watching television and reading is not as easy as it used to be, even with my glasses.' The consumer complains he is finding it more difficult to carry out his daily activities and recognise people at a distance. He also states he is starting to avoid driving at night due to the glare interrupting his vision.
HISTORY OF THE PRESENT ILLNESS	The consumer has noticed a gradual deterioration in vision over the last 12 months. His symptoms started with bilateral blurred distance vision. Consultations with an optometrist and new prescription glasses have improved but not resolved the problem. He also complains of increasing problems with glare, particularly in bright light or when driving at night, which has been getting progressively worse. The consumer denies any pain or recent injury.

>>

>>

PAST HEALTH HISTORY	MEDICAL HISTORY	Hypertension since age 48 Hyperlipidaemia since age 52
	SURGICAL HISTORY	Denies any previous ocular surgery
	ALLERGIES	Nil known
	MEDICATIONS	Hydrochlorothiazide 25 mg every morning Atorvastatin calcium 10 mg every day Denies using any ocular medications
	COMMUNICABLE DISEASES	Denies
	INJURIES AND ACCIDENTS	Previous fractured toes as a young man in Nigeria. Now is missing smallest toe from left foot
	SPECIAL NEEDS	Wears glasses for distance and near correction (bifocal lenses)
	BLOOD TRANSFUSIONS	Denies
	CHILDHOOD ILLNESSES	Chickenpox, age 12, without sequelae Measles, age 15, without sequelae
	IMMUNISATIONS	All vaccinations completed when emigrated to Australia at age 15; has yearly influenza vaccine
FAMILY HEALTH HISTORY	Family history unknown due to being orphaned as a 12-year-old.	
SOCIAL HISTORY	Widowed with 2 children	
	ALCOHOL USE	Three standard drinks per day, usually beer
	TOBACCO USE	Smoker; smokes half pack per day × 46 years (23 yr pack history); denies use of pipes and cigars
	DRUG USE	Denies
	DOMESTIC AND INTIMATE PARTNER VIOLENCE	Denies
	SEXUAL PRACTICE	Widowed, denies recent sexual partners
	TRAVEL HISTORY	Denies recent interstate or international travel in the past 10 years
	WORK ENVIRONMENT	Retired builder
	HOME ENVIRONMENT	Lives at home, with eldest daughter and her two children (aged 12 and 9); smoke detectors and safety switch fitted in home
	HOBBIES AND LEISURE ACTIVITIES	Rebuilding classic cars, gardening, watching sports
	STRESS	Denies
	EDUCATION	Bridging schooling on arriving to Australia, left at 17 to undertake building apprenticeship
	ECONOMIC STATUS	Middle class 'blue collar worker'
	MILITARY SERVICE	None
	RELIGION	Christian
	CULTURAL BACKGROUND	Nigerian descent
	ROLES AND RELATIONSHIPS	Close to children; limited extended family; several close friends from classic cars interest group
	CHARACTERISTIC PATTERNS OF DAILY LIVING	Wakes at 7 a.m., large breakfast with grandchildren most days, either works in shed on cars, or supports daughter with errands for children; lunches at home; usually has an afternoon rest; gardens most days; watches TV and goes to bed around 11 p.m.

>>

>>

HEALTH MAINTENANCE ACTIVITIES	SLEEP	7–8 hours of sleep each night; often feels tired. Poor sleeper	
	DIET	Eats traditional dishes weekly with children	
	EXERCISE	Gardening. No formal exercise program	
	STRESS MANAGEMENT	Denies any	
	USE OF SAFETY DEVICES	Uses seat belt in car; does not wear sunglasses when out of doors	
	HEALTH CHECK-UPS	Sees primary care provider every 6–9 months for management of hypertension and hyperlipidaemia; has not visited dentist in years; visits optometrist every 12–18 months for examination	

PHYSICAL EXAMINATION

EXAMINATION OF VISUAL ACUITY	INSPECTION	DISTANCE VISION (WITH GLASSES)	> 6/12 right eye, 6/9 left eye > 6/9 with both eyes
		37.2 MM	Impaired, N 8 (blurred) both eyes
		COLOUR VISION TESTING (ISHIHARA COLOUR TEST PLATES)	Normal (15/15 right and left eye)
EXAMINATION OF VISUAL FIELDS		Confrontation field testing normal, no field defects detected	
EXAMINATION OF EXTERNAL EYE AND LACRIMAL APPARATUS	INSPECTION AND PALPATION	EYELIDS, EYEBROWS AND EYELASHES	Normal, no abnormalities detected
		LACRIMAL APPARATUS	No abnormalities detected
EXAMINATION OF EXTRAOCULAR MUSCLE FUNCTION	INSPECTION	CORNEAL LIGHT REFLEX COVER/UNCOVER TEST CARDINAL FIELDS OF GAZE	Only need to be tested if the consumer is complaining of double vision (not performed on this consumer)
EXAMINATION OF ANTERIOR SEGMENT STRUCTURES	INSPECTION	CONJUNCTIVA	Transparent; no swelling, injection, foreign bodies or lesions noted
		SCLERA	No abnormalities detected
		CORNEA	Clear, no opacities or irregularities noted
		ANTERIOR CHAMBER	Clear and deep
		IRIS	No irregularities noted
		PUPIL	Size – 3 mm Symmetry – equal Reaction to light – brisk in right and left eyes to direct and consensual light
		LENS	Pearly grey clouding noted when illuminated with torch
	OPHTHALMOSCOPY WITH DIRECT OPHTHALMOSCOPE	Posterior structures appear normal. View of optic disc and retina blurred due to opacity in the ocular media (advanced practice only)	
	AMSLER GRID TESTING	> Normal > No distortion or blank spots noted > Evenly distributed slight blur	

EVALUATION AND CLINICAL REASONING FOR CASE STUDY

The assessment and clinical decisions you make should reflect your scope of practice. For example, advanced practice health professionals, such as nurse practitioners and remote area nurses with endorsement, may be able to make diagnostic decisions and prescribe medications without referring to a medical officer.

Fundamentally, all health professionals collect, evaluate and act on consumer-focused health information, which will at times include referral to, or collaboration with, other healthcare team members. Nurses assess consumer responses to interventions and determine when to escalate key changes in a consumer's condition. The clinical reasoning cycle provides health professionals with a framework to consider all this information in a meaningful way for planning consumer care. These phases are stepped out below, and draw on information presented and collected during the health history and physical examination. We then work through the cycle components that are relevant to this case study (cycle components are bolded).

For Teroma Kunle, the significant data that needs to be considered includes the following.

Collecting cues/information

Recall and Review: In the first instance you will need to reflect on what you know about cataracts, their formation and risk factors.

Chief complaint and history of present illness

> Bilateral progressive decrease in distance and near vision over the last 12 months.
> Symptoms started with bilateral blurred distance vision; for example, being unable to recognise people at a distance.
> Complains of glare, especially when driving at night – therefore has started avoiding this activity.
> Changes to his prescription glasses have improved but not resolved the problem.

Processing information

Interpret: These symptoms and details of history outline the scope of the issue for this consumer and how it is affecting his wellbeing and ability to self-manage this deviation from normal health. It is important to take the consumer's age, previous occupation and health protection practices into consideration along with the symptoms described.

Discriminate: There is an increasing impact on his activities of daily living, for example driving at night, which led him to consult an optometrist.

Relate: New glasses have improved but not resolved the issue.

Medications

> Hydrochlorothiazide 25 mg every morning
> Atorvastatin calcium 10 mg every day

Tobacco use

> Smoker for 46 years

Interpret and Discriminate: This element of the consumer history is noteworthy as smoking is associated with higher risk of developing cataracts.

Hobbies and leisure activities

> Rebuilding classic cars, gardening and watching sports

Use of safety devices

> Does not wear sunglasses when out of doors

Interpret and Discriminate: His previous work was an outdoor role and all his hobbies involve likely increased exposure to sunlight (UV light), which is associated with higher risk of developing cataracts.

Relate: As the consumer's leisure activities involve increased exposure to UV light, the non-use of UV filtering glasses is significant.

Visual acuity

> Decrease in distance and near visual acuity

Interpret and Discriminate: Visual acuity is measured using the consumer's corrective lenses if normally worn.

Infer: This rules out any refractive error; for example, myopia or hypermetropia.

Relate: Visual acuity can be decreased due to opacities in the ocular media, including the cornea, lens or vitreous.

Visual field testing

> Visual fields are normal using confrontation testing

Infer: Normal visual fields generally rule out glaucoma, retinal detachment and vision loss as the result of tumours, strokes or other neurological diseases.

Pupil examination

> Pupils are equal, round and 3 mm in diameter. They react to direct and consensual light. No relative afferent papillary defect (RAPD) is noted.

Relate: RAPD is never present in a consumer whose visual loss is due to cataract.

Examination of anterior segment structures using a torch

> Cornea – clear and regular
> Lens – pearly grey appearance in both pupils

Relate: A cloudy or pearly grey appearance of the lens when illuminated with a torch indicates opacity in the lens (cataract).

Ophthalmoscopy with direct ophthalmoscope

> Blurred view of optic disc and retina on ophthalmoscopy

Relate: Blurring of the ophthalmoscopic view into the posterior segment indicates an opacity in the ocular media, in this case the lens.

Putting it all together – synthesise information

The nurse in this case would note the significant features of the history, the presenting illness and the physical examination findings, and refer to the medical officer.

Important findings in the consumer history and history of the presenting illness include:

> Risk factors for cataract
  - Age
  - Tobacco use
  - Recreational UV light exposure related to hobbies and leisure activities
  - Non-use of UV-light-filtering sunglasses when out of doors
> Symptoms and history of presenting illness indicating senile cataract development
  - Bilateral, progressive decrease in ability to see clearly both at distance and near
  - Glare, especially when driving at night
  - Improved but not resolved with corrective lenses
  - No pain or recent injury
  - Unknown family history of eye diseases, including glaucoma, retinal detachment and macular degeneration
> Significant physical examination findings include:
  - decreased distance and near visual acuity
  - normal visual fields
  - normal pupils, no RAPD detected
  - cloudy, pearly grey appearance of lens when examined using torch; all other anterior segment structures normal
  - blurred view of the optic disc and retina on ophthalmoscopy indicating an opacity in the ocular media (in this case the lens).

Actions based on assessment findings

The nurse should also provide additional consumer education for interventions that do not require a doctor's order, such as:

1 use of safety devices such as UV-filtering sunglasses when sun exposure is likely

2 advice and strategies to aid the cessation of smoking, advice and referral to quit smoking services

3 developing an awareness of safety issues associated with decreased visual acuity; for example, safety when driving and decreased depth perception. The nurse should be aware of the vision requirements for driving and be able to advise the consumer if they do not meet these requirements.

The final step in the process is accurate documentation. The nurse must document findings, referrals, interventions, advice and education given. The consumer would then be reassessed following definitive diagnosis and medical interventions for his ongoing health maintenance.

CHAPTER RESOURCES

REVIEW QUESTIONS

For answers to these questions, see Answer section at the end of the book.

1. Which of the following is the eye structure that is the round red structure in the inner canthus and contains sebaceous glands?
   a. Limbus
   b. Cornea
   c. Sclera
   d. Caruncle

2. What are some of the normal ageing changes that can be observed during the eye examination? Select all that apply.
   a. Drusen, or small white dots in the fundus
   b. Dry eyes
   c. Loss of peripheral vision
   d. Decreasing ability to focus on near objects
   e. Lagophthalmos
   f. Arcus senilis

3. A 40-year-old consumer tells you that he has noticed his right eye is turning in towards his nose and this is not normal for him. What condition is this consumer describing?
   a. Amblyopia
   b. Myopia
   c. Esotropia
   d. Hyperopia

4. Your patient has one pupil that is 1 mm smaller than the other. This finding is called:
   a. Consensual response
   b. Anisocoria
   c. Accommodation
   d. Strabismus

5. Which non-eye specific medical history may be linked to eye pathology? Select all that apply.
   a. Renal disease
   b. Thyroid disease
   c. Long bone fractures
   d. Carpal tunnel syndrome
   e. Diabetes mellitus
   f. Surgical emphysema

6. The consumer's bulbar conjunctiva has a bright red appearance. What condition may have caused this clinical finding?
   a. Ultraviolet light
   b. Warfarin therapy
   c. Osteogenesis imperfecta
   d. Cholecystitis

7. Which of the following physical examination findings is a consumer likely to exhibit in glaucoma?
   a. Steamy, cloudy cornea
   b. Conical protrusion of the centre of the cornea
   c. Greyish, well-circumscribed ulcerated area on the cornea
   d. Tree-like configuration on the cornea
8. A yellow sclera can be seen in which of the following conditions in adults? Select all that apply.
   a. Gallstones
   b. Hepatitis
   c. Sickle cell anaemia
   d. Osteogenesis imperfecta
   e. Pterygium
   f. Bacterial conjunctivitis
9. Oculomotor nerve damage may be seen with which of the following symptoms?
   a. Fixed and dilated pupil on one side that does not react to light and does not accommodate. Ptosis and lateral deviation of the eye is also present.
   b. Fixed pinpoint pupil on one side.
   c. Pupils are bilaterally small and irregularly shaped. React to accommodation but not to light.
   d. One pupil is larger than the other, regularly shaped, reacting to light and accommodation may be absent or sluggish.

CS CLINICAL SKILLS

The following Clinical Skill is relevant to this chapter and can be found in Tollefson & Hillman, *Clinical Psychomotor Skills*, 8th edition:
> 27 Healthcare teaching.

FURTHER RESOURCES

> Eyerobics – Natural eyesight improvement site: http://eyerobics.com.au/eyesight.html
> Macular Degeneration New Zealand: http://www.mdnz.org.nz/
> Save our sight New Zealand: http://www.saveoursight.co.nz
> Vision 2020 Australia: http://www.vision2020australia.org.au/
> Vision Australia: http://www.visionaustralia.org.au
> Vision Initiative: http://www.visioninitiative.org.au

REFERENCES

Australian Department of Health and Aged Care. (2023). Eye health and vision. Retrieved 5 May 2023 from http://www.health.gov.au/internet/main/publishing.nsf/Content/eye-health

Australian Institute of Health and Welfare (AIHW). (2021a). Eye health, AIHW, Australian Government. Retrieved 5 December 2022 from https://www.aihw.gov.au/reports/eye-health/eye-health/contents/about

Australian Institute of Health and Welfare (AIHW). (2021b). Indigenous eye health measures 2021. Cat. no. IHW 242. Retrieved 5 December 2022 from https://www.aihw.gov.au/getmedia/efec3a5e-657e-412f-9e4e-d6503c8b0cf6/aihw-ihw-242.pdf%C2%A0

Australian Institute of Health and Welfare (AIHW). (2022). Australia's health 2022 in brief. Australia's health series no. 18. Cat. no. AUS 241. Canberra: AIHW, Australian Government.

Blind Low Vision New Zealand (NZ). (2022). Statistics and research: Cost of vision loss in New Zealand. Retrieved 5 December 2022 from https://blindlowvision.org.nz/news/cost-of-vision-loss-in-2021/

Centre for Eye Research Australia (CERA). (2022). Glaucoma. Retrieved 14 December 2022 from https://www.cera.org.au/conditions/glaucoma/

Chilibeck, C., Mathan, J. J., Ng, S. G., & McKelvie, J. (2020). Cataract surgery in New Zealand: access to surgery, surgical intervention rates and visual acuity. *New Zealand Medical Journal, 133*(1524), 40–9. PMID: 33119569.

Glaucoma Australia. (2022). *What is Glaucoma?* Retrieved 12 December 2022 from https://glaucoma.org.au/what-is-glaucoma

Glaucoma Research Foundation. (2022). Glaucoma worldwide: A growing concern. Retrieved 12 December 2022 from https://glaucoma.org/glaucoma-worldwide-a-growing-concern/

Hoskin, A. (2020). Eye injuries: The hidden costs revealed, mivision *The Ophthalmic Journal*. Retrieved 12 December 2022 from https://mivision.com.au/2020/04/eye-injuries-the-hidden-costs-revealed/

Kamińska, A., Pinkas, J., Wrześniewska-Wal, I., Ostrowski, J., & Jankowski, M. (2023). Awareness of common eye diseases and their risk factors – a nationwide cross-sectional survey among adults in Poland. *International Journal of Environmental Research and Public Health, 20*(4), 3594. https://doi.org/10.3390/ijerph20043594

Macular Degeneration New Zealand. (2020). Macular degeneration New Zealand. Retrieved 5 December 2022 from https://www.mdnz.org.nz/

Macular Disease Foundation Australia. (n.d.(a)). Age-related macular degeneration. Retrieved 12 December 2022 from https://www.mdfoundation.com.au/about-macular-disease/age-related-macular-degeneration/amd-overview/

Macular Disease Foundation Australia. (n.d.(b)). Diabetic retinopathy. Retrieved 12 December 2022 from https://www.mdfoundation.com.au/about-macular-disease/diabetic-eye-disease/about-diabetic-retinopathy/

Mayo Clinic (2021). Cataracts. Retrieved 8 August 2022 from https://www.mayoclinic.org/diseases-conditions/cataracts/symptoms-causes/syc-20353790

Pagano, C. G. M., de Campos Moreira, T., Sganzerla, D., Matzenbacher, A. M. F., Faria, A. G., Matturro, L., … Lutz de Araujo, A. (2021). Teaming-up nurses with ophthalmologists to expand the reach of eye care in a middle-income country: Validation of health data acquisition by nursing staff in a telemedicine strategy. *PloS One, 16*(11), e0260594–e0260594. https://doi.org/10.1371/journal.pone.0260594

Razavi, H., Burrow, S., & Trzesinski, A. (2018). Review of eye health among Aboriginal and Torres Strait Islander people. *Australian Indigenous Health Bulletin, 18*(4). Retrieved 12 December 2022 from https://healthbulletin.org.au/articles/review-of-eye-health-among-aboriginal-and-torres-strait-islander-people/

Sturrock, B. (2018) Treating depression in people with vision impairment, *InPsych, 40*(1), Australian Psychological Society. Retrieved 12 December 2022 from https://psychology.org.au/for-members/publications/inpsych/2018/feb/treating-depression-in-people-with-vision-impairm

Tolchard, B., & Stuhlmiller, C. M. (2018). Outcomes of an Australian Nursing Student-led School Vision and Hearing Screening Programme. *Child Care in Practice, 24*(1), 43–52. https://doi.org/10.1080/13575279.2017.1287058

Vision 2020. (2021). 2021–22 Pre-budget submission. Retrieved 12 December 2022 from https://www.vision2020australia.org.au/resources/2021-22-pre-budget-submission/

Vision Australia. (2022). Age-related macular degeneration. Retrieved 12 December 2022 from https://www.visionaustralia.org/services/eye-conditions/age-related-macular-degeneration

World Health Organization (WHO). (2022). Blindness and vision impairment. Retrieved 5 December 2022 from https://www.who.int/news-room/fact-sheets/detail/blindness-and-visual-impairment

Zhang, N., Wang, J., Li, Y., & Jiang, B. (2021). Prevalence of primary open angle glaucoma in the last 20 years: a meta-analysis and systematic review. *Scientific Reports, 11*, 13762. https://doi.org/10.1038/s41598-021-92971-w

UNIT 2

EARS, NOSE, MOUTH AND THROAT

LEARNING OUTCOMES

By the end of this chapter you should be able to:

1 identify the structures of the ears, nose, mouth and throat
2 describe system-specific history and normal findings in the physical examination of the ears, nose, mouth and throat
3 describe common abnormalities with pathophysiology found in the physical examination of the ears, nose, mouth and throat
4 identify health education opportunities for consumers with specific conditions
5 perform the physical examination of the ears, nose, mouth and throat
6 discuss the clinical reasoning in evaluating outcomes of health assessment and physical examination including documentation requirements for recording information, health education given and relevant health referral.

BACKGROUND

Health assessment and physical examination of the ears, nose, sinuses, mouth and throat can be linked to assessment of the neurological, respiratory, endocrine, gastrointestinal, musculoskeletal and cardiovascular systems.

Ear-related conditions include:

> *infections* (either bacterial or viral) such as otitis media (middle ear infection) and otitis externa ('tropical ear' or 'swimmer's ear'). In Australia there are between 900 000 and 2.4 million cases per year of otitis media (Veivers et al., 2022), one of the leading causes of disease in Aboriginal and Torres Strait Islander children, and a significant contributor to hearing loss (De Lacey, Dune & Macdonald, 2020). In 2018–19, 43% of Aboriginal and Torres Strait Islander children aged seven and older had measured hearing loss in one or both ears (AIHW, 2020a). Clinical presentation differs for this cohort, in that they are, on average, younger in age for first infection, have a higher frequency of infection and experience infections of greater severity and persistence, compared with non-Indigenous children (Jervis-Bardy, Carney, Duguid & Leach, 2017). In New Zealand, approximately 60% of children have experienced at least one episode of acute otitis media by age four, and 27% of children aged 0 to 4 years are affected each year (BPAC, 2022). Research indicates Māori and Pasifika children experience higher rates of middle ear infection and subsequent hearing loss than the broader New Zealand population (EMC, 2021).

> *hearing loss*, which may be due to disease processes such as Ménière's disease, age-related changes, drug-related conditions, acoustic neuroma and trauma. Hearing loss in children is significantly correlated with ear disease and infection,

which are especially prevalent among Aboriginal and Torres Strait Islander children. Self-reported ear and hearing problems in Aboriginal and Torres Strait Islander children were estimated to be over twice the rate for non-First Nations children in 2018–19; however, given that many cases go unreported, the true disparity is likely to be higher (AIHW, 2020a). Childhood hearing loss is due to preventable causes in 60% of cases (WHO, 2021), and can significantly affect the achievement of developmental milestones, many of which are associated with the acquisition of language and cognitive function (Victorian Government, 2021).

> *hearing disabilities*, which include tinnitus and hyperacusis. In New Zealand, 15% of the population experiences tinnitus (Health Navigator New Zealand, 2021), while around one in three Australians experience tinnitus at some point in their lives (Tinnitus Australia, n.d.). Hyperacusis is a form of increased sensitivity for sound that causes a low tolerance for environmental noise. Common causes are exposure to loud noise and ageing (Better Health Vic, 2019).

Nose and sinuses-related conditions are usually due to:
> infection (common cold, head cold and flu)
> allergy-related rhinitis, sinus-related infections (sinusitis)
> trauma
> nasal obstruction often due to nasal polyps.

Allergic rhinitis (hay fever) affects around 18% of the population (children and adults) in Australia and New Zealand (ASCIA, 2019). It is most prevalent in 25- to 54-year-olds (AIHW, 2020b).

Mouth-related conditions are categorised as:
> *infections* (for example: herpes, syphilis, thrush or candidiasis; and in children: viruses such as coxsackie, which causes hand, foot and mouth disease, and impetigo)
> *oral cancers* (with higher incidence of mouth and tongue cancer in smokers), which account for approximately 2% of all cancers diagnosed in New Zealand (Cancer Society NZ, 2018). In Australia there were 687 new diagnoses of mouth cancer in 2021, up from 435 in 1994 (Cancer Council, 2021).
> *loss of teeth*, which affects nutrition, systemic health, self-image, quality of life and the ability to socialise (Deutsch & Jay, 2021). In 2012, 52.2% of older adults in New Zealand had lost all of their natural teeth and 74% of people living in residential care and 87% of people living at home wore full upper and lower dentures to replace their lost teeth (CBG Health Research, 2015). This suggests a significant proportion of this cohort were not wearing full dentures, which can impact significantly on nutritional intake and all aspects of health and wellbeing. Untreated tooth decay, a precursor to tooth loss, in nursing home residents with dementia is high, with 68% of residents in an Australian aged care facility having coronal caries, and 77% having root caries (Deutsch & Jay, 2021). Preventative care such as tooth brushing with fluoridated tooth paste was a common protective measure; however prohibitive cost, lack of access, anxiety and lack of perceived need were barriers to older adults receiving regular dental health checks (Mohammed, 2019).

Throat-related conditions can be categorised into:
> *diseases* such as thyroid diseases, cancer
> *trauma*
> *infection.*

Trauma and infection may also lead to loss of vocal ability.

Hearing loss or damage can quite radically affect a consumer's life. This may be life-threatening due to the consumer's inability to use hearing for safety responses. For example, mishearing health-related advice, especially regarding medication administration, affects people who also have poor eyesight. Although loss of sense of smell or taste may not be life-threatening, links have been made to distortions in these senses being caused not only by infection, injury and side effects of drugs, but also as a symptom of depression. Loss of quality of life is usually the most common complaint that loss or distortion of these senses has for consumers experiencing these conditions.

ANATOMY AND PHYSIOLOGY

Ear

The ear has three sections: the external, the middle and the inner ear.

The external ear, which is also called the **auricle** or pinna, extends through the auditory canal to the tympanic membrane. The auricle receives sound waves and funnels them through the auditory canal to produce vibrations on the tympanic membrane. The auricle is composed of cartilage and is flared to catch sound waves and funnel them through to the middle ear. The helix is the rim of the auricle and the posterior portion of the auricle is also referred to as the lobule (**Figure 11.1**).

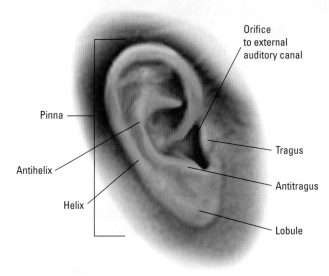

Pinna

Antihelix

Helix

Orifice to external auditory canal

Tragus

Antitragus

Lobule

FIGURE 11.1 External ear

The external auditory canal is an S-shaped tube approximately 2.5 cm in length, with the outer third made up of cartilage and the remainder of bone covered by a thin layer of skin (**Figure 11.2**). The canal is lined with tiny hairs and modified sweat glands that secrete a thick, wax-like substance called **cerumen (ear wax)**, which can vary in consistency from dry and flaky to wet and waxy. Cerumen ranges from a pale, honey colour in light-skinned individuals to dark brown or black in dark-skinned people. Colour and consistency may also change due to the presence of impurities and infections.

Middle ear

The middle ear is composed of the tympanic membrane, the ossicles and the tympanic cavity. The cavity is an air-filled compartment that separates the middle ear from the internal ear. The tympanic membrane, which is circular or oval and is about 10–15 mm in diameter, sits in an oblique position in the external canal so that it leans slightly forward. The rim of the tympanic membrane (also referred to as the ear drum) is called the annulus, the superior portion is the pars flaccida, and the tighter, largest area of the drum is the pars tensa.

The **ossicles** are three tiny bones – the malleus (hammer), the incus (anvil) and the stapes (stirrup) – that play a crucial role in the transmission of sound. Vibrations set up in the tympanic membrane by sound waves reaching it through the external auditory canal are transmitted to the inner ear by rapid movement of the ossicles.

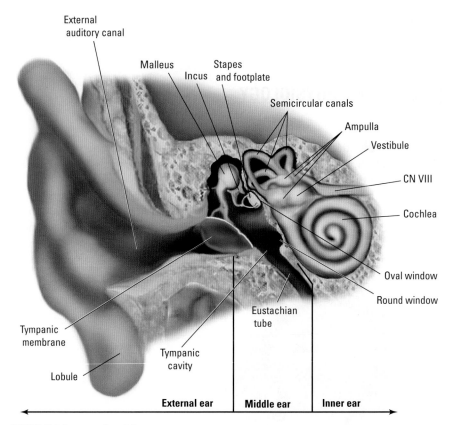

FIGURE 11.2 Cross section of the ear

External ear   Middle ear   Inner ear

Labels: External auditory canal; Malleus; Incus; Stapes and footplate; Semicircular canals; Ampulla; Vestibule; CN VIII; Cochlea; Oval window; Round window; Eustachian tube; Tympanic cavity; Tympanic membrane; Lobule

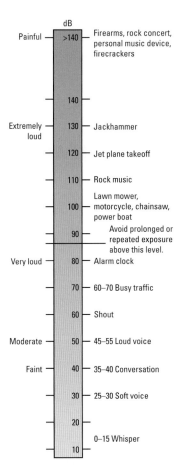

FIGURE 11.3 Decibel scale of frequently heard sounds

dB

Painful	>140	Firearms, rock concert, personal music device, firecrackers
	140	
Extremely loud	130	Jackhammer
	120	Jet plane takeoff
	110	Rock music
	100	Lawn mower, motorcycle, chainsaw, power boat
	90	Avoid prolonged or repeated exposure above this level.
Very loud	80	Alarm clock
	70	60–70 Busy traffic
	60	Shout
Moderate	50	45–55 Loud voice
Faint	40	35–40 Conversation
	30	25–30 Soft voice
	20	
	10	0–15 Whisper

The middle ear is connected to the nasopharynx by the auditory or **eustachian tube**, which serves as a channel through which air pressure within the cavity can be equalised with air pressure outside to maintain normal hearing. Equalisation of pressure is aided by yawning or swallowing, which causes the opening of valve-like flaps that cover the openings of the eustachian tubes.

Inner ear

The inner ear is a complex, closed, fluid-filled system of interconnecting tubes called the **labyrinth**, which is essential for hearing and equilibrium. The labyrinth has bony and membranous portions. The bony labyrinth is composed of the cochlea, the semicircular canals and the vestibule. The **vestibule** is located between the cochlea and the **semicircular canals** and is important in both hearing and balance. The three semicircular canals located at right angles to each other provide balance and equilibrium for the body. The **cochlea** is a snail-shaped structure made up of three compartments filled with fluid. As sound waves travel through the ear, they cause the fluid to vibrate, stimulating the thousands of hearing-receptor cells of the organ of Corti. Nearby nerve fibres transmit impulses along the cochlear branch of the vestibulocochlear nerve to the brain, allowing us to hear. The human ear is capable of hearing within a frequency range of 20 to 20 000 Hz, and a decibel range of 0 to 140. **Figure 11.3** illustrates the decibel levels of various commonly heard sounds.

Nose

The nose consists of the external or outer nose and the nasal fossae, or internal nose (see **Figure 11.4**). The outer nose is made up of bone and cartilage and is divided internally into two nasal fossae by the nasal septum, and externally by the columella. Anterior openings into the nasal fossae are nostrils, or nares. Each fossa has a lateral extended 'wing' portion, the ala nasi, on the outside and a vestibule just inside the nostril. Superior, middle and inferior meatuses or grooves are

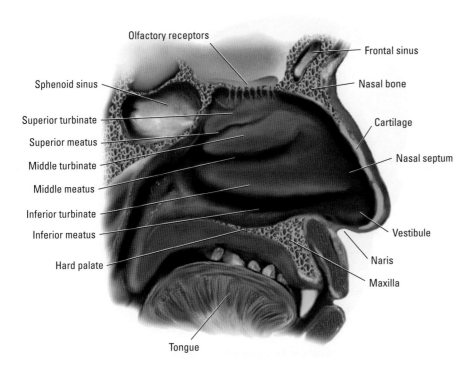

FIGURE 11.4 Lateral cross section of the nose

located on the lateral walls of the nostrils just below the corresponding conchae, or **turbinates**. The nasal turbinates are covered by mucous membranes and greatly increase the surface area of mucous membrane in the nose because of their shape. Kiesselbach's plexus is a vascular area on the nasal septum, and a common site of nosebleeds (also called epistaxis).

Air enters the anterior nares, passes through the vestibule, and enters the fossa. The vestibule contains nasal hairs and sebaceous glands. The fossae have both olfactory and respiratory functions. To protect the lungs from noxious agents, these structures of the nose clean, filter, humidify and control the temperature of inspired air. The mucous covering in the nose and sinuses traps fine dust particles, and lysosomes kill most of the bacteria. The tiny hairs of the nose (cilia) transport the mucus and the particles to the pharynx to be swallowed.

The nasal mucosa is capable of adding large amounts of water to inspired air through evaporation from its surface. The rich vascular supply to the turbinates radiates heat to the incoming air as it passes through the nasal cavity.

Sinuses

Air-filled cavities lined with mucous membranes are present in some of the cranial bones and are referred to as **paranasal sinuses** (see **Figure 11.5**). These air-filled sinuses lighten the weight of the skull and add resonance to the quality of the voice. The frontal, maxillary, ethmoid and sphenoid paranasal sinuses open into the nose. Only the frontal and maxillary sinuses can be assessed in the physical examination.

Mouth and throat

The lips are sensory structures found at the opening of the mouth (see **Figure 11.6**). The labial tubercle is the small projected area in the midline of the upper lip. The area where the upper and lower lips meet is the labial commissure. The vermilion zone is the reddish or reddish-brown area of the lips, and the area where the lips meet the facial skin is called the vermilion border. The medial groove superior to the upper lip is called the philtrum. The cheeks form the lateral walls of the mouth and are lined with buccal mucosa. The posterior pharyngeal wall is at the back of the mouth.

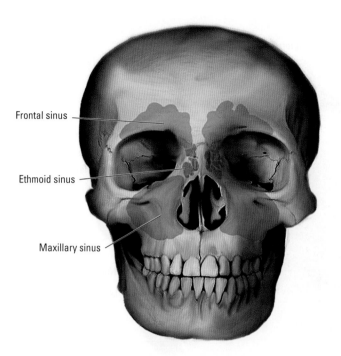

FIGURE 11.5 Location of the sinuses (sphenoid sinuses are directly behind ethmoid sinuses)

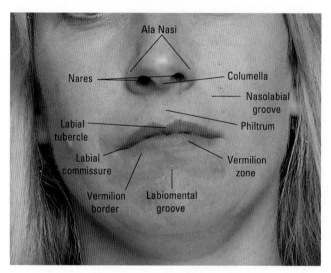

FIGURE 11.6 Landmarks of the area around the mouth

The roof of the mouth consists of the hard palate anteriorly and the soft palate posteriorly (see **Figure 11.7**). The **linear raphe** is a linear ridge in the middle of the hard palate that is formed by two palatine bones and part of the superior maxillary bone. The mucous membrane on either side of the linear raphe is thick, pale and corrugated, while the posterior mucous membrane is thin, a deeper pink, and smooth.

Situated in the floor of the mouth, the tongue is a muscular organ connected to the hyoid bone posteriorly and to the floor of the mouth anteriorly by the **fraenulum**. The tongue assists with mastication, swallowing, speech, and mechanical cleansing of the teeth.

The mucous membrane covering the upper surface of the tongue has numerous projections called **papillae**, which assist in handling food and contain taste buds. Four qualities of taste are found in taste buds distributed over the surface of the tongue. The **sulcus terminalis** is the midline depression that separates the anterior two-thirds of the tongue from the posterior one-third.

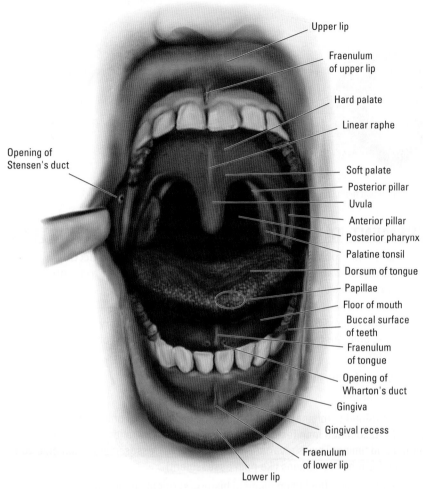

FIGURE 11.7 Structures of the mouth

Two of the three pairs of salivary glands open into the mouth on the ventral surface of the tongue. Submaxillary glands secrete fluid through **Wharton's ducts**, located on both sides of the fraenulum. Sublingual glands open into the floor of the mouth posteriorly to Wharton's ducts. The larger parotid glands are located in the cheeks and secrete their amylase-rich fluid through **Stensen's ducts**, located just opposite the upper second molars.

The salivary glands produce 1000 to 1500 mL of saliva per day to assist with digestion of food and maintenance of oral hygiene. Saliva prevents dental caries and bacterial damage of healthy oral tissue by washing away bacteria and destroying it with antibodies and proteolytic enzymes.

Gums, or gingivae, appear pink or coral in light-skinned individuals and brown with a darker melanotic line along the edges in dark-skinned individuals. Gums hold the teeth in place.

Adults have 32 permanent teeth: four incisors, two canines, four premolars and six molars in each half of the mouth (**Figure 11.8**). The teeth are well designed for chewing. Incisors provide strong cutting action, and molars provide strong grinding action.

The soft palate is suspended from the posterior border of the hard palate and extends downwards as folds, the palatine arches or pillars forming an incomplete septum between the mouth and the nasopharynx. The **uvula** is a finger-like projection of tissue that hangs down from the centre of the soft palate. Two palatine tonsils (primarily lymphoid tissue) are connected to the palatine arches; they vary greatly in size from one individual to another. Lymphoid tissue in the tonsils plays a role in the control of infection.

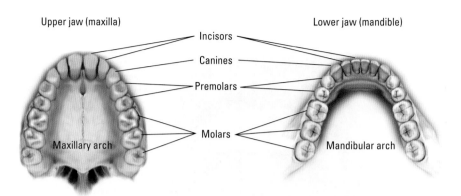

Upper jaw (maxilla)   Lower jaw (mandible)

Incisors
Canines
Premolars
Molars
Maxillary arch   Mandibular arch

FIGURE 11.8 Permanent teeth

ASSESSMENT: TAKING THE CONSUMER'S HEALTH HISTORY

Assessment is the first phase of the nursing process, and involves collecting subjective information about the consumer's health status in order to identify consumer problem areas to focus on.

> **Subjective data** is most frequently collected during a health history and serves as the starting point for the health professional to base the depth of their assessment on.
>
> The sections for the health history include:
> > **Consumer profile**
> > **Chief complaint** (explained systematically using variations of location, quality, quantity, associated manifestations, aggravating factors, alleviating factors, setting and timing. This is a variation on the OPQRST assessment mnemonic you may use for other conditions like pain assessment)
> > **Past health history** (including medical history, surgical history, allergies, medications, injuries and accidents, special needs and childhood illnesses)
> > **Family health history**
> > **Social history** (including alcohol, tobacco and drug use, sexual practice, work and home environment, hobbies and leisure activities, stress and culture).

HEALTH HISTORY

CONSUMER PROFILE	The ears, nose, mouth and throat health history provides insight into the link between a consumer's life and lifestyle and ears, nose and sinuses, mouth and throat information and pathology. Diseases or changes that are age-, sex- and race-specific for the ears, nose, mouth and throat are listed.		
	AGE	**EARS**	> Elderly consumers: • Hearing loss related to presbycusis, sensorineural degeneration or otosclerosis • Excessive or impacted cerumen
		NOSE	> Elderly consumers: • Decrease in ability to smell
		MOUTH AND THROAT	Orthodonture > Elderly consumers: • Tooth loss and gum disease • Candidiasis related to immunosuppression • Decrease in ability to taste

>>

>>

	SEX	EARS	Female: Calcifications of the ossicles
		NOSE AND SINUSES	Male: Rhinophyma, deviated septum related to trauma, polyps Female: polyps
		MOUTH AND THROAT	Male: Singer's nodule on the larynx (over 30), cancer of the larynx, leukoplakia of the tongue, gums, and buccal mucosa
	CULTURAL BACKGROUND	CHINESE	> Nasopharyngeal cancer
		INDIVIDUALS FROM MEDITERRANEAN COUNTRIES, SOUTH-EAST ASIA, INDONESIA, SOUTH AMERICA	> Rhinoscleroma
CHIEF COMPLAINT	Common chief complaints for the ears, nose, mouth and throat are defined, and information on the characteristics of each sign or symptom is provided.		
	EAR		
	1. CHANGE IN OR LOSS OF HEARING	Reduction in the perception of sound	
		LOCATION	Unilateral, bilateral
		QUALITY	Loud sounds heard, soft sounds heard
		QUANTITY	Partial or complete
		ASSOCIATED MANIFESTATIONS	Tinnitus, vertigo, drainage, swelling, fever, ear pain
		AGGRAVATING FACTORS	Loud noises, excessive or impacted cerumen, swimming
		ALLEVIATING FACTORS	Hearing aid, removal of excessive cerumen, turning up volume when possible, cupping the ear, facing the speaker
		SETTING	Work (jobs with loud background noise or machinery)
		TIMING	Constant or intermittent, after drug therapy, onset sudden, gradual, or slow
	2. OTORRHOEA	Drainage of liquid from the ear	
		LOCATION	Unilateral or bilateral
		QUALITY	Painful or nontender, watery, bloody or purulent, foul odour
		ASSOCIATED MANIFESTATIONS	Hearing loss, headache, fever, vertigo, upper respiratory infection
		AGGRAVATING FACTORS	Upright or supine position
		ALLEVIATING FACTORS	Upright or supine position
		TIMING	Following trauma, continuous, intermittent
	3. OTALGIA	Discomfort in the ear	
		LOCATION	Unilateral or bilateral, in jaw region, in pinna region
		QUALITY	Aching, dull, sharp
		ASSOCIATED MANIFESTATIONS	Drainage, tinnitus, dysphagia, sore throat, vertigo, diminished hearing
		AGGRAVATING FACTORS	Tooth infection, upper respiratory infection, perforated tympanic membrane, insect bites in the ear, upright or supine position, objects in ear, change in air pressure

>>

	ALLEVIATING FACTORS	Analgesics, upright or supine position, avoiding swimming, avoiding pressure changes, removal of objects, change in air pressure
	SETTING	Outdoors, high altitudes, noisy environments
	TIMING	Continuous, intermittent; after swimming, following trauma to the head or ear, following loud noises, after pressure changes, flying
4. TINNITUS	'Ringing' in the ears	
	LOCATION	Unilateral or bilateral
	QUALITY	Pulsatile, buzzing, high-pitched ringing
	ASSOCIATED MANIFESTATIONS	Vertigo, drainage, pain, nausea, fullness or pressure in the ears, hearing loss, upper respiratory infection, allergies, middle ear infection, inner ear lesions, eustachian tube inflammation
	AGGRAVATING FACTORS	Medications, fluid in the middle ear, perforation of the tympanic membrane, position, pressure on the neck, excessive cerumen
	ALLEVIATING FACTORS	Discontinuing medications, position change, avoiding allergens
	SETTING	Work (high noise levels), outdoors
	TIMING	Longstanding, recent; constant, intermittent; following drug therapy, after exposure to loud noises
NOSE AND SINUSES		
1. PAIN	Discomfort in the nose and sinuses	
	QUALITY	Aching, throbbing, sharp
	ASSOCIATED MANIFESTATIONS	Fever, chills, visual changes, swelling, sneezing, nasal discharge
	AGGRAVATING FACTORS	Exposure to allergens, decreased humidity indoors, cocaine use
	ALLEVIATING FACTORS	Use of medications (decongestant or antihistamine), removal of allergens, humidification of the environment, discontinuation of cocaine
	SETTING	Outdoors, dry heat, low humidity
	TIMING	Seasonal, in the morning
2. DRAINAGE/RHINITIS	Excessive discharge of nasal secretions	
	QUALITY	Unilateral or bilateral, amount, viscosity, colour, odour, blood-tinged
	ASSOCIATED MANIFESTATIONS	Fever, sneezing, pain, mouth breathing, swelling, skin irritation around drainage site, itchy eyes
	AGGRAVATING FACTORS	Allergens, infections
	ALLEVIATING FACTORS	Medication, hydration, avoiding allergens
	SETTING	Outdoors, indoors
	TIMING	In the morning, seasonal, after trauma

3. BLOCKAGE OR CONGESTION	Reduced ability to move air through the nose and sinuses secondary to obstruction	
	QUALITY	Complete, partial
	ASSOCIATED MANIFESTATIONS	Mouth breathing, snoring, pain, disfigurement, sneezing, itchy eyes, sinus infection
	AGGRAVATING FACTORS	Infection, allergens, medications, objects in nose
	ALLEVIATING FACTORS	Mouth breathing, medications, avoidance of allergens, removal of objects, immunotherapy to reduce response to allergens
	SETTING	Outdoors, indoors
	TIMING	Following drug therapy, trauma after oral intake, after nasal surgery, may be seasonal or perennial
4. LOSS OF SMELL	Loss or alteration or reduction in smell function secondary to disease or virus	
	QUALITY	Complete (anosmia), altered (dysnosmia) or partial (hyposmia)
	ASSOCIATED MANIFESTATIONS	loss of taste, with or without flu symptoms, loss of appetite, cough, congestions or rhinitis
	AGGRAVATING FACTORS	Brain injuries, COVID-19, other viral respiratory infections, radiation therapy, antidepressants, antibiotics, nasal polyps, sinusitis, cancers, Alzheimer's disease, Parkinson's disease, smoking, hypothyroidism
	ALLEVIATING FACTORS	Disease progression
	SETTING	Usually in community cases
	TIMING	Varied; for viral disease between 5 days and 6 months, for others may be permanent or fluctuate with condition and treatment

MOUTH AND THROAT

1. HALITOSIS	Unpleasant odour of the breath	
	QUALITY	Ammonia, acetone, newly mown grass or old wine odour; foul
	ASSOCIATED MANIFESTATIONS	Gum disease, caries, systemic disease, sinusitis, pharyngitis, gastro-oesophageal reflux disease (GORD), smoking
	AGGRAVATING FACTORS	Poor oral hygiene, poor nutrition, poor diabetic control, alcohol intake, decreased hydration, inadequate renal function
	ALLEVIATING FACTORS	Good oral hygiene, control of systemic diseases, breath mints, good nutrition, adequate dental care, treatment of infection
	TIMING	Associated with systemic disease or acute infectious process
2. LESIONS	Disruptions in the mucosa of the mouth or tongue	
	QUALITY	Tender, nontender
	ASSOCIATED MANIFESTATIONS	Malnutrition, odour, pain, swelling, fever, stress
	AGGRAVATING FACTORS	Eating, drinking, spices, smoking, hot or cold stimuli, alcohol, dehydration

>>

		ALLEVIATING FACTORS	Medications, avoiding eating, hydration, proper nutrition, avoiding smoking and alcohol
		TIMING	Associated with systemic disease, intermittent, continuous
	3. SWELLING	Oedema of the pharynx	
		QUALITY	Mild, moderate, severe
		ASSOCIATED MANIFESTATIONS	Dysphagia, urticaria, wheezing, pruritus, rhinorrhoea, difficulty breathing, lesions, chills, sweats, fever, sneezing, itchy eyes
		AGGRAVATING FACTORS	Exposure to allergens, heat
		ALLEVIATING FACTORS	Medications, avoiding allergens, ice, saltwater gargles
		TIMING	Following drug therapy, after eating, after an insect bite, after trauma, during or after an infectious process
	4. LOSS OF TASTE (AGEUSIA)	See loss of smell – usually loss of taste and smell occur simultaneously for the same causes	
PAST HEALTH HISTORY	The various components of the past health history are linked to ears, nose, mouth and throat pathology and ear-, nose-, mouth- and throat-related information.		
	MEDICAL HISTORY	**EAR-SPECIFIC**	Acute otitis media, acute otitis externa, serous otitis media, hearing difficulties
		NOSE- AND SINUSES-SPECIFIC	Polyps, septal deviation, sinus infection, allergic rhinitis, anosmia, epistaxis
		MOUTH- AND THROAT-SPECIFIC	Tonsillitis, caries, herpes simplex virus, *Candida* infections, streptococcal throat, frequent upper respiratory infections, tonsillar abscess
		NON-EAR-, NOSE- AND SINUSES-, MOUTH- AND THROAT-SPECIFIC	Diabetes mellitus, renal disease, atherosclerotic disease, hypertension, inflammatory processes, infections (viral or bacterial), immunosuppressive disease, dental pathology, blood dyscrasias, sexually transmitted infections, anaphylaxis, nutritional disturbances
	SURGICAL HISTORY	Neurosurgery, tonsillectomy, adenoidectomy, tumour removal, cosmetic surgery of head or neck, repair of septal deviation, oral surgery, tympanostomy tube placement	
	ALLERGIES	Pollen: sneezing, nasal congestion, watery or itchy eyes, cough Insect stings: swelling of the throat, around the eyes Animal dander: sneezing, nasal congestion, watery or itchy eyes, cough	
	MEDICATIONS	Antibiotics, antihistamines, decongestants, steroids, chemotherapy, immunotherapy, immunosuppressive drugs	
	INJURIES AND ACCIDENTS	Foreign bodies; trauma to the ears, nose, mouth, throat; noxious fumes; sports injuries to the face; motor vehicle accidents	
	SPECIAL NEEDS	Deafness, speech disorders	
	CHILDHOOD ILLNESSES	Frequent tonsillitis, frequent ear infections	
FAMILY HEALTH HISTORY	Ear, nose and sinuses, mouth and throat diseases that are familial are listed. Hearing loss, otosclerosis, neonatal blindness secondary to cataracts from mother contracting rubella in pregnancy.		

>>

SOCIAL HISTORY	The components of the social history are linked to ear, nose and sinuses, mouth and throat factors and pathology.	
	ALCOHOL USE	Predisposes the person to cancer of the oral cavity as well as decreased nutrition leading to cheilosis
	TOBACCO USE	Smoking predisposes the person to mouth, lip or throat cancer
	DRUG USE	Snorting cocaine may cause perforation of the nasal septum
	SEXUAL PRACTICE	Herpes simplex viruses I and II and gonorrhoea can be contracted from oral sex
	WORK ENVIRONMENT	Exposure to toxins, chemicals, infections, excess noise, allergens
	HOME ENVIRONMENT	Exposure to loud music may cause hearing loss
	HOBBIES AND LEISURE ACTIVITIES	Shooting without proper ear protection may cause hearing loss
	STRESS	With frequent upper respiratory infections, hearing teeth brush together or grind together can be decreased

PERSON-CENTRED HEALTH EDUCATION

When conducting a health assessment, opportunities for the provision of person-centred health education will arise. This is a significant consideration in relation to the assessment process for examination of the ears, nose, mouth and throat due to the number of health conditions that are preventable. These occasions are identified as individualised education and may generate further data that can be added to the assessment. All education given should be documented so that in future, health professionals can assess the impact of previous information provided to the consumer. (Refer to Chapter 1 for initiating health education.) Refer to the following examples.

CLINICAL REASONING

Practice tip: Risk factors for hearing loss

Consumers who fit any of the following hearing loss risk factors should be assessed for hearing damage. This is also an opportunity to provide person-centred health education about possible ways to avoid hearing loss based on the risk factor that are identified.

> Noise exposure
> Smoking
> Ototoxic drugs
> Congenital or heredity
> Cardiovascular disease
> Ageing
> Tumours

> Trauma
> Chronic infection
> Systemic disease
> Tympanic membrane perforation
> Ménière's disease
> Barotrauma

INDIVIDUALISED HEALTH EDUCATION INTERVENTIONS	
Assessing the consumer for the following health-related activities can assist in identifying the need for education about these factors. This information provides a bridge between the health maintenance activities and ears, nose, mouth and throat functions.	
Sleep	Deprivation may be associated with frequent upper respiratory infections
Diet	Deficiencies may affect integrity of nasal and oral mucosa and increase risk of oral cancers
Use of safety devices	Use of mouth guard for sports participants; face shields for sports, job or home projects; ear protection when around loud noise to prevent damage to hearing
Health check-ups	Hearing assessment, dental examination

PLANNING FOR PHYSICAL EXAMINATION

The planning phase refers to evaluating subjective data to narrow the focus on physical examination, determining what objective data needs to be gathered, as well as considering the environment and equipment that will be required.

At this time, you will identify which of the four diagnostic techniques you will need to implement the physical examination, and how you will sequence these. For the physical examination of the ears, nose, mouth and throat, you will include inspection, palpation and percussion.

> **Objective data** is:
> > collected during the physical examination of the consumer
> > usually collected after subjective data
> > information that is measured or observed by the clinician as opposed to being reported by the consumer
> > vital to the overall health assessment, to enable you to make clinical decisions that are representative of the whole consumer picture.

Evaluating subjective data to focus physical examination

Before commencing the physical examination of the consumer's ears, nose and sinuses, mouth and throat, consider what information the health history has provided. Critical consideration, linked to knowledge of anatomy and physiology, should focus the physical assessment so your examination will be more effective and efficient.

Environment

Assessment of ears, nose and sinuses, mouth and throat can be done in most physical environments in healthcare settings. Adequate privacy is required as for any health assessment, with some consideration needed for noise levels and the ability to accurately assess hearing in your environment.

Equipment

> Otoscope with earpieces of different sizes and pneumatic attachment
> Penlight
> Tuning fork, 512 Hz
> Tongue blade
> Watch
> Gauze square
> Nonsterile gloves
> Transilluminator
> Nasal speculum
> Cotton-tipped applicator

CLINICAL REASONING

Practice tip: The person with decreased hearing
Observe the consumer for signs of hearing difficulty and deafness during the health history and physical examination. Turning the head to facilitate hearing, lip reading, speaking in a loud voice, or asking you to write words are signs of hearing difficulty. If the consumer is wearing a hearing aid, ask if it is turned on, when the batteries were last changed, and if the device causes any irritation of the ear canal.

Advanced Assessment

IMPLEMENTATION: CONDUCTING THE PHYSICAL EXAMINATION

Implementation of the physical examination requires you to consider your scope of practice as well. In this section, depending on your context, you may be performing foundation assessment with aspects of advanced assessment if you are practising in a specialised area.

EXAMINATION IN BRIEF: EARS, NOSE AND SINUSES, MOUTH AND THROAT

Examination of the ear

Auditory screening
> Voice-whisper test
> Tuning fork tests
  • Weber test
  • Rinne test

Inspection
> External ear

Palpation
> Otoscopic examination

Examination of the nose

Inspection
> External nose
> Patency
> Internal nose

Examination of the sinuses

Inspection

Palpation and percussion

Transillumination of the sinuses

Examination of the mouth and throat

Examination of the breath

Examination of the lips

Inspection

Palpation

Examination of the tongue

Examination of the buccal mucosa

Examination of the gums

Examination of the teeth

Examination of the palate

Examination of the throat

Inspection

Physical examination of the ear consists of three parts:
1. Auditory screening (CN VIII)
2. Inspection and palpation of the external ear
3. Otoscopic assessment. Note that in some contexts this would be considered advanced practice.

URGENT FINDING

Cerebrospinal fluid (CSF) drainage from the ear
If the consumer has cerebrospinal fluid (clear liquid that tests positive for glucose on Dextrostix) leaking from the ear, be sure to use good hand washing technique and avoid placing any objects into the ear canal in order to prevent the development of meningitis. A consumer with this finding needs immediate referral to a qualified specialist for emergency assessment.

General approach to examination of the ears, nose and sinuses, mouth and throat
1. Greet the consumer and explain the techniques that you will be using.
2. Use a quiet room that will be free from interruptions.
3. Ensure that the light in the room provides sufficient brightness to allow adequate observation of the consumer.

4. Place the consumer in an upright sitting position on the examination table or, for consumers who cannot tolerate the sitting position, gain access to the consumer's head so that it can be rotated from side to side for assessment.
5. Visualise the underlying structures during the assessment process to allow adequate description of findings.
6. Always compare right and left ears, as well as right and left sides of the nose, sinuses, mouth and throat.
7. Use a systematic approach that is followed consistently each time the assessment is performed.

Examination of the ear
Auditory screening
Voice-whisper test

E 1. Instruct the consumer to occlude one ear with a finger.
2. Stand 60 cm behind the consumer's other ear and whisper a two-syllable word or phrase that is evenly accented.
3. Ask the consumer to repeat the word or phrase.
4. Repeat the test with the other ear.

N The consumer should be able to repeat words whispered from a distance of 60 cm.

A The consumer is unable to repeat the words correctly or states that he or she was unable to hear anything.

P This indicates a hearing loss in the high-frequency range that may be caused by excessive exposure to loud noises.

Tuning fork tests
Depending on context, this may be foundation or advanced practice.

Weber and **Rinne tests** help to determine whether the type of hearing loss the consumer is experiencing is conductive or sensorineural. In order to understand how these tests are evaluated, it is important to know the difference between air and bone conduction. Air conduction refers to the transmission of sound through the ear canal, tympanic membrane and ossicular chain to the cochlea and auditory nerve. Bone conduction refers to the transmission of sound through the bones of the skull to the cochlea and auditory nerve.

Weber test

E 1. Hold the handle of a 512 Hz (vibrates 512 cycles per second to create a specific frequency) tuning fork and strike the tines on the ulnar border of the palm to activate it.
2. Place the stem of the fork firmly against the middle of the consumer's forehead, on the top of the head at the midline (**Figure 11.9**), or on the front teeth.
3. Ask the consumer if the sound is heard centrally or towards one side.

N The consumer should perceive the sound equally in both ears or 'in the middle'.

A The sound lateralises to the affected ear.

P This occurs with unilateral conductive hearing loss because the sound is being conducted directly through the bone to the ear. Conductive hearing loss occurs when there are external or middle ear disorders such as impacted cerumen, perforation of the tympanic membrane, serum or pus in the middle ear, or a fusion of the ossicles.

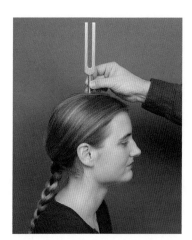

FIGURE 11.9 Weber test

E Examination **N** Normal findings **A** Abnormal findings **P** Pathophysiology

A The sound lateralises to the unaffected ear.

P This occurs with sensorineural loss related to nerve damage in the impaired ear. Sensorineural hearing loss occurs when there is a disorder in the inner ear, the auditory nerve, or the brain. Disorders include congenital defects, effects of ototoxic drugs, and repeated or prolonged exposure to loud noise.

Rinne test

E 1. Stand behind or to the side of the consumer and strike the tuning fork.
2. Place the stem of the tuning fork against the consumer's right mastoid process to test bone conduction (**Figure 11.10A**).
3. Instruct the consumer to indicate if the sound is heard.
4. Ask the consumer to tell you when the sound stops.
5. When the consumer says that the sound has stopped, move the tuning fork, with the tines facing forwards, in front of the right auditory meatus, and ask the consumer if the sound is still heard. Note the length of time the consumer hears the sound (testing air conduction) (**Figure 11.10B**).
6. Repeat the test on the left ear.

N Air conduction is heard for twice as long as bone conduction when the consumer hears the sound through the external auditory canal (air) after it is no longer heard at the mastoid process (bone). This is denoted as AC > BC, or a ⊕ Rinne.

A The consumer reports hearing the sound longer through bone conduction; that is, bone conduction is equal to or greater than air conduction. This is a ⊖ Rinne.

P This occurs when there is conductive hearing loss resulting from disease, obstruction, or damage to the outer or middle ear.

A Bone conduction is prolonged in the context of a normal tympanic membrane, patent eustachian tube, and middle ear disease.

P These findings are typical of otosclerosis.

Inspection

External ear

E 1. Inspect the ears and note their position, colour, size and shape.
2. Note any deformities, nodules, inflammation or lesions.
3. Note colour, consistency and amount of cerumen.

N The ear should match the flesh colour of the rest of the consumer's skin and should be positioned centrally and in proportion to the head. The top of the ear should cross an imaginary line drawn from the outer canthus of the eye to the occiput (see **Figure 11.11**). Cerumen should be moist and not obscure the tympanic membrane. There should be no foreign bodies, redness, drainage, deformities, nodules or lesions.

A The ears are pale, red or cyanotic.

P Vasomotor disorders, fevers, hypoxaemia and cold weather can account for various colour changes.

A The ears are abnormally large or small.

P These abnormalities can be congenitally determined or the result of trauma.

A An ear that is permanently swollen and deformed resembling a 'cauliflower' is abnormal.

P Perichondrial haematoma (cauliflower ear) is a condition common among footballers, wrestlers and boxers. It is caused by blunt trauma to the external ear resulting in a blood clot formation and fluid collection under the perichondrium, which leads to fibrosis and deformity of the external ear.

A An external ear that is erythematous, oedematous, warm to the touch, and painful is abnormal.

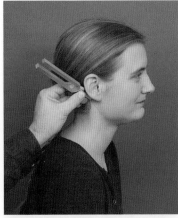

A. Assessing bone conduction

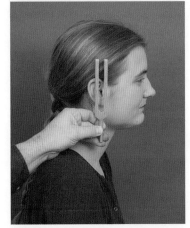

B. Assessing air conduction

FIGURE 11.10 Rinne test

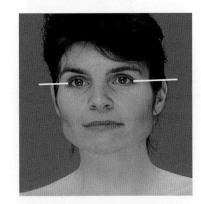

FIGURE 11.11 Normal ear alignment

E Examination **N** Normal findings **A** Abnormal findings **P** Pathophysiology

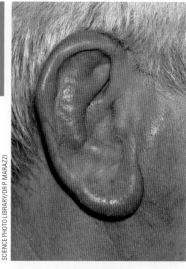

SCIENCE PHOTO LIBRARY/DR P. MARAZZI

FIGURE 11.12 Perichondritis

P Perichondritis is an inflammation of the fibrous connective tissue that overlies the cartilage of the ear (**Figure 11.12**).

A A tumour on the external ear is abnormal.

P Basal cell and squamous cell carcinomas are the most common external ear tumours. Prolonged sunlight exposure is a predisposing factor for these tumours.

A Purulent drainage is abnormal.

P Purulent drainage usually indicates an infection.

A Clear or bloody drainage is present.

P Clear or bloody drainage may be due to cerebrospinal fluid leaking as a result of head trauma or surgery.

A A haematoma behind an ear over the mastoid bone is abnormal.

P This is called Battle's sign and indicates head trauma to the temporal bone of the skull.

A A hard, painless, irregular-shaped nodule on the pinna is abnormal.

P Tophi are uric acid nodules and may indicate the presence of gout. These are usually located near the helix. Many other nodules are benign **fibromas**.

A Sebaceous cysts are abnormal.

P Sebaceous cysts or retention cysts form as a result of the blockage of the ducts to the sebaceous gland.

A Lymph nodes anterior to the tragus or overlying the mastoid are abnormal.

P Lymph nodes may be enlarged due to a malignancy or an infection such as external otitis.

Palpation

E 1. Palpate the auricle between the thumb and the index finger, noting any tenderness or lesions. If the consumer has ear pain, assess the unaffected ear first, then cautiously assess the affected ear.
2. Using the tips of the index and middle fingers, palpate the mastoid tip, noting any tenderness.
3. Using the tips of the index and middle fingers, press inwards on the tragus, noting any tenderness.
4. Hold the auricle between the thumb and the index finger and gently pull up and down, noting any tenderness.

N The consumer should not complain of pain or tenderness during palpation.

A Auricular pain or tenderness is noted.

P Auricular pain is a common finding in external ear infection and is called acute otitis externa.

A There is tenderness over the mastoid process.

P Mastoid tenderness is associated with middle ear inflammation or mastoiditis.

A The tragus is oedematous or sensitive.

P This finding may indicate inflammation of the external or middle ear.

Otoscopic examination
This may not be part of your scope of practice; please review your context's requirements.

E 1. Ask the consumer to tip the head away from the ear being assessed.
2. Select the largest speculum that will comfortably fit the consumer.
3. Hold the otoscope securely in the dominant hand, with the handle held like a pencil between the thumb and the forefinger.
4. Rest the back of the dominant hand on the right side of the consumer's head (**Figure 11.13**).

E Examination **N** Normal findings **A** Abnormal findings **P** Pathophysiology

E 5. Use the free hand to pull the right ear in a manner that will straighten the canal. In adults and in children over 3 years old, pull the ear up and back. (See Chapter 20 for the assessment of children younger than 3.)

6. If hair obstructs visualisation, moisten the speculum with water or a water-soluble lubricant.

7. If wax obstructs visualisation, it should be removed only by a skilled practitioner, either by curettement (if the cerumen is soft or the tympanic membrane is ruptured) or by irrigation (if the cerumen is dry and hard and the tympanic membrane is intact).

8. Slowly insert the speculum into the canal, looking at the canal as the speculum passes.

9. Assess the canal for inflammation, exudates, lesions and foreign bodies.

10. Continue to insert the speculum into the canal, following the path of the canal until the tympanic membrane is visualised.

11. If the tympanic membrane is not visible, gently pull the pinna slightly further in order to straighten the canal to allow adequate visualisation.

12. Identify the colour, light reflex, umbo, the short process, and the long handle of the malleus. Note the presence of perforations, lesions, bulging or retraction of the tympanic membrane, dilatation of blood vessels, bubbles or fluid.

13. Ask the consumer to close the mouth, pinch the nose closed, and blow gently while you observe for movement of the tympanic membrane.

14. Gently withdraw the speculum and repeat the process with the left ear.

N The ear canal should have no redness, swelling, tenderness, lesions, drainage, foreign bodies or scaly surface areas. Cerumen varies in amount, consistency and colour. The tympanic membrane should be pearly grey with clearly defined landmarks and a distinct cone-shaped light reflex extending from the umbo towards the anteroinferior aspect of the membrane. This light reflex is seen at 5 o'clock in the right ear and at 7 o'clock in the left ear. Blood vessels should be visible only on the periphery, and the membrane should not bulge, be retracted, or have any evidence of fluid behind it (**Figure 11.14**). The tympanic membrane should move when the consumer blows against resistance.

A A foreign body in the external auditory canal (EAC) is abnormal (**Figure 11.15**).

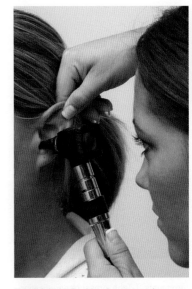

FIGURE 11.13 Position for otoscopic examination

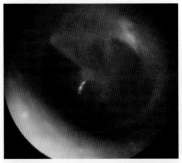

FIGURE 11.14 Normal tympanic membrane

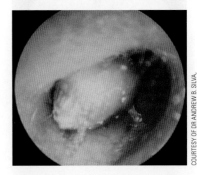

FIGURE 11.15 A foreign body (a bean) in the external auditory canal

CLINICAL **REASONING**

Practice tip: Clearing the external auditory canal (EAC) of cerumen (ear wax)
Two methods can be used to remove cerumen from the EAC in order to visualise the tympanic membrane: manual removal and irrigation with water.

> Manual removal involves the use of a plastic loop or spoon. This method is quick and does not expose the EAC to moisture; therefore it may reduce the risk of infection. However, it requires a cooperative person and skilled practitioner to reduce the risk of trauma to the EAC.

> Irrigation with water at body temperature can be performed with a 20–30 mL syringe with a plastic catheter or a bulb syringe. The water should be instilled gently, and the canal should be checked intermittently for clearance of cerumen. Oral jet irrigators are fast and portable; however, they have been associated with trauma, as has irrigation with small syringes. Do not use anything less than a 20 mL size syringe – this is to reduce the amount of pressure that is exerted in the ear canal – and be aware of where the end of the syringe is touching during irrigation so mechanical trauma does not occur. Water irrigation should be avoided in patients with tympanic membrane perforation, acute otitis media, otitis externa, myringotomy tubes, ear surgery or vertigo.

> NOTE: if you cannot be sure there is no perforation to the tympanic membrane DO NOT irrigate with water; this can cause balance loss and permanent hearing loss.

> Additionally, ears should not be irrigated if any discharge that is not normal cerumen is noted. In this case a fungal or bacterial infection may be the cause.

P Both adults and children can have foreign bodies in the EAC. Some objects are more difficult to remove than others; for instance, vegetables in the EAC can swell with time and make removal challenging.

P Tympanostomy tubes, or T-tube, grommets or PE tubes (pressure equalisation) (**Figure 11.16**), are surgically placed for prolonged otitis media with effusion (OME). The tubes allow drainage of the effusion, normal vibration of the ossicles, and equalisation of pressures across the tympanic membrane. These tubes may fall out, so the presence of the tubes (or lack of) needs to be documented upon examination.

A A painful, boil-like pustule in the EAC is abnormal (**Figure 11.17**).

P Furunculosis is an infection of a hair follicle. EAC oedema and otorrhoea may also be present.

A Black or brown spores (**Figure 11.18A**), yellow or orange spores (**Figure 11.18B**) or white fluffy hyphae in the EAC are abnormal.

P Prolonged use of aural antibiotics can cause otomycosis, or a fungal infection in the ear (other causes of otomycosis is overuse of ear cleaning buds, insects, or water in the ear canal). Different strains of fungi cause the variations in appearance.

A Bony, hard lesions in the deep EAC (see **Figure 11.19**) are abnormal.

P These are exostoses. Consumers who frequently participate in cold-water activities are at risk for developing them. If an exostosis becomes large enough, it can block the EAC and trap debris between it and the tympanic membrane. This can lead to infection.

A Severe pain accompanied by erythema deep into the EAC and on the tympanic membrane, along with serous-filled blebs (**Figure 11.20**), is abnormal.

P This describes viral bullous myringitis. This can easily be mistaken for acute otitis media.

A The appearance of chalk patches on the tympanic membrane (**Figure 11.21**) is abnormal.

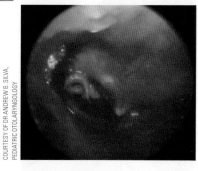

COURTESY OF DR ANDREW B. SILVA, PEDIATRIC OTOLARYNGOLOGY

FIGURE 11.16 Tympanostomy tube (grommets, T-Tube, pressure equalisation tube)

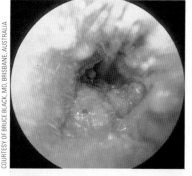

COURTESY OF BRUCE BLACK, MD, BRISBANE, AUSTRALIA

FIGURE 11.17 Furunculosis

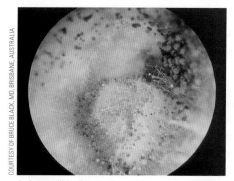

COURTESY OF BRUCE BLACK, MD, BRISBANE, AUSTRALIA

A. Aspergillus nigra
FIGURE 11.18 Otomycosis

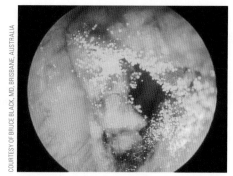

COURTESY OF BRUCE BLACK, MD, BRISBANE, AUSTRALIA

B. Aspergillus flavum

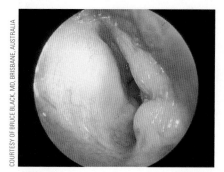

COURTESY OF BRUCE BLACK, MD, BRISBANE, AUSTRALIA

FIGURE 11.19 Exostoses

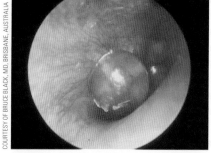

COURTESY OF BRUCE BLACK, MD, BRISBANE, AUSTRALIA

FIGURE 11.20 Bullous myringitis

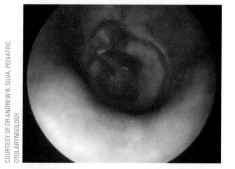

COURTESY OF DR ANDREW B. SILVA, PEDIATRIC OTOLARYNGOLOGY

FIGURE 11.21 Myringosclerosis and otitis media with effusion

E Examination **N** Normal findings **A** Abnormal findings **P** Pathophysiology

P These are calcifications found in myringosclerosis, which can occur after tympanic membrane surgery, infection or inflammation. Myringosclerosis can be associated with a gradual hearing loss. Involvement of the entire tympanic membrane is called tympanosclerosis.

A Air bubbles on the tympanic membrane (**Figure 11.22**) are abnormal.

P Conditions such as coryza and influenza and changes in extratympanic pressure (such as in scuba diving, plane travel) can lead to eustachian tube failure.

A The presence of blood in the middle ear is abnormal (**Figure 11.23**).

P Haemotympanum occurs as a result of trauma to the head. The tympanic membrane can have a bluish hue or can be red in appearance.

A A severely retracted tympanic membrane has exaggerated landmarks. Mobility of the tympanic membrane is decreased.

P Retraction of the tympanic membrane can occur when the intratympanic membrane pressures are reduced, as in eustachian tube blockage caused by otitis media with effusion or allergies. Repeated negative pressure in the middle ear sucks in the tympanic membrane and leads to retractions. Over time, keratinised epithelial debris deposits itself in these retraction pockets and leads to ossicle fixation. This leads to cholesteatoma (**Figure 11.24**). A foul-smelling ear discharge, as well as deafness, may accompany cholesteatoma.

A There is redness, swelling, narrowing and pain of the external ear (**Figure 11.25**). Drainage may be present.

P Acute otitis externa (AOM) is caused by infectious organisms or allergic reactions. Predisposing factors include excessive moisture in the ear related to swimming, trauma from cleansing the ears with a sharp instrument, or allergies to substances such as hairspray.

A Hard, dry, and very dark yellow-brown cerumen is abnormal.

P Old cerumen is harder and drier, and may become impacted if not removed.

A The tympanic membrane is red, with decreased mobility and possible bulging (**Figure 11.26**).

P This is **otitis media**, or an inflammation of the middle ear. Pain and fever may accompany the ear infection. Otalgia, fever, decreased hearing, irritability, disturbed sleep and otorrhoea may accompany the middle ear infection. *Streptococcus pneumoniae*, *Haemophilus influenzae* and *Moraxella catarrhalis* are the major pathogens that cause AOM.

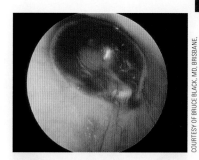
FIGURE 11.22 Barotrauma caused by scuba diving

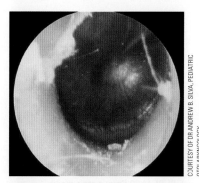
FIGURE 11.23 Haemotympanum

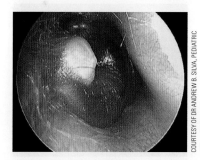
FIGURE 11.24 Cholesteatoma

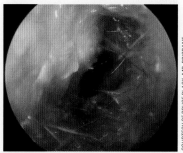
FIGURE 11.25 Acute otitis externa

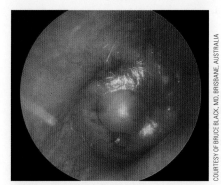
A. Early AOM. Note the bulging tympanic membrane.
FIGURE 11.26 Acute otitis media

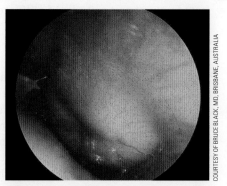
B. More advanced AOM with bleb formation. Note the bulging tympanic membrane and purulent effusion behind it. The pressure behind the membrane caused a vesicle to form on the pars tensa.

E Examination **N** Normal findings **A** Abnormal findings **P** Pathophysiology

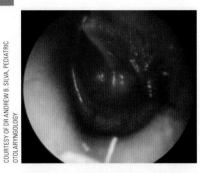

FIGURE 11.27 Otitis media with effusion

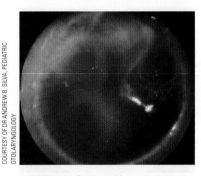

FIGURE 11.28 Serous otitis media

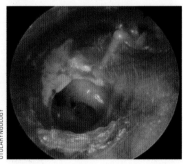

FIGURE 11.29 Tympanic membrane perforation

A Amber-yellow fluid on the tympanic membrane is abnormal. It may be accompanied by a fluid line or bubbles behind the membrane. Bulging may be present and mobility of the eardrum may be decreased (**Figures 11.27** and **11.28**). The consumer may complain of ear popping, pain and decreased hearing.

P Otitis media with effusion (OME), or serous otitis media, can be caused by allergies, infections, and a blocked eustachian tube. **Table 11.1** compares AOM, OME and otitis externa.

TABLE 11.1 Comparison of acute otitis media (AOM), otitis media with effusion (OME) and otitis externa

	ACUTE OTITIS MEDIA	OTITIS MEDIA WITH EFFUSION	OTITIS EXTERNA
Tympanic membrane colour	Diffuse red, dilated peripheral vessels	Yellowish	Within normal limits
Tympanic membrane appearance	Bulging	Bubbles, fluid line	Within normal limits
Tympanic membrane landmarks	Decreased	Retracted with prominent malleus	Within normal limits
Movement of tragus	Painless	Painless	Painful
Hearing	Within normal limits/decreased	Within normal limits/decreased	Within normal limits
External auditory canal	Within normal limits	Within normal limits	Erythematous, oedematous

A The tympanic membrane appears to have a darkened area or a hole.

P A perforated eardrum is caused by untreated ear infection secondary to increasing pressure. Trauma to the ear canal can also cause a perforation (**Figure 11.29**).

A The tympanic membrane is pearly grey and has dark patches.

P These patches are usually old perforations in the tympanic membrane.

A The tympanic membrane is pearly grey and has dense white plaques.

P These plaques represent calcific deposits of scarring of the tympanic membrane from frequent past episodes of otitis media.

CLINICAL REASONING

Practice tip: Caution in taking nasal swabs

For any client who requires nasal swabs, care should be taken as people with a history of nosebleeds (epistaxis) can have this triggered by the swabbing of the nares and nasal passages, as most nose bleeds occur in the anterior nasal passages. Alternate testing should be considered if possible. If this is not possible, the clinician needs to be prepared to treat epistaxis and also educate the client that they may experience a nose bleed post swab and what to do if this occurs after leaving the health settings.

E Examination   **N** Normal findings   **A** Abnormal findings   **P** Pathophysiology

Examination of the nose

Inspection

External nose

E Inspect the nose, noting any trauma, bleeding, lesions, masses, swelling and asymmetry.

N The shape of the external nose can vary greatly among individuals. Normally, it is located symmetrically in the midline of the face and is without swelling, bleeding, lesions or masses.

A The nose is misshapen, broken or swollen.

P The shape of the nose is determined by genetics; however, changes can occur because of trauma or cosmetic surgery.

Patency

E 1. Have the consumer occlude one nostril with a finger.
2. Ask the consumer to breathe in and out through the nose as you observe and listen for air movement in and out of the nostril.
3. Repeat on the other side.

N Each nostril is patent.

A You observe or the consumer states that air cannot be moved through the nostril(s).

P Occlusion of the nostrils can occur with a deviated septum, foreign body, upper respiratory infection, allergies or nasal polyps.

A Nasal drainage is observed from only one side of the nose.

P Unilateral nasal drainage may be a sign of nasal obstruction (on the side of no drainage).

Internal nose

Depending on context, this may be foundation or advanced practice.

E 1. Position the consumer with the head in an extended position.
2. Place the nondominant hand firmly on top of the consumer's head.
3. Using the thumb of the same hand, lift the tip of the consumer's nose.
4. Gently insert a nasal speculum or an otoscope with a short, wide nasal speculum (**Figure 11.30**). If using a nasal speculum, use a penlight to view the nostrils.
5. Assess each nostril separately.
6. Inspect the mucous membranes for colour and discharge.
7. Inspect the middle and inferior turbinates and the middle meatus for colour, swelling, drainage, lesions and polyps.
8. Observe the nasal septum for deviation, perforation, lesions and bleeding.

N The nasal mucosa should be pink or dull red without swelling or polyps. The septum is at the midline and without perforation, lesions or bleeding. A small amount of clear, watery discharge is normal.

A A nasal septum that is 'pushed' to one side can be an abnormal finding (**Figure 11.31**).

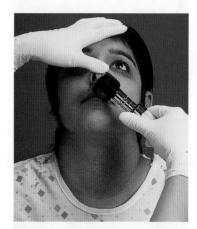

FIGURE 11.30 Internal inspection of the nose

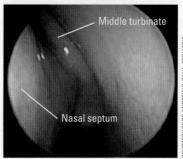

Middle turbinate

Nasal septum

COURTESY OF DR ANDREW B. SILVA, PEDIATRIC OTOLARYNGOLOGY

FIGURE 11.31 Deviated septum

E Examination   **N** Normal findings   **A** Abnormal findings   **P** Pathophysiology

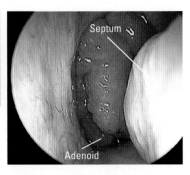

FIGURE 11.32 Nasal cavity blocked by adenoid

COURTESY OF DR ANDREW B. SILVA, PEDIATRIC OTOLARYNGOLOGY

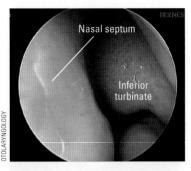

COURTESY OF DR ANDREW B. SILVA, PEDIATRIC OTOLARYNGOLOGY

FIGURE 11.33 Oedematous inferior turbinate causing almost total occlusion of the nasal cavity. Note the slight difference in colour between the septum and the turbinate. These findings can occur in consumers with allergic rhinitis.

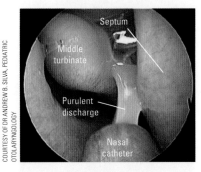

COURTESY OF DR ANDREW B. SILVA, PEDIATRIC OTOLARYNGOLOGY

FIGURE 11.34 Purulent discharge in the nasal cavity at the middle turbinate

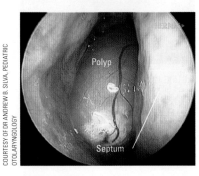

COURTESY OF DR ANDREW B. SILVA, PEDIATRIC OTOLARYNGOLOGY

FIGURE 11.35 Nasal polyp

CLINICAL **REASONING**

Practice tip: Assessing patency of the nose

This is a basic part of assessing the nose. It is important to find the reason for reduced patency. This can be easily assessed by checking for the consumer's sense of smell. The sense of smell (CN I) is evaluated during testing of cranial nerves. Refer to Chapter 7. If the consumer has a reduced sense of smell, then the clinician can check for reasons behind this reduction (e.g. physical obstruction either by foreign object, change in physiology or presence of mucus should be ruled out before considering nerve issues as the cause). Depression has also been linked to a reduction of sense of smell and taste.

P A deviated septum can be a naturally occurring finding, or it can be caused by trauma to the face and nasal area.

A A nasal septum with a hole or fissure is abnormal.

P A perforated nasal septum may be caused by nasal insufflation (snorting) of cocaine, which can lead to necrosis of the septal cartilage. Long-term intranasal corticosteroids can also result in a perforated nasal septum if an incorrect administration technique is used.

A A nasal cavity that is occluded is abnormal.

P There are many causes of an occluded nasal cavity. Foreign bodies may be present, especially in children. Trauma may induce nasal oedema, sinus infection may produce copious discharge, an adenoid may be so large that it occludes the nasal cavity (**Figure 11.32**), and allergies can lead to oedematous turbinates (**Figure 11.33**).

A The nasal mucosa is red and swollen with copious clear, watery discharge. This is rhinitis, an inflammation of the nasal mucosa.

P These findings indicate the occurrence of the common cold (coryza) when there is an acute onset of symptoms. Discharge may become purulent if a secondary bacterial infection develops.

A Nasal mucosa is pale and oedematous with clear, watery discharge.

P These findings usually indicate the presence of allergies or hay fever.

A Following trauma to the head, there is a clear, watery nasal discharge with normal-appearing mucosa. This discharge tests positive for glucose.

P These findings indicate the presence of cerebrospinal fluid. This may occur following head injury or complications of nose or sinus surgery or dental work. Immediate referral is warranted.

A Nasal mucosa is red and swollen with purulent nasal discharge (see **Figure 11.34**). These findings are usually worse on one side but may be found bilaterally.

P These are common findings in bacterial sinusitis.

A Smooth, round masses that are pale and shiny are noted protruding from the middle meatus.

P These masses are nasal polyps (see **Figure 11.35**), which may obstruct air passages. They are often seen in consumers who have chronic allergic rhinitis, asthma or cystic fibrosis. They are usually found bilaterally. A unilateral polyp is suspect for a malignancy until proven otherwise.

E Examination　**N** Normal findings　**A** Abnormal findings　**P** Pathophysiology

PUTTING IT IN CONTEXT

Allergy assessment

Jenny Adams is a 13-year-old Caucasian female attending high school. She presents to the general practice with her mother complaining of hay fever symptoms that have been worsening over the past 6 months. Mum states she notices Jenny is increasingly restless when sleeping, becoming cranky and easily upset, unable to concentrate for long, has watery eyes, sneezes up to 17 times in a row, and normal doses of antihistamines are not helping. Jenny states that sometimes her eyes are so itchy and watery that she has trouble with her vision from rubbing them so hard; she wakes up with a dry mouth and bad breath and mum reports she has been snoring lately.

On examination Jenny's visual acuity is normal, her eyes are slightly reddened, she has a small amount of periorbital oedema, and you observe her sneeze 12 times in a row. Her tonsils are normal size, with no redness or swelling in her mouth or throat. She has had a Claratyne this morning along with ibuprofen for her headache, which she states is in her temples and behind her eyes. She consistently rubs her eyes and appears tired, yawning frequently and has dark shadows under her eyes.

A skin prick test shows Jenny has a 9 times 'normal' size allergy wheal to dust mites, and within 8 minutes of the skin prick test has a red itchy line travelling up her arm to her shoulder. Jenny is diagnosed with severe allergy to dust mites. On inspection of her nasal passages, she has approximately 80% blockage on each side of her septum. Jenny starts to have trouble breathing within 14 minutes of her skin prick test and is given adrenalin for a mild anaphylactic reaction to the dust mite allergen. The nurse educates Jenny and her mum on how to modify her environment to reduce allergen levels. Jenny commences on immunotherapy to reduce her sensitivity. She is also placed on large doses of antihistamines to reduce the histamine response that her symptoms are showing.

A Bleeding is noted from an area of the lower portion of the nasal septum (also known as epistaxis).

P Kiesselbach's plexus, a vascular area on the septum, is the site of most nosebleeds (see **Figure 11.36**). Repeated nosebleeds warrant attention for blood dyscrasias, environmental causes, medication use (e.g. anticoagulants) and malignancies, among other aetiologies.

A There is unilateral purulent discharge; however, the consumer does not experience other symptoms of an upper respiratory infection. Nasal mucosa on the unaffected side appears normal.

P Unilateral purulent discharge without other findings of an upper respiratory infection indicates the development of a local infection. A common cause of localised infection is the presence of a foreign body.

A Nasal mucosa is inflamed and friable with possible septal perforation. There is no infection present.

P These findings may indicate nasal inhalation of cocaine or amphetamines, or the overuse of nasal spray.

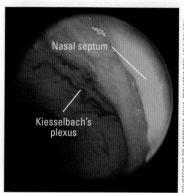

FIGURE 11.36 Kiesselbach's plexus

COURTESY OF DR ANDREW B. SILVA, PEDIATRIC OTOLARYNGOLOGY

Examination of the sinuses

Inspection

E Observe the consumer's face for any swelling around the nose and eyes.

N There is no evidence of swelling around the nose and eyes.

A Swelling is noted above or below the eyes.

P Acute sinusitis may result in swelling of the face around the eyes due to inflammation and accumulation of purulent material in the paranasal sinuses.

E Examination   **N** Normal findings   **A** Abnormal findings   **P** Pathophysiology

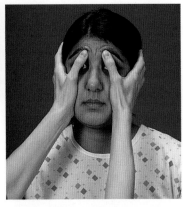

A. Palpation of frontal sinuses

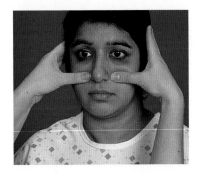

B. Palpation of maxillary sinuses

FIGURE 11.37 Palpation of sinuses

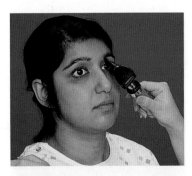

A. Frontal sinus

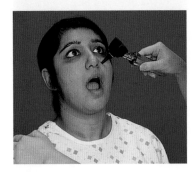

B. Maxillary sinus

FIGURE 11.38 Transillumination of sinuses

Palpation and percussion

To palpate and percuss the frontal sinuses:

E 1. Stand facing the consumer.
   2. Gently press the thumbs under the bony ridge of the upper orbits (see **Figure 11.37A**). Avoid applying pressure on the globes themselves.
   3. Observe for the presence of pain.
   4. Percuss the areas using the middle or index finger of the dominant hand (direct percussion).
   5. Note the sound.

N A P Refer to maxillary sinuses.

To palpate and percuss the maxillary sinuses:

E 1. Stand in front of the consumer.
   2. Apply gentle pressure in the area under the infraorbital ridge using the thumb or middle finger (**Figure 11.37B**).
   3. Observe for the presence of pain.
   4. Percuss the area using the dominant middle or index finger.
   5. Note the sound.

N The consumer should experience no discomfort during palpation or percussion. The sinuses should be air-filled and therefore resonant to percussion.

A The consumer complains of pain or tenderness at the site of palpation or percussion.

P Sinusitis can be due to viral, bacterial or allergic processes that cause inflammation of the mucous membranes and obstruction of the drainage pathways.

A Percussion of the sinuses elicits a dull sound.

P Dullness can be caused by fluid or cells present in the sinus cavity from an infectious or allergic process, or congenital absence of a sinus.

Transillumination of the sinuses

If palpation and percussion of the sinuses suggest sinusitis, transillumination of the frontal and maxillary sinuses may be performed by the advanced practitioner.

To evaluate the frontal sinuses:
1. Place the consumer in a sitting position facing you in a dark room.
2. Place a strong light source such as a transilluminator, penlight, or tip of an otoscope with the speculum under the bony ridge of the upper orbits (**Figure 11.38A**).
3. Observe the red glow over the sinuses and compare the symmetry of the two sides.

To evaluate the maxillary sinuses:
1. Place the consumer in a sitting position facing you in a dark room.
2. Place the light source firmly under each eye and just above the infraorbital ridge (**Figure 11.38B**).
3. Ask the consumer to open the mouth; observe the red glow on the hard palate.
4. Compare the two sides.
   - The glow on each side is equal, indicating air-filled frontal and maxillary sinuses.
   - Absence of glow is abnormal.
   - Absence of glow suggests sinus congestion or the congenital absence of a sinus.
   - An extremely bright glow is abnormal.
   - This phenomenon may be present in an elderly consumer with decreased subcutaneous fat.

E Examination   **N** Normal findings   **A** Abnormal findings   **P** Pathophysiology   Advanced Assessment

Examination of the mouth and throat

1. Physical examination of the oral cavity should include the following: breath, lips, tongue, buccal mucosa, gums and teeth, hard and soft palates, throat (oropharynx), and temporomandibular joint (see Chapters 9 and 16).
2. If the consumer is wearing dentures or removable orthodontia, ask that they be removed before the examination begins.
3. Use gloves and a good light source such as a penlight for optimum visualisation of the oral cavity and pharynx.

Examination of breath

E 1. Stand facing the consumer and about 30 cm away.
2. Smell the breath.

N The breath should smell fresh.

A The breath smells foul.

P The foul smell of halitosis can be a symptom of tooth decay, poor oral hygiene, or diseases of the gums, tonsils or sinuses, or gastrointestinal ulcers.

A The breath smells of acetone.

P Acetone or 'fruity' breath is common in consumers who are malnourished or who have diabetic ketoacidosis. The consumer may also be on a low carbohydrate diet.

A The breath smells musty.

P Foetor hepaticus is the musty smell of the breath of a consumer in liver failure and is caused by the breakdown of nitrogen compounds.

A The breath smells of ammonia.

P The smell of ammonia can be detected in a consumer in end-stage renal failure (uraemia) because of the inability to eliminate urea.

Examination of the lips

Inspection

E 1. Observe the lips for colour, moisture, swelling, lesions and other signs of inflammation.
2. Instruct the consumer to open the mouth.
3. Use a tongue blade to inspect the membranes that connect the upper and lower lips to the gums for colour, inflammation, lesions and hydration.

N The lips and membranes should be pink and moist with no evidence of lesions or inflammation.

A The lips are pale or cyanotic.

P Refer to Chapter 14.

A The lips are dry and cracked.

P Chapping or superficial cracking of the lips may be due to exposure to wind, sun, or a dry environment, dehydration of the consumer, or persistent licking of the lips.

A Swelling of the lips is noted.

P Allergic reactions to medications, insect bites, foods or other allergens can result in swelling of the lips.

A The skin at the outer corners of the mouth is atrophic, irritated and cracked.

P Angular cheilosis may be due to increased accumulation of saliva in the corners of the mouth or constant drooling from the mouth. This occurs in nutritional deficiencies (such as riboflavin), poorly fitting dentures, and deficiencies of the immune system. *Candida* infections may also be present.

E Examination   **N** Normal findings   **A** Abnormal findings   **P** Pathophysiology

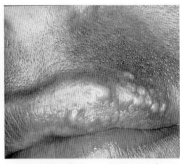

A. Fever blister (herpes simplex virus)

COURTESY OF DR JOSEPH KONZELMAN, SCHOOL OF DENTISTRY, MEDICAL COLLEGE OF GEORGIA

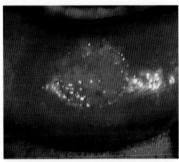

B. Chancre from primary syphilis

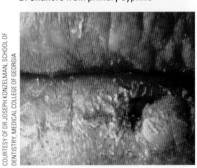

COURTESY OF DR JOSEPH KONZELMAN, SCHOOL OF DENTISTRY, MEDICAL COLLEGE OF GEORGIA

C. Squamous cell carcinoma

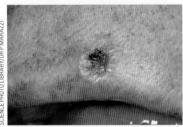

SCIENCE PHOTO LIBRARY/DR P MARAZZI

D. Basal cell carcinoma

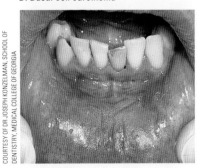

COURTESY OF DR JOSEPH KONZELMAN, SCHOOL OF DENTISTRY, MEDICAL COLLEGE OF GEORGIA

E. Leukoplakia

FIGURE 11.39 Lip abnormalities

A Vesicles on erythematous bases with serous fluid are found on the lips, gums or hard palate, either singly or in clusters. They later rupture, crust over and become painful (**Figure 11.39A**).

P These are herpes simplex lesions, which are commonly called cold sores or fever blisters. This common viral infection may be precipitated by febrile illness, sunlight, stress or allergies.

A A round, painless lesion with central ulceration (**Figure 11.39B**) is noted. This lesion may become crusted.

P This is a chancre, the primary lesion of syphilis.

A A plaque, wart, nodule or ulcer is noted, usually on the lower lip.

P This may be squamous cell carcinoma, the most common form of oral cancer, which is more frequent in males (**Figure 11.39C**).

P Basal cell carcinoma lesions can have pearly borders, crusting, and central ulcerations (**Figure 11.39D**).

A Persistent, painless, white, painted-looking patches are noted on the lips (**Figure 11.39E**). They are associated with heavy smoking and the use of chewing tobacco.

P These patches are leukoplakia and are considered premalignant lesions. They often occur at sites of chronic irritation from dentures, tobacco or excessive alcohol intake.

Palpation

E 1. Don nonsterile gloves.
2. Gently pull down the consumer's lower lip with the thumb and index finger of one hand and pull up the consumer's upper lip with the thumb and index finger of the other hand.
3. Note the tone of the lips as they are manipulated.
4. If lesions are present, palpate them for consistency and tenderness.

N Lips should not be flaccid and lesions should not be present.

A P See inspection of the lips for pathologies.

Examination of the tongue

E 1. Ask the consumer to stick out the tongue (CN XII assesses tongue movement).
2. Observe the dorsal surface for colour, hydration, texture, symmetry, fasciculations, atrophy, position in the mouth and the presence of lesions.
3. Ask the consumer to move the tongue from side to side and up and down.
4. With the consumer's tongue back in the mouth, ask the consumer to press it against the cheek. Provide resistance with your finger pads held on the outside of the cheek. Note the strength of the tongue and compare bilaterally.
5. Ask the consumer to touch the tip of the tongue to the roof of the mouth. You may also grasp the tip of the tongue with a gauze square held between the thumb and the index finger of the gloved hand (**Figure 11.40**).
6. Inspect the ventral surface of the tongue, the fraenulum and Wharton's ducts for colour, hydration, lesions, inflammation and vasculature.
7. With the gauze square, pull the tongue to the left and inspect and palpate the tongue using the finger pads.
8. Repeat with the tongue held to the right side.

E Examination   **N** Normal findings   **A** Abnormal findings   **P** Pathophysiology

N The tongue is in the midline of the mouth. The dorsum of the tongue should be pink, moist, rough (from the taste buds), and without lesions. The tongue is symmetrical and moves freely. The strength of the tongue is symmetrical and strong. The ventral surface of the tongue has prominent blood vessels and should be moist and without lesions. Wharton's ducts are patent and without inflammation or lesions. The lateral aspects of the tongue should be pink, smooth and lesion free.

A The tongue is enlarged.

P An enlarged tongue may be associated with myxoedema, acromegaly, Down syndrome or amyloidosis. Transient enlargement may be associated with glossitis, stomatitis, cellulitis of the neck, angioneurotic oedema, haematoma or abscess.

A The tongue is red and smooth with absent papillae.

P This indicates glossitis caused by a vitamin B_{12}, iron or niacin deficiency. It may also be a side effect of chemotherapy.

A There is a thick, white, curd-like coating on the tongue that leaves a raw, red surface when it is scraped off (**Figure 11.41A**).

P This is candidiasis, or thrush, which may also be red in the absence of the coating. Thrush can result from changes in the normal oral flora due to chemotherapy, radiation therapy, disorders of the immune system such as AIDS, antibiotic therapy, or excessive use of alcohol, tobacco or cocaine.

A Thin, pearly white lesions that coalesce and become thick and palpable are noted on the sides of the tongue. These white lesions are firmly attached to the underlying tissue and will not scrape off.

P This is leukoplakia. It is considered a premalignant lesion. Some leukoplakia progresses from dysplasia to a malignancy.

A A painful, small, round, white ulcerated lesion with erythematous borders is abnormal (**Figure 11.41B**).

P This is an aphthous ulcer (canker sore), which can be associated with stress, extreme fatigue, food allergies and oral trauma.

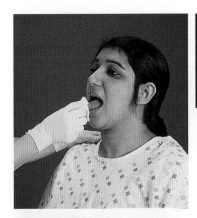

FIGURE 11.40 Tongue assessment

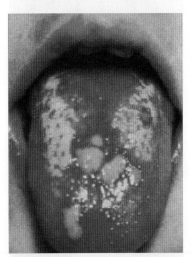

A. Candidiasis (thrush)

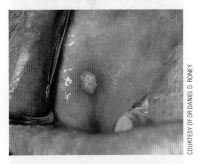

B. Aphthous ulcer (canker sore)

FIGURE 11.41 Tongue conditions

COURTESY OF DR DANIEL D. RONEY

HEALTH EDUCATION

Making connections – oral cancer

Oral cancer risk factors are important to consider for long-term health promotion and harm minimisation, especially for factors that are modifiable by a change in lifestyle choices. Consider which of these factors are modifiable and would influence your opportunistic education approaches.

> Male sex
  • Aboriginal and Torres Strait Islander peoples are 1.4 times more likely to die from cancer and have a lower five-year relative survival rate compared to non-Aboriginal and Torres Strait Islander peoples (AIHW, 2018).
> Age > 40 years
> Tobacco use (pipes, cigars, cigarettes)
> Excessive alcohol use
> Sun exposure (lips)
> History of leukoplakia
> History of erythroplasia

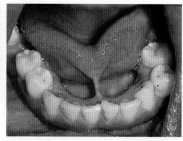

C. Ankyloglossia

COURTESY OF DR JOSEPH KONZELMAN, SCHOOL OF DENTISTRY, MEDICAL COLLEGE OF GEORGIA

COURTESY OF DR JOSEPH KONZELMAN, SCHOOL OF DENTISTRY, MEDICAL COLLEGE OF GEORGIA

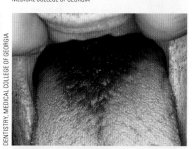

D. Oral hairy leukoplakia

COURTESY OF DR DANIEL D. RONEY

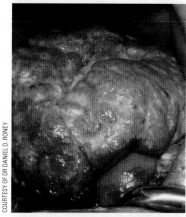

E. Carcinoma of the tongue

COURTESY OF DR JOSEPH KONZELMAN, SCHOOL OF DENTISTRY, MEDICAL COLLEGE OF GEORGIA

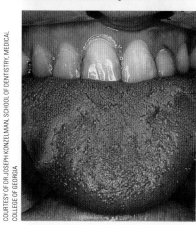

F. Geographic tongue

FIGURE 11.41 continued Tongue conditions

A A short lingual fraenulum is observed (**Figure 11.41C**).

P Ankyloglossia is a congenital abnormality (also known as tongue-tie).

A The tongue has a hairy appearance and is yellow, black or brown (**Figure 11.41D**).

P This is oral hairy leukoplakia, or hairy tongue, a benign condition that can result from antibiotic therapy. The hairy appearance is caused by elongated papillae.

A Lesions are noted on the ventral surface of the tongue.

P The ventral surface of the tongue is an area where malignancies are likely to develop, especially in consumers who drink alcohol and smoke or use smokeless tobacco.

A Indurations, or ulcerations (**Figure 11.41E**), are present on the lateral surfaces of the tongue.

P Most lingual cancers are located in this area and are associated with use of alcohol and tobacco.

A Patches of red denuded areas on the lingual surface of the tongue, frequently at the papillae, surrounded by ridges of pale yellow epithelium are abnormal (**Figure 11.41F**).

P This harmless condition, geographic tongue, has no known cause. Its name is derived from the patterns of regular and irregular surfaces on the tongue that resemble a map.

A Numerous furrows or grooves are observed, often radiating horizontally from the midline of the dorsal surface of the tongue (**Figure 11.41G**).

P This harmless and often inherited condition is fissured or scrotal tongue. It is different from syphilitic glossitis, which is characterised by longitudinal furrows.

A Engorged blood vessels of the tongue are abnormal (see **Figure 11.41H**).

P A haemangioma of the tongue is a benign overgrowth of vascular tissue.

A Deviation of the tongue toward one side (see **Figure 11.41I**), atrophy and asymmetrical shape of the tongue are abnormal.

P Unilateral paralysis of the tongue muscles will cause the tongue to deviate towards the affected side because the muscles on the paralysed side are unable to oppose the strong muscles of the unaffected side. The consumer is unable to push the tongue towards the nonparalysed side. Lesions of the hypoglossal nucleus or nerve fibre cause these unilateral symptoms.

A Atrophy of the tongue and the inability to protrude the tongue are abnormal.

P Bilateral paralysis of the tongue muscles will prevent the consumer from protruding the tongue. Syringobulbia or trauma to CN XII may cause hypoglossal nerve paralysis.

Examination of buccal mucosa

E 1. Ask the consumer to open their mouth as wide as possible.
2. Use a tongue depressor and a penlight to assess the inner cheeks and the openings of Stensen's ducts (**Figure 11.42**).
3. Observe for colour, inflammation, hydration and lesions.

N The colour of the oral mucosa on the inside of the cheek may vary according to race. Dark skinned people have a bluish hue; light-skinned people have pink mucosa. Freckle-like macules may appear on the inside of the buccal mucosa. The buccal mucosa should be moist, smooth, and free of inflammation and lesions. Some consumers may have torus mandibularis (see **Figure 11.43A**), which are bony nodules in the mandibular region.

A Leathery, painless, white, painted-looking patches are noted.

E Examination **N** Normal findings **A** Abnormal findings **P** Pathophysiology

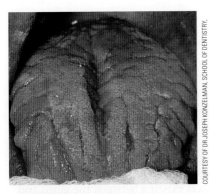

G. Fissured tongue (scrotal tongue)

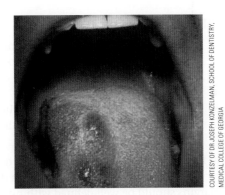

H. Haemangioma

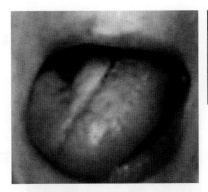

I. Cranial nerve XII (hypoglossal) palsy

FIGURE 11.41 continued Tongue conditions

P Leukoplakia may be found in the buccal mucosa.

A Yellow patches on the buccal mucosa are present.

P Fordyce spots are small sebaceous glands (see **Figure 11.43B**).

A The orifice of Stensen's duct is erythematous and oedematous. It may be tender to palpation.

P This is seen in parotitis, an inflammation of the parotid gland. The area between the ear lobule and angle of the mandible may not be visible due to the swelling of the parotid gland (see **Figure 11.43C**). Acute unilateral swelling may be seen in mumps.

A The mucosa is pale.

P This can be caused by anaemia or vasoconstriction that may occur when the sympathetic nervous system is stimulated, such as in shock.

A The mucosa is cyanotic.

P Cyanosis can indicate systemic hypoxaemia. See Chapters 8 and 14.

A The mucosa is erythematous.

P Erythema can be associated with stomatitis.

A There is excessive dryness of the mucosa.

P This is xerostomia, which occurs when salivary gland activity is decreased, when the consumer is hypovolaemic, or with mouth breathing, Sjögren's syndrome or salivary gland obstruction.

A Excessive moisture is noted in the mouth.

P This condition may be noted in the early stages of inflammation or when the consumer is hypervolaemic.

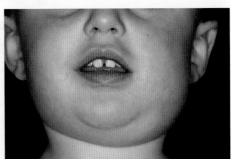

FIGURE 11.42 Assessment of the buccal mucosa

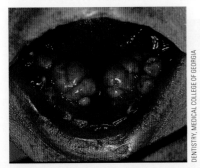

A. Torus mandibularis

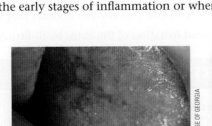

B. Fordyce spots

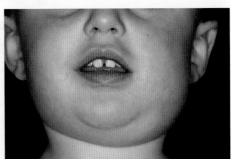

C. Left parotitis

FIGURE 11.43 Buccal mucosa

E Examination **N** Normal findings **A** Abnormal findings **P** Pathophysiology

Examination of the gums

E 1. Instruct the consumer to open the mouth.
2. Observe dentures or orthodontics for fit.
3. Remove any dentures or removable orthodontia.
4. Shine the penlight in the mouth.
5. Use the tongue depressor to move the tongue to visualise the gums.
6. Observe for redness, swelling, bleeding, retraction from the teeth or discolouration.

N In light-skinned individuals, the gums have a pale red, stippled surface. Patchy brown pigmentation may be present in dark-skinned consumers. The gum margins should be well defined with no pockets existing between the gums and the teeth and no swelling or bleeding.

A The gingiva are red, tender and swollen, and bleed easily (**Figure 11.44**).

P This describes gingivitis, which may be caused by poor dental hygiene, improperly fitted dentures, and scurvy. Gingivitis can also occur with stomatitis that occurs in mouth infections and upper respiratory tract infections.

A Gingival borders are red and there is infection of the pockets formed between receding gums and teeth. Purulent drainage may be present.

P This is periodontitis, which is an inflammation of the periodontium due to chronic gingivitis. This condition is caused by infrequent brushing of the teeth and poor oral hygiene.

A Blue lines are noted approximately 1 mm from the gingival margin.

P These are lead lines or bismuth lines caused by chronic exposure to lead or bismuth.

A The gums are brownish.

P This occurs in association with Addison's disease.

A A nontender, immobile tumour lighter than the gums is noted on the gum.

P This lesion is epulis, a fibrous tumour of the gums.

A The gums are retracted from the teeth (**Figure 11.45**), sometimes exposing the roots of the teeth.

P This recession of the gums often occurs in older individuals due to poor oral hygiene.

A Hypertrophy of gum tissue is abnormal (**Figure 11.46**).

P This is gingival hyperplasia and is usually painless; it occurs in pregnancy, in wearers of orthodontic braces, by dental plaque, or with the use of some medications such as phenytoin.

A Small ulcers or folds of excess tissue are noted on the gums under an ill-fitting denture. Inflamed and swollen nodules may be seen in the area of the palate.

P Continued irritation of the gums by ill-fitting dentures results in hyperplasia.

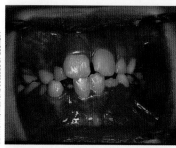
FIGURE 11.44 Gingivitis with herpes simplex

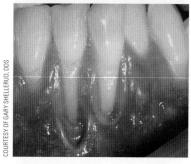
FIGURE 11.45 Gingival recession

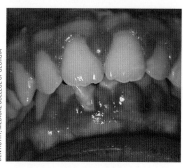
FIGURE 11.46 Gingival hyperplasia

REFLECTION IN PRACTICE

The consumer with poor oral hygiene

Mary is a 78-year-old widow who lives alone. She attends the clinic for a blood pressure check-up, but you notice that she has left her dentures out. When you ask her where her teeth are she states they are hurting her. On inspection you note multiple ulcers in her gums, remains of food particles in her gum and cheek margins and a foul smell. On further investigation you find out that she brushes her dentures every few days but does not have a cleaning regimen for her gums and mucous membranes.

> What type of education would you recommend and why?
> Would you refer Mary to anyone?
> What type of treatment may she require and why?

Examination of the teeth

E 1. Instruct the consumer to open the mouth.
2. Count the upper and lower teeth.
3. Observe the teeth for discolouration, loose or missing teeth, caries, malocclusion and malformation.

N The adult normally has 32 teeth, which should be white with smooth edges, in proper alignment, and without caries.

A Teeth are absent.

P This problem may be due to loss or failure of development. The consumer's nutritional status may be seriously impaired when the teeth are insufficient.

A There are white or black patches on the surface of a tooth. These patches may become eroded as damage progresses.

P These are dental caries, or cavities, resulting from poor oral hygiene.

A The teeth are worn at an angle.

P Biting surfaces of the teeth may become worn down by repetitive biting on hard substances or objects or grinding of teeth (bruxism), especially at night.

A A tooth is dark in colour and the consumer reports insensitivity to cold.

P This is usually a dead tooth, which results in a darkening of the enamel.

A Teeth that have serrated edges (**Figure 11.47**) are abnormal.

P These are called Hutchinson's incisors. Pregnant women with syphilis can have infants with abnormal dentition because of the effects of the disease on tooth development.

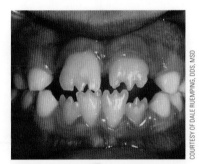

FIGURE 11.47 Hutchinson's incisors

COURTESY OF DALE RUEMPING, DDS, MSD

Examination of the palate

E 1. Ask the consumer to tilt the head back and open the mouth as wide as possible.
2. Shine the penlight in the consumer's mouth.
3. Observe both the hard and the soft palates.
4. Note their shape and colour, and the presence of any lesions or malformations.

N The hard and soft palates are concave and pink. The hard palate has many ridges; the soft palate is smooth. No lesions or malformations are noted.

A The palates are red, swollen, tender, or with lesions.

P These findings are symptoms of infection.

A A fibrous, encapsulated tissue growth on the palate is abnormal (**Figure 11.48**).

P A fibroma may be idiopathic or neoplastic in origin. Chronic trauma can also lead to fibroma formation.

A A lesion that has become eroded is noted on the palate.

P This may be a cancerous lesion in the epithelium of the hard palate.

A There is a hole in the hard palate.

P Palatine perforation is related to syphilis or radiation therapy.

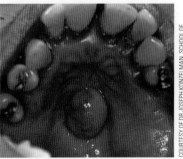

FIGURE 11.48 Fibroma

COURTESY OF DR JOSEPH KONZELMAN, SCHOOL OF DENTISTRY, MEDICAL COLLEGE OF GEORGIA

E Examination   **N** Normal findings   **A** Abnormal findings   **P** Pathophysiology

CLINICAL **REASONING**

Practice tip: Maintaining dignity during physical examination
Examining the mouth, gums and teeth of a client is important; however, please ensure you
are managing this examination with dignity. This means allowing the client to remove teeth
if they can, and ensure they are rinsed before being offered to place back in the mouth.
Do not ask questions while teeth are removed as this can be difficult and embarrassing for
the client to try and speak clearly while they have no teeth in. Handle false teeth and dental
plates gently and ensure they are not dropped.

While people of any age may have false teeth and dental plates, this is seen in higher
percentages in elderly consumers. Revisit the aged care standards (hint Standard 1)
to review examples of this. Resource link: https://www.agedcarequality.gov.au/
providers/standards

Examination of the throat
Inspection

E 1. Ask the consumer to tilt the head back and to open the mouth wide. The
consumer can either stick out the tongue or leave it resting on the floor
of the mouth.
2. With the right hand, place the tongue blade on the middle third of
the tongue.
3. With the left hand, shine a light at the back of the consumer's throat.
4. Ask the consumer to say 'ah'.
5. Observe the position, size, colour and general appearance of the tonsils
and uvula.
6. Touch the posterior third of the tongue with the tongue blade.
7. Note movement of the palate and the presence of the gag reflex.
8. Assess the colour of the oropharynx. Note the presence of swelling,
exudate or lesions.

N When the consumer says 'ah', the soft palate and the uvula should rise
symmetrically (CN IX and X). The uvula is midline. The throat is normally pink
and vascular and without swelling, exudate or lesions. Normal tonsillar size is
evaluated as 1+ to 2+. (See **Figure 11.49** for grading scale.) This indicates that both
tonsils are behind the pillars. The consumer's gag reflex should be present but is
congenitally absent in some consumers (CN IX and X).

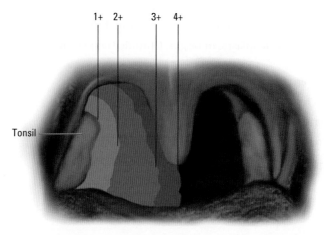

FIGURE 11.49 Grading of tonsils: 1+ tonsils are visible, 2+ tonsils are between the pillars and uvula, 3+ tonsils
are touching the uvula, 4+ tonsils extend to the midline of the oropharynx

E Examination **N** Normal findings **A** Abnormal findings **P** Pathophysiology

A The posterior pharynx is red with white patches. The tonsils are large and red with white patches, and the uvula is red and swollen.

P Viral pharyngitis and tonsillitis are common illnesses with these findings.

A Tonsils, pillars and uvula are very red and swollen, with patches of white or yellow exudate on the tonsils (**Figure 11.50**). The posterior pharynx is bright red. The consumer reports soreness of the throat with swallowing.

P These findings are typical of streptococcal pharyngitis and tonsillitis and are usually associated with significant lymphadenopathy. However, diagnosis requires throat culture.

A There is a greyish membrane covering the tonsils, uvula and soft palate.

P These findings are typical of diphtheria, acute tonsillitis or infectious mononucleosis.

A The consumer speaks with a hoarse voice and the oropharynx is red.

P Causes of hoarseness are varied and may include overuse of the voice, inflammation due to viral or bacterial infection, lesions of the larynx, foreign bodies, and pressure on the larynx from masses or an enlarged thyroid gland.

A The consumer has difficulty opening the mouth (trismus) and is noted to have unilateral tonsillar swelling. Unusual phonation is also observed.

P These findings are associated with peritonsillar abscess, which is most commonly seen in older children and young adults with a history of frequent tonsillitis.

A Chronic 3+ or 4+ tonsils (**Figure 11.51**) are abnormal.

P Large tonsils frequently lead to loud snoring and obstructive sleep apnoea.

A The consumer has a small oropharynx and history of snoring.

P Obstructive sleep apnoea occurs when muscles in the nasopharynx and pharynx relax during sleep, resulting in pauses in breathing. Typically, consumers are overweight, middle-aged men who complain of excessive daytime sleepiness.

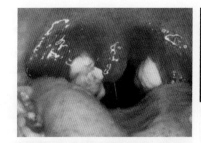

FIGURE 11.50 Streptococcal pharyngitis

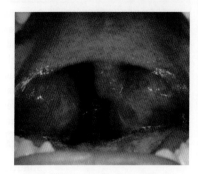

FIGURE 11.51 Left tonsil is 4+ and right tonsil is 3+

EVALUATION OF HEALTH ASSESSMENT AND PHYSICAL EXAMINATION FINDINGS

In the evaluation phase of a health assessment, the focus is on ensuring the data gathered is complete, accurate and documented appropriately (see case study as an example of the focused assessment; see Chapter 22 for a comprehensive health assessment). In evaluating the data you should:

> draw on your critical thinking and problem-solving skills to make sound clinical decisions

> act on abnormal data (include communicating findings to other health professionals)

> ensure documentation reflects the outcomes of the clinical decisions/actions taken (refer to Chapter 3, which discusses in detail why documentation is so important and how this may be undertaken in different health settings). The case study that follows steps you through this process.

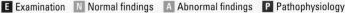

E Examination   **N** Normal findings   **A** Abnormal findings   **P** Pathophysiology

THE CONSUMER WITH ACUTE RHINOSINUSITIS

This case study illustrates the application and the objective documentation of the ears, nose, mouth and throat assessment.

Lianna Potter is a 61-year-old nurse who presents to the health clinic complaining of facial pain and frontal headache.

HEALTH HISTORY		
CONSUMER PROFILE	61-year-old Caucasian female	
CHIEF COMPLAINT	'I have had a headache and facial pressure for over 10 days.'	
HISTORY OF THE PRESENT ILLNESS	Consumer was in her usual state of health until 10 days ago, when she developed an upper respiratory infection that seems to have become worse. Her symptoms started with nasal congestion, purulent nasal discharge and mild facial pressure. After 5 days, she developed thick, green, purulent nasal discharge, bilateral frontal headache (4/10 intensity), maxillary facial pain (6/10 intensity), and bilateral maxillary toothache. She has had a low-grade fever (37.4°C) without chills, sweats, ear pain, sore throat, chest congestion, wheezing or dyspnoea. The symptoms seem to get worse when she leans over. She has been taking decongestants every 6 hours and ibuprofen 400 mg at bedtime without relief for 3 days. Consumer has been renovating downstairs bathroom and guest bedroom for the past two weeks.	
PAST HEALTH HISTORY	**MEDICAL HISTORY**	Hypertension since age 40
	SURGICAL HISTORY	Hysterectomy, age 54
	ALLERGIES	Bees – anaphylaxis
	MEDICATIONS	> Hydrochlorothiazide 25 mg every morning > Ibuprofen for headaches 200–600 mg BD PRN > Demazin Cold and Flu – paracetamol (500 mg) and phenylephrine PRN for nasal congestion (5 mg)
	COMMUNICABLE DISEASES	Has had COVID-19 in past three months
	INJURIES AND ACCIDENTS	Denies
	SPECIAL NEEDS	Denies
	BLOOD TRANSFUSIONS	Denies
	CHILDHOOD ILLNESSES	Chickenpox, age 5, without sequelae
	IMMUNISATIONS	All up to date as per employment requirements
FAMILY HEALTH HISTORY		
SOCIAL HISTORY	**ALCOHOL USE**	1–2 glasses of wine per week
	TOBACCO USE	Never smoked
	DRUG USE	Denies
	DOMESTIC AND INTIMATE PARTNER VIOLENCE	Denies
	SEXUAL PRACTICE	Monogamous relationship with husband
	TRAVEL HISTORY	Denies recent travel more than 100 km from home in past month
	WORK ENVIRONMENT	Is a nurse manager at local health service
	HOME ENVIRONMENT	Lives with husband and adult daughter and grandchild in a single-family home. Recent renovation of downstairs area to allow for Airbnb rental to supplement income, as getting ready for retirement
	HOBBIES AND LEISURE ACTIVITIES	Music, playing golf, caravanning

>>

HEALTH HISTORY

	STRESS	New home arrangement with daughter and grandchild returning home after marriage breakdown, home renovation, recent pandemic was stressful for healthcare workers
	EDUCATION	Postgraduate qualification in nursing
	ECONOMIC STATUS	Professional – middle class; husband retired
	MILITARY SERVICE	None
	RELIGION	Christian
	CULTURAL BACKGROUND	Dutch ancestors; would like to visit European cousins some day
	ROLES AND RELATIONSHIPS	Very close to her husband and children; several close friends from her social book club and neighbourhood
	CHARACTERISTIC PATTERNS OF DAILY LIVING	Wakes at 5 a.m., skips breakfast, drives 45 minutes to get to work; usually buys lunch at hospital café, often works over hours, especially during staff shortages and during the recent pandemic; goes to the gym 2–3 times a week; arrives home around 6.30 p.m., prepares dinner for family; watches TV and goes to bed around 10 p.m.
HEALTH MAINTENANCE ACTIVITIES	SLEEP	7–8 hours of sleep during the week; 8–9 hours on the weekends; does not feel well rested last 10 days and states 'just perpetually tired since COVID started with workload'. At times is woken by grandchild during night.
	DIET	Gluten free
	EXERCISE	Walks on treadmill three times weekly for 45 minutes followed by stretching; occasional spin/aerobics class
	STRESS MANAGEMENT	Talks openly with her friends and exercises regularly
	USE OF SAFETY DEVICES	Uses seat belt in car; not taking any health precautions with home remodelling equipment/masks
	HEALTH CHECK-UPS	Annual well-woman examination; sees primary care provider every 4 months for hypertension; up to date in all other areas of preventive health (mammogram and pap smear)

PHYSICAL EXAMINATION

EXAMINATION OF THE EAR	AUDITORY SCREENING	VOICE-WHISPER TEST	Intact
		TUNING FORK TESTS	> Weber test – midline without lateralisation > Rinne test – ⊕
	INSPECTION AND PALPATION	EXTERNAL EAR	Nontender, external auditory canal clear without inflammation, no mastoid tenderness
	OTOSCOPIC ASSESSMENT		Both tympanic membranes are shiny pink and mobile with visible light reflexes; without bulging or perforation
EXAMINATION OF THE NOSE	INSPECTION	EXTERNAL NOSE	Midline without swelling, bleeding, lesions or masses
		PATENCY	Each nare is patent
		INTERNAL NOSE	Mucosa is red and swollen with purulent nasal discharge bilaterally; septum deviated to the left

>>

>>

PHYSICAL EXAMINATION

EXAMINATION OF THE SINUSES	INSPECTION			Swelling noted below eyes bilaterally
	PALPATION AND PERCUSSION			Tenderness over right maxillary sinus; dullness to percussion noted over right maxillary sinus
	TRANSILLUMINATION OF THE SINUSES			Absence of glow noted over right maxillary sinus
EXAMINATION OF THE MOUTH AND THROAT	INSPECTION AND PALPATION	BREATH		Foul smell noted
		LIPS		Pink, moist without lesions No abnormalities detected
		TONGUE		Midline, pink, well papillated without fasciculations, lesions, swelling or bleeding
		BUCCAL MUCOSA		Pink, moist without lesions
		GUMS		Pink and moist without swelling or bleeding
		TEETH		32 present, no caries; in proper alignment
		PALATE		Intact, rises with phonation
		THROAT		Mildly erythematous with 1+ tonsils bilaterally and no exudates; uvula midline; gag reflex positive

EVALUATION AND CLINICAL REASONING FOR CASE STUDY

The assessment and clinical decisions you make should reflect your scope of practice. For example, advanced practice health professionals, such as nurse practitioners and remote area nurses with endorsement, may be able to make diagnostic decisions and prescribe medications without referring to a medical officer.

Fundamentally, all health professionals collect, evaluate and act on consumer-focused health information, which will at times include referral to, or collaboration with, other healthcare team members. Nurses assess consumer responses to interventions and determine when to escalate key changes in a consumer's condition. The clinical reasoning cycle provides health professionals with a framework to consider all this information in a meaningful way for planning consumer care. These phases are stepped out below, and draw on information presented and collected during the health history and physical examination. We then work through the cycle components that are relevant to this case study (cycle components are bolded).

For Lianna, the 61-year-old woman who presents to the clinic with facial pain, the significant data that needs to be considered includes the following.

Collecting cues/information

Recall and Review: In the first instance you will need to reflect on what you know about sinusitis, upper respiratory infections,

allergy responses and the role of over-the-counter medications to manage these symptoms and the effect this can have on infections and pain.

Chief complaint and history of present illness

> 10 days ago, developed an upper respiratory infection
> Symptoms started with nasal congestion, purulent nasal discharge and mild facial pressure; after 5 days, developed thick, green, purulent nasal discharge, bilateral frontal headache (4/10 intensity), maxillary facial pain, and bilateral maxillary toothache and a low-grade fever (37.4°C)
> Symptoms worse when she leans over
> Has been taking decongestants every 6 hours and ibuprofen 400 mg at bedtime without relief for 3 days
> Has been renovating house for the past two weeks

Processing information

Interpret: These symptoms and details of history outline the scope of the issue for this consumer and how it is affecting her wellbeing and ability to self-manage this deviation from normal health. So far she is taking steps to minimise the severity of her symptoms and control her temperature and pain levels.

Medications

> Hydrochlorothiazide 25 mg every AM
> Ibuprofen for headaches 200–600 mg BD PRN
> Demazin cold and flu tablets – paracetamol 500 mg and phenylephrine PRN for nasal congestion (5 mg)

Use of safety devices

> Not taking any precautions with home remodelling

Discriminate, Relate, Infer and Predict: Both use of medications and past allergies need to be accurate and considered as it will be likely that Lianna will need antibiotic therapy to combat the signs of localised infection that are evident (thick, green, purulent nasal discharge, bilateral frontal headache [4/10 intensity], maxillary facial pain, and bilateral maxillary toothache; she has had a low-grade fever [37.4°C]), along with the trigger of renovating, making it likely that this has provided a source of localised infection. As the nose is where air is first filtered, it is where small particles (such as wallpaper/glue, underlying paint or dust) have lodged. This is more likely the source of infection as no other precautions (e.g. face mask) have been used while undertaking this job.

Stress

> New home arrangement with daughter and grandchild returning home after marriage breakdown, home renovation, recent pandemic was stressful for healthcare workers

Relate: This indicates that the body is already under stress so may be more susceptible to infection.

Patency

> Each nare is patent.

Discriminate and Infer: This indicates no physical blockage causing pain or swelling, therefore most likely to be mucosal in nature.

Internal inspection

> Mucosa is red and swollen with purulent nasal discharge bilaterally; septum deviated to the left.

Interpret: Localised signs of irritation, with infected discharge

Discriminate and Infer: Of significance here is Lianna's changed physiology, often making it more difficult to clear her nostrils and airways, therefore causing pockets for mucus to sit in, and infection to develop.

Sinuses – Inspection

> Swelling noted below eyes bilaterally.

Interpret: Localised sign of mucus build-up and filled sinuses.

Palpation and percussion

> Tenderness over right maxillary sinus; dullness to percussion noted over right maxillary sinus.

Interpret and Discriminate: Localised pain can be a sign of localised infection where there is swelling, discharge and pressure.

Relate: Dullness when percussing over an area that should be filled with air indicates that air space is filled with fluid or mucus-like substance.

Transillumination of the sinuses

> Absence of glow noted over right maxillary sinus.

Interpret and Infer: An advanced skill, this finding validates that sinuses are filled with mucus or fluid rather than air.

Mouth and throat

> Breath
  • Foul smell noted.
> Throat
  • Mildly erythematous with 1+ tonsils bilaterally and no exudates; uvula midline; gag reflex positive.

Interpret and Relate: Foul-smelling breath is an indicator of infection, and throat findings show an indication of the body's immune response in trying to overcome the localised sinus infection.

Putting it all together – synthesise information

The nurse in this case would note all of these abnormalities, and refer to the medical officer. As it is likely antibiotics will be prescribed, the nurse will need to check that medication prescribed does not have contraindications or adverse interactions with Lianna's antihypertensive drugs.

Actions based on assessment findings

The nurse should also provide additional education for interventions that do not require a doctor's order, such as:

1 Inhaling steam will to help loosen secretions.
2 Reduce intake of phenylephrine products as these dry mucus production; in turn, this thickens secretions, increasing pressure in the sinuses and therefore pain and heaviness, as well as reducing the body's ability to expel infected mucus.
3 Continue use of ibuprofen for analgesia and comfort measure.
4 Use a face mask to reduce the number of particles that can be inhaled when renovating.
5 Rest and sleep as much as possible until symptoms improve; this will aid the body's immune response.

The final step in the process is accurate documentation. The nurse must document findings, referrals, interventions, advice and education given. The consumer would continue to have ongoing long-term management and follow-up by specialist medical staff in collaboration with general practitioner.

Documenting the physical examination, and clinical decisions and interventions including education may look like this in a clinic's electronic client information system.

CLINIC ENTRY

Lianna Potter, MRN: 2189960 DOB:13/07/1961

29/09/2022, 1345hs: Nursing.

PRESENTING PROBLEM: Acute

Client presents with bilateral frontal headache pain (4/10), maxillary facial pain (6/10) with bilateral maxillary toothache.
Nasal discharge – purulent green, T – 37.4C, denies chills, sweats or other pain/respiratory symptoms. Worse when bending over, symptoms appeared 10 days ago after commencing renovation on bathroom and guest room in house. Initial symptoms included nasal congestion and mild sinus pressure.
Has been self-medicating with decongestants (phenylephrine q6/24), and ibuprofen 400 mg nocte, little relief past 3 nights, poor sleep.
T- 37.4, P- 72, R- 18, BP- 135/89, SpO2- 96% RA
Wt- 74 kg
Ht- 165 cm

EXAMINATION

Ears: Intact voice whisper test, Weber-midline, no lateralisation, +ve Rhinne test. No abnormalities noted on inspection of external or internal ear.
Nose: midline, nil external abnormalities, nares patent, internal mucosa red and swollen, purulent nasal discharge
bilaterally (when blowing nose), septal deviation to the left.
Sinuses: Swelling noted bilaterally, tender on palpation over R maxillary sinus, dullness when percussed.
Transillumination- absence of glow over R maxillary sinus.
Mouth and Throat: Foul smelling breath, nil abnormalities in lips/mouth. Throat mildly erythematous, tonsils 1+ bilaterally, nil other abnormalities on inspection.

HISTORY

Medical hx: Hypertension since age 40, recent COVID-19 in past 3/12, chickenpox as child. All vaccinations up-to-date
Surgical Hx: Hysterectomy age 54
Current medication: Hydrochlorothiazide 25 mg every morning, Ibuprofen for headaches 200–600 mg BD PRN, Demazin cold and flu tablets Paracetamol 500 mg and Phenylephrine PRN for nasal congestion (5 mg)
Social & home: lives at home with husband, renovating bathroom and guest bedroom (has not been using respiratory protection devices), recent change to family arrangements, daughter and grandchild now living back at home after marriage breakdown, stress ++ at work with recent COVID-19 Pandemic.
Alcohol 1–2 units per week, non-smoker, Hobbies- music, golf caravanning with husband.
Work: works as nurse manager at local health service in acute care setting mental health.
Education: postgraduate qualification in nursing
Sleep: impaired for last 10 days, usually sleeps well
Exercise & Diet: reduced regular exercise this week due to pain, usually does gym exercise (walking and classes) 2–3 times per week. No change in diet-gluten free as usual.
Stress and wellbeing: feeling better workwise than during worst staff shortages, however still tired. Up to date with well women's checks, pap smear, routine monitoring for HTN every 4 months. Generally, uses safety precautions (seat belts etc.) just not specifically during home renovation- no mask. States good general social supports. Concerned for daughter and grandchild's new arrangements and adjusting to having them living at home again.

TREATMENT

Seen by Dr Guardian, script for Bactrim (800/16 0mg) 1 × BD for 5/7. Advised to take with food, review product information and seek health care if any concerns. Educated on following interventions to manage sinusitis.
1. Steam inhalation
2. Reduce intake of phenylephrine products while on antibiotics
3. Continue use of ibuprofen as per directed on label
4. Use respiratory/face mask when working on renovation projects
5. Increase rest/sleep where possible

Entry by P. Calleja RN RACH health clinic

COURTESY OF PAULINE CALLEJA, RN, LECTURER, SCHOOL OF NURSING, QUEENSLAND UNIVERSITY OF TECHNOLOGY, BRISBANE.

FIGURE 11.52 Documenting the physical examination

CHAPTER RESOURCES

REVIEW QUESTIONS

For answers to these questions, see Answer section at the end of the book.

1. On examination of a 44-year-old man's inner ear, you notice a darkened area or hole in his left tympanic membrane. This is likely to be:
   a. A perforated ear drum
   b. A fungal infection on the ear drum
   c. A bacterial infection on the ear drum
   d. A tumour or ear cancer

2. Acute otitis externa is a common infection among children and adults. Which of the following describes a typical examination finding of otitis externa?
   a. Thickening and clouding of the tympanic membrane
   b. Erythema and oedema of the external auditory canal
   c. Bubbles and air-fluid levels are visible
   d. Retraction and immobility of tympanic membrane

3. Jimmy Rees is a 27-year-old man who has been a carpenter in a kitchen factory. Risk factors for hearing loss are noise exposure, ageing, and which of the following?
   a. Leukoplakia
   b. Amphetamine use
   c. Excessive alcohol use
   d. Recurrent ear infections

4. During examination of the nasal mucosa, you note that the nasal mucosa is red and inflamed, and the client complains of green and yellow nasal discharge and painful sinuses/headache. These findings are most consistent with:
   a. The common cold
   b. Acute sinusitis
   c. Allergies or hay fever
   d. Presence of cerebrospinal fluid

5. During internal inspection of the nose, you note that the nasal mucosa is inflamed and friable, and there is bleeding. These findings are most consistent with which of the following? Select all that apply.
   a. Presence of a foreign body
   b. Nasal inhalation of cocaine
   c. Allergies or hay fever
   d. Bacterial sinusitis
   e. Overdose of decongestant nasal spray
   f. Epistaxis

6. The paranasal sinuses are air-filled cavities lined with mucous membranes that lighten the weight of the skull and add resonance to the quality of the voice. The sinuses that can be assessed on physical examination include:
   a. Frontal and sphenoid sinuses
   b. Frontal and ethmoid sinuses
   c. Maxillary and frontal sinuses
   d. Maxillary and sphenoid sinuses

7. During your assessment of a 28-year-old female client who presents after attending a concert, you note that she speaks with a hoarse voice and the oropharynx is red. Which condition is this most likely to be?
   a. Foetor hepaticus
   b. Overuse of voice
   c. Peritonsillar abscess
   d. Halitosis

8. During examination of your consumer's throat, you note that the consumer has difficulty opening her mouth and has 3+ swelling of the right tonsil with exudate. These findings are commonly associated with:
   a. Infectious mononucleosis
   b. Peritonsillar abscess
   c. Viral pharyngitis
   d. Diphtheria

9. During your assessment of a 15-year-old female, you note that her breath smells of acetone and has a 'fruity' odour. Acetone breath is most commonly associated with the following condition:
   a. Foetor hepaticus
   b. Uraemia
   c. Diabetic ketoacidosis
   d. Halitosis

10. During examination of your consumer's lips, you note clusters of vesicles on erythematous bases with serous fluid. They are painful. This finding is consistent with which of the following conditions?
   a. Herpes simplex lesions
   b. Aphthous ulcers
   c. Basal cell carcinoma
   d. Chancre

CS CLINICAL SKILLS

The following Clinical Skill is relevant to this chapter and can be found in Tollefson & Hillman, *Clinical Psychomotor Skills*, 8th edition:
> 27 Healthcare teaching.

FURTHER RESOURCES

> Australasian Sleep Association: http://www.sleep.org.au
> Australian and New Zealand Academy of Periodontists: http://www.perio.org.au/
> Australian Dental Association Incorporated: http://www.ada.org.au/
> Australian Hearing: http://www.hearing.com.au/
> Australian Society of Otolaryngology – Head and neck surgery: http://www.asohns.org.au/
> Health Direct Australia: http://www.healthdirect.gov.au/ear-disorders

> Hearing House: http://www.hearinghouse.co.nz
> National Foundation for the Deaf: http://www.nfd.org.nz
> New Zealand Dental Association: http://www.nzda.org.nz/pub/
> New Zealand Sleep Apnoea Association: http://www.sleepapnoeanz.org.nz/
> New Zealand Society of Otolaryngology – Head and Neck Surgery Incorporated: http://www.orl.org.nz/
> Overwhelming Daytime Sleep Society of Australia: http://www.nodss.org.au/sleep_apnoeas.html

REFERENCES

Australasian Society of Clinical Immunology and Allergy (ASCIA). (2019). Hay fever (allergic rhinitis). Retrieved on 12 December 2022 from: https://www.allergy.org.au/patients/fast-facts/hay-fever-allergic-rhinitis

Australian Institute of Health and Welfare (AIHW). (2018). Cancer in Aboriginal & Torres Strait Islander People of Australia. Cat. no. CAN 109. Canberra, Australia: AIHW.

Australian Institute of Health and Welfare (AIHW). (2020a). 1.15 Ear Heath, Aboriginal and Torres Strait Islander Health Performance Framework. Retrieved on 12 December 2022 from: https://www.indigenoushpf.gov.au/measures/1-15-ear-health

Australian Institute of Health and Welfare (AIHW). (2020b). Allergic rhinitis (hay fever). Retrieved on 12 December 2022 from: https://www.indigenoushpf.gov.au/measures/1-15-ear-health

Best Practice Advocacy Centre New Zealand (BPAC). (2022). Otitis media: a common childhood illness. Retrieved on 12 December 2022 from: https://bpac.org.nz/2022/docs/otitis-media.pdf

Better Health Vic. (2019). Hearing problems – hyperacusis. Retrieved on 12 December 2022 from: https://www.betterhealth.vic.gov.au/health/conditionsandtreatments/hearing-problems-reduced-tolerance-to-sound

Cancer Society NZ. (2018). Oral cancer. Retrieved 9 September 2018 from: https://auckland-northland.cancernz.org.nz/cancer-information/cancer-types/head-and-neck-cancers/oral-cancer/?divisionId=17&centreId=1

CBG Health Research. (2015). Our older people's oral health. Key findings of the 2012 New Zealand older people's oral health survey. Auckland, New Zealand: CBG Health Research. Retrieved 27 July 2018 from: https://www.health.govt.nz/publication/our-older-peoples-oral-health-key-findings-2012-new-zealand-older-peoples-oral-health-survey

De Lacy, J., Dune, T., & Macdonald, J. (2020). The social determinants of otitis media in Aboriginal children in Australia: are we addressing the primary causes? A systematic content review. *BMC Public Health, 20*, 492. https://doi.org/10.1186/s12889-020-08570-3

Deutsch, A., & Jay, E. (2021). Optimising oral health in frail older people. *Australian Prescriber, 44*, 153–60. https://doi.org/10.18773/austprescr.2021.037

Eisdell Moore Centre New Zealand (EMC). (2021). Equitable ear and hearing care for Tamariki in Aotearoa – A national cross-sector Kōrero. https://www.emcentre.ac.nz/2021/12/17/equitable-ear-and-hearing-care-for-tamariki-in-aotearoa-a-national-cross-sector-korero/

Health Navigator New Zealand. (2021). Tinnitus. Retrieved on 12 December 2022 from: https://www.healthnavigator.org.nz/health-a-z/t/tinnitus/

Jervis-Bardy, J., Carney, A. S., Duguid, R., & Leach, A. J. (2017). Microbiology of otitis media in Indigenous Australian children. *The Journal of Laryngology & Otology, 131*(S2), S2–S11.

Mohammed, H. (2019). Oral health of older people. PhD dissertation, University of Otago, New Zealand. Retrieved on 12 December 2022 from: https://ourarchive.otago.ac.nz/bitstream/handle/10523/9732/MohammedHamidS2019DClinDent.pdf?sequence=3&isAllowed=y

Tinnitus Australia. (n.d.). How many people have tinnitus? Retrieved on 12 December 2022 from: https://www.tinnitusaustralia.org.au/supporting-you/

Veivers, D., Williams, G., Toelle, B., Waterman, A., Guo, Y., Denison, L., … Knibbs, L. D. (2022). The indoor environment and otitis media among Australian children: A national cross-sectional study. *International Journal of Environmental Research and Public Health, 19*(3), 1551. doi: 10.3390/ijerph19031551

Victorian Government. (2021). Understanding hearing loss. Retrieved on 12 December 2022 from: https://www.vic.gov.au/understanding-hearing-loss

World Health Organization (WHO). (2021). Deafness and hearing loss. Retrieved on 12 December 2022 from: https://www.who.int/news-room/fact-sheets/detail/deafness-and-hearing-loss

CHAPTER **12**

BREASTS AND REGIONAL NODES

LEARNING OUTCOMES

By the end of this chapter you should be able to:
1   describe the anatomy and physiology of the breasts and regional lymphatics, including age-related variations
2   obtain a health history from a consumer with a breast or regional node health-related problem
3   demonstrate assessment techniques for the evaluation of the breasts and regional lymphatics
4   differentiate common variations and abnormal changes of the breasts
5   discuss the clinical reasoning in evaluating outcomes of health assessment and physical examination, including documentation, health education given and relevant health referrals.

BACKGROUND

This chapter focuses primarily on the female breast as it is a more complex structure than the male breast. However, it is also important to undertake breast assessment on males, non-binary and transgender people. Breasts are an external symbol of sexuality, femininity and nurturance in women, whereas in men, they symbolise strength, fitness and masculinity. Breast disease, specifically breast cancer and its potentially devastating effects, are well known and publicly recognised, and this attention has generated considerable research investment. Breast cancer incidence rates have increased significantly over time, and this can be directly attributed to breast screening programs. Conversely, mortality from breast cancer has decreased steadily. Long-term survival rates have a direct correlation to early detection of breast cancer (refer to **Table 12.6** for information related to the National Breast Screening Programs in Australia and New Zealand). Nurses can have a major impact on breast health by teaching breast awareness and encouraging healthy lifestyle choices, as these can diminish breast cancer risks.

These are common breast health problems in Australia and New Zealand that may be encountered when undertaking examination:
> Benign breast diseases are the most common lesions of the breast found in women. These include (though not exclusively) fibroadenomas, breast abscesses and cysts. These are found most frequently in the childbearing age, reflecting a strong association with hormones, pregnancy and lactation. Gynaecomastia is the most common benign disease found in men.
> Carcinoma of the breast is the most common cancer found in women in Australia and New Zealand. Age is the biggest risk factor in developing the disease, with over 75% of breast cancers occurring in women over 50. Most breast cancers are diagnosed in women with no family history; however, approximately 5–10% relate to hereditary factors (i.e. a breast cancer gene – BRCA1 or BRCA2) (Breast Cancer Network Australia, 2022; Breast Cancer

Foundation New Zealand, 2022; Cancer Australia, 2022). The lifetime risk for women to have a diagnosis of breast cancer by the age of 85 is one in seven in Australia and one in nine in New Zealand (Breast Cancer Trials, 2022). Breast cancer is the most commonly diagnosed cancer for First Nations women, similar to their counterparts in the wider Australian population. Although First Nations women are 0.9 times as likely to be diagnosed, they are also 1.2 times more likely to die from breast cancer (National Breast Cancer Foundation, 2022), with this higher mortality rate attributed to a combination of factors including lower participation in screening, advanced stage at diagnosis, geographic remoteness, and comorbidities (AIHW, 2021; Cancer Australia, 2022). The 5-year relative survival rate for Aboriginal and Torres Strait Islander women is also lower (81%) compared to the general population (92%) (National Breast Cancer Foundation, 2022). In New Zealand, Māori women are 37% more likely to be diagnosed with breast cancer than non-Māori women, and have a higher mortality rate (Breast Cancer Foundation New Zealand, 2022). The reasons for the higher incidence and ethnic disparities in cancer survival are complex, but likely include a range of factors related to patient demographics, tumour biology, and inequities in access, timeliness and quality of care (Tin Tin et al., 2018). Breast cancer in men is uncommon and accounts for less than 1% of all breast cancers (Breast Cancer Network Australia, 2022). Around 200 men in Australia, and around 25 men in New Zealand, are diagnosed with breast cancer each year (Cancer Australia, 2022; Breast Cancer Foundation New Zealand, 2022).

In Australia, the risk of a woman being diagnosed with breast cancer is:

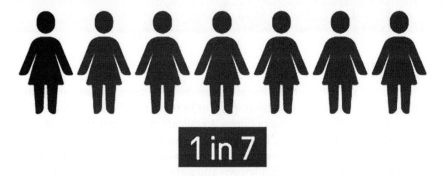

1 in 7

In New Zealand, the risk of a woman being diagnosed with breast cancer is:

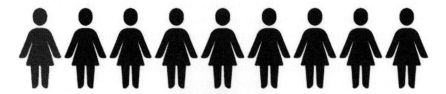

1 in 9

FIGURE 12.1 Risk of breast cancer before the age of 75

SOURCE: HTTPS://WWW.BREASTCANCERTRIALS.ORG.AU/BREAST-CANCER-RESOURCES/BREAST-CANCER-STATISTICS/

ANATOMY AND PHYSIOLOGY

The breasts and regional nodes are now discussed, as is the development of the breasts during adolescence.

Breasts

The female **breasts** are a pair of mammary glands located on the anterior chest wall, extending vertically from the second to the sixth rib and laterally from the sternal border to the axilla. Anatomically, the breast may be divided into four quadrants: the upper inner quadrant, the lower inner quadrant, the upper outer quadrant, and the lower outer quadrant (**Figure 12.2**). The upper outer quadrant extends into the axilla; this is known as the **tail of Spence**. The breasts are supported by a bed of muscles: pectoralis major and minor, latissimus dorsi, serratus anterior, rectus abdominus and external oblique muscles, which extend vertically from the deep fascia (**Figure 12.3**). **Cooper's ligaments**, which extend vertically from the deep fascia through the breast to the inner layer of the skin, provide support for the breast tissue (**Figure 12.4**).

In the centre of each breast is the **nipple**, a round, hairless, pigmented protrusion of erectile tissue approximately 0.5 to 1.5 cm in diameter. The nipple becomes more erect during sexual excitement, pregnancy, lactation, cold temperatures and certain phases of the menstrual cycle. There are 12 to 20 minute openings on the surface of the nipple. These are openings of the **lactiferous ducts** through which milk and colostrum are excreted.

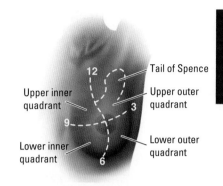

FIGURE 12.2 Quadrants of the left breast. Note the numbers on the breast. They represent the hours of a clock face that can be used to specify the location of a finding on the circular breast. The right breast clock notation is a mirror image of the left breast.

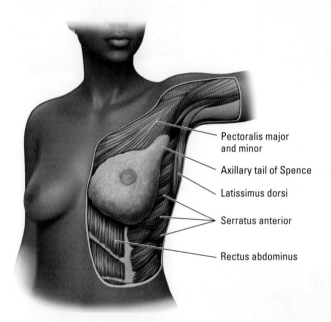

FIGURE 12.3 Muscles supporting the breast

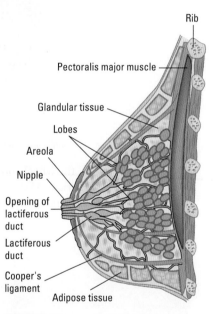

FIGURE 12.4 Cross section of the left breast

The **milk line**, or **ectodermal galactic band**, shown in **Figure 12.5A**, develops from the axilla to the groin during the fifth week of fetal development. Most of the band atrophies except in the thoracic area, where it forms a mammary ridge. Incomplete atrophy of the galactic band results in the development of extra nipples or breast tissue known as **supernumerary nipples**, shown in **Figure 12.5B**. The additional nipples or mammary tissue develop along the milk lines and are a normal variant in a small percentage of adult women.

Surrounding the nipple is the **areola**, a pigmented area approximately 2.5 to 10 cm in diameter. The size and pigmentation vary from woman to woman. Several sebaceous glands (**Montgomery's tubercles**) are present on the surface of the areola. These glands lubricate the nipple, helping to keep it supple during lactation. Hair follicles punctuate the border of the areola.

The breast is composed of glandular, connective (Cooper's ligaments) and adipose tissue. The glandular tissue is arranged radially in the form of 12 to 20 **lobes**. This disbursement is similar to a bicycle wheel; each lobe represents a spoke of

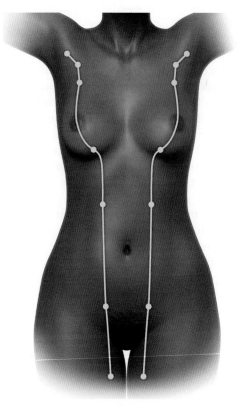

A. These bands develop in utero and later atrophy.

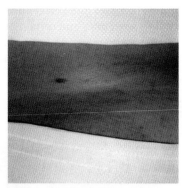

B. Supernumerary nipple

FIGURE 12.5 Ectodermal galactic bands

the wheel and extends from a central point (the nipple) to the outermost border (**Figure 12.6**). Each lobe is composed of 20 to 40 **lobules** that contain milk-producing glands called **alveoli** or **acini**. The lobules are arranged in grapelike bunches and

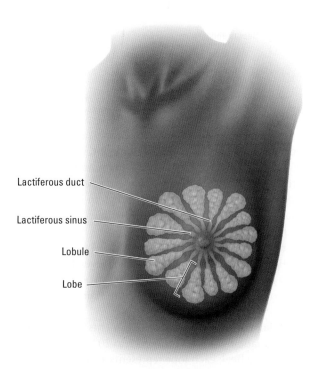

Lactiferous duct

Lactiferous sinus

Lobule

Lobe

FIGURE 12.6 Glandular tissue of the left breast

are clustered around several ducts. These ducts gradually form one main lactiferous (excretory) duct per lobe. Each lactiferous duct widens to form a sinus that acts as a reservoir for milk during lactation. The duct opens onto the surface of the nipple. The lobes are lodged in tissue composed of subcutaneous and **retromammary adipose tissue**, and it is this tissue that composes the bulk of the breast.

The function of the female breast is to produce milk for the nourishment and protection of neonates and infants. In many cultures, breasts provide sensual pleasure during sexual foreplay and breastfeeding. The breasts also provide some protection to the anterior thoracic chest wall.

The male breast is composed of a well-developed areola and a small nipple that has immature tissue underneath. **Gynaecomastia**, the enlargement of male breast tissue (**Figure 12.7**), may occur normally in adolescent and in elderly males. The condition is normally unilateral and temporary.

Regional nodes

The **lymphatic drainage** (the yellow alkaline drainage composed primarily of lymphocytes) of the breast is via a complex network of lymph vessels and nodes. It is estimated that a majority of the lymph from the breast flows to the axillary nodes. The **axillary nodes** are composed of four groups: brachial nodes (lateral), central axillary nodes (midaxillary), pectoral nodes (anterior), and subscapular nodes (posterior). The central axillary nodes receive lymph from the three other nodal groups. The lymph is then channelled from the central axillary nodes to the infraclavicular and supraclavicular nodes. The remainder of the lymph flows into the internal mammary chain or directly to the infraclavicular chain via the Rotter's nodes, deep into the chest or abdominal cavity, or to the other breast. The pattern of lymph drainage is illustrated in **Figure 12.8**.

The axillary nodes are easily accessible by palpation because of their superficial location. The internal mammary nodes are very deep in the chest wall and are inaccessible by palpation.

Breast development

Female breast development usually begins at 8 to 10 years of age and is stimulated by oestrogen release during puberty. Enhanced fat deposition increases the size of the breasts, while the ductal system, lobes and lobules increase in number and in size. Asymmetry in breast development is not abnormal. Tanner staging, or sexual maturity ratings, describe the pattern of adolescent breast development for females (see **Table 12.1**).

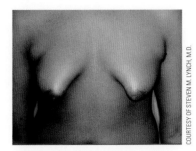

COURTESY OF STEVEN M. LYNCH, M.D.

FIGURE 12.7 Gynaecomastia

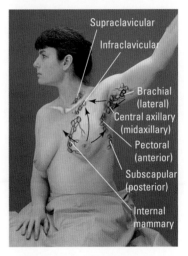

Supraclavicular
Infraclavicular
Brachial (lateral)
Central axillary (midaxillary)
Pectoral (anterior)
Subscapular (posterior)
Internal mammary

FIGURE 12.8 Regional lymphatics and drainage patterns of the left breast

TABLE 12.1 Sexual maturity rating (SMR) for female breast development

	DEVELOPMENTAL STAGE
	1 Preadolescent stage (before age 8). Nipple is small, slightly raised.
	2 Early adolescent stage. Breast bud development (after age 8). Nipple and breast form a small mound. Areola enlarges. Height spurt begins.

>>

>> **TABLE 12.1** *continued*

	DEVELOPMENTAL STAGE
	3 Adolescent stage (10–14 years). Nipple is flush with breast shape. Breast and areola enlarge. Menses begin. Height spurt peaks.
	4 Late adolescent stage (14–17 years). Nipple and areola form a secondary mound over the breast. Height spurt ends.
	5 Adult stage. Nipple protrudes; areola is flush with the breast shape.

ASSESSMENT: TAKING THE CONSUMER'S HEALTH HISTORY

Assessment is the first phase of the nursing process, and involves collecting subjective information about the consumer's health status in order to identify the consumer's problem areas to focus on.

Subjective data is most frequently collected during a health history and serves as the starting point for the health professional to base the depth of their assessment on. The sections for the health history include:

> **Consumer profile**
> **Chief complaint** (explained systematically using variations of location, quality, quantity, associated manifestations, aggravating factors, alleviating factors, setting and timing. This is a variation on the OPQRST assessment mnemonic you may use for other conditions such as pain assessment)
> **Past health history** (including medical history, surgical history, allergies, medications, injuries and accidents, special needs and childhood illnesses)
> **Family health history**
> **Social history** (including alcohol, tobacco and drug use, sexual practice, work and home environment, hobbies and leisure activities, stress and culture).

The health history example included here identifies components for questioning the consumer about their health for this specific body system (breasts and regional nodes). Further, it guides the sequencing and highlights considerations for conducting the physical examination.

HEALTH HISTORY			
CONSUMER PROFILE	The breasts and regional nodes health history provides insight into the link between a consumer's life and lifestyle and breast information and pathology. Diseases that are age-, sex- and race-specific for the breasts and regional nodes are listed.		
	AGE	> Early menarche increases the risk of breast cancer (puberty) > Gynaecomastia (adolescent and elderly males) > Fibroadenoma (20–40) > Benign breast disease (cystic hyperplasia) (30–55) > Mastitis and plugged milk ducts (childbearing years) > Increasing risk of breast cancer (first pregnancy after 30, or nulliparous) > Paget's disease (postmenopausal) > Incidence of breast cancer increases (50 or older)	
	SEX	**FEMALE**	> The incidence of breast cancer in Australia and New Zealand is increasing. It was estimated in Australia in 2022 there would be 20 741 new cases of breast cancer diagnosed in women (up from 15 902 in 2013) (AIHW, 2021). > See Table 12.2 for breast cancer risk factors.
		MALE	> The incidence of men being diagnosed with breast cancer has been stable over the last three decades, with an estimation of 173 new cases in 2022 (142 in 2013) (AIHW, 2021). > Gynaecomastia (adolescent and elderly men)
	CULTURAL BACKGROUND	Aboriginal and Torres Strait Islander and Māori breast cancer mortality rate is higher than that of Caucasian women.	
CHIEF COMPLAINT	Common chief complaints for the breasts and regional nodes are defined and information on the characteristics of each sign or symptom is provided.		
	1. BREAST MASS	Presence of a lump in the breast	
		LOCATION	Anywhere in the breast or axilla, usually in the upper outer quadrant, unilateral or bilateral
		QUALITY	Size, size in relationship to menstrual cycle, shape, consistency, mobility, delineation of borders
		QUANTITY	Number of masses
		ASSOCIATED MANIFESTATIONS	Tenderness, presence of dimpling, nipple retraction, nipple discharge, tender palpable lymph nodes
		AGGRAVATING FACTORS	Methylxanthines (found in chocolate and coffee), recent injury to breast
		ALLEVIATING FACTORS	Aspiration, biopsy, surgery, radiation, chemotherapy
		TIMING	Incidence rises with age, in relation to menses and ovulation
	2. BREAST TENDERNESS	Sensation of discomfort in the breast	
		LOCATION	Pinpoint, discrete, generalised; unilateral or bilateral
		QUALITY	Sharp, dull, pulling
		ASSOCIATED MANIFESTATIONS	Mass, dimpling, nipple retraction, breast swelling, premenstrual syndrome symptoms (see Chapter 17), induration, discharge, palpable nodes, fever, breastfeeding

>>

HEALTH HISTORY

		AGGRAVATING FACTORS	Recent injury to breast, palpation, vigorous exercise, oral contraceptives, chlorpromazine, alpha-methyldopa
		ALLEVIATING FACTORS	Warm compresses, analgesics, massage, support bras, aspiration, biopsy, surgery, breastfeeding, cessation of aggravating medications
		TIMING	In relation to menses or ovulation, pregnancy, lactation, activity
	3. BREAST DISCHARGE	Abnormal substance expressed from the breast	
		LOCATION	From the nipple or sebaceous gland, unilateral or bilateral
		QUALITY	Colour, odour, consistency
		ASSOCIATED MANIFESTATIONS	Redness, swelling, induration, mass, dimpling, nipple retraction, breast swelling, palpable nodes, lactation, headaches, history of pituitary disorders, fever
		AGGRAVATING FACTORS	Trauma to breast, breastfeeding, pituitary tumour, hyperthyroidism, chlorpromazine, alpha-methyldopa, digitalis, diuretics, oral contraceptives, papillomas, carcinomas of the ducts
		ALLEVIATING FACTORS	Breastfeeding, biopsy, surgery, cessation of medications
		TIMING	In relation to pregnancy, menses, lactation, ovulation
PAST HEALTH HISTORY	The various components of the past health history are linked to breasts and regional nodes pathology and related information.		
	MEDICAL HISTORY	**BREAST-SPECIFIC**	Benign breast disease, cysts, fibroadenomas, intraductal papillomas, mammary duct ectasia, mastitis, areas of greater density, breast cancer, masses, breast abscess, Paget's disease, inflammatory breast disease
		NON-BREAST-SPECIFIC	Thyroid disorders, pituitary tumour, chest radiation, cancer of ovary or endometrium, obesity; lifetime weight gain associated with increased risk of postmenopausal breast cancer
	SURGICAL HISTORY	Breast biopsy, lumpectomy, quadrantectomy, partial mastectomy, radical mastectomy, breast reduction or augmentation	
	ALLERGIES	Localised rashes of breast, contact dermatitis	
	MEDICATIONS	Oral contraceptives, chlorpromazine, alpha-methyldopa, diuretics, digitalis, steroids and tricyclics may precipitate nipple discharge; use of hormone replacement therapy has been linked with increased incidences of some breast cancers	
	INJURIES AND ACCIDENTS	May cause haematoma or oedema; lumps may result from previous trauma to soft tissue	
	CHILDHOOD ILLNESSES	Varicella scarring of cutaneous tissue	
FAMILY HEALTH HISTORY	Breasts and regional nodes diseases that are familial are listed. Five to ten per cent of breast cancers are thought to have a familial link via a primary relative; for example, a mother, sister, grandmother. The link is stronger if the family history includes bilateral breast cancer, BRCA1 or BRCA2 gene mutation, Cowden or Hamartoma syndrome (PTEN gene mutation), Li-Fraumeni (TP53 and CHEK2 gene mutations), Peutz-Jeghers syndrome (STK11 gene mutation), or ataxia telangiectasia (ATM). Benign breast disease		

HEALTH HISTORY		
SOCIAL HISTORY	The components of the social history are linked to breasts and regional nodes factors and pathology.	
	ALCOHOL USE	More than two drinks per day is associated with some risk; recurrent/current use increases risk rather than past use; research shows a dose–response relationship
	TOBACCO USE	Cigarette smoking of long duration plays a role in breast cancer.
	WORK ENVIRONMENT	Radiation exposure
	HOME ENVIRONMENT	Increased incidence of breast cancer noted in urban communities.
	ECONOMIC STATUS	Increased incidence of breast cancer in women of upper socioeconomic status.
	CULTURAL BACKGROUND	Incidence of breast cancer among Australian and New Zealand women is higher than that of Japanese and Middle Eastern women; it is estimated that 1 in 100 women of Ashkenazi Jewish origin are at greater risk of breast cancer due to a mutation of the BRCA1 gene.

TABLE 12.2 Breast cancer risk factors

NONMODIFIABLE FACTORS	MODIFIABLE FACTORS	RED FLAGS FOR HIGH-RISK FACTORS

> Female sex
> Age greater than 50
> Personal history of breast cancer
> Family history of breast cancer
> Prior thoracic radiation (e.g. Hodgkin's disease)
> Number and result of prior breast biopsies (e.g. atypical hyperplasia)
> Hereditary breast cancer syndromes:
  • BRCA1 and BRCA2 are the majority of breast cancer syndromes
  • Cowden or Hamartoma syndrome (PTEN gene mutation)
  • Li-Fraumeni (TP53 and CHEK2 gene mutations)
  • Peutz-Jeghers syndrome (STK11 gene mutation)
  • Ataxia telangiectasia mutated (ATM)
> Reproductive history (earlier age at menarche, nulliparity, first child after age 30, late onset of menopause)
> African American/Ashkenazi Jewish heritage
	> Increased alcohol consumption
	> Obesity
	> Physical inactivity
	> Cigarette smoking
	> Postmenopausal hormonal therapy
		> Early age of onset of breast cancer (<50 in consumer or family member)
		> Multiple family members with breast cancer
		> Autosomal dominant pattern
		> Individual with more than one primary breast cancer
		> Male breast cancer at any age
		> Family member with known hereditary mutation (e.g. BRCA1, BRCA2, TP53, PTEN)
		> Family history of breast cancer and ovarian cancer on same side of family

PERSON-CENTRED HEALTH EDUCATION

When conducting a health assessment, opportunities for the provision of person-centred health education will arise. This is a significant consideration in relation to the assessment process for examination of the breasts and regional nodes due to the intimate nature of the examination. These occasions are identified as individualised education and may generate further data that can be added to the assessment. All education given should be documented so that in future, health professionals can assess the impact of previous information provided to the consumer. (Refer to Chapter 1 for initiating health education.) Refer to the following examples.

INDIVIDUALISED HEALTH EDUCATION INTERVENTIONS	
Assessing the consumer for the following health-related activities can assist in identifying the need for education about these factors. This information provides a bridge between the health maintenance activities and breast and regional nodes function.	
Diet	No longer a correlation between a high-fat diet and incidence of breast cancer; increased incidence of benign breast disease with caffeine use
Exercise	Strong correlation between obesity and incidence of breast cancer; in multiple studies there is a breast cancer reduction with increased activity

>>

INDIVIDUALISED HEALTH EDUCATION INTERVENTIONS	
Use of safety devices	Use of restraining devices in motor vehicles to prevent chest trauma
Health check-ups	> Breast awareness starting in the 20s. > Healthcare providers should advise women to be 'breast aware' and inform them about the changes that may indicate cancer, when women are having a general check-up. > Women should discuss their individual needs and preferences with their healthcare provider as there is no evidence that clinical breast examination as a screening method is of any benefit. > Clinical breast examination may be of benefit for women who are eligible but not attending regular mammography. > Baseline mammography and annual mammography screening starting at age 45 (NZ) and age 50 (Australia) in asymptomatic women. > Women of all ages who are at high risk should have an individualised surveillance program developed by their consultant. This may include regular clinical breast examinations, mammography, ultrasound/MRI. These women should also be encouraged to be breast aware (Breast Screen Australia, 2022; NZ National Screening Unit, 2022).

HEALTH EDUCATION

Reducing the risk of breast cancer

When undertaking a woman's health history it is important to recognise the following, as these have been linked to *lowering* the risk of breast cancer:

> Breastfeeding
> Moderate to vigorous physical activity
> Healthy body weight
> Stop smoking
> Low alcohol consumption.

Incorporate health education whenever appropriate, to inform women of these modifiable risks.

PLANNING FOR PHYSICAL EXAMINATION

The planning phase refers to evaluating subjective data to narrow the focus on physical examination, determining what objective data needs to be gathered, as well as considering the environment and equipment that will be required.

At this time, you will identify which of the four diagnostic techniques you will need to implement the physical examination, and how you will sequence these. For physical examination of the female breasts and regional nodes, you will include inspection and palpation.

Objective data is:

> collected during the physical examination of the consumer
> usually collected after subjective data
> information that is measured or observed by the clinician as opposed to being reported by the consumer
> vital to the overall health assessment, to enable you to make clinical decisions that are representative of the whole consumer picture.

Evaluating subjective data to focus physical examination

In the evaluation phase of a health assessment, the focus is on ensuring the data gathered is complete, accurate and documented appropriately (see case study as an example of the focused assessment; see Chapter 22 for a comprehensive health assessment). In evaluating the data you should:

> draw on your critical thinking and problem-solving skills to make sound clinical decisions
> act on abnormal data (include communicating findings to other health professionals)
> ensure documentation reflects the outcomes of the clinical decisions/actions taken (refer to Chapter 3, which discusses in detail why documentation is so important and how this may be undertaken in different health settings). The case study that follows steps you through this process.

Environment

Breast and regional node assessment and examination can be done in most physical environments in healthcare settings that will provide the level of privacy that is required. Reassuring the consumer that privacy will be maintained during the assessment by providing screens and/or closing the door will assist them to feel more at ease during the assessment.

Equipment

> Towel
> Drape
> Centimetre ruler
> Teaching aid for breast awareness/self-examination.

IMPLEMENTATION: CONDUCTING THE PHYSICAL EXAMINATION

Implementation of the physical examination and assessment requires you to consider your scope of practice. In this section, depending on your context, you may be performing foundation assessment with aspects of advanced assessment if you are practising in a specialised area. Physical examination can produce feelings of fear, anxiety, embarrassment and loss of control in many women. These feelings may be reduced by the sensitivity of the nurse before, during and after assessment of the breasts.

EXAMINATION **IN BRIEF: BREASTS AND REGIONAL NODES**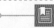

Examination of female breasts and regional nodes

Inspection

> Colour
> Vascularity
> Thickening or oedema
> Size and symmetry
> Contour
> Lesions or masses
> Discharge

Palpation

> Supraclavicular and infraclavicular lymph nodes
> Breasts: consumer in sitting position
> Axillary lymph node region
> Breasts: consumer in supine position

Examination of male breasts

Inspection and palpation

General approach to examination of female breasts and regional nodes

Prior to the assessment

1. When possible, instruct the consumer not to use creams, lotions, powders, or shave her underarms 24–48 hours before the scheduled examination. Application of toiletry products may mask or alter the nature of the surface

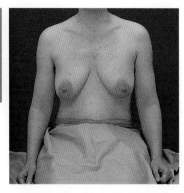

FIGURE 12.9 Position of consumer for breast inspection: arms at side

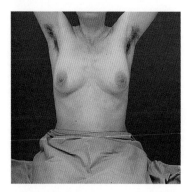

FIGURE 12.10 Position of consumer for breast inspection: arms overhead

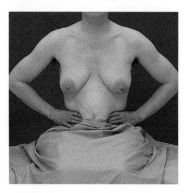

FIGURE 12.11 Position of consumer for breast inspection: hands pressed against hips

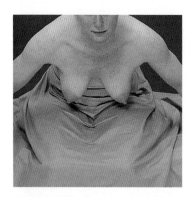

FIGURE 12.12 Position of consumer for breast inspection: leaning forwards

integument of the breasts, and shaving the underarms may cause folliculitis, which may result in pain upon palpation.

2. Encourage the consumer to express any anxieties and concerns about the physical examination. Acknowledge anxieties and validate concerns. Many women avoid having their breasts assessed because they fear social discomfort and potential adverse findings. Assure the consumer that she has taken a positive step in her own health care by having her breasts assessed.

3. Inform the consumer that the examination should not be painful but may be uncomfortable at times. This is especially true if the consumer is currently experiencing menses, ovulation or pregnancy.

4. Adopt a non-judgemental and supportive attitude.

5. Be aware of the impact of culture on breast assessment and breast self-examination. In some Asian cultures, breast self-examination may be considered a form of masturbation. In some Middle Eastern cultures, baring the breasts to a male is taboo, even if the male is a healthcare provider.

6. Instruct the consumer to remove any jewellery that might interfere with the assessment.

7. Ensure that the room is warm enough to prevent chilling, and provide additional draping material as necessary.

8. Warm your hands with warm water or by rubbing them together prior to the assessment.

9. Ensure that privacy will be maintained during the examination. Provide screens, closed doors, and door sign stating that an examination is in progress.

During the assessment

1. Inform the consumer of what you are going to do before you do it.
2. Use this time to educate the consumer about her body.
3. Offer the consumer the opportunity to ask questions about her body and sexuality.
4. Keep areas not being assessed appropriately draped.
5. Always compare right and left breasts.
6. Wear gloves if the consumer has any discharge from the breast.

After the assessment

1. Assess whether the consumer needs assistance in dressing.
2. After the consumer is dressed, discuss the experience with her, invite questions and comments, listen carefully, and provide her with information regarding the examination.

Examination of female breasts and regional nodes

Inspection

E 1. Position the consumer uncovered to the waist, seated at the edge of the examination table, and facing you.

2. Instruct the consumer to let her arms relax by her sides as shown in **Figure 12.9**.

3. Inspect the breasts, axillae, areola areas and nipples for colour, vascularity, thickening, oedema, size, symmetry, contour, lesions or masses, and exudates.

4. Repeat the above inspection sequence with the consumer's arms raised over her head (see **Figure 12.10**). This will accentuate any retraction (tissue drawn back) if present.

5. Repeat inspection sequence with consumer pressing hands into hips, which will contract the pectoral muscles (**Figure 12.11**). Once again, if retraction is present, it will be more pronounced with this manoeuvre.

6. Have the consumer lean forwards to allow the breasts to hang freely away from the chest wall as shown in **Figure 12.12**, and repeat the inspection sequence. Provide support to the consumer as necessary.

E Examination **N** Normal findings **A** Abnormal findings **P** Pathophysiology

PUTTING IT IN CONTEXT

Breast examination: Cultural factors to consider

The nurse practitioner (NP) is conducting a well-woman examination on a 28-year-old consumer. The consumer made this appointment at the insistence of her husband, who wants to start a family. She has been in New Zealand for two years and has never had a female health assessment. She comes from a culture that highly respects women's privacy and modesty. The female NP spends 10 minutes explaining the procedure and what to expect. As there are no questions, the NP gives the woman time to undress in privacy. The NP explains that the breast examination will be performed first and inspects and then palpates the consumer's breasts. The NP finds a small area she would like her 'male' colleague, working with her at the time, to also assess. The woman refuses, stating, 'Only women may see me in a state of undress in my culture.'

> What might the NP say to the consumer?
> What action would be taken?

Colour

E Inspect the breasts, areolar areas, nipples and axillae for colouration.

N The breasts and axillae are flesh-coloured and the areolar areas and nipples are darker in pigmentation. This pigmentation is normally enhanced during pregnancy. Moles and naevi are normal variants, and terminal hair may be present on the areolar areas.

A Reddened areas of the breasts, nipples or axillae need further assessment.

P Redness may be an indication of inflammation, an infection such as mastitis, or inflammatory carcinoma (See **Table 12.3** for a description of the five major types of breast cancer.)

TABLE 12.3 Breast cancer types

DUCTAL CARCINOMA IN SITU (DCIS)	Cancer cells confined to the milk ducts. DCIS may present as microcalcifications on mammography. There is no invasion to outlying tissue or lymph nodes.
INFILTRATING (INVASIVE) DUCTAL CARCINOMA (IDC)	Cancer cells have invaded tissues beyond the milk ducts. Constitutes 85–90% of all breast cancers. IDC will usually present as a discrete, solid breast mass on mammography.
INFILTRATING (INVASIVE) LOBULAR CARCINOMA (ILC)	Cancer cells that started in the lobules and milk ducts, have invaded outlying tissue. ILC represents 10% of breast cancers that may be more easily diagnosed from an MRI than mammography. This cancer may present as a thickened area rather than a mass.
INFLAMMATORY BREAST CANCER (IBC)	Cancer cells have rapid tumour growth with an erythemic, thickened skin or diffuse oedema (peau d'orange). IBC represents 1–6% of breast cancers. It is diagnosed via core biopsy or punch biopsy.
PAGET'S DISEASE	Presents as an eczematous rash on the nipple. Represents 1–3% of breast cancers. Pruritus, erythema and nipple discharge may be present. Paget's disease can coexist with DCIS or IDC.

A Striae (**Figure 12.13**) are streaks over the breasts or axillae and are abnormal. In light-skinned individuals, new striae are red and become silver to white in colouration with age. In dark-skinned individuals, new striae are a ruddy, dark brown colour, and older striae become lighter than the skin colour.

P Striae are caused by rapid stretching of the skin, which damages the elastic fibres found in the dermis. Though normal in pregnancy, striae are often also observed with obesity.

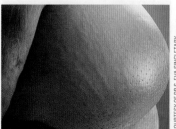

COURTESY OF DR S. EVA SINGLETARY, UNIVERSITY OF TEXAS, M.D. ANDERSON CANCER CENTER

FIGURE 12.13 Striae secondary to inflammatory breast cancer; also note peau d'orange

---

E Examination   **N** Normal findings   **A** Abnormal findings   **P** Pathophysiology

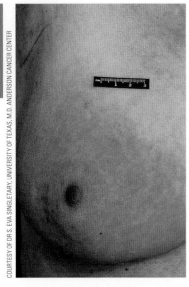

FIGURE 12.14 Erythema with abnormal vascular pattern secondary to inflammatory breast cancer

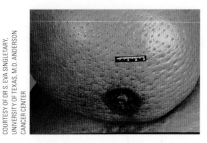

FIGURE 12.15 Peau d'orange

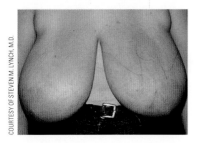

FIGURE 12.16 Massive hypertrophy of breasts

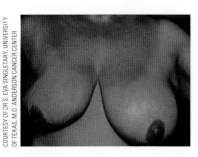

FIGURE 12.18 Asymmetry of breasts due to cancer

Vascularity

E Observe the entire surface of each breast for superficial vascular patterns.

N Normal superficial vascular patterns are diffuse and symmetrical.

A Abnormal patterns of vascularity are focal or unilateral.

P Focal or unilateral superficial vascular patterns (**Figure 12.14**) occur as the result of an increased blood supply and may indicate tumour formation, which requires increased vascularisation and an increased blood supply.

Thickening or oedema

E Observe the breasts, axillae and nipples for thickening or oedema.

N Normally, thickening or oedema is not found in the breasts, axillae or nipples.

A Thickening or oedema of the breast tissue or nipple may present itself as enlarged skin pores that give the appearance of orange rind (**peau d'orange**). It may be more prevalent in the dependent or inferior portions of the breast (**Figure 12.15**).

P This peau d'orange appearance may be indicative of obstructed lymphatic drainage due to a tumour, or inflammatory breast cancer.

Size and symmetry

E Observe the breasts, axillae, areolar areas and nipples for size and symmetry.

N It is not unusual for there to be some difference in the size of the breasts and areolar areas, with the breast on the side of the dominant arm being larger. Bilateral hypertrophy of the breasts may be normal for some consumers (**Figure 12.16**). Nipple inversion, which is present from puberty, is a normal variant and is of no clinical consequence except for difficulty in breastfeeding. Nipples should point upwards and laterally, or they may point outwards and downwards (**Figure 12.17A**). Supernumerary nipples are a variant of normal and have no pathological significance in either males or females.

A Asymmetry in the directions in which the nipples are pointed is an abnormal finding (**Figure 12.17B**).

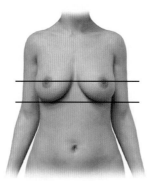

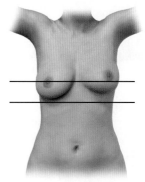

A. Symmetrical without deviation

B. Asymmetrical with deviation

FIGURE 12.17 Deviation of nipples

P Asymmetrical nipple direction is suggestive of an underlying invasive process that is contorting nipple tissue. Often the direction of nipple deviation is towards the underlying process.

A Significant differences in the size or symmetry of the breasts, axillae, areolar areas or nipples are abnormal (see **Figure 12.18**).

P Significant enlargement of one breast, axilla or areola may be indicative of tumour formation.

E Examination **N** Normal findings **A** Abnormal findings **P** Pathophysiology

A Recent inversion, flattening or depression of a nipple is abnormal.

P A sudden onset of nipple inversion, flattening or depression is indicative of nipple retraction, which is suggestive of an underlying cancer (**Figure 12.19**).

A Nipples that have been inverted since puberty and become broader or thicker are abnormal.

P Additional broadening or thickening of a previously inverted nipple may be indicative of tumour formation.

A Lack of breast tissue unilaterally is abnormal.

P Unilateral reduction of breast tissue or structures may result from trauma, mastectomy, or breast reduction.

Contour

E 1. Assess the breasts for contour.
2. Compare the breasts to each other.

N The breast is normally convex, without flattening, retractions or dimpling.

A Dimpling, retractions, flattening (**Figure 12.20**) or other changes in breast contour are abnormal.

P Changes in contour are highly suggestive of cancer. The invasive process that causes the contour changes is the result of fibrotic shortening and disablement of the Cooper's ligament. Fat necrosis and mammary duct ectasia may also cause retraction, dimpling and puckering.

Lesions or masses

E Inspect the breasts, axillae, areolar areas and nipples for lesions or masses.

N The breasts, axillae, areolar areas and nipples are free of masses, tumours, and primary or secondary lesions.

A Breast masses, tumours, nodules or cysts of any kind are abnormal.

P See **Table 12.4** for common pathologies of breast masses.

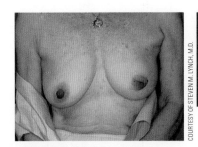

FIGURE 12.19 Nipple retraction of left breast

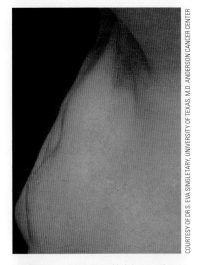

FIGURE 12.20 Dimpling of left breast tissue

TABLE 12.4 Characteristics of common breast masses

	GROSS CYST	FIBROADENOMA	CARCINOMA
Age	30–50; diminishes after menopause	Puberty to menopause; peaks between ages 20 and 30	Most common after 50 years
Shape	Round	Round, lobular or ovoid	Irregular, stellate or crab-like
Consistency	Soft to firm	Usually firm	Firm to hard
Discreteness	Well defined	Well defined	Not clearly defined
Number	Single or grouped	Most often single	Usually single
Mobility	Mobile	Very mobile	May be mobile or fixed to skin, underlying tissue or chest wall
Tenderness	Tender	Nontender	Usually nontender
Erythema	No erythema	No erythema	May be present
Retraction/dimpling	Not present	Not present	Often present

A A scaly, eczema-like erosion of the nipple, or persistent dermatitis of the areola and nipple, is abnormal.

E Examination **N** Normal findings **A** Abnormal findings **P** Pathophysiology

UNIT 2

P Persistent eczematous dermatitis of the areola and nipple region is suggestive of **Paget's disease**, a malignant neoplasm, which is usually unilateral in its involvement.

Discharge

E Observe for spontaneous discharge from the nipples or other areas of the breast.

N In the nonpregnant, nonlactating female, there should be no discharge. During pregnancy and up through the first week after birth, there may be a yellow discharge known as colostrum. During lactation, there is a white discharge of breast milk.

A The presence of a nipple discharge in the nonpregnant, nonlactating woman is abnormal.

P Nipple discharge may be caused by the use of medications such as tranquillisers and oral contraceptives, manual stimulation, pituitary tumour or infection. It may also be indicative of malignant or benign breast disease.

CLINICAL **REASONING**

Practice tip: Examining nipple discharge
If a consumer is found to have abnormal nipple discharge, the nurse should undertake the following:
1 Don gloves before proceeding with the assessment.
2 Note the colour, odour, consistency, amount of discharge, unilateral or bilateral, spontaneous or provoked.
3 With a sterile, cotton-tipped swab, obtain a sample of the discharge so that a culture and sensitivity as well as a Gram stain can be obtained.
4 Consider checking the sample for occult blood.
5 Follow your institution's guidelines for sample preparation.

Palpation

Palpation is performed in a sequential manner:

1. Supraclavicular and infraclavicular lymph node areas
2. Breasts, with the consumer in sitting position
   a Arms at side
   b Arms raised over head
3. Axillary lymph node regions
4. Breasts, with the consumer in supine position.

Supraclavicular and infraclavicular lymph nodes

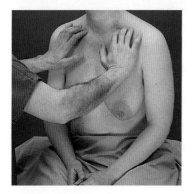

FIGURE 12.21 Palpation of supraclavicular nodes

E 1. Have the consumer seated and uncovered to the waist.
2. Encourage the consumer to relax the muscles of the head and neck because this pulls the clavicles down and allows a thorough exploration of the supraclavicular area.
3. Flex the consumer's head to relax the sternocleidomastoid muscle.
4. Standing in front of the consumer, in a bilateral and simultaneous motion, place the finger pads over the consumer's clavicles, lateral to the tendinous portion of the sternocleidomastoid muscles.
5. Using a rotary motion of the palmar surfaces of the fingers, probe deeply into the scalene triangles in order to palpate the supraclavicular lymph nodes (**Figure 12.21**).
6. Palpate the infraclavicular nodes using the same rotary motion of the palmar surfaces of the fingers (**Figure 12.22**).

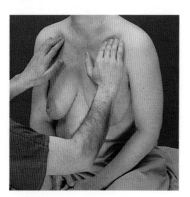

FIGURE 12.22 Palpation of infraclavicular nodes

E Examination **N** Normal findings **A** Abnormal findings **P** Pathophysiology   Advanced Assessment

N Palpable lymph nodes less than 1 cm in diameter are usually considered normal and clinically insignificant, provided that there are no additional enlarged lymph nodes found in other regions such as the axilla. Palpation should not elicit pain.

A Fixed, firm, immobile, irregular lymph nodes more than 1 cm in diameter are considered abnormal.

P These nodes are considered suspicious for metastasis from a variety of sources or primary lymphoma.

A Enlarged, painful or tender nodes that are matted together are abnormal.

P Tender, enlarged nodes may indicate systemic infection or carcinoma.

Breasts: consumer in sitting position

E 1. Place the consumer in a sitting position with arms at sides.
2. Stand to the consumer's right side, facing the consumer.
3. Using the palmar surfaces of the fingers of the dominant hand, begin the palpation at the outer quadrant of the consumer's right breast.
4. Use the other hand to support the inferior aspect of the breast.
5. In small-breasted consumers, the dominant hand can palpate the tissue against the chest wall, but if the breasts are pendulous, use a bimanual technique of palpation as shown in **Figure 12.23**.
6. Palpate in a downwards fashion, sweeping from the outer quadrants to the sternal border of each breast.
7. Repeat this sequence on the other breast.
8. Repeat the entire assessment with the consumer's arms raised over her head to enhance any potential retraction.

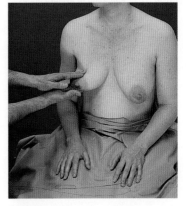

FIGURE 12.23 Bimanual palpation of the breasts while consumer is sitting

N The consistency of the breasts is widely variable, depending on age, time in menstrual cycle, and proportion of adipose tissue. The breasts may have a nodular or granular consistency that may be enhanced prior to the onset of menses. The inferior aspect of the breast will be somewhat firmer due to a transverse inframammary ridge. Palpation should not elicit significant tenderness, although the breasts and especially the nipples may become full and slightly tender premenstrually. Breasts that feel fluid-filled or firm throughout with accompanying inferior suture-line scars are indicative of breast augmentation.

A The presence of any lump, mass, thickening or unilateral granulation that is noticeably different from the rest of the breast tissue should be considered suspicious and abnormal.

P For a description of breast masses and their pathologies, see **Table 12.4**.

A Significant breast tenderness is abnormal and may indicate mammary duct ectasia.

P This is a benign condition in which lactiferous ducts become inflamed.

A Erythema and swelling of the breast with possible pitting oedema is abnormal and usually indicates mastitis.

P This condition is usually seen postpartum and is an inflammation of the breast usually caused by *Staphylococcus aureus*.

Axillary lymph node region

E 1. Stand at the consumer's right side, facing the consumer.
2. Tell the consumer to take a deep breath and relax the shoulders and arms (this relaxes the areas to be palpated).
3. Using your left hand, adduct the consumer's right arm so that it is close to the chest wall. This manoeuvre relaxes the muscles.
4. Support the consumer's right arm with your left hand.

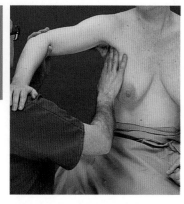

FIGURE 12.24 Palpation of axillary nodes

E 5. Using the palmar surfaces of the finger pads of your right hand, place your fingers into the apex of the axilla. Your fingers will be positioned behind the pectoral muscles.
6. Gently roll the tissue against the chest wall and axillary muscles as you work downwards.
7. Locate and palpate the four axillary lymph node groups:
    a brachial (lateral) at the inner aspect of the upper part of the humerus, close to the axillary vein
    b central axillary (midaxillary) at the thoracic wall of the axilla
    c pectoral (anterior) behind the lateral edge of the pectoralis major muscle
    d subscapular (posterior) at the anterior edge of the latissimus dorsi muscle.
8. Repeat this method of palpation with the consumer's arm abducted (i.e. instruct the consumer to remain in the same position and lift the upper arm and elbow away from the body). Support the consumer's abducted arm on your left shoulder, as shown in **Figure 12.24**.
9. Palpate the consumer's left axilla using the same technique.

URGENT FINDING

Breast mass
Any new breast mass or change in a previously benign known breast mass must be referred to an appropriate health professional for further assessment.

N Palpable lymph nodes less than 1 cm in diameter are usually considered normal and clinically insignificant provided that there are no additional enlarged lymph nodes found in other regions. Palpation should not elicit pain.

A Fixed, firm, immobile, irregular lymph nodes more than 1 cm in diameter are clinically significant.

P These nodes are considered suggestive of metastasis from a variety of sources or primary lymphoma.

A Enlarged, painful or tender nodes that are matted together are abnormal.

P Tender, enlarged nodes may be indicative of a systemic infection or carcinoma.

REFLECTION IN PRACTICE

Attitude and awareness of older women and breast cancer
You are conducting a seminar on female health to residents of an assisted living community. You review the importance of breast examination and how to be breast aware. Some of the women start to laugh and you hear comments such as:
> 'My breasts are so saggy, there's no need to worry.'
> 'I had one breast removed for cancer and the other breast is OK.'
> 'Breast cancer only occurs in young women.'
   How might you respond to these comments?
   What further breast awareness advice could you provide?

Breasts: consumer in supine position

E 1. Keep the consumer uncovered to the waist.
2. Instruct the consumer to assume a supine position. This position spreads the breast tissue thinly and evenly over the chest wall. Palpation is more accurate when there is the least amount of breast tissue between the skin and the chest wall.

E Examination **N** Normal findings **A** Abnormal findings **P** Pathophysiology Advanced Assessment

E 3. If the breasts are large, place a small towel or folded sheet under the consumer's right shoulder. This helps to flatten the breast more.

4. Stand at the right side of the consumer. Palpation can be performed with the consumer's arms at her sides or with her right arm above her head.

5. Using the palmar surfaces of the fingers, palpate the right breast by compressing the mammary tissues gently against the chest wall. Do not press too hard. You may mistake a rib for a hard breast mass. Palpation may be performed in wedge sections, concentric circles or parallel lines (**Figure 12.25**). Using two out of the three palpation methods is acceptable, in order to ensure thoroughness of palpation.

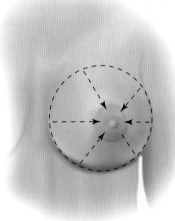

A. Wedge

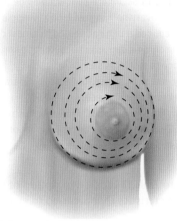

B. Concentric circles

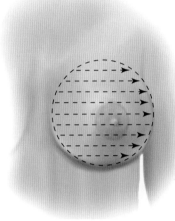

C. Parallel lines

FIGURE 12.25 Breast palpation methods

E 6. Palpation must include the tail of Spence, periphery (**Figure 12.26A**) and areola (**Figure 12.26B**).

7. Finally, don gloves and compress the nipple to express any discharge, as shown in **Figure 12.26C**. If discharge is noted, palpate the breast along the wedge radii to determine from which lobe the discharge is originating.

8. Repeat procedure on opposite breast.

N See previous section on normal breast tissue findings upon palpation. The nipple should be elastic and return readily to its previous shape. No discharge should be expressed in the nonpregnant, nonlactating consumer.

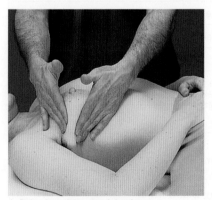

A. Palpation of the glandular tissue

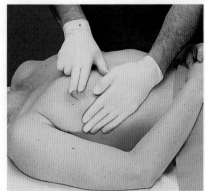

B. Palpation of the areola

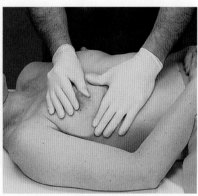

C. Compression of the nipple

FIGURE 12.26 Palpation of the breasts while consumer is supine

E Examination **N** Normal findings **A** Abnormal findings **P** Pathophysiology

HEALTH EDUCATION

Breast awareness and mammography

Your mother states that she questions the value of breast awareness and serial mammography in light of recent publicity. What health education do you think is appropriate?

You might consider explaining that it is always good to have a discussion related to health, as this enables correct facts to be shared.

In relation to breast cancer, most women do not experience any symptoms. This is why they are encouraged to be breast aware, to become familiar with the normal look and feel, so if any changes are identified, they can seek medical advice early. Regular breast screening should be encouraged, including mammography, which simply detects suspicious areas in the breast where cancer could be present. Provide facts, such as the following:

> There is overwhelming evidence (multiple robust research) that supports early detection, with reduced deaths attributed to breast cancer.
> Mammograms can assist in detecting small breast cancers, before they have had a chance to metastasise.
> Early detection allows for less toxic therapies and less extensive surgical intervention.

For further information, see:

> Australia: Breast Cancer Network Australia https://www.bcna.org.au/
> New Zealand: Breast Cancer Foundation New Zealand https://www.breastcancerfoundation.org.nz/

Refer to Table 12.4 for a description of breast masses. Table 12.5 offers a list of breast mass characteristics that are used to evaluate abnormal findings.

TABLE 12.5 Evaluation of breast mass characteristics

If a mass is noted during palpation, the following information should be obtained regarding the mass. Always note if one or both breasts are involved.	
Location	Identify the quadrant involved or visualise the breast with the face of a clock superimposed upon it. The nipple represents the centre of the clock. Note where the mass lies in relation to the nipple (e.g. 3 cm from the nipple in the 3 o'clock position).
Size	Determine size in centimetres in all three planes (height, width and depth).
Shape	Masses may be round, ovoid, matted or irregular.
Number	Note if mass is singular or multiple. Note if one or both breasts are involved.
Consistency	Masses may be firm, hard, soft, fluid or cystic.
Definition	Note if the mass borders are discrete or irregular.
Mobility	Determine if the mass is fixed or freely movable in relation to the chest wall.
Tenderness	Note if palpation elicits pain.
Erythema	Note any redness over involved area.
Dimpling or retraction	Observe for dimpling or retraction as the consumer raises arms overhead and presses her hands into her hips.
Lymphadenopathy	Note if the mass involves any of the regional lymph nodes, and indicate whether there is associated lymphadenopathy.

A Loss of nipple elasticity or nipple thickening is abnormal.

P Loss of elasticity in the nipple may indicate tumour formation.

A Milky-white discharge in a nonpregnant, nonlactating consumer may be nonpuerperal galactorrhea.

E Examination **N** Normal findings **A** Abnormal findings **P** Pathophysiology

P Nonpuerperal galactorrhea is either hormonally induced from lesions of the anterior pituitary gland or drug induced.

A Non-milky discharge from the nipple, which may be green, brown, straw coloured or grey, is abnormal.

P Non-milky discharge may be indicative of benign or malignant breast disease such as duct ectasia.

A Bleeding from the nipple is abnormal.

P Bleeding from the nipple is often seen in the benign condition of intraductal papilloma.

CLINICAL REASONING

Practice tip: The consumer who has had a mastectomy

Assessment of the mastectomy consumer will be guided by the type of mastectomy and the presence or absence of reconstructive surgery. Follow the standard assessment procedures and modify your technique to suit the amount of breast tissue and the presence, if any, of a nipple. Always begin the assessment on the unaffected breast. Women who have had a mastectomy should continue to do their monthly breast awareness examinations to detect any changes, such as a mass in the excised area. Annual clinical assessment and mammography are also recommended. The types of mastectomy procedures are as follows:

> Partial – Lumpectomy or wide local incision (also referred to as breast conserving surgery), involves removing the breast cancer as well as a small amount of surrounding tissue.
> Simple – Only the breast is removed.
> Modified radical – The breast and lymph nodes from the axilla are removed (Figure 12.27A).
> Radical – The breast, lymph nodes from the axilla, and pectoral muscles are removed (Figure 12.27B). This procedure is rarely performed.
> Subcutaneous – The skin and nipple are left intact, but the underlying breast tissue and lymph nodes are removed.

Which procedure the woman has will depend on the stage of her breast cancer and whether it involves the lymph nodes.

Reconstruction techniques include:
> synthetic implants
> tissue expansion techniques (in which a temporary device is placed in a subpectoralis-subserratus position between the anterior chest wall and skin and is then inflated with saline over a period of weeks)
> latissimus dorsi myocutaneous flap breast reconstruction. A myocutaneous flap reconstruction involves transferring skin from the back or the abdomen to the anterior chest wall.

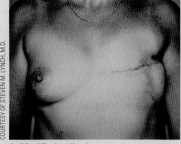

COURTESY OF STEVEN M. LYNCH, M.D.

A. Modified radical

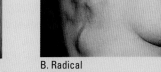

COURTESY OF STEVEN M. LYNCH, M.D.

B. Radical

FIGURE 12.27 Mastectomy consumers

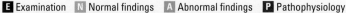

E Examination   **N** Normal findings   **A** Abnormal findings   **P** Pathophysiology

CLINICAL **REASONING**

Breast augmentation and reduction

> Breast augmentation, or augmentation mammoplasty, is a popular surgical procedure in Australia and New Zealand. There are two main types of synthetic implants: the saline implant, which is a silicone envelope filled with normal saline; and the silicon implant, a silicon envelope that is filled with an elastic gel. When assessing a consumer, ask if the breasts have been augmented and what type of implant was used. Incision sites can be found in the axillae, circumareolar areas and inframammary creases. Potential complications from augmentation include haematoma, infection, scarring, loss of nipple or skin sensation, pain from engorgement, asymmetry and malpositioning. Another rare complication is breakage of the implant, which can lead to granulomatous reaction in the breasts, where small, nodular, inflammatory lesions develop, and a capsular membrane forms over the breasts. The augmented breast will feel firmer upon palpation and remain more erect when the consumer is supine.

> Breast reduction is usually performed for women who suffer from back, neck or shoulder pain caused by breast hypertrophy. Two types of procedures may be performed to reduce the breasts: free nipple graft and dermal pedicles. The type of procedure can be ascertained from the postoperative scarring. A free nipple graft leaves scars around the nipple and at the inferior mammary fold. A dermal pedicles procedure leaves 'keyhole' scars over the breasts. Recently, breast liposuction has become popular. Potential complications from these breast reduction procedures include haematoma, infection, nipple or skin necrosis, fat necrosis, and asymmetry. Palpation results will depend on the type of procedure performed and the amount of scar tissue formed.

For both breast augmentation and breast reduction, a baseline mammogram should be performed to provide a reference for future mammography. Otherwise, the guidelines for breast awareness, clinical assessment and mammography are the same as for women who have not undergone breast surgeries.

HEALTH EDUCATION

Breast awareness

Early detection of breast cancer increases the chances of successful treatment and, ultimately, survival. Everyone is different, and breasts continually change as individuals go through the different stages of life. It is important to be familiar with the normal look, feel and shape of one's breast so that abnormal changes can be recognised. Women should be encouraged to examine their breasts at regular intervals and, if they notice a change, they should see a health professional without delay. Changes may include pain, lumps or lumpiness, size and shape changes, skin changes such as puckering or dimpling on the breast, thickened breast tissue, any area that feels different from the rest and changes to nipples such as discharge or inversion (pulling in).

Teaching breast awareness

Before you commence, reiterate that there is no right or wrong way to check one's breasts for any changes. It is important that they develop a routine and a place and time that feels comfortable to look at and feel their own breast regularly. It is also important that they check all parts of the breast, including up to the collarbone and the armpits. The following is a guide:

> The woman should examine her breasts for symmetry, retractions, dimpling, inverted nipples or nipple deviation (as shown in Figure 12.28). She may find it easier to do this in the shower, while getting dressed or lying on the bed (Figure 12.28A).

> She should stand in front of a mirror with her arms at her sides (see Figure 12.28C), then with her arms raised over her head (see Figure 12.28D), and finally with her hands pressed into her hips (see Figure 12.28E).

> She should also be instructed to become familiar with the normal feel of her breasts at different times of the month. She should feel all the breast tissue from the collarbone to below the bra line and the axilla area.

> Also instruct her to squeeze the nipple to examine for discharge (as shown in Figure 12.28F).

>>

>>

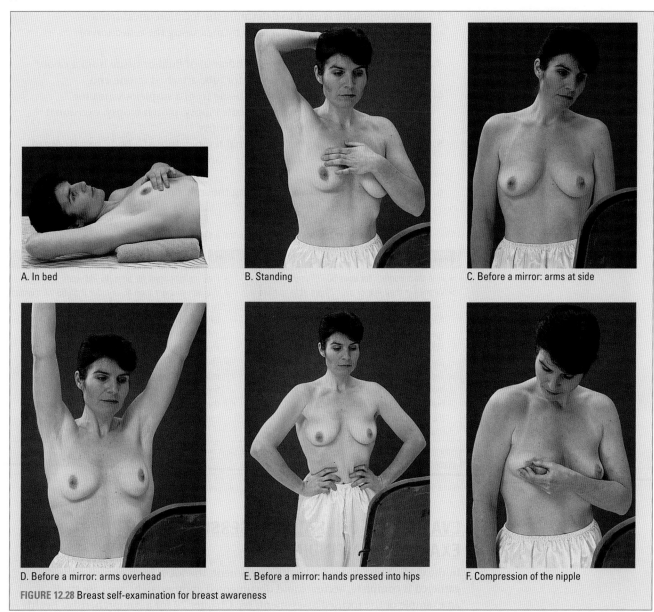

A. In bed

B. Standing

C. Before a mirror: arms at side

D. Before a mirror: arms overhead

E. Before a mirror: hands pressed into hips

F. Compression of the nipple

FIGURE 12.28 Breast self-examination for breast awareness

Examination of the male breasts

Inspection and palpation

Assessment of the male breasts is completed in essentially the same manner as that of the female breast. Modify your technique for a smaller breast with less tissue bulk. Having the consumer lean forwards is usually not necessary unless gynaecomastia is present. Males should be encouraged to be breast aware and have clinical examinations of the breast every 1 to 3 years, if identified as being at high risk, because a small percentage of all breast cancer is found in men (National Breast Cancer Foundation, 2022).

Diagnostic techniques

Aetiologic determination of breast or lymphatic masses can be accurately assessed only via a combination of the diagnostic techniques listed below.

1. Mammography is the roentgenographic examination of the breasts by means of X-rays, ultrasound or magnetic resonance imaging (MRI). Refer to **Table 12.6** for information related to the national breast screening programs in Australia and New Zealand.

2. Ultrasonography is used to determine the location, measurement and delineation of deep structures by measuring the reflection of ultrasonic waves.
3. Needle aspiration involves the withdrawal of fluid or tissue from a cavity via a hollow needle with an aspirator tube attached to one end.
4. Biopsy is the process of removing tissue from a suspicious area for examination. Methods include needle biopsy, punch biopsy, excisional biopsy, core biopsy and stereotactic biopsy.
5. Thermography measures the regional temperature of a body part or organ. Malignant lesions are often warmer than non-malignant areas and are called 'hot spots'.
6. Ductal lavage is a method of rinsing the milk duct to obtain cells for analysis of atypia.

TABLE 12.6 National breast screening programs in Australia and New Zealand

BREASTSCREEN AUSTRALIA	BREASTSCREEN AOTEAROA (NEW ZEALAND)
> Free mammogram for ages 50–74 years > Women in their 40s or over 74 are able to have a free screening mammogram through BreastScreen Australia if they wish. However, they are not specifically targeted to attend. *Why are women under 40 years not included in the free screening program?* > The tissue of younger women's breasts is usually more dense than that of older women; this makes breast lumps/changes difficult to detect. Also, the risk of breast cancer in younger women is low compared to that for older women.	> Free mammogram for ages 45–69 years > Women younger than 45 or older than 69 who wish to have a mammogram need to be referred by their GP to a private radiologist. *Why are women under 45 years not included in the free screening program?* > The tissue of younger women's breasts is usually more dense than that of older women; this makes breast lumps/changes difficult to detect. Also, the risk of breast cancer in younger women is low compared to that for older women.
Younger women who notice any unusual breast lumps, pain or nipple discharge should see their doctor immediately.	

ADAPTED FROM BREASTSCREEN AUSTRALIA PROGRAM (2022) AND BREASTSCREEN AOTEAROA (2022)

EVALUATION OF HEALTH ASSESSMENT AND PHYSICAL EXAMINATION FINDINGS

In the evaluation phase of a health assessment, the focus is on ensuring the data gathered is complete, accurate and documented appropriately (see case study as an example of the focused assessment; see Chapter 22 for a comprehensive health assessment). In evaluating the data you should:

> draw on your critical thinking and problem-solving skills to make sound clinical decisions
> act on abnormal data (include communicating findings to other health professionals)
> ensure documentation reflects the outcomes of the clinical decisions/actions taken (refer to Chapter 3, which discusses in detail why documentation is so important and how this may be undertaken in different health settings). The case study that follows steps you through this process.

THE CONSUMER WITH FIBROCYSTIC BREAST CHANGES

This case study illustrates the application and objective documentation of the breasts and regional nodes assessment. The setting is a short-stay ward for day surgery.

Ms Holly Hastings has been admitted for an excisional biopsy of a lump in her left breast.

HEALTH HISTORY

CONSUMER PROFILE	34-year-old, single woman	
CHIEF COMPLAINT	'I'm scared I have cancer. A friend was diagnosed last year with breast cancer and I can't afford to be seriously ill.'	
HISTORY OF THE PRESENT ILLNESS	Holly Hastings states that she has discovered a lump in the upper outer quadrant of her right breast. She reports that she has frequent breast tenderness, lumpiness and swelling prior to menses. She denies any nipple discharge or any other breast changes noted. She states her doctor informed her she has fibrocystic disease; however, the new lump feels different and harder than the lumpiness she usually experiences.	
PAST HEALTH HISTORY	**MEDICAL HISTORY**	History of fibrotic breast disease, denies fibroadenomas, breast cancer, endometrial or ovarian cancer. Denies hypertension, dyslipidaemia, thyroid disease, exposure to chest radiation. Her onset of menarche was age 12, suffers from severe dysmenorrhea, has never been pregnant.
	SURGICAL HISTORY	Wisdom teeth removed at 23 years of age, rhinoplasty at 26 years of age
	ALLERGIES	Penicillin and tetracycline (rash and throat swelling)
	MEDICATIONS	Levlen (contraception) Takes a multivitamin daily
	COMMUNICABLE DISEASES	Hepatitis A as a child
	INJURIES AND ACCIDENTS	Fractured wrist at age 18
	SPECIAL NEEDS	Nil identified
	BLOOD TRANSFUSIONS	States nil
	CHILDHOOD ILLNESSES	Mumps, age 5; chickenpox, age 5
	IMMUNISATIONS	Flu vaccine annually
FAMILY HEALTH HISTORY	Holly has 2 sisters; denies family history of breast disease	
SOCIAL HISTORY	**ALCOHOL USE**	2–3 glasses wine per week
	TOBACCO USE	Quit smoking 7 years ago; previously 1 pack per day for 10 years
	DRUG USE	Denies experimentation as a teenager
	DOMESTIC AND INTIMATE PARTNER VIOLENCE	Does not have a partner at the moment, denies any history of abuse
	SEXUAL PRACTICE	Heterosexual, sexually active; 3 lifetime partners, no one at present Taking contraceptive pill to assist with dysmenorrhea
	TRAVEL HISTORY	Travels regularly interstate
	WORK ENVIRONMENT	Works in social media marketing
	HOME ENVIRONMENT	5-year-old brick low-set house
	HOBBIES AND LEISURE ACTIVITIES	Reading and bushwalking

HEALTH HISTORY

	STRESS	Bills and home mortgage concerns; has a very stressful job
	EDUCATION	High school graduate, TAFE diploma (Business studies)
	ECONOMIC STATUS	Middle socioeconomic status
	RELIGION	Roman Catholic
	CULTURAL BACKGROUND	Anglo-Saxon (Born in London, UK)
	ROLES AND RELATIONSHIPS	Friend, employee; she is close to her family and sisters
	CHARACTERISTIC PATTERNS OF DAILY LIVING	Wakes at 7 a.m. (twice a week gets up at 6 a.m. to go to the gym), breakfast usually cereal and coffee, at work by 8 a.m.; usually has two more coffees before midday, eats lunch – a salad or sandwich and coffee – works until 4:30 p.m., arrives home by 6 p.m., eats dinner – meat and vegetables – occasionally walks after dinner, watches TV with cup of coffee, in bed by 11 p.m.
HEALTH MAINTENANCE ACTIVITIES	**SLEEP**	7 hours/night. Some nights not sleeping well due to worry about work
	DIET	States she tries to eat a well-balanced diet, does have take-away fast-food on a regular basis (high-fat/high-salt diet). She is aware that she should cut back on amount of coffee she has a day. Also enjoys chocolate regularly, stating she is a 'chocoholic'
	EXERCISE	Tries to get to the gym twice a week, occasional walk after dinner for 20 minutes
	STRESS MANAGEMENT	Prayer, walking, talking to mother/friend. States that she does have a lot of stress with her job
	USE OF SAFETY DEVICES	Wears seat belts, smoke detector in home
	HEALTH CHECK-UPS	Last gynae exam and clinical breast exam 8 months ago, regularly is breast aware for changes

PHYSICAL EXAMINATION

INSPECTION	**COLOUR**	Breast and axilla are flesh coloured with the areolar area and nipples darker pigmentation, no naevi
	VASCULARITY	No enhanced vascular pattern
	THICKENING OR OEDEMA	There is no appearance of thickening or oedema at present
	SIZE AND SYMMETRY	Large, pendulous breasts, appear symmetrical, no nipple inversion or distortion of nipples
	CONTOUR	Convex in shape
	LESIONS OR MASSES	Nil noted
	DISCHARGE	Nil discharge
PALPATION	**SUPRACLAVICULAR AND INFRACLAVICULAR LYMPH NODES**	Nonpalpable
	BREASTS: CONSUMER IN SITTING POSITION	A single firm well-defined and mobile palpable round mass approx. 2 cm in size is felt in the upper outer quadrant of the right breast; consumer states it is tender
	AXILLARY LYMPH NODE REGION	A palpable lymph node of <1 cm noted
	BREASTS: CONSUMER IN SUPINE POSITION	A single firm well-defined and mobile palpable round mass approx. 2 cm in size is felt in the upper outer quadrant of the right breast; consumer states it is tender, no nipple discharge

DIAGNOSTIC DATA

MAMMOGRAPHY	No abnormalities detected
STEREOTACTIC BIOPSY	No fluid is apparent on aspiration biopsy of the lesion
EXCISIONAL BIOPSY	Has now been taken, pathology report not received as yet

EVALUATION AND CLINICAL REASONING FOR CASE STUDY

The assessment and clinical decisions you make should reflect your scope of practice. For example, advanced practice health professionals, such as nurse practitioners and remote area nurses with endorsement, may be able to make diagnostic decisions and prescribe medications without referring to a medical officer.

Fundamentally, all health professionals collect, evaluate and act on consumer-focused health information, which will at times include referral to, or collaboration with, other healthcare team members. Nurses assess consumer responses to interventions and determine when to escalate key changes in a consumer's condition. The clinical reasoning cycle provides health professionals with a framework to consider all this information in a meaningful way for planning consumer care. These phases are stepped out below, and draw on information presented and collected during the health history and physical examination. We then work through the cycle components that are relevant to this case study (cycle components are bolded).

For Holly Hastings, the significant data that needs to be considered includes the following.

Collecting cues/information

Recall and Review: In the first instance you will need to reflect on what you know about breast lumps and more specifically fibrocystic breast changes. These benign changes to breasts are very common in women 30–50 years of age, rare in postmenopausal women. It is not a disease as such, as it relates to fluctuations in hormones. Women who suffer from premenstrual abnormalities, are nulliparous, have never taken the contraceptive pill and had early menarche are more susceptible to this disorder. The symptoms include swelling, pain, tenderness, lumpiness and nipple discharge (which may or may not be present) and these increase just before menstruation. On examination: one or more palpable lumps that are round, soft to firm, well defined and freely movable can be felt. Some will be cysts full of fluid, while others can be fibrous with no fluid. It should be noted that fibrocystic changes do not increase the chances of breast cancer in the majority; however, women with this disorder should have frequent clinical check-ups with the GP.

Medical management following a complete health history, examination with imaging studies, if not conclusive, a biopsy for definitive diagnosis, is usually based on palliating the symptoms. These include medication such as analgesics, diuretics, hormone therapy and antioestrogen therapy. Danazol, a synthetic androgen, can be prescribed for consumers with severe pain. Many other interventions can also be suggested to alleviate the disorder, such as diet (low salt, restrict methylxanthines found in chocolate and coffee), reduction of stress (a common contributing factor for breast disorders), stopping smoking (women who stop have reported a reduction in the lumpiness of their breasts), vitamin E therapy and/or local heat and cold therapy may assist in reducing swelling and pain. These interventions remain experimental as there has been no research as to their effectiveness; hence it is trial and error for each individual woman.

Taking all this into consideration when you are processing Holly Hastings' information will allow you to undertake the clinical reasoning cycle appropriately.

Chief complaint and history of present illness

> Consumer states she is worried she has breast cancer.
> She has discovered a lump in the upper outer quadrant of her right breast.
> She complains of frequent breast tenderness, lumpiness and swelling.
> History of fibrocystic disorder.

Processing information

Interpret: These symptoms and details of history outline the scope of the issue for this consumer and how it is affecting her wellbeing and ability to self-manage this deviation from normal health.

Medication
> Taking a multivitamin.

Relate and Discriminate: At present she appears to be treating her stress by commencing a multivitamin. It would be important to find out if she has in the past taken any analgesia for the breast tenderness and if so what type and how effective it was.

Taking Levlen (contraceptive pill).

Relate and Discriminate: Holly has reported having severe dysmenorrhea, and has recently commenced taking Levlen to assist with this.

Social history
> Not in a relationship at present and is nulliparous.
> Has a very stressful job.

Discriminate: Need to consider these things as it has been identified that women who are nulliparous and suffer from stress are more susceptible to this disorder.

Health maintenance activities
> Drinks a considerable amount of coffee.
> States she is a 'chocoholic'.

Interpret and Relate: Coffee and chocolate contain methylxanthines and it is believed that this contributes to fibrocystic changes, so it is significant information relating to her present health alteration.

Physical examination/diagnostic data

> A single firm, well-defined and mobile palpable round mass approx. 2 cm in size is felt in the upper outer quadrant of the right breast; consumer states it is tender.
> Nil abnormalities detected on mammography.
> Stereotactic biopsy, nil fluid aspirated.
> Excisional biopsy – has now been taken, awaiting results.

Infer and Predict: These findings give an indication that the lump is probably fibrocystic; however, the excisional biopsy will give a definitive diagnosis. This is significant as the consumer has not received the results yet, so she will still be quite anxious re the possibility she has breast cancer.

Putting it all together – synthesise information

The role of the nurse in this case is primarily emotional support and teaching. As Holly Hastings will be discharged before she receives the results of her test, relieving her anxieties will be paramount. Also, providing further information about contributing factors to her health alteration, so that she can self-care and use comfort measures, will aid her in managing this disorder.

Actions based on assessment findings

The nurse should provide additional information/education for interventions that do not require a doctor's order. These would include:

1 Encourage her to express any fears and anxieties that she may have in relation to her possible diagnosis of breast cancer and answer her questions honestly.

2 Give Ms Hastings further information about fibrocystic disorders – that it is a common disorder in premenopausal women, and is also more prevalent in women who suffer from premenstrual conditions (such as severe dysmenorrhea).

3 Explain that the majority of breast lumps, approx. 80%, are benign, and that fibrocystic changes do not increase the risk of breast cancer.

4 Educate her re the use of analgesia to assist her to cope with the tenderness and discomfort of her breasts pre menses, specifically with NSAIDs (commence taking as soon as breasts feel tender to maximise effect, correct dose 250–500 mg tds).

5 Encourage Holly to wear a well-fitted and supporting bra, as this will reduce feeling of weight and thus pain.

6 Discuss/encourage her to decrease/eliminate caffeine and chocolate from her diet, especially close to her menses.

7 Taking a vitamin E supplement may relieve swelling and tenderness, especially right before her menstrual period.

8 Hot or cold packs can also relieve pain and swelling.

9 As stress has been linked to breast discomforts – discuss ways to manage/decrease stress (exercise, balanced diet, work–life balance, adequate sleep etc.).

10 Encourage her to continue to be breast aware, as well as visit her GP for clinical examinations as they suggest. (Possible mammogram regularly.)

The final step in the process is accurate documentation. The nurse must document findings, referrals, interventions, and advice and education given. The consumer would be advised to make an appointment to see her surgeon as requested to discuss results and further management of her breast disorder.

CHAPTER RESOURCES

REVIEW QUESTIONS

For answers to these questions, see Answer section at the end of the book.

1. Abby, a 12-year-old female, is having a physical examination. She tells you that she began her menses at age 10 and she is 160 cm tall. On examination you see that her nipple is flush with the breast. The areola and breast are larger than a small mound. What is Abby's sexual maturity rating stage for breast development?
   a. 1
   b. 2
   c. 3
   d. 4

2. Which breast structure is a sebaceous gland that lubricates the nipple and helps to keep it supple during lactation?
   a. Montgomery's tubercles
   b. Ectodermal galactic band
   c. Cooper's ligaments
   d. Tail of Spence

3. A 16-year-old female presents to clinic with complaints of 'multiple moles' on her breast. Upon inspection, the Women's Health nurse observes an ectodermal galactic band extending from the axilla to the groin. The nurse explains to the consumer that they are not moles, but they are which of the following?
   a. Montgomery tubercles
   b. Lymph nodes
   c. Supernumerary nipples
   d. Areola

4. Which of the following conditions is found most commonly in postmenopausal women?
   a. Mastitis
   b. Paget's disease
   c. Fibroadenoma
   d. Cystic hyperplasia

5. A consumer visits the health clinic because she has been experiencing nipple discharge for a few weeks. You review her health history. Which of the following medications may have a link to breast discharge?
   a. Theophylline
   b. Chemotherapy
   c. Hormone replacement
   d. Chlorpromazine

6. Which of the following recommendations by BreastScreen Australia and the New Zealand Breast Cancer Foundation is true for breast health checks in a 35-year-old woman?
   a. Breast self-awareness
   b. Clinical breast examination
   c. Annual mammogram
   d. Baseline breast MRI

7. Which of the following are nonmodifiable risk factors for developing breast cancer? Select all that apply.
   a. Age greater than 50
   b. Family history with breast cancer
   c. Male sex
   d. Personal history of breast cancer
   e. Obesity
   f. Postmenopausal hormone therapy

8. Which type of breast cancer starts in the lobules and milk ducts and has invaded outlying tissue?
   a. Ductal carcinoma in situ
   b. Invasive ductal carcinoma
   c. Infiltrating lobular carcinoma
   d. Paget's disease

9. Which of the following would identify that a woman is at high risk of developing breast cancer?
   a. Multiple (blood) family members with a diagnosis of breast cancer
   b. Previous history of breast cancer
   c. Family (blood) member with hereditary mutation (e.g. BRCA1/BRCA2)
   d. All of the above

10. Carolyn, a 26-year-old nonlactating female, presents with a complaint of a single, nontender breast mass she found during a self-breast examination. The consumer describes the mass as firm, well defined and mobile. The nurse suspects which of the following?
    a. Cyst
    b. Fibroadenoma
    c. Mastitis
    d. Carcinoma

CS CLINICAL SKILLS

The following Clinical Skill is relevant to this chapter and can be found in Tollefson & Hillman, *Clinical Psychomotor Skills*, 8th edition:
> 27 Healthcare teaching.

FURTHER RESOURCES

> Australian Breast Cancer Research: https://www.abcr.com.au/
> Australian Government Department of Health – Breast Screen Australia Program: http://www.health.gov.au/internet/screening/publishing.nsf/Content/breast-screening-1
> Australian National Breast Cancer Foundation: https://nbcf.org.au/
> Breast Cancer Cure – New Zealand Breast Cancer Research Trust: https://www.breastcancercure.org.nz/
> Breast Cancer Network Australia: http://www.bcna.org.au
> Breast Cancer Trials: http://www.bcia.org.au
> Cancer Australia, Australian Government – Breast Cancer: https://breast-cancer.canceraustralia.gov.au/
> Inflammatory Breast Cancer Research Foundation: http://www.ibcresearch.org
> Ministry of Health, New Zealand: http://www.health.govt.nz/
> National Breast Cancer Foundation: https://nbcf.org.au/about-national-breast-cancer-foundation/about-us/
> National Screening Unit – Breastscreen Aotearoa: http://www.nsu.govt.nz/current-nsu-programmes/breastscreen-aotearoa.aspx
> New Zealand Breast Cancer Foundation: http://www.nzbcf.org.nz/

REFERENCES

Australian Institute of Health and Welfare (AIHW). (2021). Cancer in Australia 2021. Cancer series no. 133. Cat. no. CAN 144. Retrieved 12 December 2022 from https://www.aihw.gov.au/reports/cancer/cancer-data-in-australia/

Breast Cancer Foundation New Zealand. (2022). Retrieved 12 December 2022 from https://www.breastcancerfoundation.org.nz/breast-awareness/breast-cancer-facts/breast-cancer-in-nz

Breast Cancer Network Australia. (2022). Risk factors. Retrieved 12 December 2022 from https://www.bcna.org.au/breast-health-awareness/risk-factors

Breast Cancer Trials. (2022). Breast cancer statistics. Retrieved 12 December 2022 from https://www.breastcancertrials.org.au/breast-cancer-resources/breast-cancer-statistics/

BreastScreen Australia. (2022). Department of Health Australian Government. Retrieved 7 May 2022 from http://cancerscreening.gov.au/internet/screening/publishing.nsf/Content/breast-screening-1

Cancer Australia. (2022). Breast cancer. Retrieved 12 December 2022 from https://www.canceraustralia.gov.au/cancer-types/breast-cancer/statistics

National Breast Cancer Foundation. (2022). Breast cancer and Aboriginal and Torres Strait Islander peoples. Retrieved 12 December 2022 from https://nbcf.org.au/about-breast-cancer/further-information-on-breast-cancer/breast-cancer-in-aboriginal-and-torres-strait-islander-peoples

NZ National Screening Unit. (2022). Breast screening. Retrieved 6 May 2022 from https://www.timetoscreen.nz/breast-screening/

Tin Tin, S., Elwood, M., Brown, C., Sarfati D., Campbell I., Scott, N., … Lawrenson R. (2018). Ethnic disparities in breast cancer survival in New Zealand: Which factors contribute? *BMC Cancer, 18*(1), 58, doi 10.1186/s12885-017-3797-0

CHAPTER 13

RESPIRATORY

LEARNING OUTCOMES

By the end of this chapter you should be able to:

1 identify the anatomic landmarks of the thorax and the lungs
2 describe the characteristics of the most common respiratory complaints
3 obtain a health history from a consumer with a respiratory problem
4 demonstrate inspection, palpation, percussion and auscultation on a healthy adult and on a consumer with a respiratory problem
5 discuss the clinical reasoning in evaluating outcomes of health assessment and physical examination, including documentation, health education provision and relevant health.

BACKGROUND

Respiratory health problems affect a person's airways and produce symptoms such as shortness of breath, chest tightness, cough and wheezing. In the 2020–21 reference period, 1 in 3 Australians (ABS, 2022) and 1 in 7 New Zealanders (Asthma and Respiratory Foundation NZ, 2022a) reported having chronic respiratory conditions. These include asthma, chronic obstructive pulmonary disease (COPD) (encompassing emphysema and chronic bronchitis), allergic rhinitis or 'hay fever', chronic sinusitis, bronchiectasis, cystic fibrosis, occupational lung diseases and sleep apnoea (AIHW, 2022a). The Severe Acute Respiratory Syndrome Coronavirus (SARS-CoV-2) that causes coronavirus disease (COVID-19) and the subsequent worldwide pandemic has created significant challenges and changes to the respiratory health of many people. To date, Australia has experienced over 11 million cumulative cases of COVID-19 (COVID Live, 2023), and New Zealand has experienced almost 2.5 million cumulative cases of COVID-19 (Ministry of Health, 2023).

Between 2017 and 2021 the most common cause of respiratory-related deaths in Australia, and the fifth most common overall, was chronic lower respiratory disease (ABS, 2022); in New Zealand asthma and respiratory disease was the third leading cause of death (Asthma and Respiratory Foundation NZ, 2022a). In 2021 in Australia, the mortality rate from respiratory diseases was very low, at a rate of 39.1 per 100 000 people (ABS, 2022), with cancer of the lung, trachea and bronchus accounting for 8674 deaths and chronic lower respiratory disease accounting for 7805 deaths (ABS, 2022). The health measures put in place to control the spread of COVID-19 significantly reduced the spread of droplet-transmitted acute respiratory infections, such as influenza and some types of pneumonia, resulting in the second lowest mortality rate on record from respiratory illness (ABS, 2022).

To date, there have been nearly 13 500 deaths in Australia (ABS, 2023) and 2792 deaths in New Zealand attributed to COVID-19 (Ministry of Health, 2023).

COVID-19 has caused the death of over 7000 males, and 6000 females in Australia (ABS, 2023). In 2021 it was the 15th highest cause of death (ABS, 2022). Emerging data and research indicates post-COVID syndrome, also known as post-acute COVID or long COVID, is increasingly affecting the long-term health of consumers following an episode of COVID-19 (Augustin et al., 2021).

Of the non-COVID-19 respiratory diseases, asthma and COPD are singled out here for a brief exploration. Asthma is a significant global problem affecting people of all ages, and it is often under-diagnosed and under-treated (WHO, 2022). In Australia, just under 2.7 million Australians (10.7%) suffered from asthma in 2020–21 (ABS, 2022). The mortality rate for asthma in Aboriginal and Torres Strait Islander peoples in 2014–18 was 2.2 times that for non-First Nations people (AIHW, 2020). In New Zealand, one in eight people take medication for asthma (Asthma and Respiratory Foundation NZ, 2020). Hospitalisation is significantly higher for Māori (3 times higher), Pasifika people (3.2 times higher) and people from the most deprived households (nearly 3 times higher) when compared with the broader population (Asthma and Respiratory Foundation NZ, 2020). Other key respiratory problems for Māori are COPD, bronchiectasis, childhood bronchiolitis and childhood pneumonia (Asthma and Respiratory Foundation NZ, 2020).

The most significant risk factors for COPD are being a current daily tobacco smoker, obesity and being physically inactive (AIHW, 2020), with tobacco use causing the highest preventable burden for the Australian population (AIHW, 2020). Similarly, in New Zealand most cases of COPD are associated with breathing tobacco smoke (either by smoking, or indirectly from second-hand smoke) (Health Navigator New Zealand, 2021). Moreover, the effects of smoking contribute negatively to the management of asthma and other chronic respiratory disease symptoms. Of note, however, is the continued decline in smoking in New Zealand, with daily smoking for Year 10 students down to 1.1% (Asthma and Respiratory Foundation NZ, 2022b); in Australia, 97% of people aged 14 to 17 have never smoked, compared with 82% in 2001 (AIHW, 2022b).

The respiratory system is divided into the upper and lower tracts. The upper respiratory tract comprises the nose, pharynx, larynx and the upper trachea. The nose and pharynx are discussed in Chapter 11. The lower respiratory tract is composed of the lower trachea to the lungs. This chapter covers only those components of the respiratory system that are located in the thorax.

ANATOMY

The respiratory system extends from the nose to the alveoli (**Figure 13.1**). The normal air pathway is nose, pharynx, larynx, trachea, main stem bronchus, right and left main bronchi, lobar/secondary bronchi, segmental/tertiary bronchi, terminal bronchioles, respiratory bronchioles, alveolar ducts, alveolar sacs and alveoli.

Thorax

The thorax (**Figure 13.2**) is a cone-shaped structure (narrower at the top and wider at the bottom) that consists of bones, cartilage and muscles. Of these, the bones are the supportive structure of the thorax. For the anterior thorax, these bones are the 12 pairs of ribs and the sternum. Posteriorly, there are the 12 thoracic vertebrae and the spinal column.

Sternum

The sternum, or breastbone, is a flat, narrow bone approximately 13 cm long. It is located at the medial line of the anterior chest wall and is divided into three sections: the **manubrium** (the upper bone of the sternum that articulates with the clavicles and the first pair of ribs), the body, and the **xiphoid process** (a cartilaginous process at the base of the sternum that does not articulate with the ribs).

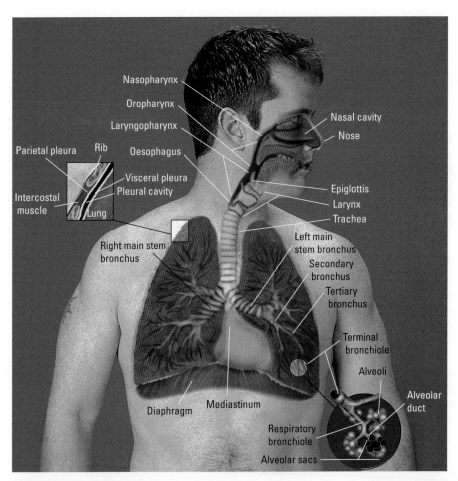

FIGURE 13.1 The respiratory tract

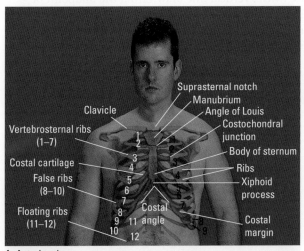

A. Anterior view

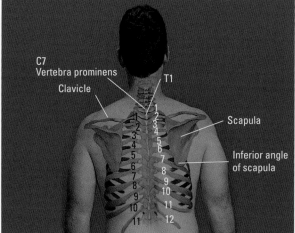

B. Posterior view

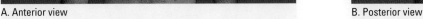

FIGURE 13.2 Thorax: rib number is shown on the consumer's right; intercostal space number is shown on the consumer's left

Ribs

The first seven pairs of ribs are articulated to the sternum via the costal cartilages and are called the **vertebrosternal** or **true ribs**. The **false ribs**, or rib pairs 8–10, articulate with the costal cartilages just above them. The remaining two pairs of ribs (11 and 12) are termed **floating ribs** and do not articulate at their anterior ends. The 10th rib is the lowest rib that can be palpated anteriorly. The 11th rib is palpated on the lateral thorax, and the 12th rib is palpated on the posterior thorax. All ribs articulate posteriorly to the vertebral column. When a rib is palpated, the costal cartilage cannot be distinguished from the rib itself (**Figure 13.2**).

Intercostal spaces

Each area between the ribs is called an **intercostal space** (ICS). There are 11 ICSs.

CLINICAL **REASONING**

Practice tip: Counting anterior intercostal spaces
Use the angle of Louis as a landmark for identifying the rib number. Count the ribs in the midclavicular line. Each ICS is named for the number of the rib directly above it. For example, the space between the third and fourth ribs would be called the third ICS.

Lungs

The lungs are cone-shaped organs that fill the lateral chamber of the thoracic cavity. The lower outer surface of each lung is concave where it meets the convex diaphragm. Likewise, the medial aspect is concave to allow room for the heart, with the left lung having a more pronounced concavity (cardiac notch). The lungs lie against the ribs anteriorly and posteriorly.

The right lung is broader than the left lung because of the position of the heart. Inferiorly, the right lung is about 2.5 cm shorter than the left lung because of the upward displacement of the diaphragm by the liver. The right lung consists of three lobes (upper, middle and lower); the left lung has two lobes (upper and lower). In the lung, the **apex** denotes the top of the lung; the **base** refers to the bottom of the lung. Anteriorly, the apices of the lung extend 2.5 to 4 cm superior to the inner third of the clavicles, and posteriorly, the apices lie near the T1 process. On deep inspiration posteriorly, the lower lung border extends to the level of T12, and to T10 on deep expiration. The anterior inferior border of the lungs is at the sixth rib at the **midclavicular line** (MCL: vertical line drawn from the midpoint of the clavicle) and at the eighth rib at the **midaxillary line** (MAL: vertical line drawn from the apex of the axilla and lying midway between the anterior and the **posterior axillary lines**) (see **Figure 13.3**).

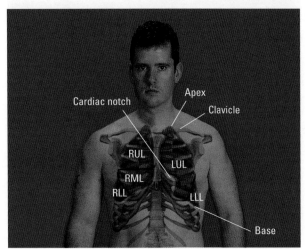

A. Anterior view

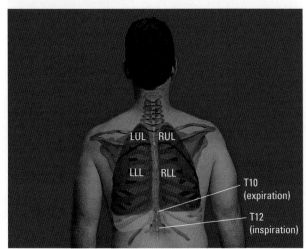

B. Posterior view

FIGURE 13.3 Lungs: RUL = right upper lobe; RML = right middle lobe; RLL = right lower lobe; LUL = left upper lobe; LLL = left lower lobe

The lobes of the right and left lungs are divided by grooves called fissures. It is important to know the locations of the fissures to describe clinical findings. **Figure 13.4** illustrates the right oblique (or diagonal) fissure, the right horizontal fissure and the left oblique (or diagonal) fissure.

CLINICAL **REASONING**

Practice tip: Thoracic anatomic topography

Additional landmarks that are useful when describing assessment findings are:

> **Anterior axillary line** – vertical line drawn from the origin of the anterior axillary fold and along the anterolateral aspect of the thorax
> **Midspinal (vertebral) line** – vertical line drawn from the midpoint of the spinous process
> **Midsternal line** – vertical line drawn from the midpoint of the sternum
> **Posterior axillary line** – vertical line drawn from the posterior axillary fold
> **Scapular line (left and right)** – vertical line drawn from the inferior angle of the scapula.

Take a look at **Figure 13.5**. Locate each of the above imaginary lines and note the anatomical locations and structures they showcase. For example, the anterior axillary line locates the mid thorax (left lower lung) and commences from the mid underarm.

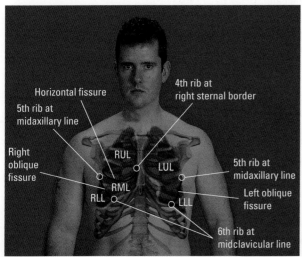

A. Anterior view

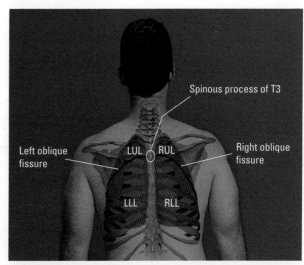

B. Posterior view

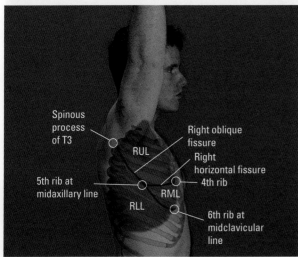

C. Right lateral view

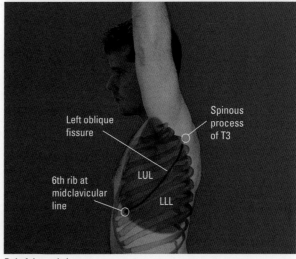

D. Left lateral view

FIGURE 13.4 Lung fissures

When assessing the thorax, it is helpful to envision it as a rectangular box, with the four sides being the anterior, posterior, right lateral and left lateral thoraxes. Figure 13.5 illustrates the imaginary thoracic lines on each of the four sides. These landmarks are helpful in discussing clinical findings.

CLINICAL **REASONING**

Practice tip: Identifying thoracic landmarks
> Anterior
  * Sternum
  * Clavicles
  * Nipples
  * **Suprasternal notch:** With the finger pad of the index finger, feel in the midsternal line above the manubrium; the depression is the suprasternal notch.
  * **Angle of Louis (or manubriosternal junction or sternal angle):** With the finger pads, feel for the suprasternal notch and move your finger pads down the sternum until they reach a horizontal ridge (the junction of the manubrium and the body of the sternum); this is the angle of Louis (or sternal angle).The second rib articulates with this landmark and serves as a convenient reference point for counting the ribs and ICSs (the first rib is difficult to palpate).
  * Costal angle: Place your right finger pads on the bottom of the consumer's anterior left rib cage (10th rib); place your left finger pads on the bottom of the anterior right rib cage (10th rib); move both hands horizontally towards the sternum until they meet in the midsternal line; the angle formed by the intersection of the ribs creates the costal angle.
> Posterior
  * **Vertebra prominens:** Flex the neck forwards; palpate the posterior spinous processes. If two processes are palpable, the superior process is C7 (vertebra prominens) and the inferior is T1; this landmark is useful in counting ribs to the level of T4. Beyond T4 the spinous processes project obliquely and no longer correspond to the rib of the same number as the vertebral process.
  * **Inferior angle of scapula:** Locate the inferior border of the scapula; this level corresponds to the seventh rib or seventh ICS.
  * Spine
  * **Twelfth rib:** Palpate the lower thorax in the scapular line. Move your hand laterally to palpate the free tip of the 12th rib.

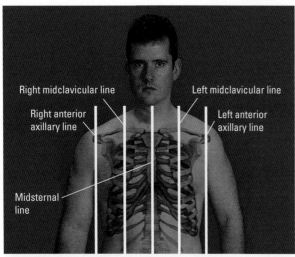

A. Anterior view

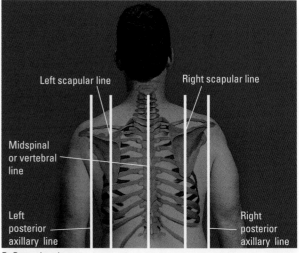

B. Posterior view

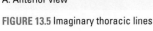

FIGURE 13.5 Imaginary thoracic lines

>> **FIGURE 13.5** *continued*

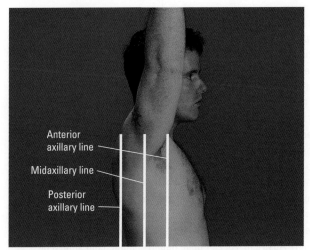

C. Right lateral view

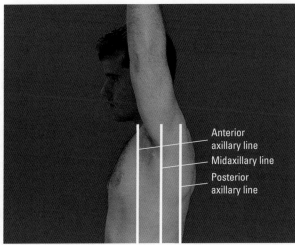

D. Left lateral view

Pleura

Each lung is encased in a serous sac, or **pleura**. The **parietal pleura** lines the chest wall and the superior surface of the diaphragm. The **visceral pleura** lines the external surface of the lungs. Usually, a small amount of fluid is found in the space between these two pleurae; this fluid prevents the pleurae from rubbing against each other and acts as a cushioning agent for the lungs.

Mediastinum

The **mediastinum**, or **interpleural space**, is the area between the right and left lungs. It extends from the sternum to the spinal column and contains the heart, great vessels, trachea, oesophagus and lymph vessels. The only respiratory structures in the mediastinum are the trachea and the pulmonary vasculature. The trachea is a fibromuscular hollow tube located in the anterior thorax in the median plane. It is 11 to 13 cm in length and 2 to 3 cm in width. The trachea lies anterior to the oesophagus.

Bronchi

The trachea bifurcates into the left and right mainstem bronchi at the level of the fourth or fifth vertebral process posteriorly and the sternal angle anteriorly. The right main bronchus is wider, shorter and more vertical than the left. This anatomic difference is critical because it makes the right main bronchus more susceptible to aspiration and endotracheal intubation. The main bronchi further divide into lobar or secondary bronchi. Each lobar bronchus supplies a lobe of the lung. The bronchi transport gases as well as trap foreign particles in their mucus. Cilia aid in sweeping the foreign particles upwards in the respiratory tract for possible elimination. Culmination of the tracheobronchial tree is in the alveoli.

PUTTING IT IN CONTEXT

Assessing for tuberculosis exposure

A new graduate from a bachelor of education course presents to your clinic for a purified protein derivative (PPD) test and physical examination in order to commence a new teaching job. He returns 48 hours later and is found to have a positive PPD. He informs you that 1 year ago, he lived in Haiti on a teaching exchange in one of the local schools. How would you proceed?

In this situation you should consider the following in the provision of your care.

>>

>>

The positive reaction assists to identify an individual who may be infected with one of the organisms of *Mycobacterium tuberculosis* complex bacilli. The reaction may be due to any of the mycobacteria infections (*M. tuberculosis*, *M. canetii*, *M. bovis* etc.) or previous vaccination with BCG – (bacille Calmette-Guérin) (Communicable Diseases Network Australia, 2022). It is thus important to assess in more detail the person's previous exposure to risk factors for tuberculosis (see Health Education box – Risk factors for tuberculosis) and determine if he has received a BCG vaccination in the past. You would undertake your usual physical examination, implementing standard and transmission-based precautions drawing on your knowledge that TB is an airborne infection (transmitted by inhalation of infectious aerosols) and that most people are unaware of possible TB infection, as they remain asymptomatic (Refer to Chapter 5: Physical examination techniques) (Australian Technical Advisory Group on Immunisation, 2018). It will be important to ensure the consumer is aware of the need to be vigilant about identifying any development of future symptoms. Ensure you emphasise that the risk of developing TB in the first 2 years is high post a positive test result (Communicable Diseases Network Australia, 2022). Public health management should be obtained from the state/territory or relevant public health authority.

Alveoli

The **alveoli** are the smallest functional units of the respiratory system. It is here that gas exchange occurs. It is estimated that approximately 300 million alveoli are present in each lung. This aerating surface is about equal to 100 times the body surface area of an adult. Each alveolus has its own blood supply and lymphatic drainage. Branches of the pulmonary artery carry blood to the capillaries surrounding the alveoli to be oxygenated. Branches of the pulmonary vein transport oxygenated blood from the alveoli to the heart.

Diaphragm and muscles of respiration

The diaphragm, which is innervated by the phrenic nerve, is a dome-shaped muscle that forms the inferior border of the thorax. Anteriorly, its right edge is located at the fifth rib – fifth ICS at the MCL. The left dome of the diaphragm is at the sixth rib – sixth ICS at the MCL. The presence of the liver below the right dome of the diaphragm accounts for the elevated border on that side. On expiration posteriorly, the diaphragm is located at the level of the 10th vertebral process, and at T12 on inspiration. Laterally, the diaphragm is found at the eighth rib at the midaxillary line. The diaphragm is the principal muscle of respiration. Contraction of the diaphragm leads to an increase in volume in the thoracic cavity.

The external intercostal muscles are located in the ICS. During inspiration, the external intercostal muscles elevate the ribs, thus increasing the size of the thoracic cavity. The internal intercostal muscles draw adjacent ribs together, thereby decreasing the size of the thoracic cavity during expiration.

Accessory respiratory muscles are used to accommodate increased oxygen demand. Exercise and some diseases lead to the use of accessory muscles. The accessory muscles are the scalene, sternocleidomastoid, trapezius and rectus abdominus (**Figure 13.6**).

CLINICAL **REASONING**

Practice tip: Preventing aspiration of fluid into the lungs
Aspiration is the inhalation of foreign material into the respiratory tract (e.g. aspiration of mucus or vomitus).

Aspiration can have significant health consequences; therefore, you should assess the risk for consumers and manage them accordingly. These points will help guide your practice:
> Place the at-risk consumer (intoxicated, unconscious) in a side-lying or upright position.
> Ensure the airway is always maintained. If the consumer is lying down and they are vomiting, ensure their head is to the side, to decrease the chance of aspiration.

>>

>>

> > Consumers receiving intermittent tube feedings should be placed in an upright position during the feeding and for 30 minutes after feeding; individuals receiving continuous tube feedings should be placed in an upright position at all times.
> > Delay tube feeding if the gastric residual is significant (amount varies per individual and per amount of usual feeding), and communicate/document this.
> > Suction oropharynx of consumers with tracheostomies prior to deflation of their cuff.

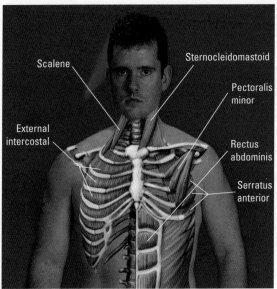

A. Anterior view.

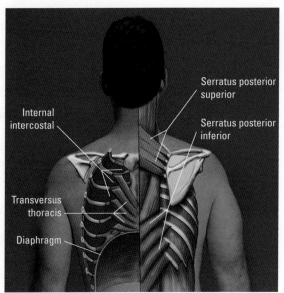

B. Posterior view.

FIGURE 13.6 Muscles of respiration

PHYSIOLOGY

Ventilation

The primary function of the respiratory system is to deliver oxygen to the lungs and to remove carbon dioxide from the lungs. The breathing process includes inspiratory and expiratory phases. During inspiration, the pressure inside the lungs becomes subatmospheric when the diaphragm and external intercostal muscles contract. The diaphragm lowers and the ribs elevate, thus increasing the intrapulmonic volume. As a result of the negative intra-alveolar pressure, atmospheric air is pulled into the respiratory tract until intra-alveolar pressure equals atmospheric pressure. The lungs increase in size with the air.

Expiration is a passive process and occurs more rapidly than inspiration. During expiration, the diaphragm and external intercostal muscles relax, decreasing the volume of the thoracic cavity. The diaphragm rises. The intrapulmonic volume decreases and the intrapulmonic pressure increases above the atmospheric pressure. The lungs possess elastic recoil capabilities that allow air to be expelled until intrapulmonic pressure equals atmospheric pressure.

External respiration

External respiration is the process by which gases are exchanged between the lungs and the pulmonary vasculature. Oxygen diffuses from the alveoli into the blood, and carbon dioxide diffuses from the blood to the alveoli. Diffusion is a passive process in which gases move across a membrane from an area of higher concentration to an area of lower concentration. In the lungs, the membrane is the alveolar–capillary network.

Internal respiration

Internal respiration is the process by which gases are exchanged between the pulmonary vasculature and the body's tissues. Oxygen from the lungs diffuses from the blood into body tissue. Carbon dioxide diffuses from the tissue into the blood and is then carried back to the right side of the heart for reoxygenation.

Control of breathing

Control of breathing is influenced by neural and chemical factors. The pons and medulla are the central nervous system structures primarily responsible for involuntary respiration. The stimulus for breathing is an increased carbon dioxide level, a decreased oxygen level, or an increased blood pH level.

HEALTH EDUCATION

Risk factors for tuberculosis

Tuberculosis (TB) is a notifiable and significant health issue that represents a global and national public health threat. In Australia and New Zealand numbers are low and relatively stable; in Australia there are approximately 1200 cases per year (Australian Technical Advisory Group on Immunisation, 2018; Australian Government Department of Health, 2018). In New Zealand incidence is also stable, with approximately 300 cases per year (Ministry of Health/Manatù Hauora, 2022b). Guidelines are available for the control of TB. It is spread airborne via droplet nuclei into the respiratory tract. The following are risk factors for contracting pulmonary tuberculosis and should be considered in gathering health assessment data:

> Living with or being in close contact with others who have active TB
> Malnourishment
> Immunosuppressed status
> Homelessness, including living in shelters
> Imprisonment, due to close living quarters
> Residing in a nursing home, hospice etc. due to close living quarters
> Working with high-risk consumers
> Chronic diseases leading to decreased resistance
> Immigration from countries with tuberculosis prevalence
> Being a migrant farming/rural worker
> Positive tuberculin skin test
   Health education is a key to minimising the spread of tuberculosis.

ASSESSMENT: TAKING THE CONSUMER'S HEALTH HISTORY

Assessment is the first phase of the nursing process, and involves collecting subjective information about the consumer's health status in order to identify consumer problem areas to focus on.

Subjective data is most frequently collected during a health history and serves as the starting point for the health professional to base the depth of their assessment on. The sections for the health history include:

> **Consumer profile**
> **Chief complaint** (explained systematically using variations of location, quality, quantity, associated manifestations, aggravating factors, alleviating factors, setting and timing. This is a variation on the PQRST assessment mnemonic you may use for other conditions such as pain assessment)

\>>

> > **Past health history** (including medical history, surgical history, allergies, medications, injuries and accidents, special needs and childhood illnesses)
> > **Family health history**
> > **Social history** (including alcohol, tobacco and drug use, sexual practice, work and home environment, hobbies and leisure activities, stress and culture).

The example health history provided identifies scope for questioning the consumer about their health for this specific body system.

HEALTH HISTORY

CONSUMER PROFILE	The respiratory health history provides insight into the link between a consumer's life and lifestyle and respiratory information and pathology. Diseases that are age-, sex- and race-specific for the thorax and lungs are listed with approximate commencing age range in years.		
	AGE	> Bronchiectasis (birth–20) > Cystic fibrosis (birth–30) > Pneumothorax (20–40) > Sarcoidosis (30–40) > Chronic bronchitis (>35) > Pneumonia (>60) > Emphysema (50–60) > Idiopathic pulmonary fibrosis (60–70) > Asthma > Lung cancer > Severe Acute Respiratory Syndromes (SARS, e.g. coronavirus)	
	SEX	**FEMALE**	Lung cancer, sarcoidosis, COPD, influenza, SARS and pneumonia
		MALE	Lung cancer, COPD, idiopathic pulmonary fibrosis, pneumothorax, influenza, SARS, pneumonia and asthma
	CULTURAL BACKGROUND	**ABORIGINAL AND TORRES STRAIT ISLANDERS, NEW ZEALAND MĀORI**	COPD, pneumonia, influenza and SARS, asthma (most common cause of hospitalisation in Māori), lung cancer, COPD, bronchiectasis
		CAUCASIAN	Cystic fibrosis
CHIEF COMPLAINT	Common chief complaints for the respiratory system are defined, and information on the characteristics of each sign or symptom is provided.		
	1. DYSPNOEA	Subjective feeling of shortness of breath (SOB)	
		QUANTITY	The number of steps that can be climbed before SOB occurs, distance that can be walked, number of pillows needed to sleep comfortably
		ASSOCIATED MANIFESTATIONS	Palpitations, leg pain, faintness, anxiety, fatigue, cough, sputum, wheezing, diaphoresis, cyanosis, pain, fever
		AGGRAVATING FACTORS	Smoking, exercise, poorly ventilated rooms, cold weather, wind
		ALLEVIATING FACTORS	Sit the consumer upright and use pillows to support (helpful with orthopnoea). Examples of well-known positions are semi-Fowler, Fowler positions. Try side-lying position, tripod position, fresh air, medications (e.g. bronchodilators), supplemental oxygen, resting
		TIMING	Night-time (paroxysmal nocturnal dyspnoea)
	2. COUGH	Stimulation of afferent vagal endings, helps clean the airway of extraneous material by producing a sudden, forceful and noisy expulsion of air from the lungs	
		QUALITY	Dry, wet, hacking, barking, congested, harsh, brassy, high-pitched, whooping, bubbling, productive/nonproductive

>>

HEALTH HISTORY

			ASSOCIATED MANIFESTATIONS	SOB, wheezing, sputum, pleuritic pain, chest pain, fever, haemoptysis, coryza, anxiety, diaphoresis, gastro-oesophageal reflux disease (GORD) symptoms, postnasal drip, hoarseness
			AGGRAVATING FACTORS	Position of consumer, exposure to noxious stimuli, exercise
			ALLEVIATING FACTORS	Medications (e.g. nebuliser, inhaler, cough suppressant medications, steroids), humidity, cool air, cool liquids
			SETTING	Temperature and humidity of environment, exertion
			TIMING	Winter, early morning, bedtime, middle of the night, after eating, prior to fainting, continuous
		3. SPUTUM		Substance produced by the respiratory tract that can be expectorated or swallowed; it is composed of mucus, blood, purulent material, microorganisms, cellular debris and, occasionally, foreign objects
			QUALITY	> Colour: white or clear, purulent, blood-tinged, yellow or green, mucoid, rust, black, pink > Consistency: thick, thin, moderate; frothy – separates into layers > Odour: malodorous
			QUANTITY	Normal daily sputum production is 60–90 mL (normally this is not expectorated); small, moderate, copious
			ASSOCIATED MANIFESTATIONS	Cough, fever, dyspnoea
			AGGRAVATING FACTORS	Exposure to allergens, smoking
			ALLEVIATING FACTORS	Medications (e.g. guaifenesin), liquids
			SETTING	When person is asleep, exposure to an allergen
			TIMING	Early morning
		4. CHEST PAIN		Pain can have a pulmonary, cardiac, gastrointestinal or musculoskeletal aetiology. Chapter 14 differentiates the types of chest pain.
PAST HEALTH HISTORY				The various components of the past health history are linked to thorax and lung pathology and related information.
	MEDICAL HISTORY		RESPIRATORY-SPECIFIC	Asthma, bronchitis, croup, frequent colds, cystic fibrosis, emphysema, epiglottitis, pleurisy, pneumonia, pneumothorax, pulmonary oedema, pulmonary embolus, lung cancer, tuberculosis, pertussis, COPD, pleural effusion, bronchiectasis, intubation, confirmed or suspected SARS
			NON-RESPIRATORY-SPECIFIC	Lupus, drug-induced respiratory pathology, rheumatoid arthritis, congenital musculoskeletal chest defects, severe scoliosis, multiple sclerosis, amyotrophic lateral sclerosis
	SURGICAL HISTORY			Lobectomy, pneumonectomy, tracheostomy, wedge resection, bronchoscopy, chest tube insertion
	ALLERGIES			Asthma is the predominant manifestation of allergies in the consumer with respiratory conditions. Hypersensitivity to drugs, food, pets, dust, cigarette smoke, perfume or pollen should be closely scrutinised. In addition, any common signs of allergies, such as cough, sneeze and sinusitis, should be closely evaluated.
	MEDICATIONS			Beta agonists, inhaled corticosteroids, anticholinergics, mast cell stabilisers, leukotriene receptor antagonists, antibiotics, bronchodilators, cough expectorant, cough suppressant, oxygen, steroids

HEALTH HISTORY

	COMMUNICABLE DISEASES	> Common cold (head cold): sneezing, coughing > Tuberculosis (TB): pulmonary fibrosis and calcification > Flu: pneumonia > AIDS: *Pneumocystis carinii* pneumonia > Hantavirus: bilateral pulmonary infiltrates, respiratory failure (low incidence in Australia) > COVID-19: cough, difficulty breathing, SOB
	INJURIES AND ACCIDENTS	Chest trauma, near drowning
	CHILDHOOD ILLNESSES	Pertussis and measles: bronchiectasis
FAMILY HEALTH HISTORY		Respiratory diseases that are familial are listed: Allergies, alpha1-antitrypsin deficiency, asthma, bronchiectasis, cancer, cystic fibrosis, emphysema, sarcoidosis, TB, pulmonary emboli, COVID-19
SOCIAL HISTORY		The components of the social history are linked to respiratory factors and pathology.
	ALCOHOL USE	Decreases efficiency of lung defence mechanisms, predisposes to aspiration pneumonia; consumers with carbon dioxide retention are more sensitive to the depressant effect of alcohol
	TOBACCO USE	Cigarette smoking is the primary risk factor for chronic bronchitis, emphysema and lung cancer, as well as other disorders
	DRUG USE	> Heroin: pulmonary oedema > Barbiturates or narcotic overdose: respiratory depression > Cocaine: tachypnoea
	TRAVEL HISTORY	> Prolonged exposure to confined space with recirculated air (e.g. aeroplane) > TB (South-East Asia): poor sanitation and rural conditions > Pneumonic plague (India): carried by nuclei droplets
	WORK ENVIRONMENT	Repeated exposure to materials in the workplace can create respiratory complications that range from minor problems to life-threatening events. Numerous categories of respiratory diseases have been identified from repeated exposure to toxic substances. These diseases are listed along with the industries and agents related to them. > Silicosis: glassmaking, tunnelling, stonecutting, mineral mining, insulation work, quarrying, cement work, ceramics, foundry work, semiconductor manufacturing > Asbestosis: mining, shipbuilding, construction > Coal worker's pneumoconiosis: coal mining > Pneumoconiosis: tin and aluminium production, welding, insecticide manufacturing, rubber industry, fertiliser industry, ceramics, cosmetic industry > Occupational asthma: electroplating, grain working, woodworking, photography, printing, baking, painting > Chronic bronchitis: coal mining, welding, fire fighting > Byssinosis: cotton mill dust, flax > Extrinsic allergic alveolitis (hypersensitivity pneumonia): animal hair, contamination of air conditioning or heating systems, mouldy hay, mouldy grains, mouldy dust, sugarcane > Toxic gases and fumes: welding, cigarette smoke, auto exhaust, chemical industries, firefighting, hair spray, sniffing glue > Pulmonary neoplasms: radon gas, mustard gas, printing ink, asbestos, chromium (from chrome plating, stainless steel welding) > Pneumonitis: furniture polish, petroleum or kerosene ingestion; mineral oil, olive oil and milk aspiration > SARS-CoV-2: airborne transmission associated with inability to physically distance, inadequate ventilation, inappropriate PPE
	HOME ENVIRONMENT	> Air pollution, cigarette smoke, wood-burning stoves, gas stoves and heaters, kerosene heaters, radon gas, pet hair and dandruff > Tropical diseases such as melioidosis, dengue haemorrhagic fever, scrub typhus, leptospirosis, salmonellosis, penicilliosis marneffei, malaria, amoebiasis, paragonimiasis, strongyloidiasis, gnathostomiasis, trinchinellosis, schistosomiasis, echinococcosis

HEALTH HISTORY

HOBBIES AND LEISURE ACTIVITIES	Birds (bird breeder's lung), mushroom growers (mushroom grower's lung), scuba diving (lung rupture, oxygen toxicity, decompression sickness), high-altitude activities (skiing, climbing: pulmonary oedema and pulmonary embolus)	
STRESS	Asthma can be exacerbated by stress.	
ECONOMIC STATUS	Poor sanitation and densely populated areas are ideal conditions for the spread of TB and COVID-19.	

Person-centred health education

When conducting a health assessment, opportunities for the provision of person-centred health education will arise. This is a significant consideration in relation to the assessment process for examination of the thorax and lungs. These occasions are identified as individualised education and may generate further data that can be added to the assessment. All education given should be documented so that in future, health professionals can assess the impact of previous information provided to the consumer. (Refer to Chapter 1 for initiating health education.) Refer to the following examples.

INDIVIDUALISED HEALTH EDUCATION INTERVENTIONS

Assessing the consumer for the following health-related activities can assist in identifying the need for education about these factors. This information provides a bridge between the health maintenance activities and respiratory function.

Sleep	Obstructive sleep apnoea: absence of inspiratory muscle activation; upper airway occlusion COPD or neuromuscular disease: nocturnal oxygen desaturation caused by hypoventilation without apnoea
Diet	Obesity: chronic hypoventilation, obstructive sleep apnoea (e.g. due to Pickwickian syndrome)
Exercise	Regular exercise improves pulmonary function
Use of safety devices	Wear a mask when exposed to toxic substances, other occupational precautions as mandated by Occupational Health and Safety workplace legislation
Health check-ups	Respiratory rate, lung auscultation, chest X-ray, sputum culture and sensitivity, pulmonary function test, TB testing, influenza and pneumococcal vaccines, immunotherapy (allergy shots), SARS-CoV-2 testing

PUTTING IT IN CONTEXT

COVID-19

On 11 March 2020, the World Health Organization declared the Severe Acute Respiratory Syndrome Coronavirus (SARS CoV-2), which causes coronavirus disease 2019 (COVID-19), a worldwide pandemic. From 2020, healthcare systems and healthcare professionals worldwide have coordinated significant changes to their environments and management of persons requiring care. The evidence to support clinical policy and practice, based on high-quality research, is still emerging. Therefore, the information included in the text is correct at the time of publication; however, we acknowledge the rapidly changing evidence related to COVID-19. Epidemiological reports suggest 80% of COVID-19 cases will experience mild or moderate disease that does not require medical intervention. However, 20% of COVID-19 cases will experience severe disease requiring hospital treatment. Severe or fatal outcomes are common in older persons, or those with co-morbid conditions.

>>

COVID-19 affects many body systems. Persons with COVID-19 may present with a wide array of symptoms. Mild symptoms may include cough, sore throat, pyrexia, diarrhoea, headache, myalgia or arthralgia, fatigue, anosmia and ageusia.

The presence of anosmia or ageusia may be a useful red flag for COVID-19 (Struyf et al., 2021).

In addition to the burden of acute COVID-19 on healthcare systems and professionals, evidence suggests large numbers of persons experience post COVID infection. Post COVID infection is known as post COVID syndrome, post-acute COVID or long COVID. There is currently no Australian or international definition for the range of symptoms experienced following an acute COVID infection.

Post COVID infection signs and symptoms may include:
> pulmonary symptoms (cough, shortness of breath)
> neurological symptoms (fatigue, headache, cognitive dysfunction, sleep disturbance, anosmia, paraesthesia)
> hair loss
> skin conditions
> renal disease
> thromboembolism
> psychological symptoms (anxiety, depression, mood swings)
> cardiac symptoms (chest pain)
> musculoskeletal symptoms (non-specific pain, myalgia)
> fever (low-grade fevers)
> reduced activity and functional level
> reduced nutritional status and weight loss
> post-intensive care syndrome (PICS).

Currently, there is limited evidence supporting effective management of post COVID infection. Goals of care currently include effective, culturally appropriate communication, coordinated primary care, support wellbeing, exclude serious complications, manage red flag symptoms (RACGP, 2021).

Australian Government Department of Health (2022); Australian National COVID-19 Clinical Evidence Taskforce (2022, 9 May, p. 770); Ministry of Health/Manatū Hauora (2022c, 6 May); RACGP (2021, December)

PUTTING IT IN CONTEXT

Inhalants

You are conducting a history on a new 19-year-old consumer in the student health centre of the local university. The consumer has a history of asthma and needs a refill of her short-acting bronchodilator. The individual denies using tobacco but admits to inhaling some substances at recent parties. You ask her to tell you more about this practice when she says, 'I have said too much. I never should have brought it up. I just want a prescription for my asthma medication and I will leave.' How should you proceed?

Such a situation may provide an opportunity for the nurse to highlight the deleterious effects of short- and long-term illegal drug use. It may be possible to provide written materials or the details of an online website/s if the person is not keen to discuss the situation. Nurses are often placed in situations that provide opportunities to deliver key health updates and this should be enacted when the situation arises.

HEALTH EDUCATION

Maintaining respiratory health

The following considerations should be noted during assessment of the consumer's respiratory health history and will depend on their context.

> Avoid smoking; encourage those living with you to stop.
> Do not smoke or allow others to smoke around infants and children.
> If you live with a smoker, ask that smoking be confined to one well-ventilated room or, preferably, undertaken outside.
> If dust and mould are allergy triggers or aggravating factors for other respiratory ailments, clean the house frequently, avoid wall-to-wall carpeting, use easily washed curtains, and avoid having a cluttered room.
> Change filters on heaters, air conditioners, exhaust systems and range hoods as the manufacturer specifies.
> Ensure chimneys are cleaned at the beginning of each season and more frequently if used heavily.
> Have home inspected for radon and take remedial steps as needed.
> Check carbon monoxide and smoke detectors monthly.
> If oxygen is used in the home, use and store away from heat; avoid contact with open flames and cigarettes.

PLANNING FOR PHYSICAL EXAMINATION

The planning phase refers to evaluating subjective data to narrow the focus on physical examination, determining what objective data needs to be gathered, as well as considering the environment and equipment that will be required.

At this time, you will identify which of the four diagnostic techniques you will need to implement the physical examination, and how you will sequence these. For the physical examination of the respiratory system comprising thorax and lungs, you will include inspection, palpation, percussion and auscultation.

Objective data is:

> collected during the physical examination of the consumer
> usually collected after subjective data
> information that is measured or observed by the clinician as opposed to being reported by the consumer
> vital to the overall health assessment, to enable you to make clinical decisions that are representative of the whole consumer picture.

Evaluating subjective data to focus physical assessment

Before commencing the physical examination of the consumer's thorax and lungs, consider what information the health history has provided. Critical consideration, linked to knowledge of anatomy and physiology, should focus the physical assessment so your examination will be more effective and efficient.

Environment

Assessing the respiratory system requires a physical environment in the healthcare setting that has:

> a flat table/surface for the consumer to lie on
> adequate lighting
> adequate privacy for the consumer.

Equipment

Assemble items before placing the consumer on the examination table; materials should be arranged in order of use and within easy reach.

> Stethoscope
> Tape measure
> Washable marker
> Watch with second hand
> Examination table
> Pen light
> Personal protective equipment (PPE).

HEALTH EDUCATION

Influenza vaccine
The following persons are STRONGLY recommended to receive influenza vaccine every year:
> Children aged <5 years
> Adults aged 65 years and over
> Aboriginal and Torres Strait Islander people
> Individuals >55 years of Māori or Pasifika ethnicity
> People aged 6 months and over with medical conditions associated with an increased risk of influenza disease and complications
> Pregnant women
> Healthcare workers, carers, household contacts of people in high-risk groups
> Teachers and support staff in schools, early childhood education
> Residents, staff, volunteers and visitors to aged care, longer-term residential care facilities
> Commercial poultry and pork industry workers
> Essential services providers
> People who are travelling during the influenza season
> Homeless people.

For further information regarding changes, dosage, administration, contraindications and adverse events, please review the government guidelines.

Sources: Australian Technical Advisory Group on Immunisation (ATAGI) (2018); Ministry of Health/Manatù Hauora (2022d) version 17a released 2022

HEALTH EDUCATION

COVID-19 vaccine
On 22 February 2021, the first doses of COVID-19 vaccine were administered in Australia and Aotearoa New Zealand. Vaccination for COVID-19 is recommended for all persons 5 years of age and over. In Australia and Aotearoa New Zealand, two doses of vaccine are currently recommended for people aged over 5 years. Up to five doses of vaccine are currently recommended for special populations. Special populations include those who are severely immunocompromised, pregnant, breastfeeding or planning pregnancy, residents of aged or disability care facilities, and Aboriginal and Torres Strait Islander people aged over 50 years. There are currently no recommendations for vaccination for neonates and children aged less than 5 years of age.

COVID-19 vaccination is strongly recommended for the following at risk groups:
> All adults aged ≥65 years
> Aboriginal and Torres Strait Islander people
> People of Māori and Pasifika ethnicity
> Pregnant and breastfeeding women
> People with cardiac disease, obesity, chronic respiratory and liver disease
> Other groups such as residents and staff of long-term and aged-care facilities, homeless people, essential service providers, carers and household contacts of those in high-risk groups.

Australian Technical Advisory Group on Immunisation (ATAGI) (2022, May). Australian Technical Advisory Group on Immunisation (ATAGI) recommended COVOD-19 vaccines and doses. https://www.health.gov.au/; Ministry of Health/Manatù Hauora (2022d, 6 May). Immunisation Handbook. http://www.health. govt.nz/

HEALTH EDUCATION

Pandemics

A pandemic is an epidemic where an infectious disease spreads worldwide, affecting a substantial number of people.

The most recent and significant pandemic outbreak, declared on 11 March 2020, was Severe Acute Respiratory Syndrome (SARS), an acute respiratory disease caused by a coronavirus (CoV). In 2022, the World Health Organization reported over 515 million cumulative cases of SARS CoV-2 causing COVID-19 worldwide. Strict national systems of surveillance are in place to monitor, manage and control communicable respiratory and like diseases. National guidelines direct individuals to safe preventative practices.

For further information go to:

> Australian Government Department of Health (2023). Coronavirus (COVID-19) pandemic. https://www.health.gov.au/health-alerts/covid-19
> Ministry of Health/Manatū Hauora (2022a). COVID-19 (novel coronavirus). https://www.health.govt.nz/covid-19-novel-coronavirus

IMPLEMENTATION: CONDUCTING THE PHYSICAL EXAMINATION

Physical examination of the respiratory system is undertaken in the one sequence of assessments. Implementation of the physical examination requires you to consider your scope of practice. In this section, depending on your context, you may be performing a foundation assessment or the addition of advanced assessment techniques if you are practising in a specialised area.

EXAMINATION IN BRIEF: RESPIRATORY (THORAX AND LUNG)

Examination of the thorax and lungs

Inspection
> Shape of thorax
> Symmetry of chest wall
> Presence of superficial veins
> Costal angle
> Angle of the ribs
> Intercostal spaces (ICS)
> Muscles of respiration

Examination of respirations

Inspection
> Rate
> Pattern
> Depth
> Symmetry
> Audibility
> Consumer position
> Mode of breathing
> Sputum

Palpation
> General palpation
> Pulsations
> Masses
> Thoracic tenderness

> Locating the site of a fractured rib
> Crepitus

Thoracic expansion
> Tactile fremitus
> Tracheal position

Percussion
> General percussion
> Diaphragmatic excursion

Auscultation
> General auscultation
> Breath sounds
> Voice sounds

Assessing consumers with respiratory supportive equipment

Oxygen

Pulse oximeter

Incentive spirometer

Endotracheal tube

Peak flow meter

Tracheostomy tube

Mechanical ventilation

Advanced Assessment

General approach to respiratory assessment
Prior to assessment:

1. Undertake a risk assessment to determine if standard or transmission-based precautions are required.
2. Greet the consumer and explain the assessment techniques that you will be undertaking.
3. Ensure that the examination room is at a warm, comfortable temperature to ensure the consumer is relaxed and comfortable.
4. Use a quiet room that will be free from interruptions.
5. Ensure that the light in the room provides sufficient brightness to adequately observe the consumer.
6. Instruct the consumer to remove all their clothes from the waist up and to don an examination gown.
7. Place the individual in an upright sitting position on the examination table.
8. Expose the entire area being assessed. Provide a drape that women can use to cover their breasts (if desired) when the posterior thorax is assessed.
9. When palpating, percussing or auscultating the anterior thorax of female or obese consumers, ask them to displace the breast tissue. Assessing directly over breast tissue is not an accurate indicator of underlying structures.
10. Visualise the underlying respiratory structures during the assessment process to accurately describe the location of any pathology.
11. Always compare the right and the left sides of the anterior thorax and the posterior thorax to each other, as well as the right lateral thorax to the left lateral thorax.
12. Use a systematic approach every time the assessment is performed. Proceed from the lung apices to the bases, right to left to lateral.

Examination of the respiratory system
Inspection
Shape of thorax

E 1. Stand in front of the consumer and observe.
2. Estimate visually the transverse diameter of the thorax.
3. Move to one side of the consumer.
4. Estimate visually the width of the anteroposterior (AP) diameter of the thorax.
5. Compare the estimates of these two visualisations.

N In the normal adult, the ratio of the AP diameter to the transverse diameter is approximately 1:2 to 5:7. In other words, the normal adult is wider from side to side than from front to back. The normal thorax is slightly elliptical in shape. A barrel chest is normal in infants and sometimes in the older adult. (See Chapter 20 for a discussion of the paediatric consumer.) Figure 13.7 illustrates the normal and abnormal cross sections of the thorax.

A With a **barrel chest**, the ratio of the AP diameter to the transverse diameter is approximately 1:1. The consumer's chest is circular or barrel-shaped in appearance (Figure 13.7B).

P The consumer with COPD has a barrel chest due to air being trapped in the alveoli and subsequent lung hyperinflation. Lung volume thus increases and the diaphragm flattens over time. The ribs are forced upwards and outwards. Collectively these changes result in the barrel chest appearance.

A **Pectus carinatum**, or pigeon chest, is a marked protrusion of the sternum. This increases the AP diameter of the thorax (Figure 13.7C).

P Pectus carinatum can result from a congenital anomaly. A consumer with severe pectus carinatum will exhibit respiratory difficulty.

E Examination **N** Normal findings **A** Abnormal findings **P** Pathophysiology

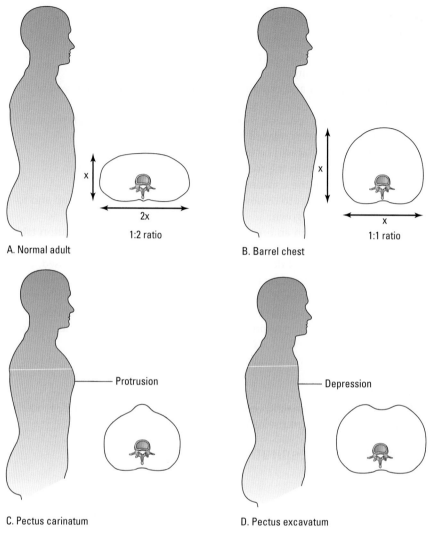

A. Normal adult

2x
1:2 ratio

x

B. Barrel chest

x
1:1 ratio

— Protrusion

C. Pectus carinatum

— Depression

D. Pectus excavatum

FIGURE 13.7 Chest configurations

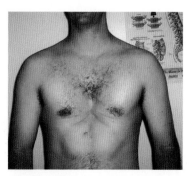

FIGURE 13.8 Pectus excavatum

P Rickets can result from a vitamin D deficiency. In this condition, the bones become demineralised and weak. The loss of bone strength allows the intercostal muscles to pull the ribs and sternum forwards, resulting in pectus carinatum.

A **Pectus excavatum**, or funnel chest (**Figures 13.7D and 13.8**), is a depression in the body of the sternum. This indentation can compress the heart and cause myocardial disturbances. The AP diameter of the chest decreases.

P Pectus excavatum results from a congenital anomaly. Respiratory insufficiency can ensue from the compression of the lungs in marked pectus excavatum.

A **Kyphosis**, or humpback, is an excessive posterior convexity of the thoracic vertebrae (**Figure 13.9A**). Gibbus kyphosis is an extreme deformity of the spine.

P Most kyphosis cases are idiopathic. Respiratory compromise is manifested only in severe cases.

A **Scoliosis** is a lateral curvature of the thorax or lumbar vertebrae (**Figure 13.9B**). See Chapter 16 for further discussion.

P Most cases of scoliosis are idiopathic, although scoliosis can also result from neuromuscular diseases, connective tissue diseases and osteoporosis. Marked scoliosis can interfere with normal respiratory function. The total lung capacity and vital capacity decline in proportion to the severity of the scoliosis.

E Examination **N** Normal findings **A** Abnormal findings **P** Pathophysiology

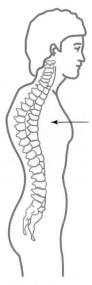
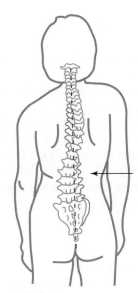

A. Kyphosis   B. Scoliosis

FIGURE 13.9 Abnormalities of the spine

Symmetry of chest wall

E 1. Stand in front of the consumer.
2. Inspect the right and the left anterior thoraxes.
3. Note the shoulder height. Observe any differences between the two sides of the chest wall, such as the presence of masses.
4. Move behind the consumer.
5. Inspect the right and the left posterior thoraxes, comparing right and left sides.
6. Note the position of the scapula.

N The shoulders should be at the same height. Likewise, the scapula should be the same height bilaterally. There should be no masses.

A Having one shoulder or scapula higher than the other is abnormal.

P The presence of scoliosis can lead to a shoulder or a scapula that is higher than its corresponding part. Marked scoliosis impairs lung function.

A The presence of a visible mass is abnormal.

P A visible chest mass is always abnormal. Likely aetiologies are mediastinal tumours or cysts. If large enough, they can compress lung tissue and impair normal lung function.

Presence of superficial veins

E 1. Stand in front of the consumer.
2. Inspect the anterior thorax for the presence of dilated superficial veins.

N In the normal adult, dilated superficial veins are not seen.

A The presence of dilated superficial veins on the anterior chest wall is an abnormal finding.

P Dilated veins on the anterior thorax may be indicative of superior vena cava obstruction. Due to the obstruction, the superficial veins and collateral vessels become engorged with blood and dilate. Venous return to the heart is diminished, compromising oxygenation. A consumer may present with dyspnoea.

E Examination **N** Normal findings **A** Abnormal findings **P** Pathophysiology

> ## CLINICAL **REASONING**
>
> **Practice tip: Assessing nail bed clubbing and capillary refill**
> The presence of nail bed clubbing provides information on a consumer's long-term oxygen status (hypoxia), and capillary refill indicates peripheral circulation. Note these findings when assessing respiratory function.
>
> You undertake a respiratory physical examination of Sharon, a 59-year-old woman, and identify she has the presence of clubbing and a barrel-shaped chest. She reports increasing fatigue, dyspnoea post exertion and coughs 'a lot'. These signs and symptoms are consistent with her recent diagnosis of COPD. For more information about the assessment techniques, normal findings and abnormal findings associated with clubbing and capillary refill, refer to Chapter 8.

Costal angle

E
1. Stand in front of the consumer.
2. In a consumer whose thoracic skeleton is easily viewed, visually locate the **costal margins** (medial borders created by the articulation of the false ribs).
3. Estimate the angle formed by the costal margins during exhalation and at rest. This is the **costal angle**.
4. In a heavy or obese consumer, place your fingertips on the lower anterior borders of the thoracic skeleton.
5. Gently move your fingertips medially to the xiphoid process.
6. As your hands approach the midline, feel the ribs as they meet at the apex of the costal margins. Visualise the line that is created by your fingers as they move up the floating ribs towards the sternum. This is the costal angle (see **Figure 13.10A**). Approximate this angle.

N The costal angle is less than 90° during exhalation and at rest. The costal angle widens slightly during inhalation due to the expansion of the thorax.

A A costal angle greater than 90° is abnormal.

P Processes in which hyperinflation of the lungs (emphysema) or dilation of the bronchi (bronchiectasis) occurs result in a costal margin angle greater than 90°. The diaphragm flattens out and the ribs are forced upwards and outwards, leading to the change in the costal margin angle.

Angle of the ribs

E
1. Stand in front of the consumer.
2. In a consumer whose thoracic skeleton is easily viewed, visually locate the midsternal area.
3. Estimate the angle at which the ribs articulate with the sternum.
4. If you are unable to visually locate the angle of the ribs, such as in an obese consumer, place your fingertips on the midsternal area.
5. Move your fingertips along a rib laterally to the **anterior axillary line**. Visualise the line that is created by your hand as it traces the rib. Approximate this angle. See **Figure 13.10B**.

N The ribs articulate at a 45° angle with the sternum.

A An angle greater than 45° is considered abnormal. Consumers with particular respiratory pathology may have ribs that are nearly horizontal and perpendicular to the sternum.

P Conditions characterised by an increased AP diameter, such as emphysema, bronchiectasis and cystic fibrosis, result in an angle greater than 45° because the lungs are forced out due to hyperinflation or dilation of the bronchi.

E Examination   **N** Normal findings   **A** Abnormal findings   **P** Pathophysiology

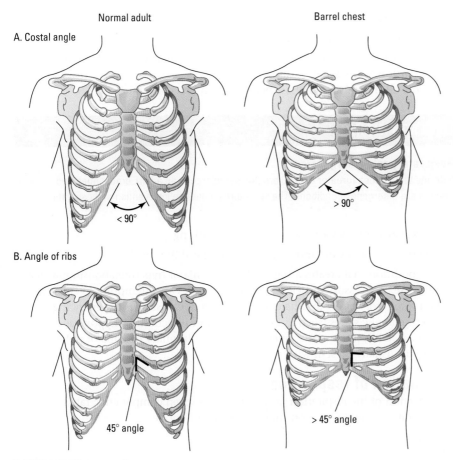

FIGURE 13.10 Rib cage angles

Intercostal spaces (ICS)

E 1. Stand in front of the consumer.
2. Inspect the ICS throughout the respiratory cycle.
3. Note any bulging of the ICS and any retractions.

N There should be an absence of retractions and of bulging of the ICS.

A The presence of retractions is abnormal. Retractions occur during inspiration.

P Conditions that obstruct the free inflow of air may lead to retractions. These include emphysema, asthma, tracheal or laryngeal obstruction, and the presence of a foreign body or tumour that compresses the respiratory tract.

URGENT FINDING

Tension pneumothorax
A tension pneumothorax occurs when air accumulates progressively in the pleural space and exerts positive pressure on mediastinal and intrathoracic structures. The person most often presents with difficulty breathing, hypoxia, tachycardia, chest pain and unexplained hypotension. A tension pneumothorax is a medical emergency and requires immediate intervention to decompress the lung.

A The presence of bulging of the ICS is abnormal. Bulging of the ICS tends to occur during expiration.

P Abnormal bulging of the ICS occurs when there is an obstruction to the free exhalation of air, such as in emphysema, asthma, an enlarged heart, aortic aneurysm, massive pleural effusion, tension pneumothorax and tumours.

E Examination   **N** Normal findings   **A** Abnormal findings   **P** Pathophysiology

Muscles of respiration

E 1. Stand in front of the consumer.
2. Observe the consumer's breathing for a few respiratory cycles, paying close attention to the anterior thorax and the neck.
3. Note all the muscles that are being used by the consumer.

URGENT FINDING

Respiratory rate emergencies
Extreme tachypnoea (greater than 30 breaths per minute in an adult), bradypnoea and apnoea are emergency conditions. These require immediate intervention and escalation.

N No accessory muscles are used in normal breathing.

A The use of the accessory muscles is a pathological finding.

P Any condition that creates a state of hypoxaemia or hypermetabolism may lead to the use of accessory muscles. Accessory muscles are attempting to create an extra respiratory effort to inhale needed oxygen. Consumers experiencing hypermetabolic states (such as exercise, fever or infection) or hypoxic events (such as COPD, pneumonia, pneumothorax, pulmonary oedema or pulmonary embolus) usually present with accessory muscle use.

Examination of respirations

The inspection of the respiration process includes seven components: rate, pattern, depth, symmetry, audibility, consumer position and mode.

Inspection

Rate

E 1. Stand in front of the consumer or to the right side.
2. Observe the consumer's breathing without stating what you are doing, because the consumer may change the respiratory rate (increase or decrease it) if aware that you are watching the chest rising and falling. This assessment can be conducted simultaneously with the pulse rate assessment.
3. Count the number of respiratory cycles that the consumer has for one full minute. A respiratory cycle consists of one inhaled and one exhaled breath.

N In the resting adult, the normal respiratory rate is 12 to 20 breaths per minute. This type of breathing is termed **eupnoea**, or normal breathing (Figure 13.11A).

A A respiratory rate greater than 20 breaths per minute is termed tachypnoea (Figure 13.11B).

P Tachypnoea is frequently present in hypermetabolic and hypoxaemic states. By increasing the respiratory rate, the body is trying to supply additional oxygen to meet the body's demands. Tachypnoea occurs in many disease states, such as pneumonia, bronchitis, asthma and pneumothorax.

P Tachypnoea is often a sign of stress. In stressful situations, the body releases catecholamines that elevate the respiratory rate to supply sufficient oxygen.

A A respiratory rate lower than 12 breaths per minute is termed bradypnoea (Figure 13.11C).

P Injury to the brain may cause bradypnoea because of excessive intracranial pressure applied to the respiratory centre in the medulla oblongata.

Respiratory distress
You are away with a couple of friends camping and enjoying sitting around the campfire.
Just as you are about to toast some marshmallows in the coals of the campfire, one of your
friends sitting next to you grabs your hand and says, 'I can't breathe.'
> What questions would you ask the person?
> What assessments would you undertake?
> How would you proceed?

P In drug overdoses (barbiturates, alcohol and opiates), bradypnoea is a sign of the drug's depressant effect on the respiratory centre.

P Bradypnoea occurs in sleep because of the lowered metabolic state of the body. The respiratory rate also slows in non-REM sleep due to changes in the response of the respiratory centre to chemical signals.

A Apnoea is the lack of spontaneous respirations for 10 or more seconds (Figure 13.11D).

P Traumatic brain injury may lead to apnoea because of herniation of the brain stem.

P Sleep apnoea can be central or obstructive in nature. In central sleep apnoea, the respiratory drive is altered, leading to periods of respiratory cessation. In obstructive sleep apnoea, enlarged upper airway anatomy leads to a physical blockage in the oropharynx.

Pattern

E 1. Stand in front of the consumer.
2. While counting the respiratory rate, note the rhythm or pattern of the breathing for regularity or irregularity (Figure 13.11).

N Normal respirations are regular and even in rhythm.

A **Cheyne-Stokes respirations** occur in **crescendo** and **decrescendo** patterns interspersed between periods of apnoea that can last 15–30 seconds (Figure 13.11E). This can be a normal finding in older adults and in young children. Cheyne-Stokes respiration is an example of a regularly irregular respiratory pattern; that is, the respirations predictably or regularly become irregular.

P Central cerebral or high brain stem lesions that occur in brain injury produce Cheyne-Stokes respirations.

P Cheyne-Stokes respirations can also appear in sleep due to alterations in the respiratory centre's ability to accurately perceive chemical and mechanical stimuli.

A **Biot's respirations**, or **ataxic respirations**, are examples of an irregularly irregular respiratory pattern (Figure 13.11F). In an irregularly irregular rhythm, there is no identifiable pattern to the respiratory cycle. There is an absence of a crescendo and decrescendo pattern. Deep and shallow breaths occur at random intervals interspersed with short and long pauses. Periods of apnoea can be long and frequent.

P Biot's breathing indicates damage to the medulla.

A **Apneustic respirations** are characterised by a prolonged gasping during inspiration followed by a very short, inefficient expiration. These pauses can last 30–60 seconds (Figure 13.11G).

P Injury to the upper portion of the pons can lead to apneustic breathing.

A **Agonal respirations** are irregularly irregular respirations (Figure 13.11H). These are of varying depths and patterns.

P Impending death, where there is little or no oxygen supplying the brain, or compression of the respiratory centre, may lead to agonal breaths.

E Examination   **N** Normal findings   **A** Abnormal findings   **P** Pathophysiology

Depth

E
1. Stand in front of the consumer.
2. Observe the relative depth with which the consumer draws a breath during inspiration.

N The normal depth of inspiration is not exaggerated, and effortless.

A In hypoventilation, or shallow respirations, the chest wall is moved minimally during inspiration and expiration. A small tidal volume is being inspired (**Figure 13.11I**).

P Obese consumers frequently have small tidal volumes due to the sheer weight of the chest wall and the effort it takes to move it with each breath.

P The consumer in pain or with a recent abdominal or thoracic incision has shallow respirations due to the discomfort of moving the rib cage, the integument and the respiratory muscles with each breath.

P Shallow respirations are also seen in conditions where lung pathology exists and breathing is painful (e.g. pulmonary embolus, pneumonia, pneumothorax).

A **Hyperpnoea** is a breath that is greater in volume than the resting tidal volume (**Figure 13.11J**). The respiratory rate is normal and the pattern is even in hyperpnoea.

P In the warm-up and cool-down periods of exercise, hyperpnoea is present. The deep breath is drawn to meet the increased metabolic needs of the body.

P Consumers in highly emotional states exhibit hyperpnoea as the body attempts to meet the increased oxygen demand.

P Consumers who are thrust into high-altitude regions will become hyperpnoeic due to the decreased partial pressure of oxygen. Deep breaths and slight tachypnoea represent an attempt to supply the oxygen needs of the body.

A **Air trapping** is an abnormal respiratory pattern with rapid, shallow respirations and forced expirations (**Figure 13.11K**).

P Consumers with COPD have difficulty with exhaling. When these consumers exercise or experience increased heart rate, they have insufficient time to fully exhale. As a result, air is trapped in the lungs and, over time, the chest overexpands. Likewise, an asthmatic consumer experiencing an acute attack has difficulty exhaling due to increased mucus and bronchial constriction. Air trapping ensues.

A **Kussmaul respirations** are characterised by extreme increased depth and rate of respirations (**Figure 13.11L**). These respirations are regular and the inspiratory and expiratory processes are both active.

P Diabetic ketoacidosis and metabolic acidosis may result in Kussmaul respirations. The body is lowering its $PaCO_2$ level, thereby raising the pH and attempting to correct the acidosis.

A **Sighing** is characterised by normal respirations interrupted by a deep inspiration and followed by a deep expiration (**Figure 13.11M**). It may be accompanied by an audible sigh. Sighing is pathological if it occurs frequently.

P Excessive sighing can occur in central nervous system lesions.

Symmetry

E
1. Stand in front of the consumer.
2. Observe the symmetry with which the chest rises and falls during the respiratory cycle.

N The healthy adult's thorax rises and falls in unison with the respiratory cycle. There is no paradoxical movement.

A Unilateral expansion of either side of the thorax is abnormal.

E Examination **N** Normal findings **A** Abnormal findings **P** Pathophysiology

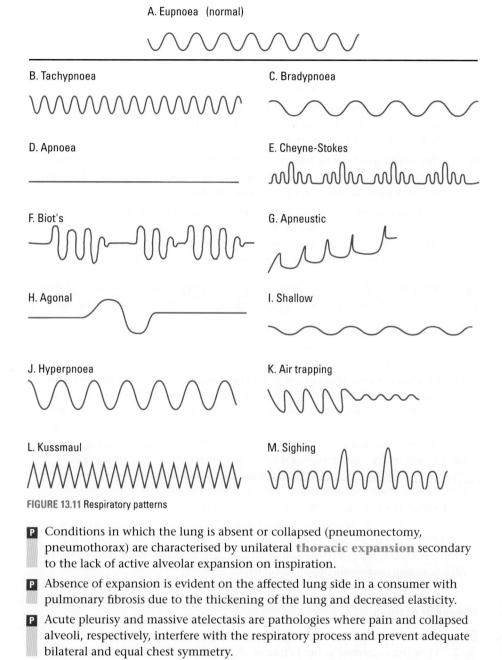

FIGURE 13.11 Respiratory patterns

P Conditions in which the lung is absent or collapsed (pneumonectomy, pneumothorax) are characterised by unilateral **thoracic expansion** secondary to the lack of active alveolar expansion on inspiration.

P Absence of expansion is evident on the affected lung side in a consumer with pulmonary fibrosis due to the thickening of the lung and decreased elasticity.

P Acute pleurisy and massive atelectasis are pathologies where pain and collapsed alveoli, respectively, interfere with the respiratory process and prevent adequate bilateral and equal chest symmetry.

A Paradoxical, or seemingly contradictory, chest wall movement is always abnormal. In paradoxical chest wall movement, the unaffected part of the thorax will rise during inspiration while the affected area will fall. Conversely, during expiration the unaffected part of the thorax will fall while the affected area will rise.

P Broken ribs from trauma to the chest wall or flail chest interferes with the normal rib cage dynamics during the respiratory process and may lead to paradoxical chest wall movement.

A Hoover's sign is the paradoxical inwards movement of the lower ICS during inspiration. This occurs when the diaphragm is flat instead of its normal dome shape. Muscle fibres are horizontal, and diaphragmatic contraction pulls the rib cage inwards rather than down.

P Broken ribs from trauma to the chest wall or flail chest interferes with the normal rib cage dynamics during the respiratory process and may lead to the presence of Hoover's sign.

E Examination   **N** Normal findings   **A** Abnormal findings   **P** Pathophysiology

UNIT 2

Audibility

E 1. Stand in front of the consumer.
   2. Listen for the audibility of the respirations.

N A consumer's respirations are normally heard by the unaided ear a few centimetres from the consumer's nose or mouth.

A It is abnormal to hear audible breathing when standing 1 metre from the consumer. Upper airway sounds may also be heard. These should not be confused with pulmonary sounds.

P Any condition in which air hunger exists has the potential to create audible and noisy breathing. The body is attempting to meet its oxygen demands. Examples of these states are exercise, COPD, pneumonia and pneumothorax.

P Loud and persistent coughing can indicate asthma, COPD and many other pulmonary conditions. Be alert to a 'whooping' sound because of the increasing incidence of pertussis. One can hear an example of an adult who has a 'whooping cough' at https://www.youtube.com/watch?v=31tnXPlhA7w.

HEALTH EDUCATION

Pertussis (whooping cough) resurgence

Whooping cough is a serious respiratory infection caused by the bacteria *Bordetella pertussis*. Whooping cough is highly contagious, spread through airborne droplets from person to person and can affect people of all ages. Symptoms commence about 7–10 days after acquiring pertussis, and include a cold, blocked or runny nose, mild fever and cough. The cough becomes worse and can be quite violent. Not everyone develops a cough with a distinctive 'whooping' sound. Current immunisation coverage does not confer long-term immunity. As a nurse you should be aware that those immunised against whooping cough can still contract the disease, especially if they have not sought out a booster dose in the previous 10 years. As some individuals may have the disease and not be aware, they may spread this to others. Susceptible groups include babies less than six months, those living in the same home as someone who is diagnosed with whooping cough, and individuals who have not had a booster for whooping cough in the previous 10 years. A pertussis booster was added in December 2017 to the Australian NIP for 18-month-old children (Australian Technical Advisory Group on Immunisation (ATAGI), 2022; Ministry of Health/Manatū Hauora, 2021; Australian Government Department of Health, 2017).

Consumer position

E 1. Ask the consumer to sit upright for the respiratory assessment.
   2. View the consumer either before or after the assessment and note the assumed position for breathing. Ask if the assumed position is required for respiratory comfort.
   3. Note if the consumer can breathe normally when in a supine position.
   4. Note if pillows are used to prop the consumer upright to facilitate breathing.

N The healthy adult breathes comfortably in a supine, prone or upright position.

A **Orthopnoea** is difficulty breathing in positions other than upright.

P COPD, heart failure and pulmonary oedema exemplify conditions where orthopnoea may be present. The upright position maximises the use of the respiratory muscles in consumers who might otherwise be unable to breathe in a supine position, secondary to fluid in the lungs. Consumers with COPD may assume the tripod position to breathe easier and make breathing look natural (**Figure 13.12**). The tripod position allows for easier use of accessory muscles.

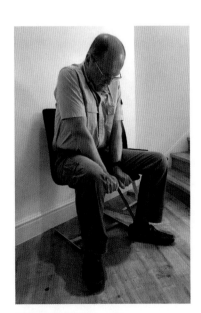

FIGURE 13.12 Tripod position

MEDICAL IMAGES/MEDICUS

Mode of breathing

E 1. Stand in front of the consumer.
   2. Note whether the consumer is using the nose, the mouth, or both, to breathe.
   3. Note for which part of the respiratory cycle each is used.

N Normal findings vary among individuals but, generally, most consumers inhale and exhale through the nose.

A Continuous mouth breathing is usually abnormal.

P Any type of nasal or sinus blockage obstructs the normal breathing passageway and leads to mouth breathing.

A Pursed-lip breathing is performed by consumers who need to prolong the expiration phase of the respiratory cycle. It appears that the consumer is trying to blow out a candle or is preparing for a kiss.

P Pursed-lip breathing is performed by consumers with COPD. It is the consumer's innate mechanism to apply positive-pressure breathing to prevent total alveolar collapse with every breath. Less energy is expended with each breath because the alveoli do not completely collapse after expiration.

A Consumers may breathe through a stoma or tracheostomy (**Figure 13.13**).

P Consumers with laryngeal cancer who have had a surgical removal of the larynx breathe initially through a tracheostomy and then through a stoma. This is their normal mode of breathing.

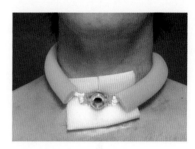

FIGURE 13.13 Tracheostomy
ALAMY STOCK PHOTO/MEDISCAN

Sputum

To ease **sputum** collection, it is best to increase the consumer's fluid intake and humidify the environment. For consumers with copious secretion, such as in cystic fibrosis, it may be helpful to first use postural drainage and chest physiotherapy. Postoperative consumers and those who have pain may benefit from splinting the painful area with a pillow during the expectoration.

E 1. Ask the consumer to expectorate a sputum sample.
   2. If the consumer is unable to expectorate, ask the consumer for a recent sputum sample from a handkerchief or tissue.
   3. Note the colour, odour, amount and consistency of the sputum.

N A small amount of sputum is normal in every individual. The colour is light yellow or clear. Normal sputum is odourless. Depending on the hydration status of the consumer, the sputum can be thick or thin.

A Abnormal colours of sputum are mucoid, yellow or green, rust or blood-tinged, black, and pink (and frothy).

P **Table 13.1** lists the pathologies that are associated with different colours of sputum.

A Foul-smelling sputum is always abnormal.

P Anaerobic infections produce foul-smelling sputum.

A A large amount of sputum can be pathological.

P Chronic bronchitis produces a large amount of sputum as a result of the irritation to the respiratory tract.

P Consumers with pneumonia expectorate large quantities of sputum. The sputum is produced in reaction to the infectious process.

E Examination **N** Normal findings **A** Abnormal findings **P** Pathophysiology

TABLE 13.1 Pathologies associated with different colours of sputum

SPUTUM COLOUR	PATHOLOGY
Mucoid	Tracheobronchitis, asthma, coryza
Yellow or green	Bacterial infection
Rust or blood-tinged	Pneumococcal pneumonia, pulmonary infarction, tuberculosis, lung cancer
Black	Black lung disease
Pink	Pulmonary oedema

P An excessive amount of sputum is found in pulmonary oedema as a result of fluid that has leaked from pulmonary capillary membranes into large airways.

A Very thick sputum can be abnormal.

P Water is a normal component of the sputum. Therefore, when a consumer is dehydrated, the sputum will be thicker because the mucus, blood, purulent material and cellular debris form the bulk of the sputum.

A Sputum that has a thin consistency can be abnormal.

P In overhydration, the extra fluid tends to dilute the remaining components of the sputum. In pulmonary oedema, the sputum is thin, pink and frothy.

Palpation
General palpation
General palpation assesses the thorax for pulsations, masses, thoracic tenderness and crepitus.

To perform anterior palpation:

E 1. Stand in front of the consumer.
2. Place the finger pads of the dominant hand on the apex of the right lung (above the clavicle).
3. Using light palpation, assess the integument of the thorax in that area.
4. Move the finger pads down to the clavicle and palpate.
5. Proceed with the palpation, moving down to each rib and ICS of the right anterior thorax. Palpate any area(s) of tenderness last.
6. Repeat the procedure on the left anterior thorax.

To perform posterior palpation:

E 1. Stand behind the consumer.
2. Place the finger pads of the dominant hand on the apex of the right lung (approximately at the level of T1).
3. Using light palpation, assess the integument of the thorax in that area.
4. Move the finger pads down to the first thoracic vertebra and palpate.
5. Proceed with the palpation, moving down to each thoracic vertebra and ICS of the right posterior thorax.
6. Repeat the procedure on the left posterior thorax.

To perform lateral palpation:

E 1. Stand to the consumer's right side.
2. Have the consumer lift the arms overhead.
3. Place the finger pads of the dominant hand beneath the right auxiliary fold.
4. Using light palpation, assess the integument of the thorax in that area.
5. Move the finger pads down to the first rib beneath the auxiliary fold.
6. Proceed with the palpation, moving down to each rib and ICS of the right lateral thorax.
7. Move to the consumer's left side.
8. Repeat steps 2–6 for the left lateral thorax.

E Examination   **N** Normal findings   **A** Abnormal findings   **P** Pathophysiology

Pulsations

N No pulsations should be present.

A The presence of pulsations on the thorax is abnormal.

P A thoracic aortic aneurysm that is large may be seen pulsating on the anterior chest wall.

Masses

N No masses should be present.

A The presence of a thoracic mass is abnormal.

P The presence of a thoracic tumour or cyst should be closely evaluated and malignancy ruled out.

Thoracic tenderness

N No thoracic tenderness should be present.

A Fractured ribs may cause thoracic tenderness.

P Blunt chest trauma can affect any component of the respiratory tract, as well as the heart and great vessels. The region involved, the type of injury and the impact of the injury dictate the amount of internal damage.

Locating the site of a fractured rib

To locate the site of a fractured rib:

E 1. Tell the consumer what you are going to do and that some pain may be involved.
2. Place the consumer in a supine or upright position. In the latter position, support the consumer's back with one hand.
3. Place your hand over the middle of the sternum and depress lightly.
4. Quickly remove your hand from the sternum.
5. Outcome: The consumer will complain of pain at the fracture site. Have the consumer point to the site of pain. This technique is not effective for the 11th and 12th pairs of ribs because of their anatomic nature and location.

Crepitus

N Crepitus should be absent.

A The presence of **crepitus**, also referred to as subcutaneous emphysema, is always an abnormal finding. Fine beads of air escape the lung and are trapped in the subcutaneous tissue. As this area is palpated, a crackling sound may be heard. This air is slowly absorbed by the body. Crepitus is usually felt earliest in the clavicular region, but it can easily be found in the neck, face and torso. It can also be described as feeling similar to bubble packing material that can be palpated and popped.

P Any condition that interrupts the integrity of the pleura and the lungs has the potential to lead to crepitus. Pathologies in which crepitus is frequently found are pneumothorax, chest trauma, thoracic surgery, mediastinal emphysema, alveolar rupture and tearing of pleural adhesions.

Thoracic expansion

Thoracic expansion assesses the extent of chest expansion and the symmetry of chest wall expansion. Anterior and posterior thoracic expansions can be assessed (**Figure 13.14**).

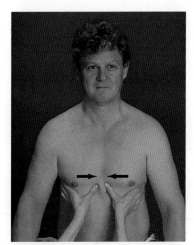

A. Anterior

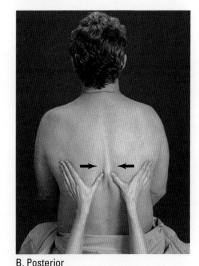

B. Posterior

FIGURE 13.14 Thoracic expansion

E Examination N Normal findings A Abnormal findings P Pathophysiology ▨ Advanced Assessment

To perform anterior thoracic expansion:

E 1. Stand directly in front of the consumer. Place the thumbs of both hands on the costal margins and pointing towards the xiphoid process. Gather a small fold of skin between the thumbs to assist with the visualisation of the results of this technique.
   2. Lay your outstretched palms on the anterolateral thorax.
   3. Instruct the consumer to take a deep breath.
   4. Observe the movement of the thumbs, both in direction and in distance.
   5. Ask the consumer to exhale.
   6. Observe the movement of the thumbs as they return to the midline.

To perform posterior thoracic expansion:

E 1. Stand directly behind the consumer. Place the thumbs of both hands at the level of the 10th spinal vertebra, equidistant from the spinal column and approximately 2.5 to 7.5 cm apart. Gather a small amount of skin between the thumbs as directed for anterior expansion.
   2. Place your outstretched palms on the posterolateral thorax.
   3. Instruct the consumer to take a deep breath.
   4. Observe the movement of the thumbs, both in direction and in distance.
   5. Ask the consumer to exhale.
   6. Observe the movement of the thumbs as they return to the midline.

N The thumbs separate an equal amount from the spinal column or xiphoid process (distance) and remain in the same plane of the 10th spinous vertebra or costal margin (direction). The normal distance for the thumbs to separate during thoracic expansion is 3 to 5 cm.

A Unilateral decreased thoracic expansion is abnormal.

P Unilateral decreased thoracic expansion on the affected or pathological side occurs in pneumothorax, pneumonia, atelectasis, lower lobe lobectomy, pleural effusion and bronchiectasis. In these conditions, the alveoli are either not present or not fully expanding on the affected side due to pathology inside or external to the lung.

A Bilateral decreased thoracic expansion is an abnormal finding.

P Bilateral disease external or internal to the lungs must be present in order for bilateral decreased thoracic expansion to be present. Hypoventilation, emphysema, pulmonary fibrosis and pleurisy exemplify diseases where the alveoli do not fully expand.

P Displacement of thumbs from the 10th spinal vertebra region (thumbs will not meet in the midline when the consumer exhales) is abnormal.

P In scoliosis, the spine is laterally deviated to a particular side. Thus, when the consumer takes a deep breath, there can be a slight or marked expansion of the lungs in an unequal fashion due to the compression of the lungs by the spine.

Tactile fremitus

Tactile or **vocal fremitus** is the palpable vibration of the chest wall that is produced by the spoken word. This technique is useful in assessing the underlying lung tissue and pleura. The anterior, posterior and lateral chest walls are assessed. Three different aspects of the hand can be used to perform this skill: the palmar bases of the fingers, the ulnar aspect of the hand, and the ulnar aspect of a closed fist (Figure 13.15). You might like to experiment with each technique and decide which is the most comfortable. It is recommended that the ulnar aspect of the hand be used initially because this exposes the least amount of surface area, and, therefore, more discrete areas can be assessed.

E Examination **N** Normal findings **A** Abnormal findings **P** Pathophysiology   Advanced Assessment

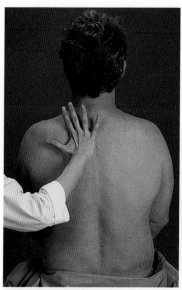

A. Using palmar base of fingers

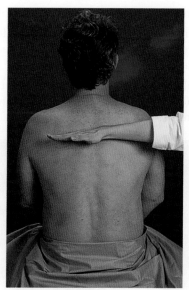

B. Using ulnar aspect of hand

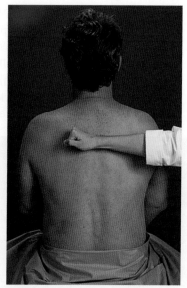

C. Using ulnar aspect of closed fist

FIGURE 13.15 Tactile fremitus

To perform tactile fremitus:

E
1. Firmly place the ulnar aspect of an open hand (or palmar base of the fingers or ulnar aspect of a closed fist) on the consumer's right anterior apex (above the clavicle).
2. Instruct the consumer to say the words '99' or '1, 2, 3' with the same intensity every time you place your hand on the thorax.
3. Feel any vibration on the ulnar aspect of the hand as the consumer phonates. If no fremitus is palpated, you may need to have the consumer speak more loudly.
4. Move your hand to the same location on the left anterior thorax.
5. Repeat steps 2 and 3.
6. Compare the vibrations palpated on the right and left apices.
7. Move the hand down 5 to 7.5 cm and repeat the process on the right and then on the left. Ensure that your hand is in the ICS in order to avoid the bony structures. Minimal or no fremitus will be felt over the ribs because they lie on top of the lungs.
8. Continue this process down the anterior thorax to the base of the lungs.
9. Repeat this procedure for the lateral chest wall and compare symmetry. Either do the entire right then the entire left thorax, or alternate right and left at each ICS.
10. Repeat this procedure for the posterior chest wall. **Figure 13.16** illustrates the progression of the assessment.

N Normal fremitus is felt as a buzzing on the ulnar aspect of the hand. The fremitus will be more pronounced near the major bronchi (second ICS anteriorly, and T1 and T2 posteriorly) and the trachea, and will be less palpable in the periphery of the lung. The diaphragm is approximately at the level of T10–T12 posteriorly and it is slightly higher on the right because of the presence of the liver.

A Increased tactile fremitus is abnormal.

P Diseases that involve consolidation, such as pneumonia, atelectasis and bronchitis, also involve increased tactile fremitus in the affected area. A compressed lung will also exhibit increased tactile fremitus because solids conduct sound better than air does.

E Examination   **N** Normal findings   **A** Abnormal findings   **P** Pathophysiology   Advanced Assessment

A Decreased or absent tactile fremitus is a pathological finding.

P Because porous materials conduct vibrations less effectively than do fluids and solids, decreased tactile fremitus will be present in pneumothorax, emphysema and asthma.

P In a pleural effusion, the exudate is external to the alveoli and therefore acts as a blockade to the transmission of sound waves. This results in decreased tactile fremitus.

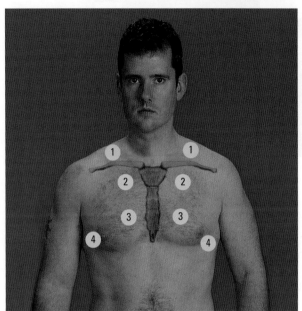

A. Anterior thorax

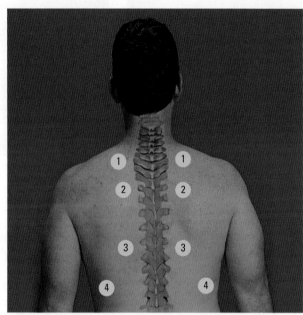

B. Posterior thorax

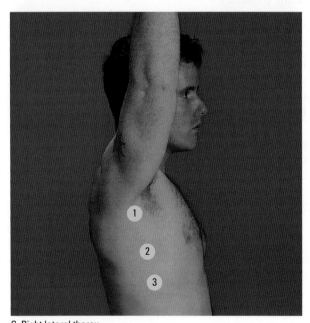

C. Right lateral thorax

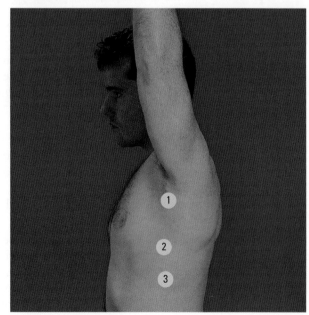

D. Left lateral thorax

FIGURE 13.16 Pattern for tactile fremitus

P A consumer with a large chest wall and an obese consumer will have decreased tactile fremitus because the sound waves are dampened as they pass through a greater distance.

A A high diaphragm level is abnormal.

P The diaphragm level is abnormally high in a consumer with a lower lobe lobectomy. Tactile fremitus will be present above the surgical site.

A There are three additional findings that can be revealed during tactile fremitus: pleural friction fremitus, tussive fremitus and rhonchal fremitus.

P **Pleural friction fremitus** is a palpable grating sensation that feels more pronounced on inspiration when there is an inflammatory process between the visceral and the parietal pleuras.

P **Tussive fremitus** is the palpable vibration produced by coughing.

P **Rhonchal fremitus** is the coarse palpable vibration produced by the passage of air through thick exudate in large bronchi or the trachea. This can clear with coughing.

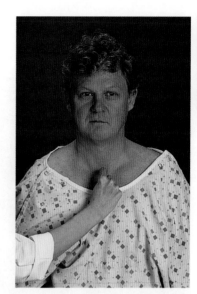

FIGURE 13.17 Assessing tracheal position

Tracheal position

To assess the position of the trachea:

E 1. Place the finger pad of the index finger on the consumer's trachea in the **suprasternal notch** (Figure 13.17).
2. Move the finger pad laterally to the right and gently move the trachea in the space created by the border of the inner aspect of the sternocleidomastoid muscle and the clavicle.
3. Move the finger pad laterally to the left and repeat the procedure.

Another method by which the trachea can be palpated is:

E 1. Gently place the finger pad of the index finger in the midline of the suprasternal notch.
2. Palpate for the position of the trachea.

N The trachea is midline in the suprasternal notch.

A Tracheal deviation to the affected side is abnormal.

P The normal midline position of the trachea is maintained by the counterbalancing forces of the air in the alveoli in the right and left lungs. In atelectasis and pneumonia, alveoli are closed to some degree or filled with exudate. Fewer aerating alveoli are present and therefore the trachea is slightly pushed by the healthy lung to the affected side, which contains less air.

P The mechanical pulling force of ventilator tubing that is attached to an endotracheal tube or tracheostomy for a prolonged period can cause tracheal deviation toward the side of the pulling.

A Tracheal deviation to the unaffected side is abnormal.

P A tension pneumothorax, pleural effusion and a tumour may each generate sufficient pressure to force the trachea towards the unaffected side.

P An enlarged thyroid may deviate the trachea via its space-occupying capacity.

Percussion

Indirect or mediate percussion is used to further assess the underlying structures of the thorax. Remember that percussion reverberates a sound that is generated from structures approximately 5 cm below the chest wall. Deep pathological conditions will not be revealed during the percussion process.

There is no harm in repeating the percussion strike in a given area if you are uncertain about the sound that was produced or if you would like to compare it to the sound from another area. Remember always to visualise the underlying structures that are being assessed.

E Examination **N** Normal findings **A** Abnormal findings **P** Pathophysiology   Advanced Assessment

General percussion

Figure 13.18 demonstrates the percussion pattern for the anterior, posterior, right lateral and left lateral thoraxes.

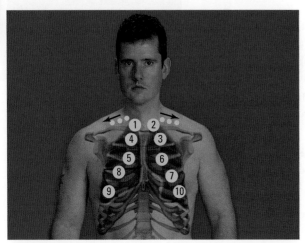

A. Anterior thorax

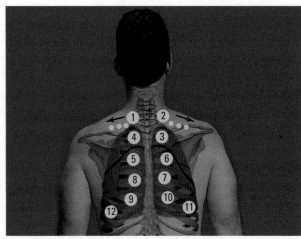

B. Posterior thorax

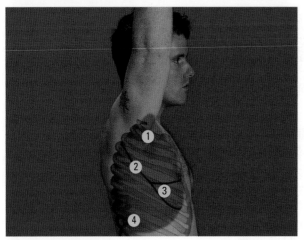

C. Right lateral thorax

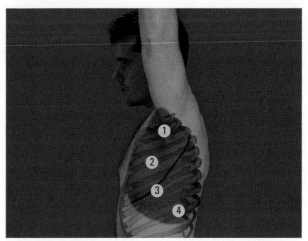

D. Left lateral thorax

FIGURE 13.18 Percussion patterns

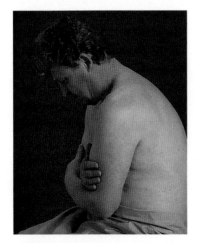

FIGURE 13.19 Consumer position for posterior percussion

To perform anterior thoracic percussion:

E
1. Place the consumer in an upright sitting position with the shoulders back.
2. Percuss two or three strikes along the right lung apex.
3. Repeat this process at the left lung apex.
4. Note the sound produced from each percussion strike and compare the sounds. If different sounds are produced or if the sound is not resonant, then pathology is suggested.
5. Move down approximately 5 cm, or every second ICS, and percuss in that area.
6. Percuss in the same position on the other side.
7. Continue to move down until the entire lung has been percussed.

To perform posterior thoracic percussion:

E
1. Place the consumer in an upright sitting position with a slight forwards tilt. Have the consumer bend the head down and fold the arms in front at the waist. These actions move the scapula laterally and maximise the lung area that can be percussed (**Figure 13.19**).
2. Percuss the right lung apex located along the top of the shoulder. Approximately three percussion strikes should be struck along this area.
3. Repeat the process on the left lung apex.

E Examination   **N** Normal findings   **A** Abnormal findings   **P** Pathophysiology

E 4. Note the sound produced from each percussion strike and compare the sounds. If different sounds are produced or if the sound is not resonant, then pathology is suggested.

5. Move down approximately 5 cm, or every second ICS, and percuss in that area.

6. Percuss in the same position on the contralateral side.

7. Continue to move down the thorax until the entire posterior lung field has been percussed.

To perform lateral thoracic percussion:

E 1. Place the consumer in an upright sitting position, with hands and arms raised directly overhead. This position allows for the greatest exposure of the thorax.

2. Either percuss the entire right lateral thorax and then the entire left lateral thorax, or alternate right and left sides. Start to percuss in the ICS directly below the axilla.

3. Note the sound produced from that strike.

4. Percuss approximately 5 cm below the original location, or about every other ICS.

5. Percuss down to the base of the lung.

N Normal lung tissue produces a resonant sound. The diaphragm and the cardiac silhouette emit dull sounds. Rib sounds are flat. Hyperresonance is normal in thin adults and in consumers with decreased musculature.

A The presence of hyperresonance in the majority of adults is abnormal.

P Hyperresonance is percussed in air-filled spaces. It can be elicited in pneumothorax, emphysema, asthma and an emphysematous bulla.

A The healthy human lung never produces a dull sound.

P Dullness is found in solid or fluid-filled structures. Pneumonia, atelectasis, pulmonary oedema, pleural effusion, pulmonary fibrosis, haemothorax, empyema and tumours are dull to percussion.

Diaphragmatic excursion

Diaphragmatic excursion provides information on the consumer's depth of ventilation. This is accomplished by measuring the distance the diaphragm moves during inspiration and expiration.

To perform diaphragmatic excursion:

E 1. Position the consumer for posterior thoracic percussion.

2. With the consumer breathing normally, percuss the right lung from the apex (resonance in healthy adults) to below the diaphragm (dull). Note the level at which the percussion note changes quality to orient your assessment to the consumer's percussion sounds. If full posterior thoracic percussion has already been performed, then this step can be eliminated.

3. Instruct the consumer to inhale as deeply as possible and hold that breath.

4. With the consumer holding their breath, percuss the right lung in the scapular line from below the scapula to the location where resonance changes to dullness.

5. Mark this location and tell the consumer to exhale and breathe normally.

6. When the consumer has recovered, instruct the consumer to inhale as deeply as possible, exhale fully, and hold this exhaled breath.

7. Repercuss the right lung below the scapula in the scapular line in a caudal direction. Mark the spot where resonance changes to dullness.

8. Measure the distance between the two marks.

9. Repeat steps 1–8 for the left posterior thorax. **Figure 13.20** illustrates diaphragmatic excursion.

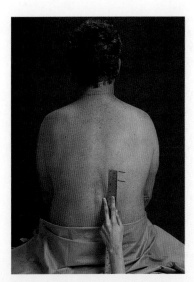

FIGURE 13.20 Diaphragmatic excursion

E Examination **N** Normal findings **A** Abnormal findings **P** Pathophysiology ▨ Advanced Assessment

N The measured distance for diaphragmatic excursion is normally 3 to 5 cm. The level of the diaphragm on inspiration is T12, and T10 on expiration. The right side of the diaphragm is usually slightly higher than the left.

A A diaphragmatic excursion that is less than 3 cm is abnormal.

P Conditions involving hypoventilation, in which the consumer is unable to inhale deeply or hold that breath, can lead to a reduction in the diaphragmatic excursion. Pain, obesity, lung congestion, emphysema, asthma and pleurisy are examples.

A A high diaphragm level suggests lung pathology.

P Surgical intervention can elevate the diaphragm. If a lower lobe lobectomy is performed, the diaphragm will move upwards to partially fill the empty space. Likewise, after a pneumonectomy the paralysed diaphragm will move upwards, leading to a high diaphragm level.

P Space-occupying states such as **ascites** and pregnancy will lead to an elevated diaphragm due to the upwards displacement of the lungs and diaphragm.

P If atelectasis or a pleural effusion is present in a lower lobe, then the diaphragm will seem abnormally high, because these conditions are dull to percussion, as is the diaphragm. The border between the diaphragm and the dull lung will thus be indistinguishable.

REFLECTION IN PRACTICE

Diaphragmatic excursion technique

You are performing diaphragmatic excursion on a consumer. Midway through performing this assessment, the consumer states, 'Are you sure you know what you are doing? You keep tapping me and I keep breathing over and over.'

> How would you respond to the consumer?
> Would you alter your assessment in any way after this comment?
> Why would you do so?

Auscultation

The aim of respiratory auscultation is to identify the presence of normal breath sounds, abnormal lung sounds, adventitious (or added) lung sounds, and adventitious pleural sounds. The anterior, posterior and lateral aspects of the chest are auscultated. A stethoscope is required for this assessment. If an acoustic stethoscope is used, the diaphragm, which transmits high-pitched sounds, is the headpiece of choice. Technological developments accelerated because of the COVID-19 pandemic, meaning that wireless stethoscopes (Zhang et al., 2021), artificial intelligence (Glangetas et al., 2021), and smartphone applications (Alkhodari & Khandoker, 2022) are being used as safe and effective tools to support respiratory diagnoses.

CLINICAL REASONING

Practice tip: Factors affecting auscultation

When auscultating you need to consider factors that may impact on the quality of your assessment. The following factors may impact on auscultation.

> Chest hair: Coarse or dense chest hair can be dampened to prevent the distortion of auscultatory findings (can sound like crackling).
> Rustling of paper gowns or drapes: Instruct the consumer to remain still while you are auscultating the lungs.
> Mechanical ventilator tubing: Water accumulation in mechanical ventilator tubing can produce a gurgling sound. Clear all tubing of moisture prior to auscultation.
> Shivering or chattering teeth: Ascertain why the consumer is shivering or chattering the teeth (e.g. hypothermia) and intervene to correct the aetiology.

E Examination **N** Normal findings **A** Abnormal findings **P** Pathophysiology Advanced Assessment

General auscultation

Watch the consumer closely for signs of hyperventilation, such as dizziness. If the consumer complains of dizziness, normal breathing should be resumed. Continue the examination when their dizziness has gone and the consumer's breathing has returned to baseline.

To perform anterior thoracic auscultation:

E 1. Place the consumer in an upright sitting position with the shoulders back.
2. Instruct the consumer to breathe only through the mouth. Mouth breathing, when compared to nasal breathing, decreases air turbulence, which can interfere with the interpretation of breath sounds. Have the consumer inhale and exhale deeply and slowly every time the stethoscope is felt or when instructed to do so.
3. Place the stethoscope on the apex of the right lung and listen for one complete respiratory cycle (one inhalation and one exhalation).
4. Note the sound that is auscultated.
5. Repeat on the left apex.
6. Note the breath sound auscultated in each area and compare one side to the other.
7. Continue to move the stethoscope down approximately 5 cm, or every second ICS, comparing contralateral sides. Remember to visualise the anatomic topography of the chest during auscultation (**Figure 13.18A**).

To perform posterior thoracic auscultation:

E 1. Place the consumer in an upright sitting position with a slight forwards tilt, head bent down, and arms folded in front at the waist, as shown in **Figure 13.19**. These actions move the scapulae laterally and maximise the lung area that can be auscultated.
2. Place the stethoscope firmly on the consumer's right lung apex. Ask the consumer to inhale and exhale deeply and slowly every time the stethoscope is felt on the back.
3. Repeat this process on the left lung apex.
4. Move the stethoscope down approximately 5 cm, or every second ICS, and auscultate in that area.
5. Auscultate in the same position on the contralateral side.
6. Continue to move inferiorly with the auscultation until the entire posterior lung has been assessed. See **Figure 13.18B** from the percussion section for the recommended stethoscope location for each auscultation site.

To perform lateral thoracic auscultation:

E 1. Place the consumer in an upright sitting position with the hands and arms directly overhead.
2. Auscultate the entire right thorax first, then the entire left thorax, or auscultate the right and left lateral thoraxes by comparing side to side. The stethoscope should initially be placed in the ICS directly below the axilla.
3. Instruct the consumer to breathe only through the mouth. Have the consumer inhale and exhale deeply and slowly every time the stethoscope is felt on the lateral thorax.
4. Note the sound that is auscultated and continue to move the stethoscope inferiorly approximately every 5 cm, or every second ICS, until the entire thorax has been auscultated (**Figures 13.18C** and **13.18D**).

Breath sounds

N Air rushing through the respiratory tract during inspiration and expiration generates different breath sounds in the normal consumer. There are three distinct types of normal breath sounds (see **Table 13.2**):

1. **Bronchial (or tubular breath sound)**
2. **Bronchovesicular**
3. **Vesicular**

E Examination   **N** Normal findings   **A** Abnormal findings   **P** Pathophysiology

TABLE 13.2 Characteristics of normal breath sounds

BREATH SOUND	PITCH	INTENSITY	QUALITY	RELATIVE DURATION OF INSPIRATORY (I) AND EXPIRATORY (E) PHASES	LOCATION
Bronchial	High	Loud	Blowing or hollow	I < E	Trachea
Bronchovesicular	Moderate	Moderate	Combination of bronchial and vesicular	I = E	Between scapulae, first and second ICS lateral to the sternum
Vesicular	Low	Soft	Gentle rustling or breezy	I > E	Peripheral lung fields

Each breath sound is unique in its pitch, intensity, quality, relative duration in the inspiratory and expiratory phases of respiration, and location. Table 13.2 depicts this information. It is abnormal to auscultate these breath sounds in locations other than where they are usually found. For example, a consumer with emphysema may have **bronchial breath sounds** in the peripheral lung parenchyma, where vesicular sounds are expected to be found. Also keep in mind that heart sounds may obscure some of the breath sounds during the anterior chest auscultation.

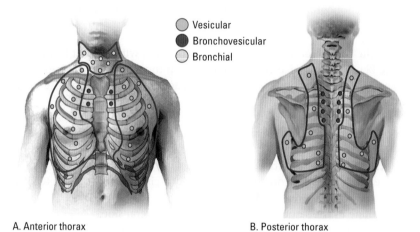

○ Vesicular
● Bronchovesicular
○ Bronchial

A. Anterior thorax

B. Posterior thorax

FIGURE 13.21 Location of breath sounds

Breath sounds that are not normal can be classified as either abnormal or adventitious breath sounds. Abnormal breath sounds are characterised by decreased or absent breath sounds. **Adventitious breath sounds** are superimposed sounds on the normal bronchial, **bronchovesicular** and **vesicular breath sounds**.

There are five adventitious breath sounds:

1. Fine crackle
2. Coarse crackle
3. Wheeze
4. **Pleural friction rub**
5. Stridor

Table 13.3 depicts general characteristics of adventitious breath sounds.

A Decreased breath sounds are abnormal.

P Decreased breath sounds may be noted when auscultating a large chest because of the distance between the lungs, where the sounds are generated, and the chest wall.

TABLE 13.3 Characteristics of adventitious breath sounds

BREATH SOUND	RESPIRATORY PHASE	TIMING	DESCRIPTION	CLEAR WITH COUGH	AETIOLOGY	CONDITIONS
Fine crackle	Predominantly inspiration	Discontinuous	Dry, high-pitched crackling, popping, short duration (roll hair near ears between your fingers to simulate this sound)	No	Air passing through moisture in small airways that suddenly reinflate	COPD, heart failure, pneumonia, pulmonary fibrosis, atelectasis
Coarse crackle	Predominantly inspiration	Discontinuous	Moist, low-pitched crackling, gurgling; long duration	Possibly	Air passing through moisture in large airways that suddenly reinflate	Pneumonia, pulmonary oedema, bronchitis, atelectasis
Wheeze	Predominantly expiration	Continuous	High pitched; musical	Possibly	Narrowing of large airways or obstruction of bronchus	Asthma, chronic bronchitis, emphysema, tumour, foreign body obstruction
Pleural friction rub	Inspiration and expiration	Continuous	Creaking, grating	No	Inflamed parietal and visceral pleura; can occasionally be felt on thoracic wall as two pieces of dry leather rubbing against each other	Pleurisy, tuberculosis, pulmonary infarction, pneumonia, lung abscess
Stridor	Predominantly inspiration	Continuous	Crowing	No	Partial obstruction of the larynx, trachea	Croup, foreign body obstruction, large airway tumour

CLINICAL REASONING

Practice tip: Upper airway sounds

If the consumer has secretions in the oropharynx (upper airway), whether from allergies, infection, coryza or some other cause, their respirations may be loud and gurgling. It may sound as if the consumer is having difficulty breathing. Ask the individual to clear the throat, then reassess the breath sounds.

P An emphysematous consumer may have decreased breath sounds due to the inability to inhale and exhale deeply.

P Conditions such as bronchial obstruction and atelectasis may lead to decreased breath sounds because a foreign object or sputum occludes some portion of the respiratory tract, thus blocking the passage of air.

A Absent breath sounds are always a pathological finding.

P A pleural effusion, tumour, pulmonary fibrosis, emphysema, haemothorax and hydrothorax lead to absent breath sounds. These states occupy or displace normal aerating lung space internally or externally to the lungs.

P A consumer with a large pneumothorax can present with absent breath sounds due to the collapse of the lung.

P Absent breath sounds occur when the lung has been removed (pneumonectomy).

P Blocked passageways in the respiratory tract explain the aetiology for absent breath sounds in pulmonary oedema, massive atelectasis and complete airway obstruction.

E Examination   **N** Normal findings   **A** Abnormal findings   **P** Pathophysiology   Advanced Assessment

---

CLINICAL **REASONING**

Lung auscultation practice
In addition to practising auscultation in the clinical setting, it is possible to refine skills on the internet. Websites such as the R.A.L.E. Repository at http://www.rale.ca and the UCLA Auscultation Assistant at http://www.wilkes.med.ucla.edu/ allow you to hear a variety of normal and pathological breath sounds.

Voice sounds

The assessment of **voice sounds** is an additional assessment not commonly practised by Australian and New Zealand Registered Nurses. Voice sounds assist to confirm or distinguish potential abnormalities. They reveal whether the lungs are filled with air, fluid, or are solid. This auscultation is performed only if an abnormality is detected during the general auscultation, percussion or palpation assessment. There are three techniques by which voice sounds can be assessed:

1. Bronchophony
2. Egophony
3. Whispered pectoriloquy

Only one of these assessments needs to be performed because they all are variations of the same physical principle and assessment technique, and they all provide the same information. The voice sound findings will parallel those obtained during tactile fremitus. Thus, voice sounds will be heard loudest over the trachea and softest in the lung's periphery.

To perform **bronchophony**:

E 1. Position the consumer for posterior, lateral or anterior chest auscultation. The area to be auscultated will be that in which an abnormality was found during percussion or palpation or in which adventitious breath sounds were heard.
2. Place the stethoscope in the appropriate location on the consumer's chest.
3. Instruct the consumer to say the words '99' or '1, 2, 3' every time the stethoscope is placed on the chest or when told to do so.
4. Auscultate the transmission of the consumer's spoken word.

To perform **egophony**:

E 1. Repeat steps 1 and 2 from the bronchophony procedure.
2. Instruct the consumer to say the sound 'ee' every time the stethoscope is placed on the chest or when told to do so.
3. Auscultate the transmission of the consumer's spoken word.

To perform **whispered pectoriloquy**:

E 1. Repeat steps 1 and 2 from the bronchophony procedure.
2. Instruct the consumer to whisper the words '99' or '1, 2, 3' every time the stethoscope is placed on the chest or when told to do so.
3. Auscultate the transmission of the consumer's spoken word.

N The normal finding when performing tests for bronchophony, egophony and whispered pectoriloquy is an unclear transmission or muffled sounds.

A > Positive (or present) voice sounds are:
- Bronchophony: clear transmission of '99' or '1, 2, 3' with increased intensity
- Egophony: transformation of 'ee' to 'ay' with increased intensity; the voice has a nasal or bleating quality
- Whispered pectoriloquy: clear transmission of '99' or '1, 2, 3' with increased intensity.

P Any type of consolidation process, such as pneumonia, will produce positive voice sounds. Remember the principle that sound is transmitted reasonably well by a fluid medium.

E Examination   **N** Normal findings   **A** Abnormal findings   **P** Pathophysiology   ▦ Advanced Assessment

A Voice sounds are absent or even more decreased than in the normal lung in conditions where the lung is more air-filled than usual.

P Air conducts sound poorly. Therefore, air-filled lungs (emphysema, asthma, pneumothorax) will produce absent voice sounds.

Table 13.4 compares physical examination findings for 12 respiratory conditions. Figure 13.22 illustrates each of these 12 respiratory conditions.

TABLE 13.4 Comparison of physical examination findings in selected respiratory conditions

INSPECTION			
CONDITION	SHAPE OF THORAX	SKIN COLOUR: LIPS AND NAILS	CLUBBING, ANGLE OF RIBS
A. Normal lung	1:2 to 5:7	Pink in light-skinned individuals; darker than normal in dark-skinned individuals	No clubbing, rib angle 45°
B. Asthma	If chronic, may have barrel chest	Pale or cyanotic in acute attack	No clubbing, rib angle 45°
C. Atelectasis (patent bronchus)	1:2 to 5:7	Pale or cyanotic	No clubbing, rib angle 45°
D. Atelectasis (obstructed bronchus)	1:2 to 5:7	Pale or cyanotic	No clubbing, rib angle 45°
E. Bronchiectasis	1:1 (barrel chest)	Pale or cyanotic if severe	Clubbing possible, rib angle >45°
F. Bronchitis	1:2 to 5:7	Possibly pale	No clubbing, rib angle 45°
G. Chronic heart failure	1:2 to 5:7	Pale or cyanotic	Clubbing possible, rib angle 45°
H. Emphysema	1:1 (barrel chest)	Pale	Clubbing, rib angle >45°
I. Pleural effusion	1:2 to 5:7	Pale or cyanotic	No clubbing, rib angle 45°
J. Pneumonia with lobar consolidation	1:2 to 5:7	Pale or cyanotic	No clubbing, rib angle 45°
K. Pneumothorax	1:2 to 5:7	Pale or cyanotic	No clubbing, rib angle 45°
L. Pulmonary oedema	1:2 to 5:7	Pale or cyanotic	No clubbing, rib angle 45°

INSPECTION			
CONDITION	CAPILLARY REFILL	RETRACTIONS OR BULGING OF ICS	RESPIRATORY RATE
A. Normal lung	Brisk	Absent	12–20/min eupnoea
B. Asthma	Sluggish in acute attack	Retractions	20/min tachypnoea
C. Atelectasis (patent bronchus)	Sluggish to moderate	Absent	>20/min tachypnoea
D. Atelectasis (obstructed bronchus)	Sluggish	Absent	>20/min tachypnoea
E. Bronchiectasis	Sluggish if severe	Retractions if severe	>20/min tachypnoea
F. Bronchitis	Sluggish to moderate	Absent	>20/min tachypnoea
G. Chronic heart failure	Sluggish	Retractions	>20/min tachypnoea
H. Emphysema	Sluggish	Both present	>20/min tachypnoea
I. Pleural effusion	Sluggish	Bulging	>20/min tachypnoea
J. Pneumonia with lobar consolidation	Sluggish	Absent	>20/min tachypnoea
K. Pneumothorax	Sluggish	Bulging	>20/min tachypnoea
L. Pulmonary oedema	Sluggish	Absent	>20/min tachypnoea

PALPATION			
CONDITION	THORACIC EXPANSION	TACTILE FREMITUS	TRACHEAL POSITION
A. Normal lung	3–5 cm	Moderate (normal)	Midline
B. Asthma	Decreased in attack	Decreased	Midline

>>

E Examination **N** Normal findings **A** Abnormal findings **P** Pathophysiology Advanced Assessment

>> **TABLE 13.4** *continued*

PALPATION			
CONDITION	**THORACIC EXPANSION**	**TACTILE FREMITUS**	**TRACHEAL POSITION**
C. Atelectasis (patent bronchus)	Decreased	Increased	Shifts to affected side
D. Atelectasis (obstructed bronchus)	Decreased	Increased	Shifts to affected side
E. Bronchiectasis	Decreased on affected side	Increased	Midline or deviated toward affected side
F. Bronchitis	Possibly decreased	Moderate or increased	Midline
G. Chronic heart failure	May be decreased	Moderate	Midline
H. Emphysema	Decreased	Decreased	Midline
I. Pleural effusion	Decreased	Decreased	Shifts to unaffected side
J. Pneumonia with lobar consolidation	Decreased	Increased	Shifts to affected side
K. Pneumothorax	Decreased	Absent or decreased	Shifts to unaffected side
L. Pulmonary oedema	Decreased	Increased	Midline

PERCUSSION		
CONDITION	**GENERAL PERCUSSION**	**DIAPHRAGMATIC EXCURSION**
A. Normal lung	Resonant	3–5 cm
B. Asthma	Hyperresonant	Decreased
C. Atelectasis (patent bronchus)	Dull	Decreased
D. Atelectasis (obstructed bronchus)	Dull	Decreased
E. Bronchiectasis	Resonant to dull	Decreased
F. Bronchitis	Resonant	Decreased if severe
G. Chronic heart failure	Resonant	Decreased
H. Emphysema	Hyperresonant	Decreased
I. Pleural effusion	Dull	Decreased
J. Pneumonia with lobar consolidation	Dull	Decreased
K. Pneumothorax	Hyperresonant	Decreased
L. Pulmonary oedema	Dull	Decreased

AUSCULTATION			
CONDITION	**BREATH SOUNDS**	**ADVENTITIOUS SOUNDS**	**VOICE SOUNDS**
A. Normal lung	Vesicular in periphery	Absent	Muffled
B. Asthma	Decreased or absent in severe obstruction	Wheezes	Decreased
C. Atelectasis (patent bronchus)	Bronchial	Crackles or wheezes	Increased or muffled
D. Atelectasis (obstructed bronchus)	Absent or decreased	Absent	Absent or muffled
E. Bronchiectasis	Vesicular or bronchial if severe	Crackles or wheezes	Muffled or decreased
F. Bronchitis	Vesicular or bronchial	Crackles or wheezes	Increased or muffled
G. Chronic heart failure	Vesicular	Crackles	Muffled
H. Emphysema	Bronchial and decreased	Wheezes	Decreased
I. Pleural effusion	Absent or decreased	Possible friction rub	Decreased or absent
J. Pneumonia with lobar consolidation	Bronchial	Crackles or occasional friction rub	Increased
K. Pneumothorax	Absent or decreased	Absent	Decreased or absent
L. Pulmonary oedema	Absent or decreased	Crackles	Increased

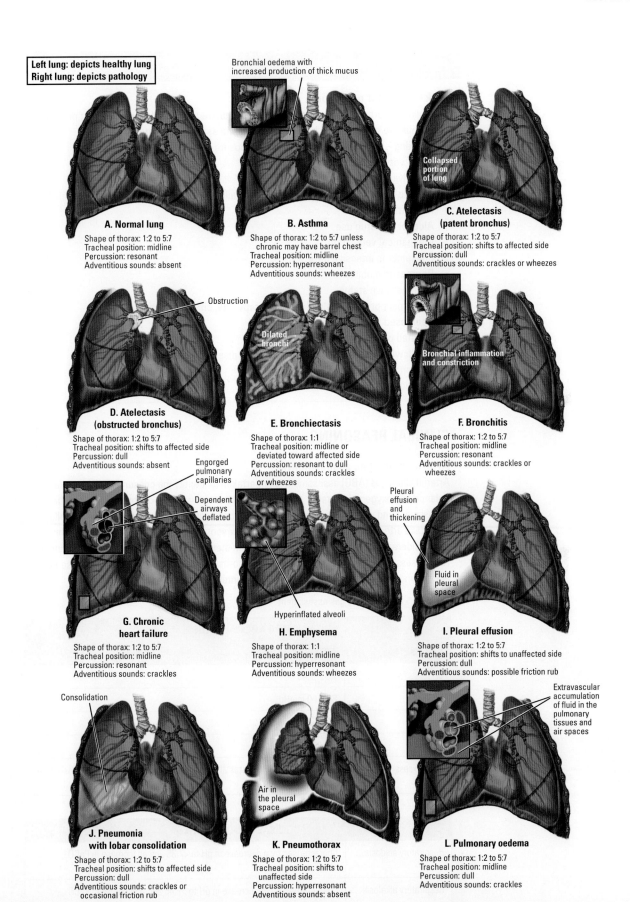

Left lung: depicts healthy lung
Right lung: depicts pathology

Bronchial oedema with
increased production of thick mucus

A. Normal lung

Shape of thorax: 1:2 to 5:7
Tracheal position: midline
Percussion: resonant
Adventitious sounds: absent

B. Asthma

Shape of thorax: 1:2 to 5:7 unless
    chronic may have barrel chest
Tracheal position: midline
Percussion: hyperresonant
Adventitious sounds: wheezes

Collapsed
portion
of lung

**C. Atelectasis
(patent bronchus)**

Shape of thorax: 1:2 to 5:7
Tracheal position: shifts to affected side
Percussion: dull
Adventitious sounds: crackles or wheezes

Obstruction

**D. Atelectasis
(obstructed bronchus)**

Shape of thorax: 1:2 to 5:7
Tracheal position: shifts to affected side
Percussion: dull
Adventitious sounds: absent

Dilated
bronchi

E. Bronchiectasis

Shape of thorax: 1:1
Tracheal position: midline or
    deviated toward affected side
Percussion: resonant to dull
Adventitious sounds: crackles
    or wheezes

Bronchial inflammation
and constriction

F. Bronchitis

Shape of thorax: 1:2 to 5:7
Tracheal position: midline
Percussion: resonant
Adventitious sounds: crackles or
    wheezes

Engorged
pulmonary
capillaries

Dependent
airways
deflated

**G. Chronic
heart failure**

Shape of thorax: 1:2 to 5:7
Tracheal position: midline
Percussion: resonant
Adventitious sounds: crackles

Hyperinflated alveoli

H. Emphysema

Shape of thorax: 1:1
Tracheal position: midline
Percussion: hyperresonant
Adventitious sounds: wheezes

Pleural
effusion
and
thickening

Fluid in
pleural
space

I. Pleural effusion

Shape of thorax: 1:2 to 5:7
Tracheal position: shifts to unaffected side
Percussion: dull
Adventitious sounds: possible friction rub

Consolidation

**J. Pneumonia
with lobar consolidation**

Shape of thorax: 1:2 to 5:7
Tracheal position: shifts to affected side
Percussion: dull
Adventitious sounds: crackles or
    occasional friction rub

Air in
the pleural
space

K. Pneumothorax

Shape of thorax: 1:2 to 5:7
Tracheal position: shifts to
    unaffected side
Percussion: hyperresonant
Adventitious sounds: absent

Extravascular
accumulation
of fluid in the
pulmonary
tissues and
air spaces

L. Pulmonary oedema

Shape of thorax: 1:2 to 5:7
Tracheal position: midline
Percussion: dull
Adventitious sounds: crackles

FIGURE 13.22 Comparison of selected respiratory conditions

HEALTH EDUCATION

Risk factors for pneumonia

The following are risk factors for consumers who are susceptible to developing pneumonia and should be considered when gathering health assessment data:

> Smoking – including passive smoking exposure
> Age – very young and very old
> Underlying lung disease
> Chronic diseases (e.g. renal failure, heart failure)
> Malnutrition
> Alcohol and drug use
> Mechanical ventilation
> Consumer in intensive care
> Decreased mobility
> Postoperative status
> Immunosuppressed status (chemotherapy, HIV, chronic diseases)
> Decreased cough reflex
> Sedated or decreased consciousness
> Swallowing disorders (stroke, Parkinson's disease, traumatic brain injury)
> Oxygen therapy
> Infectious diseases that cause SARS.

CLINICAL REASONING

Arterial blood gas assessment

Arterial blood gas (ABG) assessment is undertaken to identify the consumer's acid–base balance and oxygenation status. Often results of this test will be a definitive aspect of the assessment and will direct interventions for the consumer's respiratory support. The ability to undertake arterial ABG will be influenced by your scope of practice. For some people this will be considered advanced practice. It is important that you have some basic understanding about ABG assessment. You should be aware of the normal range of values in your clinical setting and understand common abnormalities and how to interpret and action these (Table 13.5).

TABLE 13.5 Arterial blood gas assessment

ABG NORMAL VALUES	
PARAMETER	**ARTERIAL VALUE**
pH	7.35–7.45
PaO_2	80–100 mmHg
$PaCO_2$	35–45 mmHg
HCO_3^-	22–26 (28) mmol/L
Base excess	±2 (normal is 0, + indicates alkalosis/base excess, – indicates acidosis/base deficit)
SaO_2	>95%
CLINICAL ABNORMALITIES	
Respiratory acidosis	Characterised by a decrease in pH to <7.35 and an increase in $PaCO_2$ of >45 mmHg
Respiratory alkalosis	Characterised by an increase in pH to >7.45 and a decrease in $PaCO_2$ of <35 mmHg

>>

>>

>>

>> TABLE 13.5 *continued*

CLINICAL ABNORMALITIES	
Metabolic acidosis	Characterised by a decrease in pH to <7.35 and a decrease in HCO_3^- of <22 mmol/L
Metabolic alkalosis	Characterised by an increase in pH to >7.45 and an increase in HCO_3^- of >26 mmol/L

Steps for ABG assessment
1. Check the value of each number (i.e. pH, $PaCO_2$ and HCO_3^-).
   - Does it represent acidity or alkalinity?
2. Check the pH:
   - **If >7.45 – alkalaemia.**
   - **If <7.35 – acidaemia.**
   - **If 7.40 – normal.**
3. Find the value that matches the acid–base status of the pH:
   - If $PaCO_2$ matches, the problem is respiratory.
   - If HCO_3^- matches, the problem is metabolic.
4. Determine the extent of compensation:
   - Absent – The value that doesn't match the acid–base status of the pH is normal.
   - Partial – Both the value that doesn't match the acid–base status of the pH and the pH itself are above or below normal.
   - Complete – The value that doesn't match the acid–base status of the pH is above or below normal but the pH is normal.

(Berman et al., 2018; Wotton, 2017)

Assessing consumers with respiratory supportive equipment

Supportive equipment may be necessary to support respiratory structure and function. The need for such devices automatically indicates an underlying respiratory disorder. For each type of supportive equipment, determine the reason for its use.

Oxygen
> Mode of delivery (e.g. nasal cannula/prongs [HFNO – high-flow nasal oxygen], face mask [non-rebreather mask; NIV – non-invasive ventilation])
> Non-invasive ventilation (continuous positive airway pressure [CPAP]; bilevel positive pressure support [BiPAP])
> Percentage of oxygen that is being delivered (e.g. 25%, 40%)
> Flow rate of the oxygen (e.g. 2 L/min, 4 L/min)
> Humidification provided and oxygen warmed

Pulse oximeter (Figure 13.23A)
> Determine the monitor's settings.
> The monitor's alarms are on. The appropriate limits are set.
> If using the probe on a nail, the consumer's nail polish has been removed.
> If using the probe on the ear, the skin is intact and earrings are not interfering.

Incentive spirometer
> Frequency of use
> Volume achieved (e.g. 1000 mL, 1500 mL)
> Number of times consumer reaches goal with each use

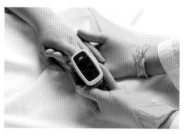

A. Pulse oximeter

SHUTTERSTOCK.COM/NEW AFRICA

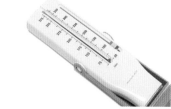

ISTOCK.COM/ABALCAZAR

B. Peak flow meter

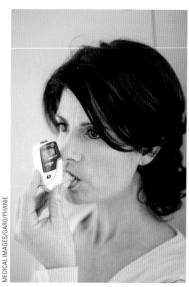

MEDICAL IMAGES/GARO/PHANIE

C. Consumer using another type of peak flow meter

FIGURE 13.23 Respiratory supportive equipment

Endotracheal tube

> Size of endotracheal tube
> Nasal or oral insertion
> Tube secured to the consumer
> Length of the endotracheal tube as it exits the nose or the mouth (e.g. 24 cm at the lips or 27 cm at the tip of the left nare)
> Cuff inflated or deflated

Peak flow meter (Figure 13.23B)

> Consumer is seated while performing the manoeuvre.
> Indicator line is lowered to the baseline level.
> Consumer exhales as deeply as possible while maintaining a firm seal with the lips around the mouthpiece (Figure 13.23C).
> Consumer does not obstruct the exhalation outlet.

Tracheostomy tube

> Size of tracheostomy tube
> Cuff present; if yes, cuff inflated or deflated
> Tracheostomy ties secure the tube

Mechanical ventilation

> Type of ventilator (e.g. Servo, Bear, Emerson)
> Fraction of inspired oxygen (FiO2) setting
> Mode used (e.g. assist, intermittent mandatory ventilation)
> Amount of positive end-expiratory pressure (PEEP) or continuous positive airway pressure (CPAP)
> Rate and tidal volume
> Peak inspiratory pressure
> Temperature of the humidification
> Alarms set

EVALUATION OF HEALTH ASSESSMENT AND PHYSICAL EXAMINATION FINDINGS

In the evaluation phase of a health assessment, the focus is on ensuring the data gathered is complete, accurate and documented appropriately (see case study as an example of the focused assessment; see Chapter 22 for a comprehensive health assessment). In evaluating the data you should:

> draw on your critical thinking and problem-solving skills to make sound clinical decisions
> act on abnormal data (include communicating findings to other health professionals)
> ensure documentation reflects the outcomes of the clinical decisions/actions taken (refer to Chapter 3 which discusses in detail why documentation is so important and how this may be undertaken in different health settings).

The case study that follows steps you through this process.

THE CONSUMER WITH COVID-19 (MODERATE DISEASE WITH DETERIORATION)

This case study illustrates the application and objective documentation of the respiratory assessment.

Aarav Maharjan is a 77-year-old male who is transported to the medical ward from a local aged care facility.

HEALTH HISTORY

CONSUMER PROFILE	77-year-old Indian male	
CHIEF COMPLAINT	'I have a headache, I have a sore throat and cough, shortness of breath.'	
HISTORY OF THE PRESENT ILLNESS	Mr Maharjan was in reasonable health until 4 days ago, when he became lethargic, lost his appetite, and began to cough. He reports clear rhinorrhoea and anosmia (loss of smell). Mr Maharjan feels increasing shortness of breath (SOB); however, breathing is slightly easier when the bed is elevated. In the aged care facility Mr Maharjan has been displaying restless, unsettled behaviour.	
PAST HEALTH HISTORY	**MEDICAL HISTORY**	> Hypertension > Cardiovascular disease > Bilateral hearing deficit > Osteoarthritis
	SURGICAL HISTORY	Coronary artery stenting (left anterior descending coronary artery)
	ALLERGIES	Nil known
	MEDICATIONS	Lisinopril 5 mg daily Acetaminophen PRN
	COMMUNICABLE DISEASES	Nil known
	INJURIES AND ACCIDENTS	Crush injury left foot >30 years ago Severed middle finger at the distal interphalangeal joint >40 years ago
	SPECIAL NEEDS	Nil noted
	BLOOD TRANSFUSIONS	Nil noted
	CHILDHOOD ILLNESSES	Chickenpox age 3 Mumps age 7 Rubella age 16
	IMMUNISATIONS	Last tetanus 10 years ago Influenza vaccination current COVID vaccination three doses
FAMILY HEALTH HISTORY	Denies family history of asthma or TB	
SOCIAL HISTORY	**ALCOHOL USE**	1–2 stubbies of beer 3–4 times per week
	TOBACCO USE	Nil
	DRUG USE	Nil noted
	DOMESTIC AND INTIMATE PARTNER VIOLENCE	Denies
	SEXUAL PRACTICE	Monogamous relationship with his wife of 57 years
	TRAVEL HISTORY	Limited travel for the last 5 years Previous biennial trips to India
	WORK ENVIRONMENT	Retired Small business owner (builder) for >50 years
	HOME ENVIRONMENT	Has lived in an aged care facility for the last seven years
	HOBBIES AND LEISURE ACTIVITIES	Member of chess club; plays bowls regularly at the facility, likes to paint, potter in the facility garden

>>

>>

HEALTH HISTORY

	STRESS	Nil noted
	EDUCATION	Building apprenticeship trade certification
	ECONOMIC STATUS	Middle class
	RELIGION	Hindu
	CULTURAL BACKGROUND	Indian
	ROLES AND RELATIONSHIPS	Married to his wife Vamika for 57 years Four children and 10 grandchildren
	CHARACTERISTIC PATTERNS OF DAILY LIVING	Routine
HEALTH MAINTENANCE ACTIVITIES	SLEEP	Sleeps for four hours per night
	DIET	Vegetarian
	EXERCISE	Bowls, walks around the facility gardens
	STRESS MANAGEMENT	Playing chess
	USE OF SAFETY DEVICES	Walking stick occasionally
	HEALTH CHECK-UPS	As required by the residential aged care facility's visiting general practitioner

PHYSICAL EXAMINATION

INSPECTION	SHAPE OF THORAX	AP diameter/transverse diameter = 5:7; kyphosis
	SYMMETRY OF CHEST WALL	Shoulder and scapula height equal; no masses present
	PRESENCE OF SUPERFICIAL VEINS	Nil noted
	COSTAL ANGLE	Less than 90°
	ANGLE OF THE RIBS	45° with sternum
	INTERCOSTAL SPACES	No bulging/retractions noted
	MUSCLES OF RESPIRATION	Minimal use of sternocleidomastoid muscles
	RESPIRATIONS	> Rate: 32/min > Pattern: regular > Depth: exaggerated, some effort required > Symmetry: paradoxical movement > Audibility: heard upon entering room > Consumer position: sitting upright > Mode of breathing: predominantly nose, occasional mouth
	SPUTUM	Nil
PALPATION	GENERAL PALPATION	> Pulsations: Nil noted > Masses: Nil noted > Thoracic tenderness: Nil reported > Crepitus: Nil noted
	THORACIC EXPANSION	Unilateral expansion: Right <2 cm, Left 5 cm
	TACTILE FREMITUS	Increased tactile fremitus Tussive fremitus
	TRACHEAL POSITION	Right side

>>

HEALTH HISTORY

PERCUSSION	GENERAL PERCUSSION	Dull
	DIAPHRAGMATIC EXCURSION	Reduced
AUSCULTATION	BREATH AUSCULTATION	Bronchial and vesicular
	ADVENTITIOUS SOUNDS	Fine and coarse crackles in RLL, posterior thorax
	VOICE SOUNDS	Increased voice sounds Asymmetric bronchophony
	SUPPORTIVE EQUIPMENT	> Pulse oximetry: SpO$_2$ 92–94% > Ventilation: non-invasive ventilation (continuous positive airway pressure [CPAP]) (or HNFO if CPAP is unavailable) > Oxygen: via CPAP

EVALUATION AND CLINICAL REASONING FOR CASE STUDY

The assessment and clinical decisions you make should reflect your scope of practice. For example, advanced practice health professionals, such as nurse practitioners and remote area nurses with endorsement, may be able to make diagnostic decisions and prescribe medications without referring to a medical practitioner.

Fundamentally, all health professionals collect, assess, synthesise, evaluate and act on person-centred health information. Person-centred health information may include referral to, or collaboration with, other healthcare team members. Nurses interpret responses to interventions and determine escalation to the broader healthcare team, based on changes in a person's condition. The clinical reasoning cycle provides health professionals with a framework to consider all this information in a meaningful way for planning person-centred care. These phases are reflected below and draw on the health history and physical examination information presented. We will work through the clinical reasoning cycle components that are relevant to this case study (clinical reasoning cycle components are bolded).

For Aarav Maharjan, the 77-year-old man who has been admitted to the medical ward from a residential aged care facility, and subsequently diagnosed with COVID-19, the significant data that needs to be considered includes the following.

Collecting Cues/Information

Recall and Review: In the first instance you will need to reflect on what you know about COVID-19. COVID-19 is an acute respiratory syndrome that leads to various respiratory and systematic conditions. Airway inflammation leads to recurrent episodes of coughing, and breathlessness. Symptoms may require conservative management or intensive invasive treatment. You will also need to consider infection control and prevention measures to ensure that Mr Maharjan does not spread COVID-19 to visitors, staff, or healthcare professionals. Additional information required to determine treatment will include blood test (full blood count, creatinine, electrolytes, liver function test, c-reactive protein), chest X-ray, blood gas, consider ECG, coagulation screening (d-dimer, ferritin) and blood cultures.

Chief complaint and history of present illness
> Headache, sore throat and cough and breathlessness
> Reports clear rhinorrhoea, and anosmia
> Reports feeling shortness of breath with mild exertion, requiring elevated bed and pillows to support upright positioning

Processing information

Interpret: These symptoms and details outline the scope of the issue for this consumer and how it will now affect his present deviation from normal health.

Health maintenance activities
> Unable to manage activities of daily living
> Feels very fatigued

Physical assessment
> Respiration rate 32 breaths/minute
> Temperature 38.7°C
> Respirations audible upon entering room; Mr Maharjan positioned upright and breathing predominantly through nose and occasionally mouth
> Adventitious breath sounds, crackles RLL, posterior thorax
> Pulse oximetry: 92–94% room air, requiring oxygen to maintain adequate O$_2$ level

Interpret, Discriminate, Infer and Predict: The significance of these findings indicates that Mr Maharjan is experiencing an acute episode of respiratory distress caused by COVID-19. According to the current guidelines, Mr Maharjan's findings put him in the moderate disease with deterioration category. Close observation will be required to determine transfer to critical care services.

Putting it all together – synthesise information

The role of the nurse in this case is to ensure Mr Maharjan is managed appropriately in the ward so that he is seen promptly by the interprofessional healthcare team. This will ensure that intervention is undertaken before any further deterioration in respiratory status occurs and to limit the possibility of invasive intervention. While the medical officer will review and prescribe medical treatment for Mr Maharjan, the nursing team will manage holistic care for the consumer and his family/whānau. Treatment focuses on relieving respiratory distress, positioning, medications, monitoring deterioration. Relief from symptoms should usually occur following supportive treatment, and medication administration. Close monitoring for deterioration for 5 to 10 days following onset of symptoms is vital.

Actions based on assessment findings

Other areas that need to be considered include:

1 Monitor the continued use of infection prevention and control strategies. Consider communication with Mr Maharjan and how he might manage his hearing impairment while staff and healthcare professionals are wearing personal protective equipment (PPE).

2 Ongoing assessment, pulse oximetry and respiratory assessments (pulmonary embolism) will be vital to detect potential deterioration.

3 Consider periods of prone positioning if tolerated until Mr Maharjan is no longer deteriorating (i.e. maintain oxygen levels above 93%).

4 Assessment for deterioration of cardiovascular (thromboembolism, arrhythmias, cardiac impairment), neurological (delirium) and renal (acute kidney injury) systems, sepsis, shock, and multi-organ dysfunction is imperative.

5 Medication management currently suggests intravenous or oral corticosteroids (dexamethasone) for up to 10 days. Baricitinib (selective immunosuppressant), low molecular weight heparin (e.g. enoxaparin 40 mg daily), and possible antibiotic therapy.

6 Close monitoring of consumer deterioration particularly 5 to 10 days after onset of symptoms.

7 Communication and holistic care: clear communication regarding symptoms and management to consumer, family/whānau or carers. The nurse should give Mr Maharjan the opportunity to communicate concerns about his condition to his family/whānau while he is in hospital. Remember that Mr Maharjan has a hearing impairment, therefore the nurse will need to implement additional strategies to facilitate effective communication.

8 Support communication between Mr Maharjan and his wife Vamika, who remains alone in the residential aged care facility while he is in hospital.

9 Liaise with pastoral care, counselling and other social support services considering his cultural beliefs and needs while he is in hospital.

10 Discharge planning: consider specialist clinic follow-up, investigations, and support. Discharge planning usually begins prior to discharge.

11 Education about post COVID infection management is critical for Mr Maharjan.

12 Post COVID infection signs and symptoms include cough, SOB, neurological symptoms, hair loss, skin conditions, renal disease, thromboembolism, psychological symptoms, cardiac and musculoskeletal symptoms, fever, reduced activity and function, altered nutrition and weight loss.

Australian National COVID-19 Clinical Evidence Taskforce (2022); Ministry of Health/Manatū Hauora (2022)

The final step in the process is accurate documentation. The nurse must document findings, referrals, interventions, and advice and education given. The consumer would then be reassessed following definitive diagnosis, and long-term management and follow-up would be facilitated.

Evaluate outcomes

Mr Maharjan was admitted to your ward with moderate COVID-19 disease, and he was deteriorating. Was the treatment and care enough to manage Mr Maharjan in the ward, or did he deteriorate and require transfer to critical care services? Were you the nurses that detected a slight change in his condition, communicated this with the team, and instigated nursing care that minimised the possibility of his transfer for invasive treatment?

Reflections

Consider Mr Maharjan's clinical presentation, and management underpinned by current and evolving evidence, and how Mr Maharjan recovered. What did you learn about the management of a person with COVID-19? What would you do the same or differently in the future? Are there additional opportunities for learning about the management of people with COVID-19?

CHAPTER RESOURCES

REVIEW QUESTIONS

For answers to these questions, see Answer section at the end of the book.

1. The nurse observes that the consumer is having difficulty breathing. Which muscles are used in a state of increased oxygen demand? Select all that apply.
   a. Diaphragm
   b. External intercostal muscles
   c. Sternocleidomastoid muscles
   d. Abdominal rectus muscles
   e. Internal intercostal muscles
   f. Trapezius muscles

2. A consumer reports that he was climbing Mount Cook and noted an increase in the depth of his respirations. This physical assessment finding is called:
   a. Biot's respirations
   b. Apneustic respirations
   c. Hyperpnoea
   d. Air trapping

3. Kussmaul respirations are respirations that:
   a. Have an increased depth and slow rate
   b. Are the body's attempt to raise its $PaCO_2$ level
   c. Are regularly irregular
   d. Are tachypnoeic and hyperpnoeic

4. The nurse suctions the consumer's endotracheal tube and notes that the secretions are pink coloured. What is a possible aetiology of this consumer's pathology?
   a. Asthma
   b. Pulmonary oedema
   c. Viral infection
   d. Pneumococcal pneumonia

5. When performing diaphragmatic excursion, you measure a distance of 2 cm. This finding suggests:
   a. A normal distance
   b. Hypoventilation
   c. Pneumonectomy
   d. High diaphragm level

6. During inspection of a consumer's thorax, you note that the consumer's ribs attach to the sternum at a 45° angle. This consumer has:
   a. A normal finding
   b. Pleural effusion
   c. Cystic fibrosis
   d. Chronic bronchitis

7. You auscultate abnormal breath sounds on the consumer's right chest at the 5th rib in the midclavicular line. In which lobe of the lung are you auscultating this sound?
   a. Right upper lobe
   b. Right middle lobe
   c. Right lower lobe
   d. Right oblique fissure

8. Which of the following consumers has the highest risk of contracting COVID-19?
   a. A 78-year-old male with chest pain and diarrhoea
   b. A 55-year-old sheep farmer who presents with a cough
   c. A 17-year-old female who has cystic fibrosis, and spends a lot of time with her grandmother in a residential aged care facility
   d. A 27-year-old person with a history of drug and alcohol abuse who recently moved to Darwin, Northern Territory, Australia

9. In which condition might you expect to see a rib angle of 45°, decreased thoracic expansion, tracheal deviation, dull percussion, tachypnoea, and increased tactile fremitus?
   a. Pneumothorax
   b. Emphysema
   c. Pneumonia
   d. Atelectasis

10. The nurse auscultates the consumer's lungs and hears fine and coarse bronchial crackles, and increased voice sounds. These sounds are heard during inspiration. What condition does the nurse suspect that the consumer is experiencing?
    a. Pneumonia
    b. Bronchitis
    c. Croup
    d. Pleurisy

CS CLINICAL **SKILLS**

The following Clinical Skills are relevant to this chapter and can be found in Tollefson & Hillman, *Clinical Psychomotor Skills*, 8th edition:
> 19 Focused respiratory health history assessment and physical assessment
> 27 Healthcare teaching.

FURTHER RESOURCES

> Asthma + Respiratory Foundation NZ: https://www.asthmafoundation.org.nz/health-professionals
> Asthma New Zealand: https://www.asthma.org.nz/
> Auscultation Assistant: http://www.wilkes.med.ucla.edu/
> Australian Asthma Handbook: https://www.nationalasthma.org.au/health-professionals/australian-asthma-handbook
> Australian Government Cancer Australia. Cancer Learning: Our Lungs, Our Mob Community Education Resource: http://cancerlearning.gov.au/resources/links/our-lungs-our-mob-community-education-resource
> Australian Government Department of Health: *The Australian immunisation handbook* (10th ed.). Australian Technical Advisory Group on Immunisation (ATAGI): https://immunisationhandbook.health.gov.au/
> Australian Government Department of Health: The Strategic Plan for Control of Tuberculosis in Australia, 2016–2020: Towards Disease Elimination: https://www1.health.gov.au/internet/main/publishing.nsf/Content/ohp-ntac-tb-strat-plan.htm
> Better Health Channel Victoria State Government: https://www.betterhealth.vic.gov.au/
> Cancer Society New Zealand: http://www.cancernz.org.nz/
> Centers for Disease Control and Prevention: http://www.cdc.gov

> Health Direct: https://www.healthdirect.gov.au/
> Health Navigator New Zealand: http://www.healthnavigator.org.nz
> Health Navigator New Zealand – COPD/Mate ia tuku: https://www.healthnavigator.org.nz/health-a-z/c/copd/
> Immunisation Advisory Centre: https://www.influenza.org.nz/
> Influenza Specialist Group: http://www.isg.org.au/index.php/vaccination/
> Lung Foundation Australia: https://lungfoundation.com.au/health-professionals/
> Mayo Clinic: http://www.mayoclinic.com
> Ministry of Health/Manatù Hauora: http://www.health.govt.nz/
> National Asthma Council Australia: https://www.nationalasthma.org.au/health-professionals
> National Immunisation Program Schedule: https://beta.health.gov.au/topics/immunisation/immunisation-throughout-life/national-immunisation-program-schedule
> R.A.L.E. Repository: http://www.rale.ca
> The Thoracic Society of Australia & New Zealand: http://www.thoracic.org.au

REFERENCES

Alkhodari, M., & Khandoker, A. H. (2022). Detection of COVID-19 in smartphone-based breathing recordings: A pre-screening deep learning tool. *PloS One, 17*(1), e0262448–e0262448. https://doi.org/10.1371/journal.pone.0262448

Asthma and Respiratory Foundation New Zealand. (2020). Key statistics. Retrieved 12 December 2022 from: https://www.asthmafoundation.org.nz/research/key-statistics

Asthma and Respiratory Foundation New Zealand. (2022a). Homepage. Retrieved 12 December 2022 from: https://www.asthmafoundation.org.nz

Asthma and Respiratory Foundation New Zealand. (2022b). Youth vaping and smoking trends moving in right direction, but sustained effort is needed. Retrieved 12 December 2022 from: https://www.asthmafoundation.org.nz/news-events/2022/youth-vaping-and-smoking-trends-moving-in-right-direction-but-sustained-effort-is-needed

Augustin, M., Schommers, P., Stecher, M., Dewald, F., Gieselmann, L., Gruell, H., ... & Lehmann, C. (2021). Post-COVID syndrome in non-hospitalised consumers with COVID-19: a longitudinal prospective cohort study. *The Lancet Regional Health-Europe, 6*, 100–22.

Australian Bureau of Statistics (ABS). (2022). Health conditions prevalence. Retrieved 12 December 2022 from: www.abs.gov.au/statistics/health/health-conditions-and-risks/health-conditions-prevalence/latest-release

Australian Bureau of Statistics (ABS). (2023). COVID-19 mortality in Australia: Deaths registered until 31 March 2023. Retrieved 5 May 2023 from: https://www.abs.gov.au/articles/covid-19-mortality-australia-deaths-registered-until-31-march-2023

Australian Government Department of Health. (2017). Clinical update: Pertussis booster for 18 month olds. Retrieved 29 June 2022 from: https://www.health.gov.au/news/clinical-update-pertussis-booster-for-18-month-olds

Australian Government Department of Health. (2018). Tuberculosis notifications in Australia annual reports. Retrieved 7 June 2022 from: http://www.health.gov.au/internet/main/publishing.nsf/content/cda-pubs-annlrpt-tbannrep.htm

Australian Government Department of Health. (2021). Australian COVID-19 vaccination policy. https://www.health.gov.au/

Australian Government Department of Health. (2022). COVID-19 management guidelines for primary care providers. https://www.health.gov.au/our-work/living-with-covid-primary-care-package/covid-19-management-guidelines-for-primary-care-providers

Australian Government Department of Health. (2023). Coronavirus (COVID-19) pandemic. https://www.health.gov.au/health-alerts/covid-19

Australian Institute for Health and Wellbeing (AIHW). (2020). Chronic obstructive pulmonary disease (COPD), associated comorbidities and risk factors. Retrieved 12 December 2022 from: www.aihw.gov.au/reports/web/105/copd-associated-comorbidities-risk-factors/contents/risk-factors-associated-with-copd

Australian Institute for Health and Wellbeing (AIHW). (2022a). Chronic respiratory conditions. Retrieved 12 December 2022 from: https://www.aihw.gov.au/reports/australias-health/chronic-respiratory-conditions

Australian Institute for Health and Wellbeing (AIHW). (2022b). Alcohol, tobacco & other drugs in Australia. Retrieved 12 December 2022 from: https://www.aihw.gov.au/reports/phe/221/alcohol-tobacco-other-drugs-australia/contents/population-groups-of-interest/young-people

Australian Technical Advisory Group on Immunisation (ATAGI). (2018). *Australian immunisation handbook.* Australian Government Department of Health, Canberra. Retrieved 7 June 2022 from: https://www.immunisationhandbook.health.gov.au.

Australian Technical Advisory Group on Immunisation (ATAGI). (2022, May). Australian Technical Advisory Group on Immunisation (ATAGI) recommended COVID-19 vaccines and doses. Retrieved 22 May 2022 from: https://www.health.gov.au/

Berman, A., Snyder, S., Levett-Jones, T., Dwyer, T., Hales, M., Harvey, N., ... & Stanley, D. (2018). *Kozier and Erb's fundamentals of nursing: Concepts, process and practice*, 4th Australian edition. Frenchs Forest, NSW: Pearson Education Australia.

Communicable Diseases Network Australia. (2022). Tuberculosis: CDNA national guidelines for public health units. Version 3.0. Australian Government, Department of Health. Retrieved 7 June 2022 from: https://www1.health.gov.au/internet/main/publishing.nsf/Content/D140EDF48C0A0CEACA257BF0001A3537/$File/DS_Tuberculosis%20(TB)%20SoNG%20V-3.0.pdf

COVID Live. (2023). COVID Live. Retrieved 5 May 2023 from: https://covidlive.com.au/.

Glangetas, A., Hartley, M. A., Cantais, A., Courvoisier, D. S., Rivollet, D., Shama, D. M., ... & Siebert, J. N. (2021). Deep learning diagnostic and risk-stratification pattern detection for COVID-19 in digital lung auscultations: clinical protocol for a case–control and prospective cohort study. *BMC pulmonary medicine, 21*(1), 1–8.

Health Navigator New Zealand. (2021). COPD | Mate ia tuku. Retrieved 12 December 2022 from: https://www.healthnavigator.org.nz/health-a-z/c/copd/

Immunisation Advisory Centre, The (2022). Influenza information for health professionals. Retrieved 4 August 2023 from: https://www.influenza.org.nz/

Ministry of Health, New Zealand. (2023). Influenza. Retrieved 4 August 2023 from: https://www.health.govt.nz/your-health/conditions-and-treatments/diseases-and-illnesses/influenza

Ministry of Health/Manatū Hauora. (2021). Whooping cough. Retrieved 29 June 2022 from: https://www.health.govt.nz/your-health/conditions-and-treatments/diseases-and-illnesses/whooping-cough

Ministry of Health/Manatū Hauora. (2022a). *COVID-19: Current cases.* Retrieved 15 May 2022 from: https://www.health.govt.nz/covid-19-novel-coronavirus

Ministry of Health/Manatū Hauora. (2022b). *Tuberculosis disease.* Retrieved 7 June 2022 from: https://www.health.govt.nz/your-health/conditions-and-treatments/diseases-and-illnesses/tuberculosis-disease

Ministry of Health/Manatū Hauora. (2022c, 6 May). *Clinical Management of COVID-19 in hospitalised adults (including in pregnancy).* New Zealand Government. Retrieved 5 May 2023 from: https://www.health.govt.nz/covid-19-novel-coronavirus/covid-19-information-health-professionals

Ministry of Health/Manatū Hauora. (2022d). *Immunisation handbook.* Retrieved 5 May 2023 from: http://www.health. govt.nz/

Ministry of Health/Manatū Hauora. (2023). COVID-19: Current-cases. Retrieved 5 May 2023 from: https://www.health.govt.nz/covid-19-novel-coronavirus/covid-19-data-and-statistics/covid-19-current-cases

National COVID-19 Clinical Evidence Taskforce. (2020). *Australian guidelines for the clinical care of people with COVID-19*, v57.1. Australian Government Department of Health, Living Guidelines. https://app.magicapp.org/#/guideline/L4Q5An

National COVID-19 Clinical Evidence Taskforce. (2020, 18 December). Care of people who experience symptoms post-acute COVID-19. https://covid19evidence.net.au/

Royal Australian College of General Practitioners (RACGP). (2021, December). *Caring for patients with post-COVID-19 conditions.* https://www.racgp.org.au

Struyf, T., Deeks, J. J., Dinnes, J., Takwoingi, Y., Davenport, C., Leeflang, M. M. G., ... & Van den Bruel A. (2021). Signs and symptoms to determine if a patient presenting in primary care or hospital outpatient settings has COVID-19. *Cochrane Database of Systematic Reviews*, Issue 2. Art. No.: CD013665. doi: 10.1002/14651858.CD013665.pub2. Retrieved 18 May 2022.

World Health Organization (WHO). (2022). Asthma, key facts. Retrieved 12 December 2022 from: https://www.who.int/news-room/fact-sheets/detail/asthma

Wotton, K. (2017). Balancing fluid, electrolyte and acid-base status. In J. Crisp, C. Douglas, G. Rebeiro & D. Waters, (Eds). *Potter and Perry's fundamentals of nursing* (5th ed., pp. 1152–240). Chatswood: Elsevier Australia.

Zhang, P., Wang, B., Liu, Y., Fan, M., Ji, Y., Xu, H., ... & Zhang, Z. (2021). Lung auscultation of hospitalized patients with SARS-CoV-2 pneumonia via a wireless stethoscope. *International Journal of Medical Science,18*(6), 1415–22. doi: 10.7150/ijms.54987. PMID: 33628098; PMCID: PMC7893566.

CHAPTER 14

CARDIOVASCULAR

LEARNING OUTCOMES

By the end of this chapter you should be able to:

1 identify the anatomic landmarks of the chest and blood vessels
2 describe the characteristics of the most common cardiovascular complaints
3 obtain a health history from a consumer with cardiovascular pathology
4 demonstrate a cardiovascular assessment on a healthy adult (refer to Chapter 20 for specific assessment of the paediatric consumer)
5 demonstrate a cardiovascular assessment on a consumer with cardiovascular pathology, and differentiate normal and abnormal findings during the assessment
6 provide evidence-based rationales for abnormal cardiovascular assessment findings
7 discuss the clinical reasoning in evaluating outcomes of health assessment and physical examination, including documentation, health education provision and relevant health referral.

BACKGROUND

The heart's primary function is to pump blood to all parts of the body. The circulating blood not only brings oxygen and nutrients to the body's tissues but also helps to remove waste products. As the heart rate regulates blood flow, vessels will expand or relax in order to distribute the blood according to the body's demands.

Cardiovascular disease (CVD) refers to a range of disorders that involve the heart and blood vessels. The major types of CVD are commonly divided into heart, stroke and blood vessel diseases. Coronary heart disease (CHD), stroke (or cerebrovascular accident, CVA) and heart failure (HF) are some of the most common and serious CVDs (AIHW, 2021a). When undertaking health assessment, the key cardiovascular health problems are CHD, also known as ischaemic heart disease (IHD), stroke, HF, and peripheral vascular diseases (PVD) (ABS, 2020, 2021, 2022; AIHW, 2021a; Heart Foundation New Zealand, 2022a).

Cardiovascular disease remains the leading cause of death in Australia, New Zealand and the world, including First Nations peoples, who are at even higher risk (ABS, 2022; AIHW, 2021a; Heart Foundation New Zealand, 2022a; National Heart Foundation of Australia, 2022a; WHO, 2021). Death due to CVD is significantly higher in Aboriginal and Torres Strait Islander people (1.6 times the mortality rate of non-First Nations Australians) (AIHW, 2021b), those from lower socioeconomic groups (AIHW, 2022a), and individuals living in regional and remote areas (AIHW, 2022b) than for any other Australians.

Congenital heart and vascular diseases constitute one of the leading causes of death for children (AIHW, 2019). Among Aboriginal and Torres Strait Islander peoples, ischaemic heart disease, hypertension and rheumatic heart disease are major problems (ABS, 2022; AIHW, 2021b; Merone et al., 2019; National Heart Foundation of Australia, 2021a).

Other considerations during the health assessment are the person's cardiovascular risk factors (See Clinical reasoning box: Risk factors for coronary heart disease). There is compelling evidence that making positive lifestyle choices can reduce the impact of further CVD development (AIHW, 2021a; Heart Foundation New Zealand, 2022b; National Heart Foundation of Australia, 2021a, b, c; Health New Zealand, 2022).

CLINICAL REASONING

Practice tip: Risk factors for cardiovascular disease

> Non-modifiable risk factors (a person cannot alter these):
>   • Increasing age, sex (men are at greater risk than pre-menopausal women, similar risk for men and women after female menopause), cultural background, family history of CVD (genetics)
> Modifiable risk factors – sometimes referred to as lifestyle risks or behaviours (an individual can significantly reduce risk of cardiovascular disease if able to control these risk factors):
>   • Smoking, elevated cholesterol, hypertension, physical inactivity, not being a healthy weight (overweight or obese), diet, alcohol consumption, and psychosocial determinants – depression, social isolation and lack of social support.

Source: National Heart Foundation of Australia, 2022b, c, d; AIHW, 2021a; Health Navigator New Zealand 2022; Heart Foundation New Zealand, 2022b.

Consider one member of your family and identify what CVD risks they might have and consider how you might support them to change these practices. How could you draw on this knowledge in clinical practice to assist a consumer?

Given the strong evidence that supports the impact of risk factors in the development of coronary heart disease, what actions could you take to support your consumer to reduce the risk? If a consumer presents with two or more risk factors, what actions could you take to support them to reduce risk?

Download and calculate your absolute cardiovascular risk, using the Australian Chronic Disease Prevention Alliance CVD Check absolute risk CVD calculator at https://www.cvdcheck.org.au/calculator.

HEALTH EDUCATION

Cardiovascular risk management

Identifying if a person is at risk of experiencing a cardiovascular event in the next five years is supported by risk identification. Table 14.1 identifies the risk, and suggests lifestyle, pharmacotherapy strategies with the target ranges and how to monitor each stage. For New Zealand readers, refer to Ministry of Health (2018) and Heart Foundation New Zealand (2018).

TABLE 14.1 CVD risk management summary

CVD RISK	LIFESTYLE	PHARMACOTHERAPY	TARGETS	MONITORING
High risk Clinically determined or calculated using FRE as >15% absolute risk of CVD events over 5 years	> Frequent and sustained specific advice and support regarding diet and physical activity > Appropriate advice, support and pharmacotherapy for smoking cessation > Advice given simultaneously with BP- and lipid-lowering drug treatment	> Treat simultaneously with lipid-lowering and BP-lowering medication unless contraindicated or clinically inappropriate. > Aspirin not routinely recommended. > Consider withdrawal of therapy for people who make profound lifestyle changes.	BP: > ≤140/90 mmHg in general or people with CKD > ≤130/80 mmHg in all people with diabetes > ≤130/80 mmHg if micro or macro albuminuria (UACR >2.5 mg/mmol in men and >3.5 mg/mmol in women) Lipids: > TC <4.0 mmol/L > HDL-C ≥1.0 mmol/L > LDL-C <2.0 mmol/L > Non HDL-C <2.5 mmol/L > TG <2.0 mmol/L. Lifestyle: > Smoking cessation (if smoker) > Consume diet rich in vegetables and fruit, low in salt and saturated and trans fats > At least 30 min moderate intensity physical activity on most or preferably every day of the week > Limit alcohol intake	> Adjust medication as required > Review absolute risk according to clinical context
Moderate risk Calculated using FRE as 10–15% absolute risk of CVD events over 5 years	> Appropriate, specific advice and support regarding diet and physical activity > Appropriate advice, support and pharmacotherapy for smoking cessation > Lifestyle advice given in preference to drug therapy	> Not routinely recommended > Consider BP lowering and/or lipid lowering medication in addition to lifestyle advice if 3–6 months of lifestyle intervention does not reduce risk or: • BP persistently ≥160/100 mmHg • Family history of premature CVD • Specific population where the FRE underestimates risk, e.g. A&TSI peoples, South Asian, Māori and Pasifika, Middle Eastern > Consider withdrawal of therapy for people who make profound lifestyle changes		> Adjust medication as required > Review absolute risk every 6–12 months
Low risk Calculated using FRE as <10% absolute risk of CVD events over 5 years	> Brief, general lifestyle advice regarding diet and physical activity > Appropriate advice, support and pharmacotherapy for smoking cessation	> Not routinely recommended > Consider BP lowering therapy in addition to specific lifestyle advice if BP persistently ≥160/100 mmHg > Consider withdrawal of therapy for people who make profound lifestyle changes		> Adjust medication as required > Review absolute risk every 2 years > Blood test results within 5 years can be used

A&TSI: Aboriginal and Torres Strait Islander peoples; BP: blood pressure; CKD: Chronic kidney disease; DBP: diastolic blood pressure; FRE: Framingham Risk Equation; HDL-C: high-density lipoprotein cholesterol; LDL-C: low-density lipoprotein cholesterol; SBP: systolic blood pressure; TC: total cholesterol; TG: triglycerides; UACR: urinary albumin : creatinine ratio

SOURCE: NATIONAL VASCULAR DISEASE PREVENTION ALLIANCE. (2012). GUIDELINES FOR THE MANAGEMENT OF ABSOLUTE CARDIOVASCULAR DISEASE RISK, 2012, P.9

ANATOMY AND PHYSIOLOGY

Heart

In a resting, healthy adult, the heart contracts 60 to 100 times while pumping 4 to 5 litres of blood per minute. An individual's heart is about the size of a clenched fist. The human heart is remarkably efficient considering its size in relation to the rest of the body.

The heart is located in the thoracic cavity between the lungs and above the diaphragm in an area known as the mediastinum **(Figure 14.1)**. The **base** of the heart is the uppermost portion that includes the left and right atria as well as the aorta, pulmonary arteries and the superior and inferior vena cava. These structures lie behind the upper portion of the sternum. The **apex**, or lower portion, of the heart extends into the left thoracic cavity, causing the heart to appear as if it is lying on its right ventricle.

Pericardium

The heart and roots of the great vessels lie within a sac called the pericardium, which is composed of fibrous and serous layers. The fibrous layer is the outermost layer and is connected to the diaphragm and sternum by ligaments and tendons. Its major role is to limit the stretching of the myocardial muscle, especially in the setting of strenuous activity or hypervolaemia.

There are two serous layers of the pericardium: the **parietal pericardium**, which lies close to the fibrous tissues, and the **visceral pericardium**, which lies against the actual heart muscle. This visceral layer is often referred to as the epicardium. Between the two serous layers is a small space that contains approximately 20 to 50 mL of pericardial fluid. This pericardial fluid serves to facilitate the movement of the heart muscle and protect it via a lubricant effect that reduces friction.

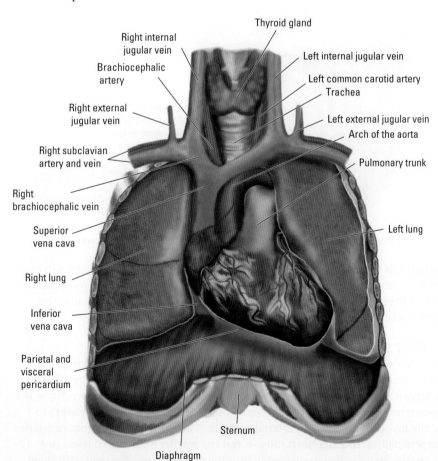

FIGURE 14.1 Position of the heart in the thoracic cavity

Chambers of the heart

The heart is divided into four chambers, which are separated laterally by walls known as the vertical **septa**. These vertical septa divide the heart into the right and the left atria (interatrial septum) and the right and the left ventricles (interventricular septum). The right atrium is the collection point for the blood returning from the systemic circulation for reoxygenation in the lungs. The left atrium receives its freshly oxygenated blood via the four pulmonary veins, which are the only veins in the body that carry oxygenated blood.

The walls of the left ventricle are three times thicker than those of the right ventricle because of its greater workload as it pumps blood through the high-pressure systemic arterial system. Left ventricular pressures are five times greater than those in the right ventricle. Figure 14.2 shows the configuration of the heart's chambers, the pressures, and normal oxygen content of the blood contained therein.

Heart valves

As blood empties into the two atria, the **atrioventricular (A-V) valves** prevent it from prematurely entering the ventricles. The A-V valve between the right atrium and the right ventricle is known as the tricuspid valve, named for its three flaps or cusps. The A-V valve between the left atrium and the left ventricle is the bicuspid valve, named for its two flaps or cusps; it is commonly known as the mitral valve. When the tricuspid and mitral valves are closed, blood cannot flow from the atria into the ventricles. In a normal heart, they open only as atrial pressures increase with progressive filling.

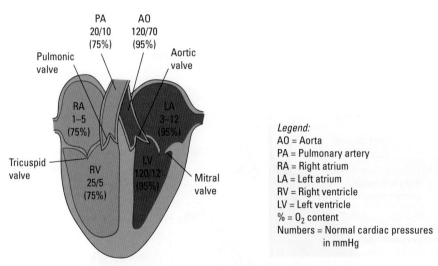

FIGURE 14.2 The configuration, normal pressures and oxygen content of the heart chambers

Blood exits the heart through semilunar valves, also known as outflow valves. Blood flows from the right ventricle to the pulmonary vasculature for oxygenation by way of the pulmonic valve. Blood is pumped from the left ventricle into the systemic and coronary circulation through the aortic valve.

Coronary circulation

The exterior surface of the heart muscle contains a very important and intricate blood supply. Two major coronary arteries arise from the small openings in the aorta known as the sinuses of Valsalva, located just behind the aortic valve. Figure 14.3 demonstrates the position of the coronary arteries as they exit from the aorta to cover the myocardium with an arterial network. The left and right coronary arteries run superficially across the heart muscle, but the smaller branches of these two main arteries actually penetrate deeply into the myocardium, carrying with them a rich, nutritive blood supply. Blood flow to the coronary arteries is greatest during diastole because the force of the ventricular contraction during systole actually impedes flow through the sinuses of Valsalva.

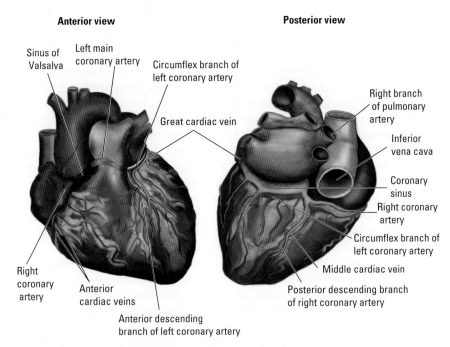

Anterior view

Posterior view

Sinus of Valsalva

Left main coronary artery

Circumflex branch of left coronary artery

Great cardiac vein

Right branch of pulmonary artery

Inferior vena cava

Coronary sinus

Right coronary artery

Circumflex branch of left coronary artery

Middle cardiac vein

Posterior descending branch of right coronary artery

Right coronary artery

Anterior cardiac veins

Anterior descending branch of left coronary artery

FIGURE 14.3 The coronary arteries and major veins of the heart (anterior and posterior views)

The myocardium is extremely dependent on a constant supply of oxygen that is delivered through the coronary arterial system. The heart's oxygen requirements increase when it is stimulated by conditions such as exercise. If the coronary blood supply is not sufficient to meet the needs of the heart, the result may be **ischaemia** (local and temporary lack of blood supply to the heart, e.g. during coronary artery spasm), injury (beyond ischaemia but still reversible), or an **infarction** (necrosis, due to acute myocardial infarction) of the heart muscle itself. Myocardial ischaemia is often manifested as chest, neck or arm pain known as **angina**.

The left main coronary artery branches into the left circumflex coronary artery and the left anterior descending (LAD) coronary artery. The left main coronary artery may be referred to as the 'widow maker', because of the lethal effect of any obstruction to blood flow prior to its branch point.

The LAD supplies blood to the anterior wall and apex of the left ventricle as well as to the anterior portion of the interventricular septum. The smaller arterial branches that supply the septum also nourish the ventricular conduction system, including the bundle of His and the right and left bundle branches. The left circumflex (LCX) branch supplies arterial blood to the left atrium and to the lateral and posterior portions of the left ventricle. In some individuals, the sinoatrial (S-A) node and the **atrioventricular (A-V) node** are also supplied by this branch.

The right coronary artery (RCA) supplies nutrients and oxygen to the right atrium, the right ventricle, and the inferior wall of the left ventricle. In most individuals, the RCA supplies the S-A and the A-V nodes as well as the posterior portion of the interventricular septum. With an inferior wall infarction, the RCA is most likely the vessel that has been occluded. With an anterior wall infarction, the LAD branch would be the most likely source of occlusion, with resulting complications in the ventricular conduction system, such as bundle branch blocks or ventricular arrhythmias.

Venous drainage from the myocardium is carried by the coronary sinus, anterior cardiac veins, and Thebesian veins. About 75% of the venous blood empties into the right atrium via the coronary sinus. The Thebesian veins carry only a small portion of the deoxygenated blood that is emptied directly into all four chambers of the heart.

Cardiac cycle

Figure 14.4 illustrates the electrical and mechanical events in the heart. Physical examination findings can be correlated with these electrophysiological mechanisms.

The cardiac cycle consists of two phases: systole and diastole. In systole, the myocardial fibres contract and tighten to eject blood from the ventricles (for the purpose of this chapter, any mention of systole will mean ventricular systole unless specifically called atrial systole). Diastole is a period of relaxation and reflects the pressure remaining in the blood vessels after the heart has pumped.

Systole is divided into three phases, beginning with the isovolumic (or isometric) contraction phase, which marks the onset of a ventricular contraction. During this phase, the pressure is increasing but no blood is entering or leaving the ventricle. As the pressure rises in the left ventricle, the mitral valve closes (similar events occur in the right ventricle with the tricuspid valve). Closure of these A-V valves produces the first heart sound, known as S_1 (depicted as '1st' on the phonocardiogram (a recording of the heart sounds) curve in **Figure 14.4**).

Once the pressure in the left ventricle exceeds that in the aorta, and the pressure in the right ventricle exceeds that in the pulmonary artery, the semilunar (aortic and pulmonic) valves open and blood is rapidly ejected. This rapid ejection phase is also referred to as early systole. It is followed by a third phase of reduced ejection, which is also known as late systole.

Ventricular diastole begins with the isovolumic, or isometric, relaxation phase. During this phase, ventricular ejection ceases and the pressure in the left ventricle is reduced to less than that in the aorta. This permits a backflow of blood from the aorta to the left ventricle, causing the aortic valve to close (similar events occur in the pulmonary artery to cause the pulmonic valve to close). The closure of the semilunar valves produces the second heart sound, known as S_2 (depicted as '2nd' on the phonocardiogram curve in **Figure 14.4**). When the A-V and semilunar valves are closed, the pressure in the left ventricle falls rapidly.

Atrial pressures then rise as a result of the large amount of blood accumulating in the atria because of the closed A-V valves. When systole is over and the ventricular pressures fall, the high pressure in the atria forces the A-V valves to open to allow for rapid ventricular filling (rapid inflow) during early diastole. Filling then slows during a phase called diastasis or mid-diastole. Seventy per cent of ventricular filling occurs in a passive manner during these early and mid-diastolic filling periods.

The final phase of diastole is known as atrial systole. The atria contract to complete the remaining 20% to 30% of ventricular filling, which is often referred to as **atrial kick**. After atrial systole, the cardiac cycle starts all over again.

The **electrocardiogram** (abbreviated as either **ECG** or **EKG**, from the German word 'Elektrokardiogramm') in **Figure 14.4** shows the P, Q, R, S and T waves. These waves are electrical voltages produced by the heart and recorded by ECG leads placed on the body. When the atria depolarise, the P wave is produced on the ECG. During this period, the pressure in the atria exceeds that in the ventricles, thus forcing the blood from the atria into the ventricles. Approximately 0.16 second after the appearance of the P wave, the QRS complex on the ECG occurs as the ventricles are electrically depolarised. As the ventricles begin to repolarise, the T wave appears on the ECG. The downslope of the T wave indicates the end of ventricular repolarisation and the beginning of a relaxation period. Note that the ECG contains an **isoelectric line**, or flat line, after the T wave, indicating a period of electrical rest.

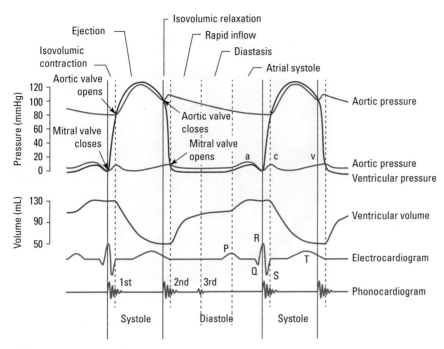

FIGURE 14.4 Events of the cardiac cycle

WIKIMEDIA COMMONS/DANIELCHANGMD (DESTINYQX, XAVAX)/CC BY-SA 2.5

Conduction system of the heart

The **sinoatrial (S-A) node** is the normal pacemaker of the heart and is located about 1 mm below the right atrial epicardium at its junction with the superior vena cava. It initiates a rhythmic impulse approximately 60 times per minute. The infranodal atrial pathways conduct the impulse initiated in the S-A node to the A-V node via the myocardium of the right atrium. The three infranodal pathways are the anterior, middle and posterior tracts. Meanwhile, the Bachmann's bundle conducts the impulse from the S-A node to the left atrium. In the absence of a signal from the S-A node, the A-V node has its own intrinsic rate of 40 to 60 impulses per minute. The A-V node, also known as the A-V junction, delays the impulse received from the atria before transmitting it to the ventricles in order to give them time to fill prior to the next systole. The impulse then travels very rapidly from the A-V node to the bundle branch system via the bundle of His. The bundle branch system is composed of the right bundle branch (RBB) and the left bundle branch (LBB). The RBB carries the impulse down the right side of the interventricular septum into the right ventricle. The LBB separates into three fascicles that relay the impulse to the left ventricle. Finally, the Purkinje fibres arising from the distal portions of the bundle branches transmit the impulse into the subendocardial layers of both ventricles. Barring interference with the connections described above, the final transmission of the impulse allows depolarisation of the ventricles to occur followed by a normal systole. **Figure 14.5** depicts the normal conduction pathways of the heart. If A-V node disease causes transmission of the electrical signal to be blocked, the intrinsic rate of the ventricles kicks in at a rate of fewer than 40 beats per minute.

Blood vessels

The circulatory system consists of arterial pathways, which are the distribution routes, and venous pathways, the collection system that returns the blood to the central pumping station, the heart. **Figure 14.6** demonstrates the journey of the blood through the systemic and pulmonary circuits.

Arterial walls are composed of three layers. The innermost layer is known as the tunica intima and is composed of the endothelium and some connective tissue. The tunica media is the middle layer and is composed of both smooth muscle and an

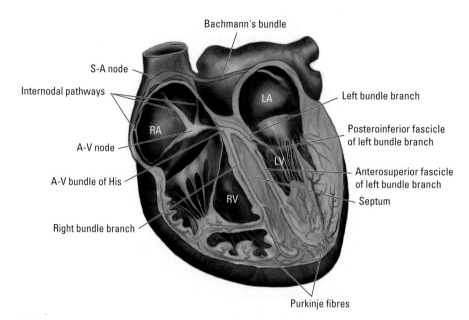

FIGURE 14.5 Conduction system of the heart. The cardiac impulse is transmitted from the S-A node to the A-V node via the internodal pathways and Bachmann's bundle, and then on to the bundle of His and down the left and right bundle branches to the Purkinje fibres, which distribute the impulse to the rest of the ventricles.

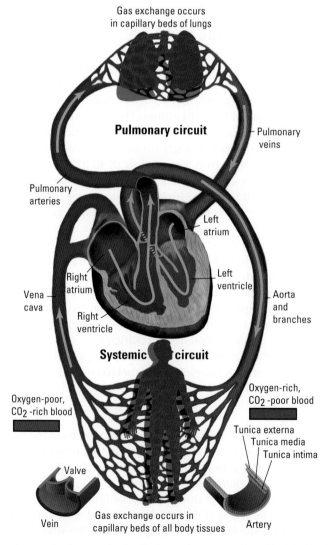

FIGURE 14.6 The systemic and pulmonary circuits. The systemic pump consists of the left side of the heart; the pulmonary circuit pump represents the right side of the heart.

elastic type of connective tissue. The outer layer, the tunica externa or adventitia, has a more fibrous connective tissue that is arranged longitudinally.

As the arterial system branches and subdivides on its way to the periphery, the diameters of the vessels decrease. Arterioles are the smallest group of arteries, with a diameter of less than 0.5 mm. It is here that the rapid velocity of blood flow found in the larger arteries begins to decrease. Blood flow becomes even slower in the capillaries arising from each arteriole. The walls of the capillaries are only one cell thick, which, coupled with the slow rate of blood flow, provides optimal conditions for the exchange of nutrients and wastes and the transfer of fluid volume between the plasma and the interstitium.

After leaving the capillaries, the blood flows into the low-pressure venous system beginning with vessels known as venules. Veins are similar in construction to arteries, but they have much less elasticity, thinner walls, and greater diameters. One-way valves are found in most veins where blood is carried against the force of gravity, such as in the lower extremities. Arteries do not have valves.

As blood passes from the arterial system through the capillaries, there is a change from the pulsatile character of arterial flow to a steady flow in the venous system. Arterial pulsations are caused by the intermittent contractions of the left ventricle. Figures 14.7 and 14.8 illustrate the arterial and venous networks of blood flow.

CLINICAL REASONING

Deterioration in the cardiovascular consumer

Consumers who experience any of the signs or symptoms noted below should be directed to follow up with a health professional. This may serve to minimise the likelihood of the development of major cardiovascular problems. Early recognition and treatment are key aspects in the management of CVD; prevention is one of the best ways to reduce complications or onset of disease.

> Change in colour of lips, face or nails
> Chest discomfort (e.g. uncomfortable pressure, squeezing, fullness or pain)
> Episode/s of a cold sweat
> Light-headedness
> Shortness of breath
> Oedema
> Extremity pain
> Fatigue
> Feeling of doom
> Numbness in the extremities
> Pain that limits self-care
> Palpitations
> Syncope
> Tingling in the extremities

Mr Marow has shortness of breath and feels light headed. Apply the clinical reasoning process to this scenario. How would you act on this situation in the community? Would your practice be different in the acute care setting? For example, in the community you would support and assess your consumer, and telephone the emergency services for urgent transport to hospital. In the acute setting you would escalate an emergency situation as per your organisation policy for a deteriorating consumer.

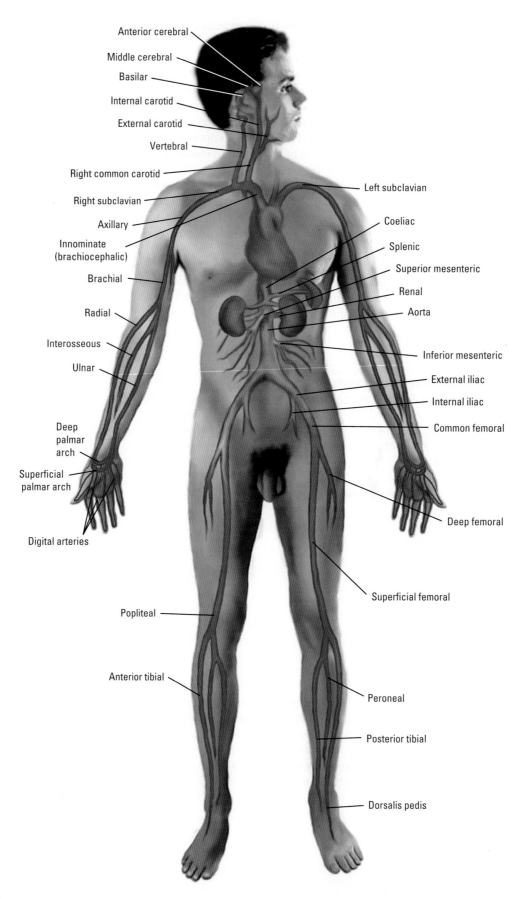

Anterior cerebral

Middle cerebral

Basilar

Internal carotid

External carotid

Vertebral

Right common carotid

Right subclavian

Axillary

Innominate
(brachiocephalic)

Brachial

Radial

Interosseous

Ulnar

Deep
palmar
arch

Superficial
palmar arch

Digital arteries

Left subclavian

Coeliac

Splenic

Superior mesenteric

Renal

Aorta

Inferior mesenteric

External iliac

Internal iliac

Common femoral

Deep femoral

Superficial femoral

Popliteal

Anterior tibial

Peroneal

Posterior tibial

Dorsalis pedis

FIGURE 14.7 Arterial system anatomy

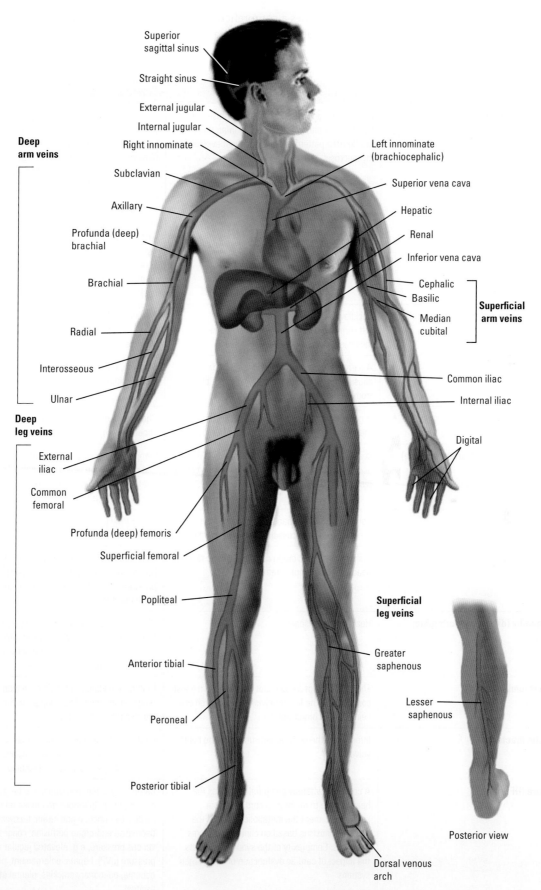

Superior
sagittal sinus

Straight sinus

External jugular

Internal jugular

**Deep
arm veins**

Right innominate

Left innominate
(brachiocephalic)

Subclavian

Superior vena cava

Axillary

Hepatic

Profunda (deep)
brachial

Renal

Inferior vena cava

Brachial

Cephalic

Basilic

**Superficial
arm veins**

Median
cubital

Radial

Interosseous

Common iliac

Ulnar

Internal iliac

**Deep
leg veins**

External
iliac

Common
femoral

Digital

Profunda (deep) femoris

Superficial femoral

Popliteal

**Superficial
leg veins**

Anterior tibial

Greater
saphenous

Peroneal

Lesser
saphenous

Posterior tibial

Posterior view

Dorsal venous
arch

FIGURE 14.8 Venous system anatomy

Table 14.2 includes a comprehensive list of key cardiovascular disorders. These are defined in the table and common assessment findings are noted for reference.

TABLE 14.2 Cardiovascular disorders

DISORDER	DEFINITION	COMMON FINDINGS
Acute coronary syndrome (ACS)	Include a broad spectrum of clinical presentation, spanning ST elevation myocardial infarction to an accelerated pattern of angina without evidence of myonecrosis	Chest pain that is similar to angina except that it is more intense and more persistent (>30 minutes), not fully relieved by rest or nitroglycerine, and accompanied by systemic symptoms (e.g. nausea, sweating, apprehension)
Aneurysm	Localised abnormal dilation of a blood vessel	Abdominal aortic aneurysm (AAA), sometimes referred to as a 'triple – A': dulled abdominal or lower back pain; nausea and vomiting; ruptured AAA – severe, sudden and continuous pain that radiates to the back Thoracic aortic aneurysm (TAA): sudden, tearing pain in chest radiating to shoulders, neck and back; dysphagia; dyspnoea
Aortic regurgitation or insufficiency	Backflow of blood from the aorta to the left ventricle during diastole because of an incompetent valve	Dyspnoea, paroxysmal nocturnal dyspnoea (PND), orthopnoea, palpitations, angina, fatigue, syncope, diastolic murmur
Aortic stenosis	A narrowing or constriction of the aortic valve causing an obstruction to the ejection of blood from the left ventricle during systole	Syncope, fatigue, weakness, palpitations, angina, systolic murmur
Arteriosclerosis	A general term used to group medical conditions that cause arteries to thicken and stiffen	Chest pain, difficulty speaking, leg, arm or shoulder pain, shortness of breath, sweating
Atherosclerosis (coronary artery disease)	Is a type of arteriosclerosis; localised accumulations of lipid-containing material, called plaque, within the blood vessels	Symptoms may vary pending affected artery, and as the plaque builds up. Angina, myocardial infarction (MI), chronic heart failure (CHF), sudden cardiac death; arrhythmias
Cardiac tamponade	Compression of the heart resulting from the accumulation of excess fluid in the pericardium	Beck's triad (hypotension, distended neck veins and distant heart sounds), pulsus paradoxus
Cardiogenic shock	A shock of cardiac origin caused by pump failure, deadly if not promptly treated	Pulmonary congestion, peripheral oedema, hypotension, tachycardia, decreased pulse pressure, cool, pale, and sweating, loss of consciousness
Cardiomyopathy (dilated, hypertrophic, restrictive)	Heart muscle disease	CHF-type symptoms; cardiomegaly with dilated form; familial history with hypertrophic form; breathlessness with or without activity; fatigue; swelling of legs, ankles and feet
Deep vein thrombosis (DVT)	The formation of a blood clot in a deep vein (most commonly in the leg or pelvis); inflammation of a vein due to a blood clot	Unilateral oedema, calf pain or tenderness, temperature and colour changes in the affected leg, cyanosis in the foot
Endocarditis (bacterial)	Infection of the endocardial surface or the heart valves	Fever, chills, fatigue, anorexia, nausea and vomiting, arthralgia, back pain, dyspnoea, splinter haemorrhages of the nails, petechiae
Heart failure (HF)	A condition whereby pump failure makes the heart unable to maintain a cardiac output sufficient to meet the metabolic needs of the body; diagnosis is based on clinical symptoms and signs. Complexity of the syndrome reflects the impact of cardiac dysfunction on body organ systems	Cardinal symptom is dyspnoea; other symptoms are fatigue, palpitations and those related to cardiac dysfunction and strain: tachycardia, decreased end-organ perfusion; congestion (high venous pressure, e.g. elevated jugular venous pressure (JVP), hepatic enlargement, peripheral oedema, pulmonary crackles, pleural effusion and ascites).

>> **TABLE 14.2** *continued*

DISORDER	DEFINITION	COMMON FINDINGS
Hypertension	Elevated blood pressure	Systolic blood pressure (SBP) >140 mmHg; diastolic blood pressure (DBP) >90 mmHg, most often asymptomatic, headaches or epistaxis (see Chapter 9 for further clarification)
Marfan syndrome (annuloaortic ectasia)	A syndrome of congenital collagen deficiency affecting the connective tissues	Consumer may be tall and thin with hyperextensive joints and long arms, legs and fingers; aortic dissection; aortic regurgitation; mitral regurgitation; arrhythmias
Metabolic syndrome (insulin-resistance syndrome)	Characterised by a group of metabolic risk factors that place consumers at greater risk for coronary artery disease, stroke, and/or peripheral vascular disease as well as type 2 diabetes mellitus	Abdominal obesity and insulin resistance or glucose intolerance are the predominant risk factors associated with this disorder; others include hyperlipidaemia, hypertension, a prothrombotic state and/or a proinflammatory state
Mitral regurgitation or insufficiency	The backflow of blood from the left ventricle to the left atrium during systole and resulting from an incompetent valve	CHF-type symptoms; history of rheumatic fever, infection, trauma, or mitral valve prolapse; systolic murmur
Mitral stenosis	A narrowing or constriction of the mitral valve causing an obstruction of blood flow from the left atrium to the left ventricle during diastole	CHF-type symptoms, history of rheumatic heart disease or congenital heart defect, diastolic murmur, thrill at apex
Myocardial infarction	Myocardial cell death due to prolonged ischaemia	Nausea and vomiting, diaphoresis, shortness of breath, abnormal heart and lung sounds, angina, arrhythmias, CHF, cardiogenic shock
Myocarditis	Inflammation of the heart's muscular tissue	History of rheumatic fever, viral or parasitic infection, irregular pulse, tenderness over the pericardium; may lead to dilated cardiomyopathy
Pericarditis	An inflammation of the pericardium; origin may be viral, malignant or autoimmune	Precordial pain that increases with inspiration or in the supine position; pain may be relieved by leaning forwards; fever, fatigue, pulsus paradoxus, pericardial friction rub
Peripheral vascular disease	Vascular disorders of the arteries (peripheral artery disease) and veins (peripheral venous disease) that supply the extremities (usually refers to arterial disease)	Changes in the skin, including decreased skin temperature, or thin, brittle, shiny skin on the legs and feet; diminished pulses in the legs and the feet; gangrene; hair loss on the legs; impotencies; restricted mobility; non-healing wounds over pressure points; numbness, weakness or heaviness in muscles; pain at rest, commonly in the toes, and at night while lying flat; pallor with elevated legs; reddish-blue discolouration of the extremities; severe pain; thickened toenails
Pulmonary regurgitation or insufficiency	The backflow of blood from the pulmonary artery to the right ventricle because of an incompetent valve	Dyspnoea on exertion, fatigue, diastolic murmur
Pulmonary stenosis	A narrowing or constriction of the pulmonary artery causing an obstruction to the ejection of blood from the right ventricle	Dyspnoea on exertion, fatigue, right-sided heart failure symptoms, systolic murmur
Rheumatic heart disease (RHD)	Damage to heart valves which arises following the development of acute rheumatic fever (acute rheumatic fever is an illness caused by a group A streptococcal (or Step A) infection	RHD is a chronic disease; symptoms may be mild and go unnoticed. Pending on the heart valve affected, type and severity of symptoms vary. Many have a heart murmur, and as the disease progresses chest pain, breathlessness, fatigue and swelling of legs can occur

>>

>> **TABLE 14.2** *continued*

DISORDER	DEFINITION	COMMON FINDINGS
Reynaud's disease	A condition caused by abnormal blood vessel spasms in the extremities, especially in response to cold temperatures	Fingers or toes become pale, cold and numb, then red, hot and tingling
Stroke (medical term cerebrovascular accident, CVA)	Brain damage that results from decreased blood flow; a stroke can have an ischaemic origin, when a blood clot blocks the supply of blood to the brain (two types: embolic and thrombotic), or a haemorrhagic cause, when the wall of a blood vessel within the brain breaks (two types: intracerebral haemorrhage (artery in the brain bursts & bleeds) and subarachnoid haemorrhage (a bleed occurs in the space surrounding the brain))	Decreased neurological function, headaches, hemiparesis, hemiplegia, aphasia, coma, abnormal cranial nerve findings The best way to remember the main symptoms of stroke are to use the word **F.A.S.T.** > Face – has their face or mouth drooped? > Arms – can they lift both arms? > Speech – is their speech slurred? Do they understand you? > Time is critical – Call triple zero (000) immediately and ask for an ambulance
Thrombus/embolus	A blood vessel blockage caused by a thrombus (a blood clot) or an embolus (a tiny mass of debris that moves through the bloodstream)	Pain, tenderness, and/or swelling around the site where the obstruction occurs
Thrombophlebitis	A blood clot in an inflamed vein; most common in the legs, but can also occur in the arms. It can result from pooling of the blood, venous wall injury, and/or altered blood coagulation	Swelling, pain, tenderness, redness, and/or warmth in the affected extremity; if a vein close to the surface of the skin is affected, the consumer may have a red, hard and/or tender cord just under the surface of the skin
Tricuspid regurgitation or insufficiency	The backflow of blood from the right ventricle to the right atrium because of an incompetent valve	Dyspnoea, fatigue, systolic murmur
Tricuspid stenosis	A narrowing or constriction of the tricuspid valve causing an obstruction of blood flow from the right atrium to the right ventricle	Dyspnoea, fatigue, diastolic murmur, right-sided HF
Ventricular aneurysm	The dilatation of a portion of necrosed ventricular wall after an MI	Tachyarrhythmias, HF-type symptoms, clot formation, arterial emboli, rupture with cardiac tamponade, systolic murmur

SOURCES: NATIONAL HEART FOUNDATION OF AUSTRALIA AND CARDIAC SOCIETY OF AUSTRALIA AND NEW ZEALAND, 2018; HEALTHDIRECT, 2022; RHDAUSTRALIA, 2022; STROKE FOUNDATION, 2022

URGENT FINDING

Chest pain
If an individual complains of chest pain, this should always be assessed immediately and treated as a priority. Use Table 14.3 to assist you to better understand the different reasons why a consumer may complain of experiencing chest pain. Escalate the situation appropriate to your area of practice. This may include consumer transfer or enacting your organisation's chest pain protocol.

REFLECTION IN PRACTICE

One-minute chest pain assessment
Undertake a 'one minute' assessment of a consumer's chest pain risk. Use the well-known acronym PQRST: **P** (precipitating), **Q** (quality), **R** (region), **S** (severity rate 1–10 scale), **T** (time). Refer to Table 14.3 for assistance with determining possible conditions that are life-threatening and require prompt action before proceeding with the consumer's health assessment. What questions have worked well for you in practice to guide this quick, important cardiovascular assessment?

Different clinical settings may use different pain assessment methods/acronyms, so look out for these.

TABLE 14.3 Differentiating chest pain

ALL OF THESE CONDITIONS (EXCLUDING MUSCULOSKELETAL) ARE LIFE-THREATENING AND REQUIRE IMMEDIATE ATTENTION.	
Myocardial ischaemia (also known as acute coronary syndrome)	**Pain:** burning, squeezing or aching, heaviness, smothering > Not reproducible by palpation of the chest wall; may be relieved with rest or oxygen if appropriate, and may or may not be accompanied by ECG changes > May lead to acute myocardial infarction; when in doubt, assume a cardiac cause and follow your institution's chest pain protocol
Aortic (thoracic) dissection	**Pain:** sudden, sharp and tearing, and radiates to shoulders, neck, back and abdomen > Neurological complications: hemiplegia, sensory deficits secondary to carotid artery occlusion > May present with a new murmur, bruits, or unequal blood pressure in upper extremities
Pericarditis	**Pain:** positional ache, dyspnoea > May also present with a pericardial friction rub or distended neck veins
Pulmonary embolus	**Pain:** sudden onset, sharp or stabbing, varies with respiration > May also present with dyspnoea, tachypnoea, fever, tachycardia, diaphoresis or DVT
Pneumothorax	**Pain:** sudden onset, tearing or pleuritic, worsened by breathing > May also have dyspnoea, tachycardia, decreased breath sounds, and a deviated trachea (refer to Chapter 13 for further information)
Pneumonia	**Pain:** stabbing that is exacerbated by coughing and deep breathing > Presents with fever, chills, productive cough, tachypnoea (refer to Chapter 13 for further information)
Oesophageal rupture	**Pain:** sudden onset upon swallowing or constant retrosternal, epigastric pain > May mimic signs and symptoms of a pneumothorax > Consider oesophageal rupture when a consumer has experienced penetrating trauma, a severe epigastric blow, or a first or second rib fracture
Musculoskeletal	**Pain:** reproducible by chest wall palpation > May be relieved by position changes
Recreational drug use (cocaine, amphetamines or stimulants)	**Pain:** Myocardial ischaemia pain (as listed above) > May produce a direct, toxic effect on the myocardium

ASSESSMENT: TAKING THE CONSUMER'S HEALTH HISTORY

Assessment is the first phase of the nursing process, and involves collecting subjective information about the consumer's health status in order to identify consumer problem areas to focus on.

Subjective data is most frequently collected during a health history and serves as the starting point for the health professional to base the depth of their assessment on. The sections for the health history include:

> **Consumer profile**

> **Chief complaint** (explained systematically using variations of location, quality, quantity, associated manifestations, aggravating factors, alleviating factors, setting and timing. This is a variation on the PQRST assessment mnemonic you may use for other conditions such as pain assessment)

> **Past health history** (including medical history, surgical history, allergies, medications, injuries and accidents, special needs and childhood illnesses)

> **Family health history**

> **Social history** (including alcohol, tobacco and drug use, sexual practice, work and home environment, hobbies and leisure activities, stress and culture).

The example health history provided identifies scope for questioning the consumer about their health for this specific body system.

Before commencing your health history, and following the introduction to your consumer, begin assessment by establishing if the consumer is in any immediate danger or is exhibiting signs of chest pain or discomfort. Establishing whether a consumer has chest pain will determine whether you proceed with gaining a health history and physical examination or whether your consumer requires prompt medical attention.

HEALTH HISTORY

CONSUMER PROFILE	colspan content
	The cardiovascular health history provides insight into the link between a consumer's life and lifestyle and heart and peripheral vasculature information and pathology. Diseases that are age- and sex-specific for the heart and blood vessel are listed. Table 14.2 differentiates the common cardiovascular disorders.

	AGE	Key age-related diseases are noted with approximate commencing/expected age range in years. > Rheumatic fever (5–15) > Reynaud's disease (18–50) > Mitral valve prolapse (20–50) > Hypertension (20–70) > Valve **stenosis** (narrowing or constriction of a diseased heart valve) or **regurgitation** (backwards flow of blood through a heart valve) (30–50) > Coronary artery disease (CAD) (40–60) > Dilated or congestive cardiomyopathy (40–60) > Myocardial infarction (MI) (40–70) > Atherosclerosis (50–70) > Cerebrovascular accident (CVA) or stroke (50–70) > Abdominal aortic aneurysm (AAA) (60–70)
	SEX	**FEMALE**	> Higher mortality rate after a severe MI, marked rise in CAD after menopause, atrial septal defect (ASD), Reynaud's disease. > Women experiencing an MI may not have the classic warning signs experienced by men. Instead, they may complain of unusual fatigue, sleep disturbance, and/or shortness of breath. > Combination hormone therapy is no longer used to prevent cardiovascular disease in healthy, postmenopausal women.
		MALE	> Marked predisposition to CAD, ventricular septal defect (VSD).
	CULTURAL BACKGROUND	**FILIPINO**	Hypertension
		ABORIGINAL AND TORRES STRAIT ISLANDER PEOPLES, MĀORI PEOPLE	> CAD, CVA > Acute rheumatic fever and rheumatic heart disease

CHIEF COMPLAINT	Common chief complaints for the heart and blood vessels are defined, and information on the characteristics of each sign or symptom is provided. Keep in mind that the following complaints can also be signs of a potential cardiovascular problem: diaphoresis; change in colour of lips, face or nails; fatigue; feeling of doom; light-headedness; peripheral oedema; shortness of breath; syncope; extremity pain; and/or tingling/numbness in the extremities.

	1. CHEST PAIN	Subjective sense of pain in the thorax; also referred to as angina if it is caused by myocardial ischaemia. Not all chest pain is angina. Table 14.3 differentiates the origins of chest pain.
		RADIATION	Arm, shoulder, neck, jaw, teeth
		QUALITY	Crushing, heavy, tight, stabbing, burning, squeezing, aching, smothering, or perceived as indigestion
		ASSOCIATED MANIFESTATIONS	Nausea and vomiting, shortness of breath (SOB), restlessness, anxiety, weakness, feeling of impending doom, diaphoresis, faintness, dizziness
		AGGRAVATING FACTORS	Exercise, stress, ingesting food
		ALLEVIATING FACTORS	Medication (e.g. nitroglycerine/glyceryl trinitrate), rest, position change
		SETTING	Most settings, sleeping (dreaming), eating, excited, stressed, exercising or resting; hot or cold environment
		TIMING	Early morning is most common, but can be any time of the day

>>

HEALTH HISTORY

2. SYNCOPE	Fainting caused by a transient decrease in cerebral blood flow	
	ASSOCIATED MANIFESTATIONS	Nausea, perspiration, palpitations, yawning, seizures, flushed face, cessation of breathing during episode, aura prior to episode
	AGGRAVATING FACTORS	Exercise, medications, fever, lack of food
	ALLEVIATING FACTORS	Rest
	SETTING	Heavy activity, hot environment, buttoning the collar of a shirt
	TIMING	Early morning, after medication, after exercise, rising from a supine or sitting position
3. PALPITATIONS	Irregular heartbeats, the sensation of a rapidly throbbing or fluttering heart	
	QUALITY	Skipped heart beats, throbbing, pounding, fluttering
	ASSOCIATED MANIFESTATIONS	Anxiety, weakness, nausea, SOB, chest pain, perspiration, fainting
	AGGRAVATING FACTORS	Smoking, caffeine, exercise
	ALLEVIATING FACTORS	Rest
	SETTING	Resting, smoking, exercising, drinking or eating food containing caffeine
	TIMING	After exercise or at rest
4. PERIPHERAL OEDEMA	Swelling of the extremities, usually the feet and hands	
	QUALITY	Imprints on swollen areas after applying pressure
	ASSOCIATED MANIFESTATIONS	Recent weight gain, pain in upper right half of abdomen, swollen abdomen, shoes tighter, rings difficult to remove from fingers
	AGGRAVATING FACTORS	Continuous standing, high salt intake
	ALLEVIATING FACTORS	Lying down or elevating the feet
5. EXTREMITY PAIN	Sense of discomfort usually occurring in the legs or feet; claudication	
	QUALITY	Temperature change in feet or leg
	ASSOCIATED MANIFESTATIONS	Swelling in the affected extremity, discolouration of the skin, tenderness, change in skin temperature
	AGGRAVATING FACTORS	Continual standing, walking, exercise, cold weather, smoking, stress
	ALLEVIATING FACTORS	Rest, elevation, dangling the extremity to a dependent position if the pain is caused by arterial insufficiency (but pain actually worsens with venous insufficiency)
	SETTING	Walking, exercise
	TIMING	Late night, early morning

>>

HEALTH HISTORY

PAST HEALTH HISTORY	The various components of the past health history are linked to heart and blood vessel pathology and related information.		
	MEDICAL HISTORY	**CARDIAC-SPECIFIC**	Angina, cardiogenic shock, cardiomyopathy, chest trauma, congenital anomalies, heart failure (HF), CAD, endocarditis, hyperlipoproteinaemia, hypertension, MI, myocarditis, pericarditis, peripheral vascular disease, rheumatic fever, valvular disease, rheumatic heart disease
		NON-CARDIAC-SPECIFIC	Bleeding or blood disorder, diabetes mellitus, gout, Marfan syndrome, phaeochromocytoma, primary aldosteronism, renal artery disease, stroke, thyroid disease
	SURGICAL HISTORY	Ablation of accessory pathways, aneurysm repair, cardiac catheterisation, chest surgery for trauma, congenital heart repair, coronary artery bypass graft, coronary stents, directional coronary atherectomy, electrophysiology studies, heart transplant, implantable or internal cardioverter/defibrillator (ICD) placement, myotomy or myectomy, percutaneous laser myoplasty, pacemaker insertion, percutaneous transluminal coronary angioplasty or other type of percutaneous coronary intervention (PCI), pericardial window, pericardiectomy, pericardiotomy, peripheral vascular grafting and bypass, valve replacement		
	ALLERGIES	Aspirin (most consumers who are recovering from an MI receive aspirin), intravenous pyelogram dye and seafood (both contain iodine compounds used in the dye that is injected during a cardiac catheterisation), latex (found in gloves used for procedures), betadine (which is used as a skin surface prep for cardiac and vascular procedures)		
	MEDICATIONS	Antianginals, antiarrhythmics, anticoagulants, antihypertensives, antilipidaemics, β-blockers, diuretics, inotropics, thrombolytic enzymes, vasodilators		
	COMMUNICABLE DISEASES	Rheumatic fever (valvular dysfunction), untreated syphilis (aortic regurgitation, aortitis, aortic aneurysm), viral myocarditis (cardiomyopathy)		
	INJURIES AND ACCIDENTS	Chest trauma (falls, motor vehicle accidents, blunt force)		
	CHILDHOOD ILLNESSES	Rheumatic fever (valvular dysfunction)		
FAMILY HEALTH HISTORY	Heart and blood vessel diseases that are familial are listed: Aneurysm, stroke, CAD, hypertension, hypertrophic cardiomyopathy, Marfan syndrome, mitral valve prolapse, acute myocardial infarction (AMI), Reynaud's disease, rheumatic fever, sudden cardiac death, long QT syndrome, congenital cardiac defects		
SOCIAL HISTORY	The components of the social history are linked to heart and blood vessel factors and pathology.		
	ALCOHOL USE	Prolonged use of alcohol can interfere with the normal pumping function and electrical activity of the heart, leading to **cardiomegaly** (enlargement of the heart), poor left ventricular contractility, ventricular dilatation, palpitations, peripheral oedema, fatigue and SOB. Thiamine deficiencies that usually occur concurrently with alcohol abuse may contribute to arrhythmias and heart failure. Excessive alcohol intake may play a role in the pathogenesis of dilated cardiomyopathy, angina, CAD, hypertension, arrhythmias, stroke, and beriberi heart disease. However, the intake of alcohol in moderation, up to 57 g a day, is inversely related to the development of CAD due to the protective effect of the increased HDL cholesterol.		
	TOBACCO USE	Nicotine increases catecholamine release, leading to elevated cardiac output, heart rate and blood pressure. Nicotine also inhibits the development of collateral circulation, causes peripheral vasoconstriction, thickens cardiac arterioles, causes platelet aggregation, leads to arrhythmias, and neutralises heparin, thus increasing the risk of thrombus formation. The tobacco habit contributes to the pathogenesis of CAD, angina and atherosclerosis.		

CHAPTER 14

>>

HEALTH HISTORY

DRUG USE	Intravenous drug use: Increased risk for contracting infective endocarditis because of the use of nonsterile needles and the embolisation of localised infections from the injection site. Amphetamines, cocaine and heroin: Tachycardia, severe hypertension, hypotension, coronary vasospasm, MI, arrhythmias, aortic rupture or dissection, coronary artery dissection, stroke, and dilated cardiomyopathy.	
SEXUAL PRACTICE	Effect of intercourse on the heart (such as exertional chest pain) or eliciting a vagal response (which may occur with anal intercourse), thus making the consumer prone to syncope and other sequelae. Consumers who use nitrate drugs should never take phosphodiesterase type 5 inhibitors.	
WORK ENVIRONMENT	Exposure to cardiotoxic substances can cause profound cardiac pathology.	
HOME ENVIRONMENT	Smoke in the environment can lead to the worsening of chest pain. Passive smoking poses an increased risk to CHD.	
HOBBIES AND LEISURE ACTIVITIES	Any activity that involves exertion may contribute to a decline in status in a consumer with cardiovascular pathology.	
STRESS	Atherosclerosis, tachycardia, hypertension, arrhythmias, sudden death	

Calculating target heart rate zone

1. Subtract the consumer's age in years from 220 to calculate the consumer's maximum heart rate.
2. The low end of the consumer's target heart rate (THR) zone is 50% of the value obtained in step 1. The high end of the consumer's THR zone is 85% of the value obtained in step 1. For example, the THR zone of a 48-year-old would be calculated as follows:

    $$(220 - 48) \times 0.50 = 86 \text{ (low end)}$$
    $$(220 - 48) \times 0.85 = 146 \text{ (high end)}$$

    Thus, the consumer's THR zone (range) would be 86–146 beats per minute.
3. If the consumer's goal is weight management and/or to burn fat, then the consumer should train to 50–65% of the maximum heart rate determined in step 1. If the consumer's goal is purely aerobic exercise, then the consumer should train to 65–85% of the maximum heart rate calculated in step 1.

HEALTH EDUCATION

Risk factors for chronic arterial insufficiency and varicose veins

When assessing consumers, consider the following risk factors related to chronic arterial insufficiency and varicose veins. Your knowledge recall about these risk factors may lead you to more in-depth questioning and assessment for consumers who display these risks. This should then be considered for planning health education and further interventions.

Risk factors for chronic arterial insufficiency

> Age (>60 years old)
> Smoking
> Sex (men more than women)
> Hypertension
> Diabetes mellitus
> Hyperlipidaemia

>>

Risk factors for varicose veins

Varicose veins affect approximately 10% of the adult population and occur four times more often in women than in men. The pathogenesis of varicose veins remains unknown; however, it is not uncommon to find varicose veins in consumers:

> who have a family history of varicose veins
> whose occupation requires long periods of standing
> who are obese
> who are pregnant.

Health professionals can intervene with consumers in assisting them to address their modifiable risk factors, using health education approaches. Areas for health education evolve around the following:

> Cease smoking
> Control blood pressure and hyperlipidaemia
> Avoid heavy lifting
> Manage diet to reduce weight gain and control diabetes mellitus
> Do not cross legs
> Wear support panty hose
> Elevate feet while sitting
> Encourage regular exercise

Person-centred health education

When conducting a health assessment, opportunities for the provision of person-centred health education will arise. This is a significant consideration in relation to the assessment process for examination of the cardiovascular system. These occasions are identified as individualised education and may generate further data that can be added to the assessment. All education given should be documented so that, in future, health professionals can assess the impact of previous information provided to the consumer. (Refer to Chapter 1 for initiating health education.)

The following table provides examples of individualised health education interventions related to cardiovascular health.

HEALTH EDUCATION

Exercise and cardiovascular health

Educate individuals about the benefits of physical activity for their heart, body and mind. The following should be considered:

> Always consult with your primary care provider before starting an exercise program. This may be determined through stress tests, bicycle tests or treadmill tests.
> Avoid activities that have caused previous cardiac problems.
> Avoid strenuous activity in extremes of temperature or after a heavy meal because this may predispose to angina.
> Stop any exercise and notify the primary care provider if dizziness, faintness, light-headedness or angina occurs (National Heart Foundation of Australia, 2021c).
> In 2019, the Heart Foundation produced the third edition of *Blueprint for an active Australia*. This blueprint has 13 action areas, detailing how to increase physical activity (National Heart Foundation of Australia, 2019).

See the Further Resources list at the end of this chapter for the Heart Foundation of Australia, 'Physical activity and your heart health', and the physical activity guidelines of the New Zealand Ministry of Health.

INDIVIDUALISED HEALTH EDUCATION INTERVENTIONS

Assessing the consumer for the following health-related activities can assist in identifying the need for education about these factors. This information provides a bridge between the health maintenance activities and the heart and blood vessel functions.

Sleep	Disturbance in sleep due to dyspnoea, orthopnoea or paroxysmal nocturnal dyspnoea
Diet	> Eating disorders (e.g. bulimia) and liquid protein diets have been associated with sudden death due to electrolyte imbalances (e.g. hypokalaemia). > Foods high in vitamin K may reduce the effectiveness of anticoagulants. > Awareness of the sodium content of the tap water in your area (home water softeners often contain sodium). > Caffeine (in coffee, tea, soft drinks, chocolate, over-the-counter medications) is a sympathomimetic amine that increases the blood pressure and heart rate, elevates the serum catecholamine level, and can lead to arrhythmias (especially premature atrial contractions). > BMI normal score should be 18.5–24.9 (see Chapter 15).
Exercise	Physical exercise may have either deleterious or beneficial effects on the heart, depending on the type and amount of activity performed, and the condition of the exerciser. The aim of an individual's cardiovascular fitness program should be the attainment of the target heart rate (THR) (also known as perceived rate of exertion; see the section Calculating target heart rate zone) to increase cardiovascular tone. In general, it is believed that aerobic exercise or sustained physical activity for at least 20 to 30 minutes per day, three to five times per week, positively affects cardiovascular conditioning.
Stress management	Exercise, time management, activities with pets, reading, listening to music, eating, biofeedback, yoga, meditation, imagery, massage, and participation in a variety of support groups are all helpful.
Use of safety devices	Consumers with pacemakers should avoid close or prolonged contact with electrical devices or devices that have strong magnetic fields. Examples include smart phones, tablets, household devices such as microwave ovens and metal detectors, as these may cause interference with pacemakers.
Health check-ups	Regular health check-ups are advised and will usually include undertaking an ECG, chest X-ray, blood pressure measurement, pulse rate, serum lipid profile, and fasting blood glucose level.

HEALTH EDUCATION

Age care standards: Consumer dignity and choice

The Australian Government, Aged Care Quality and Safety Commission in 2019 released eight Aged Care Quality Standards, to assist aged care services to implement and maintain compliance with standards. Standard 1 titled Consumer dignity and choice, recognises the significance of the consumer and their sense of self and highlights their ability to act independently, make personal choices and take part in the community.

This standard supports the need for health professionals to engage in partnership with consumers to develop individualised and realistic management plans. This is especially important for consumers with known cardiovascular disease, to ensure side effects are minimised.

The Australian Government Aged Care Quality and Safety Commission Resource Library contains a rich source of online resource to assist working with health management and the older person.

https://www.agedcarequality.gov.au/resource-library?resources%5B0%5D=topics%3A211

NYHA classification system: Patient functional capacity

The New York Heart Association (NYHA) has outlined four classifications for patients with cardiac pathologies, with a focus on a patient's functional capacity. This classification scale is used widely in health care in Australia and New Zealand.

> Class I: The consumer has no symptoms with ordinary physical activity.
> Class II: The consumer has some symptoms with normal activity and may have a slight limitation of activity.
> Class III: The consumer has symptoms with less than ordinary activity and has a marked limit of activity.
> Class IV: The consumer has symptoms with any physical activity or even at rest.

When assessing your patient's functional capacity and any changes to this, the NYHA classification system is a useful assessment tool. For example, Nina, a 94-year-old, is normally able to walk up one flight of stairs without feeling short of breath. Over the last two months she has become unable to walk up more than three steps without experiencing dyspnoea. Assessing against the NYHA scale, Nina has moved from Class I to Class III. Note that when assessing for change you will always need to know a person's normal functional activity level.

Note: The NYHA refers to the consumer as the patient in this classification system.

PLANNING FOR PHYSICAL EXAMINATION

The planning phase refers to evaluating subjective data to narrow the focus on physical examination, determining what objective data needs to be gathered, as well as considering the environment and equipment that will be required.

At this time, you will identify which of the four diagnostic techniques you will need to implement the physical examination, and how you will sequence these. For the physical examination of the cardiovascular system (heart and blood vessels) you will include inspection, palpation, percussion and auscultation.

Objective data is:

> collected during the physical examination of the consumer
> usually collected after subjective data
> information that is measured or observed by the clinician as opposed to being reported by the consumer
> vital to the overall health assessment, to enable you to make clinical decisions that are representative of the whole consumer picture.

Evaluating subjective data to focus physical examination

Before commencing the physical examination of the consumer's cardiovascular system, which includes the heart and blood vessels, consider what information the health history has provided. Critical consideration, linked to knowledge of anatomy and physiology, should focus the physical assessment so your examination will be more effective and efficient.

Environment

Assessing the heart and blood vessels requires a physical environment in the healthcare setting that has:

> a flat table/surface for the consumer to lie on
> minimal noise for accurate auscultation of heart sounds and other sounds
> adequate lighting
> adequate privacy for the consumer.

Equipment

Assemble items before placing the consumer on the examination table. Materials should be arranged in order of use and within easy reach.

> Examination table
> Stethoscope
> Sphygmomanometer
> Watch with second hand
> Tape measure
> Weighing scales
> Linen for draping.

IMPLEMENTATION: CONDUCTING THE PHYSICAL EXAMINATION

Physical examination of the cardiovascular system has two major components:

> assessment of the **precordium** (the area on the anterior surface of the body overlying the heart, great vessels, pericardium and some pulmonary tissue)
> assessment of the blood vessels (also referred to as assessment of the peripheral blood vessels or peripheral vascular system).

Implementation of the physical examination requires you to consider your scope of practice as well. In this section, depending on your context, you may be performing a foundation assessment, or the addition of advanced assessment techniques if you are practising in a specialised area.

EXAMINATION **IN BRIEF: CARDIOVASCULAR**

Examination of the precordium

Inspection
> Aortic area
> Pulmonic area
> Midprecordial area (Erb's point)
> Tricuspid area
> Mitral area

Palpation
> Aortic area
> Pulmonic area
> Midprecordial area (Erb's point)
> Tricuspid area
> Mitral area

Auscultation
> Aortic area
> Pulmonic area
> Midprecordial area (Erb's point)
> Tricuspid area
> Mitral area
> Mitral and tricuspid areas (S_3)
> Mitral and tricuspid areas (S_4)
> Murmurs
> Pericardial friction rub
> Pericardial friction rub versus pleural friction rub
> Prosthetic heart valves

Examining consumers with cardiovascular supportive equipment

Examination of the blood vessels

Inspection
> Jugular venous pressure
> Hepatojugular reflux

Palpation and auscultation
> Arterial pulses
> Examining for pulsus paradoxus

Inspection and palpation of blood vessels for peripheral perfusion
> Orthostatic hypotension assessment

Examination of the venous system

Inspection
> Homan's sign

Examination of the arterial system

Inspection
> Pallor
> Colour return and capillary refill
> Allen test
> Ankle–brachial index (ABI)

Inspection and palpation of lymph nodes

Advanced Assessment

General approach to heart assessment

Prior to the assessment:

1. Introduce yourself to the consumer and explain the assessment technique and approach that you will be using.
2. Ensure that the examination room is warm, quiet and well lit.
3. Expose the consumer's chest only as much as is needed for the assessment.
4. Position the consumer in a supine or sitting position.
5. Stand to the consumer's right side. The light should come from the side opposite where you are standing so that shadows can be accentuated.

Examination of the precordium

Inspection, palpation and auscultation should be performed in a systematic manner, using certain cardiac landmarks. Percussion has limited usefulness in the cardiovascular assessment because X-rays and other diagnostic tests provide the same information in a much more accurate manner. The cardiac landmarks (**Figure 14.9**) are defined as follows:

1. The aortic area is the second intercostal space (ICS) to the right of the sternum.
2. The pulmonic area is the second ICS to the left of the sternum.
3. The midprecordial area, Erb's point, is located in the third ICS to the left of the sternum.
4. The tricuspid area is the fifth ICS to the left of the sternum. Other terms for this area are the right ventricular area or the septal area.
5. The mitral area is the fifth ICS at the left midclavicular line. Other terms for this area are the left ventricular area or the apical area.

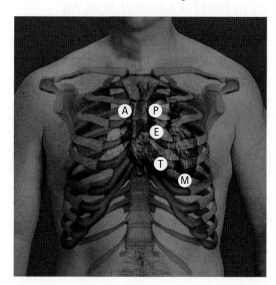

FIGURE 14.9 The cardiac landmarks: A = aortic area; P = pulmonic area; E = Erb's point; T = tricuspid area; M = mitral area

These cardiac landmarks are the locations where the heart sounds are heard best, not where the valves are actually located. The mitral area correlates anatomically with the apex of the heart; the aortic and pulmonic areas correlate anatomically with the base of the heart. Examination of the heart should proceed in an orderly fashion from the base of the heart to the apex, or from the apex of the heart to the base.

Inspection

Aortic area

E 1. Lightly place your index finger on the **angle of Louis** (see **Figure 13.2**).
   2. Move your finger laterally to the right of the sternum to the rib. This is the second rib.
   3. Move your finger down beneath the second rib to the ICS. The aortic area is located in the second ICS to the right of the sternum.

N No pulsations should be visible.

A A pulsation in the aortic area is abnormal.

P A pulsation in the aortic area may indicate the presence of an aortic root aneurysm. The aneurysm's dilation may become bigger when the consumer experiences hypertension. A rupture can occur at any time, but the risk is greater when the aneurysm becomes 5 cm or more in diameter.

Pulmonic area

E 1. Lightly place your index finger on the left second ICS.
   2. The pulmonic area is located at the second ICS to the left of the sternum.

N No pulsations should be visible.

A A pulsation or bulge in the pulmonic area is an abnormal finding.

P Pulmonary stenosis, which is usually congenital, impedes blood flow from the right ventricle into the lungs, causing a bulge. The right side of the heart then dilates and the right ventricle becomes hypertrophied in order to accommodate the load.

Midprecordial area (Erb's point)

E 1. Lightly place your index finger on the left second ICS.
   2. Continue to move your finger down the left rib cage, counting the third rib and the third ICS.
   3. The midprecordial area, or Erb's point, is located at the third ICS, left sternal border. Both aortic and pulmonic murmurs may be heard here.

N No pulsations should be visible.

A The presence of a pulsation or a systolic bulge in the midprecordial area is not normal.

P A left ventricular aneurysm can produce a midprecordial pulsation. Ventricular aneurysms can develop several weeks following an acute myocardial infarction (AMI). With an AMI, the hydraulic stress on the infarcted area may cause the damaged ventricular wall to bulge and become extremely thin during systole.

A A retraction in the midprecordial area is abnormal.

P Pericardial disease can produce retractions in this area (retractions occur when there is a pulling in of some of the tissues of the precordium, depending on the activities of the heart).

Tricuspid area

E 1. Lightly place your index finger on the left third ICS.
   2. Continue to move down the left rib cage, counting the fourth rib, the fourth ICS, and the fifth rib followed by the fifth ICS.
   3. The tricuspid area is located at the fifth ICS, left of the sternal border.

N No pulsations should be visible.

A A visible systolic pulsation in the tricuspid area is abnormal.

P A visible systolic pulsation can result from right ventricular enlargement secondary to an increased stroke volume. Anxiety, hyperthyroidism, fever and pregnancy are clinical situations that produce an increased stroke volume.

E Examination **N** Normal findings **A** Abnormal findings **P** Pathophysiology

Mitral area

E **1.** Lightly place your index finger on the left fifth ICS.
   2. Move your finger laterally to the midclavicular line. This is the mitral landmark. In a large-breasted consumer, have the consumer displace the left breast upwards and to the left so you can locate the mitral landmark.

N Normally, there is no movement in the precordium except at the mitral area, where the left ventricle lies close enough to the skin's surface that it visibly pulsates during systole. The apical impulse at the mitral landmark is generally visible in about half of the adult population. This pulsation is also known as the point of maximal impulse (but the term is used infrequently) and occurs simultaneously with carotid pulsation.

A **Hypokinetic** (decreased movement) pulsations at the mitral area are considered abnormal.

P Conditions that place more fluid between the left ventricle and the chest wall, such as a pericardial effusion or cardiac tamponade, produce a hypokinetic or absent pulsation. In obese individuals, excess subcutaneous tissue dampens the apical impulse. Low-output states such as shock produce a less palpable apical impulse as a result of the reduced blood volume and decreased myocardial contractility. Keep in mind that absent pulsations are normal in half of the adult population.

A **Hyperkinetic** (increased movement) pulsations are always abnormal when located at the mitral area.

P High-output states such as mitral regurgitation, thyrotoxicosis, severe anaemia and left-to-right heart shunts are potential causes of hyperkinetic pulsations.

Palpation

Palpation follows inspection. You must be systematic in this part of the assessment and palpate the cardiac landmarks starting at either the base or the apex of the heart. During palpation, assess for the apical impulse, pulsations, **thrills** (vibrations that feel similar to what one feels when a hand is placed on a purring cat), and **heaves** (lifting of the cardiac area secondary to an increased workload and force of left ventricular contraction; also referred to as lift). The consumer should be in a supine position for this portion of the assessment.

Palpate the cardiac landmarks for:

E **1.** pulsations: Using the finger pads, locate the cardiac landmark and palpate the area for pulsations (**Figure 14.10**).
   2. thrills: Using the palmar surface of the hand at the base of the fingers (also known as the ball of the hand), locate the cardiac landmark and palpate the area for thrills (**Figure 14.11**).
   3. heaves: Follow step 2 and palpate the area for heaves.

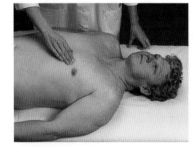

FIGURE 14.10 Palpating for pulsations

Aortic area

E Palpate the aortic area for pulsations, thrills and heaves.

N No pulsations, thrills or heaves should be palpated.

A Palpation of a thrill in the aortic area is abnormal.

P Aortic stenosis and aortic regurgitation create turbulent blood flow in the left ventricle, which may be palpated as a thrill.

Pulmonic area

E Palpate the pulmonic area for pulsations, thrills and heaves.

N No pulsations, thrills or heaves should be palpated.

A Palpation of a thrill in the pulmonic area is abnormal.

P Pulmonic stenosis and pulmonic regurgitation create turbulent blood flow in the right ventricle, which may be palpated as a thrill.

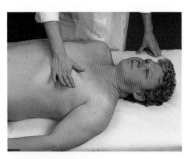

FIGURE 14.11 Palpating for thrills

E Examination **N** Normal findings **A** Abnormal findings **P** Pathophysiology

Midprecordial area (Erb's point)

E Palpate the midprecordial area for pulsations, thrills and heaves.

N No pulsations, thrills or heaves should be palpated.

A Palpation of pulsations in the midprecordial area is abnormal.

P Both a left ventricular aneurysm and an enlarged right ventricle can produce a pulsation in the midprecordial area.

Tricuspid area

E Palpate the tricuspid area for pulsations, thrills and heaves.

N No pulsations, thrills or heaves should be felt.

A Palpation of a thrill in the tricuspid area is abnormal.

P Tricuspid stenosis and tricuspid regurgitation create turbulent blood flow in the right atrium, which may be palpated as a thrill.

A Palpation of a heave in the tricuspid area is abnormal.

P Right ventricular enlargement may produce a heave in the tricuspid area secondary to an increased workload.

Mitral area

E Palpate the mitral area for pulsations, thrills and heaves. If a pulsation (apical impulse) is not palpable, turn the consumer to the left side and palpate in this position (**Figure 14.12**). This position facilitates palpation because the heart shifts closer to the chest wall.

N The apical impulse is palpable in approximately half of the adult population. It is felt as a light, localised tap that is 1 to 2 cm in diameter. The amplitude is small and it can be felt immediately after the first heart sound, lasting for about one-half of systole. This impulse may be exaggerated in young consumers. A thrill is not found in the normal adult population. A heave is absent in the healthy adult.

A A thrill palpated at the fifth ICS at the left midclavicular line is considered abnormal.

P Mitral stenosis and mitral regurgitation may produce a thrill from the turbulent blood flow found in the left atrium.

E A visible heave, or sustained apex beat, displaced laterally to the left sixth ICS at the anterior axillary line is abnormal. It is usually more than 3 cm in diameter and has a large amplitude.

P Left ventricular hypertrophy produces a laterally displaced apical impulse because of the increased size of the left ventricle in the thorax and the subsequent shifting of the heart. In addition, the hypertrophied muscle works harder during a contraction to produce a heave or sustained apex beat. This frequently occurs in conditions such as aortic stenosis, systemic hypertension and idiopathic hypertrophic subaortic stenosis (which is a form of hypertrophic cardiomyopathy).

A Hypokinetic pulsations, usually less than 1 to 2 cm in diameter and of small amplitude, are abnormal.

P Conditions that place more fluid between the left ventricle and the chest wall, such as a pericardial effusion or cardiac tamponade, produce a hypokinetic or absent pulsation. In obesity, the excess subcutaneous tissue dampens the apical impulse. Low-output states such as shock produce a less palpable apical impulse as a result of the reduced blood volume and decreased myocardial contractility.

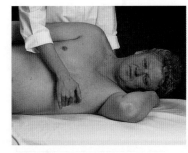

FIGURE 14.12 Palpating the apical impulse with the consumer on the left side

---

E Examination **N** Normal findings **A** Abnormal findings **P** Pathophysiology ▮ Advanced Assessment

UNIT 2

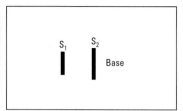

A. Normal S_2

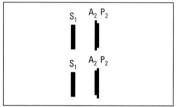

B. Intensified A_2, diminished A_2

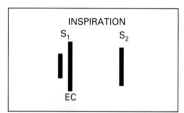

C. Ejection click

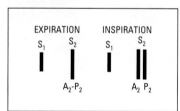

D. Normal physiological split of S_2

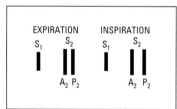

E. Wide splitting of S_2

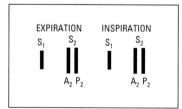

F. Fixed splitting of S_2

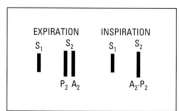

G. Paradoxical splitting of S_2

FIGURE 14.13 Summation of heart sounds

A Hyperkinetic pulsations, usually greater than 1 to 2 cm in diameter and of increased amplitude, are abnormal.

P High-output states such as mitral regurgitation, thyrotoxicosis, severe anaemia, and left-to-right heart shunts are potential causes of hyperkinetic pulsations.

Auscultation

Aortic area

E Place the diaphragm of the stethoscope on the aortic landmark and listen for S_2.

N S_2 is caused by the closure of the semilunar valves. S_2 corresponds to the 'dub' sound in the phonetic 'lub-dub' representation of heart sounds. S_2 heralds the onset of diastole. S_2 is louder than S_1 at this landmark (**Figure 14.13A**).

A The components of S_2 are A_2 (aortic) and P_2 (pulmonic). A greatly intensified or diminished A_2 is considered abnormal (**Figure 14.13B**).

P Arterial hypertension, which increases the pressure in the aorta, may be suspected in the case of a greatly intensified A_2. Aortic stenosis, in which the aortic valve is calcified or thickened, may be the cause of a diminished A_2.

A An ejection **click** is an abnormal systolic sound that is high pitched and can radiate in the chest wall. It is created by the opening of the damaged valve and it does not vary with the respiratory cycle. An ejection click follows S_1 (**Figure 14.13C**).

P An ejection click can be auscultated in aortic stenosis, in which the calcified valve produces this sound on opening.

Pulmonic area

E Place the diaphragm of the stethoscope on the chest wall at the pulmonic landmark and listen for S_2.

N S_2 is also heard in the pulmonic area. S_2 is louder than S_1 at this landmark, as depicted in **Figure 14.13A**. It is softer than the S_2 auscultated in the aortic area because the pressure on the left side of the heart is greater than that on the right. There is a normal physiological splitting of S_2 that is heard best at the pulmonic area. The components of a split S_2 are A_2 (aortic) and P_2 (pulmonic) (see **Figure 14.13D**). The aortic component occurs slightly before the pulmonic component during inspiration. The physiology of a split S_2 is that during inspiration, because of the more negative intrathoracic pressure, the venous return to the right side of the heart increases. Thus, pulmonic closure is delayed because of the extra time needed for the increased blood volume to pass through the valve. Normally, the A_2 component of the split S_2 is louder than the P_2 component because of the greater pressures in the left side of the heart.

A When a split S_2 occurs that is abnormally wide, the aortic valve closes early and the pulmonic valve closes late. There is a split on both inspiration and expiration, but a wider split on inspiration, as shown in **Figure 14.13E**.

P Delayed closure of the pulmonic valve may be due to a delay in the electrical stimulation of the right ventricle, as seen with right bundle branch block.

A Fixed splitting, a wide splitting that does not change with inspiration or expiration, is abnormal (**Figure 14.13F**). The pulmonic valve consistently closes later than the aortic valve. The right side of the heart is already ejecting a large volume, so filling cannot be increased during inspiration.

P Right ventricular failure that results in a prolonged right ventricular systole or a large atrial septal defect can lead to fixed splitting.

A In paradoxical splitting, the aortic valve closes after the pulmonic valve because of the delay in left ventricular systole. This occurs during expiration and disappears with inspiration. It is considered abnormal (**Figure 14.13G**).

E Examination **N** Normal findings **A** Abnormal findings **P** Pathophysiology Advanced Assessment

P Left bundle branch block, aortic stenosis, patent ductus arteriosus, severe hypertension and left ventricular failure are conditions in which paradoxical splitting may be auscultated.

A A pulmonic ejection click always indicates an abnormality (**Figure 14.13H**).

P A pulmonic ejection click is caused by the opening of a diseased pulmonic valve. It is heard loudest on expiration and is quieter on inspiration. It occurs early in systole and it does not radiate.

A A P$_2$ that is louder than or equal in volume to A$_2$ is abnormal, as is a greatly diminished P$_2$ (**Figure 14.13I**).

P A loud P$_2$ is expected in pulmonary hypertension, where the pressures in the pulmonary artery are abnormally high; pulmonic stenosis, in which the pulmonic valve is calcified or thickened, may be the cause of a diminished P$_2$.

Midprecordial area (Erb's point)

Erb's point is where both aortic and pulmonic murmurs may be auscultated. Refer to the discussion on murmurs later in this chapter for additional information.

Tricuspid area

E Place the diaphragm of the stethoscope on the chest wall at the tricuspid landmark to listen for S$_1$.

N S$_1$ in the tricuspid area is softer than the S$_1$ auscultated in the mitral area, because the pressure in the left side of the heart is greater than that in the right. S$_1$ is louder than S$_2$ at this landmark (see **Figure 14.13J**). There is a normal physiological splitting of S$_1$ that is best heard in the tricuspid area (see **Figure 14.13K**). This split occurs because the mitral valve closes slightly before the tricuspid valve due to greater pressures in the left side of the heart. The components of a split S$_1$ are M$_1$ (mitral) and T$_1$ (tricuspid). Physiological splitting disappears when the consumer holds their breath.

A A split S$_1$ with an abnormally wide split is pathological (**Figure 14.13L**). The split is wider than usual during inspiration and is still heard on expiration.

P A split S$_1$ is usually due to electrical malfunctions such as right bundle branch block or mechanical problems such as mitral stenosis. In mitral stenosis, the tricuspid valve can close before the mitral valve closes because of calcification of the diseased mitral valve.

Mitral area

E 1. Place the diaphragm of the stethoscope over the mitral area to identify S$_1$.
2. If you are unable to distinguish S$_1$ from S$_2$, palpate the carotid artery with the hand closest to the head while auscultating the mitral landmark. You will hear S$_1$ with each carotid pulse beat.

N S$_1$ is heard the loudest in the mitral area. S$_1$ is caused by the closure of the mitral and tricuspid valves. S$_1$ corresponds to the 'lub' sound in the phonetic 'lub-dub' representation of heart sounds. S$_1$ is louder than S$_2$ at this landmark (**Figure 14.13J**). S$_1$ also heralds the onset of systole. At normal or slow heart rates, systole (the time occurring between S$_1$ and S$_2$) is usually shorter than diastole. Diastole constitutes two-thirds of the cardiac cycle, with systole being the other third. The intensity of S$_1$ depends on:
1. the adequacy of the A-V cusps in halting the ventricular blood flow
2. the mobility of the cusps
3. the position of the cusps and the rate of ventricular contraction.

A An abnormally loud S$_1$ occurs when the mitral valve is wide open when systolic contraction begins, then slams shut (**Figure 14.13M**).

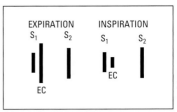
H. Pulmonic ejection click

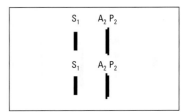
I. Intensified P$_2$, diminished P$_2$

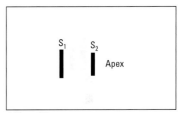
J. Normal S$_1$

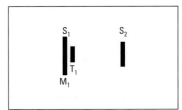
K. Normal physiological split of S$_1$

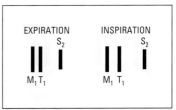
L. Wide split of S$_1$

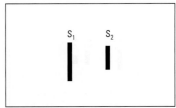
M. Loud S$_1$

FIGURE 14.13 *continued* Summation of heart sounds

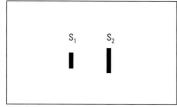

N. Soft S₁

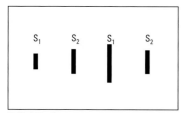

O. Variable S₁

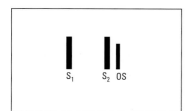

P. Opening snap

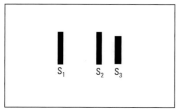

Q. S₃

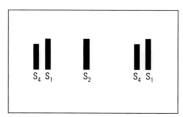

R. S₄

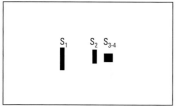

S. Summation gallop

FIGURE 14.13 *continued* Summation of heart sounds

P A loud S_1 occurs in mitral stenosis, short PR interval syndrome (0.11 to 0.13 second), or in high-output states such as tachycardia, hyperthyroidism and exercise.

A A soft S_1 is abnormal (**Figure 14.13N**).

P A soft S_1 can occur as a result of rheumatic fever, where the mitral valve has only limited motion.

P A variable abnormal S_1 occurs when diastolic filling time varies. Both a soft and a loud S_1 can be auscultated (**Figure 14.13O**).

A A variable S_1 can occur with complete heart block, in which the atria and the ventricles are beating independently, and in atrial fibrillation, in which the ventricles are beating irregularly.

A An opening snap is an early diastolic sound that is high-pitched. It is abnormal (**Figure 14.13P**).

P An opening snap is caused by the opening of a diseased valve and can be auscultated in mitral stenosis. The sound does not vary with respirations and can radiate throughout the chest. It follows S_2 and can be differentiated from an S_3 because it occurs earlier than an S_3.

A In tachycardia, the heart rate increases, diastole shortens, and systole and diastole become increasingly difficult to distinguish. Tachycardia is abnormal.

P Tachycardia can occur in exercise, fever, anxiety, pregnancy and conditions that lead to hypertrophy, such as heart failure.

Mitral and tricuspid areas (S_3)

Auscultation of the mitral and tricuspid areas is repeated for low-pitched sounds, specifically an S_3 (otherwise known as a ventricular diastolic **gallop**, or extra heart sound). An S_3 is an early diastolic filling sound that originates in the ventricles and is therefore heard best at the apex of the heart. A right-sided S_3 (tricuspid area) is heard louder during inspiration because the venous return to the right side of the heart increases with a more negative intrathoracic pressure. An S_3 sound occurs just after an S_2 (**Figure 14.13Q**).

It might help you to focus and fine tune your listening skills for detecting an S_3 additional heart sound by saying out loud or pronouncing the word *Kentucky*. It is thought that doing this resembles the beat/rhythm of the S_3 heart sound:

S_1	S_2	S_3
Ken	túc	ky

E 1. Place the bell of the stethoscope lightly over the mitral landmark. When the S_3 originates in the left ventricle, it is heard best with the consumer in a left lateral decubitus position and they are exhaling.
2. When originating in the right ventricle, an S_3 can best be heard by placing the bell of the stethoscope lightly over the third or fourth ICS at the left sternal border.
3. Auscultate for 10 to 15 seconds for a left- or right-sided S_3.

N An S_3 heart sound can be a normal physiological sound in children and in young adults. After the age of 30, a physiological S_3 is very infrequent. An S_3 can also be normal in high-output states such as the third trimester of pregnancy.

A In an adult, an S_3 heart sound may be one of the earliest clinical findings of cardiac dysfunction. A loud, persistent S_3 can be an ominous sign. The average life expectancy after a persistent S_3 sound is detected is approximately 4 to 5 years.

E Examination **N** Normal findings **A** Abnormal findings **P** Pathophysiology Advanced Assessment

P An S$_3$ is caused by rapid ventricular filling. An S$_3$ sound may occur with ventricular dysfunction, excessively rapid early diastolic ventricular filling, and restrictive myocardial or pericardial disease. It often indicates acute heart failure and fluid overload.

Mitral and tricuspid areas (S$_4$)

An S$_4$ heart sound, or atrial diastolic gallop, is a late diastolic filling sound associated with atrial contraction. An S$_4$ can be either left- or right-sided and is therefore heard best in the mitral or tricuspid areas. An S$_4$ is a late diastolic filling sound that occurs just before S$_1$ (**Figure 14.13R**).

Sometimes, the S$_3$ and S$_4$ heart sounds can occur simultaneously in mid-diastole, thus creating one loud diastolic filling sound. This is known as a summation gallop (**Figure 14.13S**).

E 1. Place the bell of the stethoscope lightly over the mitral area.
2. Place the bell of the stethoscope lightly over the tricuspid area.
3. Auscultate for 10 to 15 seconds for a left- or right-sided S$_4$.

N An S$_4$ heart sound may occur with or without any evidence of cardiac decompensation. A left-sided S$_4$ is usually louder on expiration. A right-sided S$_4$ is usually louder on inspiration.

A The presence of an S$_4$ can be indicative of cardiac decompensation.

P An S$_4$ heart sound can be auscultated in conditions that increase the resistance to filling because of a poorly compliant ventricle (e.g. AMI, CAD, HF, cardiomyopathy) or in conditions that result in systolic overload (e.g. hypertension, aortic stenosis, hyperthyroidism).

Murmurs

Murmurs are distinguished from heart sounds by their longer duration. Murmurs may be classified as innocent (which are always systolic and are not associated with any other abnormalities), functional (which are associated with high-output states) or pathological (which are related to structural abnormalities). Murmurs are produced by turbulent blood flow when there is:

1. flow across a partial obstruction
2. increased flow through normal structures
3. flow into a dilated chamber
4. backward or regurgitant flow across incompetent valves
5. shunting of blood out of a high-pressure chamber or artery through an abnormal passageway.

It might help you to focus and fine tune your listening skills for detecting an S$_4$ additional heart sound by saying out loud or pronouncing the word *Tennessee*. It is thought that doing this resembles the beat/rhythm of the S$_4$ heart sound:

S$_4$	S$_1$	S$_2$
Ten	nes	sée

When assessing for a murmur, analyse the murmur according to the following seven characteristics.

1. Location: area where the murmur is heard the loudest (e.g. mitral, pulmonic).
2. Radiation: transmission of sounds from the specific valves to other adjacent anatomic areas; for example, mitral murmurs can often radiate to the axilla.
3. Timing: phase of the cardiac cycle in which the murmur is heard. Murmurs can be either systolic or diastolic. If the murmur occurs simultaneously with the pulse, it is a systolic murmur. If it does not, it is a diastolic murmur. Murmurs can further be characterised as **pansystolic** or **holosystolic**, meaning that the murmur is heard throughout all of systole. Murmurs can also be characterised as early, mid or late systolic or diastolic murmurs.

UNIT 2

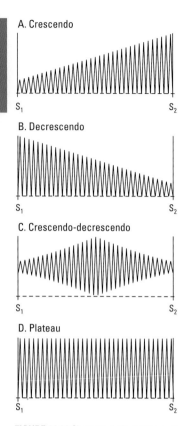

A. Crescendo

S₁   S₂

B. Decrescendo

S₁   S₂

C. Crescendo-decrescendo

S₁   S₂

D. Plateau

S₁   S₂

FIGURE 14.14 Characteristic patterns of murmurs

4. Intensity: See Table 14.4 for the six grades of loudness or intensity. The murmur is recorded with the grade over the roman numeral 'VI' to show the scale being used (e.g. III/VI).
5. Quality: harsh, rumbling, blowing or musical.
6. Pitch: high, medium or low. Low-pitched murmurs should be auscultated with the bell of the stethoscope whereas high-pitched murmurs should be auscultated with the diaphragm of the stethoscope.
7. Configuration: pattern that the murmur makes over time (Figure 14.14). The configuration of a murmur can be described as crescendo (soft to loud), decrescendo (loud to soft), crescendo-decrescendo (soft to loud to soft) or plateau (sound is sustained).

TABLE 14.4 Grading heart murmurs

GRADE	CHARACTERISTICS
I	Very faint; heard only after a period of concentration
II	Faint; heard immediately
III	Moderate intensity
IV	Loud; may be associated with a thrill
V	Loud; stethoscope must remain in contact with the chest wall in order to hear; thrill palpable
VI	Very loud; heard with stethoscope off chest wall; thrill palpable

E 1. The consumer should be in the same position for murmur auscultation as for the first auscultation (i.e. supine or sitting).
2. Auscultate each of the following cardiac landmarks for 10 to 15 seconds:
   a. Aortic and pulmonic areas, with the diaphragm of the stethoscope
   b. Mitral and tricuspid areas, with the diaphragm of the stethoscope
   c. Mitral and tricuspid areas, with the bell of the stethoscope
3. Label the murmur using the characteristics of location, radiation, timing, intensity, quality, pitch and configuration. See Table 14.4 for information on grading heart murmurs.
5. You may also have the consumer sit up, lean forwards, completely exhale, and hold his or her breath while you listen at the right and left second and third ICSs for aortic murmurs (especially aortic regurgitation).

N No murmur should be heard; however, a physiological or functional murmur in children and adolescents may be innocent. These murmurs are usually systolic, short, grade I or II, vibratory, heard at the left sternal border, and do not radiate. No cardiac symptoms accompany the murmur.

A Abnormal murmurs of stenosis can be found in each of the four valvular cardiac landmarks.

P Stenosis occurs when a valve that should be open remains partially closed. It produces an increased **afterload**, or pressure overload. Stenosis may develop from rheumatic fever, congenital defects of the valves, or calcification associated with the ageing process.

A Abnormal murmurs of regurgitation or insufficiency can be auscultated in each of the four valvular cardiac landmarks.

P Regurgitation or insufficiency occurs when a valve that should be closed remains partially open. An insufficient valve causes volume overload, or increased **preload**. Regurgitation frequently results from the effects of rheumatic fever and congenital defects of the valves.
See Table 14.5 for additional information on murmurs.

E Examination   **N** Normal findings   **A** Abnormal findings   **P** Pathophysiology   Advanced Assessment

TABLE 14.5 Murmurs and pericardial friction rub

HEART SOUND	LOCATION/ RADIATION	QUALITY/PITCH	CONFIGURATION
SYSTOLIC MURMURS			
Aortic stenosis	Second right ICS; may radiate to neck or left sternal border	Harsh/medium	Crescendo/decrescendo
Pulmonic stenosis	Second or third left ICS; radiates towards shoulder and neck	Harsh/medium	Crescendo/decrescendo
Mitral regurgitation	Apex; fifth ICS, left midclavicular line; may radiate to left axilla and back	Blowing/high	Pansystolic/plateau
Tricuspid regurgitation	Lower left sternal border; may radiate to right sternum	Blowing/high	Pansystolic/plateau
DIASTOLIC MURMURS			
Aortic regurgitation	Second right ICS and Erb's point; may radiate to left or right sternal border	Blowing/high	Decrescendo
Pulmonic regurgitation	Second left ICS; may radiate to left lower sternal border	Blowing/high	Decrescendo
Mitral stenosis	Apex; fifth ICS, left midclavicular line; may get louder with consumer on left side; does not radiate	Rumbling/low	Crescendo/decrescendo
Tricuspid stenosis	Fourth ICS, at sternal border	Rumbling/low	Crescendo/decrescendo
Pericardial friction rub	Third to fifth ICS, left of sternum; does not radiate	Leathery, scratchy, grating/high	Three components: > Ventricular systole > Ventricular diastole > Atrial systole

Timing is described as systolic or diastolic; intensity (grading) is described in **Table 14.4**.

Pericardial friction rub

E 1. Position the consumer so they are reclining in the sitting position, in the knee-chest position, or leaning forwards.
2. Auscultate from the sternum (third to fifth ICS) to the apex (mitral area) with the diaphragm of the stethoscope for 10 to 15 seconds.
3. Characterise any sound according to its location, radiation, timing, quality and pitch.

N No pericardial friction rub should be auscultated.

A A pericardial friction rub is always an abnormal finding. It is heard best during held inspiration or expiration. It does not change with the respiratory cycle. See Table 14.5 for additional information on pericardial friction rubs.

P Pericardial friction rubs are caused by the rubbing together of the inflamed visceral and parietal layers of the pericardium. They may be present in conditions such as **pericarditis** (inflammation of the pericardium) and renal failure.

Pericardial friction rub versus pleural friction rub
- A pericardial friction rub produces a high-pitched, multiphasic and scratchy (may be leathery or grating) sound that does not change with respiration. It is a sign of pericardial inflammation.
- A pleural friction rub produces a low-pitched, coarse and grating sound that does change with respiration. When the consumer holds his or her breath, the sound disappears. The consumer may also complain of pain upon breathing. It is a sign of visceral and parietal pleurae inflammation.

Prosthetic heart valves

E **N**

Prosthetic heart valves can be located in any of the four heart valves, although mitral and aortic valve replacements are the most common. Refer to the aortic and mitral valve auscultation discussions.

A Prosthetic heart valves produce abnormal heart sounds. Furthermore, mechanical prosthetic valve sounds can sometimes be heard without the use of a stethoscope.

P Mechanical prosthetic valves (caged-ball, tilting disc and bileaflet valves) produce 'clicky' opening and closing sounds. Homograft (human tissue) and heterograft (animal tissue) valves produce sounds that are similar to those of the human valves; however, they usually produce a murmur.

Examining consumers with cardiovascular supportive equipment
The consumer with cardiovascular disease may need the assistance of special equipment to maintain an optimal cardiovascular system. The presence of cardiovascular supportive equipment must be noted during the inspection process. Consider the following to assist you in observing these devices:

1. Artificial cardiac pacemaker (e.g. temporary external chest pacing, temporary internal pacing, permanent pacemaker), implantable cardiac defibrillator (ICD)
   - The pacemaker is on. Check the settings.
   - The ICD is on. Check the settings.
   - Check for external pacer wires. Wires should be protected from electrical hazards per your facility's policy.

- The insertion site is free of infection.
- Check your facility's policy for verifying and controlling the settings.
2. Haemodynamic monitoring (e.g. arterial pressure line [a-line], central venous pressure [CVP] line, right atrial pressure [RAP] line, left atrial pressure [LAP] line, pulmonary artery [PA] catheter [Swan-Ganz])
   - Check the goal of the line (e.g. fluid, monitoring).
   - The monitor's alarms are on. The appropriate limits are set.
   - The transducer level is at the consumer's right atrium (phlebostatic axis – fourth ICS, midaxillary line).
   - The pressure bag(s) is pumped to 300 mmHg.
   - Change the flush bag(s) per your facility's policy.
   - The line is safely secured to the consumer or the bed (it is not just dangling).
   - The insertion site is free of infection.
3. Antiembolic stockings
   - Determine whether the stockings are knee-high or thigh-high.
   - Ensure that they are the correct size (see the manufacturer's directions for correct sizing).
   - The consumer has palpable or audible pulses in the lower extremities.
   - The stockings have been removed at least once per day to assess the consumer's skin.
4. Chest tubes
   - Determine where the chest tube is.
   - Determine whether the chest tube is for air or fluid.
   - Ascertain whether the drainage system is wet suction or dry suction.
   - Determine whether the chest tube is on wall suction or water seal.
   - If the chest tube is on suction, the chest drainage system is bubbling and the water-seal chamber is fluctuating.
   - The chest tube connections are secured.
   - The chest tube is kink-free.
   - The insertion site is free of subcutaneous emphysema.
   - The insertion site is free of infection.
5. Electrocardiograph (ECG) monitoring
   - The consumer's skin is intact where the ECG pads are located.
   - The leads are placed correctly.
   - The monitor's alarms are on. The appropriate limits are set.
6. Intravenous (IV) catheters
   - Determine whether the catheter is inserted peripherally or centrally.
   - The insertion site is free of infection, infiltration or thrombophlebitis.
   - Determine what the fluid is.
   - Determine whether there are any additives in the fluid.
   - Determine the rate of the IV.
   - Determine when the IV can be discontinued.
   - Rotate IV site per your facility's policy.
7. Pneumatic compression stockings
   - Determine whether the consumer has some sort of stocking between the legs and the plastic enclosures.
   - The device is on.
   - The stockings have been removed at least once per day to assess the consumer's skin.

General approach to blood vessels examination

1. Explain to the consumer what you are going to do.
2. Use a drape and uncover only those areas that are necessary as the assessment is done.
3. Position the consumer in a supine or sitting position.

Examination of the blood vessels

Examination of the blood vessels is the second major component of a comprehensive cardiovascular assessment. The components of the examination of the blood vessels include:

1. inspection of the jugular venous pressure (JVP)
2. inspection of the hepatojugular reflux (advanced skill)
3. palpation and auscultation of the arterial pulses
4. inspection and palpation of peripheral perfusion.

Inspection

Jugular venous pressure

Identify the internal and external jugular veins (see Figure 14.15) with the consumer in a supine position with the head elevated to 30° or 45° so that the jugular veins are visible. Tangential lighting (lighting across the veins rather than on top of the veins) will facilitate the assessment. Both sides of the neck should be assessed. The external jugular veins are more superficial than the internal jugular veins and traverse the neck diagonally from the centre of the clavicle to the angle of the jaw. The internal jugular veins are larger and are located deep below the sternocleidomastoid muscle adjacent to the carotid arteries. The pulsations of the internal jugular veins can be difficult to identify visually because the veins are deep and the pulsations can be confused with the adjacent carotid arteries.

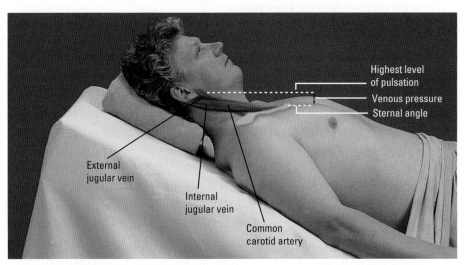

Highest level of pulsation
Venous pressure
Sternal angle
External jugular vein
Internal jugular vein
Common carotid artery

FIGURE 14.15 Inspection of jugular venous pressure

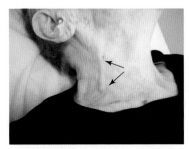

FIGURE 14.16 Positive JVP in a consumer positioned at a 45° angle. This consumer had not taken her diuretics and was complaining of SOB.

Information about the central venous pressure (CVP) can be obtained directly via a catheter inserted into one of the jugular veins (the internal jugular veins are the veins of choice for cannulation because they do not have valves and they provide a more direct route to the right atrium) or indirectly as discussed below.

E 1. To indirectly estimate a consumer's CVP, estimate the JVP (Figure 14.15):
   a. Place the consumer at a 30° to 45° angle (the highest position where the neck veins remain visible; Figure 14.16).
   b. Measure the vertical distance in centimetres from the consumer's sternal angle to the top of the distended neck vein. This will give you the JVP.
   c. Knowing that the sternal angle is roughly 5 cm above the right atrium, take the JVP measurement obtained in the previous step and add 5 cm to get an estimate of the CVP. For example, a JVP of 2 cm at a 45° angle estimated on a consumer's right side is equivalent to a CVP of 5 + 2 or 7 cm.

E Examination   **N** Normal findings   **A** Abnormal findings   **P** Pathophysiology   Advanced Assessment

E 2. Direct CVP measurements in the consumer with a central venous cannula should be obtained with the consumer in the supine position or reclining at no more than a 45° angle.

    a. Do not forget to level the transducer at the consumer's right atrium (phlebostatic axis – fourth ICS, midaxillary line) prior to obtaining any CVP reading.

    b. When recording CVP measurements, chart the angle of the consumer when the measurement was taken.

N A JVP reading less than 4 cm is considered normal. Normally, the jugular veins are:

1. most distended when the consumer is flat because gravity is eliminated and the jugular veins fill
2. 1 cm to 2 cm above the sternal angle when the head of the bed is elevated to a 45° angle
3. absent when the head of the bed is at a 90° angle.

    Normal direct CVP readings are 3–8 cm H_2O.

A A JVP greater than 4 cm is considered abnormal (**Figure 14.16**).

P An elevated JVP can be due to an increased right ventricular pressure, increased blood volume, or an obstruction to right ventricular flow.

A Bilateral jugular venous distension is abnormal.

P Jugular venous distension indicates an increased JVP, which occurs in conditions such as heart failure.

A Unilateral jugular venous distension is abnormal.

P Unilateral jugular venous distension indicates a local vein blockage.

A Jugular venous distension with the head of the bed elevated to a 90° angle is abnormal.

P Jugular venous distension at a 45° to 90° angle indicates more serious pathology, such as severe right ventricular failure, constrictive pericarditis, or cardiac tamponade.

Hepatojugular reflux

Hepatojugular reflux is a test that is very sensitive in detecting right ventricular failure. This procedure is performed if the CVP is normal but right ventricular failure is suspected.

E 1. Place the consumer flat in bed, or elevated to a 30° angle if the jugular veins are visible. Remind the consumer to breathe normally.
2. Using single or bimanual deep palpation, press firmly on the right upper quadrant for 30 to 60 seconds. Press on another part of the abdomen if this area is tender.
3. Observe the neck for an elevation in JVP (**Figures 14.17** and **14.18**).

N Normally, this pressure should not elicit any change in the jugular veins.

A A rise of more than 1 cm in JVP is abnormal.

P A rise in JVP that occurs with this technique is suggestive of right-sided (diastolic) heart failure or fluid overload. The heart simply cannot accept the increase in venous return.

Palpation and auscultation

Arterial pulses

Information concerning the function of the right ventricle is gained via the examination of the venous pulses, and assessment of the arterial pulses provides information about the left ventricle. The pulses to be evaluated are the temporal, carotid, brachial, radial, femoral, popliteal, posterior tibial and the dorsalis pedis. The radial arteries are most frequently examined due to their easy accessibility.

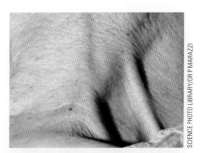

FIGURE 14.17 Elevated JVP

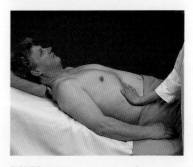

FIGURE 14.18 Hepatojugular reflux

E 1. The arterial pulse assessment is best facilitated with the consumer in a supine position with the head of the bed elevated at 30° to 45°. If the consumer cannot tolerate such a position, then the supine position alone is acceptable.

2. Using your dominant hand, palpate the pulses with the pads of the index and middle fingers. The number of fingers used will be determined by the amount of space in which the pulse is located.

3. Evaluate the pulse in terms of:
   a. rate: Determine the rate.
   b. rhythm: If there is an irregularity in the pulse rate, then auscultate the heart.
   c. amplitude (refer to Chapter 6 for scales for measuring pulse volume).
   d. symmetry: Palpate the pulses on both sides of the consumer's body simultaneously (with the exception of the carotid pulses).

4. If a peripheral pulse cannot be palpated, an amplification device can be used to detect the presence, rate and rhythm at that location (**Figure 14.19**).

5. Assess the '5 Ps' when examining a consumer with a suspected arterial occlusion: pain, pallor, pulselessness, paraesthesia and paralysis.

6. Using the bell of the stethoscope, auscultate the temporal, carotid and femoral pulses for **bruits**, which are blowing sounds heard when blood flow becomes turbulent as it rushes past an obstruction. Ask the consumer to hold his or her breath during auscultation of the carotid pulse because respiratory sounds can interfere with auscultation.

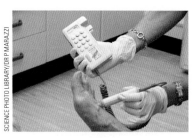

FIGURE 14.19 Use of an ultrasonic stethoscope to detect a dorsalis pedis pulse

N Refer to Chapter 6 for normal pulse rate, rhythm and amplitude. When assessing symmetry, the pulses should be equal bilaterally. No bruits should be auscultated in the temporal, carotid or femoral pulses.

A P Figure 14.20 illustrates abnormal arterial pulses with possible causes. As a foundation practitioner you would not normally be expected to recognise these pulse patterns, but the inclusion of these provides all practitioners with a reference point as well as a description for the altered waveform. These waveforms will only be visible/interpretable if the consumer is being haemodynamically monitored.

A Asymmetrical pulses are abnormal.

P Variations in the symmetry of pulses can occur because of anatomic differences in the depths and locations of the arteries.

A Absent pulses are abnormal.

P An arterial occlusion may result in an absent pulse distal to the occlusion.

A Auscultation of bruits at the temporal, carotid and femoral areas is abnormal.

P Bruits in these areas can be caused by an obstruction related to atherosclerotic plaque formation, a jugular vein–carotid artery fistula, or high-output states such as anaemia or thyrotoxicosis.

CLINICAL REASONING

Practice tip: Palpation of carotid pulses
The carotid pulses should not be palpated together because excessive stimulation can elicit a vagal response and slow down the heart. Palpating both carotid pulses at the same time could also cut off circulation to the consumer's head and brain.

Examining for pulsus paradoxus
During inspiration, the blood flow into the right side of the heart is increased, the right ventricular output is enhanced, and pulmonary venous capacitance is increased, resulting in less blood reaching the left ventricle. These mechanisms account for a decrease in both the left ventricular stroke volume and arterial pressure. An exaggerated form of this mechanism is referred to as **pulsus paradoxus**.

E Examination   **N** Normal findings   **A** Abnormal findings   **P** Pathophysiology   ▢ Advanced Assessment

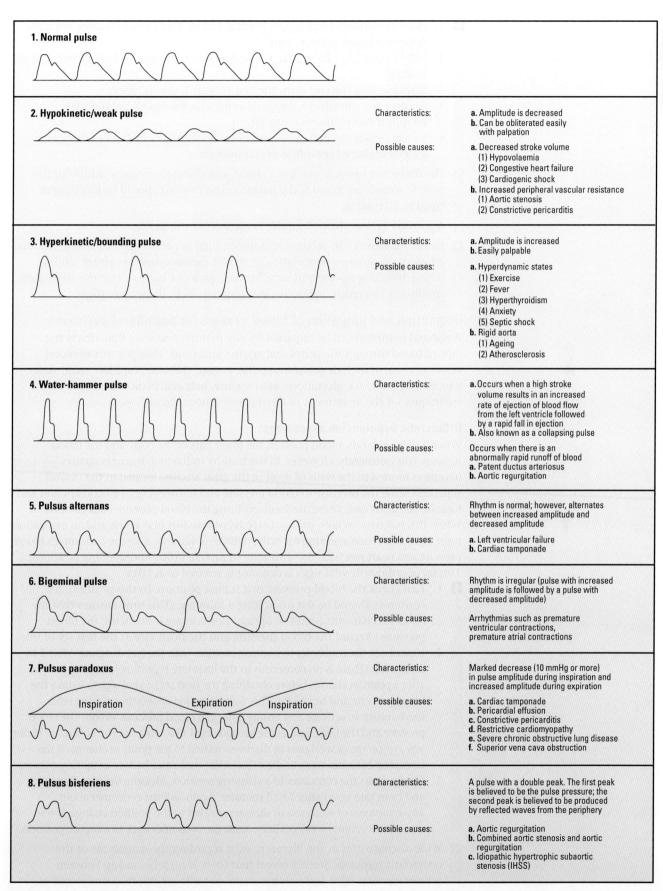

1. Normal pulse

2. Hypokinetic/weak pulse

Characteristics:
a. Amplitude is decreased
b. Can be obliterated easily with palpation

Possible causes:
a. Decreased stroke volume
(1) Hypovolaemia
(2) Congestive heart failure
(3) Cardiogenic shock
b. Increased peripheral vascular resistance
(1) Aortic stenosis
(2) Constrictive pericarditis

3. Hyperkinetic/bounding pulse

Characteristics:
a. Amplitude is increased
b. Easily palpable

Possible causes:
a. Hyperdynamic states
(1) Exercise
(2) Fever
(3) Hyperthyroidism
(4) Anxiety
(5) Septic shock
b. Rigid aorta
(1) Ageing
(2) Atherosclerosis

4. Water-hammer pulse

Characteristics:
a. Occurs when a high stroke volume results in an increased rate of ejection of blood flow from the left ventricle followed by a rapid fall in ejection
b. Also known as a collapsing pulse

Possible causes:
Occurs when there is an abnormally rapid runoff of blood
a. Patent ductus arteriosus
b. Aortic regurgitation

5. Pulsus alternans

Characteristics:
Rhythm is normal; however, alternates between increased amplitude and decreased amplitude

Possible causes:
a. Left ventricular failure
b. Cardiac tamponade

6. Bigeminal pulse

Characteristics:
Rhythm is irregular (pulse with increased amplitude is followed by a pulse with decreased amplitude)

Possible causes:
Arrhythmias such as premature ventricular contractions, premature atrial contractions

7. Pulsus paradoxus

Inspiration   Expiration   Inspiration

Characteristics:
Marked decrease (10 mmHg or more) in pulse amplitude during inspiration and increased amplitude during expiration

Possible causes:
a. Cardiac tamponade
b. Pericardial effusion
c. Constrictive pericarditis
d. Restrictive cardiomyopathy
e. Severe chronic obstructive lung disease
f. Superior vena cava obstruction

8. Pulsus bisferiens

Characteristics:
A pulse with a double peak. The first peak is believed to be the pulse pressure; the second peak is believed to be produced by reflected waves from the periphery

Possible causes:
a. Aortic regurgitation
b. Combined aortic stenosis and aortic regurgitation
c. Idiopathic hypertrophic subaortic stenosis (IHSS)

FIGURE 14.20 Alterations in arterial pulses

E 1. Place the consumer in a supine position and instruct them to breathe normally.
2. Apply the blood pressure cuff.
3. Inflate the cuff to 20 mmHg above the consumer's last systolic blood pressure reading.
4. Slowly deflate the cuff until the first systolic sound is heard.
5. Observe the consumer's respirations because the systolic sound may disappear during normal inspiration.
6. Slowly deflate the cuff again and note the point at which all of the systolic sounds are heard regardless of respirations.

N The difference between the first systolic sound and the point at which all the systolic sounds are heard is the paradox. The paradox should be less than or equal to 10 mmHg.

A A paradox greater than 10 mmHg is considered abnormal.

P Pulsus paradoxus can occur in conditions such as cardiac tamponade, pericardial effusion, constrictive pericarditis, restrictive cardiomyopathy, severe chronic obstructive lung disease and superior vena cava obstruction, because all of these conditions can result in a decreased blood return to the left ventricle.

Inspection and palpation of blood vessels for peripheral perfusion

Peripheral perfusion can be impaired by any pathological state that affects the flow of blood through the peripheral arteries and veins. Components of blood vessel assessment include peripheral pulse, colour, clubbing, capillary refill, skin temperature, oedema, ulcerations, skin texture, hair distribution, and special techniques for the assessment of arterial and venous blood flow.

Orthostatic hypotension assessment

When a person stands, blood pools in the lower part of the body and the blood pressure falls transiently. However, in the healthy individual, **baroreceptors** (receptors located in the walls of most of the great arteries) located in the carotid sinus area sense the decrease in blood pressure and initiate reflex vasoconstriction and increase the heart rate. These mechanisms bring the blood pressure back to normal. When this mechanism fails, **orthostatic hypotension** may ensue and an evaluation must be made. When assessing for orthostatic hypotension, take the consumer's blood pressure and heart rate with the consumer in supine, sitting and standing positions. This set of orthostatic vital signs is commonly referred to as **tilts**.

E 1. First check the blood pressure in a supine position. In this position, the consumer should be flat for at least 5 minutes. (This time ensures that no reflex mechanisms from the upright position are influencing the blood pressure.) Record the blood pressure and the heart rate as the first set of tilts.
2. Next, assist the consumer to a sitting position with the feet dangling. Wait 1 to 3 minutes. (There is no consensus in the literature regarding how long to wait after a position change before obtaining the next set of vital signs.) Retake the blood pressure and heart rate. This waiting period allows time for the reflex mechanisms to activate and ensure a normal blood pressure. Record the blood pressure and the heart rate as the second set of tilts. Also, ask the consumer about any symptoms of weakness or dizziness related to the position change. If the consumer becomes weak or dizzy, assist the consumer back to a supine position.
3. Finally, assist the consumer to a standing position. Measure the blood pressure and heart rate again after 1 to 3 minutes. Again, ask the consumer about any symptoms of weakness or dizziness related to the position change. If the consumer becomes weak or dizzy, assist the consumer back to a supine position.

N Wide discrepancies in the literature exist regarding the magnitude of the orthostatic response. Studies reveal that there is no relationship between orthostatic vital signs and volume status, yet tilts are still frequently used as indicators of intravascular volume status. In other words, consumers can have 'positive' tilts even though they are not hypovolaemic.

E Examination   **N** Normal findings   **A** Abnormal findings   **P** Pathophysiology   Advanced Assessment

A Orthostatic vital signs that have been considered positive in the past include a systolic or a diastolic blood pressure decrease of more than 10 mmHg or a heart rate increase of more than 20 beats per minute. However, tilts have fallen out of favour with many, for the reason previously stated.

P Orthostatic hypotension can occur in consumers who are hypovolaemic, have a neurogenic problem or are experiencing side effects from a prescribed medication.

E 1. Inspect the fingers, toes, or points of trauma on the feet and legs for ulceration. Inspect the sides of the ankles for ulceration.
2. Inspect for pallor.
3. Palpate for colour return and capillary refill.
4. Consider completing the Allen's test to assess the patency of the radial and ulnar arteries.
5. Consider determining the ankle–brachial index (ABI) to examine arterial perfusion.
6. Inspect and palpate the lymph nodes.

N Ulcerations: No ulcerations should be noted.

A Arterial ulcerations are abnormal.
1. Location: occurs at toes or points of trauma on the feet or the legs.
2. Characteristics: well-defined edges; black or necrotic tissue; a deep, pale base and lack of bleeding; hairlessness or disruption of the hair along with shiny, thick, waxy skin.
3. Pain: exceedingly painful; claudication related to chronic arterial insufficiency is relieved by rest; pain at rest is relieved by dependency.

P The location and characteristics of ulceration are due to inadequate arterial flow, such as in peripheral vascular disease and diabetes mellitus. Most distal arterial beds are prone to ulceration. The pain is caused by ischaemia.

P Arterial ulcers on the tips of the fingers, toes or nose can be caused by Reynaud's disease (**Figure 14.21**). Arteriolar spasms lead to pallor and pain in the affected area, followed by cyanosis, with numbness, tingling and burning; redness also develops. Over time, the affected area may develop an ulcer (**Figure 14.22**). Attacks occur bilaterally and last minutes to hours.

A Venous ulcerations are abnormal (**Figure 14.23**).
1. Location: occurs at the sides of the ankles.
2. Characteristics: uneven edges and ruddy granulation of tissue; thin, shiny skin that lacks the support of subcutaneous tissue; disruption of hair pattern or hairlessness.
3. Pain: deep muscular pain (associated with inadequate venous flow) with acute DVT; aching and cramping are relieved with elevation.

P Ulcers are due to inadequate venous flow that results when communication between the superficial and deep veins is compromised. Both the characteristics and the pain are related to inadequate venous blood flow.

Examination of the venous system

Inspection

Homan's sign
It is important to note that because a **Homan's sign** has a low sensitivity (an indication of the frequency of a positive test result in a population with the disease) for thrombophlebitis, the use of this test has fallen out of favour with some healthcare providers. The Homan's test is also controversial because there have been reports of the dislodging of deep vein thromboses (DVT) with the performance of the manoeuvre. In addition, conditions other than DVT could yield positive results from this test. A positive Homan's sign is present in less than one-third of consumers with a confirmed DVT (Radhakrishnan, 2022).

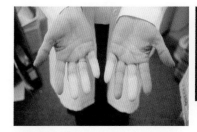

FIGURE 14.21 Reynaud's disease in the early stage. Note the pallor in the distal half of some of the fingers.

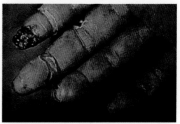

COURTESY OF MARVIN ACKERMAN, M.D., SCARSDALE, NY

FIGURE 14.22 Reynaud's disease in the late stage. Note the necrotic digit.

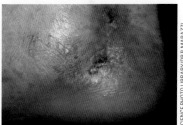

SCIENCE PHOTO LIBRARY/DR P. MARAZZI

A. Note the ulcerations at the side of the ankle.

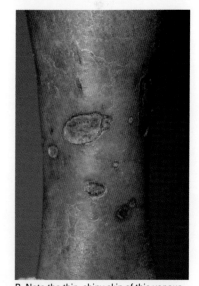

B. Note the thin, shiny skin of this venous stasis ulcer.

FIGURE 14.23 Venous ulcerations

E Examination   **N** Normal findings   **A** Abnormal findings   **P** Pathophysiology   ▮ Advanced Assessment

E   **1.** With the consumer's knee slightly bent, sharply dorsiflex the consumer's foot and ask the consumer if this manoeuvre elicits pain in the calf.
     2. Repeat this technique with the other foot.

N   There should be no complaints of calf pain when this is evaluated.

A   A positive Homan's sign may be abnormal.

P   A positive Homan's sign may indicate thrombophlebitis or DVT. Early detection of thrombophlebitis is essential because it can lead to life-threatening complications such as pulmonary embolus, which occurs when a thrombus breaks loose from the vein and travels to the lung. Three factors can disrupt the balance between blood-clotting activators and inhibitors. Known as Virchow's triad, they are stasis of blood flow, an injured venous wall, and hypercoagulability. All three factors can predispose a consumer to thrombosis. Thrombosis can occur in either deep or superficial veins.

Examination of the arterial system

Inspection

Pallor

E   **1.** Instruct the consumer to raise the extremities.
     2. Note the time it takes for pallor, or lack of colour, to develop.

N   Normally no pallor develops within 60 seconds.

A   Pallor that develops quickly in the extremities when the extremities are lifted is abnormal.

P   Pallor that develops quickly is indicative of arterial insufficiency. The quicker the pallor develops, the more severe the disease.

Colour return and capillary refill

E   **1.** Gently squeeze one of the consumer's fingers or toes (depending on the body area you are assessing). Hold this position for approximately 1 second.
     2. Release the consumer's digit.
     3. Note the time it takes for the colour to return to the digit and for the superficial veins to refill.

N   Normal capillary refill/colour return is 3 seconds or less.

A   A delayed capillary refill of greater than 3 seconds is abnormal.

P   These scores can contribute to the assessment of moderate ischaemia.

A   A delayed capillary refill of 5 seconds or more is abnormal.

P   These scores can contribute to the assessment of severe ischaemia.

CLINICAL **REASONING**

Practice tip: Capillary refill and peripheral perfusion
A delayed return of colour to the nail beds suggests that there is an impairment of blood flow in the microcirculation. A return capillary refill should occur within 3 seconds. A delayed capillary refill may occur with heart failure, shock, or peripheral vascular disease. Refer to Chapter 8 for further information on capillary refill. When decreased peripheral perfusion is noted, this should prompt the clinician to then assess for central perfusion, as central cyanosis has serious implications for the consumer's immediate health status.
Central cyanosis
When assessing a consumer's periphery, remember to look for cyanosis in the mucous membranes, the earlobes and the cheeks.

E Examination   **N** Normal findings   **A** Abnormal findings   **P** Pathophysiology   Advanced Assessment

Allen test

The Allen test is used to assess the patency of the radial and ulnar arteries (see **Figure 14.24**).

E 1. Ask the consumer to make a tight fist. If the consumer is unresponsive, raise the arm above the heart for several seconds to force blood to leave the hand.
2. Apply direct pressure on the radial and ulnar arteries to obstruct blood flow to the hand as the consumer opens and closes the fist.
3. Instruct the consumer to open the hand, while the radial artery remains compressed. If the consumer is unresponsive, keep the arm above the heart level.
4. Examine the palmar surface of the hand for a blush or pallor within 15 seconds.

N If the radial artery is compressed, the blood flow through the ulnar artery should be sufficient to maintain the normal palm colour after the consumer unclenches the fist. Also, if the ulnar artery is compressed, the blood flow through the radial artery should be sufficient to maintain the normal palm colour. This is a positive Allen test.

A If the colour does not return to normal within 6 seconds after the consumer unclenches the fist, then obstruction of either the radial or the ulnar arteries may be present. This is a negative Allen test. Thus, the radial artery should not be punctured for an arterial blood gas or invasive arterial line.

P Atherosclerosis or a thrombus can cause either artery to be not patent.

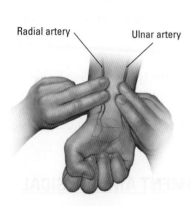

A. Pallor is initiated by compressing the radial and ulnar arteries with the fist clenched.

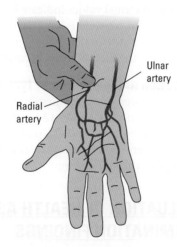

B. A patent ulnar artery reveals the return of palm perfusion despite radial artery compression.

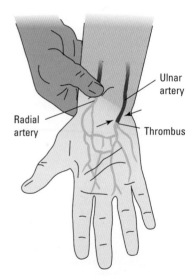

C. An occluded ulnar artery results in continued pallor of the hand while the radial artery is still compressed.

FIGURE 14.24 The Allen test

Ankle–brachial index (ABI)

The ankle–brachial index examines arterial perfusion in consumers who have leg ulcers. ABI is an easy, dependable and inexpensive test used in the assessment of peripheral vascular disease (PVD), sometimes called peripheral artery disease. Consumers are usually evaluated annually or on acute admission, to note the progression of the disease as well as their response to treatment.

E 1. Have the consumer remove socks and shoes, as well as roll up sleeves and/or pants legs (but do not obstruct blood flow).
2. Consumer should rest in a supine position for 5 minutes prior to taking the readings.
3. Place blood pressure cuff snugly on the consumer's arm and above the ankles.

E Examination **N** Normal findings **A** Abnormal findings **P** Pathophysiology Advanced Assessment

E 4. Apply a small amount of gel to the first brachial artery site and place the Doppler probe at the point with the loudest signal.

5. Inflate the BP cuff to 20 mmHg above the occlusion pressure.

6. Deflate the cuff at approximately 2 mmHg per second, listening for the blood flow sound to return (this is the systolic pressure). Rapidly deflate the cuff after auscultating this systolic pressure and record the results.

7. Repeat this process for the other arm and record the results.

8. Use either the posterior tibial or dorsalis pedis for auscultation when obtaining the ankle pressures. Again, apply a small amount of gel to the first site and place the Doppler probe at the point with the loudest signal.

9. Inflate the BP cuff to 20 mmHg above the occlusion pressure.

10. Deflate the cuff at approximately 2 mmHg per second, listening for the blood flow sound to return. Rapidly deflate the cuff after auscultating the systolic pressure and record the results.

11. Repeat this process for the other ankle and record the results.

12. For the left-side ABI, divide the left ankle systolic pressure by the higher of the two brachial systolic pressures and record the results. Repeat this process for the right-side ABI, using the right ankle systolic pressure divided by the higher of the two brachial systolic pressures. For example, if the left ankle systolic pressure was 148 and the higher brachial systolic pressure was 152, then the ABI is 0.97 (148 ÷ 152).

N An ABI range of 1.0 to 1.4 is considered normal.

A An ABI less than 0.90 is abnormal.

P These abnormal values indicate PVD. Note that the ABI reading may not be accurate for consumers who have diabetes or kidney disease, or for some older consumers as they may have rigid blood vessels, which make it difficult to compress the BP cuff to get accurate readings.

Inspection and palpation of lymph nodes

Refer to Chapter 9 for examination techniques on the lymphatic vessels that drain the head and neck, Chapter 12 for the regional lymphatics of the breast, including axillary lymph nodes, and Chapter 15 on the spleen and appendix. Examination of the thymus and bone marrow require specialty diagnostic testing and are outside the scope of this discussion.

EVALUATION OF HEALTH ASSESSMENT AND PHYSICAL EXAMINATION FINDINGS

In the evaluation phase of a health assessment, the focus is on ensuring the data gathered is complete, accurate and documented appropriately (see case study as an example of the focused assessment; see Chapter 22 for a comprehensive health assessment). In evaluating the data you should:

> draw on your critical thinking and problem-solving skills to make sound clinical decisions

> act on abnormal data (include communicating findings to other health professionals)

> ensure documentation reflects the outcomes of the clinical decisions/actions taken (refer to Chapter 3, which discusses in detail why documentation is so important and how this may be undertaken in different health settings).

The case study that follows steps you through this process.

THE CONSUMER WITH HYPERTENSION

This case study illustrates the application and objective documentation of the cardiovascular assessment. The setting is in the hospital medical ward.

Mrs Kathleen Luck is a 66-year-old female who recently arrived on the medical ward.

HEALTH HISTORY

CONSUMER PROFILE	66-year-old Caucasian female	
CHIEF COMPLAINT	'I think my blood pressure is up and I need this looked at by a professional. I have been getting headaches the last 2 days.'	
HISTORY OF THE PRESENT ILLNESS	Consumer states she is generally well but notes she has experienced headaches over the last 2 days. She has recently moved interstate, and had been referred to hospital after her first appointment with a new general practitioner.	
PAST HEALTH HISTORY	**MEDICAL HISTORY**	Hypertension for 15 years Arthritis for 6 years
	SURGICAL HISTORY	Left knee repair 10 years ago (consumer unsure what surgery was done) Right knee repair last year (consumer unsure what surgery was done, feels much better than before surgery)
	ALLERGIES	States she is allergic to shellfish and she comes out in hives and has difficulty breathing
	MEDICATIONS	Paracetamol for arthritis 1000 mg four times per day
	COMMUNICABLE DISEASES	Has not experienced any
	INJURIES AND ACCIDENTS	Other than a fractured wrist many years ago while playing netball, states no major events
	SPECIAL NEEDS	No longer needs a walking stick since her right knee has been repaired, but she still finds it hard to ascend and descend stairs
	BLOOD TRANSFUSIONS	Nil noted
	CHILDHOOD ILLNESSES	Measles, mumps, chickenpox
	IMMUNISATIONS	Last tetanus booster was 7 years ago. Annual flu vaccination for the past 10 years. COVID-19 vaccinations and booster completed.
FAMILY HEALTH HISTORY	No significant history of cardiovascular disease	
SOCIAL HISTORY	**ALCOHOL USE**	Enjoys a 'sherry every night'
	TOBACCO USE	Has never smoked
	DRUG USE	States has never consumed any form of drugs
	DOMESTIC AND INTIMATE PARTNER VIOLENCE	Husband died 14 years ago
	SEXUAL PRACTICE	Has been widowed for 14 years
	WORK ENVIRONMENT	Retired journalist
	HOME ENVIRONMENT	Relates that she was unable to keep up with the day-to-day management of her own home. Recently relocated to the area to live with her daughter's family. The family have built her a granny flat; they are relieved to have her close so they do not have to worry about her living on her own, so far away from them.

>>

HEALTH HISTORY

	HOBBIES AND LEISURE ACTIVITIES	Reads books and watches a lot of television; misses her lifelong friends in her previous neighbourhood
	STRESS	Appears a little resentful that she left her home of 40 years and had to move interstate. (She states 'My daughter said I had to come here because I can't live by myself anymore'.)
	EDUCATION	Completed secondary school and university Bachelor of Arts
	ECONOMIC STATUS	States she is financially comfortable and that her income is derived from her pension benefits and her husband's superannuation fund
	MILITARY SERVICE	None
	RELIGION	Anglican
	CULTURAL BACKGROUND	Caucasian
	ROLES AND RELATIONSHIPS	Cares for granddaughters one afternoon a week; helps cook and eats dinner with the family on Sunday night. Otherwise, she has meals in her flat watching the television.
	CHARACTERISTIC PATTERNS OF DAILY LIVING	Rises at 7 a.m. and eats breakfast. Spends most of the day in recliner watching television. Eats lots of snacks during the day, followed by large dinner in the evening. Retreats to recliner for evening television shows. Retires to bed around 11 p.m.
HEALTH MAINTENANCE ACTIVITIES	SLEEP	Sleeps from 11 p.m. to 7 a.m. every day; however, has to 'go to the bathroom' several times throughout the night. Will sometimes nap in the recliner prior to dinner. 'I'm always tired.'
	DIET	Coffee and a muffin when she wakes. Fruit, biscuit and a diet soft drink in the afternoon. Dinner meal consists of frozen meals, tinned food and snack foods as she gets so tired and does not like to stand and prepare meals for long periods of time. Often at night snacks on lollies. 'I have a sweet tooth.'
	EXERCISE	Limited exercise as often tired and 'bad knees limit me doing too much', although there has been improvement since the surgery
	STRESS MANAGEMENT	Loves her cat, which is great company for her
	USE OF SAFETY DEVICES	No specific devices in use
	HEALTH CHECK-UPS	Usually 2–3 times per year and as needed
	IDENTIFIABLE RISK FACTORS	NONMODIFIABLE — Age, family history
		MODIFIABLE — Hypertension, elevated lipid profile, physical inactivity, being overweight
CONSUMER CLASSIFICATION (CLINICAL SEVERITY PROGNOSIS)	NYHA I (refer to previous information about classifications of consumer's functional capacity by the New York Heart Association, page 461)	

PHYSICAL EXAMINATION

EXAMINATION OF THE PRECORDIUM	INSPECTION	AORTIC AREA	Negative
		PULMONIC AREA	Negative
		MIDPRECORDIAL AREA	Negative
		TRICUSPID AREA	Negative
		MITRAL AREA	Negative

>>

HEALTH HISTORY			
	PALPATION	**AORTIC AREA**	Negative
		PULMONIC AREA	Negative
		MIDPRECORDIAL AREA	Negative
		TRICUSPID AREA	Negative
		MITRAL AREA	Negative
	AUSCULTATION	**AORTIC AREA**	$+ S_2$
		PULMONIC AREA	$+ S_2$
		MIDPRECORDIAL AREA	−ve for murmurs
		TRICUSPID AREA	$+ S_1, -ve\ S_3$
		MITRAL AREA	$+ S_1, -ve\ S_3$
		MITRAL AND TRICUSPID AREAS (S_3)	Absent
		MITRAL AND TRICUSPID AREAS (S_4)	Absent
		MURMURS	Absent
		PERICARDIAL FRICTION RUB	Absent
		BP	168/90 mmHg
EXAMINATION OF THE BLOOD VESSELS	**INSPECTION**	**JUGULAR VENOUS PRESSURE**	No distension
		HEPATOJUGULAR REFLUX	No change in jugular veins
	PALPATION AND AUSCULTATION	**ARTERIAL PULSE**	> Rate: 84 > Rhythm: Regular > Pulse (strength): normal all +2 **Scale = 0 to +4** Stick figure peripheral pulse documentation > Symmetry: All symmetrical > Bruits: None
		EXAMINING FOR PULSUS PARADOXUS	No pulsus paradoxus

HEALTH HISTORY

	INSPECTION AND PALPATION	**PERIPHERAL PERFUSION**	Colour: Normal Clubbing: None Capillary refill: Less than 2 seconds Skin temperature: Warm Oedema: Nil present Ulcerations: None Skin texture: Smooth, even. No varicose veins noted. Hair distribution: Even
		ORTHOSTATIC HYPOTENSION ASSESSMENT	Negative
	EXAMINATION OF THE VENOUS SYSTEM	**HOMAN'S SIGN**	Not present
	EXAMINATION OF THE ARTERIAL SYSTEM	**PALLOR**	Absent
		COLOUR RETURN AND CAPILLARY REFILL	2 seconds
		ALLEN TEST	Not completed
		ANKLE–BRACHIAL INDEX (ABI)	Not completed
	INSPECTION AND PALPATION	**LYMPH NODES**	Not palpable

DIAGNOSTIC DATA

Chest X-ray	Normal
ECG	Normal
Echocardiogram	Normal
Height, weight, body mass index (BMI)	> Height: 165 cm > Weight: 90 kg > BMI: 33.1 (normal limits = 18.5–24.9)
Further diagnostic data that has been collected: laboratory	> Non-fasting blood glucose level: 5.5 mmol/L > LDL cholesterol (LDL-C)l: 4.6 mmol/L > HDL cholesterol (HDL-C)l: 0.8 mmol/L > Triglycerides: 3 mmol/L > Serum creatinine: 95 micromol/L > Urinalysis: 1+ proteinuria, trace + of glucose

EVALUATION AND CLINICAL REASONING FOR CASE STUDY

The assessment and clinical decisions you make should reflect your scope of practice. For example, advanced practice health professionals. such as nurse practitioners and remote area nurses with endorsement. may be able to make diagnostic decisions and prescribe medications without referring to a medical officer.

Fundamentally, all health professionals collect, evaluate and act on consumer-focused health information, which will at times include referral to, or collaboration with, other healthcare team members. Nurses assess consumer responses to interventions and determine when to escalate key changes in a consumer's condition. The clinical reasoning cycle provides health professionals with a framework to consider all this information in a meaningful way for planning consumer care. These phases are stepped out below, and draw on information presented and collected during the health history and physical examination. We then work through the cycle components that are relevant to this case study (cycle components are bolded).

For Kathleen Luck, the 66-year-old woman who has presented to a hospital medical ward, the significant data that needs to be considered includes the following.

Collecting cues/information

Recall and Review: In the first instance you will need to reflect on what you know about hypertension. Hypertension is defined inconsistently internationally; however, high blood pressure or hypertension refers to high pressure (BP) or tension in the arteries of the body. It is a chronic medical condition in which the systemic arterial blood pressure is elevated. In those diagnosed with hypertension, the BP stays abnormally high even at rest and, in the majority of cases, the exact cause is unknown. Arteries in the body become narrowed and the heart is forced to pump harder to move blood through the narrower arterial channels, thus raising the BP (referred to as primary hypertension). In a percentage of individuals, elevated BP may be the result of other comorbidities, or it may be medication-induced or as a result of hereditary factors (referred to as secondary hypertension).

The diagnosis and classification of hypertension is confirmed by a medical doctor and is derived from taking the consumer's BP measurements a number of times on different occasions.

Chief complaint and health history of present illness (subjective data)

> Consumer states that she has experienced headaches over the last 2 days
> Recently moved house, started with new general practitioner
> Appears resentful she has had to leave her own home of 40 years
> Hypertension diagnosed for 30 years
> Consumes a sherry every night

Processing information

Interpret: These symptoms and details of history outline the scope of the issue for this consumer and how it is affecting her wellbeing and ability to self-manage this deviation from normal health.

Medications

Paracetamol for arthritis to reduce pain and swelling.

Discriminate: At present she has continued to take paracetamol for her arthritis and in hope that this will reduce her headaches. It would be important at this point to find out exactly how often she takes paracetamol medication to ensure she is not overusing this, as there are deleterious side effects.

Health maintenance activities

> Finds she is always tired, wakes several times during the night to go to the toilet.
> Consumes a poor diet, high in salt (frozen and tinned foods) and eats lots of snacks. Unable to stand for long periods of time to prepare meals.
> Undertakes limited exercise due to arthritis/previous surgery to both knees, also has problems ascending and descending stairs. Sits in the recliner often and watches a considerable amount of television.

Discriminate: This information indicates the significance of her present health alteration affecting her quality of life and is important information that the nurse must acknowledge.

Physical assessment/diagnostic data (objective data)

> BP 168/90 mmHg
> BMI 33.1
> Serum lipid levels: LDL–Cl: 4.6 mmol/L, HDL–C: 0.8 mmol/L
  • Triglycerides: 3.0 mmol/L
  • Serum creatinine: 95 micromol/L

> Non-fasting glucose: 5.5 mmol/L
  • Urinalysis: 1+ proteinuria, trace glucose

Interpret and Infer: These findings give support for her medical diagnosis (exacerbation of hypertension).

Putting it all together – synthesise information

The nurse in this case would note all of these abnormalities, and refer Kathleen to the medical doctor on duty for further review and medical treatment. It is likely that she will undergo further investigations for her reports of headaches and documented elevated blood pressure. Likely she will commence on antihypertensive therapy to control the raised BP. Given her raised serum lipid profile, she will likely be commenced on lipid-lowering medications. Also, her history of urinary frequency, trace of glucose in urine and other lifestyle risks would warrant further investigations for possible onset of diabetes mellitus, renal or cardiac problems.

Actions based on assessment data

The nurse should also provide additional education for interventions that do not require a doctor's order, such as:

1 Education on correct use of antihypertensive agent; note a combination of medications is often needed for consumers with diagnosed hypertension. Emphasise regular medication consumption as per order; knowing common side effects and use of a medication-dispensing device should assist the consumer.
2 Education to manage lifestyle cardiovascular risk factors would include setting healthy targets such as importance of daily exercise, become more active even 10-minute sessions spread 3 times across the day (target 30 minutes moderate-intensity physical activity at least 5 times a week), reduction of weight with a focus on reducing waist measurement. Need to reduce kilojoule intake and increase physical activity at the same time. Need to restrict salt in the diet, by consuming low-salt/salt-reduced foods.
3 Education regarding behavioural modification to support the management of hypertension. Need to minimise alcohol intake, to one standard drink per day and aim to have two alcohol-free days during the week.
4 Referral to a dietitian may also be helpful. Educating the consumer in cooking preparation, preparing a balanced diet, using reduced salt and sugar products.
5 May require referral or psychosocial support given concerns expressed about change in her living circumstances. Kathleen's daughter should be encouraged to be involved in this intervention. You might like to refer to the National Heart Foundation's 2016 guidelines for management of hypertension; see the Further resources list at the end of the chapter.

The final step in the process is accurate documentation. The nurse must document findings, referrals, interventions, and advice and education given. Once Kathleen has undergone investigations and her BP has stabilised, as part of her follow-up she would be directed to make an appointment with her GP, or she may need ongoing management by a general medical specialist.

CHAPTER RESOURCES

REVIEW QUESTIONS

For answers to these questions, see Answer section at the end of the book.

1. Which of the following heart chambers pumps deoxygenated blood to the lungs?
   a. Left atrium
   b. Right atrium
   c. Left ventricle
   d. Right ventricle

2. What is the average adult heart rate per minute when the impulse is initiated by the ventricles of the heart?
   a. 50
   b. >60
   c. 40
   d. <40

3. Assessment of aortic heart sounds should be checked:
   a. On the left side of the sternum, fifth intercostal space, midclavicular line
   b. On the left side of the sternum, fifth intercostal space
   c. Within 5 cm of the xyphoid process
   d. On the right side of the sternum, second intercostal space

4. What is the best location to auscultate the mitral valve of the heart?
   a. On the left side of the sternum, fifth intercostal space, midclavicular line
   b. On the left side of the sternum, fifth intercostal space
   c. Within 5 cm of the xyphoid process
   d. On the right side of the sternum, second intercostal space

5. An S_4 heart sound is often associated with which of the following conditions?
   a. Pericardial disease
   b. Myocardial infarction
   c. Fluid overload
   d. Tachycardia

6. A systolic blowing/high heart murmur auscultated on the left side of the sternum, fifth intercostal space, midclavicular line is indicative of:
   a. Aortic stenosis
   b. Pulmonic regurgitation

   c. Tricuspid stenosis
   d. Mitral regurgitation

7. Which of the following is a modifiable risk factor for cardiovascular disease?
   a. Family history
   b. Alcohol consumption
   c. Cultural background
   d. Sex

8. The sudden onset of intense, sharp, deep muscle pain in the lower leg that increases with dorsiflexion of the foot, and a lower leg that is warm to the touch, and has swelling present, makes the nurse suspect what condition?
   a. Varicose veins
   b. Thrombophlebitis
   c. Deep vein thrombosis
   d. Arterial ulceration of the leg

9. When checking carotid pulses, it is important to check them:
   a. Simultaneously
   b. One at a time
   c. Along with the apical pulse
   d. For 90 seconds

10. The Allen test is a technique used to assess the arterial system by testing for:
    a. The development of pallor in the extremities
    b. The return of colour to the consumer's legs
    c. The patency of the radial and ulnar arteries
    d. Thrombophlebitis

CS CLINICAL SKILLS

The following Clinical Skills are relevant to this chapter and can be found in Tollefson & Hillman, *Clinical Psychomotor Skills*, 8th edition:
> 17 Focused cardiovascular health history and physical assessment
> 18 12-lead electrocardiogram
> 27 Healthcare teaching
> 64 Chest drainage system assessment and management
> 71 Caring for a person with a central venous access device.

FURTHER RESOURCES

> Anatomy Atlases: http://www.anatomyatlases.org
> Auscultation Assistant: http://www.wilkes.med.ucla.edu
> Australian absolute disease risk calculator: https://www.cvdcheck.org.au/calculator
> Australian Government. (2022). Aged Care Quality and Safety Commission: Resource Library. https://www.agedcarequality.gov.au/resource-library?resources%5B0%5D=topics%3A211
> Australian Resuscitation Council: https://resus.org.au/guidelines/
> Chew, D. P., Aroney, C. N., Aylward, P. E., Kelly, A. M., White, H. D., Tideman, P. A., ... & Ruta, L. A. (2011). 2011 addendum to the

National Heart Foundation of Australia and Cardiac Society of Australia and New Zealand guidelines for the management of acute coronary syndromes (ACS) 2006. *Heart Lung and Circulation, 20,* 487–502. doi: 10.1016/j.hlc.2011.03.008
> Chew, D. P., Scott, I. A., Cullen, C., French, J. K., Briffa, T. G., Tideman, P. A., ... & Aylward, P. E. G. (2016). Guideline summary: National Heart Foundation of Australia and Cardiac Society of Australia and New Zealand: Australian clinical guidelines for the management of acute coronary syndromes 2016. *Medical Journal of Australia, 205*(3), 128–33. doi: 10.5694/mja16.0036

> DermNet NZ. All about the skin: https://www.dermnetnz.org/topics/leg-ulcer/
> Haigh, K., Bingley, J., Golledge, J., & Walker, P. (2013). Peripheral arterial disease screening in general practice. *Australian Family Physician, 42*(6), 391–5.
> Hall, J. E. (2016). *Guyton and Hall Textbook of Medical Physiology* (13th ed.). London: Surgical Neurology International.
> Heart Foundation. Physical activity and your heart health: https://www.heartfoundation.org.au/heart-health-education/physical-activity-and-exercise#:~:text=Regular%20physical%20activity%20is%20one,heart%20disease%20and%20heart%20attacks
> Mayo Clinic: http://www.mayoclinic.com
> Ministry of Health – New Zealand Health Survey: https://www.health.govt.nz/nz-health-statistics/national-collections-and-surveys/surveys/new-zealand-health-survey#2020-21
> Ministry of Health. Physical activity: https://www.health.govt.nz/our-work/preventative-health-wellness/physical-activity
> National Heart Foundation of Australia. Blueprint for an active Australia: https://www.heartfoundation.org.au/activities-finding-or-opinion/physical-activity-blueprint
> National Heart Foundation of Australia: http://www.heartfoundation.org.au
> National Heart Foundation of New Zealand: https://www.heartfoundation.org.nz/professionals/health-professionals
> National Institute of Nursing Research: http://www.ninr.nih.gov
> National Institutes of Health: http://www.nih.gov
> Nursing and Midwifery Board of Australia: http://www.nursingmidwiferyboard.gov.au/
> RHDAustralia (acute rheumatic fever & rheumatic heart disease): https://www.rhdaustralia.org.au/arf-rhd-guideline
> Stroke Foundation: https://strokefoundation.org.au/
> Wounds Australia – Australian and New Zealand Clinical Practice Guideline for Prevention and Management of Venous Leg Ulcers. (2011). Approved by NHMRC & The NZ Guideline Group. www.woundsaustralia.com.au/Web/Resources/Publications/Publications_Users_Only/Australian_and_New_Zealand_Clinical_Practice_Guideline_for_Prevention_and_Management_of_Venous_Leg_U.aspx

REFERENCES

Australian Bureau of Statistics (ABS). (2020). Causes of death, Australia 2019. Retrieved 6 December 2022 from: https://www.abs.gov.au/statistics/health/causes-death/causes-death-australia/2019

Australian Bureau of Statistics (ABS). (2021). Causes of death, Australia 2020. Retrieved 6 December 2022 from: https://www.abs.gov.au/statistics/health/causes-death/causes-death-australia/2020#australias-leading-causes-of-death-2020

Australian Bureau of Statistics (ABS). (2022). Causes of death, Australia 2021. Retrieved 6 December 2022 from: https://www.abs.gov.au/statistics/health/causes-death/causes-death-australia/latest-release

Australian Government. (2022). Aged Care Quality and Safety Commission: Resource library. Retrieved 2 May 2022 from: https://www.agedcarequality.gov.au/resource-library?resources%5B0%5D=topics%3A211

Australian Institute of Health and Welfare (AIHW). (2019). Congenital heart disease in Australia, AIHW, Australian Government. Retrieved 6 December 2022 from: https://www.aihw.gov.au/reports/heart-stroke-vascular-diseases/congenital-heart-disease-in-australia/summary

Australian Institute of Health and Welfare (AIHW). (2021a). Heart, stroke and vascular disease: Australian facts. AIHW, Australian Government. Retrieved 6 December 2022 from: https://www.aihw.gov.au/reports/heart-stroke-vascular-diseases/hsvd-facts/contents/about

Australian Institute of Health and Welfare (AIHW). (2021b). Better cardiac care measures for Aboriginal and Torres Strait Islander people: Sixth national report 2021. Cat. no. IHW 263. Canberra. Retrieved 13 December 2022 from: https://www.aihw.gov.au/getmedia/b7a73a21-4d2a-49fc-82dd-4759a5d3638c/aihw-ihw-263.pdf.aspx?inline=true

Australian Institute of Health and Welfare (AIHW). (2022a). Health across socioeconomic groups. Retrieved 13 December 2022 from: https://www.aihw.gov.au/reports/australias-health/health-across-socioeconomic-groups

Australian Institute of Health and Welfare (AIHW). (2022b). Rural and remote health. Retrieved 13 December 2022 from: https://www.aihw.gov.au/reports/rural-remote-australians/rural-and-remote-health

Health New Zealand. (2022). Cardiovascular disease. Retrieved 3 May 2023 from: https://www.health.govt.nz/our-work/diseases-and-conditions/cardiovascular-disease

Healthdirect. (2022). Stroke. Retrieved 25 April 2022 from: https://www.healthdirect.gov.au/stroke

Health Navigator New Zealand. (2022). Risk factors for heart disease. Retrieved 3 May 2023 from: https://www.healthnavigator.org.nz/health-a-z/h/heart-disease-risk-factors/

Heart Foundation New Zealand (NZ). (2018). Cardiovascular disease risk assessment and management. Retrieved 3 May 2023 from: https://www.heartfoundation.org.nz/professionals/health-professionals/cvd-consensus-summary

Heart Foundation New Zealand. (2022a). Statistics. Retrieved 6 December 2022 from: https://www.heartfoundation.org.nz/statistics

Heart Foundation New Zealand. (2022b). What is a heart check?. Retrieved 6 December 2022 from: https://www.heartfoundation.org.nz/wellbeing/managing-risk/your-risk

Merone, L., Burns, J., Poynton, M., & McDermott, R. (2019). Review of cardiovascular health among Aboriginal and Torres Strait Islander people. *Australian Indigenous Health Bulletin, 19*(4). Retrieved 13 December 2022 from: https://healthbulletin.org.au/articles/review-of-cardiovascular-health-among-aboriginal-and-torres-strait-islander-people/

Ministry of Health. (2018). *Cardiovascular disease risk assessment and management for primary care.* Wellington: Ministry of Health. Retrieved 3 May 2023 from: https://www.health.govt.nz/publication/cardiovascular-disease-risk-assessment-and-management-primary-care

National Heart Foundation of Australia. (2016). Guidelines for the diagnosis and management of hypertension in adults 2016. Melbourne: National Heart Foundation of Australia. Retrieved 20 May 2022 from: https://www.heartfoundation.org.au/Conditions/Hypertension

National Heart Foundation of Australia and Cardiac Society of Australia and New Zealand. (2018). Guidelines for the prevention, detection, and management of heart failure in Australia 2018. *Heart Lung and Circulation, 27*(10), 1123–208. Retrieved 24 April 2022 from: https://www.heartlungcirc.org/article/S1443-9506(18)31777-3/fulltext#secsect0025

National Heart Foundation of Australia. (2019). Blueprint for an active Australia. Retrieved 24 April 2022 from: https://www.heartfoundation.org.au/activities-finding-or-opinion/physical-activity-blueprint

National Heart Foundation of Australia. (2021a). Aboriginal and Torres Strait Islander peoples: Are you at risk of heart disease? Retrieved 13 December 2022 from: https://www.heartfoundation.org.au/bundles/your-heart/aboriginal-health-risk-of-heart-disease

National Heart Foundation of Australia. (2021b). CVD risk calculators. Retrieved 6 December 2022 from: https://www.heartfoundation.org.au/bundles/heart-health-check-toolkit/cardiovascular-disease-risk-calculators

National Heart Foundation of Australia. (2021c). Physical activity and your heart health. Retrieved 6 December 2022 from: https://www.heartfoundation.org.au/heart-health-education/physical-activity-and-exercise

National Heart Foundation of Australia. (2022a). Key statistics: Heart disease. Retrieved 20 April 2022 from: https://www.heartfoundation.org.au/Activities-finding-or-opinion/Australia-Heart-Disease-Statistics

National Heart Foundation of Australia. (2022b). Key statistics: Risk factors for cardiovascular disease. Retrieved 20 April 2022 from: https://www.heartfoundation.org.au/activities-finding-or-opinion/key-statistics-risk-factors-for-heart-disease

National Heart Foundation of Australia. (2022c). Absolute CVD risk clinical guidelines. Retrieved 20 April 2022 from: https://www.heartfoundation.org.au/conditions/fp-absolute-cvd-risk-clinical-guidelines

National Heart Foundation of Australia. (2022d). Heart online: Heart education assessment rehabilitation toolkit. Retrieved 20 April 2022 from: https://www.heartonline.org.au/

Radhakrishnan, N. (2022). Genesis, pathophysiology and management of venous and lymphatic disorders. Elsevier. https://doi.org/10.1016/C2020-0-03522-X

RHDAustralia (ARF/RHD writing group). (2022). The 2020 Australian guideline for prevention, diagnosis and management of acute rheumatic fever and rheumatic heart disease (3.2 edition, March 2022); 2020. Retrieved 2 May 2022 from: https://www.rhdaustralia.org.au/system/files/fileuploads/arf_rhd_guidelines_3.2_edition_march_2022.pdf

Stroke Foundation. (2022). What is a stroke? Retrieved 2 May 2022 from: https://strokefoundation.org.au/about-stroke/learn/what-is-a-stroke

World Health Organization (WHO). (2021). Cardiovascular diseases (CVDs). Retrieved 6 December 2022 from: https://www.who.int/en/news-room/fact-sheets/detail/cardiovascular-diseases-(cvds)

CHAPTER 15

GASTROINTESTINAL

LEARNING OUTCOMES

By the end of this chapter you should be able to:
1 identify the physiological function of the gastrointestinal organs
2 describe key recommendations of the dietary guidelines for Australian and New Zealand adults, children and adolescents
3 obtain the health history of a consumer with a gastrointestinal problem, including nutritional history
4 demonstrate gastrointestinal assessment, and differentiate normal and abnormal findings during the assessment
6 discuss the clinical reasoning in evaluating outcomes of health assessment and physical examination, including documentation, health education provision and relevant health referral.

BACKGROUND

Nutrition, or the processes by which the body metabolises and utilises nutrients, affects every system in the body. Nutrition is essential to sustain life, but the type and quantity are key considerations when assessing a person's nutritional health. We must also understand how the body digests and absorbs nutrients to meet daily nutritional requirements, and work collaboratively with allied health disciplines to ensure consumers have comprehensive nutritional assessment and support (e.g. nutritionists and dietitians). Psychological, social, environmental, financial and cultural issues must also be considered during a nutritional assessment, especially when considering the impact of a nutritional imbalance.

In this chapter the assessment of the gastrointestinal system and a consumer's nutritional status requires an understanding of nutritional requirements and normal gastrointestinal function. Examination of the gastrointestinal system provides significant information about the various functions of organs within the gastrointestinal and cardiovascular systems. This is augmented by assessment of the consumer's nutritional status, understanding of nutritional needs and current dietary habits. While abdominal and nutritional assessment are addressed together in this chapter, complex nutritional assessment would require referral to a dietitian or nutritionist and this will depend on your context.

There are a number of common gastrointestinal health problems that are encountered in the Australian and New Zealand population which relate to this assessment chapter. In 2021, cancers of the colon, sigmoid, rectum and anus were the sixth leading cause of death in Australia, and diabetes was the seventh, with bowel cancer being the most common form of gastrointestinal cancer (ABS, 2022).

For Aboriginal and Torres Strait Islanders, diabetes was the second leading cause of death, and cirrhosis and other diseases of the liver the ninth leading cause of death (ABS, 2022). In 2019, diabetes was the fifth leading cause of death and bowel cancer the seventh for Māori people (Health New Zealand, 2019).

Key gastrointestinal health conditions include irritable bowel, diverticulitis, ulcerative colitis and constipation. Gastric ulcers, *Helicobacter pylori* infection and gastritis are common health conditions that affect the stomach. Other gastrointestinal health problems pertain to the individual abdominal organs such as the gall bladder (gall stones), appendix (appendicitis) and peritoneum (peritonitis). Although the appendix appears a small and insignificant organ, appendicitis can occur in any age group; however, it is more commonly observed in the older child and young adult. Appendicitis can be difficult to diagnose as it mimics a number of other illnesses. Interestingly, the most common abdominal surgical emergency is acute appendicitis, with an incidence of almost 100 per 100 000 across the developed world (Danwang et al., 2020).

Obesity is an epidemic, with worldwide rates nearly tripling between 1975 and 2021 (WHO, 2021). In most developed countries, being overweight or obese is a significant modifiable risk factor that is associated with, and further complicates, many chronic diseases (Boutari & Mantzoros, 2022) (Table 15.1). Of particular concern is the number of children and young people who are obese. Children who are overweight or obese are more likely to remain so in adulthood. In 2017–18 in Australia, an estimated 1.2 million children and adolescents aged 2–17, or 1 in 4, and 67% of adults (75% of men and 60% of women) were either overweight or obese (AIHW, 2022).

TABLE 15.1 Obesity in adults, children and adolescents in New Zealand, 2021

ADULTS	CHILDREN AND ADOLESCENTS
One in three adults were obese (34.3%).	One in eight children (aged 2–14 years) were obese (12.7%).
51% of Māori adults were obese.	18% of Māori children were obese.
71% of Pasifika adults were obese.	35% of Pacific Islander children were obese.
Adults living in socioeconomically deprived areas were 1.6 times as likely to be obese as those in the least deprived areas.	Children living in socioeconomically deprived areas were 2.5 times as likely to be obese as those in the least deprived areas.

MINISTRY OF HEALTH, 2021.

The effects of obesity are wide-ranging. Common consequences include social and economic impacts as well as health-related issues such as musculoskeletal problems, cardiovascular disease, some cancers, sleep apnoea, type 2 diabetes mellitus, stroke, gall bladder and liver disease (AIHW, 2022). Additionally, being overweight contributes to other issues such as heat intolerance, breathlessness on exertion, tiredness and development of flat feet. The majority of these illnesses and issues can be prevented with appropriate diet and physical activity, and as such are a modifiable health risk. Nurses can take an active role in the education and support of the whole community, including themselves.

ABDOMEN AND NUTRITION ASSESSMENT

Nutrients

To perform a proper nutritional assessment, you must have a clear understanding of the various nutrients and food sources needed to provide an adequate diet. **Nutrients** are the substances found in food that are nourishing and useful to the body. Carbohydrates, proteins, fats, vitamins, minerals and water are the nutrients essential for life.

Carbohydrates, proteins and fats supply the body with energy, which is measured in units called kilojoules (Australia and New Zealand) or calories (USA). Kilojoules (kJ) and calories both define the energy value of food (or the amount of chemical energy that may be released as heat when food is metabolised). Australian foods are all packaged with reference to kilojoules. But if you have used calories as a measure before, one calorie is equivalent to 4.2 kJ.

Weight loss or gain is influenced by the balance between a person's energy intake and energy expended. There are advances being made in understanding of nutritional health and particularly in relation to obesity and obesity management. A current belief about weight loss and gain is that energy intake higher than energy expenditure usually results in excess body fat, with the reverse causing body fat loss. Approximately two-thirds of the required daily kilojoule intake is needed to maintain base functions; for example, to keep the blood pumping, heart beating, brain and nerves firing, lungs breathing, and for the repair and maintenance of cells. This is called the **basal metabolic rate (BMR)**, the number of kilojoules burned at rest – basically the amount of energy needed by the body to maintain itself.

Those who are physically active (either due to exercise or a job requiring physical energy) have a higher basal metabolic rate and burn more kilojoules. For example, a person in a sedentary job (computer work or office work) may use about 9000 kJ per day, a manual worker lifting materials may burn approximately 12 500 kJ per day, and a heavy labourer or athlete may use up to 17 000 kJ per day. This will change across the lifespan.

Carbohydrates

The major source of energy for the various functions of the body is **carbohydrates**. Each gram of carbohydrate contains 16.8 kJ. Adults require 50–60% of their daily intake in the form of carbohydrates to prevent ketosis and protein breakdown of muscles.

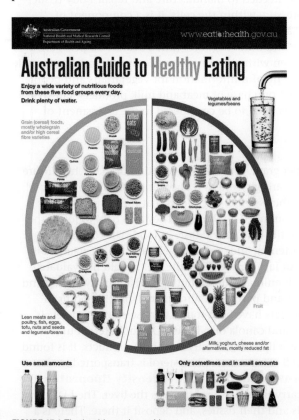

FIGURE 15.1 The healthy eating guide

© COMMONWEALTH OF AUSTRALIA 2016

Carbohydrates help form adenosine triphosphate (ATP), which is needed to transfer energy within the cells. Carbohydrates supply fibre and assist in metabolising fat. The primary sources of carbohydrates are bread, potatoes, pasta, corn, rice, dried beans and fruits. Dietary deficiency of carbohydrates can result in electrolyte imbalance, fatigue and depression. However, an excess of carbohydrates may produce obesity and tooth decay, and may adversely affect those with diabetes mellitus.

> ## REFLECTION IN PRACTICE
>
> **Assessing a consumer's diet and the link to disease prevention – your role**
> Diets high in fibre have been shown to be beneficial in disease prevention. The possible benefits are decreased weight and decreases in the risks of colon cancer, rectal cancer, heart disease (through decreasing serum cholesterol levels), dental caries, constipation and diverticulosis. Consider how much knowledge you have about diet and nutrition. Nurses are often in a position to provide a referral or start an education process around diet and nutrition linked to disease treatment and prevention. Consider how well you can start this process with your current knowledge. What else can you do to increase this and ensure you use the most appropriate resources for the consumer's benefit?

Proteins

There are 16.8 kJ in every gram of protein, but foods usually are a combination of protein and fat (meats, milk) or protein and carbohydrates (legumes). Adults require 0.8 g/kg/day of protein, or approximately 10–20% of their daily food intake. **Protein** is required to give the body the nine essential amino acids that the body is unable to synthesise. These are needed to form the basis of all cell structures in the body. Protein is needed to manufacture and repair body tissue, it helps to maintain osmotic pressure within the cells, it is a component of antibodies, and it is ultimately a source of energy. The major sources of protein are meat, poultry, fish, eggs, cheese and milk. Legumes (dried beans and peas) are a good source of protein when eaten with corn or wheat (e.g. beans and rice provide a good source of protein). This is helpful information for vegetarians and people whose incomes will not cover the purchase of meat and milk products. Lifestyle choices and socioeconomic status need to be considered in the assessment of nutritional status.

Fats

Lipids, or fats, contain 37.8 kJ per gram. The recommendation of many healthcare experts is to use fats in the diet sparingly, and to reduce fat to 20–30% of the total calories consumed. **Fats** supply the essential fatty acids that form a part of the structure of all cells and must be supplied by the diet. They also help to lower the serum cholesterol. Fats influence the texture and taste of food. The food sources of fat are animal fat (butter, shortening and lard) and vegetable fat (vegetable oil, margarine and nuts). The types of fats consumed in the diet should be evaluated. **Saturated fats** come from both animal sources (butter, lard and fatty meats) and vegetable sources (coconut, palm and partially hydrogenated oils that occur in some processed foods). Saturated fats have been found to raise cholesterol levels. **Monounsaturated fats** (olive and canola oils) lower LDL cholesterol but not HDL cholesterol. **Cholesterol** is a lipid found only in animal products. It is found in muscle, red blood cells and cell membranes. Cholesterol is transported in the blood by **high-density lipoproteins (HDL)** and **low-density lipoproteins (LDL)**. The HDL are useful in carrying cholesterol towards the liver. The LDL carry the cholesterol towards the cells and then tissues, and deposit it there. There is a strong association between high levels of LDL and coronary artery disease (CAD). In contrast, high levels of HDL protect against CAD.

Triglycerides account for most of the lipids stored in the body's tissues. In the bloodstream, triglycerides produce energy for the body. An elevated triglyceride level occurs in hyperlipidaemia, a risk factor for CAD.

A deficiency of fat in the diet can cause a decrease in weight, lack of satiety, and skin and hair changes. An excess of fat in the diet contributes to obesity and is linked to CAD. There has also been a correlation between high-fat diets and certain cancers (colon and prostate, in particular).

Vitamins

Vitamins are organic substances needed to maintain the function of the body. They are not synthesised by the body in sufficient amounts and must be obtained from dietary sources. Vitamins stored in dietary fat and absorbed in the fat portions of the body's cells are **fat-soluble vitamins**. These are vitamins A, D, E and K. **Water-soluble vitamins** include C, thiamine (B_1), riboflavin (B_2), niacin (B_3), pyridoxine (B_6), folacin (folate), cobalamin (B_{12}), pantothenic acid and biotin. These vitamins are not stored in the body but excreted in the urine. Various disease conditions occur when a vitamin source is lacking.

HEALTH EDUCATION

Hypervitaminosis

Hypervitaminosis is a toxic amount of vitamins in the body. It occurs with both water-soluble and fat-soluble vitamins. Vitamins that have been shown to cause serious toxic effects include vitamins A, K, C and B_6 (pyridoxine).

Encourage consumers to obtain proper nutrients through a healthy diet rather than through supplements. If your consumer insists on taking supplements, the consumer should use the recommended dietary intake (RDI) as a guide. It is important to stress that vitamin supplements should not replace a healthy diet (see https://www.nhmrc.gov.au/guidelines-publications/n35-n36-n37).

Minerals

Minerals are inorganic elements that regulate body processes and build body tissue. These processes are fluid balance; acid–base balance; nerve cell transmission; vitamin, enzyme and hormonal activity; and muscle contractions. Minerals are divided into two classifications. **Macrominerals**, or major minerals, are needed by the body in large amounts. **Microminerals**, or trace minerals, are needed in smaller amounts by the body.

The most common nutrient deficiency in the world is that of iron. This is particularly prevalent among infants, adolescents, and pregnant and menstruating women. It can result in iron-deficiency anaemia, which can significantly impact on general health and wellbeing and can require various levels of intervention.

HEALTH EDUCATION

Preventing iron-deficiency anaemia
> Identify those consumers at risk (e.g. children under 2 years of age, adolescents, women with heavy menstrual flow, pregnant women, and individuals with malabsorption syndromes, gastrointestinal bleeding, and gross dietary deficiencies).
> Perform a complete nutritional assessment on these high-risk consumers.
> Encourage consumers to eat foods high in iron. These include lean meats, poultry, fish, fortified cereals, dark green leafy vegetables and dried fruits.

UNIT 2

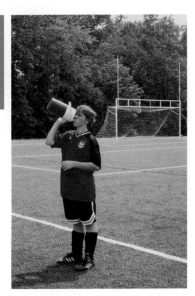

FIGURE 15.2 Hydration is essential to body function, especially when engaged in strenuous activities.

Water

Water is essential to life; we cannot survive more than a few days without it. Water accounts for 50–60% of the body's weight. The daily amount needed depends on the size of the person, the climate, and the amount of activity. The average adult needs six to eight glasses of water a day; athletes and those living in hot, dry climates require more. Thirst may not always be an adequate indicator of water intake needs, especially in infants or very ill individuals who may have a poor thirst mechanism. Those who engage in intense physical activity may have a decreased thirst sensation as well (see Figure 15.2).

In addition, it is important to determine the source of the water intake. Tap water is usually safe in most areas of Australia and New Zealand. However, for people who live in less populated areas and only have access to well or bore water, the safety risk may be high depending on environmental factors. In some rural and remote areas, particularly in outback Australia and remote areas of New Zealand, rusty water pipes with unknown pathogens may be the only source of water. In other areas, local streams and rivers may be the only source of water.

URGENT FINDING

Dehydration

Dehydration is an urgent finding across the lifespan, but becomes life-threatening in vulnerable populations such as children and elderly consumers. Consumers with persistent debilitating diarrhoea require fluid and electrolyte replacement therapy to restore homeostasis to the body. If the consumer is vomiting, there is a risk of dehydration and electrolyte imbalance. If this is not treated, the consumer will continue to decline and enter a state of hypovolaemic shock.

Dehydration can cause electrolyte imbalance and when severe can impact on cardiac function on a cellular level. It can cause delirium, and is often associated with other conditions such as viral or bacterial infection. Immediate management of dehydration needs to be undertaken once identified to reduce further deterioration.

Signs and symptoms of dehydration:
> Health history reveals inadequate intake of fluids
> Decrease in urine output
> Urine specific gravity >1.035
> Weight loss (% body weight): 3–5% for mild, 6–9% for moderate, and 10–15% for severe dehydration
> Eyes appear sunken; tongue has increased furrows and fissures
> Oral mucous membranes are dry
> Decreased skin turgor
> Sunken fontanelles in infants
> Inability to produce tears
> Changes in neurological status may occur with moderate to severe dehydration.
Remember to assess skin turgor, mucous membranes and orthostatic blood pressure.
See Chapters 8, 11 and 14.

Dietary guidelines

The guidelines for healthy eating for Australia and New Zealand have moved away from earlier 'food pyramids'. Guidelines have become more simplified in Australia since 2010. In Australia and New Zealand some variations exist in these guidelines; for example, see Table 15.2.

TABLE 15.2 Comparison of nutritional guidelines for Australia and New Zealand (adults and children)

DIETARY GUIDELINES FOR AUSTRALIAN ADULTS: A GUIDE TO HEALTHY EATING*	NEW ZEALAND FOOD AND NUTRITION GUIDELINE STATEMENTS FOR ADULTS**
Australians need to eat more: > vegetables, legumes and fruits > cereals (including breads, rice, pasta and noodles), preferably wholegrain > lean meat, fish, poultry and/or alternatives > reduced-fat milks, yoghurts, cheeses and/or alternatives; reduced-fat varieties should be chosen except for infants and children > drink plenty of water and take care to: > limit saturated fat and moderate total fat intake > choose foods low in salt > limit the alcohol intake if they choose to drink > consume only moderate amounts of sugars and foods containing added sugars > prevent weight gain: be physically active and eat according to energy needs > care for food: prepare and store it safely > encourage and support breastfeeding.	1. Enjoy variety of nutritious foods daily including plenty of fruits and vegetables, wholegrain foods and foods naturally high in fibre, some milk and dairy (reduced fat), some legumes, nuts, seeds, lean meats, fish and seafood, eggs. 2. Choose/prepare foods with unsaturated fats, low in salt, low or no added sugar, mostly whole or less processed. 3. Make plain water your choice over other drinks. 4. If drinking alcohol, limit intake. Cease intake during or when preparing for pregnancy. 5. Purchase, prepare, cook and store food to ensure food safety. **Activity statements:** 1. Sit less and move more. Do not sit for long periods. 2. Undertake at least 2.5 hours of moderate or 1.25 hours of vigorous activity throughout the week. 3. For extra benefits, aim for 5 hours of moderate or 2.5 hours of vigorous activity in the week. 4. Do muscle strengthening activities twice per week. 5. Doing some activity is better than nothing.
DIETARY GUIDELINES FOR CHILDREN AND ADOLESCENTS IN AUSTRALIA: A GUIDE TO HEALTHY EATING*	**FOOD AND NUTRITION GUIDELINES FOR HEALTHY CHILDREN AND YOUNG PEOPLE (AGED 2–18 YEARS): A BACKGROUND PAPER*****
Enjoy a wide variety of nutritious foods. Children and adolescents should be encouraged to: > eat plenty of vegetables, legumes and fruits > eat plenty of cereals (including breads, rice, pasta and noodles), preferably wholegrain > include lean meat, fish, poultry and/or alternatives > include milks, yoghurts, cheeses and/or alternatives (reduced-fat milks are not suitable for young children under 2 years, because of their high-energy needs, but reduced-fat varieties should be encouraged for older children and adolescents) > choose water as a drink and care should be taken to: > limit saturated fat and moderate total fat intake (low-fat diets are not suitable for infants) > choose foods low in salt > consume only moderate amounts of sugars and foods containing added sugars.	1. Eat a variety of foods from each of the four major food groups each day: • vegetables and fruit, including different colours and textures • breads and cereals, increasing wholegrain products as children increase in age • milk and milk products or suitable alternatives, preferably reduced or low-fat options • lean meat, poultry, fish, shellfish, eggs, legumes, nuts and seeds. 2. Eat enough for activity, growth and to maintain a healthy body size. • Have regular meals, including snacks. 3. Prepare foods or choose pre-prepared foods, snacks and drinks that are: • low in fat, especially saturated fat • low in sugar, especially added sugar • low in salt (if using salt, use iodised salt). 4. Drink plenty of fluid each day, preferably water or low-fat milk. • Limit use of drinks such as cordial, juice, fizzy drinks (including diet drinks), sports drinks and sports water. • Energy drinks or energy shots are not recommended for children or young people. • Do not give children less than 13 years of age coffee or tea. If young people choose to drink coffee or tea, limit to one to two cups per day. 5. Alcohol is not recommended for children or young people. 6. Eat meals with family or whānau as often as possible. 7. Purchase, prepare, cook and store food in ways that ensure food safety.
Encourage and support breastfeeding. Children and adolescents need sufficient nutritious foods to grow and develop normally: > Growth should be checked regularly for young children. > Physical activity is important for children and adolescents. > Care for your child's food: prepare and store it safely.	8. Be physically active. • Take part in regular physical activity, aiming for 60 minutes or more of moderate to vigorous activity each day. • Spend less than two hours a day (out of school time) in front of television, computers and gaming consoles. • Be active in as many ways as possible, e.g. through play, cultural activities, dance, sport and recreation, jobs and going from place to place. • Be active with friends and whānau, at home, school, and in your community.

*Sourced from Australian Government, National Health and Medical Research Council & Department of Health and Ageing. (2013). *Eat for health: Australian dietary guidelines* summary. Canberra: Commonwealth of Australia.

** Sourced from Ministry of Health. (2020). Eating and activity guidelines for New Zealand adults. Wellington: Ministry of Health. https://www.health.govt.nz/publication/eating-and-activity-guidelines-new-zealand-adults

***Sourced from Ministry of Health New Zealand. (2012). Food and Nutrition Guidelines for Healthy Children and Young People (Aged 2–18 Years): A background paper. Wellington: Ministry of Health. https://www.health.govt.nz/publication/food-and-nutrition-guidelines-healthy-children-and-young-people-aged-2-18-years-background-paper

Nutrition through the life cycle

Assessment of the consumer's developmental needs must always be included with a nutritional assessment. Nutritional needs change throughout the life cycle and are affected by both physical and developmental changes. A clear understanding of those changes, how they affect the consumer, and what **anticipatory guidance** is indicated are needed to conduct a nutritional assessment. Additionally, there may be specific foods and food preparation approaches to avoid or be aware of. For example, if you preserve your own food, you will need to ensure cooking temperatures, container and sterilisation levels are adequate to avoid food contamination with bacteria such as botulism. Another consideration is to avoid giving honey to babies under 12 months old – adults and children older than 12 months can manage this usually because of the natural defences established in their gastrointestinal system (NSW Health, 2018).

Cultural differences

It is not possible to have knowledge of all cultural differences, but an open and understanding attitude and acceptance of various religious and cultural beliefs is imperative. Certain foods may have special meanings and memories for individual consumers, or may be traditional among many with the same cultural backgrounds, such as the imperative for meat to be butchered with Halal methods for those complying with Islamic law, or the use of dugong and sea turtles to celebrate special events for Torres Strait Islander peoples. There may also be regional considerations, food preferences and religious beliefs that restrict certain foods and their consumption. An understanding of the food practices for various cultural groups is needed to provide appropriate nutritional assessment and education. Be sure to inquire about various cultural and religious influences on dietary practices during the nutritional assessment. In many cases, referral to or collaboration with a dietitian can assist the consumer to address dietary approaches in line with both health and cultural or religious requirements.

PUTTING IT IN CONTEXT

Culturally based nutritional practices
> Your Islamic consumer has been fasting during Ramadan. He is diabetic and continues to become hypoglycaemic. What would be your plan of care? How would you help him balance his religious and nutritional needs?
> LoAn is a pregnant Vietnamese female who is HIV positive. She incorporates the observance of *yin* and *yang* into her daily rituals. LoAn confides that she is looking forward to breastfeeding her child. You realise that pregnancy is a *yang* condition and lactation is a *yin* condition, which is in line with LoAn's beliefs.
>   • What information would you discuss with LoAn, knowing that a female who is HIV positive is advised against breastfeeding?
>   • Consider how collaborating with a dietitian or nutritionist may assist you in supporting these consumers with their health management plans related to diet.

ANATOMY AND PHYSIOLOGY

Abdominal cavity

The abdomen is the largest cavity of the body. It is located between the diaphragm and the symphysis pubis. It is oval-shaped and contains several vital organs. The posterior wall of the cavity includes the lumbar vertebrae, the sacrum and the coccyx. The iliac bones and the lateral portion of the ribs shape the sides of the abdominal cavity (**Figures 15.3** and **15.4**). These bony structures are held together by muscular tissue that surrounds the entire abdominal cavity. The muscles of the

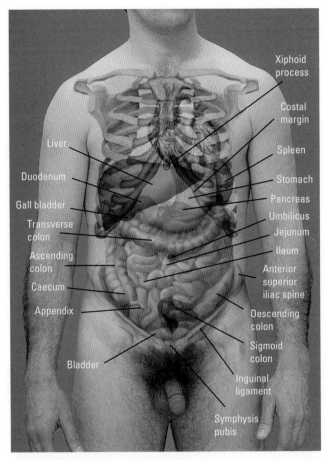

FIGURE 15.3 Structures of the abdomen: Anterior view

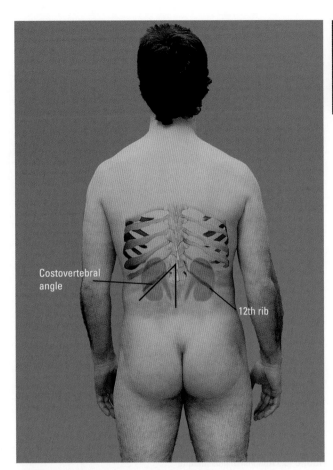

FIGURE 15.4 Structures of the abdomen: Posterior view

abdomen include the rectus abdominis, transversus abdominis, external oblique and internal oblique. The **linea alba**, a tendinous tissue that extends from the sternum to the symphysis pubis in the midline of the abdomen, is situated between the rectus abdominis muscles (see **Figure 15.5**).

Peritoneum

The endothelial lining of the abdominal cavity consists of membranes called peritoneal serous membranes. The serous layer that lines the walls of the cavity itself is called the parietal peritoneum, and that which covers the organs is called the visceral peritoneum. The potential space between the two layers is referred to as the peritoneal cavity. In the male, this cavity is completely closed, whereas in the female, openings exist for the fallopian tubes.

The organs covered with peritoneum and held in place by mesentery are referred to as intraperitoneal organs. The intraperitoneal organs are the spleen, gall bladder, stomach, liver, bile duct, small intestine and large intestine. In contrast, the organs situated behind the peritoneum and without mesenteric attachment are known as retroperitoneal organs. The retroperitoneal organs are the pancreas, kidneys, ureters and bladder.

Abdominal vasculature

The aorta is the largest artery in the body. Below the level of the diaphragm, the descending aorta becomes the abdominal aorta, giving rise to arterial vessels that supply the abdominal wall and gastrointestinal organs with blood (see **Figure 15.6**). At about the fourth lumbar vertebra, the aorta bifurcates to become the right and left common iliac arteries.

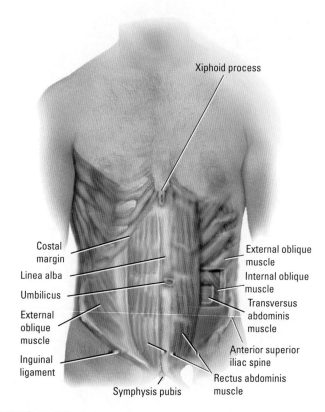

FIGURE 15.5 Abdominal musculature

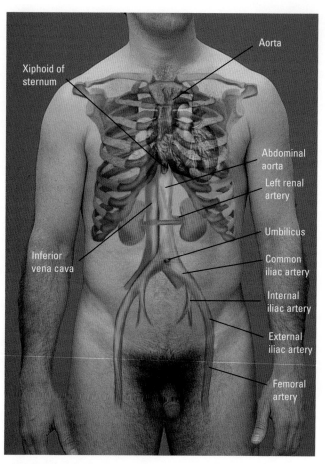

FIGURE 15.6 Abdominal vasculature

Anatomic mapping

Anatomic maps serve as a frame of reference during assessment of the abdomen. The abdominal cavity can be subdivided using two methods: quadrants or nine regions.

The most commonly used assessment approach in clinical practice is the four-quadrant technique (see **Figure 15.7**). For accuracy in documentation, the abdominal surface is divided into four sections by imaginary vertical and horizontal lines intersecting at the umbilicus. Commit to memory the location of abdominal organs according to quadrants (see **Figure 15.7**). **Table 15.3** lists pathologies by the quadrant or region in which the pain is perceived.

Another strategy for pinpointing the location of abdominal assessment findings is via nine abdominal anatomic regions (see **Figure 15.8**). You can also use the anatomic landmarks in **Figure 15.9**.

Abdominal viscera (organs)

Stomach

The stomach is a J-shaped, pouch-like organ located in the left upper quadrant of the abdomen beneath the diaphragm; it lies to the right of the spleen and is partially covered by the liver.

The stomach functions as a reservoir in which the complex mechanical and chemical processes of digestion occur. Hydrochloric acid and digestive enzymes are secreted by the stomach to aid digestion. Little absorption of foodstuffs occurs in the stomach. Foodstuffs are liquified via gastric secretions into a semisolid substance called chyme. The usual capacity of the stomach is 1–1.5 L. In a regulated manner, chyme is released into the small intestine's duodenum for further digestion and absorption.

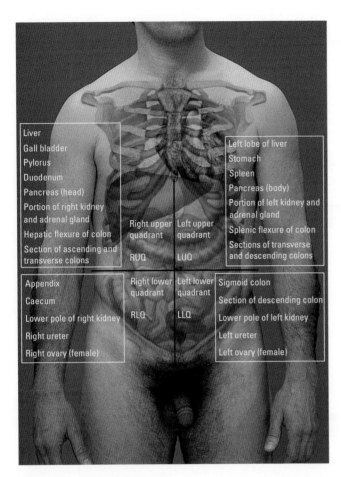

Liver
Gall bladder
Pylorus
Duodenum
Pancreas (head)
Portion of right kidney and adrenal gland
Hepatic flexure of colon
Section of ascending and transverse colons

Right upper quadrant — RUQ

Left lobe of liver
Stomach
Spleen
Pancreas (body)
Portion of left kidney and adrenal gland
Splenic flexure of colon
Sections of transverse and descending colons

Left upper quadrant — LUQ

Appendix
Caecum
Lower pole of right kidney
Right ureter
Right ovary (female)

Right lower quadrant — RLQ

Sigmoid colon
Section of descending colon
Lower pole of left kidney
Left ureter
Left ovary (female)

Left lower quadrant — LLQ

FIGURE 15.7 Abdominal quadrants

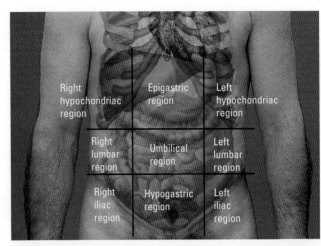

Right hypochondriac region | Epigastric region | Left hypochondriac region
Right lumbar region | Umbilical region | Left lumbar region
Right iliac region | Hypogastric region | Left iliac region

FIGURE 15.8 Nine abdominal anatomic regions

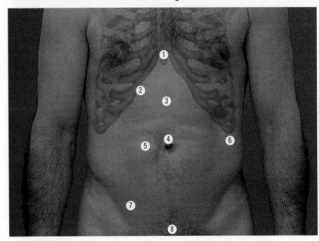

FIGURE 15.9 Abdominal assessment landmarks. When describing pathology of the abdomen, it is useful to use these anatomic landmarks: 1. Xiphoid process; 2. Costal margin; 3. Abdominal midline; 4. Umbilicus; 5. Rectus abdominis muscle; 6. Anterior superior iliac spine; 7. Inguinal ligament (Poupart's ligament); 8. Symphysis pubis.

TABLE 15.3 Causes of abdominal pain: Anatomical regions perceived

RIGHT UPPER QUADRANT	EPIGASTRIUM	LEFT UPPER QUADRANT
Biliary stone	Abdominal aortic aneurysm	Colitis
Cholecystitis	Appendicitis (early)	Gastric ulcer
Cholelithiasis	Biliary stone	Gastritis
Colitis	Cholecystitis	Myocardial infarction
Duodenal ulcer	Cholelithiasis	Nephrolithiasis
Gastric ulcer	Diverticulitis	Pneumonia
Hepatic abscess	Gastro-oesophageal reflux disease/gastritis	Pulmonary embolus
Hepatitis	Hiatus hernia	Pyelonephritis
Hepatomegaly	Myocardial infarction	Splenic enlargement
Nephrolithiasis	Pancreatitis	Splenic rupture
Pancreatitis	Peptic ulcer disease	
Pneumonia		
Pulmonary embolus		
Pyelonephritis		

>>

>>

	PERIUMBILICAL	
	Abdominal aortic aneurysm and dissection Appendicitis (early) Diverticulitis Intestinal obstruction Irritable bowel syndrome Mesenteric ischaemia Pancreatitis Peptic ulcer Recurrent abdominal pain (in children) Small bowel obstruction Volvulus	
RIGHT LOWER QUADRANT		**LEFT LOWER QUADRANT**
Appendicitis Diverticulitis Ectopic pregnancy (ruptured) Endometriosis Hernia (strangulated) Inflammatory bowel disease Irritable bowel syndrome Mittelschmerz Ovarian cyst Pelvic inflammatory disease Renal calculi Salpingitis Uterine fibroids		Diverticulitis Ectopic pregnancy (ruptured) Endometriosis Hernia (strangulated) Inflammatory bowel disease Irritable bowel syndrome Mittelschmerz Ovarian cyst Pelvic inflammatory disease Renal calculi Salpingitis Uterine fibroids
	DIFFUSE	
	Gastroenteritis Herpes zoster Muscle strain Peritonitis	

Small intestine

The small intestine is a tubular-shaped organ extending from the pyloric sphincter to the ileocaecal valve at the opening of the large intestine. The majority of food is digested and absorbed in the small intestine. The convoluted loops of intestine are relatively mobile and can measure from 3 to 9 metres, depending on the degree of muscular relaxation of the intestinal wall and the size of the individual. Portions of the small intestine can be found in all four abdominal quadrants. The three segments of the small intestine are the duodenum, the jejunum and the ileum. The duodenum is the first and shortest section. It plays a significant role in digestion because hormonal secretions are released and both the common bile and main pancreatic ducts open into the duodenum. The jejunum, the second component, is composed of circular mucosal folds that provide surface area for nutrient absorption. The ileum absorbs bile salts and vitamin B$_{12}$. The ileum terminates at the ileocaecal valve.

URGENT FINDING

Haematemesis

Haematemesis, or the vomiting of blood, may be attributed to gastrointestinal ulcers or oesophageal varices. Active bleeding is a medical emergency, and the consumer should be promptly treated, as active bleeding from varices is difficult to control and can lead to hypovolaemic shock and death from uncontrolled bleeding. Urgent escalation of care is required.

Large intestine

The large intestine is a tubular-shaped organ extending from the ileocaecal valve to the anus. It has a greater diameter than the small intestine and can vary considerably in length, depending on the size of the individual, but generally is 1.5 metres in length.

The four segments of the large intestine are the ascending, transverse, descending and sigmoid colons. The caecum is the blind pouch that is continuous with the ascending colon, the large intestine located in the lower right quadrant of the abdomen.

The work of the large intestine is to form stool from cellulose, indigestible fibres, fat, bacteria, cellular debris and inorganic materials, and then carry these intestinal contents to the end of the gastrointestinal tract. An additional function of the large intestine is the absorption of water and electrolytes. Water absorption occurs primarily in the ascending colon under the influence of the osmotic pressure gradient produced by sodium ions. The large intestine has limited digestive function.

Liver

The liver is the largest solid organ in the body. It lies directly below the diaphragm. The liver is located in the right upper quadrant but extends across the midline into the left upper quadrant. In the right upper quadrant, the superior aspect of the liver is at the fifth rib, or at the nipples. The lower border does not extend more than 1 to 2 cm below the right costal margin.

The functions of the liver are complex and varied, and can be divided into:

> storage (carbohydrates, amino acids, vitamins, minerals and blood)
> detoxification and filtration (drugs, hormones and bacteria)
> metabolism (carbohydrates, proteins, fat, ammonia to urea)
> synthesis and secretion (bile production – 600 to 1000 mL/day, formation of lymph, bile salts, plasma proteins, fibrinogen, blood-clotting substances and antibodies).

Gall bladder

The gall bladder is a pear-shaped sac located in the right upper quadrant of the abdomen. It is attached to the inferior surface of the liver.

The primary role of the gall bladder is to store and concentrate the bile produced by the liver. Bile contributes to fat digestion and absorption. The gall bladder stores approximately 30 to 50 mL of bile and releases bile in the presence of cholecystokinin, pancreozymin, and parasympathetic stimulation. As the gall bladder contracts, bile is released through the cystic duct into the common bile duct, which drains into the duodenum.

Pancreas

The pancreas is an elongated accessory organ of digestion. It lies in a transverse position along the posterior abdominal wall. It is located in the upper right and upper left quadrants of the abdomen. The pancreas is both an exocrine gland that secretes bicarbonate and pancreatic enzymes (which aid in digestion), and an endocrine gland that secretes the hormones insulin, glucagon and gastrin.

Spleen

The spleen is the largest lymph organ in the body. It is oval in shape and is composed of white, pulpy lymphoid tissue and red pulp containing capillaries and venous sinuses. It is located behind the fundus of the stomach, below the diaphragm and above the left kidney and splenic flexure. The spleen is found in the left upper quadrant of the abdomen.

The spleen is part of the reticuloendothelial system and serves the body as a filter and a reservoir for red blood cell mass. During events that can cause vasoconstriction, such as haemorrhage or exercise, the spleen contributes needed blood to the general circulation. As a filter, the spleen rids the body of old or deformed red blood cells and platelets.

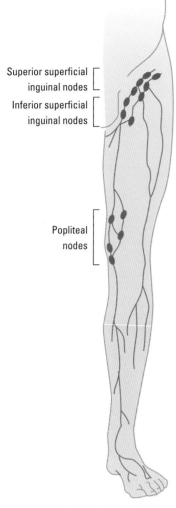

Superior superficial inguinal nodes

Inferior superficial inguinal nodes

Popliteal nodes

FIGURE 15.10 Inguinal and lower limb lymph nodes

Vermiform appendix

The vermiform appendix extends off the lower caecum in the right lower quadrant. This finger-like appendage fills with digestive materials from the caecum. The vermiform appendix frequently does not empty completely, causing obstruction and subsequent infection.

ASSESSMENT: TAKING THE CONSUMER'S HEALTH HISTORY

Assessment is the first phase of the nursing process, and involves collecting subjective information about the consumer's health status in order to identify consumer problem areas to focus on.

Subjective data is most frequently collected during a health history and serves as the starting point for the health professional to base the depth of their assessment on. The sections for the health history include:

> **Consumer profile**

> **Chief complaint** (explained systematically using variations of location, quality, quantity, associated manifestations, aggravating factors, alleviating factors, setting and timing. This is a variation on the OPQRST assessment mnemonic you may use for other conditions such as pain assessment)

> **Past health history** (including medical history, surgical history, allergies, medications, injuries and accidents, special needs and childhood illnesses)

> **Family health history**

> **Social history** (including alcohol, tobacco and drug use, sexual practice, work and home environment, hobbies and leisure activities, stress and culture).

The example health history provided identifies scope for questioning the consumer about their health for this specific body system.

Lymph nodes

The inguinal area contains deep and superficial lymph nodes. Only the superficial nodes are palpable. These lymph nodes are grouped into superior and inferior chains. The superior chain of lymph nodes is located horizontally near the inguinal ligament. The inferior chain of lymph nodes lies vertically below the junction of the saphenous and femoral veins (**Figure 15.10**). See Chapter 14 for further lymph node information.

HEALTH HISTORY		
CONSUMER PROFILE	The abdominal health history provides insight into the link between a consumer's life and lifestyle and abdominal information and pathology. Diseases that are age- and sex-specific for the abdomen are listed first. Diseases that are age- and sex-specific for nutrition are listed second.	
	AGE	> Recurrent abdominal pain (2–15) > Appendicitis (young child–30) > Peptic ulcer disease (>30, with an increased incidence in the elderly) > Cholecystitis (40–50) > Diabetes mellitus, type 2 (>45) > Diverticulitis (>50) > Bladder cancer (>65) > Pernicious anaemia (older adult) > Mesenteric arterial insufficiency or infarct (more prevalent in older adults, especially those with atherosclerotic disease) > Bulimia (adolescents)

HEALTH HISTORY

	SEX	**FEMALE**	Gall bladder disease, Mittelschmerz (ovulatory pain), coeliac disease Over 90% of consumers with anorexia nervosa are female
		MALE	Pancreatic cancer, stomach cancer, cancer of the kidney and bladder, cirrhosis, duodenal ulcer, diverticulitis
CHIEF COMPLAINT	Common chief complaints for the abdomen are defined and information on the characteristics of each sign or symptom is provided.		
	1. NAUSEA	An uncomfortable sensation in the stomach and abdominal region	
		QUALITY	Retching (dry heaves)
		ASSOCIATED MANIFESTATIONS	Vomiting, medication use, fever, chills, foods eaten, fluids consumed, diarrhoea, pregnancy
		AGGRAVATING FACTORS	Noxious odours
		ALLEVIATING FACTORS	Flat soft drink, dry biscuits, sleep, antiemetics
		TIMING	Early morning, bedtime, middle of the night, after eating, after missed menstrual period
	2. VOMITING	Expulsion of contents from the upper gastrointestinal tract via contraction of abdominal wall muscles and relaxation of the oesophageal sphincter	
		QUALITY	Colour (bright red: fresh blood; coffee grounds appearance: 'old' blood that has had time to mix with digestive juices; dark brown or black: bile; other colours may occur secondary to food intake), projectile
		ASSOCIATED MANIFESTATIONS	Nausea, medications, fever, chills, abdominal pain, headache, foods eaten, fluids consumed, diarrhoea, pregnancy
		AGGRAVATING FACTORS	Noxious odours
		ALLEVIATING FACTORS	Flat soft drink, dry biscuits, sleep, antiemetic medications
		TIMING	Early morning, bedtime, middle of the night, after eating, after missed menstrual period
	3. DIARRHOEA	Frequent watery stools resulting in the loss of essential electrolytes	
		QUALITY	Colour; presence of blood, mucus or fat; odour
		ASSOCIATED MANIFESTATIONS	Abdominal cramping, pain, physical weakness, weight loss, fever, stress
		AGGRAVATING FACTORS	Food, medications, stress
		ALLEVIATING FACTORS	Diet (bananas, rice, apples, toast), medications, fluids with electrolyte supplement, physical rest
		TIMING	Recent travel, especially to areas with non-potable water; recent antibiotic use
	4. CONSTIPATION	Infrequent stools resulting in the passage of dry, hard faecal waste	
		QUALITY	Colour, odour, appearance of blood
		ASSOCIATED MANIFESTATIONS	Physical discomfort, rectal fullness, nausea, bloating, pain with defecation
		AGGRAVATING FACTORS	Food, medications (e.g. iron, narcotics), stress
		ALLEVIATING FACTORS	High-fibre diet, medications (e.g. laxatives, stool softeners, enemas), physical activity, increased fluid intake

>>

UNIT 2

HEALTH HISTORY			
5. ABDOMINAL DISTENSION	Protuberance of the abdomen		
	QUANTITY	Degree of distension and frequency (may need to measure abdomen)	
	ASSOCIATED MANIFESTATIONS	Constipation, abdominal discomfort, ascites, enlarged liver, enlarged spleen	
	AGGRAVATING FACTORS	Food, medications, stress	
	ALLEVIATING FACTORS	Diet, medications, physical activity	
6. ABDOMINAL PAIN	Discomfort in the abdomen; may be visceral, parietal, or referred pain (see Table 15.4)		
	QUALITY	Dull, burning, sharp, gnawing, stabbing, cramping (severe cramping is referred to as colic pain), aching	
	ASSOCIATED MANIFESTATIONS	Bleeding, flank pain, weight loss, nausea and vomiting, eructation, fever or chills, changes in bowel habits, flatus, prolonged immobility, menstrual cycle	
	AGGRAVATING FACTORS	Position, stress, eating, smoking, medications (e.g. aspirin, steroids, NSAID), alcohol or drug use	
	ALLEVIATING FACTORS	Antacids, proton pump inhibitors, histamine-2 antagonists, rest, diet, stress management, position change	
	SETTING	Home environment, work environment, mealtimes, social occasions involving alcohol or drug use	
	TIMING	Pre- or postprandial, night-time, seasonal, stressful situations, menstruation, gradual, sudden	
7. INCREASED ERUCTATION	Belching, or the oral expulsion of air (gas) from the stomach		
	QUANTITY	Marked increase over consumer's normal status	
	ASSOCIATED MANIFESTATIONS	Ingestion of milk products, certain foods, carbonated beverages, beer	
8. INCREASED FLATULENCE	Passage of excess gas via the rectum		
	QUANTITY	Marked increase over consumer's normal status	
	ASSOCIATED MANIFESTATIONS	Ingestion of certain foods (onions, cabbage, beans, cauliflower, corn, wheat, barley, rye)	
	AGGRAVATING FACTORS	Food or medications	
	ALLEVIATING FACTORS	Avoidance of particular foods that are fermentable	
	TIMING	Following meals	
9. ANOREXIA	Lost or decreased interest in and desire for food		
	ASSOCIATED MANIFESTATIONS	Physical weakness, fatigue, nausea, cramps, dietary intolerances, weight loss, abdominal distension, abdominal fullness, anxiety, depression	
	AGGRAVATING FACTORS	Smoking, sleeplessness, odours, pain, emotional status, cardiorespiratory distress	
	TIMING	Early morning, afternoon, bedtime, continuous; days, weeks, months; during pregnancy	

>>

HEALTH HISTORY

	10. DYSPHAGIA	Difficulty swallowing; associated with damage to the 9th or 10th cranial nerve, causing paralysis of the swallowing mechanism or disorders of the throat, neck or oesophagus	
		ASSOCIATED MANIFESTATIONS	Weight loss, choking, or difficulty breathing when swallowing
		AGGRAVATING FACTORS	Solid or liquid foods
		ALLEVIATING FACTORS	Position, throat lozenges
		TIMING	Associated with specific times and meals during the day
	11. WEIGHT GAIN	Number of kilograms gained above usual weight	
		ASSOCIATED MANIFESTATIONS	Use of medications (corticosteroids, insulin, oral contraceptive pill, antidepressants), pregnancy, sedentary lifestyle, high-calorie diet, high-fat diet, increased appetite
		SETTING	Stress, depression, negative body image
		TIMING	Over what period of time
	12. WEIGHT LOSS	Number of kilograms lost below usual weight	
		ASSOCIATED MANIFESTATIONS	Nausea, vomiting, diarrhoea, use of laxatives or diuretics, medication side effects, decreased appetite, increase in exercise, malabsorption diseases, diseases increasing demand of nutrients
		SETTING	Stress, depression, and negative body image, following a particular diet, participating in a structured weight-loss program (e.g. Weight Watchers)
		TIMING	Over what period of time
PAST HEALTH HISTORY	The various components of the past health history are linked to abdominal pathology and abdomen-related information.		
	MEDICAL HISTORY	**ABDOMEN-SPECIFIC**	Malignancies, peritonitis, cholecystitis, appendicitis, pancreatitis, small bowel obstruction, ulcerative colitis, hepatitis, hiatus hernia, diverticulitis, peptic ulcer disease, Crohn's disease, acute renal failure, chronic renal failure, gall stones, kidney stone, irritable bowel syndrome, gastro-oesophageal (GORD) reflux disease, parasitic infections, food poisoning, cirrhosis, infectious mononucleosis, hyper- or hypoadrenalism, malabsorption syndromes
		NON-ABDOMEN-SPECIFIC	Pulmonary tuberculosis, malaria, heart disease, thyroid or parathyroid disease, pneumonia, upper respiratory infections, allergies, postnasal discharge, sinusitis, stress, sexually transmitted infection (STI), puberty, menopause, diabetes, ketoacidosis, ectopic pregnancy, cystic fibrosis, endometriosis, lupus, sickle cell anaemia
		NUTRITION-SPECIFIC	Obesity, malnutrition, malabsorption diseases, anorexia nervosa, bulimia nervosa, dysphagia, weight cycling, metabolic syndrome
		NON–NUTRITION-SPECIFIC	Diabetes mellitus, coronary artery disease, increased cholesterol level, burns, cerebrovascular accident, hypertension, cancer, diverticulosis, muscular dystrophy, multiple sclerosis, Parkinson's disease, Crohn's disease, ulcerative colitis, gout, pancreatitis, cholelithiasis, dental disease, dialysis, cystic fibrosis, Wilson disease, phenylketonuria

>>

HEALTH HISTORY

	SURGICAL HISTORY	Cholecystectomy, gastrectomy, ileostomy, colostomy, appendectomy, colectomy, pancreatectomy, ileal conduit, portacaval shunt, splenectomy, hiatus hernia repair, umbilical hernia repair, femoral or inguinal hernia repair, liver transplant, bariatric surgery Gastric reduction (bypass, lap band, stapling), jaw wiring to reduce intake of food in morbid obesity, any surgical procedure that would alter food intake from postsurgical complications, nausea, or normal recovery
	ALLERGIES	Ingestion of certain food types or medications may cause gastric irritation, nausea and vomiting; lactose intolerance Gastrointestinal disturbances may occur with medication, food and environmental allergies; infants may manifest allergies as dietary disturbances (lactose intolerance)
	MEDICATIONS	Histamine-2 antagonists, protein pump inhibitors, antibiotics, lactulose, antacids, vitamins, antiparasitics, anticholinergics, tranquillisers, steroids, antidiarrhoeals, electrolytes, laxatives, stool softeners, insulin, antiemetics, antiflatulents Review all medications for actual or potential side effects that may affect appetite or growth (antibiotics may cause gastrointestinal disturbances, methylphenidate may cause anorexia, long-term steroid use may affect linear growth), vitamins, supplements, orlistat, sibutramine
	COMMUNICABLE DISEASES	STI, HIV infection, hepatitis, tuberculosis, infectious mononucleosis, intestinal parasites Children with AIDS: failure to thrive Adults with AIDS: wasting syndrome HIV-opportunistic infections: enteric pathogens – Cryptosporidium causes weight loss from malabsorption syndrome and persistent debilitating diarrhoea. Kaposi's sarcoma lesions can cause bowel occlusion, leading to constipation
	INJURIES AND ACCIDENTS	Abdominal trauma such as ruptured or bruised organs, gunshot wounds or knife stabbings; swallowing of foreign bodies Affect eating or the ability to self-feed, such as facial or mouth trauma; need for nasogastric tube feeding, gastrostomy
	SPECIAL NEEDS	Hepatitis A and hepatitis B vaccines
	CHILDHOOD ILLNESSES	Affect ability to cut, handle, chew or swallow food
FAMILY HEALTH HISTORY		Abdominal diseases and disorders that are familial are listed first; nutritional diseases that are familial are listed second. Malignancies of the stomach, liver, pancreas or colon; peptic ulcer disease, diabetes mellitus, familial polyposis, inflammatory bowel disease, irritable bowel syndrome, colitis, malabsorption syndromes (coeliac disease), cystic fibrosis Food allergies and intolerances, eating disorders, obesity, as well as any medical conditions that may contribute to nutritional problems (e.g. diabetes mellitus, hyperlipidaemia, hypertension, CAD, coeliac disease, cancer, gout, osteoporosis, alcoholism)
SOCIAL HISTORY		The components of the social history which are linked to abdomen factors and pathology are listed first and those that are linked to nutritional factors and pathologies are listed second.
	ALCOHOL USE	Altered nutrition, impaired gastric absorption, at risk for upper and lower gastrointestinal bleeding, cirrhosis of liver Alcohol has very little nutrient value, and abuse may lead to nutritional deficiencies. These include an inadequate intake of food, decreased sense of taste and smell, altered metabolism of nutrients (by decreasing storage and increasing excretion of nutrients), and decreased absorption through intestinal mucosa. There is also an increased excretion of calcium with alcohol consumption, which increases the risk of osteoporosis. In a pregnant woman, chronic alcohol consumption can lead to a low-birthweight baby and fetal alcohol syndrome in a newborn.
	TOBACCO USE	Smoking is associated with decreased oestrogen levels in women, which increases their risk of osteoporosis. Tobacco is also an appetite suppressant that may stimulate weight gain when the person quits smoking. Tobacco may also alter the senses of taste and smell.

>>

>>

HEALTH HISTORY

	DRUG USE	Opioids reduce peristalsis and are associated with the development of constipation. Drug abuse alters nutrition due to the consumer's increased dependence on the substance and decreased intake of proper nutrients. Many drugs alter food intake by causing anorexia (e.g. amphetamines) and decreasing sense of smell and taste (e.g. cocaine).
	TRAVEL HISTORY	Infectious diarrhoea may be produced by bacteria such as *Escherichia coli,* and parasites that may not be indigenous to the consumer's usual environment. Recent travel may cause gastrointestinal disturbances. It may also temporarily change the normal dietary habits of the consumer.
	HOME ENVIRONMENT	Public water versus tank/well water; lead-based paint used.
	WORK ENVIRONMENT	Improper food preparation and handling, water contamination, and poor sanitation can lead to hepatitis and *Escherichia coli* infections.
	HOBBIES AND LEISURE ACTIVITIES	Sports such as hockey, all forms of football, and boxing are often associated with traumatic injuries. Food-related hobbies or food activities (gourmet cooking), or the amount of physical activity
	EDUCATION	Education level may not necessarily translate into an adequate knowledge of nutritional needs.
	ECONOMIC STATUS	Bacterial and parasitic diseases from poor sanitation Resources for purchase of adequate food and transportation to grocery store
	RELIGION	Religious restrictions on diet
	CULTURAL BACKGROUND	Ethnic considerations regarding diet

TABLE 15.4 Differentiating abdominal pain

	VISCERAL PAIN	PARIETAL PAIN	REFERRED PAIN
Origin	Originates in the abdominal organs	Originates in the parietal peritoneum	Originates from abdominal organs to nonabdominal locations (e.g. chest, spine, or pelvis); refer path to abdominal region
Cause	Hollow structures become painful when they contract forcefully or when distended (e.g. intestines); solid organs become painful when stretched	Inflammation	Nerve innervation
Characteristics	Deep, dull, poorly localised; usually begins as dull pain, but when it becomes intense, is associated with nausea, vomiting, pallor and diaphoresis	Sharp, precisely localised; usually severe from the onset and intensifies with movement	Well localised; pain is from a disorder in another site, for example: > duodenal pain: back and right shoulder > pancreatic pain: back and left shoulder

CLINICAL **REASONING**

Bristol stool chart

It can be difficult for a consumer to describe the exact nature of stools. To assist in identifying stools, it is practical to show the consumer the Bristol Stool Chart (Figure 15.11) (Lewis & Heaton, 1997). This can provide the nurse with clues on colon transit time. Types 1 and 2 can be classified as constipation and the consumer usually needs to strain with defecation. Types 3 and 4 are the most comfortable stools to pass. Stool types 5, 6 and 7 are associated with urgency, with 7 constituting diarrhoea. Type 1 stool spends the most time in the colon and type 7 the least.

>>

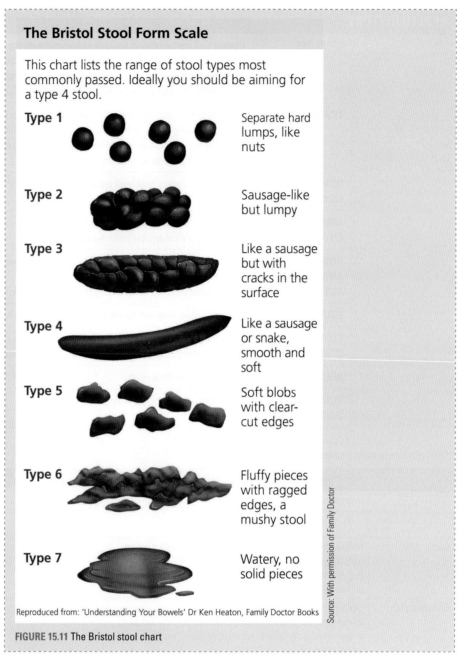

The Bristol Stool Form Scale

This chart lists the range of stool types most commonly passed. Ideally you should be aiming for a type 4 stool.

Type 1 — Separate hard lumps, like nuts

Type 2 — Sausage-like but lumpy

Type 3 — Like a sausage but with cracks in the surface

Type 4 — Like a sausage or snake, smooth and soft

Type 5 — Soft blobs with clear-cut edges

Type 6 — Fluffy pieces with ragged edges, a mushy stool

Type 7 — Watery, no solid pieces

Reproduced from: 'Understanding Your Bowels' Dr Ken Heaton, Family Doctor Books

Source: With permission of Family Doctor

FIGURE 15.11 The Bristol stool chart

PERSON-CENTRED HEALTH EDUCATION

When conducting a health assessment, opportunities for the provision of person-centred health education will arise. These occasions are identified as individualised education and may generate further data that can be added to the assessment. All education given should be documented so that in future, health professionals can assess the impact of previous information provided to the consumer. (Refer to Chapter 1 for initiating health education.)

INDIVIDUALISED HEALTH EDUCATION INTERVENTIONS

Assessing the consumer for the following health-related activities can assist in identifying a need for education about these factors. This information provides a bridge between the health maintenance activities and abdominal function and nutrition. Education opportunities for the abdomen are listed first and those for nutrition are listed second.

Sleep	Nocturnal pain with peptic ulcer disease; hiatus hernia discomfort in recumbent position. Stress increases when a consumer is sleep deprived, which may contribute to nutritional problems.
Diet	Healthy diet as a means of avoiding problems (fruits, vegetables, fibre, alcohol in moderation, decreased intake of fat and prepared foods); gall bladder attacks after fatty meals; caffeinated beverages, coffee, tea and alcohol exacerbate GORD.
Exercise	Regular exercise facilitates gastrointestinal functioning. Consumers with anorexia nervosa may exercise to excess.
Stress management	High stress levels are associated with stress ulcers, increasing or decreasing food consumption.
Use of safety devices	Shoulder and lap restraints in all forms of transport to prevent abdominal injuries; appropriate sports safety equipment to protect abdominal region.
Health check-ups	> Blood chemistry: elevated glucose and HbA1c might indicate onset of diabetes mellitus > Blood count: anaemia could reflect silent gastrointestinal bleeds > Urinalysis: dark colour may signify bilirubin in urine > Faecal occult blood test: results need to be investigated > Colonoscopy: reason for procedure, results > Lipid panel results, fasting serum glucose, weight, height, waist circumference, anthropometric measurements, blood pressure, and any other laboratory or diagnostic results

CLINICAL **REASONING**

Referred abdominal pain

Abdominal pain can be difficult to assess because the location of the abdominal pain may not be directly attributive to the area of the causative factors. In referred pain, the sensory cortex perceives pain via nerve fibres where the internal abdominal organs were located in fetal development. Pain originating from the liver, spleen, pancreas, stomach and duodenum may be referred (see Figure 15.12).

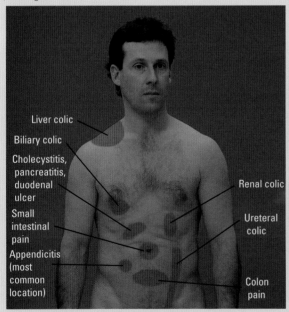

A. Anterior view

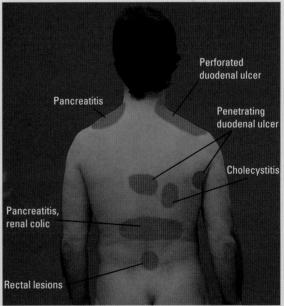

B. Posterior view

FIGURE 15.12 Areas of referred pain

PLANNING FOR PHYSICAL EXAMINATION

The planning phase refers to evaluating subjective data to narrow the focus on physical examination, determining what objective data needs to be gathered, as well as considering the environment and equipment that will be required.

At this time, you will identify which of the four diagnostic techniques you will need to implement the physical examination, and how you will sequence these. For the physical examination of nutrition and the abdomen, you will include inspection, palpation, percussion and auscultation.

Objective data is:

> collected during the physical examination of the consumer

> usually collected after subjective data

> information that is measured or observed by the clinician as opposed to being reported by the consumer

> vital to the overall health assessment, to enable you to make clinical decisions that are representative of the whole consumer picture.

Evaluating subjective data to focus physical assessment

Before commencing the physical examination of the consumer's nutrition and abdomen, consider what information the health history has provided. Critical consideration linked to knowledge of anatomy and physiology should focus the physical assessment so your examination will be more effective and efficient.

Environment

Assessing the nutritional status and abdomen requires a physical environment in the healthcare setting that has:

> a flat table/surface for the consumer to lie on

> minimal noise for accurate auscultation of specific sounds

> adequate lighting

> adequate privacy for the consumer.

Equipment

Assemble items before placing the consumer on the examination table; materials should be arranged in order of use and within easy reach.

> Drapes

> Small pillow for under the knees

> Tape measure or ruler with centimetre markings

> Pencil

> Lamp for tangential lighting

> Stethoscope

> Sterile safety pin or sterile needle

> Weighing scales

> Tape measure for waist and hip circumference

> Height tape measure (attached to wall preferably)

> Skinfold calipers (note: this is not often used by nurses, but is more widely used by dietitians and nutritionists).

IMPLEMENTATION: CONDUCTING THE PHYSICAL EXAMINATION

Implementation of the physical examination requires you to consider your scope of practice as well. In this section, depending on your context, you may be performing foundation assessment, with aspects of advanced assessment if you are practising in a specialised area.

EXAMINATION IN BRIEF: NUTRITIONAL AND ABDOMINAL

Examination of nutrition and abdomen

The nutritional history

Anthropometric measurements
> Height
> Weight
> Body mass index (BMI)
> Waist circumference and waist to hip ratio

Examination of the abdomen

Inspection
> Contour
> Symmetry
> Rectus abdominis muscles
> Pigmentation and colour
> Scars
> Striae
> Respiratory movement
> Masses and nodules
> Visible peristalsis
> Pulsation
> Umbilicus

Auscultation
> Bowel sounds
> Vascular sounds

Percussion
> General percussion
> Stomach
> Assessing for ascites: shifting dullness

Palpation
> Light palpation
> Abdominal muscle guarding
> Liver
  • Bimanual method
  • Hook method
> Inguinal lymph nodes

Examining for abdominal inflammation: rebound tenderness

Examining for appendicitis
> Rovsing's sign
> Iliopsoas muscle test

Examining inguinal lymph nodes

Examining consumers with abdominal tubes and drains

Tubes
> Enteral tubes
> Nasogastric suction tubes
> Intestinal tubes
> Gastrostomy

Drains
> Abdominal cavity drain
> Biliary drain (T-tube)

Intestinal diversions
> Colostomy
> Ileostomy

General approach to abdomen and nutrition assessment

Due to consumer comfort levels, it may be best to undertake the nutritional examination first; that is, height, weight, BMI and waist and hip measurement (and, for advanced practice, **skinfold thickness**). The order of abdominal examination is inspection, auscultation, percussion and palpation. Auscultation is performed second because palpation and percussion can alter bowel sounds.

Prior to the assessment:
1. Introduce yourself to the consumer and explain the assessment technique.
2. Ensure that the room is at a warm, comfortable temperature to prevent consumer chilling and shivering.
3. Use a quiet room that will be free from interruptions.
4. Utilise an adequate light source. This includes both a bright overhead light and a freestanding lamp for tangential lighting.
5. Ask the consumer to urinate before the exam.
6. Ask consumer to remove shoes prior to height measurement. Have older children or adults remove heavy clothing (an adult may wear a hospital gown). Undertake height, weight, BMI index, and hip and waist measurement.
7. Drape the consumer from the xiphoid process to the symphysis pubis, then expose the consumer's abdomen.
8. Position the consumer comfortably in a supine position with knees flexed over a pillow, and the arms either folded across the chest or at the sides, to ensure abdominal relaxation.

9. Stand to the right side of the consumer for the examination.
10. Visualise the underlying abdominal structures during the assessment process in order to accurately describe the location of any pathology.
11. Have the consumer point to tender areas; assess these last. Mark these and other significant findings (e.g. scars, dullness) on the body diagram in the consumer's chart.
12. Watch the consumer's face closely for signs of discomfort or pain.
13. Help the consumer relax by using an unhurried approach and by diverting attention with questions.
14. Ensure that your hands and the stethoscope are warm to promote consumer comfort.

Examination of nutrition and abdomen

Certain physical signs may indicate poor nutrition. See Table 15.5 for a list of signs and symptoms of poor nutritional status.

TABLE 15.5 Physical signs and symptoms of poor nutritional status

	SUBJECTIVE	OBJECTIVE
1. General appearance	Fatigue, poor sleep, change in weight, frequent infections	Dull affect, apathetic, increased weight, decreased weight
2. Skin	Pruritus, swelling, delayed wound healing	Dry, rough, scaling, flaky, oedema, lesions, decreased turgor, changes in colour (pallor, jaundice), petechiae, ecchymoses, xanthomas (slightly elevated yellow nodules)
3. Hair	Easily falls out, brittle	Less shiny, dry, changes in colour pigment
4. Nails	Brittle	Dry, splinter haemorrhages, spoon-shaped, pale
5. Eyes	Vision changes, night blindness, eye discharge	Hardening and scaling of cornea, conjunctiva pale or red
6. Mouth	Mouth sores	> Lips: cracked, dry, swollen, fissures around corners > Gums: recessed, swollen, bleeding, spongy > Tongue: smooth, beefy red, magenta, pale, fissures, sores, increased or decreased in size, increased or decreased papillae > Teeth: missing, caries
7. Head and neck	Headaches, decreased hearing	Xanthelasma, irritation and crusting of nares, swollen cheeks (parotid gland enlargement), goitre
8. Heart and peripheral vasculature	Palpitations, swelling	Cardiac enlargement, changes in blood pressure, tachycardia, heart murmur, oedema
9. Abdomen	Tender, changes in appetite, nausea, changes in bowel habits	Oedema, hepatosplenomegaly, vomiting, diarrhoea
10. Musculoskeletal system	Weakness, pain, cramping, frequent fractures	Muscle tone is decreased, flabby muscles, muscle wasting, bowing of lower extremities
11. Neurological system	Irritable, changes in mood, numbness, paraesthesia	Slurred speech, unsteady gait, tremors, decreased deep tendon reflexes, loss of position and vibratory sense, paraesthesia, decreased coordination
12. Female genitalia	Changes in menstrual pattern	None

The nutritional history

The first step in the nutritional assessment is the nutritional history. A comprehensive history (Table 15.6) is warranted when the consumer has a chronic medical condition or an unexplained weight loss or gain. Specific diet information is obtained via the diet history if required (Table 15.7). Once the food intake history is recorded, the nurse can evaluate the diet by comparing against national recommendations, to determine if the consumer requires referral to a dietitian or nutritionist. People at different stages of the life span need to have their nutritional assessment tailored to their development stage. Refer to specific chapters (e.g. Chapter 20: The paediatric consumer, Chapter 21: The older adult) for these details.

TABLE 15.6 Comprehensive nutritional assessment

PHYSICAL ASSESSMENT	
NUTRITIONAL HISTORY (REFER TO HEALTH HISTORY)	
1. General appearance	**7.** Head and neck
2. Skin	**8.** Heart and peripheral vasculature
3. Hair	**9.** Abdomen
4. Nails	**10.** Musculoskeletal system
5. Eyes	**11.** Neurological system
6. Mouth	**12.** Female genitalia
ANTHROPOMETRIC MEASUREMENTS	
Height: cm	Body mass index (BMI)
Weight: kg	
Waist circumference: cm	Waist/hip ratio
LABORATORY DATA	
Haematocrit (Hct)	Total lymphocyte count
Haemoglobin (Hgb)	**Antigen skin testing**
Cholesterol	**Prealbumin**
HDL	**Albumin**
Triglycerides	Glucose
LDL	HbA1c
Transferrin	CHI
TIBC	Nitrogen balance
Iron	Vitamins D, A
DIAGNOSTIC DATA	
X-rays	DEXA scanA

TABLE 15.7 Diet history

PART 1: GENERAL DIET INFORMATION
Do you follow a particular diet?
What are your food likes and dislikes?
Do you have any especially strong cravings?
How often do you eat fast food?
How often do you eat at restaurants?
Do you have adequate financial resources to purchase your food?
How do you obtain, store and prepare your food?
Do you eat alone or with a family member or other person?
Do you consume any food supplements (e.g. high-kJ beverages)?
In the last 12 months have you:
> experienced any change in weight?
> had a change in your appetite?
> had a change in your diet?
> experienced nausea, vomiting or diarrhoea from your diet?
> changed your diet because of difficulty in feeding yourself, eating, chewing or swallowing?
PART 2: FOOD INTAKE HISTORY (24-HOUR RECALL, 3-DAY DIARY, DIRECT OBSERVATION)
Time
Food and drink
Amount
Method of preparation
Eating location

Anthropometric measurements

Anthropometric measurements are the various measurements of the human body, including height, weight and body proportions. They measure growth patterns in children and changes in nutritional status in adults.

Measurements are easily obtained and can assist in an objective assessment that can be compared over time. Standardised charts should be used to compare the specific measurements with expected norms.

Height

A standing height is obtained for consumers 3 years and older (see **Figure 15.13**).

E 1. Have the consumer stand erect with back and heels against the wall or measuring device.

2. Place the headboard at a right angle to the wall and along the crown of the consumer's head.

3. Record height to the nearest 1 mm.

N Compare to standardised weight vs height chart (**Table 15.8**). Bear in mind that consumers will reflect familial growth patterns along with access to adequate nutrition. Also compare to the consumer's height and weight at the last visit if this data is available.

A Insufficient growth is abnormal.

P Chronic malnutrition may result in a decrease in height because the body does not have the nutrients necessary for proper growth.

P A consumer with osteoporosis may demonstrate a decrease in height due to thinning of the bones and possible vertebral compression fractures. A consumer with degenerative disc disease may also lose stature due to the nature of the musculoskeletal changes.

A Excessive growth is abnormal.

P Hormone abnormalities may cause excessive growth, as in acromegaly, gigantism, and precocious puberty.

P Genetic and metabolic syndromes that affect growth are Marfan syndrome and Klinefelter syndrome.

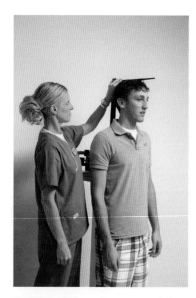

FIGURE 15.13 Measuring consumer height

Weight

E 1. Have the consumer stand on scales, facing the weights (**Figure 15.14**).

2. Slide the weight until balanced.

3. Read and record to the nearest 100 g (10 g for infants).

N Compare weight to standardised charts (see **Table 15.8**).

A Obesity is abnormal. Mild obesity occurs when the consumer is 20–40% above the ideal body weight (IBW); moderate obesity occurs when the consumer is 40–100% above the IBW; and morbid obesity occurs when a consumer is more than 100% above the IBW.

P Obesity occurs when there is excess body fat because of increased food intake, decreased activity level, or both.

P Some medications may contribute to weight gain (e.g. steroids).

P Some disease processes, such as hypothyroidism, may contribute to weight gain because of decreased metabolic rate.

P Genetics may influence weight gain.

A A weight under 90% of IBW is termed undernutrition. A weight between 80% and 90% of IBW is mild undernutrition, between 70% and 80% is moderate undernutrition, and below 70% is severe undernutrition.

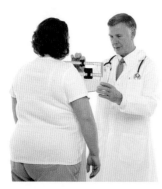

FIGURE 15.14 Measuring consumer weight
GETTY IMAGES/SCIENCE PHOTO LIBRARY

P Decreased food intake may occur with dental problems, depression, medications, alcoholism, anorexia nervosa and poverty.

P Inadequate nutrition may occur with impaired absorption, as present in malabsorption diseases (e.g. coeliac disease), AIDS and small bowel disease.

P There may be a loss of nutrients with diarrhoea, vomiting and diabetes mellitus.

P Increased demand for nutrients may be present in malignancies, fever, burns and hyperthyroidism. This increased demand may account for the weight loss that occurs early in cancer even when calories are not decreased. If this continues, the consumer exhibits signs of extreme malnutrition and wasting, which is called cachexia.

Body mass index

Body mass index (BMI) is a measurement that indicates body composition; however, as this test was developed using Europeans it may not be applicable for all people. The degree of overweight or obesity, as well as the degree of underweight, can be determined; however, it can be inaccurate in athletes (e.g. body builders) who have a higher percentage of muscle to fat ratio. The BMI can be associated with increased mortality at specific levels with consumers with known chronic diseases and those without a chronic disease.

The BMI takes into account a person's height as well as weight. The formula to determine BMI is:

$$BMI = Weight (in kg)/m^2$$

The BMI can be difficult to calculate because few people know their height in metres squared.

E Calculate the consumer's weight, divided by their height in metres squared (height in metres × height in metres).

For example: For a consumer who is 75 kg and is 167 cm tall:

Step 1: 75 kg must be divided by height in metres squared, so first work out your height in metres squared: 167 cm is 1.67 m. Square this: 1.67 m × 1.67 m = 2.7889.

Step 2: 75 kg divided by 2.7889.

BMI = 26.89

N A BMI of 20 to 25 is considered within normal limits.

A A BMI of 25 to 29.9 is considered overweight. A BMI of 30 to 34.9 is considered obese (Obesity Class I), 35 to 39.9 is moderately obese (Obesity Class II), and greater than 40 is extremely obese (Obesity Class III).

P A BMI greater than 25 is associated with an increased morbidity and mortality from cardiovascular disease, cancer and other diseases.

A A BMI less than 20 is abnormal.

P A BMI less than 20 is underweight and can be associated with possible malnutrition. A BMI less than 18 is associated with definite malnutrition. The malnutrition can be self-induced (e.g. anorexia nervosa, bulimia), caused by illness (e.g. cancer, AIDS) or it can be from a lack of available adequate nutrition.

Waist circumference and waist to hip ratio

Body fat distribution is linked to morbidity and mortality. This is frequently referred to as the 'pears' and 'apples' distribution. Women tend to deposit fat more in their hips and buttocks, giving them a pear-shaped appearance. Men, on the other hand, tend to deposit fat around the abdominal midline, thus giving them an apple-shaped appearance. The latter is usually connected more with the adverse effects associated with obesity. The waist circumference and waist to hip ratio is a simple method to determine one's body fat distribution.

TABLE 15.8 Suggested weights for adults

METRIC MEASUREMENT	
HEIGHT WITHOUT SHOES	HEALTHY WEIGHTS (MIN–MAX)
148 cm	44–55 kg
150 cm	45–56 kg
152 cm	46–58 kg
154 cm	47–59 kg
156 cm	49–61 kg
158 cm	50–62 kg
160 cm	51–64 kg
162 cm	52–66 kg
164 cm	54–67 kg
166 cm	55–69 kg
168 cm	56–71 kg
170 cm	58–72 kg
172 cm	59–74 kg
174 cm	61–76 kg
176 cm	62–77 kg
178 cm	63–79 kg
180 cm	65–81 kg
182 cm	66–83 kg
184 cm	68–85 kg
186 cm	69–86 kg
188 cm	71–88 kg
190 cm	72–90 kg
192 cm	74–92 kg
194 cm	75–94 kg
196 cm	77–96 kg
198 cm	78–98 kg
200 cm	80–100 kg
202 cm	82–102 kg
204 cm	83–104 kg

E Examination **N** Normal findings **A** Abnormal findings **P** Pathophysiology

E 1. Measure the waist in centimetres around the narrowest point of the waist between the 12th rib and the iliac crest. This is the waist circumference.

2. Measure the hips at the widest point.

3. Divide the waist measurement by the hip measurement. This is the waist to hip ratio. For example:

Waist = 84 cm, hips = 120 cm
Waist to hip ratio is 84 ÷ 120 = 0.7

N A waist circumference ≤88 cm in women and ≤102 cm in men is considered within normal limits. A waist to hip ratio <0.8 is normal in women. A waist to hip ratio <1.0 is normal in men.

A A waist to hip ratio >0.8 in women and >1.0 in men is abnormal.

A A waist circumference >88 cm in women and >102 cm in men is abnormal.

P These measurements are associated with the adverse morbidity and mortality of obesity, cardiovascular disease and diabetes.

Examination of the abdomen

Inspection

Contour

E View the contour of the consumer's abdomen from the costal margin to the symphysis pubis.

N In the normal adult, the abdominal contour is flat (straight horizontal line from costal margin to symphysis pubis) or rounded (convexity of abdomen from costal margin to symphysis pubis). See **Figure 15.15**.

A Assessment reveals a large convex symmetrical profile from the costal margin to the symphysis pubis.

P A large convex abdomen can result from one of the 5 Fs. Refer to the following Clinical reasoning box: The five Fs of abdominal distension.

A A convex abdomen that has a marked increase at the height of the umbilicus is abnormal.

P A protuberant abdomen results from a wide range of disorders. Taut stretching of the skin across the abdominal wall may occur. Refer to the following Clinical reasoning box: The five Fs of abdominal distension.

A A concave symmetrical profile from the costal margin to the symphysis pubis is abnormal.

P A scaphoid abdomen reflects a decrease in fat deposits, a malnourished state, or flaccid muscle tone.

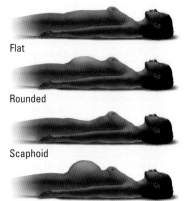

Flat

Rounded

Scaphoid

Protuberant

FIGURE 15.15 Abdominal configurations

Symmetry

E 1. View the symmetry of the consumer's abdomen from the costal margin to the symphysis pubis.

2. Move to the foot of the examination table and recheck the symmetry of the consumer's abdomen.

N The abdomen should be symmetrical bilaterally.

A Assessment reveals an asymmetrical abdomen.

P Asymmetry may be caused by a tumour, cysts, bowel obstruction, enlargement of abdominal organs, or scoliosis. Bulging at the umbilicus can indicate an umbilical hernia.

P If the abdomen is asymmetrical at the site of a surgical incision or scar, suspect an incisional hernia.

Rectus abdominis muscles

E 1. Instruct the consumer to raise the head and shoulders off the examination table.

2. Observe the rectus abdominis muscles for separation.

N The symmetry of the abdomen remains uniform; no ridge is observed parallel to the umbilicus or between the rectus abdominis muscles.

A A ridge between the rectus abdominis muscles is observed.

P This abnormality is known as diastasis recti abdominis and is attributed to marked obesity or past pregnancy. The observed separation of rectus abdominis muscles is caused by increased intra-abdominal pressure and is not considered to be harmful or ominous.

Pigmentation and colour

E View the colour of the consumer's abdomen from the costal margin to the symphysis pubis.

N The abdomen should be uniform in colour and pigmentation.

A Uneven skin colour or pigmentation is abnormal.

P The presence of jaundice suggests liver dysfunction. The yellow discolouration of the skin in light-skinned consumers is due to the accumulation of bilirubin in the blood. The average level for visible jaundice is >5 µmol/L.

A In light-skinned individuals, the observation of a blue tint at the umbilicus suggests free blood in the peritoneal cavity, known as **Cullen's sign**. Such bleeding can occur either following rupture of a fallopian tube secondary to an ectopic pregnancy or with acute haemorrhagic pancreatitis.

P Irregular patches of tan skin pigmentation (café au lait spots) may be attributed to von Recklinghausen disease (**Figure 15.16**), a familial condition associated with the formation of neurofibromas.

A Engorged abdominal veins are abnormal.

P The appearance of engorged or dilated veins around the umbilicus is called **caput medusae**. It is associated with circulatory obstruction of the superior or the inferior vena cava. In some instances, this condition is related to obstruction of the portal vein or to emaciation.

A A network of dilated veins on the abdomen is abnormal.

P This occurs in portal hypertension, cirrhosis, and vena cava obstruction secondary to increased venous pressures.

Scars

E Inspect the abdomen for scars from the costal margin to the symphysis pubis.

N There should be no abdominal scars present.

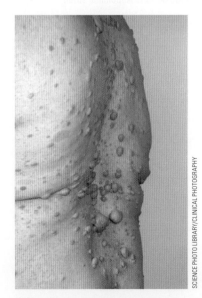

FIGURE 15.16 von Recklinghausen disease

E Examination **N** Normal findings **A** Abnormal findings **P** Pathophysiology

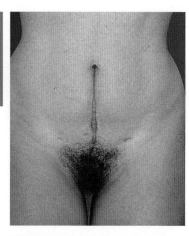

FIGURE 15.17 Abdominal scar from a hysterectomy

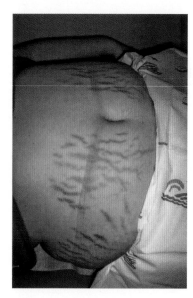

FIGURE 15.18 Abdominal striae

A Scars are present (**Figure 15.17**).

P The site of the scars discloses useful information about the consumer's surgical history. Dense, irregular, collagenous scars are keloids, which are more common in dark-skinned individuals and may be associated with traumatic injuries or burns. The presence of surgical scars may indicate internal adhesions.

Striae

E Observe the abdominal skin for **striae**, or abdominal atrophic lines or scars.

N No evidence of striae is present.

A Striae are present (**Figure 15.18**).

P Striae, atrophic lines or streaks, occur when there has been rapid or prolonged stretching of the skin. Abdominal striae may be caused by Cushing syndrome, abdominal tumours, obesity, ascites or pregnancy. Following pregnancy, striae are a normal finding.

CLINICAL **REASONING**

Abdominal scars
The most common scars are from an appendectomy, a hysterectomy or a caesarean section. Always observe a new scar for abnormalities, including bleeding or discharge. Whenever an abdominal scar is located, document the location, size and condition in a diagram in the consumer's chart.

Respiratory movement

E Observe the abdomen for smooth, even respiratory movement.

N There is no evidence of respiratory retractions. Normally, the abdomen rises with inspiration and falls with expiration.

A Abnormal respiratory movements and retractions are observed.

P The origin of abnormal respirations due to an abdominal disorder may include appendicitis with local peritonitis, pancreatitis, biliary colic or a perforated ulcer.

Masses and nodules

E Observe the abdominal skin for nodules and masses.

N No masses or nodules are present.

A Abdominal masses or nodules are present.

P The presence of abdominal masses or nodules may indicate tumours, metastases of an internal malignancy, or pregnancy.

P A bulge over an abdominal incision could possibly indicate an incisional hernia.

URGENT FINDING

Risk for aortic rupture (aortic aneurysm)
Do not palpate an aorta that you suspect has an aneurysm or has a pulsating sensation under the skin. Notify the consumer's doctor or call for emergency transport to an emergency setting immediately if you suspect an abdominal aortic aneurysm because it may dissect and cause renal failure, loss of limbs and, eventually, death if left untreated. Therefore, aorta palpation should be undertaken with caution; it is usually performed by an advanced practitioner. Risk factors for rupture include symptoms such as pain, age, sex (men are more likely), diastolic hypertension, aneurysm diameter (larger more likely), and active smoking (Antonello, Bonvini & Colacchio, 2022).

E Examination   **N** Normal findings   **A** Abnormal findings   **P** Pathophysiology

Visible peristalsis

E Observe the abdominal wall for surface motion.

N Ripples of peristalsis may be observed in thin consumers. Peristalsis movement slowly traverses the abdomen in a slanting, downward direction.

A Strong peristaltic contractions are observed.

P Peristaltic waves may indicate intestinal obstruction.

Pulsation

E Inspect the epigastric area for pulsations.

N In the consumer with a normal build, a nonexaggerated pulsation of the abdominal aorta may be visible in the epigastric area. In heavier consumers, pulsation may not be visible.

A Marked, strong abdominal pulsations are observed.

P Widened pulse pressure and strong epigastric pulsations may indicate an aortic aneurysm. An exaggerated pulsation can also occur in aortic regurgitation and in right ventricular hypertrophy.

Umbilicus

E 1. Observe the umbilicus in relation to the abdominal surface.
   2. Ask the consumer to flex the neck and perform the Valsalva manoeuvre.
   3. Observe for protrusion of the intestine through the umbilicus.

N The umbilicus is depressed and beneath the abdominal surface.

A The umbilicus protrudes above the abdominal surface (**Figure 15.19**).

P Umbilical hernia in the adult is the protrusion of part of the intestine through an incomplete umbilical ring. Umbilical hernia is confirmed by inserting the index finger into the navel and feeling an opening in the fascia. It can often be seen when the consumer's intra-abdominal pressure increases when coughing, sneezing, laughing and straining occur.

P The umbilicus that appears as a nodule may be the manifestation of abdominal carcinoma with metastasis to the umbilicus. This physical finding is known as a Sister Mary Joseph nodule and is often an indicator of widespread internal malignancy (Mudugal et al., 2020).

P Intra-abdominal pressure from ascites, masses or pregnancy can cause the umbilicus to protrude.

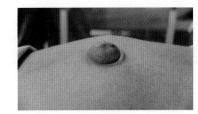

FIGURE 15.19 Umbilical hernia
SHUTTERSTOCK.COM/CASA NAYAFANA

Auscultation

Bowel sounds

E 1. Place the diaphragm lightly on the abdominal wall beginning at the RLQ.
   2. Listen to the frequency and character of the bowel sounds. It is necessary to listen for at least 5 minutes in an abdominal quadrant before concluding that bowel sounds are absent.
   3. Move diaphragm to RUQ, LUQ, LLQ (**Figure 15.20**).

CLINICAL **REASONING**

Who is at risk for bowel cancer (colorectal cancer)?
Everyone is at risk of developing bowel cancer or colorectal cancer. The risk, however, significantly increases over the age of 50. You are also at greater risk if you have:
> a previous history of polyps in the bowel
> a previous history of bowel cancer

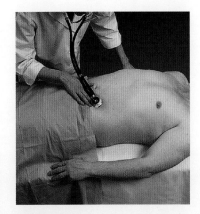

FIGURE 15.20 Technique of abdominal auscultation

>>

E Examination **N** Normal findings **A** Abnormal findings **P** Pathophysiology

UNIT 2

>>

> chronic inflammatory bowel disease (e.g. Crohn's disease)
> a strong family history of bowel cancer
> increased insulin levels or type 2 diabetes
> familial adenomatous polyposis or hereditary non-polyposis colorectal cancer (Lynch syndrome)
> excess body fat and physical inactivity
> high intake of specific foods (such as processed meat)
> high alcohol consumption
> smoking
> some gene mutation.

See https://bowel-cancer.canceraustralia.gov.au/risk-factors for more information.

(Cancer Australia, 2018)

CLINICAL REASONING

Bowel cancer screening

In Australia, since 2006, a population-based screening program for bowel cancer called the National Bowel Cancer Screening program has been in existence (Australian Government Department of Health, 2016). This program is offered to people turning 50, 55 or 65 years of age. An immunochemical sample of faecal occult blood (test) or FOBT is screened. If the FOBT is positive, further testing is required. Screening is advised every two years.

In New Zealand, a population screening program was introduced in March 2019 and closely resembles the Australian process (Ministry of Health/Manatu Hauora, 2023, National Bowel Screening Programme): https://www.health.govt.nz/our-work/preventative-health-wellness/screening/national-bowel-screening-programme

From the Cancer Council of Australia. *Understanding your FOBT (faecal occult blood test).* Retrieved 10 May 2023, from https://www.cancer.org.au/cancer-information/causes-and-prevention/early-detection-and-screening/bowel-cancer-screening

REFLECTION IN PRACTICE

Bowel sounds

You auscultate Ms Enriquez's bowel sounds and do not hear any after listening for 30 seconds in the RLQ. You are aware that you should auscultate the abdomen for 5 minutes in each quadrant if necessary. How would you proceed? What actions would you take next?

N Bowel sounds are heard as intermittent gurgling sounds throughout the abdominal quadrants. Usually, they are high-pitched sounds and occur 5 to 30 times per minute. Bowel sounds result from the movement of air through the gastrointestinal tract. Normally, bowel sounds are always present at the ileocaecal valve area (RLQ).

Normal hyperactive bowel sounds are called **borborygmi**. They are loud, audible, gurgling sounds. Borborygmi may be due to hyperperistalsis ('stomach growling') or the sound of flatus in the intestines.

A Absent bowel sounds are abnormal.

P Absent bowel sounds are indicative of late intestinal obstruction, both mechanical and non-mechanical in nature. Mechanical obstruction of the bowel may result from extraluminal lesions such as adhesions, hernias and masses. In non-mechanical obstruction, the gastrointestinal lumen remains unobstructed, but the muscles of the intestinal wall cannot move its contents. This type of obstruction can be caused by physiological, neurogenic or chemical imbalances that result in paralytic ileus.

E Examination   N Normal findings   A Abnormal findings   P Pathophysiology

A Hypoactive bowel sounds are abnormal.

P Hypoactive or diminished bowel sounds indicate decreased motility of the bowel and can occur with peritonitis and non-mechanical obstruction. Other causes include inflammation, gangrene, electrolyte imbalances and intraoperative manipulation of the bowel.

A Hyperactive bowel sounds are abnormal.

P Hyperactive or increased bowel sounds signify increased motility of the bowel and can result from gastroenteritis, diarrhoea, laxative use and subsiding ileus.

P Auscultation of high-pitched, tinkling hyperactive bowel sounds is indicative of partial obstruction. These sounds are caused by the powerful peristaltic action of the bowel segment attempting to eject its contents through a narrow, constricted area. Frequently, consumers complain of abdominal cramping.

Vascular sounds

E 1. Place the bell of the stethoscope over the abdominal aorta, renal arteries, iliac arteries, and femoral arteries (see **Figure 15.21**).

2. Listen for bruits over each area (see **Figure 15.22**).

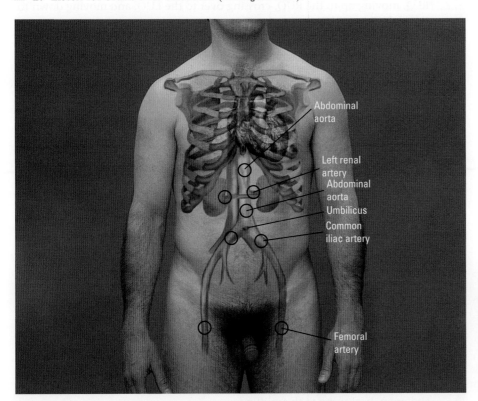

FIGURE 15.21 Stethoscope placement for auscultating abdominal vasculature

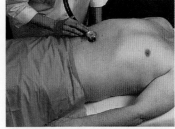

FIGURE 15.22 Auscultation of aortic bruits with the bell of the stethoscope

N No audible bruits are auscultated.

A Audible bruits are auscultated.

P A bruit over an abdominal vessel indicates turbulence of blood flow and suggests a partial obstruction. Bruits can occur with abdominal aortic aneurysm, renal stenosis, and femoral stenosis.

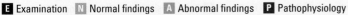

E Examination **N** Normal findings **A** Abnormal findings **P** Pathophysiology

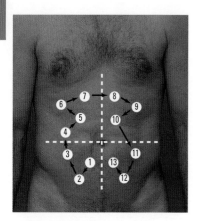

FIGURE 15.23 Direction of pattern of abdominal percussion

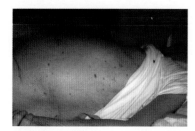

FIGURE 15.24 Ascites

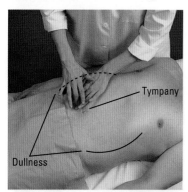

Tympany

Dullness

A. Patient supine

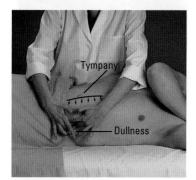

Tympany

Dullness

B. Patient on left side

FIGURE 15.25 Percussion for ascites: Shifting dullness

HEALTH EDUCATION

Risk factors for stomach cancer

Risk factors for stomach cancer include (Australian Government, Cancer Australia, 2020):

> *Helicobacter pylori* (*H. pylori*)
> age – >60 years
> diet (high in smoked foods, salted fish/meat, pickled vegetables)
> tobacco use
> chronic stomach problems such as polyps or gastritis
> family history of stomach cancer.

Consider which of these can be modified. Any modifiable risks that your consumers possess can be considered a priority focus for health education interventions or referral.

Percussion

General percussion

E 1. Percuss all four quadrants in a systematic manner. Begin percussion in the RLQ, moving up to the RUQ, crossing over to the LUQ, and moving down to the LLQ (**Figure 15.23**).

2. Visualise each organ in the corresponding quadrant; note when tympany changes to dullness.

N Tympany is the predominant sound heard because air is present in the stomach and in the intestines. It is a high-pitched sound of long duration. In obese consumers it may be difficult to elicit tympany due to the quantity of adipose tissue. Dullness is normally heard over organs such as the liver or a distended bladder. Dull sounds are high-pitched and of moderate duration.

A Dullness over areas where tympany normally occurs, such as over the stomach and intestines, is considered abnormal.

P Dullness may be caused by a mass or tumour, pregnancy, ascites or a full intestine.

Stomach

E Percuss for a gastric air bubble in the LUQ at the left lower anterior rib cage and left epigastric region.

N The tympany of the gastric air bubble is lower in pitch than the tympany of the intestine.

A An increase in size of the gastric air bubble is abnormal.

P This increase in size accompanied by gastric distension can suggest gastric dilation.

Assessing for ascites: shifting dullness

Assess the consumer for ascites (**Figure 15.24**), or excess accumulation of fluid in the abdominal cavity.

E 1. Standing to the right, with the consumer supine, percuss over the top of the abdomen, beginning at the midline.

2. Percuss outwards towards the right side of the consumer, following a downwards direction (**Figure 15.25A**).

3. Mark on the abdomen where percussion changes from tympany to dullness, because this change is indicative of settled fluid in the flanks of the abdominal cavity.

4. Turn the consumer onto the right side.

5. Repercuss the upper side of the abdomen, moving downwards.

6. If the percussion sound changes from tympany to dullness above the prior-marked fluid line, this **shifting dullness** is positive for ascites.

7. Repeat the same assessment technique on the left side of the consumer. Change the consumer's position from the right to the left side (**Figure 15.25B**).

8. Mark where the percussion changes from tympany to dullness.

N There should be no change from tympany to dullness.

A There is a marked change from tympany to dullness as you percuss outwards and downwards. Ascites is present in the abdominal cavity.

P Ascitic fluid sinks with gravity, which accounts for the dullness in dependent areas. Ascites is found in cirrhosis and in other liver diseases.

CLINICAL **REASONING**

Monitoring ascites
It is often helpful to monitor the amount of ascites by measuring the consumer's abdomen at its largest diameter. To promote consistency among nurses, it is advised that marks be drawn on the consumer's abdomen showing placement of the tape measure and comments made in consumer chart indicating movement above or below the original marks drawn. A more accurate and acceptable way of monitoring is the daily weight of the consumer.

Palpation

Light palpation

E 1. With your hands and forearm on a horizontal plane, use the pads of the fingers to depress the abdominal wall 1 cm (see **Figure 15.26**).

2. Avoid short, quick jabs.

3. Lightly palpate all four quadrants in a systematic manner.

N The abdomen should feel smooth with consistent softness.

A Light palpation reveals changes in skin temperature, tenderness or large masses.

P Tenderness and elevated skin temperature can be due to inflammation. Large masses can be due to tumours, faeces, or enlarged organs.

Abdominal muscle guarding
To determine whether muscle guarding is involuntary:

E 1. Perform light palpation of the rectus muscles during expiration.

2. Note muscle tensing.

N Muscle guarding, or tensing of the abdominal musculature, is absent during expiration. The abdomen is soft. Normally during expiration, the consumer cannot exercise voluntary muscle tensing.

A Muscle guarding of the rectus muscles occurs during expiration.

P Involuntary muscle guarding suggests irritation of the peritoneum, as in peritonitis.

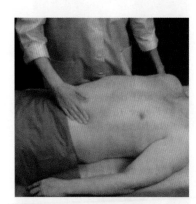
FIGURE 15.26 Light palpation of the abdomen

CLINICAL **REASONING**

Abdominal palpation
> Ensure that your hands are warm to promote consumer comfort and to prevent muscle guarding.
> Initially, avoid areas of known tenderness. Palpate these areas last.
Before beginning the palpation, ask the consumer to cough. Coughing can elicit a sharp twinge of pain if peritoneal irritation is present. Palpate this area and other known areas of pain or tenderness last.
> Instruct the consumer to take slow, deep breaths through the mouth.
> Begin with gentle pressure and gradually increase it.
> If the consumer is very ticklish, have the consumer perform self-palpation with your hand over the consumer's hand. Gradually remove the consumer's hand when the ticklishness is gone.
> Observe the consumer's face while performing abdominal palpation for changes in expression that can indicate pain or discomfort.

E Examination **N** Normal findings **A** Abnormal findings **P** Pathophysiology   Advanced Assessment

Liver

Liver palpation can be performed by one of two methods: the bimanual method or the hook method.

Bimanual method

E 1. Stand at the consumer's right side, facing the consumer's head.
2. Place the left hand under the consumer's right flank at about the 11th or 12th rib.
3. Press upwards with the left hand to elevate the liver towards the abdominal wall.
4. Place the right hand parallel to the midline at the right midclavicular line below the right costal margin or below the level of liver dullness.
5. Instruct the consumer to take a deep breath.
6. Push down deeply and under the costal margin with your right fingers. On inspiration, the liver will descend and contact the hand (**Figure 15.27A**).
7. Note the level of the liver.
8. Note the size, shape, consistency and presence of any masses.

Hook method

E 1. Stand at the consumer's right side, facing the consumer's feet.
2. Place both hands side by side on the right costal margin below the border of liver dullness.
3. Hook the fingers in and up towards the costal margin and ask the consumer to take a deep breath and hold it.
4. Palpate the liver's edge as it descends (**Figure 15.27B**).
5. Note the level of the liver.
6. Note the size, shape, consistency and presence of any masses.

N A normal liver edge presents as a firm, sharp, regular ridge with a smooth surface. Normally, the liver is not palpable, although it may be felt in extremely thin adults.

A If the liver is palpable below the costal margin both medially and laterally, it is abnormal.

P An enlarged liver can be due to congestive heart failure, hepatitis, encephalopathy, cirrhosis, cysts or cancer.

A A liver that is enlarged, has an irregular border and nodules, and is hard, is abnormal.

A These findings suggest liver malignancy. Tenderness may or may not be present.

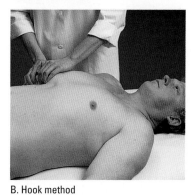

A. Bimanual method

B. Hook method

FIGURE 15.27 Palpation of the liver

E Examination **N** Normal findings **A** Abnormal findings **P** Pathophysiology

URGENT FINDING

Risk for spleen rupture when palpating
Palpate the spleen gently because an enlarged spleen will be very tender and may rupture (Wint & Sethi, 2019). For this reason, palpation of the spleen is usually advanced practice.

REFLECTION IN PRACTICE

Hepatitis risks
A 29-year-old man who recently emigrated from Sudan is seeking follow-up care for abdominal pain. On the first visit you completed his health history and physical examination, and obtained laboratory data. Your clinical suspicion is confirmed with the results of the laboratory tests: he has hepatitis B. This man is sexually active with his wife. You inform him of the importance of his wife being clinically evaluated. He tells you that it is too expensive for both of them to be seen by a specialist or for testing if he is not admitted to hospital. How would you respond? What information would you give to him?

CLINICAL **REASONING**

Hepatitis risk factors
Hepatitis is a serious health condition that causes an inflammation of the liver; there are a number of different types of hepatitis. An awareness of the risk factors for hepatitis is an important consideration when undertaking a health assessment.

Hepatitis A virus
> Risk factors (infectious hepatitis)
  * Overcrowded living quarters or institutional environments (such as correctional centres)
  * Poor personal hygiene (poor hand washing, especially after defecation)
  * Poor sanitation (sewage disposal) or those working with sewage
  * Food and water contamination
  * Ingestion of shellfish caught in contaminated water
  * Travel to endemic area such as in a developing country
  * Those in close personal contact with infected individual (oral and anal sex)
> People who have anal sex
> Illegal drug use (injectable and noninjectable agents)
> People with clotting factor disorders
> Those who live in remote communities
> People who have liver disease or have had a liver transplant
> People who have hepatitis B or C
> Child care, aged care and other day care or respite care centres (especially where children wear nappies)

Hepatitis B virus
> Risk factors for hepatitis B virus
  * IV drug use with shared needles
  * Receipt of multiple transfusions of blood and blood products (oncology and haemodialysis consumers, haemophiliacs); this is now rare in Australia
  * Exposure to blood and blood products, contaminated body fluids, needle exposure (e.g. needlestick injury, tattoo or piercing in facility with poor hygiene)
  * Sexual contact with infected individual (both heterosexual and homosexual)
  * High-risk sexual activity (multiple partners)
  * Perinatal transmission
  * Travel to endemic areas or people born in areas where the virus is endemic (e.g. China)

>>

>>

- Due to increased risk of contact with blood and body fluids
- Sharing personal items with hep B infected persons (e.g. razor, toothbrush)
- Living with a hepatitis B infected person
- Working with/residing with developmentally disabled persons who are at a care facility

Hepatitis C virus

> Risk factors for hepatitis C

- Exposure to blood and blood products, contaminated body fluids, needle exposure (e.g. needlestick injury, tattoo or piercing in facility with poor hygiene)
- IV drug use
- High-risk sexual activity
- Sexual contact with infected individual (both heterosexual and homosexual)
- Household contact with infected individual
- People with HIV
- Long-term haemodialysis
- Children born to hepatitis C infected mother
- Sharing personal care items with hepatitis C infected persons (e.g. razor, toothbrush)
- Blood transfusion in Australia prior to 1990 or in a country with a high rate of hepatitis C

Hepatitis D virus and hepatitis E virus

> Both hepatitis D and hepatitis E viruses are uncommon in Australia and New Zealand.

Source: Healthdirect Australia (2022).

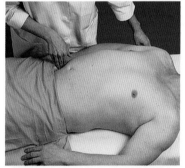

A. Apply firm pressure to the abdomen

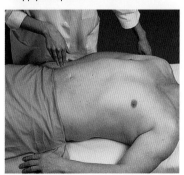

B. Quickly release the pressure

FIGURE 15.28 Rebound tenderness

Examining for abdominal inflammation: rebound tenderness

Rebound tenderness is assessed if pain has been elicited during palpation, or the consumer has reported pain. Rebound tenderness is an abnormal finding frequently associated with peritoneal inflammation or appendicitis. Be prepared to recognise that rebound tenderness assessment could elicit a strong pain response from the consumer. It is imperative to test for rebound tenderness away from the site where pain is initially determined and to conclude abdominal assessment with this test. If other tests are positive, omit this assessment.

E 1. Apply several seconds of firm pressure to the abdomen, with the hand at a 90° angle (perpendicular to the abdomen) and the fingers extended (**Figure 15.28A**).

2. Quickly release the pressure (**Figure 15.28B**).

N Pain is not elicited.

A As the abdominal wall returns to its normal position, the consumer complains of pain at the pressure site (direct rebound tenderness) or at another site (referred rebound tenderness).

P Rebound tenderness may indicate peritoneal irritation. The rebound effect of the internal structures indented by this technique causes sharp pain in the area of inflammation.

A Pain in the RLQ can indicate appendicitis. This location is known as **McBurney's point.**

Examining for appendicitis

Rovsing's sign

Rovsing's sign is a differential technique to elicit referred pain, reflective of peritoneal inflammation secondary to appendicitis.

E 1. Press deeply and evenly in the LLQ for 5 seconds.

2. Note the consumer's response.

N No pain should be elicited.

E Examination **N** Normal findings **A** Abnormal findings **P** Pathophysiology   Advanced Assessment

A Abdominal pain felt in the RLQ is abnormal and is a positive Rovsing's sign.

P This sign is based on the concept that changes in intraluminal pressure will be transmitted through the intestine when the ileocaecal valve is competent. Pressing the LLQ traps air within the large intestine and increases the pressure in the caecum. When the appendix is inflamed, this increase in pressure causes pain.

Iliopsoas muscle test
When a consumer presents with acute abdominal pain, an inflamed or perforated appendix may be distinguished via irritation of the lateral iliopsoas muscle.

E 1. Place your hand over the right thigh and push downwards as the consumer raises the leg, flexing at the hip (**Figure 15.29**).

2. Observe for pain response in the RLQ as described by the consumer.

N Normally, the consumer should experience no pain.

A The consumer experiences pain in the RLQ.

P This pain indicates an inflammation of the iliopsoas muscle in the groin and is caused by an inflamed appendix.

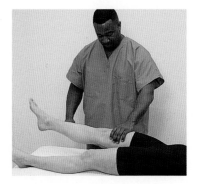

FIGURE 15.29 Iliopsoas muscle test when assessing for appendicitis

Examining inguinal lymph nodes

E 1. Place the consumer in a supine position, with the knees slightly flexed.

2. Drape the genital area.

3. Using the finger pads of the second, third and fourth fingers, apply firm pressure and palpate with a rotary motion in the right inguinal area.

4. Palpate for lymph nodes in the left inguinal area.

N It is normal to palpate small, movable nodes less than 1 cm in diameter. Palpable nodes are nontender.

A Presence of inguinal lymph nodes greater than 1 cm in diameter or elicitation of non-movable, tender lymph nodes is abnormal.

P Large, palpable nodes can be attributed to localised or systemic infections. More serious pathology includes processes associated with cancer or lymphomas.

Examining consumers with abdominal tubes and drains
For all tubes, drains and intestinal and urinary diversions, note colour, odour, amount, consistency, and the presence of blood in any drainage. Check for an obstruction if there is no drainage. The skin around the device should be intact without excoriation.

Tubes

Enteral tubes
> Nasogastric, nasoduodenal or nasojejunal
> Check the residual amount on a frequent basis. If greater than 100 mL, stop the feeding; restart the feeding based on further inspection of residual amounts.

Nasogastric suction tubes
> Levin or Salem sump
> Ensure that the suction setting (intermittent or continuous) is set at the appropriate suction level.

Intestinal tubes
> Miller-Abbott, Cantor, Johnston or Baker
> Ensure that the tube is advancing with peristalsis as expected.
> Ensure that the suction setting is at the appropriate suction level.

Gastrostomy
> Continuous versus intermittent feeding
> With intermittent feedings, clamp is applied when not in use.

E Examination **N** Normal findings **A** Abnormal findings **P** Pathophysiology   Advanced Assessment

> Tube should be secured to abdomen.
> Check that dressing is applied.

Drains

Abdominal cavity drain

> To self-suction or wall suction; if wall suction, ensure that it is set at appropriate level.

Biliary drain (T-tube)

> Tube is below insertion site.

Intestinal diversions

Colostomy

> Stoma is pink.
> Skin barrier should be used around stoma if appliance is worn.
> Evacuation method: natural or irrigation.

Ileostomy

> Stoma is pink.
> Skin barrier is used and appliance is worn.
> If consumer has Kock pouch, nipple valve is pink; frequency of drainage.

EVALUATION OF HEALTH ASSESSMENT AND PHYSICAL EXAMINATION FINDINGS

In the evaluation phase of a health assessment, the focus is on ensuring the data gathered is complete, accurate and documented appropriately (see case study as an example of the focused assessment; see Chapter 22 for a comprehensive health assessment). In evaluating the data you should:

> draw on your critical thinking and problem-solving skills to make sound clinical decisions
> act on abnormal data (include communicating findings to other health professionals)
> ensure documentation reflects the outcomes of the clinical decisions/actions taken (refer to Chapter 3, which discusses in detail why documentation is so important and how this may be undertaken in different health settings).
   The case study that follows steps you through this process.

Advanced Assessment

THE CONSUMER WITH INFLAMMATORY BOWEL DISEASE

This case study illustrates the application and the objective documentation of the assessment.

Isaac Standais is a 20-year-old university student who presents to the university health clinic with abdominal discomfort, changed bowel patterns and fatigue.

HEALTH HISTORY	
CONSUMER PROFILE	Isaac, 20-year-old male, university student, Caucasian of Jewish ancestry
CHIEF COMPLAINT	'I have had a sore stomach and diarrhoea on and off for a while. Also, I have been really tired this year.'
HISTORY OF THE PRESENT ILLNESS	Isaac has been unwell on and off for the past year. He presents to the university health clinic feeling unwell and tired, reporting abdominal pain and diarrhoea. He states that he has had these symptoms several times in the past year and they seem to coincide with assessment being due or examination period. He has an exam period coming up in a week. His abdominal pain is in the lower (L) quadrant and is somewhat relieved when he goes to the toilet. He states that he never really feels as though he has gone to the toilet properly, yet sometimes it comes out with urgency. He describes that he is always looking to make sure he knows where the nearest toilet is on campus.

>>

>>

HEALTH HISTORY

PAST HEALTH HISTORY	MEDICAL HISTORY	Skin rashes that he has used cortisone cream for, for as long as he can remember
	SURGICAL HISTORY	Circumcision at birth; appendectomy at 13 years
	ALLERGIES	Nil reported
	MEDICATIONS	Cortisone used 1% when rash is severe
	COMMUNICABLE DISEASES	Nil reported; says he practises safe sex techniques
	INJURIES AND ACCIDENTS	Nil
	SPECIAL NEEDS	Nil
	BLOOD TRANSFUSIONS	Not known
	CHILDHOOD ILLNESSES	Cannot recall, will have to ask his mother
	IMMUNISATIONS	All childhood vaccines completed; hepatitis B completed 2 years ago; completed hepatitis A series last year; annual flu vaccine – has not had this year's yet
FAMILY HEALTH HISTORY		Isaac describes his father as having high blood pressure and his sister (30 years) has inflammatory bowel disease and has to eat carefully. He is one of two children. He is unsure about his mother's health and states 'She seems healthy'.
SOCIAL HISTORY	ALCOHOL USE	Drinks beer with his mates at the weekend. Does not have much during the week because of study
	TOBACCO USE	Nil
	DRUG USE	I had a go when I was younger
	DOMESTIC AND INTIMATE PARTNER VIOLENCE	No girlfriend, has lots of friends he goes out with
	SEXUAL PRACTICE	Safe sex practice
	TRAVEL HISTORY	Travels home to Israel and Poland
	WORK ENVIRONMENT	University student, works in university breaks in family retail business
	HOME ENVIRONMENT	Lives in shared accommodation with 4 other students, has his own room, shares shopping and cooking with housemates, but eats out frequently
	HOBBIES AND LEISURE ACTIVITIES	Likes music and attends all the university concerts on campus, member of the university volleyball team
	STRESS	Exams pending and preparing for inter-university games for volleyball
	EDUCATION	Enrolled in a Bachelor of Business Administration degree; has HSC
	ECONOMIC STATUS	Student, good family support, with a small scholarship stipend for books and IT-related expenses
	MILITARY SERVICE	None
	RELIGION	Jewish
	CULTURAL BACKGROUND	Jewish, has visited Israel and Poland as a young child
	ROLES AND RELATIONSHIPS	Has a great relationship with parents and loves his sister who he says 'indulges him' and gives him special chocolaty treats. Good friends with all housemates, two he went to school with
	CHARACTERISTIC PATTERNS OF DAILY LIVING	Wakes at 7.30 a.m., has a glass of orange juice and leaves for the gym for strength training. Spends most of the day at university where he gets some food from the refectory, such as a pie or a burger, and attends volleyball practice from 4 p.m. to 6 p.m. most nights because of the approaching tournament. Usually eats at about 8 p.m. with housemates. Puts in some study time after dinner

>>

>>

HEALTH HISTORY		
HEALTH MAINTENANCE ACTIVITIES	**SLEEP**	7–8 hours of sleep during the week; 8–9 hours on the weekends; describes 'crashing on Sunday' and has an afternoon nap, yet reports feeling tired when he wakes up
	DIET	Eats what is available to him; however, describes feeling quite unwell after having cappuccino and chocolate milkshakes
	EXERCISE	Attends gym and volleyball
	STRESS MANAGEMENT	Has a good group of friends and family support. Enjoys the team atmosphere and the work of volleyball practice and games
	USE OF SAFETY DEVICES	Uses his skateboard to get to and from university without protective gear and reports that the road has a good surface
	HEALTH CHECK-UPS	Mother made him have one before he left home to come to university 2 years ago. Nothing was reported and the doctor checked his skin and gave him his hepatitis immunisations. Does not perform testicular or any other self-examination

PHYSICAL EXAMINATION			
EXAMINATION OF THE ABDOMEN	**INSPECTION**	Skin rash evident	
		CONTOUR	Flat
		SYMMETRY	Symmetrical
		RECTUS ABDOMINIS MUSCLES	Intact, separation
		PIGMENTATION AND COLOUR	Uniform pigmentation
		SCARS	Appendectomy
		RESPIRATORY MOVEMENT	Retractions
		MASSES OR NODULES	Nil of note
		VISIBLE PERISTALSIS	Some abdominal surface movement noted
		PULSATION	Slight visible in epigastrium
		UMBILICUS	Umbilicus depressed
	AUSCULTATION	**BOWEL SOUNDS**	Audible gas sounds in 4 quadrants
		VASCULAR SOUNDS	Nil audible bruits noted
	PERCUSSION	**GENERAL PERCUSSION**	Tympany
		LIVER SPAN	No hepatomegaly
		SPLEEN	Unable to percuss
		STOMACH	Tympany
		BLADDER	Dull to symphysis pubis
	PALPATION	**LIGHT PALPATION**	Smooth, warm, LLQ constant dull ache reported
		ABDOMINAL MUSCLE GUARDING	Abdominal pain and tenderness, reports more pronounced pain in the LLQ

EVALUATION AND CLINICAL REASONING FOR CASE STUDY

The assessment and clinical decisions you make should reflect your scope of practice. For example, advanced practice health professionals, such as nurse practitioners and remote area nurses with endorsement, may be able to make diagnostic decisions and prescribe medications without referring to a medical officer.

Fundamentally, all health professionals collect, evaluate and act on consumer-focused health information, which will at times include referral to, or collaboration with, other healthcare team members. Nurses assess consumer responses to interventions and determine when to escalate key changes in a consumer's condition. The clinical reasoning cycle provides health professionals with a framework to consider all this information in a meaningful way for planning consumer care. These phases are stepped out below, and draw on information presented and collected during the health history and physical examination. We then work through the cycle components that are relevant to this case study (cycle components are bolded).

For Isaac Standais, the significant data that needs to be considered includes the following.

Collecting cues/information

Recall and Review: In the first instance, you will need to reflect on what you know about the different forms of inflammatory bowel diseases, irritable bowel syndrome, and the effect of lifestyle including diet and stress.

Chief complaint and history of present illness

> Symptoms started some months ago with Isaac experiencing fatigue, intermittent diarrhoea and abdominal pain and persistent flatus.
> 10 days ago, he developed persistent abdominal pain and explosive diarrhoea.
> He has been unwell on and off for the past year.
> Skin rashes are evident on torso, elbows and heels.
> He has abdominal pain in the lower left quadrant (LLQ).
> He reports incomplete evacuation, increased defecation and hypervigilance.
> He has an exam period coming up in a week.

Processing information

Interpret: These symptoms and details of history outline the scope of the issue for Isaac and how it is affecting his wellbeing and the ability to self-manage this deviation from normal health. The nurse uses interpretation skills to consider Isaac's symptoms.

Relate and Infer: Grouped together these symptoms may indicate irritable bowel syndrome (IBD), or possibly Crohn's disease, considering his age, family history and ethnicity (you are more likely to develop Crohn's disease before age 30, if you have a close family relative with IBD, and higher risk if of Jewish ancestry).

Predict: Consumer history and physical assessment show the likelihood of Isaac's issues being caused by Crohn's disease.

Home environment

Lives in shared accommodation with four other students, has his own room, shares shopping and cooking with housemates, though eats out frequently.

Stress

Exams pending and preparing for inter-university games for volleyball.

Roles and relationships

Has a great relationship with parents and loves his sister who he says 'indulges him' and gives him special chocolaty treats.

Characteristic patterns of daily living

Wakes at 7.30 a.m., has a glass of orange juice and leaves for the gym for strength training. Spends most of the day at university

where he gets some food from the refectory, like a pie or a burger, and attends volleyball practice from 4 p.m. to 6 p.m. most nights because of the approaching tournament. Usually eats at about 8 p.m. with housemates. Puts in some study time after dinner.

Diet

Eats what is available to him; however, describes feeling quite unwell after having cappuccino and chocolate milkshakes.

Discriminate: The impact of stress, diet and environmental factors are relevant information to the consumer's presenting complaint.

Infer: Student stress at university with upcoming exams is likely to be higher at this time, and increased stress can trigger IBD. Often, specific items will trigger IBD symptoms and these may be different depending on the individual.

Sleep

7–8 hours of sleep during the week; 8–9 hours on the weekends; describes 'crashing on Sunday' and has an afternoon nap, yet reports feeling tired when he wakes up.

Infer: Recurrent fatigue and bowel symptoms over a period of time may indicate a relationship of bowel symptoms impacting on fatigue and poorer recovery.

Physical assessment

Skin rashes that he has used cortisone cream for, for as long as he can remember. Skin rash evident at present.

Relate: There is a relationship between IBD and skin rashes.

Putting it all together – synthesise information

The nurse in this case would note all these abnormalities, and refer Isaac to a medical specialist for further review and medical treatment. It is likely that Isaac will have to undergo specific testing to identify which form of inflammatory bowel disease he has developed, although it is likely to be Crohn's disease, considering all the above information.

Isaac may need to undertake a number of tests:
> Common laboratory tests
  • Full blood count for anaemia
  • ESR for inflammation
  • otassium
  • Vitamin B_{12}
  • Liver function tests
  • Stool studies to rule out infection
> Direct visual examination
> Endoscopy and X-ray series to evaluate the cause of abdominal pain and diarrhoea

Actions based on assessment findings

While waiting for further diagnostic examinations, the nurse should consider the following:
1 A complete set of observations: vital signs T, P, R, BP; weight; stool examination; identify allergies
2 Process of referral to the doctor and nutritionist with all information gathered recorded

3 Health promotion: wellbeing strategies for stress, coping with exams, addressing fatigue and sleep, strategies for social occasions, nutritional recommendations for a healthy tolerated diet, skin care (rashes and excoriation)

4 Refer to university Study Skills Support for examination and study strategies to help manage stress levels.

The final step in the process is accurate documentation. The nurse must document findings, referrals, interventions, and advice and education given. The consumer would then be reassessed following definitive diagnosis and medical interventions for his injuries.

CHAPTER RESOURCES

REVIEW QUESTIONS

For answers to these questions, see Answer section at the end of the book.

1. The emergency room nurse examines a consumer with pain in the right upper abdominal region. The nurse recalls that which of the following structures are located in this abdominal quadrant? Select all that apply.
   a. Gall bladder
   b. Liver
   c. Bladder
   d. Stomach
   e. Sections of the sigmoid and descending colons
   f. Sections of the ascending and transverse colons

2. After assessing a consumer's abdomen, you suspect that she may be experiencing pancreatitis. In which abdominal area is the consumer most likely experiencing pain?
   a. Epigastrium
   b. Right upper quadrant
   c. Periumbilical
   d. Left lower quadrant

3. A woman attends the clinic stating she has a number of symptoms you suspect are associated with constipation. Which is the most accurate description of symptoms and associated factors associated with this type of condition?
   a. Bowel movement frequency increased, blood in stool, increased foul smell, pain on defecation, recent oral codeine products for analgesia, nausea and bloating
   b. Bowel movement frequency increased, green-coloured stool, increased foul smell, pain on defecation, nausea and bloating
   c. Bowel movement frequency reduced, on reduced dietary intake for cultural reasons, increased fluid intake, nil discomfort
   d. Bowel movement frequency reduced, blood in stool, increased foul smell, pain on defecation, recent oral codeine products for analgesia, nausea and bloating

4. A consumer with pancreatitis complains of pain in the back and left shoulder. This abdominal pain is best described as:
   a. Visceral pain
   b. Parietal pain
   c. Referred pain
   d. Nociceptive pain

5. A consumer is admitted to the hospital with a diagnosis of liver cirrhosis. Which of the following might the nurse find on physical examination? Select all that apply.
   a. Visible peristalsis
   b. Venous hum
   c. Diastasis recti
   d. Liver span of 14 cm
   e. Exaggerated abdominal aortic pulsation
   f. Liver edge 2 cm below the right costal margin at rest

6. Which of the following consumers meet the criteria for the metabolic syndrome?
   a. A 32-year-old male with high HDL, high triglycerides, high fasting serum glucose
   b. A 75-year-old woman with high blood pressure, high LDL, abdominal obesity
   c. A 21-year-old male with high cholesterol, high HbA1c, high blood pressure
   d. A 44-year-old woman with abdominal obesity, high blood pressure, high triglycerides

7. A 39-year-old woman is 181 cm tall and weighs 68 kg. What conclusion do you make about her BMI?
   a. Normal BMI
   b. Overweight
   c. Obese
   d. Moderately obese

8. A consumer presents complaining of pain, swelling and discharge from an abdominal wound, seven days post appendectomy. When assessing and documenting the wound, the nurse will need to note the following:
   a. A description of the shape, size and colour of the wound and colour of ooze
   b. A description of the wound ooze (including colour, odour, amount, consistency, time commenced), pain score, shape, size, colour of the wound, alignment of wound borders, tracking colour, if surrounding skin is warm/hot to touch
   c. A description of the wound ooze (including colour, amount, consistency, time commenced), pain score, size, colour of the wound, alignment of wound borders, tracking colour, if surrounding skin is warm/hot to touch
   d. A description of the wound ooze (including colour, odour, amount, consistency, time commenced), pain score, shape, size, colour of the wound, alignment of wound borders

9. A 14-year-old female consumer attends the clinic with her mother. Her mother is concerned with her daughter's increased weight loss and refusal to eat a full 'normal' meal with her family. What actions would you take next?
   a. None. It is normal for teenagers to become picky with food.
   b. Undertake a full physical and nutritional assessment of the consumer; conditions such as anorexia and bulimia often first appear in teenage years.
   c. Refer consumer to a dietitian.
   d. Undertake a focused assessment on nutritional intake only, the most important thing is to see how much this consumer is eating.

10. The most common theme between Australian and New Zealand nutrition guidelines are:
    a. To encourage breastfeeding
    b. Eat a wide variety of foods from the food groups
    c. To snack often on health food
    d. To eat at least 10 serves of vegetables and fruit each day

CS CLINICAL SKILLS

The following Clinical Skills are relevant to this chapter and can be found in Tollefson & Hillman, *Clinical Psychomotor Skills,* 8th edition:
> 14 Blood glucose measurement
> 22 Focused gastrointestinal health history and abdominal physical assessment
> 27 Healthcare teaching
> 72 Assisting with stoma care.

FURTHER RESOURCES

> Australian and New Zealand Obesity Society: https://anzos.com/
> Bowel Cancer Australia: http://www.bowelcanceraustralia.org
> Bowel Cancer New Zealand: https://bowelcancernz.org.nz/
> Cancer Council Australia: http://www.cancer.org.au
> Cancer Society of New Zealand: http://www.cancernz.org.nz/
> Centers for Disease Control and Prevention: http://www.cdc.gov
> Coeliac New Zealand: http://www.coeliac.org.nz/
> Colorectal Surgical Society of Australia and New Zealand: http://www.cssanz.org/
> Crohns and Colitis Australia: http://www.crohnsandcolitis.com.au/
> Crohns and Colitis New Zealand: http://www.crohnsandcolitis.org.nz/

> Gastroenterological Nursing College of Australia: http://www.genca.org/
> Gastroenterological Society of Australia: http://www.gesa.org.au/
> GI Cancer Institute: http://www.gicancer.org.au/
> Healthdirect Australia: http://www.healthdirect.gov.au/
> New Zealand Ministry of Health: http://www.health.govt.nz/
> New Zealand Society of Gastroenterology: http://www.nzsg.org.nz/
> Nutrition Australia: http://www.nutritionaustralia.org/
> Weight Watchers: http://www.weightwatchers.com.au

REFERENCES

Antonello, M., Bonvini, S., & Colacchio, E. C. (2022). Chapter 8. How to approach elective and urgent thoracic aortic aneurysms. In P. Settembrini, A.M. Settembrini (Eds.), *Vascular surgery*. Academic Press. https://doi.org/10.1016/B978-0-12-822113-6.00007-3.

Australian Bureau of Statistics (ABS). (2022). Causes of death, Australia. Retrieved 13 December 2022 from: https://www.abs.gov.au/statistics/health/causes-death/causes-death-australia/2021

Australian Government, Cancer Australia. (2020). Stomach cancer. Retrieved from https://www.canceraustralia.gov.au/cancer-types/stomach-cancer/awareness

Australian Government, Cancer Australia. (2022). Liver cancer. Retrieved from https://www.canceraustralia.gov.au/cancer-types/liver-cancer/awareness

Australian Government, Department of Health (2016). National bowel cancer screening program. Fact Sheet. Retrieved 23 March 2018 from: http://www.health.gov.au/internet/screening/publishing.nsf/Content/3DB3253DE5782154CA257D720005CA06/$File/NBCSP%20fact%20sheet.pdf

Australian Government, National Health and Medical Research Council & Department of Health and Ageing. (2013). Eat for Health: Australian Dietary Guidelines, summary. Canberra: Commonwealth of Australia.

Australian Institute of Health and Wellbeing (AIHW). (2022). Overweight and obesity. Retrieved 13 December 2022 from: https://www.aihw.gov.au/reports/australias-health/overweight-and-obesity

Boutari, C., & Mantzoros, C. (2022). A 2022 update on the epidemiology of obesity and a call to action: as its twin COVID-19 pandemic appears to be receding, the obesity and dysmetabolism pandemic continues to rage on. *Metabolism, 133*, 155217. doi: 10.1016/j.metabol.2022.155217

Cancer Australia. (2018). Bowel cancer also known as colorectal cancer. Retrieved 25 March 2018 from: https://bowel-cancer.canceraustralia.gov.au/risk-factors

Cancer Council of Australia. (n.d.). A guide to: Bowel cancer screening. Retrieved 10 May 2023 from: https://www.cancer.org.au/cancer-information/causes-and-prevention/early-detection-and-screening/bowel-cancer-screening

Cancer Council of Australia. (n.d.). Understanding your FOBT results. Retrieved 10 May 2023 from: https://www.cancer.org.au/cancer-information/causes-and-prevention/early-detection-and-screening/understanding-your-fobt-results

Danwang, C., Bigna, J. J., Tochie, J. N., Mbonda, A., Mbanga, C. M., Nzalie, R. N. T., Guifo, M. L., & Essomba A. (2020). Global incidence of surgical site infection after appendectomy: A systemic review and meta-analysis. *BMJ Open, 10*(2). doi:10.1136/bmjopen-2019-034266

Healthdirect Australia. (2022). Hepatitis. Retrieved 31 October 2022 from: http://www.healthdirect.gov.au/hepatitis

Health New Zealand. (2019). Mortality summary 2019. Retrieved 13 December 2022 from: https://minhealthnz.shinyapps.io/mortality-web-tool/

Lewis, S. J., & Heaton, K. W. (1997). Stool form scale as a useful guide to intestinal transit time. *Scandinavian Journal of Gastroenterology, 32*(9), 920–4.

Ministry of Health New Zealand. (2012). Food and nutrition guidelines for healthy children and young people (aged 2–18 years): A background paper. Wellington. Retrieved 13 December 2022 from: https://www.health.govt.nz/publication/food-and-nutrition-guidelines-healthy-children-and-young-people-aged-2-18-years-background-paper

Ministry of Health/Manatu Hauora. (2021). Obesity statistics. Retrieved 13 December 2022 from: https://www.health.govt.nz/nz-health-statistics/health-statistics-and-data-sets/obesity-statistics

Ministry of Health/Manatu Hauora. (2023). National Bowel Screening Programme. Retrieved 10 May 2023 from: https://www.health.govt.nz/our-work/preventative-health-wellness/screening/national-bowel-screening-programme

Mudugal, R. Beniwal, R., Singh, & S., Khera, S. (2020). Violaceous papules and nodules over the umbilicus: The harbinger of occult intra-abdominal malignancy. *Indian Dermatology Online Journal, 11*(5), 852–3. doi: 10.4103/idoj.IDOJ_68_20

NSW Health. (2018). Botulism fact sheet. NSW Government. Retrieved from https://www.health.nsw.gov.au/Infectious/factsheets/Pages/botulism.aspx#:~:text=Avoid%20giving%20honey%20to%20babies,or%20detergent)%20and%20running%20water.

Wint, C., & Sethi, S. (2019). What you should know about an enlarged spleen. *Healthline*. Retrieved from https://www.healthline.com/health/splenomegaly

World Health Organization (WHO). (2021). Obesity and overweight, key facts. Retrieved 13 December 2022 from: https://www.who.int/news-room/fact-sheets/detail/obesity-and-overweight

CHAPTER 16

CHAPTER 16

MUSCULOSKELETAL

LEARNING OUTCOMES

By the end of this chapter you should be able to:

1 identify the anatomical landmarks of the musculoskeletal system
2 describe the characteristics of the most common musculoskeletal complaints
3 obtain a health history from a consumer with a musculoskeletal complaint
4 demonstrate inspection and palpation of the musculoskeletal system
5 explain evidence-based rationale(s) for abnormal musculoskeletal assessment findings
6 discuss the clinical reasoning in evaluating outcomes of health assessment and physical examination, including documentation, health education provision and relevant health referrals.

BACKGROUND

A musculoskeletal disorder (MSD) is defined as an injury or disorder that impacts on a person's body movement or musculoskeletal system (muscles, tendons, ligaments etc.). Musculoskeletal disorders are highly prevalent, affecting almost 1 in 3 Australians and 1 in 4 New Zealanders. Although rarely fatal, they contribute significantly to illness, pain and disability in Australia and New Zealand (AIHW, 2022a; Ministry of Health, 2020). These disorders place a high economic and personal burden on the community, with an estimated 11% ($12.5 billion) of recurrent disease expenditure in the Australian health system attributed to the musculoskeletal conditions group (AIHW, 2019).

Risk factors such as obesity (being overweight places pressure on joints) and sedentary lifestyles further contribute to the burden of disease (AIHW, 2022b). Work-related MSDs account for the majority of workers' compensation costs, adding to the social and economic burden (Safe Work Australia, 2019). Addressing musculoskeletal conditions nationally is an Australian Government priority (Department of Health and Aged Care, 2020).

There are more than 150 types of musculoskeletal conditions (Department of Health and Aged Care, 2020); however, the most common conditions are back problems, arthritis (mainly osteo and rheumatoid) and osteoporosis. Data shows that of the nearly 6.9 million people (27% of all Australians) with chronic MSDs, 3.9 million (16%) had back problems, 3.1 million (12%) had arthritis and 889 000 (3.6%) had osteoporosis (ABS, 2022).

Arthritis (joint inflammation) is often referred to as a single disease, but there are numerous conditions that affect joints and surrounding tissue. Arthritis affects both sexes and people of all ages; however, some forms of arthritis are more prevalent in women.

> Osteoarthritis (degenerative condition) is the most common type of arthritis, affecting 9% of the Australian population (1 in 11 people) (AIHW, 2020b) and 10.6% of the New Zealand population (Lao et al., 2019). It is more common in older people, particularly women, with two out of three people affected being female. Osteoarthritis is the predominant condition that leads to hip and knee replacement surgery (AIHW, 2020b; Arthritis NZ, 2018).

> Rheumatoid arthritis, RA (an autoimmune chronic disease of the joints), affects 2% of the population, with rates slightly higher for women (2.3%) than men (1.5%) (AIHW, 2020c; Arthritis NZ, 2018). Over a long period of time RA can cause bone erosion and joint deformity.

> Juvenile idiopathic arthritis (juvenile onset chronic autoimmune disease) is an umbrella term that includes several different kinds of arthritis that occur in children under the age of 16. It affects one in 1000 children (0 to 15 years), causing significant pain, disability and restrictions in school activities (AIHW, 2020d).

Osteoporosis is a common condition in older adults that causes a decrease in bone density. Bones leach minerals such as calcium too quickly for the body to replace, causing bones to become porous, weak and fragile and, therefore, more susceptible to fracture. An estimated 924 000 Australians have osteoporosis (AIHW 2020e), with more women affected than men. Across Australian and New Zealand populations, data shows that 29% of women aged 75 have osteoporosis, compared with 10% of men (AIHW 2020e; Osteoporosis NZ, n.d.).

Back problems include a range of disorders affecting the spine and muscles of the cervical, thoracic and lumbar spine. Contributing factors include injuries, osteoarthritis and posture. It is estimated that 16% of the population report a back problem (1 in 6 people) (AIHW 2020a).

Falls are a major health issue in the community. About 30% of adults over 65 experience at least one fall per year (Australian and New Zealand Falls Prevention Society, 2022) and falls are Australia's number one cause of injury hospitalisation and death, representing 42% of injury hospitalisations and 40% of injury deaths (AIHW, 2022b). Neck of femur fractures (often referred to as a fractured hip) are the most common type of injury associated with falls. In many older adults, neck of femur fractures can result in death due to post-operative complications and the consequences of the injury. For those who survive, many never regain complete mobility, due to developing a post fall syndrome (loss of confidence, hesitancy and tentativeness with resultant loss of mobility and independence). After a fall, 48% of older people report a fear of falling, with 25% curtailing activities as a result. Falls are commonly cited as a contributing reason for an older person requiring admission to a nursing home (Australian and New Zealand Falls Prevention Society, 2022).

HEALTH EDUCATION

Risk factors for osteoarthritis

Osteoarthritis (OA) is not fully understood; however, research has identified some things that can put individuals at more risk of developing this MSD. These should be identified to frame future health education strategies when assessing the musculoskeletal system:

> Excessive weight or obesity
> Family history
> Age > 40–50
> Joint injury or abnormality
> Overuse of joint – for example repetitive heavy lifting.

ANATOMY AND PHYSIOLOGY

The musculoskeletal system consists of an intricate framework of bones, joints, skeletal muscles and supportive connective tissue (cartilage, tendons and ligaments). Although the primary purpose of the musculoskeletal system is to support body position and promote mobility, it also protects underlying soft organs and allows for mineral storage. In addition, it produces select blood components (platelets, red blood cells, and white blood cells). Only those aspects of the musculoskeletal system that are responsible for body position and mobility are discussed in this chapter.

Bones

The adult human skeleton is composed of 206 bones (**Figure 16.1**). Bone is ossified connective tissue. The skeleton is divided into the central **axial skeleton** (facial bones, skull, auditory ossicles, hyoid bone, ribs, sternum, vertebrae) and the peripheral **appendicular skeleton** (limbs, pelvis, scapula, clavicle). Bone size and shape are directly related to the mobility and weight-bearing function of that bone. In some cases, bone size and shape are also related to the protection of underlying internal organs and tissues (e.g. the ribs in relation to the lungs, heart and thoracic aorta).

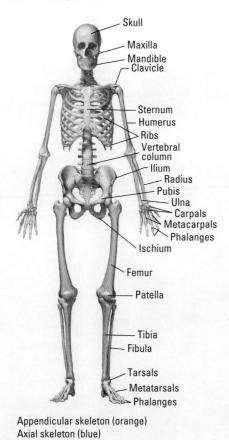

Appendicular skeleton (orange)
Axial skeleton (blue)

FIGURE 16.1 Adult skeleton: anterior view

Shape and structure

Bones have long, short, flat, rounded and irregular shapes. The long bone is a shaft (**diaphysis**) with two large ends (**epiphyses**). The two epiphyses each articulate with another bone to form a joint. A 1 to 4 mm layer of cartilage covers each epiphysis in order to minimise stress and friction on the bone ends during movement and weight bearing. The thickness of the cartilage layer varies, depending on the amount of stress placed on that joint. The interior of the diaphysis is the **medullary cavity**, which contains the bone marrow.

Short bones are found in the hands (carpals) and feet (tarsals). Flat bones, such as those of the skull and parts of the pelvic girdle, are associated with the protection of nearby soft body parts. Rounded, or sesamoid, bones such as the patella are often encased in the fascia or in a tendon near a joint.. Irregular bones include the mandible, the vertebrae, and the auditory ossicles of the inner ear.

Muscles

There are over 600 muscles in the human body, and they can be characterised as one of three types. Cardiac and smooth muscles are involuntary, meaning that the individual has no conscious control over the initiation and termination of the muscle contraction. The largest type of muscle, and the only type of voluntary muscle, is called skeletal muscle. Skeletal muscle provides for mobility by exerting a pull on the bones near a joint. In addition, skeletal muscle provides for body contour and contributes to overall body weight. **Figure 16.2** illustrates the major muscles. It is estimated that approximately 40% of adult body weight is due to the weight of the skeletal muscles. Muscles vary in size and strength in every person, and are affected by age, sex, exercise and nutrition.

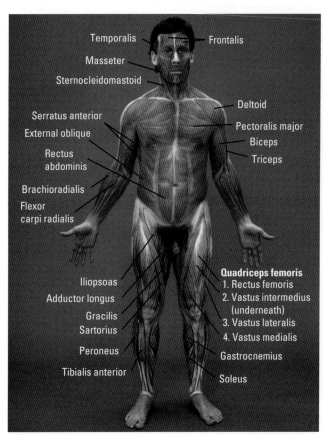

A. Anterior view

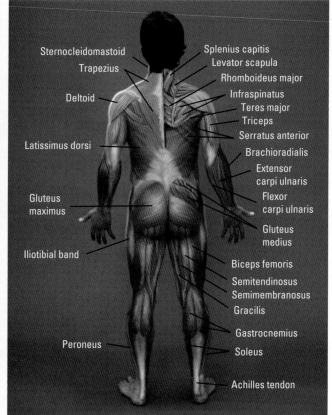

B. Posterior view

FIGURE 16.2 Muscles of the body

Tendons

A strong connective tissue sheath (**epimysium**) acts as the outer covering of the muscle belly. The ends of the epimysium extend beyond the muscle belly to form the **tendons** of the muscle. The tendon attaches the muscle to a bone (**Figure 16.3**).

Cartilage

Cartilage is an avascular, dense, connective tissue that covers the ends of opposing bones. Its resilience allows it to withstand increased pressure and tension.

Ligaments

Ligaments are composed of strong, fibrous connective tissue. They connect bones to each other at the joint level, and encase the joint capsule. Ligaments may be seen as oblique to or parallel to a joint (e.g. the knee) or encircling the joint (e.g. the hip). Ligaments support purposeful joint movement and prevent joint movement that is detrimental to that type of joint.

Bursae

Bursae are sacs filled with fluid. They act as cushions between two nearby surfaces (e.g. between tendon and bone or between tendon and ligament) to reduce friction. Bursae can also develop in response to prolonged friction or pressure.

Joints

A **joint** is a union between two bones. Joints secure the bones firmly together but allow for some degree of movement between the two bones. Contraction of overlying skeletal muscle will act to alter the angle of the two bones by pulling the distal bone towards or away from the proximal bone. Terms used for joint range of motion are described in **Table 16.1**.

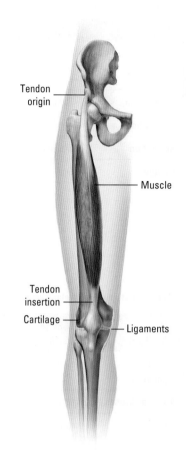

FIGURE 16.3 Connective tissue structures of the leg

TABLE 16.1 Terminology used for joint range of motion

TERM	DESCRIPTION	CHANGE IN JOINT ANGLE
Flexion	Bending of a joint so that the articulating bones on either side of the joints are moved closer together	Decreased
Extension	Bending of a joint so that the articulating bones on either side of the joint are moved further apart	Increased
Hyperextension	Extension beyond the neutral position	Increased beyond the angle of extension
Adduction	Moving the extremity medially and towards the midline of the body	Decreased
Abduction	Moving the extremity laterally and away from the midline of the body	Increased
Internal rotation	Rotating the extremity medially along its own axis	No change
External rotation	Rotating the extremity laterally along its own axis	No change
Circumduction	Moving the extremity in a conical fashion so that the distal aspect of the extremity moves in a circle	No change
Supination	Rotating the forearm laterally at the elbow so that the palm of the hand turns laterally to face upwards	No change
Pronation	Rotating the forearm medially at the elbow so that the palm of the hand turns medially to face downwards	No change
Opposition	Moving the thumb to touch the little finger of the same hand	No change
Eversion	Tilting the foot (outwards) with the medial side of the foot lowered	No change
Inversion	Tilting the foot (inwards) with the medial side of the foot lowered	No change
Dorsiflexion	Flexing the foot at the ankle so that the toes move towards the chest	Decreased

>> **TABLE 16.1** *continued*

TERM	DESCRIPTION	CHANGE IN JOINT ANGLE
Plantar flexion	Moving the foot at the ankle so that the toes move away from the chest	Increased
Elevation	Raising a body part in an upwards direction	No change
Depression	Lowering a body part	No change
Protraction	Moving a body part anteriorly along its own axis (parallel to the ground)	No change
Retraction	Moving a body part posteriorly along its own axis (parallel to the ground)	No change
Gliding	One joint surface moves over another joint surface in a circular or angular manner	No change

Of the three classifications of skeletal joints found in the adult human skeleton (diarthroses, amphiarthroses, synarthroses), only the synovial joint (diarthroses) is considered freely movable. Examples of each joint are provided in Table 16.2. Table 16.3 shows categories of the major synovial joints. The synovial joint allows body movement.

TABLE 16.2 Categories of skeletal joints

CATEGORY	DEGREE OF MOVEMENT	EXAMPLES
Diarthroses (synovial)	Freely movable	Shoulder, elbow, wrist, thumb, hip, knee, ankle, proximal cervical vertebrae
Amphiarthroses	Slightly movable	Vertebrae, manubriosternal joint, distal radioulnar joint, symphysis pubis
Synarthroses	Immovable	Epiphyseal growth plate (adult), skull sutures (child), between the distal ends of the radius and ulna, between the distal ends of the tibia and fibula, the attachment of the root of a tooth to the alveolar process of the maxilla or mandible

TABLE 16.3 Categories of synovial joints

CATEGORY	DESCRIPTION	EXAMPLES
UNIAXIAL JOINTS		
Hinge joint	Angular movement in one axis and in one plane	Elbow, fingers, knee
Pivot joint (trochoid)	Rotary movement in one axis; a ring rotates around a pivot, or a pivotlike process rotates within a ring	Proximal radioulnar joint, atlanto-odontal joint of the first and second cervical vertebrae
BIAXIAL JOINTS		
Saddle joint (sellar)	Articulating surface of one bone is convex and articulating surface of second bone is concave	Metacarpal bone of thumb, trapezium bone of carpus
Condyloid joint	Angular motion in two planes without axial rotation	Wrist between the distal radius and the carpals
MULTIAXIAL JOINTS		
Ball and socket (spheroidal) joint	Round end of bone fits into cuplike cavity of another bone; provides movement around three or more axes, or in three or more planes	Shoulder, hip
Gliding joint	Gliding movement	Vertebrae, tarsal bones of ankle

A synovial membrane lines the interior of the joint space (**Figure 16.4**). The primary purpose of the synovial membrane is to secrete fluid for joint lubrication, nourishment and waste removal. Normally, the joint space contains only 1 to 3 mL of synovial fluid. Excessive synovial joint fluid is called a **synovial effusion**.

ASSESSMENT: TAKING THE CONSUMER'S HEALTH HISTORY

Assessment is the first phase of the nursing process and involves collecting subjective information about the consumer's health status in order to identify consumer problem areas to focus on.

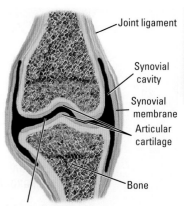

FIGURE 16.4 Synovial joint

> **Subjective data** is most frequently collected during a health history and serves as the starting point for the health professional to base the depth of their assessment on. The sections for the health history include:
>
> > **Consumer profile**
> > **Chief complaint** (explained systematically using variations of location, quality, quantity, associated manifestations, aggravating factors, alleviating factors, setting and timing. This is a variation on the OPQRST assessment mnemonic you may use for other conditions such as pain assessment)
> > **Past health history** (including medical history, surgical history, allergies, medications, injuries and accidents, special needs and childhood illnesses)
> > **Family health history**
> > **Social history** (including alcohol, tobacco and drug use, sexual practice, work and home environment, hobbies and leisure activities, stress and culture).

The example health history provided identifies scope for questioning the consumer about their health for this specific body system.

HEALTH HISTORY		
CONSUMER PROFILE		The musculoskeletal health history provides insight into the link between a consumer's life and lifestyle and musculoskeletal information and pathology. Diseases that are age-, sex- and race-specific for the musculoskeletal system are listed.
	AGE	> Osteosarcoma (10–20 and 50–60) > Ankylosing spondylitis (20–40) > Bursitis (20–40) > Rheumatoid arthritis (onset 20–40 unless juvenile form of the disease) > Systemic lupus erythematosus (SLE) (25–35) > Low back pain (30–50) > Fractures (16–100) > Gout (onset over 30, postmenopausal female) > Osteoporosis (menopausal female) > Carpal tunnel syndrome (pregnant or menopausal female) > Degenerative joint disease or osteoarthritis (onset after 55 in the female and before 45 in the male) > Multiple myeloma (50–70) > Paget's disease (50–70) > Fibromyalgia (40–75)

>>

HEALTH HISTORY			
SEX	**FEMALE**	Osteoporosis, rheumatoid arthritis, scoliosis, carpal tunnel syndrome, SLE, postmenopausal gout, polymyalgia rheumatica, scleroderma, myasthenia gravis, multiple sclerosis (MS), senile kyphosis, fibromyalgia	
	MALE	Ankylosing spondylitis, gout, Paget's disease, Reiter syndrome, Dupuytren's contracture, psoriatic arthritis, muscular dystrophy (MD), amyotrophic lateral sclerosis (ALS), low back pain	
CULTURAL BACKGROUND	**CAUCASIAN**	Rheumatoid arthritis, primary osteoarthritis, polymyalgia rheumatica, osteoporosis, Paget's disease, Dupuytren's contracture, ALS, ankylosing spondylitis	
	INDIGENOUS	SLE, rheumatoid arthritis	
CHIEF COMPLAINT	Common chief complaints for the musculoskeletal system are defined and information on the characteristics of each sign or symptom is provided.		
	1. PAIN	The subjective sense of discomfort in the axial or appendicular skeleton	
		LOCATION	Muscle, bone, tendon, ligament, joint
		QUANTITY	Degree of interruption in the consumer's usual activities of daily living (ADL) (changes in ambulation, bathing, dressing, food preparation, working, sitting, transfer to a sitting or standing position, climbing stairs, lifting, pushing, pulling)
		ASSOCIATED MANIFESTATIONS	Inflammation, skin abrasion, laceration, bruising, haematoma, stiffness, deformity, muscle spasm, paraesthesia, decreased joint mobility, restriction of weight bearing and movement, excessive weakness or fatigue, mental depression, insomnia, guarding of the painful area, crying, moaning, facial grimacing, anxiety, social withdrawal, agitation, restlessness, diaphoresis, tachycardia, elevated blood pressure, tachypnoea
		AGGRAVATING FACTORS	Muscle contraction, muscle spasm, joint movement, partial or full weight bearing, obesity, dependent position, cold and damp weather, noncompliance to physio- or occupational therapy guidelines
		ALLEVIATING FACTORS	Restriction of movement, position change, non-weight bearing, limb elevation and rest, ice, heat, analgesics, anti-inflammatory agents, steroids, muscle relaxants, local anaesthetic agents, whirlpool therapy, transcutaneous electrical nerve stimulation (TENS), acupuncture, acupressure, supportive equipment for use during weight bearing and mobility, splints
		SETTING	Recent untreated streptococcal infection
		TIMING	Sudden, insidious, intermittent, continuous
	2. WEAKNESS	The subjective sense of an overall decrease in strength and endurance	
		LOCATION	Local or diffuse, central or peripheral
		QUANTITY	Effect on ADL
		ASSOCIATED MANIFESTATIONS	Fatigue, muscle atrophy, decreased sensation, decreased joint mobility, decreased muscle strength, discomfort, decreased ability to do ADL
		AGGRAVATING FACTORS	Overexertion, fatigue, immobility, noncompliance to physio- or occupational therapy guidelines, physical or emotional stress
		ALLEVIATING FACTORS	Rest, adequate nutrition and hydration, electrolyte replacement therapy, physiotherapy and occupational therapy geared towards muscle-strengthening exercises and adaptive techniques

>>

>>

HEALTH HISTORY			
	3. LIMITED MOVEMENT	Decrease in mobility caused by a problem with impulse transmission to the muscle, stimulation of a muscle, the ability of that muscle to contract sufficiently to move the joint, or bone stability	
		LOCATION	Diffuse, or localised to a specific joint
		QUANTITY	Range of joint motion compared to maximum potential or previous measurement
		ASSOCIATED MANIFESTATIONS	Pain, inflammation, stiffness, muscle atrophy, weakness, deformity, crepitus, joint effusion
		AGGRAVATING FACTORS	Overexertion, immobility, excessive weight gain, noncompliance to medication regimen (e.g. anti-inflammatory agents), noncompliance to physio- and occupational therapy guidelines
		ALLEVIATING FACTORS	Physiotherapy and occupational therapy, anti-inflammatory agents, analgesics, ice, heat, rest, reduction of fractures, correction of dislocation or subluxation
	4. STIFFNESS	The subjective sense of inflexibility	
		LOCATION	Diffuse, or localised to a specific joint
		QUANTITY	Effect on ADL
		ASSOCIATED MANIFESTATIONS	Joint inflammation, muscle atrophy, deformity, contracture, immobility, pain, palpable joint crepitus, limited range of joint motion
		AGGRAVATING FACTORS	Immobility, ageing, overexertion (especially without adequate warming-up and cooling-down sessions during exercise), noncompliance to medication regimen (e.g. anti-inflammatory agents), noncompliance to physio- and occupational therapy guidelines
		ALLEVIATING FACTORS	Physiotherapy and occupational therapy, exercise, anti-inflammatory agents, analgesics, heat, rest, massage, muscle relaxants
		SETTING	Cold and damp environment
		TIMING	Sudden or insidious, time of day (e.g. morning stiffness for more than 30 minutes is associated with rheumatoid arthritis), in relation to vigorous or excessive physical exercise
	5. DEFORMITY	The congenital or acquired alteration in the configuration of the axial or appendicular skeleton	
		LOCATION	General (e.g. decreased overall body size) or localised (e.g. disruption in limb length and alignment due to a fracture)
		QUALITY	Degree of cosmetic alteration, degree of musculoskeletal dysfunction (adverse changes in mobility, weight bearing, and the ability to maintain body posture and position)
		ASSOCIATED MANIFESTATIONS	Enlarged skull, jaw protrusion, forehead protrusion, abnormal joint angle, limb malalignment, missing or extra digits, missing limb, discrepancy in limb length or width, abnormal posture, muscle atrophy, joint contractures
		AGGRAVATING FACTORS	Certain body positions or movements
		ALLEVIATING FACTORS	Surgery, skeletal or skin traction, manual reduction of a fracture or dislocation, limb elevation, ice, physiotherapy splint, cast, brace
		TIMING	Sudden or insidious, temporary or permanent

>>

HEALTH HISTORY			
PAST HEALTH HISTORY	The various components of the past health history are linked to musculoskeletal pathology and musculoskeletal-related information.		
	MEDICAL HISTORY	**MUSCULOSKELETAL-SPECIFIC**	Rheumatoid arthritis, osteoarthritis, osteoporosis, Paget's disease, gout, ankylosing spondylitis, osteogenesis imperfecta, loosening or malfunction of joint prosthesis, aseptic necrosis, chronic low back pain, herniated nucleus pulposus, chronic muscle spasms or cramps, scoliosis, poliomyelitis, polymyalgia rheumatica, osteomalacia, rickets, Marfan syndrome, scleroderma, spina bifida, congenital deformity, MD, MS, myasthenia gravis, ALS, Guillain-Barré syndrome, Reiter syndrome, carpal tunnel syndrome, paralysis
		NON-MUSCULOSKELETAL-SPECIFIC	Immunosuppression, necrotising fasciitis, gas gangrene, tetanus, sickle cell anaemia, SLE, Lyme disease, blood dyscrasias (including haemophilia), multiple myeloma, diabetes mellitus with or without peripheral neuropathy, hypo- or hypercalcaemia, hypo- or hyperpituitarism, hyper- or hypoparathyroidism, hyper- or hypothyroidism, peripheral vascular disease with or without claudication, malnutrition, obesity, menopause
	SURGICAL HISTORY		Joint aspiration, therapeutic joint arthroscopy, joint arthroplasty, joint replacement, synovectomy, meniscectomy, arthrodesis, open reduction and internal fixation, discectomy, laminectomy, spinal fusion, Harrington rod placement or other spinal instrumentation, repair of torn rotator cuff, debridement, limb or digit amputation or reattachment
	MEDICATIONS		Narcotic analgesics, non-narcotic analgesics, anti-inflammatory agents, anti-gout agents, muscle relaxants, steroids, calcitonin, calcium and vitamin D supplements, intra-articular injections, bisphosphonates, selective oestrogen receptor modulator, human parathyroid hormone
	COMMUNICABLE DISEASES		Poliomyelitis
	INJURIES AND ACCIDENTS		Fracture, dislocation, subluxation, tendon tear, tendonitis, muscle contusion, joint strain or sprain, spinal cord injury, torn rotator cuff, traumatic amputation of a digit or limb, crush injury, back injury (including herniated vertebral disc), sports-related injury (e.g. golf elbow, pitcher's shoulder), cartilage damage. See Table 16.4 for age-related trauma.
	SPECIAL NEEDS		Amputation, hemiplegia, paraplegia, quadriplegia, need for brace or splint, limb in a cast, need for supportive devices, muscle atrophy
	CHILDHOOD ILLNESSES		Poliomyelitis, juvenile arthritis
FAMILY HEALTH HISTORY	Musculoskeletal diseases that are familial are listed. Rheumatoid arthritis, osteoporosis, ankylosing spondylitis, gout, Paget's disease, Dupuytren's contracture, SLE, Marfan syndrome, osteomalacia, congenital defect		
SOCIAL HISTORY	The components of the social history are linked to musculoskeletal factors and pathology		
	ALCOHOL USE		Increased use associated with increased risk of osteoporosis
	TOBACCO USE		Increased use associated with increased risk of osteoporosis
	WORK ENVIRONMENT		Manual movement of heavy objects (lifting, pushing, pulling), duties requiring repetitive motions (e.g. keyboard use), duties requiring prolonged standing or ambulation, use of hazardous equipment, availability and use of safety equipment (e.g. lifting equipment, availability of back support vest or brace)

>>

HEALTH HISTORY

	ROLES AND RELATIONSHIPS	Decreased self-esteem, decreased independence, isolation secondary to immobility or pain
	HOME ENVIRONMENT	Design of home (e.g. number of floors, width of doorways, stairs, location of bedroom and bathroom), elevated toilet seat, rail in bathtub or shower, access ramp
	HOBBIES AND LEISURE ACTIVITIES	Basketball, wrestling, gymnastics, hockey, ballet, aerobics, use of free weights and exercise machines, baseball, football, lacrosse, rugby, cycling, running, horseback riding, skiing, hiking, tennis, squash, swimming, camping, gardening, painting, needlework, carpentry, rollerblading, skateboarding
	STRESS	Stress can be deleterious to consumers with autoimmune chronic diseases affecting the musculoskeletal system, such as MS, SLE and rheumatoid arthritis. During times of stress, these consumers may experience additional discomfort, stiffness, loss of mobility and fatigue.

TABLE 16.4 Common age-related trauma

AGE RANGE	COMMON TRAUMA
10–20	Sports-related injuries, motorcycle accidents, high-energy falls (e.g. downhill skiing or cycling)
20–50	Sports-related injuries, stress or overuse injuries (e.g. stress fractures, tendonitis), pedestrian accidents
50–65	Recreation-related injuries, falls, pathological fractures, pedestrian accidents

PERSON-CENTRED HEALTH EDUCATION

When conducting a health assessment, opportunities for the provision of person-centred health education will arise. This is a significant consideration in relation to the assessment process for examination of the musculoskeletal system due to health, safety and maintenance activities factors. These occasions are identified as individualised education and may generate further data that can be added to the assessment. All education given should be documented so that in future, health professionals can assess the impact of previous information provided to the consumer. (Refer to Chapter 1 for initiating health education.) Refer to the following examples.

INDIVIDUALISED HEALTH EDUCATION INTERVENTIONS

Assessing the consumer for the following health-related activities can assist in identifying the need for education about these factors. This information provides a bridge between the health maintenance activities and musculoskeletal system.

Sleep	Sleeping positions, need for pillow support, need for firm mattress
Diet	Intake of dairy products and protein, use of dietary supplements or vitamins (especially calcium and vitamin D)
Exercise	Prevents disuse atrophy, promotes bone growth (especially weight-bearing exercise), can aggravate existing musculoskeletal conditions and cause musculoskeletal trauma
Use of safety devices	Use of back support vest or lifting equipment for movement of heavy objects (e.g. Hoyer lift, forklift), safety shields when using hazardous equipment, protective padding (wrist or knee guards), helmet, use of gait belt for adult assistance/moving
Health check-ups	Immunisations up to date, especially polio and tetanus, bone mineral density screening

UNIT 2

PLANNING FOR PHYSICAL EXAMINATION

The planning phase refers to evaluating subjective data to narrow the focus on physical examination, determining what objective data needs to be gathered, as well as considering the environment and equipment that will be required.

At this time, you will identify which of the four diagnostic techniques you will need to implement the physical examination, and how you will sequence these. For the physical examination of the musculoskeletal system you will include inspection and palpation.

Objective data is:

> collected during the physical examination of the consumer
> usually collected after subjective data
> information that is measured or observed by the clinician as opposed to being reported by the consumer
> vital to the overall health assessment, to enable you to make clinical decisions that are representative of the whole consumer picture.

Evaluating subjective data to focus physical assessment

Before commencing the physical examination of the consumer's musculoskeletal system, consider what information the health history has provided. Critical consideration, linked to knowledge of anatomy and physiology, should focus the physical assessment so your examination will be more effective and efficient.

Environment

Assessment of the musculoskeletal system can be undertaken in most physical environments in healthcare settings. Adequate privacy is required as for any health assessment, with some consideration needed for safety issues related to a consumer's mobility and pain. Use caution when assessing the consumer with limited ability, poor coordination, poor balance, or a sensory deficit (e.g. visual loss, hearing loss, limb amputation, peripheral neuropathy, hemiplegia). Some of the positions and movements that are necessary may place the individual at increased risk for falling during the assessment. Be prepared to support the consumer to prevent a fall. If necessary, omit those components of the musculoskeletal assessment that would place the individual at high risk for injury, or seek the assistance of a second health professional.

To provide safe and quality care for people over the age of 65, the Australian Commission on Safety and Quality in Health Care has developed *Best practice guidelines for preventing falls and harm from falls in older people.* These can be accessed from their website: https://www.safetyandquality.gov.au/sites/default/files/migrated/Guidelines-HOSP.pdf

Equipment

> Measuring tape: cloth tape measure that will not stretch
> Goniometer: protractor-type instrument with two movable arms to measure the angle of a skeletal joint during range of motion
> Sphygmomanometer and blood pressure cuff
> Felt tip pen

<u>IMPLEMENTATION: CONDUCTING THE PHYSICAL EXAMINATION</u>

Implementation of the physical examination requires you to consider your scope of practice as well. In this section, depending on your context, you may be performing a foundation assessment or the addition of advanced assessment techniques, if you are practising in a specialised area.

EXAMINATION **IN BRIEF: MUSCULOSKELETAL SYSTEM**

Examination of the musculoskeletal system

General assessment
> Overall appearance
> Posture
> Gait and mobility

Inspection
> Muscle size and shape
> Joint contour and periarticular tissue
> Measuring limb circumference

Palpation
> Muscle tone
> Joints

Range of motion (ROM)
> Assessing joint ROM: Using a goniometer

Muscle strength

Examination of joints

Temporomandibular joint
> Assessing for neuroexcitability: Chvostek sign

Cervical spine

Shoulders
> Assessing for rotator cuff damage: Drop arm test

Elbows
> Assessing for neuroexcitability: Trousseau sign

Wrists and hands
> Assessing for carpal tunnel syndrome: Tinel's sign
> Assessing for carpal tunnel syndrome: Phalen's sign

Hips
> Assessing for hip dislocation: Trendelenburg test

Measuring limb length

Knees
> Assessing for small effusions: Bulge sign
> Assessing for large effusions: Patellar ballottement
> Assessing for meniscal tears: Apley's grinding sign
> Assessing for meniscal tears: McMurray sign
> Assessing the cruciate ligaments: Drawer test
> Assessing the anterior cruciate ligament: Lachman test
> Assessing the lateral collateral ligament: Varus stress test
> Assessing the medial collateral ligament: Valgus stress test

Ankles and feet
> Assessing for ankle sprain: Anterior drawer test
> Assessing for ankle sprain: Talar tilt test
> Assessing for ruptured Achilles tendon: Thompson squeeze test

Spine
> Assessing for scoliosis: Adams forwards bend test and use of the scoliometer
> Assessing for herniated disc: Straight leg raising test (Lasègue's test)
> Assessing for herniated disc: Milgram test

Assessing status of distal limbs and digits

Assessing consumers with musculoskeletal supportive equipment
> Crutches
> Walking stick
> Walker
> Brace, splint, immobiliser
> Cast

Advanced Assessment

The complete musculoskeletal assessment described in this chapter is designed for consumers who have musculoskeletal complaints or disease, or who have difficulty with activities of daily living (ADL). The screening, or musculoskeletal mini-assessment, is conducted on all other consumers and should include only general assessment: inspection and palpation of major muscles and joints, inspection of range of motion (ROM) as the individual moves through the examination, and muscle strength of the arms and legs.

General approach to the musculoskeletal system assessment

1. Assist the consumer to a comfortable position.
2. Offer pillows or folded blankets to support a painful body part.
3. If necessary because of a painful body part or limited mobility, provide the individual assistance in disrobing. Allow the consumer extra time to remove clothing.
4. To maximise consumer comfort during the physical assessment, maintain a warm temperature in the examination room.
5. Be clear in your instructions to the individual if you are asking them to perform a certain body movement or to assume a certain position. Demonstrate the desired movement if necessary.
6. Notify the consumer before touching or manipulating a painful body part.
7. Inspection, palpation, range of motion, and muscle testing are performed on the major skeletal muscles and joints of the body in a cephalocaudal, proximal-to-distal manner. Always compare paired muscles and joints.
8. Examine non-affected body parts before examining affected body parts.
9. Avoid unnecessary or excessive manipulation of a painful body part. If the individual complains of pain, stop the aggravating motion.
10. If necessary because of a painful body part or limited mobility, provide the consumer assistance in dressing after the physical assessment. Allow the individual extra time to get dressed.
11. Some MSDs may affect the individual more during certain parts of the day. Arrange for the follow-up appointment to be during the consumer's time of optimal function.

CLINICAL **REASONING**

Obesity and the musculoskeletal system – when to refer
Obesity adversely affects multiple body systems including a range of musculoskeletal conditions. The more weight that is on a joint, the more stressed the joint becomes, and the more likely it will wear down and be damaged. As the prevalence of obesity increases, so too does the societal burden of disability, health-related quality of life, and associated healthcare costs. Musculoskeletal disorders such as arthritis, gout, lupus, fibromyalgia and other joint diseases and conditions are impacted significantly if a person is obese. Weight reduction is important in improving some of the manifestations of MSDs and improving function.

When you are assessing the musculoskeletal system of an individual who is obese, discuss the option of referral to an appropriate program that will support them with a diet and exercise intervention. Further MSD aspects to include are their ability to rise from a seated position, stair climbing and weight transfer and balance.

Examination of the musculoskeletal system

General assessment

Overall appearance

E 1. Obtain height and weight. Refer to Chapter 15.

2. Observe the consumer's ability to tolerate weight bearing on the lower limbs during standing and ambulation. Assess the amount of weight bearing placed on each of the lower limbs. See **Table 16.5** for a description of weight-bearing terms.

3. Identify obvious structural abnormalities (e.g. atrophy, scoliosis, kyphosis, amputated limbs, contractures) (**Figure 16.5**).

4. Note indications of discomfort (e.g. restricted weight bearing or movement, frequent shifting of position, facial grimacing, excessive fatigue).

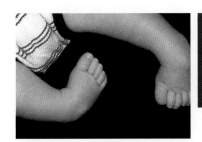

FIGURE 16.5 The musculoskeletal examination begins with assessing the consumer's general appearance. The infant in this photo has an obvious deformity (Talipes equinovarus).

ALAMY STOCK PHOTO/MEDISCAN

TABLE 16.5 Weight-bearing status

DEGREE OF WEIGHT BEARING	DESCRIPTION
Non-weight bearing	The individual does not bear weight on the affected extremity. The affected extremity does not touch the floor.
Touch down weight bearing	The individual does not place any weight on the affected extremity; however, they use the toes to touch the floor to maintain balance only.
Partial weight bearing	The individual bears a small amount of their body weight (30% to 50%) on the affected extremity.
Weight bearing as tolerated	The individual bears as much weight as can be tolerated on the affected extremity without undue strain or pain. The amount of weight is dependent on the circumstances.
Full weight bearing	The individual bears their full body weight on the affected extremity.

ADAPTED FROM ANDERSON & DUONG, 2022

N Body height and weight should be appropriate for age and sex (see Chapter 15). The consumer should be able to enter the assessment area via independent ambulation. Structural defects should be absent. There should be no outward indications of discomfort during rest, weight bearing or joint movement. There should be a distinct and symmetrical relationship among the limbs, torso and pelvis.

A An excessively tall or short, or overweight or underweight consumer is abnormal.

P Marfan syndrome affects multiple systems. The musculoskeletal changes are increased height for age due to an increased length of the distal limbs, extra digits, joint instability, pectus excavatum and kyphosis.

P Dwarfism, a congenital disorder, is manifested by a decrease in body size. It is regarded as proportionate if both limb and trunk size are smaller than average. The decrease in size may affect only the limbs, which then appear out of proportion to the torso size.

P Severe osteoporosis and ankylosing spondylitis can result in height loss due to vertebral compression fractures and thoracic kyphosis.

P Obesity is considered to be a factor in both degenerative joint disease and low back pain.

A Any weight-bearing status other than full weight bearing is abnormal.

P Low back pain may cause an individual to lean forwards or towards the affected side.

E Examination **N** Normal findings **A** Abnormal findings **P** Pathophysiology

A Structural defects are abnormal.

P Acromegaly, due to hyperpituitary function, may result in an enlarged skull with jaw protrusion, and an increase in the size of the hands, feet and long bones. The increased length of the long bones can contribute to increased height.

P A missing limb can be due to a congenital defect, surgery or trauma.

P Pectus excavatum and pectus carinatum are abnormal findings. See Chapter 13.

P Scoliosis and kyphosis are abnormal findings. They are discussed later in this chapter in the section entitled Spine.

Posture

E 1. Stand in front of the consumer.
   2. Instruct the consumer to stand with the feet together.
   3. Observe the structural and spatial relationship of the head, torso, pelvis and limbs. Assess for symmetry of the shoulders, scapulae and iliac crests.
   4. Ask the consumer to sit; observe posture.

N In the standing position, the torso and head are upright. The head is midline and perpendicular to the horizontal line of the shoulders and pelvis. The shoulders and hips are level, with symmetry of the scapulae and iliac crests. The arms hang freely from the shoulders. The feet are aligned and the toes point forwards. The extremities are proportional to the overall body size and shape, and the limbs are also symmetrical with each other. The knees face forwards, with symmetry of the level of the knees. There is usually less than a 5 cm interval between the knees when the consumer stands with the feet together, facing forwards. When full growth is reached, the arm span is equal to the height. In the sitting position, both feet should be placed firmly on the floor surface, with toes pointing forwards.

A Forward slouching of the shoulders produces a false thoracic kyphosis.

P These findings can be caused by poor posture habits.

HEALTH EDUCATION

Nutritional considerations for musculoskeletal health

A diet that is lacking in calcium, phosphorus, vitamin D and/or protein can promote adverse changes in the musculoskeletal system, such as osteoporosis and osteomalacia. When assessing the musculoskeletal system, discuss nutritional considerations (see Chapter 15 for detailed information), and the importance of safe exposure to sunlight.

The key points to consider are that protein builds healthy muscle, and calcium and phosphorus are the primary components of healthy bones. Vitamin D, however, is essential for the absorption of calcium and phosphorus from the gastrointestinal tract. Recently there has been a significant increase in vitamin D deficiency, especially where vigilant sun protection strategies are used, which means children, the elderly in aged care facilities, women who veil themselves, and people with dark skin pigmentation are most at risk for vitamin D deficiency. Safe exposure to sunlight promotes vitamin D production in the body.

The routine use of a combined calcium and vitamin D supplement for those at risk is strongly recommended by the Australian and New Zealand Bone and Mineral Society, Osteoporosis Australia and the Endocrine Society of Australia. Supplemental vitamins and minerals may also be necessary for the person with lactose intolerance, who cannot consume these essential elements easily through dietary intake of dairy products.

E Examination **N** Normal findings **A** Abnormal findings **P** Pathophysiology

The consumer with osteoporosis and bone metastasis
Bone weakened by osteoporosis and metastases has a low bone mineral density and is vulnerable to breakage during what is otherwise considered to be minor trauma. Fragility fractures are common among the elderly, and often affect the wrist, vertebrae and hip.

Healthcare providers must take caution when assessing individuals with osteoporosis or bone metastasis. Consumers with fragile bones are more susceptible to pathological fractures with even minor stress/pressure.

Fall precautions, physical therapy, proper use of supportive equipment, medications to strengthen bone, and avoidance of medications that can induce postural hypotension can reduce the risk of falls and fragility fractures.

Gait and mobility

E 1. Instruct the consumer to walk normally across the room.
2. Ask the individual to walk on the toes and then on the heels of the feet.
3. Ask the individual to walk by placing one foot in front of the other, in a 'heel-to-toe' fashion (tandem walking).
4. Instruct the person to walk forwards, then backwards.
5. Ask the individual to side-step to the left, then to the right.
6. Instruct the individual to ambulate forwards a few steps with the eyes closed.
7. Observe the consumer during transfer between the standing and sitting positions.

N Walking is initiated in one smooth, rhythmic fashion. The foot is lifted 2.5 to 5 cm off the floor and then propelled 30–45 cm forwards in a straight path. As the heel strikes the floor, body weight is shifted onto the ball of that foot. The heel of the foot is then elevated off the floor before the next step forwards. The consumer remains erect and balanced during all stages of gait. Step height and length are symmetrical for each foot. The arms swing freely at the side of the torso but in opposite direction to the movement of the legs. The lower limbs are able to bear full body weight during standing and ambulation. Prior to turning, the head and neck turn towards the intended direction, followed by the rest of the body. The individual should be able to transfer easily to various positions.

A Indications of gait disturbance include hesitancy or multiple attempts to initiate ambulation, unsteadiness, staggering, grasping for external support, high stepping, foot scraping due to inability to raise the foot completely off the floor, persistent toe or heel walking, excessive pointing of the toes inwards or outwards, asymmetry of step height or length, limping, stooping during walking, wavering gait, shuffling gait, waddling gait, excessive swinging of the shoulders or pelvis, and slow or rapid step speed. **Table 16.6** provides examples of abnormal gait patterns.

P Causes of abnormal gait include muscle weakness, joint deterioration, malalignment of the lower limbs, paralysis, lack of coordination or balance, fatigue and pain.

P Limited mobility due to stiffness is associated with degenerative joint disease, rheumatoid arthritis, Paget's disease and Parkinson's disease.

P Severe thoracic kyphosis will alter the body's centre of gravity and affect balance during both standing and ambulation.

P Pathological fracture of the femoral shaft during the stress of weight bearing may occur during standing or ambulation. Pathological fracture can occur if the bone has been significantly weakened by malignancy, osteoporosis, Paget's disease or osteomalacia.

E Examination   **N** Normal findings   **A** Abnormal findings   **P** Pathophysiology

A When rising from or sitting in a chair, the consumer may have to lean on the armrest for external support. The individual may also tend to rock forwards and push off from the armrest for propulsion upwards into the standing position. Discomfort felt while bearing the body's weight in the standing position may be reduced in the sitting position. **Table 16.7** describes techniques that will assist you in documenting the type of consumer transfer.

TABLE 16.6 Examples of abnormal gait patterns

TYPE OF ABNORMAL GAIT	AETIOLOGY	DESCRIPTION
Antalgic	Degenerative joint disease of the hip or knee	Limited weight bearing is placed on an affected leg in an attempt to limit discomfort.
Short leg	Discrepancy in leg length, flexion contracture of the hip or knee, congenital hip dislocation	A limp is present during ambulation unless shoes have been adapted to compensate for length discrepancy.
Spastic hemiplegia	Cerebral palsy, unilateral upper motor neurone lesion (e.g. stroke)	Extension of one lower extremity with plantar flexion and foot inversion; arm is flexed at the elbow, wrist and fingers. The consumer walks by swinging the affected leg in a semicircle. The foot is not lifted off the floor. The affected arm does not swing with the gait.
Scissors	Multiple sclerosis, bilateral upper motor neurone disease	Adduction at the knee level produces short, slow steps. Gait is uncoordinated, stiff and jerky. The foot is dragged across the floor in a semicircle.
Cerebellar ataxia	Cerebellar disease	Gait is broad-based and uncoordinated, and the consumer appears to stagger and sway during ambulation.
Sensory ataxia	Disorders of peripheral nerves, dorsal roots and posterior column that interfere with proprioceptive input	Stance is broad-based. Consumer lifts feet up too high and abruptly slaps them on the floor, heel first. The consumer watches the floor carefully to help ensure correct foot placement because they are unaware of their position in space.
Festinating	Parkinson's disease	Decreased step height and length, but increased step speed, resulting in 'shuffling' (feet barely clearing the floor). Consumer's posture is stooped and consumer appears to hesitate both in initiation and in termination of ambulation. Rigid body position, with flexion of the knees during standing and ambulation.
Steppage or foot-drop	Peroneal nerve injury, paralysis of the dorsiflexor muscles, damage to spinal nerve roots L5 and S1 from poliomyelitis	Hip and knee flexion are needed for step height in order to lift the foot off the floor. Instead of placing the heel of the foot on the floor first, the whole sole of the foot is slapped on the floor at once. May be unilateral or bilateral.
Apraxic	Alzheimer's disease, frontal lobe tumours	Consumer has difficulty with walking despite intact motor and sensory systems. The consumer is unable to initiate walking, as if stuck to the floor. After walking is initiated, the gait is slow and shuffling.
Trendelenburg	Developmental dysplasia of hip, muscular dystrophy	During ambulation, pelvis of the unaffected side drops when weight bearing is performed on the affected side. When both hips are affected, a 'waddling' gait may be evident.

ADAPTED FROM *ORTHOPEDIC NURSING* (3RD ED.), BY A. MAHER, S. SALMOND, & T. PELLINO, PHILADELPHIA: ELSEVIER, COPYRIGHT 2002.

E Examination **N** Normal findings **A** Abnormal findings **P** Pathophysiology

TABLE 16.7 Safe consumer handling

TECHNIQUE	DESCRIPTION
Independent	The consumer is safe with transfers and requires no assistance.
Supervise	The consumer is basically independent but may need verbal cues or observation.
Safeguard of 1	The consumer transfers well with hands-on contact by a nurse. This method is used if the person's judgement is questionable or for individuals with slightly decreased balance.
Minimal assistance of 1	The consumer requires minimal physical assistance from a nurse to stand or sit (e.g. for lower extremity placement on footrest of wheelchair).
Maximal assistance of 1	The consumer requires maximal physical assistance and many verbal cues from a nurse to transfer (e.g. for extremity placement, trunk placement).
Maximal assistance of 2	Same as for the previous example but requires two nurses. This necessitates good body mechanics and often calls for supportive equipment (e.g. Hoyer lift, total lift).

ADAPTED FROM *ORTHOPEDIC NURSING* (3RD ED.), BY A. MAHER, S. SALMOND, & T. PELLINO, PHILADELPHIA: ELSEVIER, COPYRIGHT 2002.

P Because of stiffness and discomfort, the consumer with degenerative disease of the hip joint often has difficulty rising from a sitting position without assistance.

Inspection

Muscle size and shape

E 1. Survey the overall appearance of the muscle mass.
   2. Ask the consumer to contract the muscle without inducing movement (isometric muscle contraction), relax the muscle, and then repeat the muscle contraction.
   3. Look for any obvious muscle contraction.

N Muscle contour will be affected by the exercise and activity patterns of the individual. Muscle shape may be accentuated in certain body areas (e.g. the limbs and upper torso) but should be symmetrical. There may be hypertrophy in the dominant hand. During muscle contraction, you should be able to visualise sudden tautness of the muscle area. Muscle relaxation will be associated with termination of muscle tautness. There is no involuntary movement.

Hypertrophy refers to an increase in muscle size and shape due to an increase in the muscle fibres. Hypertrophy is detected as a unilateral or bilateral increase in the contour of the muscle. During contraction, the borders of the muscle will become accentuated. An increase in muscle strength will accompany the increase in muscle size. Bilateral hypertrophy is common among athletes involved in weightlifting or other activities that require repetitive motion against opposing resistance. Hypertrophy of the proximal arms is often seen in consumers who are dependent on a wheelchair for mobility yet are able to propel the wheelchair manually.

A **Atrophy** describes a reduction in muscle size and shape. Atrophy is evidenced by the appearance of thin, flabby muscles. The contour of the skeletal muscle is less distinct than usual. The muscle will appear relaxed, even during voluntary isometric contraction. Atrophy may be local or diffuse.

P Generalised atrophy is directly related to prolonged immobility of the body as a whole (**disuse atrophy**), unless isometric exercises were routinely performed during the period of immobility. It is accentuated by poor nutrition.

P Generalised atrophy may be noted in grossly obese consumers who lead sedentary lifestyles.

P Local atrophy is often detected in the limb or limbs affected by hemiparesis, paraplegia or quadriplegia. It is also seen following the removal of a limb cast or splint.

A There is involuntary muscle movement.

P See **Table 16.8** for a description of involuntary muscle movements.

E Examination **N** Normal findings **A** Abnormal findings **P** Pathophysiology

TABLE 16.8 Involuntary muscle movements

TYPE	DESCRIPTION
Fasciculation	Visible twitching of a group of muscle fibres that may be stimulated by the tapping of a muscle.
Fibrillation	Ineffective, uncoordinated muscle contraction that resembles quivering.
Spasm	Sudden muscle contraction. A cramp is a muscle spasm that is strong and painful. Clonic muscle spasms are contractions that alternate with a period of muscle relaxation. A tonic muscle spasm is a continuous involuntary muscular contraction.
Tetany	Paroxysmal tonic muscle spasms, usually of the extremities. The face and jaw may also be affected by spasm. Tetany may be associated with discomfort.
Chorea	Rapid, irregular and jerky muscle contractions of random muscle groups. It is unpredictable and without purpose. It can involve the face, upper trunk and limbs. Sometimes, the consumer tries to incorporate the movement into voluntary movement, which may appear grotesque and exaggerated. The individual may have difficulty with chewing, speaking and swallowing.
Tremors	A period of continuous shaking due to muscle contractions. Although the quality of the tremors will be influenced by the cause, the amplitude and the frequency should remain the same. Tremors may be fine or coarse, rapid or slow, continuous or intermittent. They may be exacerbated during rest and attempts at purposeful movements, or by certain body positions.
Tic	Sudden, rapid muscle spasms of the upper trunk, face or shoulders. The action is often repetitive and may decrease during purposeful movement. It can be persistent or limited in nature.
Ballism	Jerky, twisting movements due to strong muscle contraction.
Athetosis	Slow, writhing, twisting type of movement. The consumer is unable to sustain any part of the body in one position. The movements are most often in the fingers, hands, face, throat and tongue, although any part of the body can be affected. The movements are generally slower than in chorea.
Dystonia	Similar to athetosis but differing in the duration of the postural abnormality, and involving large muscles such as the trunk. The consumer may present with an overflexed or overextended posture of the hand, pulling of the head to one side, torsion of the spine, inversion of the foot, or closure of the eyes, along with a fixed grimace.
Myoclonus	A rapid, irregular contraction of a muscle or group of muscles, such as the type of jerking movement that sometimes occurs when drifting off to sleep.
Tremors at rest	Asymmetrical and coarse movements that disappear or diminish with action. They tend to diminish or cease with purposeful movement.
Action tremors	Symmetrical or asymmetrical movements that increase in states of fatigue, weakness, drug withdrawal, hypocalcaemia, uraemia or hepatic disease. This type of tremor may be induced in a normal individual when he or she is required to maintain a posture that demands extremes of power or precision. Action tremors are also called postural tremors.
Intention tremors	These tremors may appear only on voluntary movement of a limb and may intensify on termination of movement.
Asterixis	This is a variant of a tremor. The rate of limb flexion and extension is irregular, slow and of wide amplitude. The outstretched limb temporarily loses muscle tone.

Joint contour and periarticular tissue

E 1. Observe the shape of the joint while the joint is in its neutral anatomic position.
   2. Visually inspect the 5 to 7.5 cm of skin and subcutaneous tissue surrounding that joint. Assess the periarticular area for erythema, swelling, bruising, nodules, deformities, masses, skin atrophy or skin breakdown.

N Joint contour should be somewhat flat in extension, and smooth and rounded in flexion. You should be unable to detect any difference between periarticular tissue, the skin and the subcutaneous tissue. Bilateral joints should be symmetrical in position and appearance. There should be no observable erythema, swelling, bruising, nodules, deformities, masses, skin atrophy or skin breakdown.

Measuring limb circumference

Limb circumference is measured when a limb looks larger or smaller than its counterpart during inspection.

E Examination **N** Normal findings **A** Abnormal findings **P** Pathophysiology

E During muscle relaxation or non-weight bearing, measure the limbs at exactly the same distance from a nearby joint (e.g. the knee or elbow) at the site of maximal limb diameter (**Figure 16.6**).

N Bilateral measurements should be within 1 to 3 cm of each other. A slight increase in the girth of the dominant arm is normal.

A A discrepancy in limb girth of 3 cm or more is abnormal.

P Atrophy results from disuse of a limb, as may occur in stroke.

P Swelling following trauma to soft tissue or bone (e.g. crush injury or fracture) results in an increased limb circumference.

P Unilateral hypertrophy can result from selected activities that use one side of the body more than the other (e.g. tennis arm).

P Unilateral hypertrophy may also be the result of compensating for a deficit in the corresponding limb. For example, a consumer with hemiparesis of a limb will present with some degree of hypertrophy of the nonaffected arm muscles.

P A unilateral increase in calf girth may indicate a deep vein thrombosis. Calf girth alters prior to the development of a positive Homan's sign.

A Enlargement of the joint is an abnormal finding.

P Joint inflammation can result from inflammatory disorders such as rheumatoid arthritis and gout (**Figure 16.7**).

P Trauma to the joint and its extra-articular structures will also result in joint inflammation.

A Deformity of the joint capsule is an abnormal finding.

P Immobility results in joint contractures, which cause the joint to be permanently fixated in one position. The acquired joint position may be one within its normal range of joint motion or an abnormal joint position.

P Joint destruction due to rheumatoid arthritis may result in a joint becoming fixated in one position.

P Joint dislocation or subluxation will alter the normal contour of a joint. **Dislocation** refers to a complete dislodgement of one bone out of the joint cavity. **Subluxation** is a partial dislodgement of a bone from its place in the joint cavity.

A Alteration in periarticular skin and subcutaneous tissue is an abnormal finding.

P Trauma to the joint results in inflammation and bruising of the periarticular tissue. Joint trauma may include strain, sprain, contusion, dislocation, subluxation or fracture within or near the joint capsule.

P The consumer with rheumatoid arthritis often presents with periarticular skin atrophy and subcutaneous nodules near a joint (e.g. elbow).

P Synovial effusion within the joint capsule may cause a bulging appearance that extends into the periarticular area.

Palpation

Muscle tone

E 1. Palpate the muscle by applying light pressure with the finger pads of the dominant hand. Note any tenderness.
2. Note the change in muscle shape as the muscle belly (wide central aspect of the muscle) tapers off to become a tendon.
3. Ask the consumer to alternately perform muscle relaxation and isometric muscle contraction. Note the change in palpable muscle tone between relaxation and isometric contraction.
4. Palpate the muscle belly during contraction induced by voluntary movement of a nearby joint.
5. Perform passive range of motion to all extremities and note whether these movements are smooth and sustained.

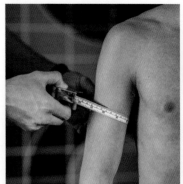

FIGURE 16.6 Measuring limb circumference

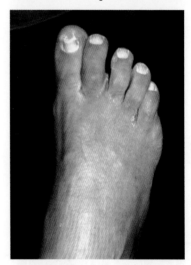

FIGURE 16.7 Joint inflammation of gout. Note the erythema and oedema of the right 2nd metatarsal interphalangeal joint.

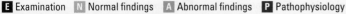

E Examination **N** Normal findings **A** Abnormal findings **P** Pathophysiology

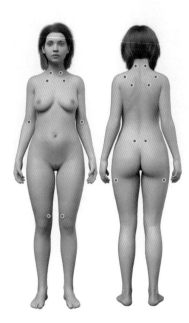

FIGURE 16.8 Fibromyalgia trigger

N Muscle tone refers to the partial muscle contraction state that is maintained in order for the muscle to respond quickly to the next stimulus. On palpation, the muscle should feel smooth and firm, even during the phase of muscle relaxation. There should be no pain. Normal muscle tone provides light resistance to passive stretch. During muscle contraction, especially against moderate external resistance to nearby joint movement, you will be able to palpate a significant overall increase in the firmness of the muscle belly. Muscle tone increases during anxiety or excitable states. Tone decreases during rest and sleep. You will be able to palpate the muscle belly and detect a change in its shape as it tapers down to become a tendon. The hypertrophied muscle will have a distinctive contour. You will detect muscle tautness even during the phase of relaxation.

A **Hypotonicity** (flaccidity) is a decrease in muscle tone. When the muscle is palpated, it feels flabby and soft to the touch. When a flaccid limb is held away from the body and then released, it falls quickly with gravity.

P Aetiology of flaccidity may include diseases involving the muscles, anterior horn cells or peripheral nerves.

A **Spasticity** refers to an increase in muscle tension on passive stretching (especially rapid or forced stretching of the muscle). It is often noted with extreme flexion or extension.

P Upper motor neurone dysfunction is associated with spasticity.

A The atrophied muscle will feel small and flabby, even during the phase of muscle contraction.

P Refer to the description of atrophy in the earlier section Muscle size and shape.

A A muscle spasm represents persistent muscle contraction without relaxation. The muscle belly will feel taut and the consumer may complain of discomfort over the muscle area. The spasm may also result in involuntary joint movement or a change in body position.

P Spasm follows fracture and may alter the distance between the bone fragments. Spasm is also common in the affected limbs of consumers with paralysis, electrolyte imbalance, peripheral vascular disease and cerebral palsy.

A Muscle pain may occur with or without palpation.

P Moderate to severe muscle pain of the neck, shoulders or proximal thigh is associated with fibromyalgia. Pain and tenderness upon palpation of at least 11 out of 18 trigger points located on the back of the neck, upper chest, trunk, low back and lower extremities is consistent with fibromyalgia (**Figure 16.8**). Palpation will often result in burning and gnawing pain.

A Crepitus refers to a grating or crackling sensation caused by two rough musculoskeletal surfaces rubbing together. Crepitus is more commonly detected with joint movement than it is with muscle contraction.

P Crepitus detected during palpation of muscle contraction, especially in a non-articulating area, may indicate shaft fracture due to trauma or loss of bone density. Muscle spasm following fracture may bring bone fragments in contact with each other, resulting in crepitus.

A Muscle masses detected on palpation are to be considered an abnormal finding.

P Muscle rupture (e.g. of the long head of the biceps muscle) will present as an inappropriate muscle mass above the joint. The muscle mass may be accentuated by muscle contraction.

P Tendon rupture may also result in an inappropriate muscle mass. An example is a complete rupture of the Achilles tendon, resulting in a mass noted in the calf area.

P Displaced fracture (e.g. of the femoral shaft near the hip joint) will often result in palpation of the displaced bone near a muscle.

E Examination   **N** Normal findings   **A** Abnormal findings   **P** Pathophysiology

P Complete dislocation (e.g. of the hip joint) will also result in palpation of the displaced bone near a muscle.

Joints

E 1. With the joint in its neutral anatomic position, begin palpating the joint by applying light pressure with the finger pads of the dominant hand 5 to 7 cm away from the centre of the joint.
  2. Palpate from the periphery inwards to the centre of the joint.
  3. Note any swelling, pain, tenderness, warmth or nodules.

N When the major skeletal joints are palpated in their neutral anatomic positions, the external joint contour will feel smooth, strong and firm. The shape of the joint corresponds to that specific joint type. The area surrounding the joint (periarticular tissue) is free from swelling, pain, tenderness, warmth and nodules. As the joint is moved through its normal range of motion, it should be able to articulate in proper alignment without any visible or palpable deformity. Palpation of joint movement produces a smooth sensation, without tactile detection of grating or popping. A synovial membrane is not palpable under normal circumstances.

A Bony enlargement or bony deformities of the joint are considered abnormal findings.

P Urate deposits associated with gout will result in a reactive synovitis, producing joint enlargement. Urate crystals accumulate in the joint as a result of a prolonged elevation of serum uric acid. The affected joint will be extremely warm and tender to the touch. Although the great toe is most commonly affected, gout can also affect other joints.

A Subcutaneous nodules detected in the periarticular area are abnormal.

P Rheumatoid arthritis is associated with subcutaneous nodules over the bony prominences and extensor joint surfaces (e.g. olecranon process of the elbow). These nodules are painless, firm but movable, and of normal skin colour. They are more of a cosmetic concern than a threat to nearby joint function, although the overlying skin is at risk for breakdown due to irritation or pressure.

P Tophi nodules may be detected in the consumer with chronic gout, and they represent soft tissue reaction to uric acid crystal deposition. They are often found on the great toes.

A Palpable, audible, severe crepitus that presents as more of a coarse than a fine sensation is abnormal.

P Crepitus is often palpated in joints affected by acute rheumatoid arthritis and degenerative joint disease due to the contact of bone surfaces.

P Bony overgrowth, muscle contracture, dislocation and subluxation are associated with joint crepitus.

A Any tenderness felt on light touch or joint palpation is considered abnormal. You must differentiate between tenderness on palpation of the joint at rest versus palpation during joint movement.

P Joint pain due to septic arthritis can occur 10 to 14 days after an untreated streptococcal pharyngitis or tonsillitis.

P Increased joint capsule pressure with a significant joint effusion may induce discomfort with light touch or pressure to the joint in the neutral position.

P Localised joint tenderness may be detected in the presence of joint contusion, infection or synovitis.

A Periarticular warmth, with temperature exceeding overall body temperature, indicates an underlying problem.

E Examination **N** Normal findings **A** Abnormal findings **P** Pathophysiology

Range of motion (ROM)

E 1. Ask the consumer to move the joint through each of its various ROM movements.
2. Note angle of each joint movement.
3. Note any pain, tenderness or crepitus.
4. If the individual is unable to perform active ROM, then passively move each joint through its ROM.
5. Always stop if the individual complains of pain, and never push a joint beyond its anatomic angle.
6. For the advanced practitioner: Use a goniometer to determine exact ROM in joints with limited ROM. Refer to the advanced technique on using a goniometer.

HEALTH EDUCATION

Risk factors for sports injuries

Exercise has proven benefits for health and wellbeing, and to maintain mobility. Noncompliance to recommended exercise guidelines can increase the risk of injury during exercise. Identification of risk factors for sports injury should be included in the nursing assessment to guide health education tailored to the individual's needs. These include, but are not limited to:

> the lack of medical clearance prior to the initiation of any aggressive exercise program following a period of prolonged sedentary activity
> aggressive cardiovascular activity not accompanied by adequate warm-up (before) or cool-down (after) periods
> the lack of adequate and appropriate instruction on the use of all exercise equipment such as treadmill and weight machines
> not using a 'spotter' assistant during gymnastic movements and heavy weightlifting
> incorrectly fitting and unsecured protective equipment such as bicycle helmets, equestrian helmets, a mouthpiece, eye goggles and shin pads
> incorrectly fitting and unsupportive running shoes
> the lack of 'rest days' between long-distance runs (e.g. 35 km during marathon training).

Assessing joint ROM: using a goniometer

E 1. With the joint in its neutral position, place the centre of the goniometer over the joint so that the two distal arms of the goniometer are in alignment with the proximal and distal bones adjacent to that joint.
2. Move the joint through its ROM and note the degree of the joint angle visible on the centre of the goniometer (**Figure 16.9**).

N Refer to the specific sections on joints for the ROM for each joint movement.

A Abnormalities of joint function are indicated by the inability of the consumer to voluntarily and comfortably move a joint in the directions and to the degrees that are considered the norms for that joint.

P Degenerative joint disease, rheumatoid arthritis and joint trauma are some of the many MSDs that prevent the affected joint from moving through its normal ROM.

P Joint inflammation (e.g. due to acute rheumatoid arthritis or recent trauma) and gout produce significant joint warmth because of the increased localised perfusion associated with the inflammatory process.

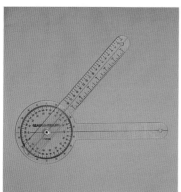

A. Goniometer

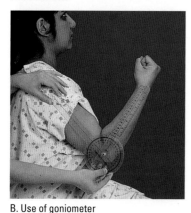

B. Use of goniometer

FIGURE 16.9 Goniometer and its use

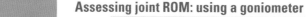

E Examination **N** Normal findings **A** Abnormal findings **P** Pathophysiology Advanced Assessment

Muscle strength

Each muscle group is assessed for strength via the same movements performed in range of motion.

E 1. Note whether muscle groups are strong and equal.
   2. Always compare right and left sides of paired muscle groups.
   3. Note involuntary movements.

N Normal muscle strength allows for complete voluntary range of joint motion against both gravity and moderate to full resistance. Muscle strength is equal bilaterally. There is no observed involuntary muscle movement. Muscle strength can be assessed indirectly by reviewing the consumer's ability to perform daily activities that involve lifting, pushing, pulling, grasping, walking, climbing stairs and transferring to a sitting position. Muscle strength can be assessed directly using the muscle strength grading scale (Table 16.9).

TABLE 16.9 Muscle strength grading scale

FUNCTIONAL ABILITY DESCRIPTION	SCALE (%)	0–5/5 SCALE
Complete range of joint motion against both gravity and full manual resistance from the health professional.	100%	5/5 Normal (N)
Complete range of joint motion against both gravity and moderate manual resistance from the health professional.	75%	4/5 Good (G)
Complete range of joint motion possible only without manual resistance from the health professional.	50%	3/5 Fair (F)
Complete range of joint motion possible only with the joint supported by the nurse to eliminate the force of gravity and without any manual resistance from the health professional.	25%	2/5 Poor (P)
Muscle contraction detectable but insufficient to move the joint even when the forces of both gravity and manual resistance have been eliminated.	10%	1/5 Trace (Tr)
Complete absence of visible and palpable muscle contraction.	0%	0/5 None (0)

A A decrease in skeletal muscle strength is significant if the complete range of joint motion is either impossible or possible only without resistance or gravity.

P Local decrease in muscle strength will accompany muscle atrophy of the limbs secondary to disuse.

P Diffuse reduction in muscle strength is associated with general atrophy, severe fatigue, malnutrition, muscle relaxant medications, long-term steroid use and deteriorating neuromuscular disorders. These deteriorating neuromuscular diseases include but are not limited to ALS, MD, MS, myasthenia gravis and Guillain-Barré syndrome.

A One-sided muscle weakness or paralysis is considered abnormal.

P Unilateral weakness or paralysis is indicative of **hemiparesis (hemiplegia)** from a cerebrovascular accident, brain tumour or head trauma.

Examination of joints

Temporomandibular joint

E 1. Stand in front of the consumer.
   2. Inspect the right and left temporomandibular joints (see **Figure 16.10**).
   3. Palpate the temporomandibular joints (see **Figure 16.11**).
      a. Place your index and middle fingers over the joint.
      b. Ask the consumer to open and close the mouth.
      c. Feel the depression into which your fingers move with an open mouth.
      d. Note the smoothness with which the mandible moves.
      e. Note any audible or palpable click as the mouth opens.

E Examination **N** Normal findings **A** Abnormal findings **P** Pathophysiology

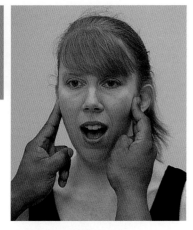

FIGURE 16.11 Palpation of the temporomandibular joint

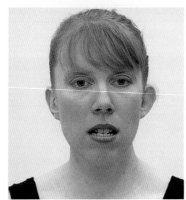

A. Pushing out the lower jaw

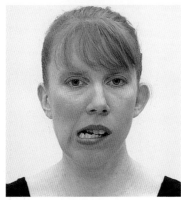

B. Moving the jaw from side to side

FIGURE 16.12 Range of motion of the temporomandibular joint

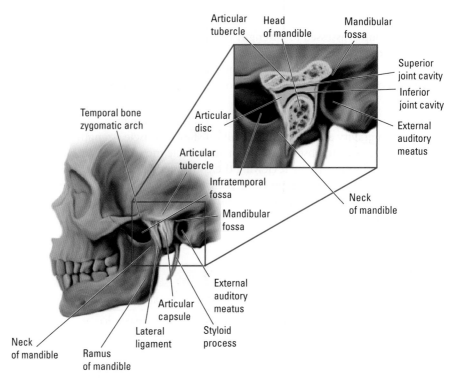

FIGURE 16.10 Anatomy of the temporomandibular joint (sagittal section)

E 4. Assess ROM (see **Figure 16.12**). Ask the consumer to:
   a. Open the mouth as wide as possible
   b. Push out the lower jaw
   c. Move the jaw from side to side.
5. Palpate the strength of the masseter and temporalis muscles as the consumer clenches their teeth. This assesses cranial nerve V.

N It is normal to hear or palpate a click when the mouth opens. The mouth can normally open 3 to 6 cm with ease. The lower jaw protrudes without deviating to the side and moves 1 to 2 cm with lateral movement.

A Pain, limited ROM, and crepitus can occur in temporomandibular joint dysfunction.

P Temporomandibular joint dysfunction can occur secondary to malocclusion, arthritis, dislocation, poorly fitting dentures, myofacial dysfunction and trauma.

Assessing for neuroexcitability: Chvostek sign

E 1. The consumer can be assessed in the standing, sitting or supine position.
2. While the consumer is facing forwards, tap the side of the face just below the temple area, using the middle or index finger (**Figure 16.13**).
3. Observe for ipsilateral changes in facial expression immediately after tapping the face.
4. Repeat the procedure on the other side of the face.

N There will be no change in the consumer's facial expression when the temple area is stimulated.

A A positive Chvostek sign, indicated by ipsilateral muscle spasm of the mouth and cheek, is abnormal. The muscle spasm will occur in an upwards direction, towards the temple.

E Examination   **N** Normal findings   **A** Abnormal findings   **P** Pathophysiology   ▨ Advanced Assessment

CHAPTER 16

P A positive Chvostek sign is suggestive of neuroexcitability associated with hypocalcaemia and tetanus infection.

Cervical spine

E 1. Stand behind the consumer.
2. Inspect the position of the cervical spine.
3. Palpate the spinous processes (see **Figure 16.14**) of the cervical spine and the muscles of the neck.
4. Stand in front of the consumer.
5. Assess the ROM of the cervical spine (see **Figure 16.15**). Ask the consumer to:
   a. Touch the chin to the chest (flexion)
   b. Look up at the ceiling (hyperextension)
   c. Move each ear to the shoulder on its respective side without elevating the shoulder (lateral bending)
   d. Turn the head to each side to look at the shoulder (rotation).
6. Assess strength of the cervical spine by repeating the movements in step 5d while applying opposing force. This also assesses the function of cranial nerve XI.

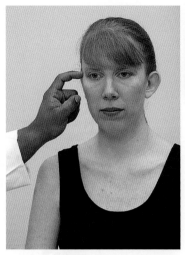

FIGURE 16.13 Assessing for Chvostek sign

N The cervical spine's alignment is straight and the head is held erect. The normal ROM for the cervical spine is flexion 45°, hyperextension 55°, lateral bending 40° to each side, and rotation 70° to each side. Hypertrophy of the neck muscles due to weightlifting exercises will produce the appearance of a thick neck.

A A neck that is not erect and straight is abnormal.

P Degenerative joint disease of the cervical vertebrae may result in lateral tilting of the head and neck.

P Torticollis is discussed in Chapter 9.

A A change in the size of the neck is abnormal.

P Klippel-Feil syndrome is the congenital absence of one or more cervical vertebrae along with fusion of the upper cervical vertebrae and bilateral elevation of the scapulae, resulting in a shortened neck appearance. It may be accompanied by a low hairline, webbing of the neck and decreased neck mobility.

A Inability of the consumer to perform ROM, and pain and tenderness on palpation are abnormal.

P Osteoarthritis, neck injury, disc degeneration (among ageing consumers or from occupational stress) and spondylosis can cause these cervical spine signs or symptoms.

Shoulders

E 1. Stand in front of the consumer.
2. Inspect the size, shape and symmetry of the shoulders (**Figure 16.16**).
3. Move behind the consumer and inspect the scapula for size, shape and symmetry.
4. Palpate the shoulders and surrounding muscles.
   a. Move from the sternoclavicular joint along the clavicle to the acromioclavicular joint.
   b. Palpate the acromion process, subacromial area, greater tubercle of the humerus, the anterior aspect of the glenohumeral joint and the bicipital groove.

E Examination **N** Normal findings **A** Abnormal findings **P** Pathophysiology   Advanced Assessment

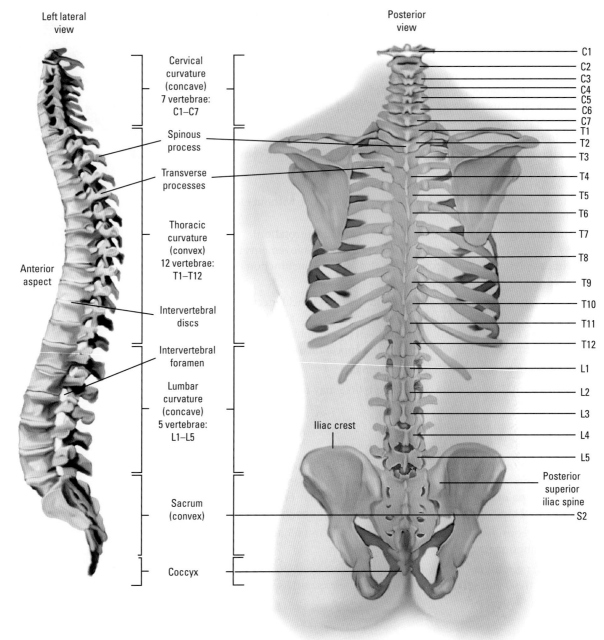

Left lateral view

Posterior view

Cervical curvature (concave)
7 vertebrae: C1–C7

Spinous process

Transverse processes

Thoracic curvature (convex)
12 vertebrae: T1–T12

Anterior aspect

Intervertebral discs

Intervertebral foramen

Lumbar curvature (concave)
5 vertebrae: L1–L5

Iliac crest

Sacrum (convex)

Posterior superior iliac spine

S2

Coccyx

C1
C2
C3
C4
C5
C6
C7
T1
T2
T3
T4
T5
T6
T7
T8
T9
T10
T11
T12
L1
L2
L3
L4
L5

FIGURE 16.14 Anatomy of the spine

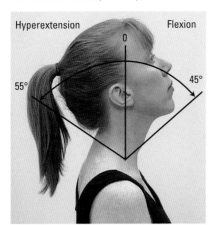

Hyperextension   Flexion
0
Right
55°   45°

A. Flexion, hyperextension

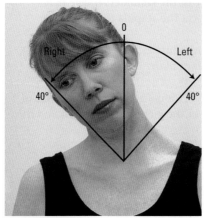

0
Right   Left
40°   40°

B. Lateral bending

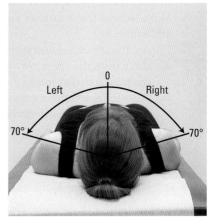

0
Left   Right
70°   70°

C. Rotation

FIGURE 16.15 Range of motion of the cervical spine

URGENT FINDING

Suspected cervical injury in trauma cases – Airway management
In any emergency primary survey, Airway, Breathing, Circulation, Disability is the accepted
form for assessment. Current guidelines state that the possibility of spinal injury must
be considered in the overall management of all trauma victims, alongside the Airway
assessment. More than half of spinal injuries in trauma cases occur in the cervical region,
and injury must be suspected in any victim with injuries above the shoulders. The potential
for cervical spine injury makes airway management more complex, particularly if the victim
is unconscious. **However, airway management takes precedence over any suspected
spinal injury.** Careful manual handling, with attention to spinal alignment, is vital to harm
minimisation. In casualties who are not breathing, use manoeuvres that are least likely to
result in movement of the cervical spine – the head tilt–chin lift will open the airway in
most consumers.

Adapted from ANZCOR. (2016). Guideline 9.1.6 Management of suspected spinal injury

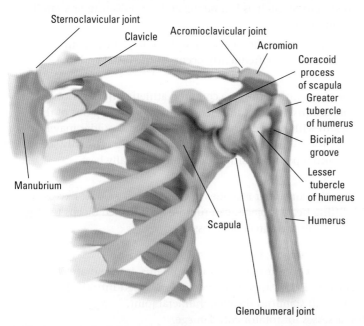

FIGURE 16.16 Anatomy of the shoulder joint

E 5. Assess ROM of the shoulders (see **Figure 16.17**). Ask the consumer to:
  a. Place arms at the side, elbows extended, and move the arms forwards in
     an arc (forward flexion)
  b. Move the arms backwards in an arc as far as possible (hyperextension)
  c. Place arms at side, elbows extended, and move both arms out to the sides
     in an arc until the palms touch together overhead (abduction)
  d. Move one arm at a time in an arc towards the midline and cross it as far
     as possible (adduction)
  e. Place hands behind the back and reach up, trying to touch the scapula
     (internal rotation)
  f. Place both hands behind the head with elbows flexed (external rotation)
  g. Shrug the shoulders. This assesses cranial nerve XI function.
  6. Assess strength of the shoulders by applying opposing force to the ROM
     movement in step 5g.

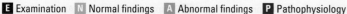

E Examination   **N** Normal findings   **A** Abnormal findings   **P** Pathophysiology

N The shoulders are equal in height. There is no fluid palpable in the shoulder area. Crepitus is absent. The normal ROM for the shoulder is forward flexion 180°, hyperextension 50°, abduction 180°, adduction 50°, internal rotation 90° and external rotation 90°.

A Increased outwards prominence of the scapula (winging) is an abnormal finding.

P Scapular winging is indicative of serratus anterior muscle injury or weakness.

A Decreased movement, pain with movement, swelling from fluid, and asymmetry are abnormal.

P These findings are associated with immobility, osteoarthritis and injury. Swelling from fluid is usually best seen anteriorly.

P A significant decrease in shoulder ROM is seen in frozen shoulder (adhesive capsulitis). In frozen shoulder, the glenohumeral joint gradually loses function, especially abduction and external rotation. Stroke with loss of shoulder movement and rotator cuff pathology are common aetiologies.

P Bursitis of the shoulder can result from overuse of the shoulder in repetitive activity (either a new activity such as leaf raking and car polishing or a familiar activity such as swimming).

P An acromioclavicular joint separation (separated shoulder) causes pain in the acromioclavicular joint. Swelling frequently occurs at the distal end of the clavicle.

P Shoulder subluxation and dislocation are common athletic injuries. Consumers with recurrent subluxations may feel the glenohumeral joint pop out of the socket and pop back in without medical intervention. The shoulder may lose its usual rounded contour. With an anterior dislocation, fluid is usually seen anteriorly, whereas with a posterior dislocation, fluid is usually best seen posteriorly.

P In biceps tendonitis, the consumer is tender in the bicipital groove. Excessive straining, as with lifting heavy objects, can rupture an inflamed biceps tendon. This can lead to a bulge in the antecubital fossa.

Assessing for rotator cuff damage: Drop arm test

The rotator cuff is composed of four muscles (supraspinatus, infraspinatus, teres minor and subscapularis) and their tendons. The tendons insert into the humeral tuberosities. The rotator cuff stabilises the glenohumeral joint.

The drop arm test assesses for rotator cuff damage.

E 1. Manually abduct the consumer's affected arm.
  2. Ask the consumer to slowly lower the raised arm to the side while maintaining extension of the arm.
  3. Observe the speed at which the individual lowers the arm.

N The consumer will be able to slowly lower the arm to the side while maintaining the arm in extension.

A An abnormal drop arm test is manifested by the inability of the consumer to slowly lower the arm to the side (e.g. the arm quickly falls to the side of the torso), or by severe pain occurring in the shoulder while the arm is slowly lowered to the side.

P An abnormal drop arm test is indicative of a rotator cuff tear. It is caused by trauma to the shoulder.

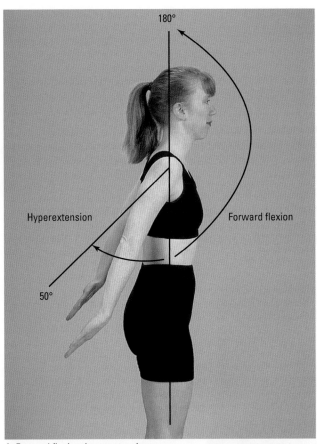

A. Forward flexion, hyperextension

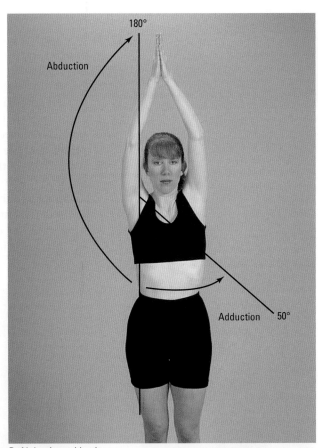

B. Abduction, adduction

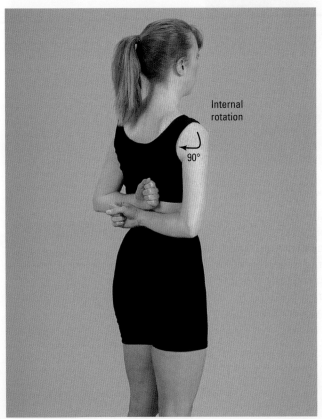

C. Internal rotation

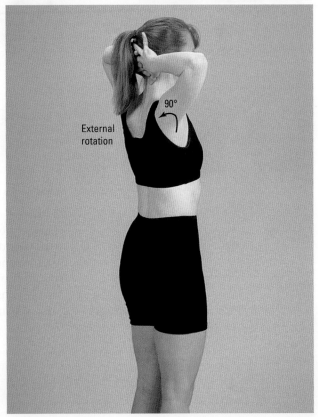

D. External rotation

FIGURE 16.17 Range of motion of the shoulder joint

Elbows

E 1. Stand to the side of the elbow being examined.
2. Support the consumer's forearm on the side that is being examined (approximately 70°).
3. Inspect the elbow in flexed and extended positions. Note the olecranon process and the grooves on each side of the olecranon process (**Figure 16.18**).
4. Using your thumb and middle fingers, palpate the elbow. Note the olecranon process, the olecranon bursa, the groove on each side of the olecranon process and the medial and lateral epicondyles of the humerus.
5. Assess ROM of the elbows (**Figure 16.19**). Ask the consumer to:
   a. Bend the elbow (flexion)
   b. Straighten the elbow (extension)
   c. Hold the arm straight out, bent at the elbow, and turn the palm upwards towards the ceiling (supination)
   d. Turn the palm downward towards the floor (pronation).

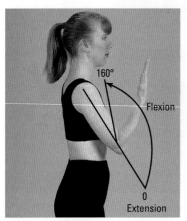

A. Flexion, extension

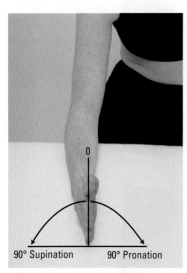

90° Supination   90° Pronation

B. Supination, pronation

FIGURE 16.19 Range of motion of the elbow joint

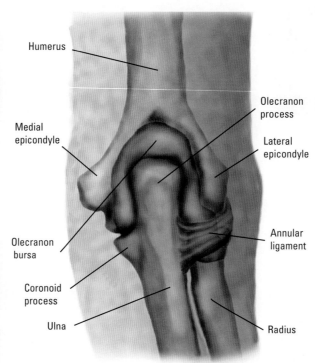

FIGURE 16.18 Anatomy of the elbow joint (posterior view, right elbow)

E 6. Assess strength of the elbow:
   a. Stabilise the consumer's arm at the elbow with your nondominant hand. With your dominant hand, grasp the consumer's wrist.
   b. Ask the consumer to flex the elbow (pulling it towards the chest) while you apply opposing resistance (see **Figure 16.20**).
   c. Ask the consumer to extend the elbow (pushing it away from the chest) while you apply opposing resistance.

Complications of joint fractures

Any fractures within a joint can have extended complications beyond that of simple fractures, due to possible nerve and tendon impingement. An example of this is a suspected radial head fracture. Any consumer, particularly an elderly person, who complains of elbow pain after suffering a fall must be carefully assessed for a radial head fracture, as there could be nerve damage to the median and ulnar nerves, and vascular involvement, especially the brachial artery.

N The elbows are at the same height and are symmetrical in appearance. The normal ROM for the elbow is flexion 160°, extension 0°, supination 90° and pronation 90°.

A Elbows that are not symmetrical are abnormal. The forearm is not in its usual alignment. Pain is present.

P These findings occur in a dislocation or a subluxation of the elbow. They usually occur from sports-related injuries, falls or motor vehicle accidents.

A Localised tenderness and pain with elbow flexion, extension or both are abnormal.

P Epicondylitis occurs from repetitive motions such as swinging a tennis racquet, hammering, using a screwdriver, tight gripping, and other activities involving repetitive movements of the forearm. Lateral epicondylitis (tennis elbow) is caused by injury to the extensor tendon at the lateral epicondyle, and medial epicondylitis (golfer's elbow) is caused by injury to the flexor tendon at the medial epicondyle.

P Radial head fractures usually result from falls. Frequently, the elbow is flexed in a 90° position.

P A flexion contracture of the elbow may be seen in a consumer with hemiparesis following a cerebrovascular accident.

A Red, warm, swollen and tender areas in the grooves beside the olecranon process are abnormal. Synovial fluid may be palpable and is soft or boggy.

P Inflammatory processes such as gouty arthritis, rheumatoid arthritis and SLE can cause these clinical manifestations.

P Olecranon bursitis (**Figure 16.21**) is classified as an overuse syndrome. It usually results from repetitive motions rather than from an acute injury. ROM is usually not affected.

Assessing for neuroexcitability: Trousseau sign
E 1. Place the consumer in a sitting or a supine position.
2. Apply a blood pressure cuff to the consumer's upper arm.
3. Inflate the blood pressure cuff to 10 mmHg above the consumer's systolic blood pressure for 1 to 3 minutes.
4. Observe for twitching of the hand and fingers on the side being tested.

N There will be no visible twitching of the hand and fingers during cuff inflation.

A A positive Trousseau sign, indicated by visible ipsilateral twitching of the hand and fingers during cuff inflation, is abnormal.

P A positive Trousseau sign is suggestive of neuroexcitability associated with hypocalcaemia and tetanus infection.

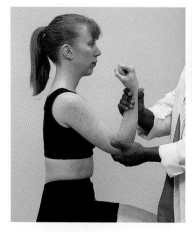
FIGURE 16.20 Muscle strength of the elbow

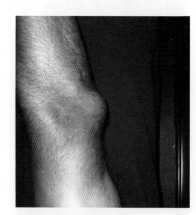
FIGURE 16.21 Olecranon bursitis

  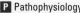

E Examination   N Normal findings   A Abnormal findings   P Pathophysiology   Advanced Assessment

Wrists and hands

E 1. Stand in front of the consumer.

2. Inspect the wrists and the palmar and dorsal aspects of the hands. Note the shape, position, contour and number of fingers (see **Figure 16.22**).

3. Inspect the **thenar eminence** (the rounded prominence at the base of the thumb).

4. Support the consumer's hand in your two hands, with your fingers underneath the consumer's hands and your thumbs on the dorsum of the consumer's hand.

E 5. Palpate the joints of the wrists by moving your thumbs from side to side. Feel the natural indentations (**Figure 16.23**).

6. Palpate the joints of the hand:

   a. Use your thumbs to palpate the metacarpophalangeal joints, which are immediately distal to and on each side of the knuckle (**Figure 16.24A**).

   b. Between your thumb and index finger, gently pinch the sides of the proximal and distal interphalangeal joints (**Figure 16.24B**).

E 7. Assess the ROM of the wrists and hands (**Figure 16.25**). Ask the consumer to:

   a. Straighten the hand (extension) and bend it up at the wrist towards the ceiling (hyperextension)

   b. Bend the hand down at the wrist towards the floor (flexion)

   c. Bend the fingers up at the metacarpophalangeal joint towards the ceiling (hyperextension)

   d. Bend the fingers down at the metacarpophalangeal joint towards the floor (flexion)

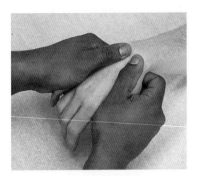

FIGURE 16.23 Palpating the wrist joint

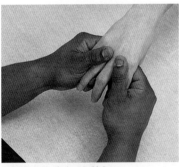

A. Metacarpophalangeal joint

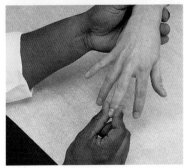

B. Interphalangeal joint

FIGURE 16.24 Palpating the hand joints

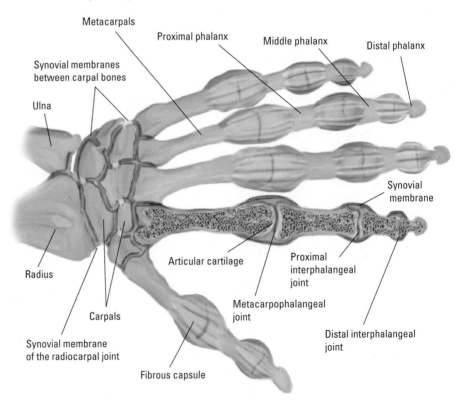

FIGURE 16.22 Anatomy of the wrist and hand

E   e. Place the hands on a flat surface and move them side to side (radial deviation is movement towards the thumb, and ulnar deviation is movement towards the little finger) without moving the elbow
   f. Make a fist with the thumb on the outside of the clenched fingers
   g. Spread the fingers apart
   h. Touch the thumb to each fingertip. Touch the thumb to the base of the little finger.

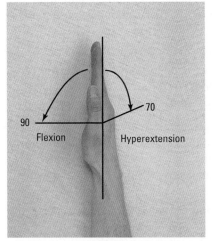
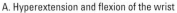

A. Hyperextension and flexion of the wrist

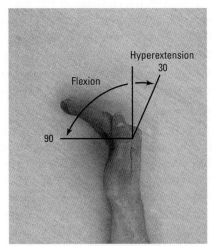

B. Flexion and hyperextension of the fingers

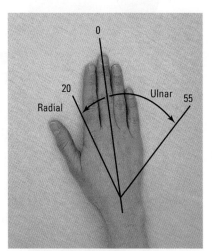

C. Radial and ulnar deviation of the wrist

FIGURE 16.25 Range of motion of the wrist and hand joints

E 8. Assess the strength of the wrists. Ask the consumer to:
   a. Place their arm on a table with the forearm supinated. Stabilise the forearm by placing your nondominant hand on it
   b. Flex the wrist while you apply resistance with your dominant hand (**Figure 16.26**)
   c. Extend the wrist while you apply resistance.
  9. Assess the strength of the fingers. Ask the consumer to:
   a. Spread the fingers apart while you apply resistance (**Figure 16.27**)
   b. Push the fingers together while you apply resistance.

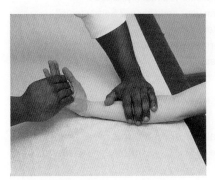

FIGURE 16.26 Muscle strength of the wrist

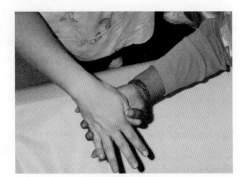

FIGURE 16.27 Muscle strength of the fingers

E Examination   **N** Normal findings   **A** Abnormal findings   **P** Pathophysiology

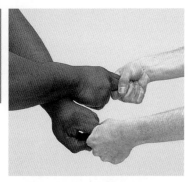

FIGURE 16.28 Muscle strength of the hand grasp

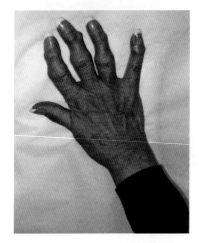

FIGURE 16.29 Bouchard's nodes and Heberden's nodes

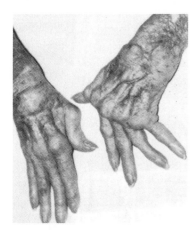

FIGURE 16.30 Ulnar deviation

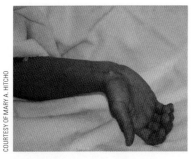

COURTESY OF MARY A. HITCHO

FIGURE 16.31 Ganglion cyst

E **10.** Assess the strength of the hand grasp. Ask the consumer to:
  a. Grasp your dominant index and middle fingers in their dominant hand and your nondominant index and middle fingers in their nondominant hand (**Figure 16.28**)
  b. Squeeze your fingers as hard as possible
  c. Release the grasp.

N There are five fingers on each hand. The normal range of motion for the wrists is extension 0°, hyperextension 70°, flexion 90°, radial deviation 20° and ulnar deviation 55°. The normal range of motion for the metacarpophalangeal joints is hyperextension 30° and flexion 90°.

A Extra fingers, loss of fingers, or webbing between fingers is abnormal.

P **Polydactyly** is the congenital presence of extra digits. **Syndactyly** is the congenital webbing or fusion of fingers or toes.

A Bony enlargement or bony deformities of the joints of the hand are abnormal.

P Osteoarthritis is associated with bony enlargement of the proximal interphalangeal joint (**Bouchard's node**) and the distal interphalangeal joint (**Heberden's node**) of the finger. These enlargements are hard and nontender. Bony enlargement may be masked by subcutaneous swelling. Bony enlargement is usually symmetrical (**Figure 16.29**).

P Rheumatoid arthritis results in ulnar deviation (**Figure 16.30**), swan-neck deformity and boutonniere deformities of the fingers. In ulnar deviation, the fingers deviate to the ulnar side of the body. In swan-neck deformity, there is flexion of the metacarpophalangeal joint, hyperextension of the proximal interphalangeal joint, and flexion of the distal interphalangeal joint. In other words, the finger appears to go up, down and up again. In boutonniere deformity, there is flexion of the proximal interphalangeal joint with hyperextension of the distal interphalangeal joint. The consumer frequently complains of pain, especially early in the morning. The joints may feel boggy on palpation. ROM may be restricted.

REFLECTION IN PRACTICE

Living with rheumatoid arthritis
Look at the hand of the person in **Figure 16.29**. How would you feel if you had a condition such as this? What would the impact be on your body image? Self-esteem? What environmental challenges might you encounter? What types of biases might you experience? How would the side effects of the pharmacological treatment impact on you? What resources are available in the community to assist you?

A A round, cystic growth near the tendons of the wrist or joint capsule is abnormal.

P A **ganglion** is a benign growth that is usually nontender and more prominent on the dorsum of the hand and wrist (**Figure 16.31**). Its aetiology is unknown.

A Flexion of the fingers is abnormal.

P Dupuytren's contracture is a flexion contracture that affects the little finger, ring finger and middle finger. Pain does not normally accompany this disorder. It is caused by the progressive contracture of the palmar fascia from an unknown aetiology (**Figure 16.32**).

A Muscular atrophy of the thenar eminence is abnormal.

E Examination **N** Normal findings **A** Abnormal findings **P** Pathophysiology

P This disorder occurs in median nerve compression such as in **carpal tunnel syndrome**.

A Severe flexion ankylosis of the wrist is abnormal.

P Ankylosis can be caused by rheumatoid arthritis or severe disuse (**Figure 16.33**).

A Tenderness over the distal radius is abnormal.

P This can occur in Colles fracture or fracture of the distal radius. This is the most common type of wrist fracture.

A Wrist drop, demonstrated by the inability of the consumer to extend the fisted hand at the wrist, is abnormal.

P Radial nerve injury may cause wrist drop.

A Inability of the consumer to prevent moving of spread fingers together is abnormal.

P Ulnar nerve injury causes weakness of the fingers.

A Weakness of opposition of the thumb and ipsilateral finger against resistance is abnormal.

P Median nerve disorders, such as carpal tunnel syndrome, affect thumb opposition. Weak thumb opposition usually occurs from injuries where the hand is outstretched during a fall or from a twisting motion.

Assessing for carpal tunnel syndrome: Tinel's sign

The median nerve lies within the carpal tunnel of the wrist (**Figure 16.34**). Compression of the tunnel leads to median nerve neuropathy. The consumer may complain of paraesthesias and burning, especially in the first three fingers, pain in the wrist and forearm, and a decreased ability to grasp objects due to a weak grip.

E 1. Place the consumer in a sitting position with the arm flexed at the elbow and the palm facing up.
   2. Using the index or middle finger of the dominant hand, briskly tap the centre of the consumer's wrist (median nerve) (**Figure 16.35**).
   3. Ask the individual to describe the sensations that occur in the forearm, hands, thumb or fingers.
   4. Repeat the technique on the other wrist.

N There will be no tingling or burning noted in the hand, thumb or fingers.

A A positive Tinel's test, indicated by a tingling or pricking sensation that occurs in the hand, thumb and index and middle fingers when the median nerve is tapped, is abnormal.

P A positive Tinel's test is indicative of median nerve compression (carpal tunnel syndrome).

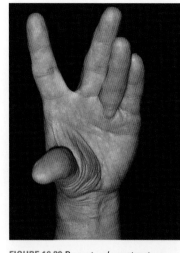

FIGURE 16.32 Dupuytren's contracture

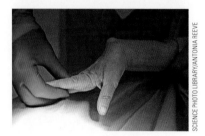

FIGURE 16.33 Flexion ankylosis

SCIENCE PHOTO LIBRARY/ANTONIA REEVE

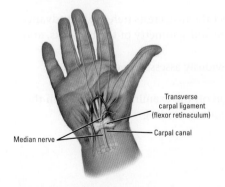

FIGURE 16.34 Anatomy of the carpal tunnel

Transverse carpal ligament (flexor retinaculum)

Carpal canal

Median nerve

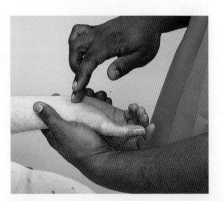

FIGURE 16.35 Assessing for Tinel's sign

E Examination   **N** Normal findings   **A** Abnormal findings   **P** Pathophysiology   Advanced Assessment

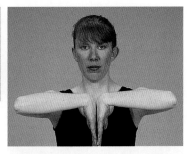

FIGURE 16.36 Assessing for Phalen's sign

Assessing for carpal tunnel syndrome: Phalen's sign

E 1. Place the consumer in a sitting position with the arms flexed at the elbow and the backs of the hands pressed together (Figure 16.36).
   2. Ask the individual to maintain the wrist flexion of 90° for at least 1 minute.
   3. Ask the individual to describe the sensations that occur in the hands and fingers.

N There will be no change in the sensation of the hands and fingers.

A A positive Phalen's test, indicated by sensations of numbness and paraesthesia in the palmar aspect of the hand and in the fingers (especially the first three fingers), is abnormal. These sensations disappear when the wrist joint is returned to its neutral anatomic position.

P A positive Phalen's test is indicative of carpal tunnel syndrome.

HEALTH EDUCATION

Risks for osteoporosis

When assessing the musculoskeletal system, identifying risk factors for osteoporosis is essential for person-centred care:

> Increased age (50), especially postmenopausal women
> Asian and Caucasian races
> Slender body build
> Smoking
> Family history
> Decreased physical activity
> Increased alcohol intake
> High caffeine intake
> Malabsorption syndromes
> Malnutrition, including decreased calcium and vitamin D intake
> Increased stress
> Diabetes mellitus
> Blood disorders
> Anorexia and bulimia
> Surgical removal of ovaries
> Hyperparathyroidism
> Medications (steroids, anticonvulsants, lithium, tamoxifen, thyroxine, thiazide diuretics)
  If the consumer has any of these risk factors identified, undertake joint decision-making with them, for possible referral for further investigation.

Hips

E 1. While the consumer is standing, inspect the iliac crests (refer to the advanced practice for the Trendelenburg test), size and symmetry of the buttocks, and number of gluteal folds (Figure 16.37).
   2. Observe the consumer's gait, if not previously assessed (see General assessment).
   3. Assist the consumer to a supine position on the examination table with the legs straight and the feet pointing towards the ceiling.
   4. Palpate the hip joints.

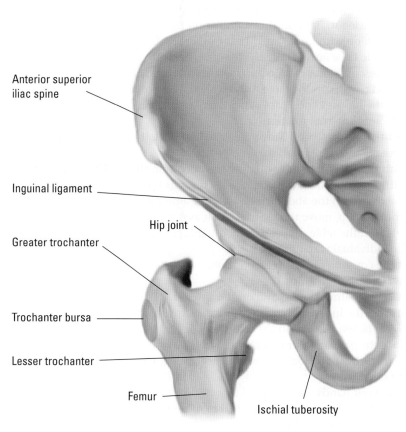

Anterior superior iliac spine

Inguinal ligament

Hip joint

Greater trochanter

Trochanter bursa

Lesser trochanter

Femur

Ischial tuberosity

FIGURE 16.37 Anatomy of the hip joint

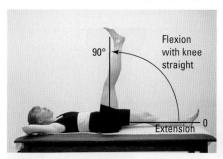

A. Flexion with knee straight

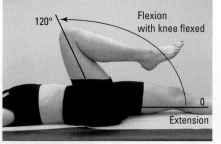

B. Flexion with knee flexed

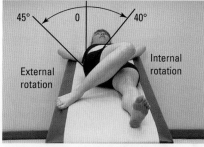

C. Internal and external rotation

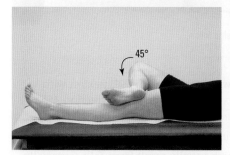

D. Position of the leg for full external rotation

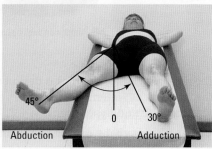

E. Abduction and adduction

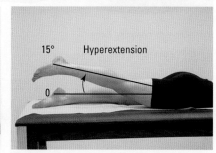

F. Hyperextension

FIGURE 16.38 Range of motion of the hip joint

E 5. Assess ROM of the hips (**Figure 16.38**). Ask the consumer to:
   a. Raise the leg straight off the examination table with the knee extended (hip flexion with knee straight); the other leg should remain on the table
   b. With the knee flexed, raise the leg off the examination table towards the chest as far as possible (hip flexion with knee flexed). The other leg should remain on the table; this is called the Thomas test
   c. Flex the hip and knee. Move the flexed leg medially as the foot moves outwards (internal rotation)
   d. Flex the hip and knee. Move the flexed leg laterally as the foot moves medially (external rotation)
   e. With the knee straight, swing the leg away from the midline (abduction)
   f. With the knee straight, swing the leg towards the midline (adduction)
   g. Roll over onto the abdomen and assume a prone position
   h. From the hip, move the leg back as far as possible while maintaining the pelvis on the table (hyperextension). This can also be performed while the individual is standing.
6. Assist the consumer to a supine position.
7. Assess strength of the hips.
   a. Place the palm of your hand on the anterior thigh, above the knee. Instruct the individual to raise the leg against your resistance (**Figure 16.39A**). Repeat on the other leg.
   b. Place the palm of your hand posteriorly above and behind the knee. Instruct the individual to lower the leg against your resistance. Repeat on the other leg.
   c. Place your hands on the lateral aspects of the consumer's legs at the level of the knee. Instruct the individual to move the legs apart against your resistance (**Figure 16.39B**).
   d. Place your hands on the medial aspects of the consumer's legs just above the knee. Instruct the individual to move the legs together against your resistance.

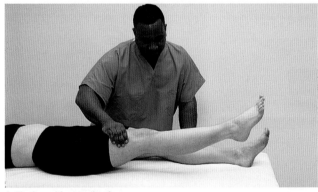

A. Flexion with opposing force

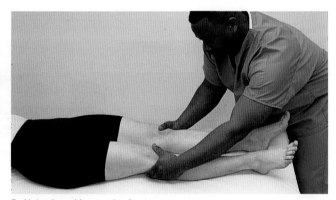

B. Abduction with opposing force

FIGURE 16.39 Muscle strength of the hip

N The normal ROM for the hips is flexion with knee straight 90°, flexion with knee flexed 120°, internal rotation 40°, external rotation 45°, abduction 45°, adduction 30° and hyperextension 15°.

A A leg that is externally rotated and painful on movement is abnormal.

P These findings occur in hip fractures, which usually result from falls (especially in elderly persons). The affected leg may also be shorter. See the advanced technique for guidelines on measuring limb length.

A A positive Thomas test, when the consumer is unable to flex one knee and hip while simultaneously maintaining the other leg in full extension, is abnormal. There may be slight to moderate hip and knee flexion of the extended leg.

E Examination   **N** Normal findings   **A** Abnormal findings   **P** Pathophysiology

HEALTH EDUCATION

Bone mineral density/Dual-energy X-ray absorptiometry (DEXA) screening – Screen recommendations

Dual-energy X-ray absorptiometry (DEXA or DXA) screening is a painless procedure for measuring bone mineral density and for detecting bone density loss. Results can quantify bone as normal, osteopenic or osteoporotic. Using a low level of radiation (or ultrasound waves in portable DEXA screening), the bones of the lower spine, hip, wrist, fingers or heel can be scanned. The Royal Australian College of General Practitioners and Osteoporosis Australia recommend screening in the following individuals:

> Females 65 years old and older
> Females on HRT for extended periods of time
> Males 65 years old and older
> Individuals with fragility fractures
> Individuals with a disease associated with osteoporosis (e.g. eating disorder, hyperparathyroidism, coeliac disease, chronic liver disease, irritable bowel disease, male hypogonadism)
> Individuals on medications associated with osteoporosis (e.g. steroids, anticonvulsants, androgen deprivation treatment such as leuprolide)
> Individuals with a condition associated with osteoporosis (e.g. menopause before age 45, X-ray findings of vertebral abnormality)
> Individuals being treated for osteoporosis to monitor the effects of treatment
  DEXA scans are usually repeated no more than every 2 years, as treatment protocols do not have short-term results.

Adapted from RACGP. (2022). Osteoporosis prevention, diagnosis and management in postmenopausal women and men over 50 years of age

P Flexion contractures of the hip joint, such as in long-term degenerative joint diseases, will result in a positive Thomas test. This test will identify hip flexion contractures that are masked by lumbar lordosis.

Assessing for hip dislocation: Trendelenburg test

E 1. Ask the consumer to stand on one foot, with the knee of the non-weight bearing leg flexed to raise the foot off the floor.
2. Assess the symmetry of the iliac crests while the individual is standing on one leg.
3. Repeat this technique on the other leg.

N The iliac crest on the side opposite the weight-bearing leg elevates slightly.

A It is abnormal for the iliac crest on the non-weight bearing leg to drop.

P This finding is a positive Trendelenburg test and is indicative of hip dislocation. The weakness of the gluteus medius muscle causes the hip on the unaffected side to drop.

Measuring limb length

E 1. Place the consumer in a supine position on the examination table with the legs extended.
2. Measure the leg from the anterior superior iliac spine to the medial malleolus (**Figure 16.40**).
3. Repeat on the other limb.
4. Compare measurements.

N Limb length measurements should be within 1 to 3 cm of each other.

A A difference in limb length of more than 3 cm is abnormal.

P Unilateral discrepancy in lower limb length may be a congenital defect.

E Examination **N** Normal findings **A** Abnormal findings **P** Pathophysiology Advanced Assessment

UNIT 2

P Sudden unilateral decrease in limb length occurs with fracture and dislocation of the hip and leg.

P A displaced proximal femoral shaft fracture (hip fracture) can result in limb shortening and internal or external rotation. Internal rotation is common if the consumer fell forwards during the fall, and external rotation is common if the individual fell onto the buttocks. The consumer is unable to straighten the leg into its neutral anatomic position.

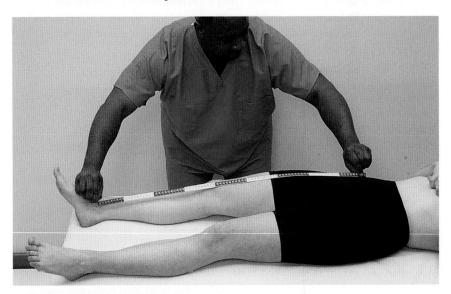

FIGURE 16.40 Measuring limb length

PUTTING IT IN CONTEXT

Missed diagnosis

Huyen, a 45-year-old Vietnamese woman, is brought in by her son to be evaluated for hip and leg pain. Huyen's son informs you that she was seen at a medical clinic three days ago after she fell down seven steps. At that time she was told she had strained muscles and needed to rest. Since then Huyen has had increasingly severe leg and hip pain. After conducting the health history and physical examination you suspect that she has a hip fracture.

> What focused questions would you ask the consumer and her son?
> What focused physical examination would you perform?
> Why might a 45-year-old woman sustain a hip fracture?
> Consider the individual's safety requirements on following up the missed diagnosis outcomes (documenting, informing other clinicians involved, educating the consumer, local consumer safety reporting requirements).

Knees

E 1. With the consumer standing, note the position of the knees in relation to each other and in relation to the hips, thighs, ankles and feet.
2. Ask the individual to sit on the examination table with the knees flexed and resting at the edge of the table.
3. Inspect the contour of the knees. Note the normal depressions around the patella (**Figure 16.41**).

E Examination **N** Normal findings **A** Abnormal findings **P** Pathophysiology

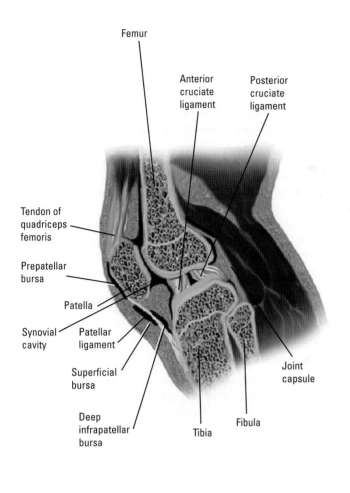

Femur
Anterior cruciate ligament
Posterior cruciate ligament
Tendon of quadriceps femoris
Prepatellar bursa
Patella
Synovial cavity
Patellar ligament
Superficial bursa
Deep infrapatellar bursa
Tibia
Fibula
Joint capsule

A. Sagittal section

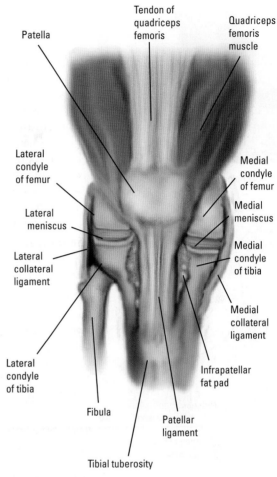

Patella
Tendon of quadriceps femoris
Quadriceps femoris muscle
Lateral condyle of femur
Lateral meniscus
Lateral collateral ligament
Lateral condyle of tibia
Fibula
Patellar ligament
Tibial tuberosity
Medial condyle of femur
Medial meniscus
Medial condyle of tibia
Medial collateral ligament
Infrapatellar fat pad

B. Anterior view

FIGURE 16.41 Anatomy of the right knee joint

E 4. Inspect the suprapatellar pouch and the prepatellar bursa.
5. Note the quadriceps muscle, located on the anterior thigh.
6. Palpate the knees. The consumer may assume a supine position if this is more comfortable.
   a. Grasp the anterior thigh approximately 10 cm above the patella, with your thumb on one side of the knee and the other four fingers on the other side of the knee (**Figure 16.42**).
   b. As you palpate, gradually move your hand down the suprapatellar pouch.
7. Palpate the tibiofemoral joints. It is best to have the knee flexed to 90° when performing this assessment.
   a. Place both thumbs on the knee, with the fingers wrapped around the knee posteriorly.
   b. Press in with the thumbs as you palpate the tibial margins (**Figure 16.43**).
   c. Palpate the lateral collateral ligament.

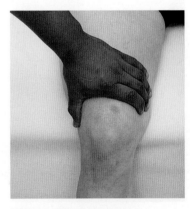

FIGURE 16.42 Palpating the knee

E Examination   **N** Normal findings   **A** Abnormal findings   **P** Pathophysiology   Advanced Assessment

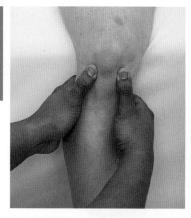

FIGURE 16.43 Palpating the tibiofemoral joint

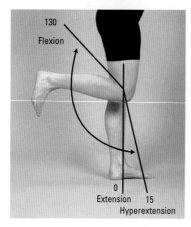

FIGURE 16.44 Range of motion of the knee joint: flexion, extension and hyperextension

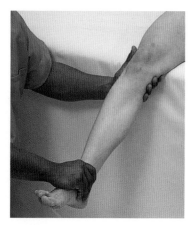

FIGURE 16.45 Strength of knee joint

E 8. If knee fluid is suspected, test for the bulge sign and ballottement. See the advanced techniques on Bulge sign and Patellar ballottement.

9. Assess ROM of the knees (**Figure 16.44**). Ask the consumer to stand and:
   a. Bend the knee (flexion)
   b. Straighten the knee (extension). The consumer may also be able to hyperextend the knee during this movement.

10. Assess strength of the knees with the consumer seated and the legs hanging off the table.
    a. Ask the consumer to bend the knee. Place your nondominant hand under the knee and place your other hand over the ankle.
    b. Instruct the consumer to straighten the leg against your resistance (**Figure 16.45**).
    c. Ask the consumer to place the foot on the bed and the knee at approximately 45° of flexion. Place one hand under the knee and place the other hand over the ankle.
    d. Instruct the consumer to maintain the foot on the table despite your attempts to straighten the leg.

N The knees are in alignment with each other and do not protrude medially or laterally. The normal ROM for the knees is flexion 130°, extension 0°; in some cases, hyperextension is possible up to 15°.

A Alteration in lower limb alignment is considered an abnormal finding.

P **Genu valgum** (knock knees) is inwards deviation towards the midline at the level of the knees (**Figure 16.46**). Both legs are usually affected by the disorder. It is detected as an increased distance between the medial malleoli when the femoral condyles are close together and the patellae are facing forwards. The knees appear closer together than is normal. Genu valgum can be congenital or acquired (rickets).

P **Genu varum** (bow legs) is outwards deviation away from the midline at the level of the knees (**Figure 16.47**). Both legs are usually affected by the disorder. It is detected as an increased distance between the femoral condyles when the medial malleoli are close together and the patellae are facing forwards. The knees appear farther apart than is normal. Genu varum can be congenital or acquired. This syndrome is common in horse jockeys due to the stretching of the nearby ligaments. It may also be seen in rickets, rheumatoid arthritis and osteomalacia due to the body's attempt to bend bone shape in order to tolerate the weight of the upper body.

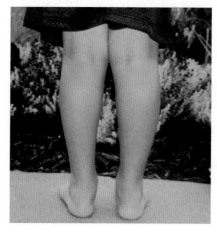

FIGURE 16.46 Genu valgum

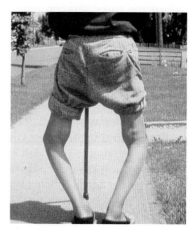

FIGURE 16.47 Genu varum

E Examination   **N** Normal findings   **A** Abnormal findings   **P** Pathophysiology   Advanced Assessment

A A knee effusion is present.

P A knee effusion can be associated with a Baker's cyst (see **Figure 16.48**). A Baker's cyst is a cystic mass in the medial popliteal fossa. If large enough, it can decrease the anatomic ROM of the knee. It is often detected in consumers with rheumatoid arthritis.

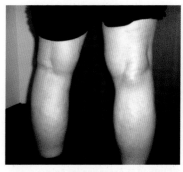

FIGURE 16.48 Baker's cyst in the right popliteal fossa

Assessing for small effusions: Bulge sign

The bulge sign tests for small effusions (4 to 8 mL) in the knee.

E 1. Place the consumer in a supine position with the legs extended.
   2. Firmly milk upwards the medial aspect of the patella several times. This displaces any fluid (**Figure 16.49A**).
   3. Press or tap the lateral aspect of the knee.
   4. Observe the hollow on the medial aspect of the knee for a bulge of fluid (**Figure 16.49B**).

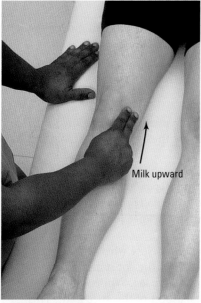

Milk upward

A. Milking the patella

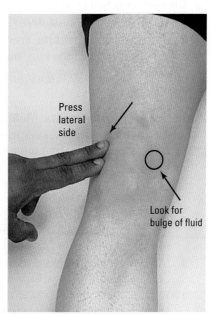

Press lateral side

Look for bulge of fluid

B. Observing for fluid

FIGURE 16.49 Assessing for bulge sign

N Normally there is no fluid return to the knee. This is a negative bulge sign.

A The return of fluid to the medial aspect of the patella is abnormal.

P A positive bulge sign is present in joint effusion.

Assessing for large effusions: Patellar ballottement

Ballottement is performed to detect large effusions in the knee.

E 1. Place the consumer either in a supine position with the legs extended or sitting up with the knees flexed at 90° and hanging over the edge of the examination table.
   2. Firmly grasp the thigh (with your thumb on one side and the four fingers on the other side) just above the patella. This compresses fluid out of the suprapatellar pouch.
   3. With your other hand, push the patella back towards the femur (see **Figure 16.50**).
   4. Feel for a click.

N There is no palpable click. Normally, the patella is close to the femur because there is no excess fluid.

A A palpable click is abnormal.

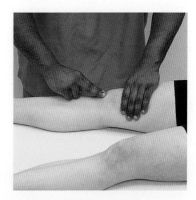

FIGURE 16.50 Patellar ballottement

E Examination **N** Normal findings **A** Abnormal findings **P** Pathophysiology   Advanced Assessment

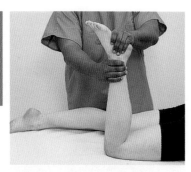

FIGURE 16.51 Assessing for Apley's grinding sign

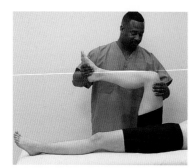

FIGURE 16.52 Assessing for McMurray sign

P When fluid is present between the femur and the patella, the patella 'floats' on top of the femur. As the patella is pushed back, fluid is displaced and a palpable click is felt when the patella hits the femur.

Assessing for meniscal tears: Apley's grinding sign

This test is performed to identify meniscal tears.

1. Place the consumer into a prone position on the examination table.
2. Manually flex the affected knee to a 90° angle so that the lower leg is perpendicular to the table.
3. With the dominant hand, apply firm downwards pressure on the foot while simultaneously rotating the lower leg inwards and then outwards (**Figure 16.51**).
4. Assess for limited knee joint movement or audible clicks during knee joint movement.

N The consumer will be able to flex the knee joint to a 90° angle, and no audible clicks will be heard during joint movement.

A A positive Apley's sign of the knee joint is indicated by limited movement of the knee joint (locking of the knee joint) or audible clicks.

P A positive Apley's sign is suggestive of torn meniscal cartilage within the knee joint.

Assessing for meniscal tears: McMurray sign

This test is performed to assess the integrity of the meniscus of the knee.

E 1. Place the consumer in a supine position on the examination table and stand on the affected side.
2. Manually flex the hip and knee. Hold the consumer's heel with one hand and stabilise the knee with the other hand (**Figure 16.52**).
3. Using the hand that is holding the heel, internally rotate the leg while applying resistance to the medial aspect of the knee joint. This assesses the medial meniscus.
4. Move the knee to a position of full extension. Note whether full extension of the knee joint can be achieved or tolerated by the consumer.
5. Flex the hip and knee and externally rotate the leg. While stabilising the knee joint, apply resistance to the lateral aspect of the knee joint. This assesses the lateral meniscus.
6. Assess for an audible or palpable click of the knee joint.

N The consumer will be able to extend the leg at the knee joint and there will be no audible or palpable click detected.

A A positive McMurray sign is indicated when the consumer is unable to extend the leg at the knee joint or when an audible or palpable click is detected.

P A positive McMurray sign is suggestive of torn meniscus cartilage of the knee. The consumer may also state that full extension of the knee joint is impossible, that the knee joint 'locks into place', or that 'it feels like something is in the knee joint'. If the torn meniscus cartilage is obstructing the articulating function of the joint, knee joint extension will be limited.

Assessing the cruciate ligaments: Drawer test

This test is performed to assess the stability of the anterior and posterior cruciate ligaments of the knee.

E 1. Assist the consumer to a supine position on the examination table.
2. Instruct the consumer to flex the right knee to 90° and to flex the right hip joint to 45°, placing the right foot flat on the examination table.
3. Sit on the consumer's right foot to stabilise it in place.
4. Observe for 'sagging' of the tibia resulting in visible concavity below the patella (gravity drawer test, or 'sag' sign).

E Examination **N** Normal findings **A** Abnormal findings **P** Pathophysiology   Advanced Assessment

E 5. Place both hands on the consumer's right tibia, with the thumb of the right hand on the medial aspect of the knee, and the left thumb on the lateral aspect of the knee (**Figure 16.53**).

6. Attempt to move the tibia forwards (anterior drawer test) and then backwards (posterior drawer test).

7. Repeat on the left leg. Compare results.

N You will not be able to pull the tibia forwards more than 6 mm or to move the tibia backwards at all. Concavity should not be detected distal to the patella.

A An abnormal result is indicated by the ability to move the tibia forwards more than 6 mm or to move the tibia backwards.

P Forwards movement of the tibia more than 6 mm indicates a tear in the anterior cruciate ligament of the knee. A false positive result may occur if the consumer has instability of the posterior cruciate ligament of the knee.

P Sagging of the tibia or backwards movement of the tibia indicates a tear in the posterior cruciate ligament of the knee.

Assessing the anterior cruciate ligament: Lachman test

This test is performed to assess for stability of the anterior cruciate ligament of the knee. It is considered the most reliable assessment technique for detecting instability of the anterior cruciate ligament.

E 1. Place the consumer in a supine position on the examination table with the unaffected knee flexed to approximately 30°. The affected leg should be fully extended and in contact with the examination table.

2. Stabilise the femur of the affected leg by holding the leg above the knee joint with the right hand.

3. Grasp the affected lower leg beneath the knee with the left hand and move the tibia forwards.

4. Note any changes in the infrapatellar slope.

N When the tibia is moved forwards, the infrapatellar tendon slope should still be noticeable.

A It is abnormal for the infrapatellar tendon slope to be no longer noticeable when the tibia is moved forwards.

P A positive Lachman test is indicative of damage to the anterior cruciate ligament of the knee.

Assessing the lateral collateral ligament: Varus stress test

E 1. Place the consumer in a supine position on the examination table.

2. Slightly abduct the affected leg.

3. Place your left hand on the medial aspect of the affected knee.

4. Place your right hand on the lateral aspect of the same ankle.

5. Apply varus stress (lateral movement) to the knee and push the right hand at the ankle medially (**Figure 16.54**).

6. Note pain with movement.

N There should be no pain when varus stress is applied.

A Pain with varus stress is abnormal.

P Pain with varus stress may indicate a tear in the lateral collateral ligament.

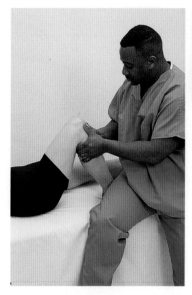
FIGURE 16.53 Drawer test

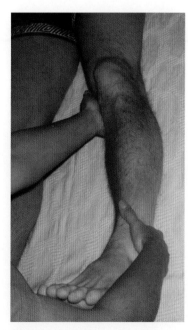
FIGURE 16.54 Varus stress test

E Examination   **N** Normal findings   **A** Abnormal findings   **P** Pathophysiology   Advanced Assessment

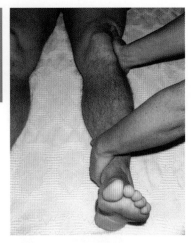

FIGURE 16.55 Valgus stress test

Assessing the medial collateral ligament: Valgus stress test

E
1. Place the consumer in a supine position on the examination table.
2. Slightly abduct the affected leg.
3. Place your right hand on the lateral aspect of the affected knee.
4. Place your left hand on the medial aspect of the same ankle.
5. Apply valgus stress (medial movement) to the knee and push the left hand at the ankle laterally (**Figure 16.55**).
6. Note pain with movement.

N There should be no pain when valgus stress is applied.

A Pain with valgus stress is abnormal.

P Pain with valgus stress may indicate a tear in the medial collateral ligament.

CLINICAL **REASONING**

Considering all possible cues

Clinicians should consider all sources for cues about consumer's health status, and this can include a variety of aspects. For example, examine the consumer's shoes and observe for wear in unusual areas. This provides information on the consumer's weight bearing that should inform further the direction of your health assessment. Keep this in mind as you watch the individual stand and walk.

Ankles and feet

E
1. Inspect the ankles and feet (see **Figure 16.56**) as the consumer stands, walks and sits (bearing no weight).
2. Inspect the alignment of the feet and toes with the lower leg.
3. Inspect the shape and position of the toes.
4. Assist the consumer to a supine position on the examination table.
5. Stand by the consumer's feet.

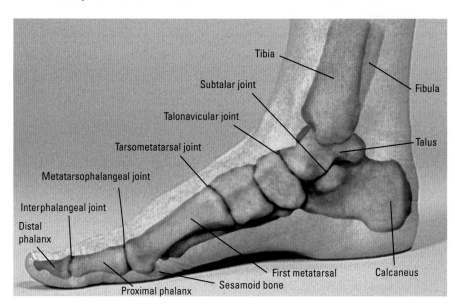

FIGURE 16.56 Anatomy of the ankle and foot

E Examination **N** Normal findings **A** Abnormal findings **P** Pathophysiology Advanced Assessment

CHAPTER 16

E 6. Palpate the ankle and foot (see **Figure 16.57**).
   a. Grasp the heel with the fingers of both hands. Palpate the posterior aspect of the heel at the calcaneus.
   b. Use your thumbs to palpate the medial malleolus (bony prominence on the distal medial aspect of the tibia) and the lateral malleolus (bony prominence on the distal lateral aspect of the fibula).
   c. Move your hands forwards and palpate the anterior aspects of the ankle and foot, particularly at the joints.
   d. Palpate the inferior aspect of the foot over the plantar fascia.
   e. Use your finger pads to palpate the Achilles tendon.
   f. Palpate each metatarsophalangeal joint with your thumb and index finger.
   g. Between your thumb and index finger, palpate the medial and lateral surfaces of each interphalangeal joint.

7. Assess ROM of the ankles and feet (**Figure 16.58**). Ask the consumer to:
   a. Point the toes towards the chest by moving the ankle (dorsiflexion)
   b. Point the toes towards the floor by moving the ankle (plantar flexion)
   c. Turn the soles of the feet outwards (eversion)
   d. Turn the soles of the feet inwards (inversion)
   e. Curl the toes towards the floor (flexion)
   f. Spread the toes apart (abduction)
   g. Move the toes together (adduction).

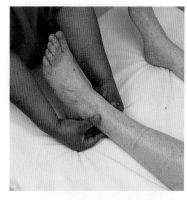

FIGURE 16.57 Palpation of the ankle

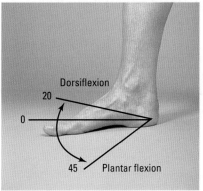

A. Plantar flexion and dorsiflexion

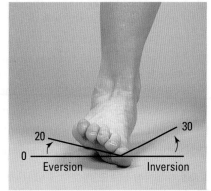

B. Eversion and inversion

FIGURE 16.58 Range of motion of the ankle and foot

E 8. Assess strength of the ankles and feet.
   a. Assist the consumer to a supine position on the examination table with the legs extended and the feet slightly apart.
   b. Stand at the foot of the examination table.
   c. Place your left hand on top of the consumer's right foot and place your right hand on top of their left foot.
   d. Ask the individual to point the toes towards the chest (dorsiflexion) despite your resistance.
   e. Place your left hand on the sole of the consumer's right foot and place your right hand on the sole of their left foot.
   f. Ask the consumer to point the toes down (plantar flexion) despite your resistance. This technique can also be performed one foot at a time as demonstrated in **Figure 16.59**.

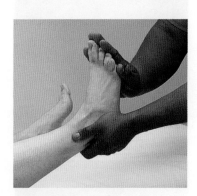

FIGURE 16.59 Strength of the ankle and foot

N The foot is in alignment with the lower leg. The foot has a longitudinal arch. There is no pain over the plantar fascia. The normal ROM for the ankles and feet is dorsiflexion 20°, plantar flexion 45°, eversion 20°, inversion 30°, abduction 30° and adduction 10°.

E Examination **N** Normal findings **A** Abnormal findings **P** Pathophysiology

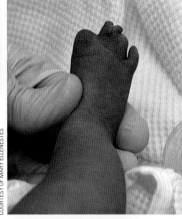

COURTESY OF MARY ELLENESTES

A. Congenital loss of the right big toe. Also note the syndactyly.

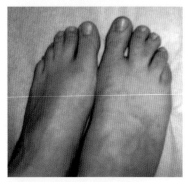

B. Syndactyly in the 2nd and 3rd metatarsals of the right foot.

FIGURE 16.60 Toe abnormalities

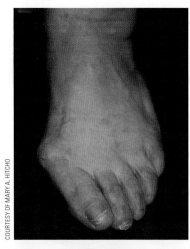

COURTESY OF MARY A. HITCHO

FIGURE 16.61 Hallux valgus

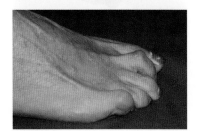

FIGURE 16.62 Hammer toe with corn

A Extra toes or webbing between the toes are congenital. Loss of toes can be congenital or acquired (**Figure 16.60A**).

P Polydactyly is the presence of extra digits. Syndactyly is the congenital webbing or fusion of toes (**Figure 16.60B**).

A An alteration in the shape and the position of the foot is considered abnormal.

P **Pes varus** describes a foot that is turned inwards towards the midline.

P **Pes valgus** occurs when the foot is turned laterally away from the midline.

P **Pes planus** (flat foot) refers to a foot with a low longitudinal arch.

P **Pes cavus** refers to a foot with an exaggerated arch height.

P In **hallux valgus** (bunion), the big toe is deviated laterally while the first metatarsal is deviated medially (**Figure 16.61**). The metatarsophalangeal joint enlarges and becomes inflamed from the pressure. A bursa may form at this point. Hallux valgus can be congenital or caused by narrow shoes and arthritis.

P Tight shoes can also cause **hammer toe**. In hammer toe, there is a flexion of the proximal interphalangeal joint and hyperextension of the distal metatarsophalangeal joint. A corn or callus can develop from undue pressure at the point of flexion (**Figure 16.62**).

P A **corn** is a conical area of thickened skin. It extends into the dermis and can be painful. Corns are caused by pressure on the affected area, particularly over bony prominences. Tight shoes and hammer toe can cause corns.

P A **callus** is a thickening of the skin due to prolonged pressure (**Figure 16.63**). It usually occurs on the sole of the foot and is not painful.

A Pain over the plantar fascia is abnormal.

P Plantar fasciitis (heel-spur syndrome) is an inflammation of the plantar fascia where it attaches to the calcaneus. The pain tends to be worse first thing in the morning, and with prolonged standing, sitting or walking.

A A swollen, red, warm and painful metatarsophalangeal joint is abnormal.

P The first metatarsophalangeal joint is usually affected in acute gouty arthritis.

A Decreased ROM of the ankle is abnormal.

Assessing for ankle sprain: Anterior drawer test

E 1. Have the consumer sit with the feet hanging freely.
2. Grasp the heel of the foot with the injured ankle with the left hand.
3. Place the right hand over the anterior aspect of the tibia on the affected side and firmly grasp the leg about 6 cm above the joint line (**Figure 16.64**).
4. Firmly hold the tibia as you apply an anterior forwards motion with your left hand.
5. Note any movement of the ankle.

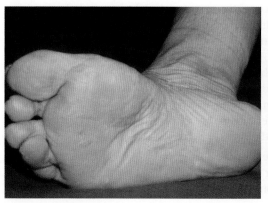

FIGURE 16.63 Callus

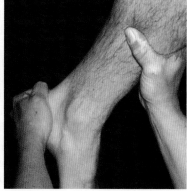

FIGURE 16.64 Anterior drawer test of the ankle

E Examination   **N** Normal findings   **A** Abnormal findings   **P** Pathophysiology

CHAPTER **16**

N There should be no forwards movement of the ankle.

A It is abnormal to have anterior movement of the ankle.

P Anterior movement of the ankle indicates a possible tear in the anterior talofibular ligament (see **Figure 16.65**)

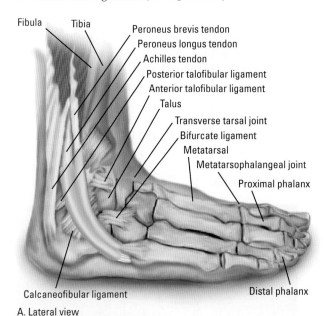

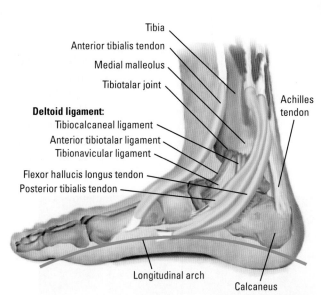

FIGURE 16.65 Ligaments of the ankle

Assessing for ankle sprain: Talar tilt test

E 1. Have the consumer sit with the feet hanging freely.
   2. Place your hands around the ankle of the affected leg so that the thumbs are inferior to the malleoli.
   3. Passively invert and evert the ankle through the range of motion (**Figure 16.66**).
   4. Note the movement of the ankle.
   5. Compare with the unaffected ankle.

N Normally, there should be an equal talar tilt, or range of motion, through inversion and eversion of both ankles.

A It is abnormal if the injured ankle has a talar tilt that is more than 5–10° compared to the unaffected ankle (most normal ankles have a tilt of approximately 5° or less).

P A talar tilt greater than 5–10° may indicate a tear in the calcaneofibular ligament.

P The consumer with an ankle sprain or fracture secondary to injury or trauma complains of pain on palpation and ROM. Crepitus may be present in an ankle fracture. Ankle sprain cannot always be differentiated from ankle fracture without the use of X-rays. Refer these consumers to an orthopaedic surgeon.

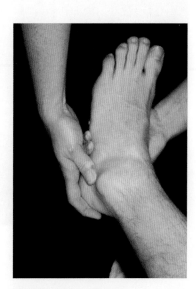

FIGURE 16.66 Talar tilt test

Assessing for ruptured Achilles tendon: Thompson squeeze test

E 1. Assist the consumer to a prone position with the feet hanging over the edge of the examination table.
   2. Manually squeeze the calf muscles of the leg.
   3. Observe for plantar flexion of the foot being examined.

E Examination   **N** Normal findings   **A** Abnormal findings   **P** Pathophysiology   ▨ Advanced Assessment

N When the calf muscles are squeezed, you should be able to visualise plantar flexion of the foot on the leg being examined.

A A positive Thompson test is manifested by the absence of plantar flexion when the calf muscles are squeezed.

P A positive Thompson test is suggestive of a ruptured Achilles tendon.

Spine

E 1. Ask the consumer to stand and to leave the back of the gown open.
2. Stand behind the individual so that you can visualise the posterior anatomy.
3. Inspect the position and alignment of the spine from a posterior and a lateral position.
4. Draw an imaginary line:
   a. From the head down through the spinous processes (see **Figure 16.67A**)
   b. Across the top of the scapula (see **Figure 16.67B**)
   c. Across the top of the iliac crests
   d. Across the bottom of the gluteal folds.

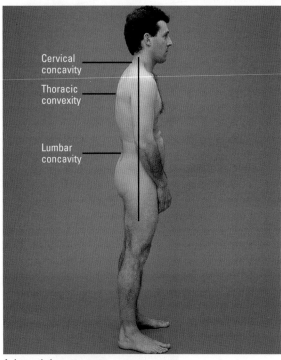

Cervical concavity

Thoracic convexity

Lumbar concavity

A. Lateral view

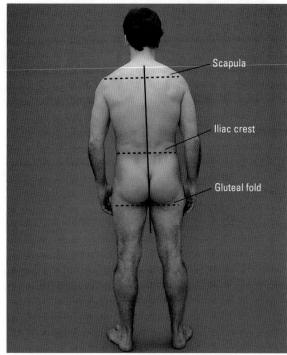

Scapula

Iliac crest

Gluteal fold

B. Posterior view

FIGURE 16.67 Alignment of spinal landmarks

E 5. Palpate the spinous processes with your thumb.
6. Palpate the paravertebral muscles.
7. Assess ROM of the spine (see **Figure 16.68**). Ask the consumer to bend forwards from the waist and touch the toes (flexion).
8. If necessary, stabilise the consumer's pelvis with your hands during the ROM assessment. Ask the consumer to:
   a. Bend to each side (lateral bending)
   b. Bend backwards (hyperextension)
   c. Twist the shoulders to each side (rotation).

N The normal spine has a cervical concavity, a thoracic convexity, and a lumbar concavity. An imaginary line can be drawn from the head straight down the spinous processes to the gluteal cleft. The imaginary lines drawn from the scapula, iliac crests and gluteal folds are parallel to each other. The normal ROM of the spine is flexion 90°, hyperextension 30°, lateral bending 35° and rotation 30°. As the consumer flexes forwards, the concavity of the lumbar spine disappears and the entire back assumes a convex C shape.

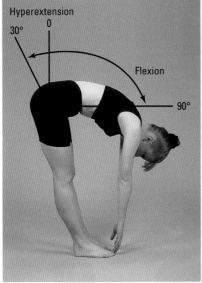

A. Flexion and hyperextension

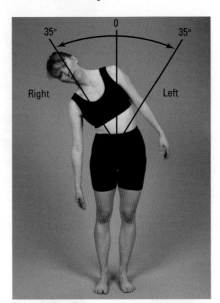

B. Lateral bending

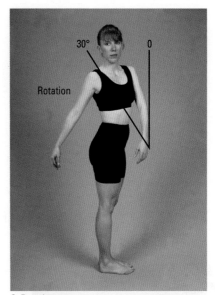

C. Rotation

FIGURE 16.68 Range of motion of the spine

CLINICAL **REASONING**

Screening for scoliosis

Scoliosis is the abnormal or exaggerated curve of the spine, which becomes a 'C' or 'S' shape, bending sideways from the middle. Sometimes it is congenital, but the majority of cases are idiopathic. Scoliosis can occur at any age; however, it tends to appear more in young adolescents, especially females, with approximately 2.5% of girls (aged 11–13) at risk of developing a significant scoliosis. In the early stages there are no symptoms to identify this condition, hence the need to examine and look. Early detection and treatment results in better long-term outcomes.

The National Self-Detection Program for Scoliosis is recommended by the Spine Society of Australia for girls in years 7–9. This entails the distribution by schools of an information brochure to the target age group, which describes scoliosis and what to look for. If, after reading the brochure, a girl and her carer think she may have a curvature, then follow-up with the family doctor is recommended.

Look at Figure 16.69. Can you identify any of the following:
> Shoulders that are uneven
> Waist creases that are uneven
> One shoulder blade that sticks out more than the other
> One hip higher than the other
> An obvious exaggerated curve of the spine.

If you do identify any of these possible signs of scoliosis, it is imperative that you refer the consumer to a medical practitioner for further assessment.

Source: Scoliosis Australia (2022). https://www.scoliosis-australia.org/policies-programs/the-nationalself-detection-program-for-scoliosis/

>>

E Examination **N** Normal findings **A** Abnormal findings **P** Pathophysiology

>>

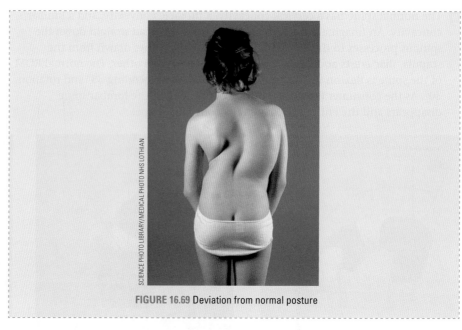

FIGURE 16.69 Deviation from normal posture

A From a posterior view, scoliosis (lateral curvature of the thoracic or lumbar vertebrae) may be detectable (**Figure 16.70**) and is an abnormal finding.

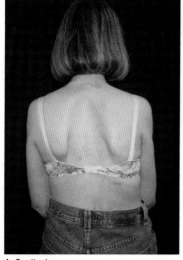

A. Scoliosis

FIGURE 16.70 Abnormalities of the spine

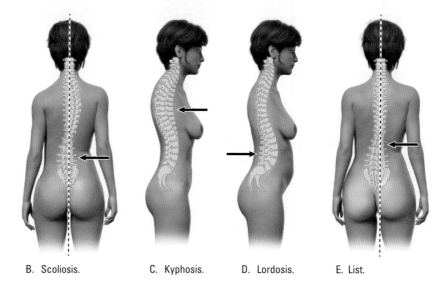

B. Scoliosis.   C. Kyphosis.   D. Lordosis.   E. List.

A The curvature is visible despite voluntary attempts at proper posture. This is structural scoliosis. The curvature becomes accentuated on forwards flexion from the waist. Scoliosis may also be accompanied by asymmetry of the clavicles, uneven shoulder and iliac crest levels, and a visible prominence of a scapula. If the lateral curvature is allowed to progress beyond 55°, cardiopulmonary problems can occur. Surgery may be indicated if the curve exceeds 40°.

P Structural scoliosis occurs most frequently in adolescence, especially in females.

A Functional scoliosis, which manifests itself only in a standing position, is abnormal.

P Functional scoliosis is due to unequal leg length or poor posture. Limb length should be measured.

E Examination   **N** Normal findings   **A** Abnormal findings   **P** Pathophysiology

Ⓐ Kyphosis, an excessive convexity of the thoracic spine (Figure 16.70C), is abnormal. The consumer with kyphosis presents with the chin tilted downwards onto the chest and with abdominal protrusion. There is also a decrease in the interval between the lower rib cage and the iliac crests. This appearance is due to forwards and downwards hunching of the head, neck, shoulders and upper back.

Ⓟ Kyphosis is seen in elderly consumers and in individuals with osteoporosis, ankylosing spondylitis or Paget's disease.

Ⓐ **Lordosis**, an excessive concavity of the lumbar spine (see Figure 16.70D), is abnormal.

Ⓟ Lordosis is accentuated in obesity and pregnancy due to the change in the centre of gravity.

Ⓐ A **list**, a leaning of the spine (see Figure 16.70E), is abnormal. If an imaginary line is drawn straight down from T1, the gluteal cleft is lateral to it. (In scoliosis, the imaginary line rests in the gluteal cleft, and the spine deviates from this straight line.)

Ⓟ A list can result from a herniated vertebral disc and painful paravertebral muscle spasms.

Ⓐ It is abnormal to have iliac crests that are unequal in height.

Ⓟ Scoliosis and congenital or acquired limb length discrepancies lead to iliac crests that are not equal in height.

Ⓐ Decreased ROM is abnormal. This is usually accompanied by pain.

Ⓟ These clinical findings are found in back injury, osteoarthritis and ankylosing spondylitis.

Assessing for scoliosis: Adams forwards bend test and use of the scoliometer

Ⓔ 1. Instruct the consumer to disrobe to their underclothing.
   2. Have the individual stand upright with the feet together.
   3. Stand behind the consumer.
   4. Ask the individual to bend forwards from the waist with the hands held downwards towards the feet and palms together (similar to a diving position). The head should be down, with the person looking at the floor.
   5. Inspect and palpate the progression of the spinous processes, starting at the cervical spine and progressing in an inferior direction to the sacral area.
   6. Draw an imaginary line through the spinous processes (or use a felt-tip marker to connect the spinous processes).
   7. Place the scoliometer (Figure 16.71A) on the thoracic vertebrae in the midspinal line. Measure the angle of trunk rotation on the scoliometer.
   8. Place the scoliometer on the lumbar vertebrae (Figure 16.71B) in the midspinal line and measure the angle of trunk rotation.

Ⓝ The imaginary (or real) line drawn through the spinous processes should be straight or with minimal deviation. The angle of the trunk rotation reading on the scoliometer should be less than 7°.

Ⓐ It is abnormal to have moderate to severe lateral deviation of the spine. An angle of trunk rotation reading greater than 7° indicates scoliosis.

Ⓟ Structural scoliosis usually develops in adolescence.

Assessing for herniated disc: Straight leg raising test (Lasègue's test)

Ⓔ 1. Assist the consumer to a supine position on the examination table.
   2. Place one hand on the heel of the right foot and place the other hand behind the upper calf area of the same leg.

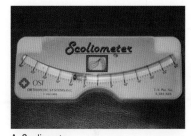

A. Scoliometer

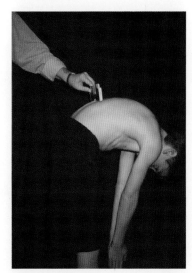

B. Use of scoliometer

FIGURE 16.71 Scoliometer and its use

 Examination   Normal findings 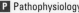 Abnormal findings Ⓟ Pathophysiology ▨ Advanced Assessment

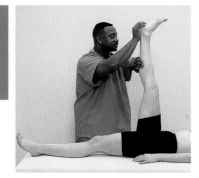

FIGURE 16.72 Straight leg raising test

E 3. Maintain the foot in its neutral anatomic position.
4. Raise the leg to the angle at which low back pain occurs.
5. With the extended leg still raised to its maximum height, manually dorsiflex the foot (Figure 16.72).
6. Repeat the technique on the left leg.

N The consumer will be able to flex the hip joint and raise the straight leg to a hip flexion angle of 90°. There will be no low back pain with lifting of the extended leg or with dorsiflexion of the foot while the leg is raised.

A A positive straight leg raising test is abnormal. The individual will be unable to raise the extended leg to a 90° angle of hip joint flexion. Low back pain will occur with any lifting of the straight leg, and this discomfort will increase when the foot is dorsiflexed while the leg is in the raised position.

P Irritation of the nerve roots of the lumbosacral area causes pain in the sciatic nerve. Pain at less than 40° generally means an irritated nerve root caused by a herniated vertebral disc in the lumbosacral area. Pain may also occur in the other leg.

Assessing for herniated disc: Milgram test

E 1. Place the consumer in a supine position on the examination table with both legs fully extended and resting on the table.
2. Instruct the consumer to raise both legs at least 5 cm off the examination table while maintaining the legs in extension for at least 30 seconds.

N The individual will be able to hold the extended legs in the raised position for at least 30 seconds.

A The inability to maintain the straight legs in the raised position for at least 30 seconds is suggestive of pressure on the spinal nerves and is abnormal.

P A positive Milgram test is often indicative of a herniated intervertebral disc.

Assessing status of distal limbs and digits

E When you suspect distal limb or digit hypoperfusion due to trauma, injury or pathology, conduct the following assessment.
1. Uncover the distal aspects of both limbs being assessed. A bilateral assessment allows for comparison of the affected and unaffected limbs. When assessing an injured limb, assess the limb areas proximal and distal to the site of injury.
2. Assess for swelling.
3. Assess the vascular status of the distal limb and its digits (peripheral pulses, skin colour, skin temperature, capillary refill).
4. Ask the consumer to perform specific movements of the distal limb on command.
   a. To assess the ulnar nerve, ask the consumer to perform abduction of the fingers.
   b. To assess the radial nerve, ask the consumer to perform hyperextension of the thumb or wrist.
   c. To assess the median nerve, ask the individual to perform opposition of the thumb to the little finger of the same hand.
   d. To assess the peroneal nerve, ask the individual to perform dorsiflexion of the toes and ankle.
   e. To assess the tibial nerve, ask the individual to perform plantar flexion of the toes and ankle.

E 5. When assessing sensation, instruct the consumer to close the eyes to prevent biased results. Use the thumb and index finger of the dominant hand to pinch certain areas of the distal limb.

  a. To assess the ulnar nerve, pinch the finger pad of the little finger.

  b. To assess the radial nerve, pinch the web space between the thumb and the index finger.

  c. To assess the median nerve, pinch the distal aspect of the index finger.

  d. To assess the peroneal nerve, pinch the lateral aspect of the great toe and the medial surface of the second toe.

  e. To assess the tibial nerve, pinch the medial and lateral surfaces of the sole of the foot.

N The individual with normal perfusion to the limbs and digits will appear comfortable during rest and muscle contraction. Pain will not occur with movement of the distal limb or digits. Limb perfusion will be manifested by strong peripheral pulses, warm skin temperature and a brisk capillary refill. There will be complete motor and sensory function of the distal limb and digits. The consumer will not experience any numbness or tingling.

A Neurovascular deterioration, manifested by the '5 Ps' (Pain, Paralysis, Paraesthesia, Pulses, Pallor) is abnormal.

P Neurovascular deterioration can occur in compartment syndrome. It is a severe complication of musculoskeletal trauma in which swelling is limited due to a confined space. Pain is the most significant and the earliest clinical manifestation of acute compartment syndrome. It occurs distal to the site of injury and is induced by the contraction of the muscle compartment being compressed. Pain results from stretching of a muscle that is experiencing vascular compromise.

P Inadequate arterial flow is a complication of digit or limb replantation following traumatic amputation.

P Arterial occlusion may also be detected as a complication of fracture or dislocation.

P Inadequate venous flow from the distal limb or digits, manifested by cyanosis, mottling, skin temperature that is warmer than usual, immediate capillary refill, and a distended or tense tissue turgor, is abnormal.

P Inadequate venous flow is a complication of digit or limb replantation following traumatic amputation.

URGENT FINDING

Compartment syndrome

Compartment syndrome is a serious complication of limb injury with extensive soft tissue trauma that can develop quickly and needs urgent management. The lower leg and forearm are vulnerable to this complication. Increasing oedema or haemorrhage within a muscle compartment reaches the point where it can no longer be accommodated by the elasticity of the fascia and skin. The continuing oedema redirects itself inwards, compressing muscle, nerves and blood vessels. Muscular necrosis can result from lack of perfusion and cause sequelae of systemic complications that can lead to multiple organ dysfunction and death.

Clinical manifestations include increased and uncontrolled pain despite narcotic analgesia, with pain aggravated by passive movement of the distal limb. Other manifestations include increased limb girth; shiny, tight skin; slow capillary refill; skin pallor; and decreased digit sensation and movement. Decreased peripheral pulse volume is a late indicator of compartment syndrome. In high-risk trauma cases, the pressure within the muscle compartment can be measured using various invasive monitoring devices (ACI Musculoskeletal Network, 2018).

E Examination **N** Normal findings **A** Abnormal findings **P** Pathophysiology

Assessing consumers with musculoskeletal supportive equipment

Supportive equipment may be necessary to support musculoskeletal structure and function. The need for such devices automatically indicates an underlying musculoskeletal disorder. For each piece of supportive equipment, determine the reason for its use.

Crutches

Determine the following:

1. Amount of weight bearing allowed on affected lower limb
2. Appropriate crutch height
3. Type of crutch gait and appropriateness for the amount of weight bearing on affected leg: two-point crutch gait (partial weight bearing), three-point crutch gait (partial or non-weight bearing), four-point alternate crutch gait (partial or full weight bearing), swing gait (non-weight bearing)
4. Condition of crutches (padded handles, rubber tips)
5. Ease of transfer into and out of a chair
6. Ease of stair climbing with the crutches
7. Consumer wearing flat, properly fitted shoes with non-skid surfaces
8. Signs or symptoms of skin breakdown or distal limb hypoperfusion.

Walking stick

Determine the following:

1. Shape of handle (C or T)
2. Number of points on contact surface
3. Appropriateness for consumer's height
4. Walking stick used on unaffected side.

Refer to steps 4–8 in the section on crutches.

Walker

Determine the following:

1. Amount of weight bearing allowed on the lower limb
2. Type of walker (e.g. rolling or pick-up walker)
3. Appropriateness for consumer's height
4. Consumer's ability to grip and propel the walker forwards with rolling walker; consumer's ability to grip, lift and propel the walker forwards with pick-up walker (**Figure 16.73**).

Refer to steps 4–8 in the section on crutches.

Brace, splint, immobiliser

Determine the following:

1. Location of device (e.g. limb, neck, torso, lower back or pelvis)
2. Joint position maintained by device (e.g. extension, flexion or abduction)
3. Joint motion allowed by device
4. If a movable device is used, whether the hinge joint of the device is aligned with the skeletal joint
5. Padding under pressure points of device
6. Amount of weight bearing allowed on the affected leg (lower leg device).

Refer to steps 7 and 8 in the section on crutches.

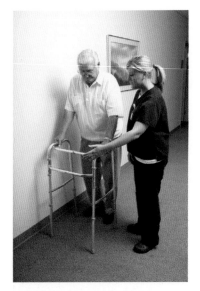

FIGURE 16.73 The nurse assesses the consumer's ability to use the walker correctly.

CHAPTER **16**

Cast

Determine the following:

1. Plaster or non-plaster cast (e.g. synthetic, fibreglass)
2. Location of cast
3. Joint position maintained (e.g. extension, flexion or abduction)
4. Joint motion allowed
5. Neurovascular observations (5 Ps: Pain, Paralysis, Paraesthesia, Pulses, Pallor)
6. Signs or symptoms of skin breakdown or distal limb hypoperfusion
7. Edges of the cast covered ('petaled') with tape to prevent skin irritation
8. Amount of weight bearing allowed (lower leg cast)
9. Damage to cast (e.g. cracked, flaking or crumbling, dented, wet, softening)
10. Visible discolouration on the cast (e.g. from underlying wound drainage or bleeding)
11. Significant odour around the cast (e.g. a musty or foul smell).

CLINICAL **REASONING**

Female athlete triad

Health concerns can also be found in fit athletes. Competitive physical activities that require small body size and heavy training can lead to a phenomenon called the female athlete triad. Premature osteoporosis can occur concurrently with an eating disorder and unexplained absence of the menstrual cycle for more than 6 months (secondary amenorrhoea). Due to premature osteoporosis, these females are at high risk for decreased bone mineral density and resulting stress fractures (multiple and/or recurrent). Restoration of oestrogen levels associated with menses provides hormone stability to optimise bone status but cannot replace existing bone loss. High-risk sports include but are not limited to running, gymnastics, ballet and figure skating.

Consider your perceptions of health and wellness in fit individuals, and the impact these may have on how you perceive their health alterations.

EVALUATION OF HEALTH ASSESSMENT AND PHYSICAL EXAMINATION FINDINGS

In the evaluation phase of a health assessment, the focus is on ensuring the data gathered is complete, accurate and documented appropriately (see case study as an example of the focused assessment; see Chapter 22 for a comprehensive health assessment). In evaluating the data you should:

> draw on your critical thinking and problem-solving skills to make sound clinical decisions

> act on abnormal data (include communicating findings to other health professionals)

> ensure documentation reflects the outcomes of the clinical decisions/actions taken (refer to Chapter 3, which discusses in detail why documentation is so important and how this may be undertaken in different health settings).

The case study that follows steps you through this process.

THE CONSUMER WITH MUSCULOSKELETAL PAIN RELATED TO OSTEOARTHRITIS

This case study illustrates the application and objective documentation of the musculoskeletal assessment. The setting is in an emergency department.

Adrianne De-Lloyd has increasing knee pain and swelling after a country hike 3 days ago and presents to the emergency department for evaluation and treatment.

HEALTH HISTORY

CONSUMER PROFILE	68-year-old female	
CHIEF COMPLAINT	'My knees hurt and are stiff.'	
HISTORY OF THE PRESENT ILLNESS	Consumer transported to the emergency department (ED) by spouse, presenting with bilateral knee pain and swelling that has occurred since a long country hike 3 days ago. She states there were hills, gullies and uneven ground on the 4-hour walk, and she did not report falling and does not remember twisting her knees. She noted her knees were painful going downhill and that she usually has soreness and stiffness after completing walking activities, so was not particularly bothered. However, the next morning on waking her knees were very stiff and swollen. Over the next 3 days they have become increasingly more painful, making getting in and out of the car more difficult. She denies subjective fevers. Her airway is patent, breathing non-laboured, limbs are warm and perfused, no bleeding wounds or pallor; she is alert but limping in obvious discomfort. Temperature 36.2°C; HR 78 BPM; RR 18 per min; BP 137/78 mmHg; BGL 4.5 mmol/L	
PAST HEALTH HISTORY	MEDICAL HISTORY	Fracture of the right tibial plateau at age 56 after a fall Gastro-oesophageal reflux Osteoarthritis of both knees for 10 years Denies having had gout or other joint pains other than her knees
	SURGICAL HISTORY	Hysterectomy aged 55 for fibroids. No complications or adverse effects of procedure
	ALLERGIES	No medication allergies Denies bee sting/insect or environmental allergies
	MEDICATIONS	Panadol osteo 665 mg orally 2–3 times per day for knee pain (last taken 1 hour before coming to emergency but 'they are not working') Ibuprofen 400 mg when her knees pain plays up (last taken 2 hours before coming to emergency but 'they are not working') Pantoprazole 20 mg daily for reflux Melatonin 2 mg MR nightly as needed to re-establish sleep routine
	COMMUNICABLE DISEASES	Denies any history
	INJURIES AND ACCIDENTS	Past 'bad' right knee ligament tear 12 years ago when she broke her tibia – no intervention other than splint and crutches were needed; but has had a 'niggly right knee after prolonged exercise since'
	SPECIAL NEEDS	Denies
	BLOOD TRANSFUSIONS	Denies
	CHILDHOOD ILLNESSES	Childhood diseases include measles, mumps, chickenpox
	IMMUNISATIONS	Consumer is fully immunised against childhood illnesses for her age group. She received her annual flu shot 4 weeks ago, and four COVID vaccinations have been completed.

>>

>>

HEALTH HISTORY

FAMILY HEALTH HISTORY		Family history of osteoarthritis (mother and father), gout (father). Denies first degree family history of rheumatoid arthritis or diabetes mellitus or hypertension
SOCIAL HISTORY	**ALCOHOL USE**	4–5 red wines per week; a few whisky shots on weekends
	TOBACCO USE	Never smoked
	DRUG USE	Denies illegal drug use or overuse of prescription drugs
	SEXUAL PRACTICE	No history of STIs. Monogamous, life partner of 40 years
	TRAVEL HISTORY	No recent travel in the last 3 years
	WORK ENVIRONMENT	Retired, was a full-time factory supervisor. Adrianne had worked at her job for 15 years prior to retirement; it was a job that required standing for long periods
	HOME ENVIRONMENT	Married. Lives with husband in a low-set house with 2 steps to enter; one small dog
	HOBBIES AND LEISURE ACTIVITIES	Walking group weekly, card night weekly; reading
	STRESS	Recently retired and knees have intermittently stopped her going with the walking group, which is stressful socially as she really looks forward to these outings
	EDUCATION	Grade 12 schooling and worked her way up to become a supervisor at the canning factory
	ECONOMIC STATUS	Adrianne is retired using superannuation; her husband works part time as an accountant
	RELIGION	Both Adrianne and spouse identify as Christian and attend a weekly online church service, which started during the first COVID lockdown
	CULTURAL BACKGROUND	Both Adrianne and spouse are Caucasian
	ROLES AND RELATIONSHIPS	Both immediate and extended family live nearby and they have monthly family gatherings. Family members and neighbours are willing to help in times of need.
	CHARACTERISTIC PATTERNS OF DAILY LIVING	Wakes at 6 a.m. to walk 4 km five times per week. Gets home in time to get her husband off to work. Tries to cook healthy meals, but once a week eats fast food for convenience. Attends card games with neighbours weekly; usually in bed by 10 p.m.
HEALTH MAINTENANCE ACTIVITIES	**SLEEP**	7.5–8 hours per night. No routine use of sedatives to induce sleep; however, occasionally uses melatonin for a week to restore normal sleep patterns when she is out of routine; reads during day but seldom naps
	DIET	Tries to avoid high-fat fried foods
	EXERCISE	Regular walking 5 times per week, when able
	STRESS MANAGEMENT	Experiencing some stress since retired, especially when her knees play up, as this stops her going on group outings
	USE OF SAFETY DEVICES	Routinely wears a seat belt while driving. When her right knee is stiff and sore, she drives less as it is difficult to get in and out of the car; no walking aids required
	HEALTH CHECK-UPS	Has annual check-up with GP. Normal lipids

>>

>>

PHYSICAL EXAMINATION

GENERAL ASSESSMENT	**OVERALL APPEARANCE**		Height: 172 cm, weight: 78 kg BMI = 26.5 (overweight but not obese) Mild valgus deformity of the knees, but no other obvious structural defects of the musculoskeletal system. All limbs and digits are present and in proportion to overall body size. Adrianne is alert and oriented to time, place and person, but appears uncomfortable on weight bearing. There are no visible grazes or ecchymosis on the limbs. There is no visual dislocation of the knees or patellas. Right knee is more swollen that the left. There is no redness to either knee. No rash noted.
	POSTURE		Adrianne is sitting, uses husband's support to get her out of the chair due to discomfort affecting her ability to do so independently.
	GAIT AND MOBILITY		Mobile with antalgic gait. Spouse reports no problem with gait or mobility prior to the hike 3 days ago.
INSPECTION	**MUSCLE SIZE AND SHAPE**		Firm and contoured calf muscles No indication of muscle wasting of the thighs. No obvious involuntary muscle movement.
	JOINT CONTOUR AND PERIARTICULAR TISSUE		Joint contour of the knees within normal range in the extension position but with minor valgus bilaterally. Patellas are centrally located. No ecchymosis or redness. Mild left knee swelling and moderate right knee swelling.
PALPATION	**MUSCLE TONE**		Normal tone associated over the thighs and calfs bilaterally.
	JOINTS		Bilaterally tender over the medial joint lines. Some crepitus over the right knee. There is no joint subluxation or dislocation of the knees or patellas. There is no laxity when stressing the knee joints. The joints are not hot to touch.
	RANGE OF MOTION		Straight leg raise intact bilaterally. Flexion to 90° both knees. Can fully extend/flex at the hips and ankles.
	MUSCLE STRENGTH		5/5 strength of the knee and hip flexor and extension mechanisms. Neurovascular observations normal lower limbs.

EVALUATION AND CLINICAL REASONING FOR CASE STUDY

The assessment and clinical decisions you make should reflect your scope of practice. For example, advanced practice health professionals, such as nurse practitioners and remote area nurses with endorsement, may be able to make diagnostic decisions and prescribe medications without referring to a medical officer.

Fundamentally, all health professionals collect, evaluate and act on consumer-focused health information, which will at times include referral to, or collaboration with, other healthcare team members. Nurses assess individual's responses to interventions and determine when to escalate key changes in a consumer's condition. The clinical reasoning cycle provides health professionals with a framework to consider all this information in a meaningful way for planning consumer care. These phases are stepped out below, and draw on information presented and collected during the health history and physical examination. We then work through the cycle components that are relevant to this case study (cycle components are bolded).

For Adrianne De-Lloyd, the significant data that needs to be considered includes the following.

Collecting cues/information

Recall and Review: In the first instance you will need to reflect on what you know about joint conditions. The assessment data that has been collected thus far indicates that Adrianne has a possible flare-up of her knee osteoarthritis (OA). Now you will need to consider what you know about osteoarthritis and other joint conditions such as gout, rheumatoid arthritis, psoriatic arthritis, or a joint infection.

Osteoarthritis is the leading cause of disability in older adults, and can lead to decreased quality of life. Worldwide estimates are that 9.6% of men and 18% of women older than 60 years have symptomatic OA. Ageing is the single greatest risk factor for the development of OA, followed by knee joint injury or surgery, and it is the main reason for knee replacement surgery (Abramoff & Caldera, 2020).

Osteoarthritis is a complex process composed of inflammatory and metabolic factors. It is a whole joint disease involving structural alteration in the articular cartilage, inflammation of ligaments, synovitis, capsular distension with effusion, and changes to the periarticular structures such as tendon, fascia, bursa, nerves (Hunter & Bierma-Zeinstra, 2019). The cardinal symptom of osteoarthritis is pain, which is provoked by load bearing and relieved by rest, followed by stiffness after resting (Katz, Arant & Loeser, 2021).

Obesity and injury are important modifiable risk factors. A 10% reduction in body weight significantly decreases the load in knee joints. Non-modifiable risk factors are older age, female sex, and family history of osteoarthritis (Abramoff & Caldera, 2020). Occupational tasks such as standing are associated with the risk for developing OA of the knees (Allen, Thoma & Golightly, 2022). Valgus joint alignment likely plays a role in the progression of OA. One or more comorbidities or chronic diseases such as diabetes or cardiovascular disease are predictive of faster worsening of pain, or of faster deterioration (Hunter & Bierma-Zeinstra, 2019).

Clinical diagnosis is made on the basis of symptoms (pain, brief morning stiffness, functional limitations) and physical examination findings of crepitus, restricted painful movement, joint tenderness and eventually bony enlargement. If the diagnosis is uncertain, then more serious joint conditions are considered for the consumer coming to emergency, such as gout or septic joint, then further tests may be needed (Abramoff & Caldera, 2020).

Neurovascular and pain assessment are significant in detecting early signs of possible joint infection. An X-ray is required but may not solely provide definitive diagnosis, as radiological findings poorly correlate to symptoms. Further tests such as FBC/Chem 20 and inflammatory markers (C-reactive protein) may be necessary to inform if a joint aspiration is indicated to exclude more serious joint pathology and therefore definitive diagnosis (Abramoff & Caldera, 2020; ACSQHC, 2017).

Chief complaint and history of present illness

> Mechanism of injury: prolonged hiking on uneven hilly terrain 3 days prior
> Consumer reports that 'My knees hurt and are stiff'.
> Gradual onset after excessive exercise
> Antalgic gait (pain on weight bearing)
> Has had flares of OA knee pain before; age >65 years; and is overweight

Processing information

Interpret: These symptoms and details outline the scope of the issue for this consumer and how it will now affect her present deviation from normal health.

Social history

> Consumer retired 3 years ago and feels socially isolated when her knees flare up.

Discriminate and Predict: It is noteworthy that Adrianne has experienced stress previously with knee pain since retiring and this may impact further on her coping abilities.

Physical assessment

> No redness to the knees and not hot to touch
> Mild to moderate swelling to both knees associated with moderate pain on weight bearing
> Valgus knee joint alignment
> Consumer is currently sitting, and finding it hard to get in and out of the chair
> Neurovascular observations – normal
> Afebrile

Infer: The significance of these findings indicates that Adrianne De-Lloyd has pain in two weight-bearing joints with a history of OA and is therefore less likely to have a more serious condition such as gout or a joint infection.

Putting it all together – synthesise information

The assessment and physical examination indicate that Adrianne has a history of OA that is exacerbated by her weight, and she has had an acute flare-up due to the recent walking activities she has been involved in. The role of the nurse in this case is to continue close observation for any deviations from normal to ensure Adrianne is triaged appropriately, based on presenting assessment data. Adrianne De-Lloyd will require further observation while her assessment is expanded with a more focused approach.

Actions based on assessment findings

While waiting for further diagnostic examinations the nurse should consider the following:

1 Repeat vital signs to check for onset of fever
2 Repeat neurovascular assessment – (5 Ps: Pain, Paralysis, Paraesthesia, Pulses, Pallor)
3 Pain assessment and management – To alleviate discomfort, the nurse should administer prescribed medications. Applying ice to the swelling may also assist in decreasing pain.
4 Apply tubular bandages to assist in reducing pain and swelling.
5 Reduce anxiety and the inevitable disruption to life this flare-up will have. The nurse should give Adrianne the opportunity to express her feelings and ensure she and her husband are consistently informed about her condition. May need to consider referral to physiotherapy to optimise physical function, asses the need for a temporary walking aid, and consider referral to dietitian for weight management.

The final step in the process is accurate documentation. The nurse must document findings, referrals, interventions, and advice and education given. The consumer would then be reassessed following definitive diagnosis and medical interventions for her pain.

CHAPTER RESOURCES

REVIEW QUESTIONS

For answers to these questions, see Answer section at the end of the book.

1. Following total hip-joint replacement, the consumer is instructed to avoid turning his affected leg and hip inwards towards midline or crossing the affected leg over the nonaffected leg. What are these movements called?
   a. External rotation, adduction
   b. Internal rotation, abduction
   c. Internal rotation, adduction
   d. External rotation, abduction

2. A 49-year-old male presented with severe pain in his right big toe that is swollen and hot to touch. He states that he has not injured himself and that he has had this pain in the same toe several times in the past, and it was determined he had gout. The pain has been relieved with indomethacin. What additional physical examination finding is likely?
   a. Muscle atrophy
   b. Flexion contracture
   c. Hallux valgus
   d. Tophi nodules

3. Malcolm is a 46-year-old male who enjoys long-distance running. He has been running 5 days a week for over 20 years. This year he has experienced increasing pain and stiffness in his knees, especially his right knee, which is his lead leg. David is most likely experiencing which musculoskeletal change?
   a. Rheumatoid arthritis
   b. Osteoarthritis
   c. Osteomyelitis
   d. Osteoporosis

4. Painful involuntary muscle contraction near an area of acute bony deformity following trauma may represent which involuntary muscle movement?
   a. Asterixis
   b. Tremor
   c. Fasciculation
   d. Spasm

5. Mandy is a data entry officer and attends the health clinic complaining of pain in her right wrist and forearm, with tingling sensations in the first three fingers of her right hand. She also reports that her grip in her right hand has been poor and she has been dropping things. While Mandy is in the sitting position, she is asked to have her right arm flexed at the elbow with the palmar surface of her right hand facing up. The examiner then taps the median nerve over the centre of the wrist. Mandy could have carpal tunnel syndrome if she reports what sensation?
   a. Sudden onset of numbness in the thumb
   b. Burning wrist pain that radiates to the elbow
   c. Tingling sensation of the thumb, index and middle fingers
   d. Sudden onset of numbness of the little finger

6. Sarah is a 63-year-old consumer who is awaiting surgery to repair a fractured wrist following a crush injury. Sarah is complaining of increased pain and paraesthesia. When you examine her, you notice a pale hand, a decreased radial pulse and capillary refill, and a loss of strength in the fingers. You know this is most likely caused by which of the following?
   a. Neurovascular compromise
   b. Anxiety due to surgery
   c. Rapid onset of infection
   d. Muscle and tendon rupture

7. What could be used as a quantitative technique for measuring grip strength in the conscious and cooperative consumer?
   a. Instruct the consumer to squeeze the examiner's hand.
   b. Instruct the consumer to squeeze a caliper held in the examiner's hand.
   c. Instruct the consumer to squeeze the examiner's finger.
   d. Instruct the consumer to squeeze a rolled-up and slightly inflated blood pressure cuff.

8. Mila is a 13-year-old girl undergoing annual screening by the school nurse. Following assessment of height, weight, visual acuity and hearing, the nurse asks Mila to bend forwards from the waist and touch her toes. What disorder is characterised by lateral curvature of the spine in this position?
   a. Kyphosis
   b. Scoliosis
   c. Lordosis
   d. List

9. Immediately following plaster cast application to a lower leg for immobilisation of a reduced fracture, what assessment foci should the nurse monitor frequently?
   a. Neurovascular status – 5 Ps: pain, pallor, pulse, paraesthesia and paralysis
   b. Limb girth, limb length and limb colour
   c. Cast odour, quantity of blood on the cast and time until the plaster cast sets
   d. Amount of weight bearing allowed on the cast

10. A 66-year-old man who is an avid golf player arrives at the clinic complaining of sudden pain and decreased mobility in his right shoulder. You manually abduct the affected arm and ask him to slowly lower the arm while maintaining extension. You note that the consumer's arm quickly falls to his side. What injury does this man most likely have?
    a. Adhesive capsulitis
    b. Rotator cuff damage
    c. Biceps tendonitis
    d. Shoulder subluxation

CS CLINICAL SKILLS

The following Clinical Skills are relevant to this chapter and can be found in Tollefson & Hillman, *Clinical Psychomotor Skills,* 8th edition:
> 20 Focused neurological health history and physical assessment

> 21 Neurovascular observations
> 24 Focused musculoskeletal health history and physical assessment and range of motion exercises
> 27 Healthcare teaching
> 58 Assisting a person to mobilise.

FURTHER RESOURCES

> Arthritis Australia: http://www.arthritisaustralia.com.au
> Arthritis New Zealand: http://www.arthritis.org.nz/
> Australian and New Zealand Bone and Mineral Society: http://www.anzbms.org.au/
> Australian and New Zealand Falls Prevention Society: http://www.anzfallsprevention.org/
> Australian and New Zealand Orthopaedic Nurses Association: http://www.anzona.net/
> Australian Commission on Safety and Quality in Health Care, Falls prevention: https://www.safetyandquality.gov.au/our-work/comprehensive-care/related-topics/falls-prevention
> Australian Institute of Health and Welfare (AIHW). (2022). Australian Burden of Disease Study: Impact and causes of illness and death in Aboriginal and Torres Strait Islander people 2018. https://www.aihw.gov.au/reports/burden-of-disease/illness-death-indigenous-2018/summary

> Australian Rheumatology Association: https://rheumatology.org.au/
> Healthy Bones Australia: https://healthybonesaustralia.org.au/
> Lin, I., & Coffin, J. (2017). Myths about musculoskeletal pain and Aboriginal Australians prevent high quality care. https://theconversation.com/myths-about-musculoskeletal-pain-and-aboriginal-australians-prevent-high-quality-care-76390
> Ministry of Health New Zealand. (2015). Health and Independence Report, 2022. https://www.health.govt.nz/publication/health-and-independence-report-2020
> Occupational Exposures of Australian Nurses: https://www.safeworkaustralia.gov.au/system/files/documents/1702/occupationalexposures_australiannurses_methodologyreport_2008_pdf.pdf
> Osteoporosis New Zealand: http://www.bones.org.nz/

REFERENCES

Abramoff, B., & Caldera, F. E. (2020). Osteoarthritis: Pathology, diagnosis, and treatment options. *Medical Clinics of North America, 104*(2), 293–311. https://doi.org/10.1016/j.mcna.2019.10.007

ACI Musculoskeletal Network. (2018). Neurovascular Assessment Guide. Retrieved 10 August 2022 from: https://aci.health.nsw.gov.au/__data/assets/pdf_file/0004/458185/ACI-Muscolskeletal-Neurovascular-assessment.pdf

Allen, K. D., Thoma, L. M., & Golightly, Y. M. (2022). Epidemiology of osteoarthritis. *Osteoarthritis and Cartilage, 30*(2), 184–95. https://doi.org/10.1016/j.joca.2021.04.020

Anderson, T.B., & Duong H. (2022). Weight Bearing. [Updated 8 May 2022]. In: StatPearls [Internet]. Treasure Island (FL): StatPearls Publishing; Jan 2022. Retrieved 7 August 2022 from: https://www.ncbi.nlm.nih.gov/books/NBK551573/)

ANZCOR. (2016). Australian and New Zealand Committee on Resuscitation, Guideline 9.1.6 – Management of Suspected Spinal Injury. Australian Resuscitation Council. Retrieved 23 February 2018 from: https://survive-student-resource.austererisk.com/trauma/anzcor_9_1_6_spinal_injury.html

Arthritis New Zealand. (2018). Economic cost of arthritis in New Zealand in 2018. Retrieved 6 December 2022 from: https://www.arthritis.org.nz/wp-content/uploads/Economic-Cost-of-Arthritis-in-New-Zealand-2018.pdf

Australian and New Zealand Falls Prevention Society. (2022). Information about falls. Retrieved 6 December 2022 from: https://www.anzfallsprevention.org/info/

Australian Bureau of Statistics (ABS). (2022). Health conditions prevalence. Retrieved 6 December 2022 from: https://www.abs.gov.au/statistics/health/health-conditions-and-risks/health-conditions-prevalence/2020-21#arthritis-and-osteoporosis

Australian Commission on Safety and Quality in Health Care (ACSQHC). (2017). Osteoarthritis of the knee clinical care standard. Clinical fact sheet. www.safetyandquality.gov.au/css

Australian Institute of Health and Welfare (AIHW). (2019). Musculoskeletal conditions and comorbidity in Australia. Retrieved 6 December 2022 from: https://www.aihw.gov.au/getmedia/e719c18d-d76d-46d2-b70a-a0b3c489afb4/aihw-phe-241.pdf.aspx?inline=true

Australian Institute of Health and Welfare (AIHW). (2020a). Back problems. Retrieved 6 December 2022 from: https://www.aihw.gov.au/reports/arthritis-other-musculoskeletal-conditions/back-problems/what-are-back-problems

Australian Institute of Health and Welfare (AIHW). (2020b). Osteoarthritis. Retrieved 6 December 2022 from: https://www.aihw.gov.au/reports/chronic-musculoskeletal-conditions/osteoarthritis/contents/about

Australian Institute of Health and Welfare (AIHW). (2020c). Rheumatoid arthritis. Retrieved 6 December 2022 from: https://www.aihw.gov.au/reports/chronic-musculoskeletal-conditions/rheumatoid-arthritis/contents/who-gets-rheumatoid-arthritis

Australian Institute of Health and Welfare (AIHW). (2020d). Juvenile arthritis. Retrieved 6 December 2022 from: https://www.aihw.gov.au/reports/phe/258-1/juvenile-arthritis/contents/summary

Australian Institute of Health and Welfare (AIHW). (2020e). Osteoporosis. Retrieved 12 December 2022 from: https://www.aihw.gov.au/reports/chronic-musculoskeletal-conditions/osteoporosis/contents/what-is-osteoporosis

Australian Institute of Health and Welfare (AIHW). (2022a). Chronic musculoskeletal conditions. Retrieved 6 December 2022 from:

UNIT 2

https://www.aihw.gov.au/reports-data/health-conditions-disability-deaths/chronic-musculoskeletal-conditions/overview

Australian Institute of Health and Welfare (AIHW). (2022b). Falls. Retrieved 6 December 2022 from: https://www.aihw.gov.au/reports/injury/falls

Department of Health and Aged Care (DHAC). (2020). What we're doing about musculoskeletal conditions. Australian Government. Retrieved 6 December 2022 from: https://www.health.gov.au/topics/chronic-conditions/what-were-doing-about-chronic-conditions/what-were-doing-about-musculoskeletal-conditions

Hunter, D. J., & Bierma-Zeinstra, S. (2019). Osteoarthritis. *The Lancet* (British Edition), *393*(10182), 1745–59. https://doi.org/10.1016/S0140-6736(19)30417-9

Katz, J. N., Arant, K. R., & Loeser, R. F. (2021). Diagnosis and treatment of hip and knee osteoarthritis: A review. *Journal of the American Medical Association*, *325*(6), 568–78. https://doi.org/10.1001/jama.2020.22171

Lao, C., Lees, D., Patel, S., White, D., & Lawrenson, R. (2019). Geographical and ethnic differences of osteoarthritis associated hip and knee replacement surgeries in New Zealand: a population-based cross-sectional study. *BMJ Open, 9*(9), e032993. doi:10.1

Ministry of Health. (2020). Health and Independence Report 2019: The Director-General of Health's Annual Report on the State of Public Health. Wellington: Ministry of Health. Retrieved 7 December 2022 from: https://www.health.govt.nz/publication/health-and-independence-report-2019

Osteoporosis NZ. (n.d). Retrieved 7 December 2022 from: https://osteoporosis.org.nz/osteoporosis-fractures/who-is-affected/

Royal Australian College of General Practitioners (RACGP). (2022). Osteoporosis prevention, diagnosis and management in postmenopausal women and men over 50 years of age. Retrieved 10 August 2022 from: https://www.racgp.org.au/clinical-resources/clinical-guidelines/key-racgp-guidelines/view-all-racgp-guidelines/osteoporosis

Safe Work Australia. (2019). Work-related musculoskeletal disorders in Australia. Retrieved 6 December 2022 from: https://www.safeworkaustralia.gov.au/system/files/documents/1912/work-related_musculoskeletal_disorders_in_australia_0.pdf

Scoliosis Australia. (2018). The National Self-Detection Program for Scoliosis. Retrieved 16 March 2018 from: https://www.scoliosis-australia.org/policies-programs/the-national-self-detection-program-for-scoliosis/

CHAPTER **17**

GENITOURINARY AND REPRODUCTIVE GENITALIA

LEARNING OUTCOMES

By the end of this chapter you should be able to:

1 describe the anatomy and physiology of female and male genitourinary and reproductive organs, including age-related changes
2 describe the techniques necessary for assessment of the genitourinary and reproductive systems
3 identify anatomic landmarks for genitourinary and reproductive systems
4 identify pathophysiological changes and explain possible aetiologies
5 identify health education opportunities for consumers in regard to specific genitourinary and reproductive health problems
6 discuss the clinical reasoning in evaluating outcomes of health assessment and physical examination including documentation, health education provision and relevant health referrals.

BACKGROUND

In this chapter male and female genitalia are presented and discussed under the construct of genitourinary and reproductive systems. The female will be explored first, then the male. The urinary system will be overviewed for both males and females, and includes focus on the kidneys, ureters and bladder.

FEMALE GENITALIA

In Australia and New Zealand, the common health problems of the female genitalia that may be encountered when undertaking an examination are:

> **vaginal infections** – the most common are bacterial vaginosis (BV) and Candida vaginosis (thrush) (Family Planning Australia, 2018). For both these infections, approximately 50% of women are asymptomatic.
> **sexually transmitted infections (STIs)** – most common are chlamydia, trichomoniasis, genital human papillomavirus (HPV) and genital herpes (herpes simplex virus). Chlamydia is the most common sexually transmitted infection in both Australia and New Zealand (HealthDirect, 2021; Health Navigator New Zealand, 2022a), and it can result in dramatic effects on a woman's health, such as pelvic inflammatory disease (PID), infertility and ectopic pregnancy. It is worth noting that the majority of STIs are asymptomatic or produce only mild symptoms. Women who are affected often find out they have an infection through routine screening.
> **cancers** – gynaecological cancers account for approximately 9 to 10% of female cancers in Australia and New Zealand (Cancer Council Australia, 2022a;

Allanson & Ayres, 2022). Benign tumours, known as leiomyomas or fibroids of the uterine muscle, are very common, especially in females over 60. Uterine cancer (endometrial adenocarcinoma) is the most common gynaecological cancer, with the incidence increasing in recent times, due to the ageing population and growing rate of obesity (Cancer Council, n.d.). With early detection the 5-year survival rate is 87%. Ovarian cancer is the second most commonly diagnosed gynaecological cancer and has the highest mortality rate. This is due to the fact that diagnosis often occurs when cancer is at an advanced stage and has metastasised, making it difficult to treat. Nevertheless, in the period 2014–18 the 5-year relative survival rate had increased significantly from 33% to 49% (Cancer Council Australia, 2022b).

The third most commonly diagnosed gynaecological cancer is cervical cancer, which has the lowest mortality rates, credited to the success of the National Cervical Screening Programs (NCSP – now using the HPV test) for early diagnosis. Further, it has been identified that most cervical cancers are caused by the infectious human papillomavirus (HPV), which can now be prevented through immunisation (Ministry of Health/Manatū Hauora, 2021a; Cancer Council, n.d.). In Australia, however, the success of the NCSP has not been as significant among the Aboriginal and Torres Strait Islander population (Cancer Council Australia, 2022c). This has been attributed to low screening participation and compliance with follow-up screenings.

Assessment of female genitalia is an area in which the nurse can have a major impact on consumer health through practices such as routine screening, education and integrating the consumer in the process of self-care. Assessment of the genitalia is often the last step in a woman's physical assessment and this process can be divided into *external examination* and *internal examination*. In most organisations, only advanced nurse practitioners examine the internal genitalia. However, general nurses may assist in these processes. Some women can be apprehensive about this examination procedure, especially if they have had a previous painful or embarrassing experience. By using therapeutic communication skills and by showing respect and understanding, as well as some basic techniques to reduce discomfort, these feelings can be diminished.

MALE GENITALIA

In Australia and New Zealand, the momentum continues to maintain public awareness about the recognition and prevention of male health problems. The release of the first Australian National Male Health Policy occurred in 2010 and included recognition of the unique needs of Aboriginal and Torres Strait Islander males (Australian Government Department of Health and Aged Care, 2010). Subsequent funding and initiatives to improve male health have continued through 'Healthy Male' and 'Spanner in the Works?' programs, as well as dedicated men's health portals on websites such as Your Health Link, which provide links to web-based resources selected by health professionals (AMSA, 2019; Healthy Male, 2022; Your Health link, 2022). In New Zealand, although the current public health agenda does not specifically address the needs of men (Xiao, Doolan-Noble, Liu, White & Baxter, 2022), best practice guidelines continue to be developed and updated (Centre for Men's Health, 2022). The health of New Zealand men is relatively high, and through improvements in the awareness of prostate and testicular cancers, antismoking campaigns and the promotion of healthy diet and exercise, it will continue to improve (Health Navigator New Zealand, 2022b).

Injuries to male genitalia can occur easily as the scrotum and penis are not protected by bones. Problems occur more commonly during recreation, such as sporting events, or during work activities that involve exposure to chemicals or hazards such as fall risk. Many of the male reproductive health issues can be supported by nurses through consumer health education, health screening and secondary prevention programs.

Assessment of the male genitalia is often the final part of the comprehensive health assessment. The majority of the assessment can be undertaken by any nurse, with a number of areas being identified for the advanced practitioner. Some men may be apprehensive about this examination, so it is important to utilise therapeutic communication skills, show respect and understanding, and have a sound, organised approach to your assessment.

In Australia and New Zealand, the common health problems of the male genitalia that may be encountered when undertaking an examination are:

> genital infections – prostatitis, epididymitis, **balanitis**
> sexually transmitted infections (STIs) – the most common are *Chlamydia trachomatis* infection, genital herpes (herpes simplex virus or HSV), genital warts and human papillomavirus (HPV). Chlamydia is the most common bacterial sexually transmitted infection. In Australia and New Zealand, the notification rate increased between 2015 and 2019, then declined in 2021; however, this is likely due to the COVID-19 pandemic and may not reflect the overall trend (Institute of Environmental Science and Research, 2021; Kirby Institute, 2022). Gonorrhoea, hepatitis A and B, and human immunodeficiency virus (HIV) that may result in acquired immune deficiency syndrome (AIDS) are other STIs of note (Kirby Institute, 2022; Ministry of Health/Manatù Hauora, 2021b)
> genital conditions – prostate cancer, testicular cancer, erectile dysfunction, **cystitis**, torsion of a testicle, hydrocoele and inguinal hernia.

Urinary system

The most common renal system health issues include the following conditions.

> Kidney infections and urinary tract infections (UTIs) are some of the most common renal system presentations for seeking medical attention. Aboriginal and Torres Strait Islander people are twice as likely to be affected. The prevalence of UTIs increases with age, with women aged over 65 more at risk (Australian Government Department of Health and Aged Care, 2019; Ministry of Health/ Manatù Hauora, 2017).
> Incontinence, which is described as accidental loss of urine, is also a significant issue affecting men and woman of all ages. (See Table 17.6.)
> Urinary stones (calculi) affect 1 in 10 people; they are hardened mineral deposits that form in the kidney and can grow in size. If they fail to pass through the urinary tract, they can grow too large to pass and can cause obstruction to the urinary drainage. Kidney stones (ureteric colic) affects 4 to 8 of 100 Australians (Kidney Health Australia, 2022).
> Renal system cancer: The risk of being diagnosed with bladder cancer is estimated as 1 in 97, with men three times more likely than women to be diagnosed, and individuals aged 85 years and over at greater risk. Kidney cancer affects 1 in 67 individuals by the age of 85 (Kidney Health Australia, 2022; ABS, 2018).
> Chronic kidney disease (CKD) refers to all conditions with reduced filtration by the kidney and/or by the leakage of protein or albumin in the urine. Diabetes mellitus and cardiovascular disease are the most common risk factors. Early stages of CKD are often underdiagnosed as many individuals have no signs or symptoms, so CKD is often diagnosed at advanced stages when symptoms are evident. The risk of kidney disease increases rapidly with age, affecting around 4 in 10 (42%) people aged 75 and over, with Aboriginal and Torres Strait Islander people twice as likely to have CKD than non-Indigenous Australians. End-stage kidney disease (ESKD) is the most severe form of CKD and people usually require kidney replacement therapy (KRT) – a kidney transplant – or dialysis to survive (AIHW, 2022; Ministry of Health/Manatù Hauora, 2023).

ANATOMY AND PHYSIOLOGY

Female

External female genitalia

The components of the external female genitalia are collectively referred to as the vulva. They consist of the mons pubis, labia majora, labia minora, clitoris, vulval vestibule and its glands, urethral meatus and vaginal introitus (**Figure 17.1**).

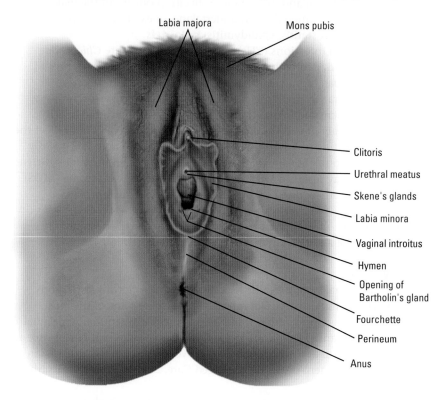

FIGURE 17.1 External female genitalia

The **mons pubis** is a pad of subcutaneous fatty tissue lying over the anterior symphysis pubis. At puberty, a characteristic triangular pattern of coarse, curly hair known as **escutcheon** develops over the mons pubis. The function of the mons pubis is to protect the pelvic bones, especially during coitus.

The **labia majora** are two longitudinal folds of adipose and connective tissue. They extend from the clitoris anteriorly and gradually narrow to merge and form the posterior commissure of the perineum. The outer surface of the labia majora becomes pigmented, wrinkled and hairy at puberty. The inner surface is smoother and softer, and contains sebaceous glands. The function of the labia majora is to protect the vulva components that it surrounds.

Within the labia majora are the **labia minora**, which enclose the vestibule. They are two thin folds of skin that extend to form the prepuce, or hood, of the clitoris anteriorly and a transverse fold of skin forming the **fourchette**, or frenulum, posteriorly. The labia minora contain sebaceous glands, erectile tissue, blood vessels and involuntary muscle tissue, but no adipose tissue or hair follicles. The secretions of the sebaceous glands are bactericidal and aid in lubricating the vulval skin and protecting the skin from urine. Both the labia majora and the labia minora contain genital corpuscles that transmit erotic sensation.

The **clitoris** is a cylinder-shaped erectile body approximately 2.5 cm in length and 0.5 cm in diameter, but normally less than 2.0 cm of the body is visible on inspection. It is located at the superior aspect of the vulva and between the labia minora. The clitoris contains erectile tissue and has a significant supply of nerve endings.

The **vestibule** is the area between the two skin folds of the labia minora. The vestibule is a boat-shaped area that contains the urethral meatus, the openings of the Skene's glands, the hymen, the openings of the Bartholin's glands and the vaginal introitus.

The external urethral meatus is located in the superior aspect of the vestibule, approximately 2.5 cm inferior to the clitoris. It is characterised as an elongated dimple or slit. Surrounding the urethral meatus are **Skene's glands**, also known as paraurethral glands, which provide lubrication to protect the skin. These tiny glands open in a posterolateral position to the urethral meatus, but they are not readily visible.

The **vaginal introitus** or orifice is situated at the inferior aspect of the vulval vestibule and is the entrance to the vagina. The size and shape of the vaginal introitus may vary. Surrounding the vaginal introitus is the **hymen**, an avascular, thin fold of connective tissue. It may be annular or crescentic in shape. The hymen may be broken by first-time sexual intercourse, strenuous physical activity, the use of tampons, masturbation or menstruation, or it may be congenitally absent. Once the hymenal ring is perforated, small, irregular tags of tissue may be visible at the vaginal opening.

In the cleft between the labia minora and the hymenal ring lie **Bartholin's glands**, also known as the greater vestibular glands. Bartholin's glands are small, pea-shaped glands located deep in the perineal structures. The ductal openings are not usually visible. The glands secrete a clear, viscid, odourless, alkaline mucus that improves the viability and motility of sperm along the female reproductive tract.

The **perineum** is located between the fourchette and the anus. Its composition of muscle, elastic fibres, fascia and connective tissue gives it an exceptional capacity for stretching during childbirth. The **anal orifice** is located at the seam of the gluteal folds, and it serves as the exit to the gastrointestinal tract.

Internal female genitalia

The components of the internal female genitalia are the vagina, uterus, fallopian tubes and ovaries (see **Figure 17.2**).

The **vagina** is a pink, hollow, muscular tube extending from the cervix to the vulva. It is located posterior to the bladder and anterior to the rectum, and it slopes backwards at an angle of approximately 45° with the vertical plane of the body. The cervix projects into the vagina. This projection creates pouch-like recesses around the cervix. These recesses are divided into anterior, posterior and lateral **fornices**. Abdominal organs such as the uterus, ovaries, appendix, caecum, colon, ureters and distended bladder can be palpated through the thin walls of these fornices.

The vaginal walls consist of an outer layer of longitudinal and circular muscle fibres and a stratified squamous epithelium arranged in folds called rugae. Lactic acid is formed by the normal vaginal flora from glycogen, which is contained in the superficial cells of the vagina. This maintains the vaginal pH and assists in the prevention of vaginal infections.

The **uterus** is an inverted, pear-shaped, hollow, muscular organ in which an impregnated ovum develops into a fetus. The inferior aspect is the **cervix**; the superior aspect is the **fundus**. The most common position of the uterus is anteverted, but it may also be anteflexed, retroverted, retroflexed or in midplane position (see **Figure 17.3**). The mature, nonpregnant uterus weighs about 60 g and is approximately 5.5 to 8.0 cm long, 3.5 to 4.0 cm wide and 2.0 to 2.5 cm thick. The uterus of a parous consumer, or one who has given birth, may be enlarged by 2 to 3 cm in any of the above dimensions.

UNIT 2

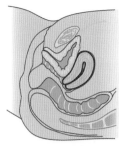

Anteverted
(most common)

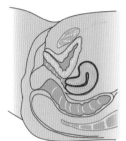

Anteflexed

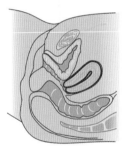

Midposition
(midplane)

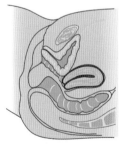

Retroverted
(palpable only during
rectovaginal exam)

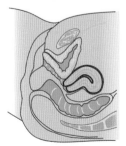

Retroflexed
(palpable only during
rectovaginal exam)

FIGURE 17.3 Positions of the uterus

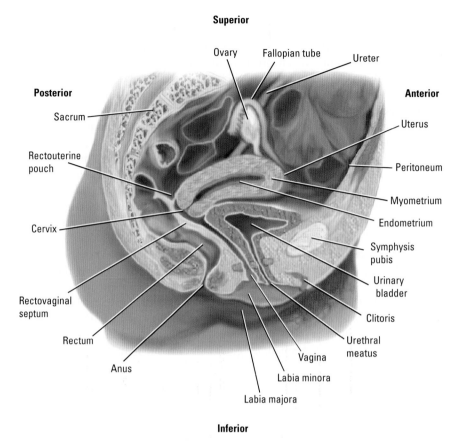

FIGURE 17.2 Left-sided sagittal section at midline of internal pelvic organs

Anatomically, the uterus can be divided into three parts: the body, the isthmus and the cervix (see **Figure 17.4**). The body consists of the fundus (a raised, dome-shaped area on the superior portion of the uterus) and the cornu (the points of insertion of the fallopian tubes). The uterine body has three layers: an outer layer of perimetrium; a middle layer of muscle called the myometrium; and the endometrium, an inner layer of columnar epithelium, mucous glands and stroma. It is this innermost layer that is shed and regenerated under normal hormonal influence during the menstrual cycle. The outer layer of the peritoneum forms a deep recess called the **rectouterine pouch**, or pouch of Douglas. It is the lowest point in the pelvic cavity and encompasses the lower posterior wall of the uterus, the upper portion of the vagina, and the intestinal surface of the rectum.

The **isthmus** is a constricted area between the body of the uterus and the cervix. The cervix is an open-ended canal approximately 2 to 3 cm in length and diameter. Its internal os (opening) is at the isthmus and its external os extends into the vagina. The os of the **nulliparous** woman, one who has not given birth, will be closed and tight. The os of a **parous** woman, one who has given birth to one or more neonates, may be open by 1 cm and the orifice may be elongated and irregular. The endocervical canal is lined with mucus-secreting columnar epithelium. The ectocervix, which protrudes into the vagina, is covered with the same squamous epithelial cells that line the vagina. The point at which the two types of cells merge is the **squamocolumnar junction**. Its exact location varies with age, but it is clinically important because it is the point at which most cervical cancer originates.

The **adnexa** of the uterus consists of the fallopian tubes, the ovaries, and their supporting ligaments. The **fallopian tubes** extend from the cornu of the uterus to the ovaries, and are supported by the broad ligaments. The tubes are approximately 8 to 14 cm long. The distal, funnel-shaped end of the fallopian tube is called the

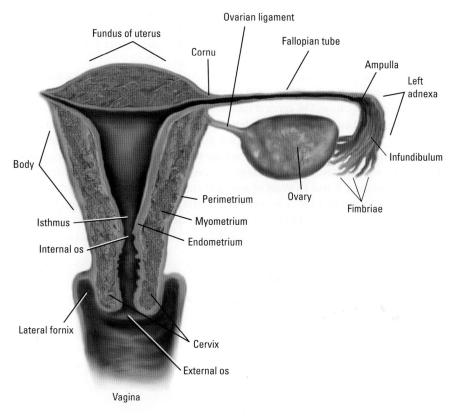

FIGURE 17.4 Coronal section of uterus and adnexal structures

infundibulum. It has moving, finger-like projections called fimbriae, which help direct ova from the ovary into the tube, where fertilisation takes place. The fallopian tubes are lined with ciliated squamous epithelium. The movement of the cilia and the peristaltic waves of the muscular layer of the tube propel the ovum towards the uterus, where implantation occurs.

The **ovaries** are a pair of almond-shaped glands, approximately 3 to 4 cm in length, in the upper pelvic cavity. **Oogenesis**, the development and formation of an ovum, and hormone production are the principal functions of the ovaries.

The **rectovaginal septum** separates the rectum from the posterior aspect of the vagina.

The female reproductive cycle

The female reproductive cycle consists of two interrelated cycles called the ovarian and the menstrual cycles. These cycles occur synchronously under neurohormonal control from the hypothalamus and the anterior pituitary gland.

The ovarian cycle consists of two phases: the follicular phase and the luteal phase. During the follicular phase, the actions of follicle-stimulating hormone (FSH) and luteinising hormone (LH) from the anterior pituitary gland stimulate the ripening of one ovarian follicle called a Graafian follicle. The remaining follicles are suppressed by LH. Ovulation occurs when high levels of LH cause the release of the ovum from the Graafian follicle. During the luteal phase, LH stimulates the development of the corpus luteum, a yellow pigmented body that fills the Graafian follicle and produces high levels of progesterone and low levels of oestrogen. The basal body temperature rises, indicating that ovulation has occurred.

The menstrual cycle begins if implantation does not occur. The corpus luteum degenerates and the levels of progesterone and oestrogen decrease, causing the endometrium to degenerate and shed. The menstrual flow lasts from 2 to 7 days and the cycles continue every 25 to 34 days, with the average being 28 days. The first day of the cycle is the first day of menstruation. The menstrual flow consists of blood and mucus and normally does not exceed 150 mL. Menstrual blood lacks fibrin; therefore, it does not clot. If clots do occur, they usually form in the vagina and are a combination of red blood cells, glycoproteins and mucus. Cyclic changes associated with the menstrual cycle are shown in **Figure 17.5**.

The proliferative phase of the menstrual cycle occurs when the endometrial lining begins to regenerate under the influence of oestrogen. Changes in the cervical mucosa also occur during this phase. The cervical mucus becomes clearer, thinner and thread-like.

If conception and implantation of the fertilised ovum occur, the corpus luteum is maintained by the presence of human chorionic gonadotropin (HCG), which is secreted by the implanting blastocyst. HCG is the hormone tested for in at-home pregnancy kits.

The female reproductive cycle begins at **menarche**, the onset of menstruation, which occurs between 9 and 16 years of age, and ends at menopause, which occurs between 45 and 55 years of age. The onset of puberty, which occurs between the ages of 8 and 9, is marked by significant increases in oestrogen production and the development of secondary sex characteristics such as breast enlargement, hair

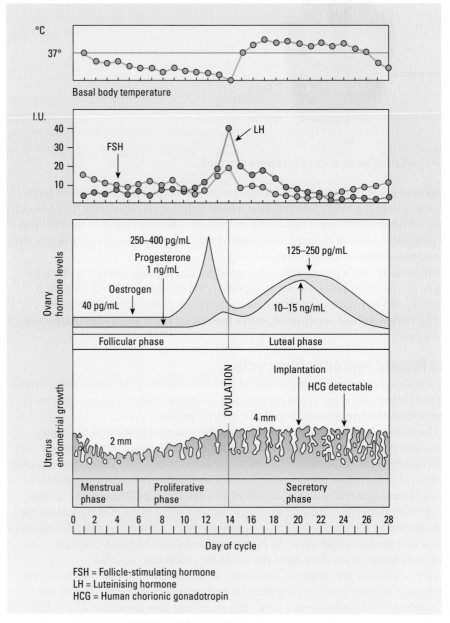

FSH = Follicle-stimulating hormone
LH = Luteinising hormone
HCG = Human chorionic gonadotropin

FIGURE 17.5 Cyclic changes associated with the menstrual cycle

distribution on the mons pubis, and contour changes of the hips and abdomen. Tanner's stages of pubic hair development provide objective criteria for the evaluation of developmental changes in the appearance of female genitalia (Table 17.1).

TABLE 17.1 Sexual maturity rating (SMR) for female genitalia

Stage 1	**Preadolescent stage** (before age 8) No pubic hair, only body hair (vellus hair)
Stage 2	**Early adolescent stage** (ages 8 to 12) Sparse growth of long, slightly dark, fine pubic hair, slightly curly and located along the labia
Stage 3	**Adolescent stage** (ages 12 to 13) Pubic hair becomes darker, curlier, and spreads over the symphysis
Stage 4	**Late adolescent stage** (ages 13 to 15) Texture and curl of pubic hair is similar to that of an adult but not spread to thighs
Stage 5	**Adult stage** Adult appearance in quality and quantity of pubic hair; growth is spread to inner aspect of thighs and abdomen

HEALTH EDUCATION

Consumer education on the reproductive cycle

Educating women about the reproductive cycle and its effects on the body assists them in improving their health literacy and empowers them to understand their body's functioning. It assists individuals in planning for gynaecological examinations and birth control measures.

This education should include:

> providing information about how to identify when ovulation is occurring – cervical mucus becomes clearer, thinner and thread-like

> explaining how she can perform her own **spinnbarkeit test**, the point at which the mucus can be drawn to maximal length, by stretching vaginal mucus between her thumb and index finger.

Inform the woman that:

> it is normal to feel low abdominal or flank pain when the ovum is released during ovulation

> a rise in basal body temperature indicates that ovulation has occurred

> occasionally spotting may be present after ovulation.

CLINICAL REASONING

Late onset of menarche

Late onset of menarche can result from a multiplicity of pathologies. You should evaluate the consumer for the following, and document findings. This is to ensure that there is baseline assessment data, as these types of delays may be linked to other health conditions in the future:

1. Pregnancy
2. Inadequate nutrition or eating disorders
3. Chronic diseases such as Crohn's disease, thyroid disease
4. Environmental stressors
5. Intensive athletic training
6. Use of opiates or steroids
7. Polycystic ovary syndrome
8. Autoimmune diseases
9. Anatomic obstruction to menstrual flow
10. Genetic or chromosomal syndromes
11. Hypothalamic–pituitary–ovarian axis disorders

Male reproductive system

The male reproductive system includes essential and accessory organs, ducts and supporting structures (see Figure 17.6). The essential organs are the testes, or male gonads. The accessory organs include the seminal vesicles and bulbourethral glands. There are also several ducts, including the epididymis, ductus (vas) deferens, ejaculatory ducts and urethra. The supporting structures include the scrotum, penis and spermatic cords. The prostate is discussed in Chapter 18.

Organs, ducts, supporting structures and sexual development are discussed.

Essential organs

The **testes**, or testicles, are two oval glands located in the scrotum. Each measures about 5 cm in length and 2.5 cm in width. The testes are partially covered by a serous membrane called the tunica vaginalis (see Figure 17.7). This membrane separates the testes from the scrotal wall. Interior to the tunica vaginalis is a dense, whitish membrane covering each testicle called the tunica albuginea. This membrane enters the testes and divides each testis into sections called lobules, which contain the tightly coiled seminiferous tubules. These coiled structures are the main components of testicular mass, and they produce sperm by spermatogenesis.

Accessory organs

The **seminal vesicles** are two pouches located posteriorly to and at the base of the bladder. They contribute about 60% of the volume of semen. The fluid secreted by the seminal vesicles is rich in fructose and helps provide a source of energy for sperm metabolism. Prostaglandins, which contribute to sperm motility and viability, are also produced by the seminal vesicles.

The **bulbourethral glands**, or Cowper's glands, are pea-sized glands located just below the prostate. Secretions are emptied from the bulbourethral glands at the time of ejaculation. The bulbourethral glands secrete an alkaline substance that protects sperm by neutralising the acidic environment of the vagina. These glands also provide lubrication at the end of the penis during sexual intercourse.

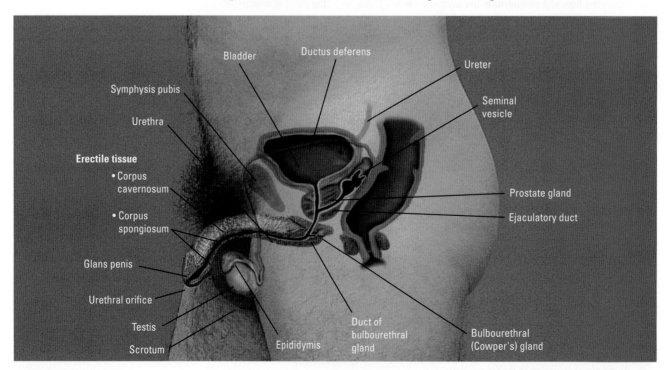

FIGURE 17.6 Male genitalia

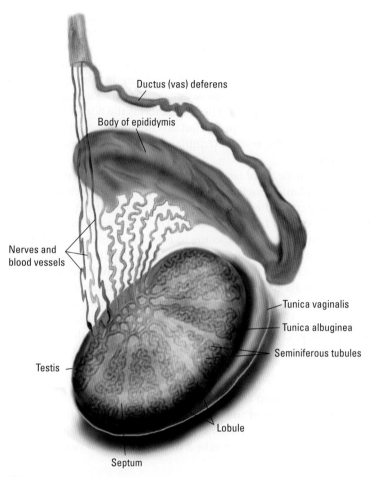

Ductus (vas) deferens

Body of epididymis

Nerves and blood vessels

Tunica vaginalis

Tunica albuginea

Seminiferous tubules

Testis

Lobule

Septum

FIGURE 17.7 Testicle

Ducts

The **epididymis** is a comma-shaped, tightly coiled tube that is located on the top and behind the testis and inside the scrotum. Each epididymis is composed of three parts: the head, which is connected to the testis; the body; and the tail, which is continuous with the vas deferens. Sperm mature and develop the power of motility as they pass through the epididymis.

The **ductus (vas) deferens** is an extension of the tail of the epididymis. Each duct ascends from the scrotum and permits sperm to exit from the scrotal sac upwards into the abdominal cavity. The ductus deferens loops over the side and down the posterior surface of the bladder. This is where the duct enlarges into the ampulla of the vas deferens and joins the duct from the seminal vesicles to form the ejaculatory ducts.

The **ejaculatory ducts** are two short tubes posterior to the bladder. They descend through the prostate gland and terminate in the urethra. The ducts eject spermatozoa into the prostatic urethra just prior to ejaculation.

The **urethra** is the terminal duct of the seminal fluid passageway. It measures about 20 cm in length, passes through the prostate gland and penis, and terminates at the external urethral orifice.

Supporting structures

The **scrotum** is a pouch-like supporting structure for the testes. It consists of rugated, deeply pigmented, loose skin. Inside, the scrotum is divided by a single septum into two sacs, each containing a single testis. The production and survival of sperm requires a temperature that is 1°C cooler than normal body temperature (37°C). This is achieved by the scrotum's exposed location.

The **penis**, or male organ of copulation and urination, is hairless, slightly pigmented, and cylindrical in shape. It consists of three compartments of erectile tissue. The corpus spongiosum surrounds the urethra and is located ventromedially. The two corpora cavernosa are located on the dorsolateral sides of the corpus spongiosum. Distally, the corpus spongiosum expands to form the **glans penis**, or the bulbous end of the penis. In the uncircumcised male, a fold of loose skin, the **prepuce** (foreskin), covers the glans penis. The corona forms the border between the glans penis and the penile shaft. The penis contains the urethra, a slit-like opening on the tip of the glans. The urethra terminates at the urethral meatus and is the passageway for urine.

The **spermatic cord** is made up of testicular arteries, autonomic nerves, veins that drain the testicles, lymphatic vessels and the cremaster muscle. Each testicle is suspended by a spermatic cord. The left spermatic cord is longer than the right, causing the left testicle to be lower in the scrotal sac. The cremaster muscles elevate the testes during sexual stimulation and exposure to cold. They also surround the testicles. The spermatic cord and ilioinguinal nerves pass through the inguinal canal into the abdomen. The inguinal canal is an oblique passageway in the anterior abdominal wall. The canal is about 4 to 5 cm long. It originates at the deep inguinal ring. The distal opening of the inguinal canal is called the external inguinal ring and is accessible to palpation. Superior to the inguinal canal lies the inguinal ligament, or Poupart's ligament. The inguinal ligament extends from the anterior iliac spine to the pubic tubercle.

Sexual development

Sexual development can be assessed according to the five stages described by Tanner (1962) (see Table 17.2). Most of the changes in the male genitalia occur during puberty, starting between 9½ and 13½ years of age. The development of male genitalia to adult size and shape can take 2 to 5 years, with 3 years being the average.

Spermatogenesis

The primary function of the male reproductive system is to produce sperm to fertilise eggs. For this to be achieved, there are several essential features of male reproduction that must take place. These are the manufacture of sperm and the deposition of sperm into the female genital tract.

The testes produce sperm by a process called **spermatogenesis**. Specialised cells found between the seminiferous tubules, called the interstitial cells of Leydig, secrete the male hormone testosterone. Testosterone is sometimes called an androgen and is responsible for the development of secondary sexual characteristics and the attainment of reproductive capacity. Testosterone is responsible for male sexual feelings and performance as well as muscle development. The testes prepare for sperm production at approximately 13 years of age.

Male sexual function

The male sexual act consists of four stages: erection, lubrication, emission and ejaculation. Erection of the penis is the first stage and is achieved through either physical or psychogenic stimulation of sensory nerves in the genital area. Parasympathetic impulses from the sacral portion of the spinal cord cause a vascular effect. The arterioles dilate and blood fills the corpora cavernosa, causing the penis to expand and become rigid. The corpora cavernosa can hold from 20 to 50 mL of blood. The veins from the tissue are compressed to occlude venous outflow.

At the same time, parasympathetic impulses cause the bulbourethral glands to secrete mucus, which provides lubrication during intercourse. When the sexual stimulus reaches a critical intensity, the reflex centres of the spinal cord send sympathetic impulses to the genital organs, and an orgasm occurs. Emission begins

TABLE 17.2 Sexual maturity rating (SMR) for male genitalia

DEVELOPMENTAL STAGE	PUBIC HAIR	PENIS	SCROTUM
1.	No pubic hair, only fine body hair (vellus hair)	Preadolescent; childhood size and proportion	Preadolescent; childhood size and proportion
2.	Sparse growth of long, slightly dark, straight hair	Slight or no growth	Growth in testes and scrotum; scrotum reddens and changes texture
3.	Becomes darker and coarser; slightly curled and spreads over symphysis	Growth, especially in length	Further growth
4.	Texture and curl of pubic hair is similar to that of an adult but not spread to thighs	Further growth in length; diameter increases; development of glans	Further growth; scrotum darkens
5.	Adult appearance in quality and quantity of pubic hair; growth is spread to medial surface of thighs	Adult size and shape	Adult size and shape

Source: Tanner, J.M. (1962). Growth at adolescence (2nd ed.). Oxford: Blackwell Science.

with contraction of the epididymis and the vas deferens, causing expulsion of sperm into the internal urethra. Ejaculation follows with contractions of the penile urethra.

Anatomy and physiology of the urinary system

Kidneys, ureters and bladder

The kidneys are bean-shaped organs that lie tucked against the posterior abdominal wall (Figure 17.8). The left kidney is slightly larger in some individuals. Because of the superior placement of the liver over the right kidney, that kidney tends to hang about 1.5 cm lower than the left, between T12 and L3.

The primary function of the kidneys is to rid the body of waste products and to maintain homeostasis through regulation of the acid–base balance, fluid and electrolyte balance, and arterial blood pressure.

Urine leaves the kidneys via the ureters. Peristaltic waves move the waste products to the bladder. The bladder stores the urine. Normally the bladder holds 200 to 400 mL of urine; however, its capacity is greater.

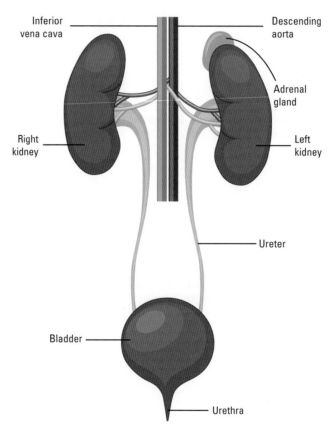

FIGURE 17.8 Urinary system

ASSESSMENT: TAKING THE CONSUMER'S HEALTH HISTORY

Assessment is the first phase of the nursing process and involves collecting subjective information about the consumer's health status in order to identify consumer problem areas to focus on.

Subjective data is most frequently collected during a health history and serves as the starting point for the health professional to base the depth of their assessment on. The sections for the health history include:

> **Consumer profile**

>>

>>

> > Chief complaint (explained systematically using variations of location, quality, quantity, associated manifestations, aggravating factors, alleviating factors, setting and timing. This is a variation on the PQRST assessment mnemonic you may use for other conditions such as pain assessment)
>
> > Past health history (including medical history, surgical history, allergies, medications, injuries and accidents, special needs and childhood illnesses)
>
> > Family health history
>
> > Social history (including alcohol, tobacco and drug use, sexual practice, work and home environment, hobbies and leisure activities, stress and culture).

The example health history provided identifies scope for questioning the consumer about their health for this specific body system. Female health history will be presented first, followed by the male health history.

HEALTH HISTORY – FEMALE			
CONSUMER PROFILE	Diseases that are age- and ethnic-specific for the female genitalia are listed.		
	AGE	> Sexually transmitted infections (STIs), (increased incidence 15–25) > Uterine myomas (30–50) > Cervical cancer (40–60) > Vulval cancer (postmenopause) > Uterine prolapse (postmenopause) > Cystocoele (postmenopause) > Rectocoele (postmenopause) > Atrophic vaginitis (postmenopause) > Endometrial cancer (diagnosis is usually made between 55 and 69) > Vaginal cancer (over 60) > Ovarian cancer (risk increases with age; highest rates are between 65 and 84)	
CHIEF COMPLAINT	Common chief complaints for the female genitalia are defined and information on the characteristics of each sign or symptom is provided.		
	1. UTERINE BLEEDING	The presence of bleeding from the endometrium	
		QUALITY	Odour, consistency, colour, clotting
		QUANTITY	Amount (number and size of tampons or pads used in 24 hours), duration and frequency of flow
		ASSOCIATED MANIFESTATIONS	Abdominal pain or cramping, passage of clots or tissue
		AGGRAVATING FACTORS	Stress, anxiety, medications (aspirin, NSAIDs), rapid weight loss or gain, obesity, sexual intercourse
		ALLEVIATING FACTORS	Medication, dilatation and curettage, surgery
		SETTING	Traumatic abortion or dilatation and curettage
		TIMING	Relationship to menses (intermenstrual, oligomenorrhoea, polymenorrhoea, menometrorrhagia, metrorrhagia); use of intrauterine device (IUD); perimenopausal
	2. VAGINAL DISCHARGE	The presence of a leaky discharge of fluid from the vagina	
		QUALITY	Colour, consistency, odour
		QUANTITY	Number and size of tampons or pads used in 24 hours
		ASSOCIATED MANIFESTATIONS	Itching, presence of discharge in sexual partner, **dyspareunia** (painful sexual intercourse), dysuria, abdominal pain or cramping, spotting
		AGGRAVATING FACTORS	Tight pants, wet swimming costume, antibiotics, birth control pills, diet, pregnancy, deodorant, tampons, bubble bath, chemical douches, lubricated condoms, contraceptive creams, pre-existing disease such as diabetes mellitus, increased number of sexual partners, semen, vaginal films, latex products

>>

>>

HEALTH HISTORY – FEMALE

		ALLEVIATING FACTORS	Position, loose-fitting pants, cotton underpants and pantyhose with cotton crotch, medication
		TIMING	Postcoital, while taking antibiotics
3. URINARY SYMPTOMS		Changes in the normal voiding pattern and in characteristics of the urine	
		QUALITY	Colour: straw, amber; microscopic or macroscopic haematuria; consistency: clear, cloudy; presence of particles; odour
		QUANTITY	Polyuria, oliguria or anuria
		ASSOCIATED MANIFESTATIONS	Flank pain, abdominal pain or cramping, dysuria, abdominal distension, vaginal discharge, urgency and frequency in voiding, stress incontinence, pneumaturia, fever
		AGGRAVATING FACTORS	Douches, intravaginal devices, traumatic coitus, alcohol, caffeine, spices, delaying urination
		ALLEVIATING FACTORS	Medication, warm baths, hydration
		SETTING	Postcoital, nocturia
		TIMING	At beginning, throughout, or end of stream
4. DYSURIA		Painful urination	
		LOCATION	Suprapubic, near urinary meatus, costovertebral angle
		QUALITY	Burning, stabbing
		ASSOCIATED MANIFESTATIONS	Lower abdominal/suprapubic/lower back pain, fever, chills, current bacterial infection, haematuria, urinary leakage/burning, decreased urinary flow, urgency, hesitancy, nocturia, recent sexual intercourse
		AGGRAVATING FACTORS	Presence of renal calculi, decreased oral fluid intake
		ALLEVIATING FACTORS	Use of non-pharmacological pain management, such as heat pack on lower abdomen; medications (antibiotics, analgesics/urinary alkaliser such as Ural), passage or surgical removal of stone, increased oral fluid intake (some of these alleviators will depend on the cause of dysuria; for example, urinary alkalisers and frequent bladder emptying for urinary tract infection)
		SETTING	New sexual partner in the last 6 months, a sexual partner known to have other sexual partners, unprotected intercourse, wiping genitalia back to front (female)
		TIMING	At start of urination, midstream, throughout stream, sense of urgency, pregnancy
5. NOCTURIA		Night arousal to void	
		ASSOCIATED MANIFESTATIONS	Hesitancy, decrease in force of urinary stream, postvoid dribbling, urge incontinence
		AGGRAVATING FACTORS	Diabetes mellitus, diuretics, urinary tract infection, alcohol ingestion, anticholinergic medications, decongestants and cough medicines
		ALLEVIATING FACTORS	Adrenergic antagonists, 5-alpha-reductase inhibitors, transurethral resection of prostate, elimination of causative medications
6. URINARY INCONTINENCE		Any involuntary or abnormal urine loss	
		QUALITY	Constant, intermittent, dribbling, large volumes, hesitancy
		QUANTITY	Frequency, urgency, number of pads used
		ASSOCIATED MANIFESTATIONS	Recent surgery, coughing, sneezing, crying, laughing, heavy lifting, activity, medications, urinary tract infection, constipation, spinal cord lesions, neurological disease
		AGGRAVATING FACTORS	Medications, caffeine intake, alcohol intake

>>

HEALTH HISTORY – FEMALE

		ALLEVIATING FACTORS	Pelvic floor muscle rehabilitation, bladder training, biofeedback, anti-incontinence devices, medications
		SETTING	Accessibility of toilet, distance to toilet, adequate lighting to toilet, handrails by toilet, height of toilet seat
		TIMING	Nocturia
	7. PELVIC PAIN	The subjective sense of discomfort in the pelvis	
		QUALITY	Stabbing, burning, cramping, aching, throbbing, drawing, pulling
		ASSOCIATED MANIFESTATIONS	Abdominal distension, pelvic fullness, vaginal discharge or bleeding, gastrointestinal symptoms, menstruation, fever, ectopic pregnancy, pelvic inflammatory disease (PID)
		AGGRAVATING FACTORS	Exercise, sexual activity, cultural perception
		ALLEVIATING FACTORS	Rest, medication, surgery, heating pad, NSAIDs
		SETTING	During coitus, ovulation
		TIMING	Sudden or gradual onset, association with activity, duration, recurrence, relation to menstrual cycle
PAST HEALTH HISTORY	The various components of the past health history are linked to female genitalia pathology and female genitalia-related information.		
	MEDICAL HISTORY	FEMALE GENITALIA-SPECIFIC	See Table 17.3: Female reproductive health history
		NON-FEMALE-GENITALIA SPECIFIC	Diabetes mellitus, thyroid disease, incontinence, constipation, urinary tract infections
	SURGICAL HISTORY	Hysterectomy, myomectomy, salpingectomy, oophorectomy, dilatation and curettage, laparoscopy, vulvectomy, tubal ligation, colpotomy, caesarean section, colposcopy, cryotherapy, uterine cryoablation, hysteroscopy	
	ALLERGIES	Numerous feminine hygiene products may cause allergic reactions or increase the incidence of Candida vaginosis. Be aware of any latex allergies; condoms and diaphragms are usually made of latex. The spermicide nonoxynol-9 may also cause allergic reactions	
	MEDICATIONS	Antibiotics may increase incidence of Candida vaginosis and lessen the effectiveness of oral contraceptives	
	COMMUNICABLE DISEASES	STI: gonorrhoea, syphilis, herpes, HIV/AIDS, hepatitis, chlamydia, human papillomavirus, hepatitis B and C, trichomoniasis, chancroid, molluscum contagiosum	
	INJURIES AND ACCIDENTS	Abdominal trauma, rape, sexual abuse, vaginal trauma or injuries, pelvic fractures, lumbar spine, sacrococcygeal injuries	
	SPECIAL NEEDS	Paraplegic and quadriplegic consumers are at increased obstetric risk depending on level of injury, tone of uterus, and competency of cervix	
	CHILDHOOD ILLNESSES	Fetal diethylstilboestrol (DES) exposure	
	IMMUNISATIONS	Gardasil (HPV vaccine)	
FAMILY HEALTH HISTORY	Female genitalia diseases that are familial are listed: Cancers of the reproductive organs, mother received DES while pregnant with consumer, transfer of STIs during delivery, placental transfer of hepatitis B and hepatitis C, HIV/AIDS, multiple pregnancies, congenital anomalies		
SOCIAL HISTORY	The components of the social history that are linked to female genitalia factors and pathology		
	ALCOHOL USE	There is a significant positive correlation between alcohol use and date rape in the young adult population.	

HEALTH HISTORY – FEMALE

TOBACCO USE		There is an increased incidence of strokes and thrombotic events in women who concurrently smoke and use hormonal therapy. Smoking is a risk factor for cervical cancer.
SEXUAL PRACTICE		Often, sexual favours are exchanged for narcotics, leading to increased rates of STIs. Prostitution increases the risk of STIs, HIV/AIDS, hepatitis and cervical carcinoma (an increase in the number of partners increases the risk of human papillomavirus, which can lead to dysplasia and possible cervical cancer).
HOME ENVIRONMENT		Poor sanitation may lead to numerous forms of vaginitis and infections; overcrowding is an ideal condition for mite infestation.
HOBBIES AND LEISURE ACTIVITIES		Wearing a wet swimming costume for extended periods of time may increase the likelihood of Candida vaginosis. Strenuous equestrian sports and off-road cycling increase the likelihood of external genitalia trauma from saddle injuries. Female athletes may suffer from **amenorrhoea** (absent menses).
STRESS		Stress can have significant effects on menstruation, causing amenorrhoea and exacerbating genital herpes simplex.

TABLE 17.3 Female reproductive health history

Menstrual history	Age of menarche, last menstrual period (LMP), length of cycle, regularity of cycle, duration of menses, amenorrhoea, menorrhagia, presence of clots or vaginal pooling, number and type of tampons or pads used during menses, dysmenorrhoea, spotting between menses, missed menses
Reproductive medical history	Vaginal infections, yeast infections, salpingitis, endometritis, endometriosis, cervicitis, fibroids, ovarian cysts, cancer of the reproductive organs, infertility, HPV test records
Obstetric history	See Chapter 19
Premenstrual syndrome (PMS)	Symptoms occur from 3 to 7 days before the onset of menses, with cessation of symptoms after second day of cycle. Symptoms include breast tenderness; bloating; moodiness; cravings for salt, sugar or chocolate; fatigue; weight gain; headaches; joint pain; nausea and vomiting
Menopause history	Menopause (cessation of menstruation), spotting, associated symptoms of menopause (such as hot flushes, palpitations, numbness, tingling, drenching sweats, mood swings, vaginal dryness, itching), treatment for symptoms (including oestrogen replacement therapy), feelings about menopause
Vaginal discharge	See Chief complaint section
History of uterine bleeding	See Chief complaint section
Sexual functioning	Sexual preference, number of partners, interest, satisfaction, dyspareunia, anorgasmia
Method of birth control	Type, frequency of use, methods to prevent STIs, any associated problems with birth control or STI-prevention methods, such as a reaction to the spermicides used with the vaginal sponges, diaphragms and condoms

HEALTH EDUCATION

Menstruation – the unmentionable

Millions of girls around the world are stigmatised simply because they menstruate. Social norms and stigma about the female body and roles can set off early patterns of linking a natural process to being dirty and shameful.

Many girls and young adults from vulnerable communities can face significant challenges to manage their menstrual cycle safely and confidently. This is related to a combination of factors such as lack of education, cost of products, and uncertainty of how to use products. This situation is known as period poverty, as it creates a sense of shame and embarrassment to talk about periods, resulting in many not participating in school, work or other aspects of daily life (Connory & WhyHive, 2021).

Research has found more than 1 in 5 people who menstruate, improvise by using items including toilet paper and socks due to cost of pads or tampons. These improvisations can cause dangerous physical health impacts such as vaginal and urinary tract infections, severe reproductive health conditions and toxic shock syndrome.

Menstrual Hygiene Day is a global annual awareness day on 28 May, aimed at reducing the stigma surrounding menstruation and educating on the importance of good menstrual hygiene management.

As a healthcare professional, consider:

> decreasing the menstrual taboo by normalising conversations about menstruation, including raising awareness about the challenges regarding access to menstrual products and period-friendly sanitation facilities.
> empowering young girls through education to manage their periods as a natural process devoid of social judgement. Education should include what menstrual products are available and what suits an individual's budget. Also be cognisant of personal situations and the possibility of period poverty.
> being an advocate in the health community to encourage awareness of sustainable and affordable menstrual products. Of note, Australia and New Zealand have commenced providing free menstrual products in some schools.

Further information:

Share the dignity: https://www.sharethedignity.org.au/

Menstrual Hygiene Day: https://menstrualhygieneday.org/about/about-mhday/

HEALTH EDUCATION

Menstrual products and sustainability

Many disposable sanitary products have a negative impact on the environment due to plastic waste culminating in oceans and landfills. Sustainable menstruation is being mindful of the negative effects of these products and focuses on the access to sustainable menstruation products that are affordable.

There are several sustainable products that a menstruating person can consider:

> Menstrual cups – bell-shaped devices that are inserted into the vagina and collect menstrual blood. These are the most environmentally friendly product and cost-effective option.
> Period underwear – reusable underwear that has many lining layers, to absorb menstrual blood. These can be rinsed, washed and re-used. There are also options for period swimwear, leotards and athletic shorts.
> Sustainable options for disposable menstrual products – these products are more environmentally friendly and include disposable pads that are non-chlorine bleached, and tampons made with organic cotton and without harmful chemicals.

HEALTH HISTORY – MALE

CONSUMER PROFILE	The male genitalia health history provides insight into the link between a consumer's life and lifestyle and male genitalia information and pathology. Diseases that are age- and ethnic-specific for the male genitalia are listed.	
	AGE	> *Chlamydia trachomatis* (14–35) > Testicular torsion (12–25 + 40–50) > Varicocele (15–35) > Testicular cancer (16–39) > Gonococcal urethritis (<35) > Epididymitis, sexually associated (<35) > Epididymitis, urinary pathogens (<35) > Hydrocoele (>30) > Spermatocoele (>30) > Testicular lymphoma (50+) > Erectile dysfunction (50+) > Bacteriuria (>65)

>>

HEALTH HISTORY – MALE

		CULTURAL BACKGROUND	CAUCASIAN	Testicular cancer
CHIEF COMPLAINT		Common chief complaints for the male genitalia are defined and information on the characteristics of each sign or symptom is provided.		

	1. URETHRAL DISCHARGE	Excretion of substance from the urethra	
		QUALITY	Colour: clear, white, purulent, blood-tinged, green, yellow, pink; consistency: thin, moderate, thick, mucoid; foul odour
		QUANTITY	Absent, scant, mild, moderate, copious
		ASSOCIATED MANIFESTATIONS	Dysuria, painful ejaculation, fever, urethral meatal discharge, change in frequency of urination, pruritus, conjunctivitis, arthritis, dermatological rash, STI
		AGGRAVATING FACTORS	Urethral trauma
		ALLEVIATING FACTORS	Medications (antibiotics, analgesics)
		SETTING	A new sexual partner in the last 6 months, multiple partners, a partner known to have other partners, unprotected intercourse
		TIMING	More prominent in the morning before urinating
	2. PALPABLE MASS	A lump in the male genitalia	
		QUALITY	Firm, smooth, stellate, soft, mobile, nonmobile, well circumscribed, poorly circumscribed, 'bag of worms', hard, heavy, transilluminating, non-transilluminating, fluctuant, separate from testes
		ASSOCIATED MANIFESTATIONS	Pain, scrotal enlargement, absence of pain, vague back or abdominal pain, gynaecomastia (if mass produces oestrogen or human chorionic gonadotropin), nausea, vomiting, generalised oedema
		AGGRAVATING FACTORS	Positioning, palpation or pressure, obesity, lifting, oedema
		ALLEVIATING FACTORS	Medications, surgical removal or repair, positioning
		SETTING	Post-trauma, recurrent testicular pain
		TIMING	Mumps orchitis present 7–10 days following parotitis
	3. SCROTAL PAIN	Discomfort in the scrotal sac	
		QUALITY	Dull, sharp, heavy
		ASSOCIATED MANIFESTATIONS	Scrotal swelling, groin pain, lower abdominal pain, flank pain, dysuria, urinary frequency, fever, nausea, vomiting, pyuria, urethral discharge, scrotal oedema, erythema, infertility
		AGGRAVATING FACTORS	Sexual encounter, urinary tract infection, scrotal trauma
		ALLEVIATING FACTORS	Medications (antibiotics, analgesics), bed rest, scrotal elevation, surgery
		SETTING	New sexual partner months prior, unprotected intercourse, recent urinary instrumentation
		TIMING	Epididymitis may present months following a new or unprotected sexual encounter; it may also present shortly after a urinary tract infection
	4. ERECTILE DYSFUNCTION	The inability or decrease in ability to achieve and maintain a penile erection or to ejaculate seminal fluid	
		QUALITY	Inability to achieve erection (failed nocturnal tumescence test), ability to achieve with failure to maintain erection, inability to achieve complete erection, inability to ejaculate
		ASSOCIATED MANIFESTATIONS	Anxiety, systemic disease (diabetes mellitus, hypertension, coronary artery disease), decreased libido, phimosis, decreased or absent cremasteric reflex, decreased femoral pulses, trauma, recent transurethral resection of the prostate or prostatectomy surgery, testicular atrophy

HEALTH HISTORY – MALE

		AGGRAVATING FACTORS	Medications (beta blockers, diuretics, reserpine, monoamine oxidase inhibitors, selective serotonin re-uptake inhibitors, diazepam, alprazolam, chemotherapeutic agents, codeine, oxycodone), anxiety, unsupportive partner, alcohol, smoking, elevated blood glucose, hyperthyroidism, hypothyroidism
		ALLEVIATING FACTORS	Medications (hormone therapy, anxiolytics, phosphodiesterase type 5 inhibitors, alprostadil), injections, implants, vascular surgery, sex counselling, avoiding alcohol, smoking cessation, change in diet (avoiding foods high in saturated fat or cholesterol), maintaining ideal body weight, reducing tension and stress, vacuum erectile device
		SETTING	Uncomfortable physical environment, stress
		TIMING	Nocturnal tumescence
	5. PENILE LESION	A growth on the penis	
		QUALITY	Colour: erythematous, hyperpigmented, hypopigmented, pink, brown, black Presentation: flat, raised, indurated, papular, macular; multiple, isolated, ulcerated; warty, exudative (clear, purulent, bloody drainage)
		ASSOCIATED MANIFESTATIONS	Fever, malaise, inguinal lymphadenopathy, pain, prodromal numbness and tingling at lesion site, myalgias, headache, pruritus, immunosuppression, systemic illness, recurrent herpes simplex virus (HSV), human papillomavirus (HPV)
		AGGRAVATING FACTORS	Stress, systemic illness, immunosuppression
		ALLEVIATING FACTORS	Medications (antivirals, antibiotics), surgical removal, lifestyle changes
		SETTING	Unprotected intercourse, multiple sexual partners
		TIMING	Lymphogranuloma venereum: papule appears 1–3 weeks after inoculation; primary HSV: lesions appear 2–7 days after inoculation, vesicles ulcerate in 3–4 days; recurrent HSV: lesions appear a few hours to days after prodromal symptoms, lesions last approximately 10 days
	6. URINARY SYMPTOMS	Changes in the normal voiding pattern and in characteristics of the urine	
		QUALITY	Colour: straw, amber; microscopic or macroscopic haematuria; consistency: clear, cloudy; presence of particles; odour
		QUANTITY	Polyuria, oliguria, anuria terminal dribbling, urinary retention
		ASSOCIATED MANIFESTATIONS	Dysuria, abdominal pain or cramping, abdominal distension, erectile disfunction penile discharge, urgency and frequency in voiding, benign prostatic hyperplasia; stress incontinence, fever
		AGGRAVATING FACTORS	STIs (Chlamydia and gonorrhoea), prostate problems – enlarged prostate; prostatitis, diabetes and medical conditions that can affect immune system, traumatic coitus, alcohol, caffeine, spices, delaying urination
		ALLEVIATING FACTORS	Antibiotics, medication hydration, pelvic floor exercises and muscle/bladder training
		SETTING	Postcoital, nocturia
		TIMING	At beginning, throughout, or end of stream
	7. DYSURIA	Painful urination	
		LOCATION	Suprapubic, near urinary meatus, costovertebral angle lower abdomen and lower back
		QUALITY	Burning, stabbing, stinging
		ASSOCIATED MANIFESTATIONS	Abdominal/flank/testicular pain, fever, chills, current bacterial infection, haematuria, dribbling, urethral discharge, decreased urinary flow, urgency, hesitancy, nocturia, recent sexual intercourse

>>

HEALTH HISTORY – MALE

		AGGRAVATING FACTORS	Presence of prostatic stones or renal calculi, decreased oral fluid intake
		ALLEVIATING FACTORS	Medications (antibiotics, analgesics), passage or surgical removal of stone, transurethral resection of the prostate, increased oral intake (some of these alleviators will depend on the cause of dysuria; for example, urinary alkalisers and frequent bladder emptying for urinary tract infection)
		SETTING	New sexual partner in the last 6 months, a sexual partner known to have other sexual partners, unprotected intercourse
		TIMING	At start of urination, midstream, throughout stream, sense of urgency
	8. NOCTURIA	Night arousal to void	
		ASSOCIATED MANIFESTATIONS	Hesitancy, decrease in force of urinary stream, postvoid dribbling, urge incontinence
		AGGRAVATING FACTORS	Enlarged prostate, diabetes mellitus, diuretics, urinary tract infection, alcohol ingestion, anticholinergic medications, diuretics, decongestants and cough medicines
		ALLEVIATING FACTORS	Adrenergic antagonists, 5–alpha-reductase inhibitors, transurethral resection of prostate, elimination of causative medications
	9. URINARY INCONTINENCE	Any involuntary or abnormal urine loss	
		QUALITY	Constant, intermittent, dribbling, large volumes, hesitancy
		QUANTITY	Frequency, urgency, number of pads used
		ASSOCIATED MANIFESTATIONS	Recent surgery, coughing, sneezing, crying, laughing, heavy lifting, activity, medications, urinary tract infection, constipation, spinal cord lesions, neurological disease
		AGGRAVATING FACTORS	Medications, caffeine intake, alcohol intake
		ALLEVIATING FACTORS	Pelvic floor muscle rehabilitation, bladder training, biofeedback, anti-incontinence devices, medications
		SETTING	Accessibility of toilet, distance to toilet, adequate lighting to toilet, handrails by toilet, height of toilet seat
		TIMING	Nocturia
PAST HEALTH HISTORY	The various components of the past health history that are linked to male genitalia pathology and male genitalia-related information		
	MEDICAL HISTORY	**MALE GENITALIA–SPECIFIC**	Prior history of sexually transmitted infection (STI), prostatitis, urinary tract infection, nephrolithiasis, cryptorchidism, trauma, cancer, benign prostatic hypertrophy (BPH), congenital or acquired deformity (epispadias, hypospadias), premature ejaculation, impotence, infertility
		NON–MALE GENITALIA–SPECIFIC	Mumps, rashes, joint pain, conjunctivitis, viral illness, renal disease, congestive heart failure, spinal cord injury, pelvic fracture, diabetes mellitus, hypertension, tuberculosis, multiple sclerosis, depression, anxiety
	SURGICAL HISTORY	Prostatectomy, transurethral prostatectomy, circumcision, orchiectomy, correction of malposition of testes, vasectomy, lesion or nodule removal, epispadias repair, hypospadias repair, hernia repair	
	ALLERGIES	Contact dermatitis from topical preparations, condoms, nonoxynol-9 or other spermicides	
	MEDICATIONS	Antibiotics, hormone replacements, 5-alpha-reductase inhibitors, antihypertensives, psychotropic agents	
	COMMUNICABLE DISEASES	HSV, HPV, molluscum contagiosum, condyloma acuminata, syphilis, penile lesion, chlamydia, gonorrhoea, ureaplasma	
	INJURIES AND ACCIDENTS	Trauma, testicular torsion	
	SPECIAL NEEDS	Urinary incontinence, indwelling or intermittent urinary catheter, penile prosthesis, suprapubic urinary catheter	
	CHILDHOOD ILLNESSES	Mumps: orchitis, infertility	

>>

HEALTH HISTORY – MALE		
FAMILY HEALTH HISTORY	Male genitalia diseases that are familial are listed: Varicocele, testicular cancer, hypospadias, infertility, mother's use of hormones (diethylstilboestrol [DES]) during pregnancy	
SOCIAL HISTORY	The components of the social history that are linked to male genitalia factors and pathology	
	ALCOHOL USE	Impairs gonadotropin release and accelerates testosterone metabolism, causing impotence and loss of libido; large doses can acutely depress the sexual reflexes; chronic alcoholism causes high levels of circulating oestrogens, which decrease libido; alcohol intoxication may impair judgement, decreasing incidence of safe-sex practices and increasing risk of exposure to STIs
	TOBACCO USE	Cigarette smoking increases risk of atherosclerotic disease, which may decrease penile blood flow; it is also associated with an increased risk of bladder cancer
	DRUG USE	May impair judgement, increasing the risk for unsafe sex practices and STI exposure Cocaine: priapism with chronic abuse, impotence, increased sexual excitability Barbiturates: impotence Amphetamines: increased libido and delayed orgasm in moderate users, impotence in chronic users
	SEXUAL PRACTICE	Multiple partners, partner with multiple partners, new sexual partner, condom use (frequency and accuracy of use), sexual orientation, anal or oral intercourse
	WORK ENVIRONMENT	Radiation exposure has been linked to cancer of the male genitalia
HEALTH MAINTENANCE ACTIVITIES	This information provides a bridge between the health maintenance activities and male genitalia function.	
	SLEEP	Nocturia secondary to urethritis
	DIET	Erectile dysfunction: foods high in saturated fat or cholesterol
	EXERCISE	Trauma to the testicle may cause a hydrocoele
	USE OF SAFETY DEVICES	Condoms used for vaginal and anal intercourse; supportive device worn while participating in sports
	HEALTH CHECK-UPS	Testicular examination

REFLECTION IN PRACTICE

Gaining confidence with the male genitalia examination
Female nurses may feel anxious about examining male genitalia. Before you can help your consumer talk comfortably about his concerns, you need to work through your own feelings to reach a level of comfort about sexuality and reproduction. Work through any reluctance you may have about discussing sexual situations by role-playing with a colleague:
> Practise phrasing questions.
> Practise interviewing a male friend or fellow student.
> Practise using correct terminology.
> Familiarise yourself with common lay and slang terms used in men's health.

PERSON-CENTRED HEALTH EDUCATION

When conducting a health assessment, opportunities for the provision of person-centred health education will arise. This is a significant consideration in relation to the assessment process for examination of the female genitalia due to the intimate nature of the examination. It is also a consideration in relation to the assessment of the male genitalia, due to the sensitivity and embarrassment that may affect some males. These occasions are identified as individualised education and may generate further data that can be added to the assessment. All education given should be documented so that in future, health professionals can assess the impact of previous information provided to the consumer. (Refer to Chapter 1 for initiating health education.)

FEMALE INDIVIDUALISED HEALTH-EDUCATION INTERVENTIONS

Assessing the consumer for the following health-related activities can assist in identifying need for education about these factors. This information provides a bridge between the health maintenance activities and female genitalia.

Sleep	Lack of sleep or extreme fatigue can lead to amenorrhoea.
Diet	Increased levels of refined sugars, salt and caffeine enhance PMS symptomatology. Extreme dieting can affect menstruation and lead to amenorrhoea. Elevated sugar and lactose can lead to vaginal candidiasis.
Exercise	Exercise may diminish dysmenorrhoea (pain or cramping during menses) and menorrhagia (heavy menses).
Use of safety devices	Condom use
Health check-ups	Date of last HPV test and results, and last STI screen

HEALTH EDUCATION

Maintaining gynaecological health

There are myths associated with maintaining gynaecological health, so you should encourage consumers to adopt these healthy practices:

> Avoid douches and feminine hygiene sprays or films, or use sparingly, because both products disrupt the natural vaginal flora and increase the vaginal pH.
> Do not leave tampons in the vagina for longer than 8 hours at a time because of the increased risk of toxic shock syndrome.
> Always wash and wipe the vaginal area from front to back to prevent contamination of the vagina and urethra with faecal material.
> Thoroughly wash diaphragms, pessaries (device used to maintain the position of the uterus/bladder) and sexual aid devices before and after each use.
> Void immediately after coitus.

REFLECTION IN PRACTICE

Gynaecological assessments for women after a hysterectomy

Some women feel that it is unnecessary to have gynaecological examinations after a hysterectomy. Many of these women had surgery because of malignancy and therefore are at risk for recurrence. All women who have had this type of surgery must be encouraged to continue seeking annual gynaecological examinations. Yearly monitoring helps to determine if malignancy has returned or if other pathologies have developed; for instance, women whose ovaries were not removed in the hysterectomy are still at risk for ovarian cancer.

> How can you get this topic out into the public arena? How can you increase women's awareness of the need for annual gynaecological check-ups even if they have had a hysterectomy?

The following table provides examples of health-education interventions related to male genitalia.

MALE INDIVIDUALISED HEALTH EDUCATION INTERVENTIONS

Assessing the consumer for the following health-related activities can assist in identifying need for education about these factors. This information provides a bridge between the health maintenance activities and male genitalia function.

Sleep	Nocturia secondary to urethritis
Diet	Foods high in saturated fat or cholesterol are associated with erectile dysfunction
Exercise	Trauma to testicle may cause a hydrocoele
Use of safety devices	Condoms used for vaginal and anal intercourse; supportive device worn while participating in sports
Health check-ups	Testicular examination – regular palpation of testes

PLANNING FOR PHYSICAL EXAMINATION

The planning phase refers to evaluating subjective data to narrow the focus on physical examination, determining what objective data needs to be gathered, as well as considering the environment and equipment that will be required.

At this time, you will identify which of the four diagnostic techniques you will need to implement the physical examination, and how you will sequence these. For the physical examination of female and male genitalia you will include inspection and palpation; for the bladder you will also incorporate percussion.

Objective data is:

> collected during the physical examination of the consumer

> usually collected after subjective data

> information that is measured or observed by the clinician as opposed to being reported by the consumer

> vital to the overall health assessment, to enable you to make clinical decisions that are representative of the whole consumer picture.

Evaluating subjective data to focus physical assessment

Before commencing the physical examination of the consumer's genitalia, consider what information the health history has provided. Critical consideration, linked to knowledge of anatomy and physiology, should focus the physical assessment so your examination will be more effective and efficient.

Environment

Genitalia assessment can be done in most physical environments in healthcare settings that provide the level of privacy that is required for this very personal examination. Reassuring the consumer that privacy will be maintained during the assessment, by providing screens and/or closing the door, will assist them to feel more at ease during the assessment.

Equipment

Assemble items before placing the consumer on the examination table. Materials should be arranged in order of use and within ease of reach.

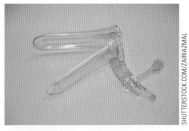

A. Speculums come in various sizes

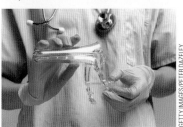

B. Graves' speculum

FIGURE 17.9 Vaginal specula

FEMALE GENITOURINARY EQUIPMENT	MALE GENITOURINARY EQUIPMENT

> Examination table
> Large hand mirror
> Gooseneck lamp
> Nonsterile gloves
> Linens for draping
> Vaginal specula (**Figure 17.9**):
  • Graves' bivalve specula, sizes medium and large, useful for most adult sexually active women
  • Pederson bivalve specula, sizes small and medium, useful for nonsexually active women, children, menopausal women
> Specimen collection materials (**Figure 17.10**):
  • Ayre spatulas
  • Cervical broom
  • Cytobrushes
  • Cotton-tipped applicators
	> Nonsterile gloves
	> Penlight
	> Stethoscope
	> Culture tube
	> Sterile cotton swabs
	> Plastic sheet
	> 2.5–3 cm gauze wrap
	> 5% acetic acid solution in spray bottle
	> Culture medium (agar plate)
	> Gen probe
	> ×10 power magnifying lens

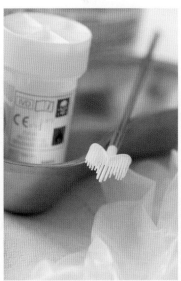

FIGURE 17.10 Specimen collection materials needed for gynaecological examination

>>

>>

FEMALE GENITOURINARY EQUIPMENT	MALE GENITOURINARY EQUIPMENT
• Liquid-based preparation vials • Microscope slides, cover slips, culture probes labelled with the consumer's name, identification number, and date specimen was collected • Cytology fixative spray • Warm water • Water-soluble lubricant	

PUTTING IT IN CONTEXT

Liquid-based cervical sampling

Liquid-based cervical sampling is used for HPV testing and for the detection of squamous epithelial abnormalities (Figure 17.11). The sample is placed in a preservative vial, and the specimen is first tested for HPV; if positive then further cell testing is carried out on the same specimen.

If you are working in women's health, you should ensure you are up to date with this investigation and the implications and follow-up of the outcomes.

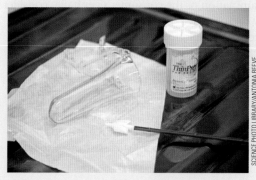

FIGURE 17.11 Liquid-based cervical cytology preparations

IMPLEMENTATION: CONDUCTING THE PHYSICAL EXAMINATION OF THE FEMALE

EXAMINATION IN BRIEF: BLADDER AND FEMALE GENITALIA

Examination of the bladder

Inspection

Palpation

Percussion

Examination of the external genitalia

Inspection
> Pubic hair
> Skin colour and condition
  • Mons pubis and vulva
> Clitoris
> Urethral meatus
> Vaginal introitus
> Perineum and anus

Palpation
> Labia
> Urethral meatus and Skene's glands
> Vaginal introitus
> Perineum

Speculum examination of the internal genitalia
> Cervix
  • Colour
  • Position
  • Size
  • Surface characteristics
  • Discharge
  • Shape of the cervical os
> Endocervical smear
> Cervical smear

Advanced Assessment

>>

>>

Classifications

Culture specimens
> Vaginal culture
> Anal culture

Examination of the vaginal wall

Inspection
Bimanual examination

Palpation
> Vagina
> Cervix

> Fornices
> Uterus
> Adnexa

Rectovaginal examination
Examining consumers with urinary diversions

Urinary diversions
> Ileal conduit
> Ureteral stents
> Indwelling catheters
> Suprapubic catheters

> If you have not performed a gynaecological examination:
  • Ask another nurse to assist you with the first few examinations.
  • Review the anatomy and physiology of the female genitalia; visualise the underlying structures of the anatomic landmarks.
  • Review and practise any procedures to be done. Some nurses find it difficult to prepare slides and cultures without assistance, if they are unfamiliar with these procedures.
> If you are an advanced practitioner developing these skills:
  • Familiarise yourself with the equipment.
  • Practise opening and closing the speculum. Plastic specula make significant audible clicking sounds when opening and closing, so you should prepare the consumer for this event.
  • Know your institution's policies regarding the option of having a female nurse present if a male nurse is performing the gynaecological exam.

General approach to female genitalia assessment
Prior to the assessment:
1. Ensure that the woman will not be menstruating at the time of the examination for optimal cytological specimen collection.
2. If the consumer is having an HPV test or swab taken, instruct her not to use vaginal sprays, douche, or have coitus 24 to 48 hours before the scheduled physical assessment. The products of coitus and commercial sprays and douches may affect the HPV smear and other vaginal cultures.
3. Encourage the individual to express any anxieties and concerns about the physical assessment. Reassure them by acknowledging anxieties and validating concerns. Women who have not had sexual intercourse need reassurance that the pelvic assessment should not affect the hymen.
4. Show the speculum and other equipment to the woman and allow her to touch and explore any items that do not have to remain sterile.
5. Inform the woman that the assessment should not be painful but might be uncomfortable at times, and tell her to inform you if she is experiencing any pain.
6. Instruct the woman to empty her bladder and then to undress from the waist to the ankles.
7. Ensure that the room is warm enough to prevent chilling, and provide additional draping material as necessary.
8. Warm your hands with warm water prior to gloving.
9. Ensure that privacy will be maintained during the assessment. Provide screens and a closed door.
10. Warm the speculum with warm water or a warming device before insertion.
During the assessment:
1. Inform the consumer of what you are going to do before you do it. Tell her she may feel pressure when the speculum is opened and a pinching sensation when the sample is taken.
2. Adopt a non-judgemental and supportive attitude.

Advanced Assessment

UNIT 2

3. Maintain eye contact with the woman as much as possible to reinforce a caring relationship.
4. Use a mirror to show the woman what you are doing and to educate her about her body. If possible, help her with positioning the mirror during the examination so she will feel comfortable using this technique at home to assess her genitalia.
5. Offer the consumer the opportunity to ask questions about her body and sexuality.
6. Encourage the consumer to use relaxation techniques such as deep breathing or guided imagery to prevent muscle tension during the assessment.

After the assessment:

1. Assess whether the consumer needs assistance in dressing.
2. Offer tissues with which to wipe excess lubrication.
3. After the woman is dressed, discuss the experience with her, invite questions and comments, listen carefully, and provide her with information regarding the assessment and any laboratory information that is available.
4. Tell the woman she may experience a small amount of spotting following the specimen collection.

Implementation of the physical examination requires you to consider your scope of practice. Depending on your context, you may be performing a foundation assessment with aspects of advanced assessment if you are practising in a specialised area. Assessment of the female reproductive system consists of inspection and palpation only, and includes assessment of the abdomen (see Chapter 15), inspection of the external genitalia, palpation of the external genitalia, speculum assessment of the internal genitalia, collection of specimens for laboratory analysis, inspection of the vaginal walls, bimanual examination, and rectovaginal assessment (see Chapter 18 for the complete rectal examination). The assessment process necessitates an uncomfortable positioning for the consumer; therefore, it should be completed as quickly and as efficiently as possible.

Examination of the bladder

You may see clinically that the order of bladder palpation and percussion varies; this may occur concurrently or out of sequence.

1. With the consumer sitting on the examination bed, provide a drape to cover the individual's torso and thighs.
2. Assist the woman in assuming a dorsal recumbent position.

Inspection

See Chapter 15 for abdominal assessment inspection.

Palpation

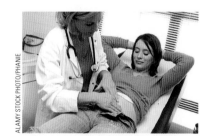

FIGURE 17.12 Palpation of the bladder

E 1. Using deep palpation, palpate the abdomen at the midline, starting at the symphysis pubis and progressing up to the umbilicus (**Figure 17.12**).
2. If the bladder is located, palpate the shape, size and consistency.

N An empty bladder is not usually palpable. A moderately full bladder is smooth and round, and it is palpable above the symphysis pubis. A full bladder is palpated above the symphysis pubis, and it may be close to the umbilicus.

A A bladder that is nodular or asymmetrical to palpation is abnormal.

P A nodular bladder may indicate a malignancy. An asymmetrical bladder may result from a tumour in the bladder or an abdominal tumour that is compressing the bladder.

A It is abnormal to palpate a bladder that has been recently emptied.

P Women may be unable to completely empty their bladder due to bladder muscle dysfunction and obstruction due to uterine prolapse.

E Examination **N** Normal findings **A** Abnormal findings **P** Pathophysiology

P Various types of urinary incontinence, due to altered mental status, muscle function, medications and other causes, can lead to incomplete bladder emptying. See **Table 17.6** for additional information on urinary incontinence.

Percussion

E 1. Percuss upwards from the symphysis pubis to the umbilicus.
2. Note where the sound changes from dullness to tympany.

N A urine-filled bladder is dull to percussion. A recently emptied bladder should not be percussible above the symphysis pubis.

A It is abnormal to percuss a bladder that has recently been emptied. The urine that remains in the bladder after urination is called residual urine. A bladder may also be dull to percussion when the individual has difficulty voiding.

P The inability to completely empty the bladder occurs in the elderly; in postoperative, bedridden and acutely ill consumers; and in consumers with neurogenic bladder dysfunction.

P Difficulty voiding can occur for a variety of conditions including urinary tract infections, bladder muscle dysfunction, prolapsed bladder, and effects of menopause and pregnancy.

Examination of the external genitalia

1. Assist the woman to re-position with her knees flexed and thighs externally rotated. (When assisting her, ask her to bend her knees, place her heels together and allow her knees to relax to the side.)
2. If able, raise the head of the examination table slightly to elevate her head and shoulders. This also prevents abdominal muscle tension.
3. Readjust the drape to cover the abdomen, thighs and knees.
4. Stand at the side of the individual, ensuring you have eye contact with her during the procedure.
5. Adjust your lighting source.
6. Finally, remember to inform her of each step of the assessment process before it is performed, and be gentle.

CLINICAL **REASONING**

Positional variations for the gynaecological examination

Some consumers have difficulty assuming a dorsal recumbent or lithotomy position because of illness or disability. You need to adapt your health assessment approaches to account for these individual cases. For example, you may need to place the consumer in a left lateral or Sims' position with the buttocks near the edge of the examination table and with the right knee flexed, if they are unable to lie on their back. Remember to limit questioning of the individual in this position, because this position often causes discomfort and embarrassment.

Some examination tables have stirrups that may be used to assist in positioning the woman for examination.

> How would you identify if a consumer's position needs to be adapted?

Inspection

Pubic hair

E 1. Observe the pattern of pubic hair distribution.
2. Note the presence of nits or lice.

N The distribution of the female pubic hair should be shaped like an inverse triangle. There may be some growth on the abdomen and upper inner thighs. A diamond-shaped pattern from the umbilicus may be due to cultural or familial differences. There are no nits or lice.

E Examination **N** Normal findings **A** Abnormal findings **P** Pathophysiology

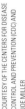

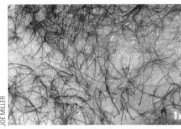

FIGURE 17.13 Pubic lice, or *Phthirus pubis.* Note the reddish-brown crab lice faeces.

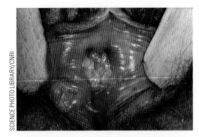

FIGURE 17.14 Syphilitic chancre

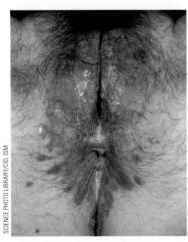

FIGURE 17.15 Secondary syphilis (condyloma latum); (note: with consumer assistance to assess)

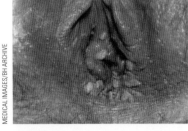

FIGURE 17.16 Genital warts (condyloma acuminatum)

🅐 A diamond-shaped pattern from the umbilicus, not associated with cultural or familial differences, is abnormal.

🅟 This distribution pattern may occur with hirsutism, which is indicative of an endocrine disorder.

🅐 Hair distribution is sparse or hair is absent at the genitalia area. This is called **alopecia** and it is abnormal.

🅟 Alopecia in the genital area may result from genetic factors, ageing, or local or systemic disease. These include developmental defects and hereditary disorders, infection, neoplasms, physical or chemical agents, endocrine diseases, deficiency states (nutritional or metabolic), destruction, damage to the follicles and obesity. Note: This variant may be expected if the consumer shaves or waxes this region.

🅐 The presence of nits or lice is abnormal.

🅟 Pubic lice (pediculosis pubis) is the infestation of the hairy regions of the body, usually the pubic area (**Figure 17.13**), but it sometimes involves the hairy aspects of the abdomen, chest and axillae.

Skin colour and condition

Mons pubis and vulva

🅔 1. Observe the skin colouration and condition of the mons pubis and vulva.
   2. Inform the consumer that you will touch the inside of her thigh before you touch her genitals.
   3. With gloved hands, separate the labia majora using the thumb and index finger of the dominant hand.
   4. Observe both the labia majora and the labia minora for colouration, lesions or trauma.

🅝 The skin over the mons pubis should be clear except for naevi and normal hair distribution. The labia majora and minora should appear symmetrical with a smooth to somewhat wrinkled, unbroken, slightly pigmented skin surface. There should be no ecchymosis, excoriation, nodules, swelling, rash or lesions. An occasional sebaceous cyst is within normal limits. These cysts are nontender, yellow nodules that are less than 1 cm in diameter.

🅐 Ecchymosis over the mons pubis or labia is abnormal.

🅟 This may be due to blunt trauma that may have resulted from an accident or intentional abuse.

🅐 Oedema or swelling of the labia is an abnormal finding.

🅟 This may be due to haematoma formation, Bartholin's cyst, or obstruction of the lymphatic system.

🅐 Broken areas on the skin surface are abnormal.

🅟 These may be due to ulcerations or abrasions secondary to infection or trauma.

🅐 Rash over the mons pubis and labia is abnormal.

🅟 Rashes have multiple aetiologies including contact dermatitis and infestations.

🅐 A nontender, reddish, round ulcer with a depressed centre, and raised, indurated edges (**chancre**) is an abnormal finding (**Figure 17.14**).

🅟 A chancre appears during the primary stages of syphilis at the site where the treponema enters the body. The chancre lasts for 4 weeks and then disappears.

🅐 Flat or raised, round, wart-like papules that have moist surfaces covered by grey exudate (condyloma latum) are abnormal (**Figure 17.15**).

🅟 These lesions occur during the secondary stage of syphilis.

🅐 White, dry, cauliflower-like growths that have narrow bases are suggestive of condyloma acuminatum (see **Figure 17.16**) and are abnormal.

🅔 Examination   🅝 Normal findings   🅐 Abnormal findings   🅟 Pathophysiology

P These warts are caused by the human papillomavirus and may be dysplastic.

A A painless mass that may be accompanied by pruritus or a mass that develops into a cauliflower-like growth is an abnormal finding.

P This type of mass is highly suggestive of malignancy.

A Venous prominences of the labia may be abnormal.

P Varicose veins may develop due to a congenital predisposition, prolonged standing, pregnancy or ageing.

For other abnormal findings see Advanced practice below.

E For the advanced practitioner, further inspection may reveal these abnormalities.

N Normal as per foundation information at N above.

A Small, swollen, red vesicles that fuse together to form a large, burning ulcer that may be painful and itchy (see **Figures 17.17 A and Figure 17.17 B**) are abnormal.

P These ulcers are indicative of herpes simplex virus (HSV). Primary HSV (or genital herpes) outbreaks can last up to 21 days. Recurrent HSV outbreaks are usually shorter in duration and last about 2 weeks (see **Figure 17.17B**). Serologic testing must be performed to determine if an outbreak is HSV-1 or HSV-2 (see **Figure 17.18**).

A Firm, painless, papular, granular lesions that are beefy red are abnormal.

P Granuloma inguinale is caused by the bacteria *Calymmatobacterium granulomatis*. It is also referred to as donovanosis and granuloma venereum. This STI tends to occur on the external genitalia, inguinal region and the anus.

Clitoris

E 1. Using the dominant thumb and index finger, separate the labia minora laterally to expose the prepuce of the clitoris (**Figure 17.19**).
2. Observe the clitoris for size and condition.

N The clitoris is approximately 2.0 cm in length and 0.5 cm in diameter and without lesions.

A Hypertrophy of the clitoris is an abnormal finding.

P This may indicate female pseudohermaphroditism due to androgen excess.

A A reddish, round ulcer with a depressed centre and raised, indurated edges (chancre) is an abnormal finding.

P Refer to the chancre discussion (see **Figure 17.14**).

A Excision of the clitoris is a post-surgical finding.

P Female genital mutilation (clitoridectomy), a practice in some cultures, can result in this finding.

Urethral meatus

E 1. Using the dominant thumb and index finger, separate the labia minora laterally to expose the urethral meatus. Do not touch the urethral meatus; this may cause pain and urethral spasm.
2. Observe the shape, colour and size of the urethral meatus.

N The urethral opening is slit-like in appearance and midline. It is free of discharge, swelling or redness and is about the size of a pea.

A Discharge of any colour from the meatus is an abnormal finding.

P Discharge indicates possible urinary tract infection.

A Swelling or redness around the urethral meatus is an abnormal finding.

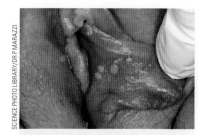

A. Genital herpes simplex virus

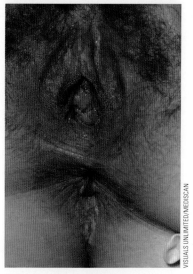

B. Primary herpes simplex virus, first episode. Serology tests are negative for HSV.

FIGURE 17.17 Examples of genital herpes

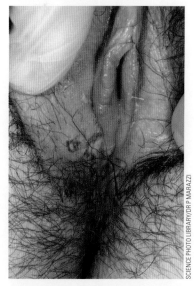

FIGURE 17.18 Nonprimary herpes simplex virus, first episode. Serology tests are positive for HSV (type 1 or type 2), meaning the consumer has had previous exposure to the virus at another body site.

E Examination **N** Normal findings **A** Abnormal findings **P** Pathophysiology Advanced Assessment

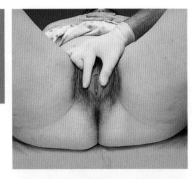

FIGURE 17.19 Inspection of the clitoris

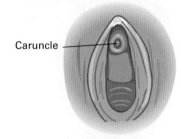

Caruncle

FIGURE 17.20 Urethral caruncle

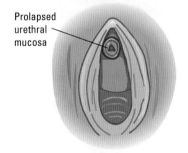

Prolapsed urethral mucosa

FIGURE 17.21 Prolapse of the urethral meatus

P Swelling indicates possible infection of the Skene's glands, urethral caruncle (small, red growth that protrudes from the meatus, shown in **Figure 17.20**), urethral carcinoma, or prolapse of the urethral mucosa (**Figure 17.21**).

Vaginal introitus

E 1. Keep the labia minora retracted laterally to inspect the vaginal introitus.
2. Ask the consumer to bear down.
3. Observe for patency and bulging.

N The introitus mucosa should be pink and moist. Normal vaginal discharge is clear to white and free of foul odour; some white clumps may be seen that are mass numbers of epithelial cells. The introitus should be patent and without bulging.

A Pale colour and dryness of the introitus are abnormal.

P Possible aetiologies include atrophy from topical steroids, the ageing process and oestrogen deficiency.

A A foul-smelling discharge that is any colour other than clear to slightly pale white is abnormal. Malodorous white, yellow, green or grey discharge that may be purulent are some possible findings.

P Gonorrhoea, chlamydia, Candida vaginosis, trichomonas vaginitis, bacterial vaginosis, atrophic vaginitis and cervicitis are possible infectious processes or vectors (see **Table 17.4**).

HEALTH EDUCATION

Risk for developing Candida vaginosis

Candida vaginosis (commonly known as thrush) is a condition that is estimated to affect 3 out of 4 women in their lifetime. Candida is one of the normal vaginal flora that is usually balanced with the more acidic pH (3.8–4.5) of vaginal secretions. The acidic environment assists in providing a natural barrier to infection and irritation; however, if the vaginal pH changes and becomes more alkaline (pH > 4.5), normal flora (such as candida) and bacteria can flourish, causing infection and discomfort. This imbalance can be caused by some medications (antibiotics), hormonal changes during pregnancy and menopause, and certain illnesses (such as diabetes or poorly functioning immune system). Candida vaginosis is not considered an STI; however, sexual activity can affect the pH balance. Further, anything that changes the vaginal environment to a warm moist one (synthetic clothing, douching etc.) will change the pH, and increase the chance of infection.

Some women are asymptomatic, while many will experience increased vaginal discharge that is thick white and creamy, and there is odour, itchiness and redness around the vagina and vulva, discomfort during sexual intercourse, and burning on urination. Treatment involves inserting antifungal (such as Clotrimazole/Miconazole etc.) pessaries or cream into the vagina, or oral medication, which can be bought over the counter from a pharmacy. Women should seek health advice if the infection reoccurs, or does not respond to the treatment (Sheppard, 2020).

> What advice would you give a woman to reduce the chances of getting Candida vaginosis (thrush)?

E Examination **N** Normal findings **A** Abnormal findings **P** Pathophysiology

TABLE 17.4 Description of vaginal discharges

DISCHARGE	NORMAL PHYSIOLOGICAL DISCHARGE	BACTERIAL VAGINOSIS	TRICHOMONAS	CANDIDA	GONOCOCCAL
Colour	White	Grey	Greyish yellow	White	Greenish yellow
Odour	Absent	Fishy	Fishy	Absent	Absent
Consistency	Nonhomogeneous	Homogeneous	Purulent, often with bubbles	Cottage cheese-like	Mucopurulent
Location	Dependent	Adherent to walls	Often pooled in fornix	Adherent to walls	Adherent to walls
Vaginal pH	4	5–6	5–6	4–4.5	—
ANATOMIC APPEARANCE					
Vulva	Normal	Normal	Oedematous	Erythematous	Erythematous
Vaginal mucosa	Normal	Normal	Usually normal	Erythematous	Normal
Cervix	Normal	Normal	May show red spots	Patches of discharge	Pus in os

HEALTH EDUCATION

Risk factors related to vaginal infection
When reviewing consumer data from your health assessment, consider the following risk factors related to vaginal infections:
> Underlying skin diseases
> Increasing age
> Antibiotic use
> Immunodeficiency
> Oral contraceptive use
> Oestrogen deficiency
> High sugar or milk intake
> Diabetes mellitus
> Steroid use
> Menses
> Douches
> Alkalinisation from semen or chemical products
> Pregnancy
> Increased number of sexual partners
> Sexual abuse
> Hygiene
Where appropriate, counsel the consumer regarding changes to their health behaviours.

E For the advanced practitioner, further inspection may reveal these abnormalities.

N Normal as per Foundation information.

A An external tear or impatency of the vaginal introitus is abnormal.

P Possible causes include trauma and fissure of the introitus. An external tear may indicate trauma from sexual activity or abuse, and a fissure may indicate a congenital malformation or childbirth trauma.

A Bulging of the anterior vaginal wall indicates a **cystocoele** (Figure 17.22) and is abnormal.

P The upper two-thirds of the anterior vaginal wall along with the bladder push forwards into the introitus, due to weakened supporting tissues and ligaments.

A Closure of the vaginal introitus is abnormal.

P Trauma to the area and possible female genital mutilation are potential aetiologies.

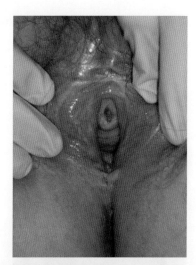
FIGURE 17.22 Cystocoele. Also note the dry, pale appearance of the labia and the prominence of the urinary meatus.

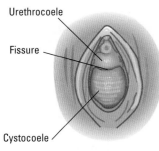

Urethrocoele

Fissure

Cystocoele

FIGURE 17.23 Cystourethrocoele

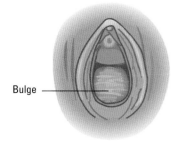

Bulge

FIGURE 17.24 Rectocoele

A Bulging of the anterior vaginal wall, bladder and urethra into the vaginal introitus indicates a cystourethrocoele (**Figure 17.23**) and is abnormal.

P The aetiology is usually a weakening of the entire anterior vaginal wall. A fissure may define the urethrocoele and cystocoele.

A Bulging of the posterior vaginal wall with a portion of the rectum indicates a rectocoele (**Figure 17.24**) and is abnormal.

P This is caused by a weakening of the entire posterior vaginal wall.

Perineum and anus

E 1. Observe the texture and colour of the perineum.
2. Observe for colour and shape of the anus.

N The perineum should be smooth and slightly darkened. A well-healed episiotomy scar is normal after vaginal delivery. The anus should be dark pink to brown and puckered. Skin tags are not uncommon around the anal area.

A A fissure or tear of the perineum is an abnormal finding.

P Possible causes include trauma, abscess and unhealed episiotomy.

A Venous prominences of the anal area indicate external haemorrhoids and are abnormal.

P An external haemorrhoid is the varicose dilatation of a vein of the inferior haemorrhoidal plexus and is covered with modified anal skin.

Palpation

Labia

E 1. Palpate each labium between the thumb and the index finger of your dominant hand.
2. Observe for swelling, induration, pain or discharge from a Bartholin's gland duct.

CLINICAL **REASONING**

The sexually abused consumer

No consumer, regardless of age, should be excluded from evaluation for sexual abuse. Physical signs of sexual abuse in women include bruising of the mons pubis, labia or perineum, and vaginal or rectal tears. The presence of STIs in the very young or the very old consumer may suggest abuse. Emotional signs such as extreme anxiety or guarding during the assessment, or refusing to assume certain positions (ensure you use culturally safe practices), may all indicate a history of abuse. Document all signs of suspected sexual abuse. Know your institution's and state's policies regarding the reporting of sexual abuse, and the locally available community support services. There are mandatory reporting policies for sexual abuse in children and teenagers. Some jurisdictions require mandatory reporting of abuse in the elderly. Consider the whole consumer situation, including immediate safety concerns, especially as many abusive partners restrict women's ability to access health services independently.

N The labium should feel soft and uniform in structure with no swelling, pain, induration or purulent discharge.

A Swelling, redness, induration or purulent discharge from the labial folds with hot, tender areas are abnormal findings (see **Figure 17.25**).

P These findings indicate a probable Bartholin's gland infection. Causative organisms include gonococci, *Chlamydia trachomatis* and syphilis.

A A firm mass that is possibly painful in the labia majora is abnormal.

P This might indicate an inguinal hernia. If this is suspected, re-palpate the mass with the consumer in a standing position.

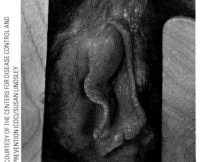

FIGURE 17.25 Bartholinitis

E Examination **N** Normal findings **A** Abnormal findings **P** Pathophysiology Advanced Assessment

Urethral meatus and Skene's glands

E 1. Insert your dominant index finger into the vagina.
2. Apply pressure to the anterior aspect of the vaginal wall and milk the urethra (see **Figure 17.26**).
3. Observe for discharge and consumer discomfort.

N Milking the urethra should not cause pain or result in any urethral discharge.

A Pain on contact and discharge from the urethra are abnormal findings.

P These findings indicate a Skene's gland infection or urinary tract infection.

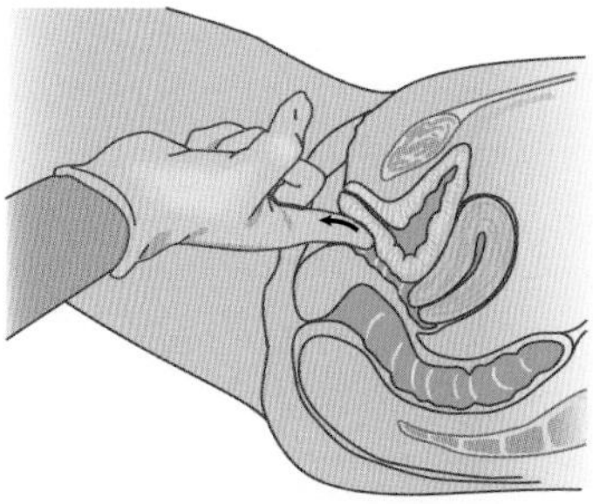

FIGURE 17.26 Milking the urethra

HEALTH EDUCATION

Cystitis – a common urinary tract infection in women

One-third of women develop cystitis (bladder inflammation) during their lifetime, due to the anatomical factors of the female urethra being less than 5 cm and its close proximity to the anus, which increases the chances of bacteria ascending the urinary tract. It can also be attributed to hormone changes during the menstrual cycle, as the pH of vaginal secretions changes and this reduces the natural barrier to infections around the vagina and urethral meatus. It is more common in late teens and older women. Risk factors include:

> sexual intercourse – especially a new sexual partner
> contraception – diaphragms, spermicides
> pregnancy – the ureters widen, so urine does not drain as quickly or the growing uterus can block the drainage of urine from the bladder
> antibiotic use (can alter the normal perineal flora)
> a family history of repeated UTIs
> post-menopausal – mechanical and/or physiologic factors that can affect bladder emptying (urinary incontinence, cystocoele, atrophic vaginitis, history of UTIs).

Many women can be asymptomatic; however, common symptoms of cystitis include:

> a burning sensation when passing urine
> frequent urge to urinate but only be able to pass a small amount
> traces of blood in the urine
> dark, cloudy or strong-smelling urine
> pain above the pubic bone and/or lower back.

The elderly may have an altered mental status and may be slightly febrile.

History and symptoms are usually adequate to identify cystitis, but a urine dipstick analysis on a midstream urine sample collected for microscopy, culture and sensitivity (MCS) will confirm infection and causative organism. The consumer should be referred to their health professional for correct antibiotic treatment.

When caring for women, you should take the opportunity to provide education to them about how to prevent cystitis:

> When feel the urge, empty bladder as soon as practical, rather than holding on.
> Keep well hydrated, to flush the urinary system.
> Wipe from front to back (urethra to anus) after going to the toilet.
> Urinate after sexual intercourse.
> Avoid wearing nylon underwear, pantyhose, tight pants or tight jeans.
> Avoid the use of perfumed soaps, talcum powder or any type of deodorant around genitals.

Continence Foundation of Australia, 2021

Vaginal introitus

E 1. While your finger remains in the vagina, ask the consumer to squeeze the vaginal muscles around your finger.

2. Evaluate muscle strength and tone.

E Examination   **N** Normal findings   **A** Abnormal findings   **P** Pathophysiology   Advanced Assessment

N Vaginal muscle tone in a nulliparous woman should be tight and strong; in a parous woman, it will be diminished.

A Significantly diminished or absent vaginal muscle tone and bulging of vaginal or pelvic contents are abnormal findings.

P Weakened muscle tone may result from injury, age, childbirth or medication. Bulging results from cystocoele, rectocoele or uterine prolapse (**Figure 17.27**).

Perineum

E 1. Withdraw your finger from the introitus until you can place your dominant index finger posterior to the perineum and place the dominant thumb anterior to the perineum.

2. Assess the perineum between the dominant thumb and index finger for muscular tone and texture.

Prolapse of the uterus

Normal anatomy

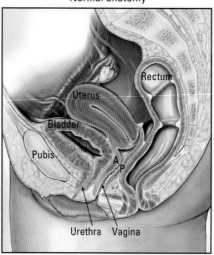

First-degree prolapse

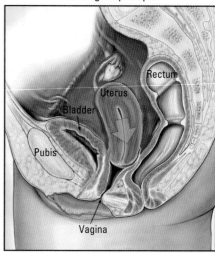

Second-degree prolapse

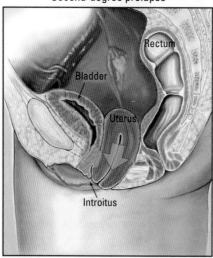

Third-degree prolapse

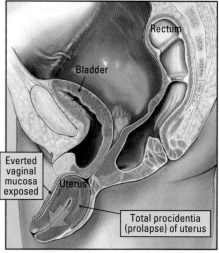

© 2023 MediVisuals

FIGURE 17.27 Uterine prolapse. In first-degree prolapse, the cervix is contained within the vagina with straining. In second-degree prolapse, the cervix is at the introitus with straining, and in third-degree prolapse, complete prolapse, the cervix, uterus and vagina are outside the introitus, even without straining.

E Examination N Normal findings A Abnormal findings P Pathophysiology Advanced Assessment

The perineum should be smooth, firm and homogeneous in the nulliparous woman, and thinner in the parous woman. A well-healed episiotomy scar is also within normal limits for a parous woman.

A A thin, tissue-like perineum, fissures or tears are abnormal.

P A thin perineum is indicative of atrophy, and fissures and tears may indicate trauma or an unhealed episiotomy.

HEALTH EDUCATION

Hormone replacement therapy
You may note that some women have a fear of hormone replacement therapy (HRT), as it has been identified that this treatment can raise the risk of breast cancer, myocardial infarction, cerebral vascular accident, and venous thromboembolisms. According to the NHMRC, for otherwise healthy women with moderate to severe symptoms, the benefits of short-term HRT are likely to outweigh the risks. The use of HRT should be tailored to the needs and desires of the individual and be reviewed every 12 months. Discuss with your consumer the benefits and risks of HRT, and refer to specialist services for further consultation.

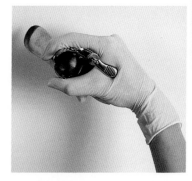
FIGURE 17.28 Holding the speculum

Speculum examination of the internal genitalia
Cervix

E 1. Select the appropriate-sized speculum. This selection should be based on the consumer's history, size of vaginal introitus, and vaginal muscle tone.
2. Lubricate and warm the speculum by rinsing it under warm water. Do not use other lubricants because they may interfere with the accuracy of cytological samples and cultures.
3. Hold the speculum in your dominant hand with the closed blades between the index and middle fingers. The index finger should rest at the proximal end of the superior blade. Wrap the other fingers around the handle, with the thumbscrew over the thumb (**Figure 17.28**).
4. Insert your nondominant index and middle fingers, ventral sides down, just inside the vagina and apply pressure to the posterior vaginal wall. Encourage the consumer to bear down. This will help to relax the perineal muscles.
5. Encourage the consumer to relax by taking deep breaths. Be careful not to pull on pubic hair or pinch the labia.
6. When you feel the muscles relax, insert the speculum at an oblique angle on a plane parallel to the examination table until the speculum reaches the end of the fingers that are in the vagina (see **Figure 17.29A**).
7. Withdraw the fingers of your nondominant hand.
8. Gently rotate the speculum blades to a horizontal angle and advance the speculum at a 45° downwards angle against the posterior vaginal wall until it reaches the end of the vagina (see **Figures 17.29B** and **17.29C**).
9. Using your dominant thumb, depress the lever to open the blades and visualise the cervix (see **Figure 17.29D**).
10. If the cervix is not visualised, close the blades and withdraw the speculum 2 to 3 cm and re-insert it at a slightly different angle to ensure that the speculum is inserted far enough into the vagina.
11. Once the cervix is fully visualised, lock the speculum blades into place. This procedure varies with the type of speculum being used.
12. Adjust your light source so that it shines through the speculum.
13. If any discharge obstructs the visualisation of the cervix, clean it away with a cotton-tipped applicator.
14. Inspect the cervix and the os for colour, position, size, surface characteristics such as polyps or lesions, discharge and shape.

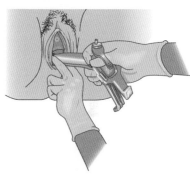
A. Opening of the vaginal introitus

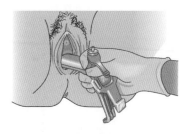
B. Oblique insertion of the speculum

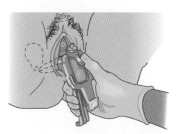
C. Final advancement of the speculum

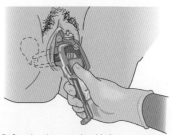
D. Opening the speculum blades

FIGURE 17.29 Speculum examination

 Examination Normal findings Abnormal findings  Pathophysiology   Advanced Assessment

HEALTH EDUCATION

Risk factors related to female genitalia cancer

Consider the following risk factors related to female genitalia cancer, when reviewing the data. Counsel the consumer in their health behaviours, to assist them to reduce their risk factors. Suspected carcinoma of the female genitalia requires an immediate referral for emergency care.

> Cervical cancer risk factors
  - Early age at first intercourse
  - Multiple sex partners or male partners who have had multiple partners
  - Prior history of herpes simplex virus
  - Current or prior history of human papillomavirus or condylomata, or both
  - Family history
  - Tobacco use
  - Drug use
  - HIV
  - Immunosuppression
  - History of STIs
  - Women of lower socioeconomic status
> Endometrial cancer risk factors
  - Early or late menarche (before age 11 or after age 16)
  - History of infertility
  - Failure to ovulate
  - Unopposed oestrogen therapy
  - Use of tamoxifen
  - Obesity
  - Family history of nonpolyposis colon cancer
> Ovarian cancer risk factors risk factors
  - Advancing age
  - Nulliparity
  - History of breast cancer
  - Family history of ovarian cancer
  - Infertility treatment
> Vaginal cancer risk factors
  - Daughters of women who ingested DES during pregnancy
  - Prior human papillomavirus
  - DES exposure – most consumers with DES exposure were born prior to 1971. These consumers are at greater risk for carcinoma of the upper vagina.

Colour

N The normal cervix is a glistening pink; it may be pale after menopause or blue (**Chadwick's sign**) during pregnancy.

A Cyanosis not associated with pregnancy is abnormal.

P Possible causes include venous congestion of the area or systemic hypoxia as in congestive heart failure.

A Redness or a friable appearance is an abnormal finding.

P Possible causes include infection and inflammation, such as chlamydia or gonorrhoea.

Position

N The cervix is located midline in the vagina with an anterior or posterior position relative to the vaginal vault and projecting approximately 2.5 cm into the vagina.

A Lateral positioning of the cervix may present as an abnormal finding.

P Possible causes include tumour or adhesions that would displace the cervix.

A Projection of the cervix into the vaginal vault greater than normal limits is suspect.

P Uterine prolapse is caused by weakened vaginal wall muscles and pelvic ligaments, and may push the cervix into the vaginal vault.

Size

N Normal size is 2.5 cm.

A Cervical size greater than 4 cm is indicative of hypertrophy and is abnormal.

P Inflammation or tumour could result in the morbid enlargement of the cervix.

Surface characteristics

N The cervix is covered by the glistening pink squamous epithelium, which is similar to the vaginal epithelium, and the deep pink to red columnar epithelium, which is a continuation of the endocervical lining.

A A reddish circle around the os may be abnormal.

P This is known as **ectropion** or **eversion**. It occurs when the squamocolumnar junction appears on the ectocervix. It results from lacerations during childbirth or, possibly, from congenital variation.

A Small, cystic, yellow lesions on the cervical surface indicate nabothian cysts (**Figure 17.30**), which are abnormal.

P These benign cysts result from the obstruction of cervical glands.

A A bright red, soft protrusion through the cervical os indicates a cervical polyp (**Figure 17.31**) and is abnormal.

P Polyps originate from the endocervical canal; they are usually benign but tend to bleed if abraded.

A Haemorrhages dispersed over the surface and known as strawberry spots are abnormal. There may also be a foul-smelling, frothy, green or yellow discharge (**Figure 17.32**).

P These may be seen in conjunction with trichomonal infections.

A Mucopurulent discharge, erythema and friability of the cervix are abnormal (**Figure 17.33**).

P Many women with *Chlamydia trachomatis* are asymptomatic; others can have pelvic pain, fever and dysuria. Consumers infected with this STI frequently have gonorrhoea.

A Irregularities of the cervical surface that may look cauliflower-like are an abnormal finding.

P Carcinoma of the cervix may manifest as a cauliflower-like overgrowth (see **Figure 17.34**).

A Columnar epithelium covering most of the cervix and extending to the vaginal wall (vaginal adenosis) and a collar-type ridge between the cervix and the vagina are abnormal (see **Figure 17.35**).

P This denotes fetal exposure to DES.

Discharge

E Note characteristics of any discharge.

N A P See **Table 17.4**.

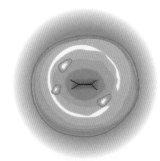

FIGURE 17.30 Nabothian cysts

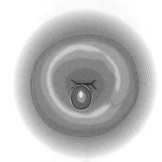

FIGURE 17.31 Cervical polyp

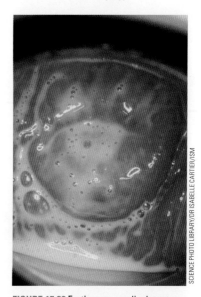

FIGURE 17.32 Frothy creamy discharge of vaginal fluid growing the *Trichomonas vaginalis* parasite

SCIENCE PHOTO LIBRARY/DR ISABELLE CARTIER/ISM

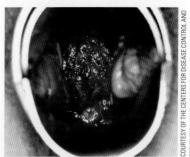

FIGURE 17.33 This woman's cervix is erythematous due to chlamydia.

COURTESY OF THE CENTERS FOR DISEASE CONTROL AND PREVENTION (CDC)/DR LOURDES FRAW, JIM PLEDGER.

 E Examination   **N** Normal findings   **A** Abnormal findings **P** Pathophysiology ▨ Advanced Assessment

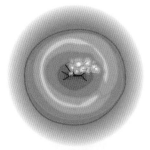

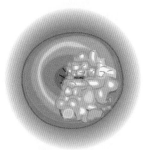

FIGURE 17.34 Carcinoma of the cervix

Shape of the cervical os

N In the nulliparous woman, the os is small and either round or oval. In the parous woman who has had a vaginal delivery, the os is a horizontal slit (**Figure 17.36**).

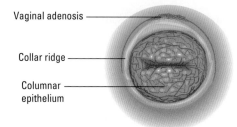

Vaginal adenosis

Collar ridge

Columnar epithelium

FIGURE 17.35 Fetal exposure to DES

A A unilateral transverse, bilateral transverse, stellate or irregular cervical os is abnormal (**Figure 17.36**). A reddish circle around the os may be abnormal.

P Possible causes include cervical tears that have occurred during rapid second-stage childbirth delivery, forceps delivery and trauma.

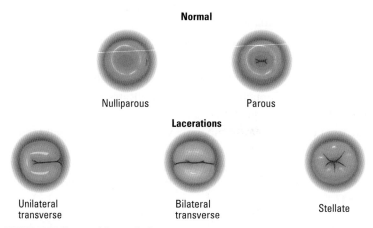

Normal

Nulliparous

Parous

Lacerations

Unilateral transverse

Bilateral transverse

Stellate

FIGURE 17.36 Shapes of the cervical os

Collecting specimens for cytological smears and cultures

After inspection of the cervix and the cervical os, obtain any laboratory specimens that are indicated. Collect the HPV sample first if other vaginal smears are required; for example, gonococcal. There are many accepted variations among laboratories regarding the collection and fixing of vaginal specimens. It is essential to identify the procedure recommended by the laboratory testing the specimens. See **Table 17.5**, which relates to national cervical screening programs for Australia and New Zealand.

HEALTH EDUCATION

Cervical screening: HPV test

Australia and New Zealand have updated the guidelines for the National Cervical Screening Program for HPV test. This change is due to the recognition that the oncogenetic human papilloma virus (HPV) causes the vast majority of cervical cancers.

There are approximately 40 different HPV types that cause infection of the genital tract and are common in sexually active women. These infections go unnoticed as they have no symptoms, are generally transient and clear up without intervention within 1 to 2 years. However, a number of HPV types are oncogenic, capable of causing cancer of the cervix, especially types 16 and 17. Screening women for HPV infection can identify those at high risk of developing cervical cancer early, enabling closer monitoring for cytological changes that precede invasive cervical cancer.

E Examination N Normal findings A Abnormal findings P Pathophysiology   Advanced Assessment

>>

The HPV test differs from the Pap smear, as it looks for the virus that causes the cell changes in the first place, rather than examining the cervical cells themselves.

This population screening program complements the publicly funded HPV vaccination program, with strong evidence that there will be a further 30% reduction in the incidence of cervical cancer over time. The test is effective for women who have had the HPV vaccine as well as those who have not. See Table 17.5 for guidelines.

As a health professional, can you identify opportunities when you could provide education to a woman about the HPV test?

Australian Government Department of Health and Aged Care (2022a); National Screening Unit (2022)

TABLE 17.5 National HPV cervical screening program guidelines

When to start	25 years of age > An invitation for a woman's first HPV test will be sent around her 25th birthday
Frequency and follow-up	> Five-yearly cervical screening using a primary HPV test with partial HPV genotyping and reflex liquid-based cytology (LBC) triage (for women who have positive results); for women HPV vaccinated and unvaccinated, 25–69 years of age, with exit testing of women up to 74 years of age > Women who test positive for high-risk HPV genotypes (i.e. HPV 16, 18) will proceed directly to colposcopy, irrespective of the LBC result.
Self-collection option	> Anyone who is eligible for cervical screening has the choice of HPV testing on a self-collected vaginal sample or on a clinician-collected sample. > Cervical screening on a self-collected vaginal sample needs to be ordered and overseen by a healthcare professional.
When to stop	74 years of age > Women will be invited and sent reminders for follow-ups until the age of 69 years, and exit communications will be sent to women 70–74 years of age.
Post-total hysterectomy	> Discontinue HPV test if hysterectomy for benign reasons and no prior history of high-grade cervical intraepithelial neoplasia (CIN).* However annual vaginal examinations are still recommended.

* Adapted from: Australian Government Department of Health and Aged Care (2022b); Cancer Council Australia (2022d); Ministry of Health/Manatū Hauora, National Screening Unit (2021c)

Endocervical smear

E 1. Using your dominant hand, insert the cytobrush or cervical broom through the speculum into the cervical os approximately 1 cm. Many consumers find that this procedure causes a cramping sensation, so forewarn your consumer that she may feel discomfort during this element of the assessment.

2. Rotate the cytobrush between your index finger and thumb 360° clockwise, then anticlockwise. Keep the cytobrush in contact with the cervical tissue (Figure 17.37).
Note: If you have to use a cotton-tipped applicator instead of a cytobrush, leave the applicator in the cervical os for 30 seconds to ensure saturation. If you use the cervical broom, rotate the broom 6 times clockwise and place the broom in the liquid-based preparation container.

3. Remove the cytobrush and, using a rolling motion, spread the cells on the slide.

4. Do not press down hard or wipe the cytobrush back and forth because doing so will destroy the cells.

5. Discard the brush.

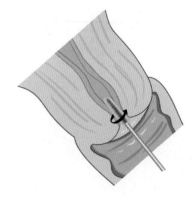

FIGURE 17.37 Endocervical smear

Cervical smear

E 1. Insert the bifurcated end of the Ayre spatula through the speculum base. Place the longer projection of the bifurcation into the cervical os. The shorter projection should be snug against the ectocervix.

2. Rotate the spatula 360° one time only (Figure 17.38). Make sure the transformation zone is well sampled.

3. Remove the spatula and gently spread the specimen on the section of the slide.

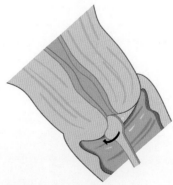

FIGURE 17.38 Cervical smear

E Examination   **N** Normal findings   **A** Abnormal findings   **P** Pathophysiology   Advanced Assessment

Classifications

N Normal classifications for all cervicovaginal tests should refer to the National Cervical Screening Program guidelines for the management of abnormal HPV/ liquid-based cytology (LBC). See www.cancerscreening.gov.au.

A A report finding of benign cellular changes is abnormal.

P Benign cellular changes have a multiplicity of causes including fungal, bacterial, protozoan or viral infections.

A A report finding of 'atypical squamous cells of undetermined significance' is abnormal.

P Causes of this finding include inflammatory or infectious processes, a preliminary lesion, or an unknown phenomenon.

A A report finding of epithelial cell abnormalities is aberrant.

Culture specimens

Vaginal culture

E 1. Insert a sterile cotton swab applicator 1 cm into the cervical os.
   2. Hold the applicator in place for 20 to 30 seconds.
   3. Remove the swab.
   4. Place the swab in a viral culture transport tube or microscope slide appropriate to the culture being tested.
   5. Dispose of the cotton swab applicator.
   6. Submit the specimens to the appropriate laboratory per your institution's guidelines for culture specimens

N Cervicovaginal tissues are normally free of abnormal bacteria such as *Neisseria gonorrhoeae* and *Chlamydia trachomatis*, and of HPV.

A It is abnormal to find a large number of Gram-negative diplococci present in cervicovaginal secretions.

P This finding is indicative of squamous intraepithelial lesion, which may or may not be transient; squamous cell carcinoma; or glandular cell abnormalities that are seen in postmenopausal women who are not on hormone replacement therapy.

A Cervicovaginal tissues are normally free of *Neisseria gonorrhoeae*.

P *N. gonorrhoeae* are Gram-negative diplococci organisms that prefer to invade columnar and stratified epithelium.

A It is abnormal to find *C. trachomatis*, serotypes D to K, or obligate, intracellular bacteria in cervicovaginal secretions.

P Trachomatis may invade the cervix or fallopian tubes, but it is often asymptomatic in women.

A Cervicovaginal tissues are normally free of *Candida albicans* except in a small percentage of women. There should be no odour.

P The presence of budding yeast is indicative of an overgrowth of *Candida*.

A An odour is abnormal.

P A fishy odour ('the whiff test') indicates bacterial vaginosis.

A Cervicovaginal tissues are normally free of human papillomavirus (HPV).

P The presence of HPV indicates genital warts, known to increase the risk of cervical cancer.

E Examination   **N** Normal findings   **A** Abnormal findings   **P** Pathophysiology   Advanced Assessment

HEALTH EDUCATION

HPV vaccination for infection prevention for teenagers
Australia and New Zealand publicly fund Gardasil 9 as the vaccine to help protect against the common types of high-risk HPV (types 16, 18, 31, 33, 45, 52 and 58). These have been identified as causing up to 90% of cervical cancers. The vaccine is also effective in protecting against two common types of low-risk HPV (types 6 and 11), which cause up to 90% of genital warts, but do not cause cervical cancer. The vaccine is included in the National Immunisation Schedule for girls and boys aged 12–13. This was a two-dose vaccine over a six-month period (Australian Government Department of Health and Aged Care, 2022a; Ministry of Health/Manatū Hauora, 2021a) but is now changing to a single dose (Australian Government Department of Health and Aged Care, 2023). Consider this information when exploring vaccination history, to guide further individualised education about vaccinations to prevent infections.

Anal culture
E 1. Insert a sterile cotton swab applicator 1 cm into the anal canal.
2. Hold the applicator in place for 20 to 30 seconds.
3. Remove the swab. If faecal material is collected, discard the applicator and start again.
4. Roll and rotate the swab in a large 'Z' pattern over a Thayer-Martin culture plate.
5. Dispose of the swab.

N Anal tissues are normally free of *Neisseria gonorrhoeae*

A The presence of a large number of Gram-negative diplococci is abnormal.

P This is indicative of *N. gonorrhoeae* infection.

Examination of the vaginal wall
Inspection
E 1. Disengage the locking device of the speculum.
2. Slowly withdraw the speculum but do not close the blades.
3. Rotate the speculum into an oblique position as you retract it to allow full inspection of the vaginal walls.
4. Observe vaginal wall colour and texture.

N The vaginal walls should be pink, moist, deeply rugated, and without lesions or redness.

A Spots that appear as white paint on the walls are abnormal.

P A possible cause is leukoplakia from *Candida albicans*. Repeated occurrences even after treatment may indicate HIV infection.

A Pallor of the vaginal walls is abnormal.

P Possible causes include anaemia and menopause.

A Redness of the vaginal walls is abnormal.

P Possible causes include inflammation, hyperaemia, and trauma from tampon insertion or removal.

A Vaginal lesions or masses are abnormal findings.

P Possible causes include carcinoma, tumours and DES exposure.

Examining the consumer with an STI

You are a women's health nurse in a small community and your first consumer for the day has presented complaining of vaginal discharge. She tells you that she has noticed an odourless, greenish discharge from her vagina during the past 2 weeks. When you are taking her health history she informs you that she has been married for 37 years and has not had any sexual partners other than her husband during that time. She shares her concerns that her husband may be having extra-marital relations. On inspection and examination you observe that her vulva is erythematous, and there is pus in her cervical os.

> How would you further assess this individual?

> What additional questions would you ask?

> What anticipatory guidance would you provide?

Bimanual examination

E 1. Observe the woman's face for signs of discomfort during the assessment process.

2. Inform the woman of the steps of the bimanual assessment, and warn her that the lubricant gel may be cold.

3. Squeeze water-soluble lubricant onto the fingertips of your dominant hand.

4. Stand between the legs of the individual as she remains in the lithotomy position, and place your nondominant hand on her abdomen and below the umbilicus.

5. Insert your dominant index and middle fingers 1 cm into the vagina. The fingers should be extended with the palmar side up. Exert gentle posterior pressure.

6. Inform the woman that pressure from palpation may be uncomfortable. Instruct her to relax the abdominal muscles by taking deep breaths.

7. When you feel the woman's muscles relax, insert your fingers to their full length into the vagina. Insert your fingers slowly so that you can simultaneously palpate the vaginal walls.

8. Remember to keep your thumb widely abducted and away from the urethral meatus and clitoris throughout the palpation in order to prevent pain or spasm.

Palpation

Vagina

E Complete steps 1–8 of the bimanual examination.

9. Rotate the wrist so that the fingers are able to palpate all surface aspects of the vagina.

N The vaginal wall is nontender and has a smooth or rugated surface with no lesions, masses or cysts.

A The presence of lesions, masses, scarring or cysts is abnormal.

P These findings may be indicative of benign lesions such as inclusion cysts, myomas or fibromas. The most common site for malignant lesions of the vagina is the upper one-third of the posterior vaginal wall.

Cervix

E 1. Position the dominant hand so that the palmar surface faces upwards.
2. Place the nondominant hand on the abdomen approximately one-third of the way down between the umbilicus and the symphysis pubis.
3. Use the palmar surfaces of the dominant hand's finger pads, which are in the vagina, to assess the cervix for consistency, position, shape and tenderness.
4. Grasp the cervix between the fingertips and move the cervix from side to side to assess mobility (Figure 17.39).

N The normal cervix is mobile without pain, smooth and firm, symmetrically rounded and midline.

A The presence of pain on palpation or the assessment of mobility is a positive Chandelier sign and is abnormal.

P This is indicative of possible pelvic inflammatory disease or ectopic pregnancy.

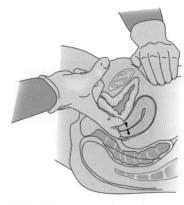

FIGURE 17.39 Assessment of cervical mobility

A Softening of the cervix (Goodell's sign) is a significant finding.

P This sign is seen at the fifth to sixth week of pregnancy.

A Irregular surface, immobility, or nodular surface structure of the cervix indicates abnormality.

P Possible causes include malignancy, fibroids, nabothian cysts and polyps.

Fornices

E 1. With the fingertips and palmar surfaces of the fingers, palpate around the fornices.
2. Note nodules or irregularities.

N The walls should be smooth and without nodules.

A The presence of nodules or irregularities is abnormal.

P Possible causes include malignancy, polyps and herniations if the walls of the fornices are impatent.

Uterus

E 1. With the dominant hand, which is in the vagina, push the pelvic organs out of the pelvic cavity and provide stabilisation while the nondominant hand, which is on the abdomen, performs the palpation (Figure 17.40).
2. Press the hand that is on the abdomen inwards and downwards towards the vagina, and try to grasp the uterus between your hands.
3. Evaluate the uterus for size, shape, consistency, mobility, tenderness, masses and position.
4. Place the fingers of the intravaginal hand into the anterior fornix and palpate the uterine surface.

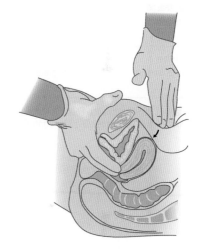

FIGURE 17.40 Uterine palpation

N The size of the uterus varies depending on parity. It should be pear-shaped in the nongravid consumer and more rounded in the parous consumer. The uterus should be smooth, firm, mobile, nontender and without masses. For uterine positions, see Figure 17.3. A uterus may be nonpalpable if it is retroverted or retroflexed. The uterus in these positions can be assessed only via rectovaginal examination. A nonpalpable uterus in the older woman may be a normal finding secondary to uterine atrophy.

A Significant exterior enlargement and changes in the shape of the uterus are abnormal.

P Uterine enlargement indicates possible intrauterine pregnancy or tumour.

A Presence of nodules or irregularities indicates leiomyomas.

P Leiomyomas are tumours containing muscle tissue.

A Inability to assess the uterus may be abnormal.

P A hysterectomy may account for a nonpalpable uterus.

E Examination   **N** Normal findings   **A** Abnormal findings   **P** Pathophysiology   Advanced Assessment

TABLE 17.6 Types of urinary incontinence

Incontinence is a common symptom and is described as accidental or involuntary loss of urine from the bladder affecting men and women of all ages, with 1 in 3 women, 1 in 10 men and 1 in 5 children impacted. It should be noted that some health conditions and circumstances increase the risk of developing urinary incontinence and relate to the following.

TYPE	DEFINITION	CAUSE
Stress	Stress incontinence is involuntary leakage of urine that occurs during exertion, such as playing sport, lifting, laughing and coughing	Childbirth, pregnancy, previous abdominal surgery, prostate surgery, radiation therapy
Urge	Urge incontinence is sudden feeling of needing to pass urine, with the individual unable to make it to the bathroom, resulting in an involuntary loss of urine	Stroke, dementia, multiple sclerosis, Parkinson's disease, brain tumour, urinary tract tumours, urinary tract infections (see Chapter 18)
Overflow	Involuntary loss of urine due to an overextended bladder; incontinence occurs when bladder pressure exceeds urethral pressure; usually small amount of urine occurs during dribbling; may be some hesitancy and frequency	Faecal impaction, diabetic neuropathy, obstruction of the bladder or urethra (due to prostate cancer, benign prostatic hypertrophy)
Functional	Involuntary loss of urine due to the inability to reach the toilet because of physical, cognitive or environmental impairments	Immobility, dementia, inaccessible toilet, inappropriate lighting, physical restraints
Increased frequency	Increased frequency is the need to empty the bladder more regularly than what is considered normal for the individual, especially during the night	Changes in muscles/nerves that affect bladder function. Infection, diseases, injury: irritation of the bladder. Conditions that increase urine production, such as diabetes insipidus
Urinary retention	Urinary retention occurs when an individual is unable to empty their bladder completely, resulting in overflow and regular leaking of urine	Benign prostatic / hyperplasia /enlarged prostate; bladder obstruction, such as urethral stricture or scar tissue in the bladder neck; pelvic organ prolapse; constipation

Adapted from Continence Foundation of Australia. https://www.continence.org.au/types-incontinence/urinary-incontinence; Continence NZ https://www.continence.org.nz/pages/Bladder-Control-Problems-in-Women/39/

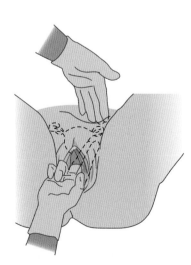

FIGURE 17.41 Palpation of the left adnexa

Adnexa

Fallopian tubes are rarely palpable, and palpation of the ovaries depends on consumer age and size. Many times, the ovaries are not palpable, and this procedure can be painful to the consumer during the luteal phase of the menstrual cycle (postovulation) or due to normal visceral tenderness.

E 1. Move the intravaginal hand to the right lateral fornix, and the hand on the abdomen to the right lower quadrant just inside the anterior iliac spine. Press deeply inwards and upwards towards the abdominal hand.
2. Push inwards and downwards with the abdominal hand and try to catch the ovary between your fingertips.
3. Palpate for size, shape, consistency and mobility of the adnexa.
4. Repeat the above manoeuvres on the left side (see **Figure 17.41**).

N The ovaries are normally almond-shaped, firm, smooth and mobile without tenderness.

A Presence of enlarged ovaries that are irregular, nodular, painful, with decreased mobility, or pulsatile indicate pathology.

P Abnormal adnexal presentation may indicate ectopic pregnancy, ovarian cyst, pelvic inflammatory disease or malignancy.

Rectovaginal examination

E 1. Withdraw your dominant hand from the vagina and change gloves. Apply lubricant to the fingertips of your dominant hand.
2. Tell the woman you will be inserting one finger into her vagina and one finger into her rectum. Remind her that the lubricant jelly will feel cold and that the rectal examination will be uncomfortable.
3. Insert the dominant index finger back into the vagina.

E Examination   **N** Normal findings   **A** Abnormal findings   **P** Pathophysiology   Advanced Assessment

E 4. Ask the woman to strain down as if she is having a bowel movement, in order to relax the anal sphincter. Assess anal sphincter tone.

5. Insert the middle finger of the dominant hand into the woman's rectum as she strains down (see **Figure 17.42**). If the rectum is full of stool, carefully remove the stool digitally from the rectum.

6. Advance the rectal finger forwards while using the nondominant hand to depress the abdomen. Assess the rectovaginal septum for patency, the cervix and uterus for anomalies such as posterior lesions, and the rectouterine pouch for contour lesions.

7. On completion of the assessment, withdraw the fingers from the vagina and rectum, and if any stool is present on the glove, test for occult blood.

8. Clean the woman's genitalia and anal area with a tissue and assist her back to a sitting position.

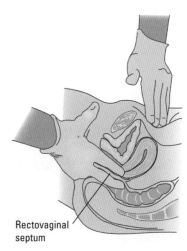

Rectovaginal septum

FIGURE 17.42 Rectovaginal examination

N The rectal walls are normally smooth and free of lesions. The rectal pouch is rugated and free of masses. Anal sphincter tone is strong. The cervix and uterus, if palpable, are smooth. The rectovaginal septum is smooth and intact. Refer to Chapter 18 for further information on the complete rectal examination.

A The presence of masses or lesions indicates pathology.

P Possible causes include malignancy and internal haemorrhoids.

A Lax sphincter tone is an abnormal finding.

P Possible causes include perineal trauma from childbirth or anal intercourse, and neurological disorders.

HEALTH EDUCATION

Maintaining sexual function in the menopausal woman

It is a myth that post-menopausal woman do not have or enjoy sexual activities. When assessing an older woman, the following advice may be beneficial in helping her to continue to be sexually active:

> Use water-soluble lubricant if vaginal secretions are decreased.
> Extend foreplay in order to attain orgasm.
> Remember that there is no risk of pregnancy.

Examining consumers with urinary diversions

For all tubes, drains and intestinal and urinary diversions, note colour, odour, amount, consistency, and the presence of blood in any drainage. Check for an obstruction if there is no drainage. The skin around the device should be intact without excoriation.

Urinary diversions

Ileal conduit

> Stoma is pink.
> Skin barrier is used with appliance.

Ureteral stents

> Stent is secured to collection bag.
> No bleeding from insertion site.

Indwelling catheter and suprapubic catheter

> Balloon is inflated.
> Catheter is secured to consumer to prevent dislodgement.
> Urinary collecting bag is closed.
> Drainage tube is below level of bladder and without kinks

IMPLEMENTATION: CONDUCTING THE PHYSICAL EXAMINATION OF THE MALE

Implementation of the physical examination requires you to consider your scope of practice. Depending on your context, you may be performing a foundation assessment, or the addition of advanced assessment techniques if you are practising in a specialised area.

EXAMINATION IN BRIEF: BLADDER AND MALE GENITALIA

Examination of the bladder

Inspection

Palpation

Percussion

Examination of the male genitalia

Inspection
> Sexual maturity rating
> Pubic hair distribution
> Penis
> Acetowhitening: examining for human papillomavirus (HPV)
> Scrotum
> Urethral meatus
> Inguinal area

Palpation
> Penis
> Urethral meatus
> Urethral swab: identifying penile pathogens
> Scrotum
> Examining for testicular torsion (Prehn's sign)
> Inguinal area
> Transillumination of the scrotum: assessing for a scrotal mass

Auscultation
> Scrotum

Examining consumers with urinary diversions
> Urinary diversions
> Ileal conduit
> Ureteral stents
> Indwelling catheters and suprapubic catheters

General approach to examination of the male genitalia

Physical assessment of the male genitalia is undertaken together in the one sequence of assessment.

1. Prior to the assessment, make sure you introduce yourself to the consumer and explain the assessment techniques that you will be using.
2. Ensure the examination room is at a warm, comfortable temperature to prevent consumer chilling and shivering.
3. Use a quiet room that will be free from interruptions.
4. Ensure that the light in the room provides sufficient brightness to adequately observe the consumer.
5. Assess the individual's apprehension level about the assessment and address this with him, reassuring him that this is normal.
6. Instruct the consumer to remove his pants and underpants.
7. Assist the consumer onto the examination table in the supine position with the legs spread slightly, and cover with a drape sheet. Stand to the consumer's right side or have the consumer stand in front of you while you are sitting.
8. Don nonsterile gloves.
9. Expose the entire genital and groin area.

REFLECTION IN PRACTICE

Sensitivity during genitalia examination

Before beginning the genitalia examination, consider the consumer's cultural background and what beliefs or attitudes he may have about having the examination. Does the individual's culture prohibit a female nurse from examining a male consumer? Does the individual's culture prohibit a male nurse from examining a female consumer?

Reflect on how you provide culturally safe practice. How does the above clinical encounter impact on how you will practise in the future?

    Advanced Assessment

Examination of the bladder
Inspection
See Chapter 15 for abdominal examination.

Palpation
You may see clinically the order of bladder palpation and percussion varies; this may occur concurrently or out of sequence.

E 1. Using deep palpation, palpate the abdomen at the midline, starting at the symphysis pubis and progressing up to the umbilicus (**Figure 17.43**).
2. If the bladder is located, palpate the shape, size and consistency.

N An empty bladder is not usually palpable. A moderately full bladder is smooth and round, and it is palpable above the symphysis pubis. A full bladder is palpated above the symphysis pubis, and it may be close to the umbilicus.

A A bladder that is nodular or asymmetrical to palpation is abnormal.

P A nodular bladder may indicate a malignancy. An asymmetrical bladder may result from a tumour in the bladder or an abdominal tumour that is compressing the bladder.

A It is abnormal to palpate a bladder that has been recently emptied.

P Specific to men with benign prostatic hypertrophy – they may be unable to completely empty their bladder because of the pressure that the enlarged prostate places on the bladder.

P Various types of urinary incontinence, due to altered mental status, muscle function, medications and other causes, can lead to incomplete bladder emptying. See **Table 17.6** for additional information on urinary incontinence.

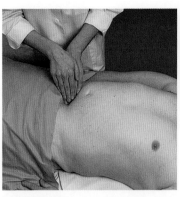
FIGURE 17.43 Palpation of the bladder

Percussion
E 1. Percuss upwards from the symphysis pubis to the umbilicus.
2. Note where the sound changes from dullness to tympany.

N A urine-filled bladder is dull to percussion. A recently emptied bladder should not be percussible above the symphysis pubis.

A It is abnormal to percuss a bladder that has recently been emptied. The urine that remains in the bladder after urination is called residual urine. A bladder may also be dull to percussion when the consumer has difficulty voiding.

P The inability to completely empty the bladder occurs in the elderly; in postoperative, bedridden and acutely ill consumers; and in consumers with neurogenic bladder dysfunction.

P Difficult voiding can occur in conjunction with benign prostatic hypertrophy (see Chapter 18 for additional information), urethral pathology and some medications (antipsychotics: phenothiazine; anticholinergics: atropine; antihypertensives: hydralazine).

Examination of the male genitalia
Inspection
Sexual maturity rating
E 1. Using the Tanner stages in **Table 17.2** (on page 655), assess the developmental stage of the pubic hair, penis and scrotum.
2. Determine the sexual maturity rating (SMR).

N Males usually begin puberty between the ages of 9½ and 13½ years. The average male proceeds through puberty in about 3 years, with a possible range of 2 to 5 years.

A An SMR that is less than expected for a male's age is abnormal.

P Delayed puberty may be familial or caused by chronic illnesses.

E Examination **N** Normal findings **A** Abnormal findings **P** Pathophysiology

A A normally formed but diminutive penis is abnormal. There is a discrepancy between the penile size and the age of the individual.

P A **microphallus** can result from a disorder in the hypothalamus or pituitary gland. It may be secondary to primary testicular failure due to partial androgen insensitivity. Maternal DES exposure has teratogenic effects caused by defects in nonandrogen-dependent regulatory agents. Microphallus can also be idiopathic in nature.

A It is abnormal when the penis appears larger than what is generally expected for the stated age. This condition is usually evident only before the age of normal puberty.

P Hormonal influence of tumours of the pineal gland or hypothalamus, tumours of the Leydig cells of the testes, tumours of the adrenal gland and precocious genital maturity may cause penile hyperplasia.

A A testicle that is smaller and softer than normal (less than 5 cm × 2.5 cm) is abnormal.

P An atrophic testicle may be the result of Klinefelter syndrome (hypogonadism), hypopituitarism, oestrogen therapy or orchitis.

HEALTH EDUCATION

Hygiene for the uncircumcised male
During the penis examination, it is important to review proper hygiene. Instruct the consumer to retract the foreskin daily so that the underlying skin can be washed with soap and warm water. The skin should also be dried thoroughly and the foreskin returned to its original position. How would you approach the provision of opportunistic education while examining a paediatric child, aged 11 years old?

Pubic hair distribution
E 1. Note hair distribution pattern.
2. Note the presence of nits or lice.

N Pubic hair is distributed in a triangular form. It is sparsely distributed on the scrotum and inner thigh and absent on the penis. Genital hair is coarser than scalp hair. There are no nits or lice.

A Hair distribution is sparse or hair is absent at the genitalia area. This is called alopecia and it is abnormal.

P Alopecia in the genital area may result from genetic factors, ageing, or local or systemic disease. These include developmental defects and hereditary disorders, infection, neoplasms, physical or chemical agents, endocrine diseases, deficiency states (nutritional or metabolic), or destruction of or damage to the follicles.

A The presence of nits or lice is abnormal.

P See Chapter 8 for further information related to skin and hair.

HEALTH EDUCATION

Risk factors for penile cancer
When reviewing your assessment data, consider the following risk factors related to penile cancer and, where appropriate, provide education to increase awareness for your consumer.
> Over 50 years of age
> Intact foreskin, especially with phimosis
> Poor hygiene and smegma build-up
> History of HPV types 16, 18 and 31
> Smoking
> AIDS

E Examination **N** Normal findings **A** Abnormal findings **P** Pathophysiology

Penis

E 1. Inspect the glans, foreskin and shaft for lesions, swelling and inflammation. If the consumer is uncircumcised, ask him to retract the foreskin so that the underlying area can be inspected. After the assessment, replace the foreskin.
2. Inspect the anterior surface of the penis first. Then lift the penis to check the posterior surface.
3. Note the shape of the penis.

N Skin is free of lesions and inflammation. The shaft skin appears loose and wrinkled in the male without an erection. The glans is smooth and without lesions, swelling or inflammation. The foreskin retracts easily and there is no discharge. There may be a small amount of **smegma**, a white, cottage cheese-like substance, present. The dorsal vein is sometimes visible. The penis is cylindrical in shape. The glans penis varies in size and shape and may appear rounded or broad.

A Inflammation of the glans penis is abnormal.

P This inflammation is called balanitis. The prepuce may also be affected. This is a bacterial infection that is associated with phimosis and is seen in diabetic men.

P Balanitis can occur with sexually transmitted diseases. The consumer in **Figure 17.44** had balanitis of the glans penis from a chlamydial infection (nongonococcal urethritis) caused by *Chlamydia trachomatis*.

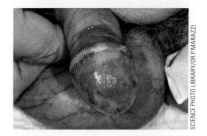

FIGURE 17.44 Balanitis of the glans penis

HEALTH EDUCATION

Unsafe sexual practices

If you identify any of the following situations while undertaking the male genitalia assessment, take the opportunity, if appropriate, to provide individualised education about the following potentially harmful practices:

> Has shared injection needles and syringes
> Has had sex without a condom with an HIV-positive partner
> Has had a sexually transmitted infection, such as chlamydia or gonorrhoea
> Had a blood transfusion or received a blood clotting factor between 1978 and 1985
> Has sex with someone who is paid to have sex
> Has sex while under the influence of drugs or alcohol
> Has had anal intercourse
> Has had multiple sex partners
> Has had sex with someone who has done any of the above

A A small lesion that enlarges and undergoes superficial necrosis to produce a sharply marginated ulcer on a clean base is abnormal.

P The chancre is the lesion of primary syphilis (**Figure 17.45**). It contains a multitude of *Treponema pallidum* spirochaetes and is highly infectious. The tissue reacts to the organism with infiltration of lymphocytes, fibroblasts and plasma cells that cause swelling and proliferation of the endothelial tissue, manifesting as a chancre.

A A tender, painful, ulcerated, exudative, popular lesion with an erythematous halo, surrounding oedema and a friable base is abnormal (**Figure 17.46**).

P **Chancroid** is caused by inoculation of *Haemophilus ducreyi* through small breaks in epidermal tissue. Acute inflammatory response causes bubo formation. This is usually accompanied by inguinal adenopathy.

A A penile lesion that ranges from a relatively subtle induration to a small papule, pustule, warty growth, or exophytic lesion is abnormal. The distribution of lesions is most commonly on the glans and prepuce.

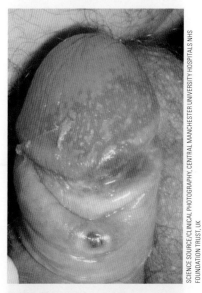

FIGURE 17.45 Syphilitic chancre

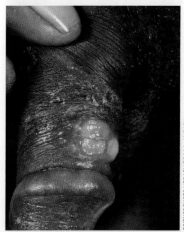

FIGURE 17.46 Chancroid of the penis with right inguinal lymphadenopathy

E Examination   **N** Normal findings   **A** Abnormal findings   **P** Pathophysiology

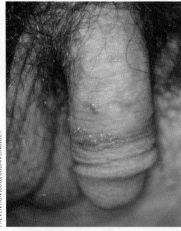

COURTESY OF THE CENTERS FOR DISEASE CONTROL AND PREVENTION (CDC)/SUSAN LINDSLEY

FIGURE 17.47 Genital warts

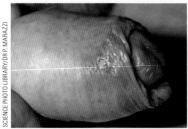

SCIENCE PHOTO LIBRARY/DR P. MARAZZI

A. Close-up of a penis affected by herpes simplex

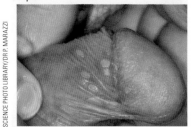

SCIENCE PHOTO LIBRARY/DR P. MARAZZI

B. Genital herpes on the penis

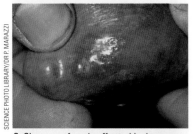

SCIENCE PHOTO LIBRARY/DR P. MARAZZI

C. Close-up of penis affected by herpes simplex

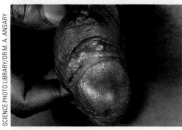

SCIENCE PHOTO LIBRARY/DR M. A. ANSARY

D. Genital ulceration caused by herpes simplex virus-2

FIGURE 17.48 Vesicular lesions

P Penile carcinoma usually begins with a small lesion that gradually extends to involve the entire glans, shaft and corpora. Circumcision has been well established as a prophylactic measure that will eliminate the occurrence of penile carcinoma.

A Pinhead papules to cauliflower-like groupings of filiform, skin-coloured, pink or red lesions are abnormal (**Figure 17.47**).

P **Condyloma acuminatum** or genital warts are caused by HPV infection of the epithelial cells. HPV may remain dormant for months to years after infection. There is a high incidence of recurrence of condyloma following appropriate treatment because of the persistence of latent HPV in normal-appearing skin. Lesions may be visualised by using acetowhitening. Refer to the advanced practice 'Acetowhitening: examining for human papillomavirus (HPV)'.

A Multifocal maculopapular lesions that are tan, brown, pink, violet or white are abnormal.

P This describes intraepithelial neoplasia. Infection by HPV oncogenic types 16, 18, 31 and 33 causes epidermal proliferation and koilocytotic, dyskeratotic cells. Female partners may have a history of cervical intraepithelial neoplasm (CIN). The majority of lesions are distributed on the glans penis and prepuce. Changes of squamous cell carcinoma in situ are seen on histological examination.

A Erythematous, painful ulcers developing into vesicular lesions that may become pustular, are abnormal (**Figure 17.48**).

P This describes genital herpes simplex virus infection. Skin-to-skin contact infection of HSV 1 and 2 causes epidermal degeneration, acanthosis and intraepidermal vesicles. Lesions become ulcerated and eroded and are moist or crusted. Epithelial changes resolve in 2 to 4 weeks and hyper- or hypopigmentation of these areas is common. Post-inflammatory scarring is rare. Recurrent herpes lesions are smaller. Diagnosis may be confirmed by Tzanck test for microscopic acanthocytes, viral culture or serology for HSV antibodies.

CLINICAL **REASONING**

Male sexual assault

Male sexual assault is forced intercourse or sexual contact that occurs without consent. Male sexual assault includes fondling, forced anal sex, forced oral sex, stimulation of an erection, stimulation of ejaculation, and oral-to-anal contact. Consumers may present with genital injuries, lacerations to the anal sphincter, rectal tears, fissures or haematomas. Non-genital injuries may include a black eye, fractured jaw, cerebral concussion or facial contusions/lacerations. Male sexual assault victims may experience confusion about their sexual orientation, have nightmares, suicidal ideation and self-blame. As a health professional you will need to explore with them the supports available and whether referral is an option they wish to pursue. It is important to protect the consumer's rights and allow them to make informed decisions; however, support them with considerations of the impact that the assault has had on them. You may need to offer the consumer referral to a trained therapist or counsellor.

A Multiple, discrete, flat pustules with slight scaling and surrounding oedema are abnormal.

P Candida is a superficial mycotic infection of moist cutaneous sites. Predisposing factors include moisture, diabetes mellitus, antibiotic therapy, and deficiencies in systemic immunity.

A Erythematous plaques with scaling; papular lesions with sharp margins, and occasionally clear centres; and pustules are abnormal.

P Tinea cruris is a fungal infection of the groin, usually caused by *Epidermophyton floccosum* or *Trichophyton rubrum*. Predisposing factors are a warm, humid environment, tight clothing and obesity.

E Examination **N** Normal findings **A** Abnormal findings **P** Pathophysiology

A An unusually long foreskin or one that cannot be retracted over the glans penis is abnormal.

P **Phimosis** occurs in uncircumcised males (**Figure 17.49**). Inability to retract the foreskin is normal in infancy. In later years, an acquired constricting circumferential scar may follow healing of a split foreskin.

A It is abnormal when the retracted foreskin develops a fixed constriction proximal to the glans (**Figure 17.50**). The penis distal to the foreskin may become swollen and gangrenous.

P This is called **paraphimosis**. If the foreskin is retracted and not returned to its original position, paraphimosis can ensue (e.g. a consumer's penis is cleansed for indwelling catheter insertion and the foreskin remains retracted). The foreskin acts as a circulatory constrictor, causing decreased blood flow, oedema and potential tissue necrosis.

A A continuous and pathological erection of the penis is abnormal.

P The cause of **priapism** is unclear in most consumers; however, it does not occur as the result of sexual desire. Some of the cases are associated with leukaemia, metastatic carcinoma, sickle cell anaemia, intracavernous injection, alcohol abuse, genital trauma and neurologic disorders. Some drugs, such as antihypertensives, antipsychotics and antidepressants, have also been associated with prolonged erections. The consumer may also present after having used a medication for erectile dysfunction. Priapism is created by the positive imbalance between the arterial blood supply and its return, created by venous drainage.

A Penile curvature, or chordee, is either a ventral or a dorsal curvature of the penis and is abnormal.

P Curvature is usually congenitally caused by a fibrous band along the usual course of the corpus spongiosum. Ventral chordee is seen mostly with **epispadias** (see **Figure 17.51**), when the urethral meatus opens dorsally on the glans. In cases of congenital penile curvature without epispadias or **hypospadias** (when the urethral meatus opens ventrally on the glans), there is no additional tissue on or in any portion of the corpora cavernosa (**Figure 17.52**). This is caused by congenital maldevelopment of the tunica albuginea of the corpora.

A Peyronie's disease is a condition of penile curvature that occurs with erection (**Figure 17.53**). The dorsal surface of the corpora cavernosa becomes hardened with palpable, nontender plaques. Its cause is unknown.

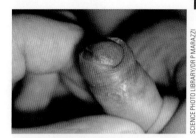

FIGURE 17.49 Phimosis

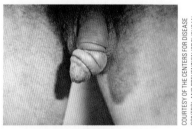

FIGURE 17.50 Paraphimosis

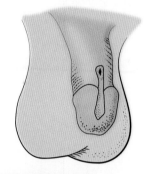

FIGURE 17.51 Epispadias

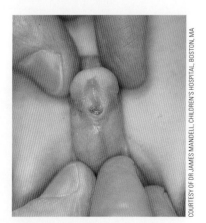

FIGURE 17.52 Hypospadias

CLINICAL **REASONING**

Signs of STIs in the male consumer

Although some STIs have recognisable symptoms associated with them, many do not. This means that a person may not be aware of transferring the infection to another. Consider the following symptoms, which you should identify through the genital assessment. Think of the ways that you might be able to assess your consumer to identify when there is no symptom recognisable/identifiable, yet the person is diagnosed with an STI.

> Urethral discharge, bloody or purulent
> Scrotal or testicular pain
> Burning or pain during urination
> Penile lesion

For example, if you noted a penile lesion, you would gain permission for further examination and take a swab of the lesion. You would then follow this up, provide education such as on safe sexual practices until formal results were available, and then ensure a referral is booked. Pending your scope of practice (i.e. as an RN versus an NP), you may be able to prescribe antibiotics or further investigations.

E Examination **N** Normal findings **A** Abnormal findings **P** Pathophysiology

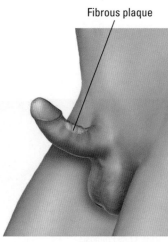

Fibrous plaque

FIGURE 17.53 Dorsal curvature of the penis in Peyronie's disease

Acetowhitening: examining for human papillomavirus (HPV)

The purpose of acetowhitening is to identify warty skin lesions that are not easily seen by the naked eye. It is indicated with a history of warts or HPV, of sexual contact with a partner with warts or HPV, of high-risk sexual behaviour or of STI. The goal of treatment is the removal of exophytic warts and the elimination of signs and symptoms, not the eradication of HPV.

Equipment

> Nonsterile gloves
> ×10 power magnifying lens
> Plastic sheet
> 2.5–3 cm gauze wrap
> Scissors
> 5% acetic acid solution (white vinegar) in spray bottle

E
1. Explain the procedure to the consumer.
2. Have the consumer undress from the waist down and sit on plastic sheet at the edge of the examination table.
3. Wash hands. Don gloves.
4. Have the consumer lie supine.
5. Wrap the penis and the scrotal area with gauze wrap that has been impregnated with 5% acetic acid solution.
6. Allow the area to soak in the saturated gauze for 5 minutes.
7. Remove the gauze from the penis and scrotal areas.
8. Examine the penis and scrotum with a magnifying lens.

N The penis and scrotal area should be free of any whitish-appearing areas.

A *Condyloma acuminatum* (HPV) appears as tiny white papules identified with a ×10 hand lens.

P The 'acetowhite' lesions are not always due to HPV, and the consumer should be referred for a biopsy to confirm the diagnosis.

P Refer to the prior discussion on HPV infection.

Scrotum

E
1. Displace the penis to one side in order to inspect the scrotal skin.
2. Lift up the scrotum to inspect the posterior side.
3. Observe for lesions, inflammation, swelling and nodules.
4. Note size and shape.
5. The consumer should then stand with legs spread slightly apart.
6. Have the consumer perform the Valsalva manoeuvre.
7. Observe for a mass of dilated testicular veins in the spermatic cords above and behind the testes.

N Scrotal skin appears rugated and thin and more deeply pigmented than body colour. The skin should hug the testicles firmly in the young male and become elongated and flaccid in the elderly male. All skin areas should be free of any lesions, nodules, swelling or inflammation. Scrotal size and shape vary greatly from one individual to another. The left scrotal sac is lower than the right. There should be no dilated testicular veins.

A **P** *Condyloma acuminatum*, *tinea cruris* and candida are abnormal findings. See prior discussion.

A Enlargement of or masses within the scrotum are abnormal.

P Scrotal masses can arise from benign or malignant conditions. Scrotal swelling is seen with inguinal hernia, hydrocoele, varicocele, spermatocoele, tumour and oedema.

E Examination   **N** Normal findings   **A** Abnormal findings   **P** Pathophysiology   Advanced Assessment

A A large, pear-sized mass in the scrotum is abnormal (**Figure 17.54**). The scrotal skin is stretched, shiny and erythematous, which may give the penis a shortened appearance.

P A **hydrocoele** is created by the accumulation of fluid between the two layers of the tunica vaginalis. Hydrocoeles may be idiopathic or due to trauma, inguinal surgery, epididymitis or testicular tumour.

A A well-defined cystic mass on the superior testis or in the epididymis is abnormal. It is usually <2 cm in diameter (**Figure 17.55**). Multiple masses may be present.

P This is called **spermatocoele**. Blockage of the efferent ductules of the rete testis causes formation of sperm-filled cysts at the top of the testis or in the epididymis.

A In light-skinned individuals, a scrotal mass with a bluish discolouration is abnormal (**Figure 17.56**).

P Dilated veins in the pampiniform plexus of the spermatic cord cause **varicocele** formation and are usually accompanied by a decreased sperm count. Most appear in the left hemiscrotum; the remainder are bilateral. A right-sided varicocele may be indicative of an obstruction at the vena cava. Acute onset of a right-sided varicocele may be pathognomonic of a renal tumour extending into the renal vein or compression of the renal vein. It may increase in size with the Valsalva manoeuvre and decrease or disappear with supine positioning.

A Round, firm, cystic nodules confined within the scrotal skin are abnormal.

P A sebaceous cyst contains sebum, an oily, fatty matter secreted by the sebaceous glands. The cyst may result from a decrease in localised circulation and closure of sebaceous glands or ducts.

Urethral meatus

E 1. Note the location of the urethral meatus.
  2. Observe for discharge.
  3. Obtain a culture of any discharge (see advanced practice on urethral culture).
  4. If the consumer complains of penile discharge but none is present, ask the consumer to milk the penis from the shaft to the glans. This manoeuvre may express a discharge that can then be cultured.

N The urethral meatus is located centrally. It is pink and without discharge.

A Erythema and swelling at the urethral meatus are abnormal.

P Urethritis is a localised tissue inflammation resulting from bacterial, viral or fungal infection as well as from urethral trauma.

A It is abnormal for the urethral meatus to be displaced dorsally (see **Figure 17.51**).

P Epispadias is a congenital abnormality caused by a complete or partial dorsal fusion defect of the urethra.

A It is abnormal for the urethral meatus to open on the ventral aspect of the glans penis (see **Figure 17.52**). The urethral meatus may also open at the perineum.

P Hypospadias is a congenital abnormality, usually associated with chordee. Complications of this defect include urethral meatal stenosis, inability to direct the urine stream and sexual dysfunction.

Inguinal area

E 1. If the consumer is supine, ask the consumer to stand.
  2. Stand facing the consumer.
  3. Observe for swelling or bulges.
  4. Ask the consumer to bear down.
  5. Observe for swelling or bulges.

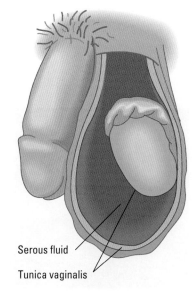

Serous fluid

Tunica vaginalis

FIGURE 17.54 Hydrocoele

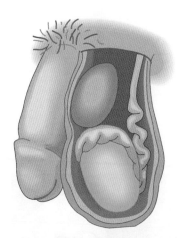

FIGURE 17.55 Spermatocoele

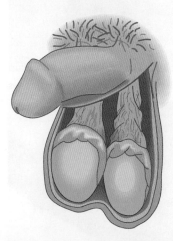

FIGURE 17.56 Varicocele

E Examination **N** Normal findings **A** Abnormal findings **P** Pathophysiology

N The inguinal area is free of any swelling or bulges.

A A bulge in the inguinal area is abnormal.

P Hernia pathology is discussed further in the section on palpation.

Palpation

Penis

E 1. Stand in front of the consumer's genital area.
2. Don nonsterile gloves.
3. With the thumb and the first two fingers, palpate the entire length of the penis (Figure 17.57).
4. Note any pulsations, tenderness, masses or plaques.

N Pulsations are present on the dorsal sides of the penis. The penis is nontender. No masses or firm plaques are palpated.

A It is abnormal to palpate fibrotic plaques or ridges along the dorsal shaft.

P Plaques develop from perivascular inflammation between the tunica albuginea and the underlying spongy erectile tissue.

A Vascular insufficiency is evidenced by diminished or absent palpable pulse or pulsations and is abnormal.

P Systemic disease, localised trauma and localised disease may adversely affect normal blood flow in the penis.

A It is abnormal for the penis to be enlarged in a nonerect state. Generalised penile swelling may be present.

P Fluid accumulation in the loose tissue of the penile integument results from anasarcic (general swelling of the whole body) states. Obstruction of the penile veins or inflammation of the penis results in local oedema. Trauma to the penis may cause swelling secondary to penile contusion and extravasation of blood. Gentle finger pressure may cause pitting.

Urethral meatus

E 1. Stand in front of the consumer's genital area.
2. Grasp the glans between the thumb and forefinger and gently squeeze to expose the meatus (Figure 17.58).
3. If discharge is seen, or if the consumer complains of a urethral discharge, a culture should be taken.

N The urethral meatus is free of discharge and drainage.

A A urethral discharge of pus and mucus shreds is abnormal (Figure 17.59). The discharge may vary in colour, consistency and amount.

P Bacterial infection of the genitourinary tract causes inflammation and formation of a liquid composed of albuminous substances, leucocytes, shedding tissue cells, and bacteria.

Urethral swab: identifying penile pathogens

Equipment

> Sterile cotton swabs
> Culture tube
> Agar plate

E 1. Explain to the consumer what you are going to do and that some discomfort may be involved.
2. Place the consumer in the supine position.
3. Note the colour, consistency and odour of the discharge.
4. With the nondominant hand, hold the penis. With the dominant hand, roll a sterile cotton swab in the discharge.

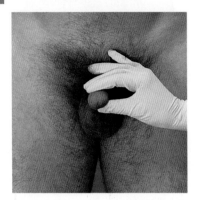

FIGURE 17.57 Palpation of the penis

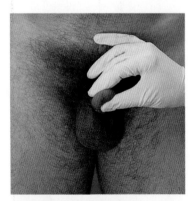

FIGURE 17.58 Palpation of the urethral meatus

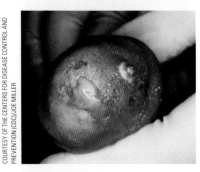

FIGURE 17.59 Purulent penile discharge from gonorrhoea

COURTESY OF THE CENTERS FOR DISEASE CONTROL AND PREVENTION (CDC)/JOE MILLER

E Examination   N Normal findings   A Abnormal findings   P Pathophysiology   Advanced Assessment

5. Place the swab in a culture tube.
6. With a second sterile cotton swab, obtain another specimen for a gonorrhoeal culture.
7. Roll the swab over a laboratory culture medium (agar plate) in a 'Z' pattern.
8. Label both cultures and send them to the laboratory for analysis.

Scrotum

E 1. With the thumb and the first two fingers, gently palpate the left testicle (**Figure 17.60**).
2. Note the size, shape, consistency and presence of masses.
3. Palpate the epididymis (**Figure 17.61**).
4. Note the consistency and presence of tenderness or masses.
5. With the thumb and the first two fingers, palpate the spermatic cord from the epididymis to the external ring.
6. Note the consistency and presence of tenderness or masses.
7. Repeat on the right side.

The scrotum contains, on each side, a testicle and an epididymis. The testicles should be firm but not hard, ovoid, smooth and equal in size bilaterally. They should be sensitive to pressure but not tender. The epididymis is comma-shaped and should be distinguishable from the testicle. The epididymis should be insensitive to pressure. The spermatic cord should feel smooth and round.

A A unilateral mass palpated within or about the testicle is abnormal (**Figure 17.62**).

P Intratesticular masses should be considered malignant until proven otherwise. They are nodular and associated with painless swelling. The majority of intratesticular masses arise from germinal elements. Extratesticular tumours are uncommon and usually are benign. They can arise from any of the surrounding structures, including the epididymis, the testicular tunica vaginalis and the spermatic cord. Testicular cancer should be suspected if a hard, fixed nodule is palpated.

P Inguinal hernia is discussed in the section entitled Inguinal area.

P Refer to the section on scrotal inspection for a description of spermatocoele.

A A large, pear-shaped mass that has a smooth wall is abnormal.

P Refer to the section on scrotal inspection for a description of hydrocoele. The entire testicle must be palpated because underlying malignancies cause a small percentage of all hydrocoeles. Sonography must be performed if the entire testicle is not palpable.

A A soft testis is abnormal.

P This might indicate hypogonadism.

A Palpation of a scrotal mass superior to the testis that reveals a 'bag of worms' is abnormal.

P Refer to the section on scrotal inspection for a description of varicocele.

A It is abnormal for the testicle to be enlarged, retracted, in a lateral position and extremely sensitive (**Figure 17.63**). Sometimes it is difficult to distinguish between testicular torsion and epididymitis. Refer to the advanced practice 'Examining for testicular torsion (Prehn's sign)'.

P Testicular torsion is a surgical emergency. Twisting or torsion of the testis causes venous obstruction, secondary oedema and eventual arterial obstruction. Doppler ultrasonography reveals absence of perfusion to the testicle.

A Palpation reveals an indurated, swollen tender epididymis (see **Figure 17.64**).

P Epididymitis results from the retrograde spreading of pathogenic organisms from the urethra to the epididymis. The majority of infections are caused by bacterial pathogens such as *Chlamydia trachomatis* and *Neisseria gonorrhoeae*. An associated hydrocoele may be present. The testis may also be enlarged and tender.

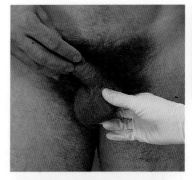

FIGURE 17.60 Palpation of the testicle

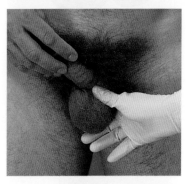

FIGURE 17.61 Palpation of the epididymis

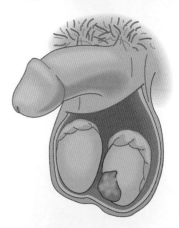

FIGURE 17.62 Testicular tumour

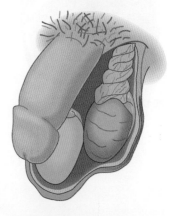

FIGURE 17.63 Testicular torsion

E Examination   **N** Normal findings   **A** Abnormal findings   **P** Pathophysiology   Advanced Assessment

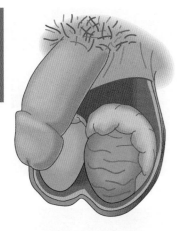

FIGURE 17.64 Epididymitis

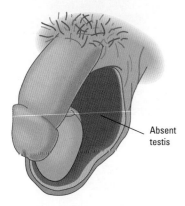

Absent testis

FIGURE 17.65 Cryptorchidism

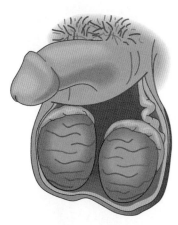

FIGURE 17.66 Orchitis

A It is abnormal for one or both testes to be undescended (**Figure 17.65**).

P The causes of **cryptorchidism** are not established, but may be multiple and related to testicular failure, deficient gonadotrophic stimulation, mechanical obstruction or gubernacular defects. The undescended testis is usually smaller than its normally descended mate. Unilateral cryptorchidism is more common than is bilateral. The undescended testicle is usually located in the inguinal canal or, less commonly, intra-abdominally. Spontaneous descent is unusual after 1 year of age.

A An acute, painful onset of swelling of the testicle along with warm scrotal skin is abnormal (**Figure 17.66**). The consumer may complain of heaviness in the scrotum.

P **Orchitis** can be caused by mumps, coxsackievirus B, infectious mononucleosis and varicella. Involvement of the testes is via the haematogenous route. Orchitis is unilateral in the majority of cases, but onset in the second testicle may occur up to 1 week after that in the first.

A In light-skinned individuals, it is abnormal for the scrotum to be enlarged, taut with pitting oedema, and reddened (**Figure 17.67**).

P Scrotal oedema accompanies oedema associated with the lower half of the body, such as in congestive heart failure (CHF), renal failure and portal vein obstruction. Scrotal oedema may also be the result of local inflammation. Scrotal contents are usually nonpalpable.

HEALTH EDUCATION

Risk factors for testicular cancer
When reviewing your assessment data, consider the following risk factors related to testicular cancer and where appropriate provide education to increase awareness for your consumer.
> Age 20–34 years is the most common
> Caucasian ethnicity
> HIV infection
> Cancer of the other testicle
> History of cryptorchidism (even if previously repaired)

A Acute, painful, scrotal swelling may occur with a history of trauma. This is abnormal.

P Trauma is a major cause of acute scrotal swelling. Scrotal or testicular haematoma formation as well as testicular rupture may be present. A small percentage of all diagnosed testicular tumours are diagnosed through medical attention for trauma; therefore, any intratesticular haematoma must be followed to rule out neoplasm.

Examining for testicular torsion (Prehn's sign)
E 1. Elevate the scrotum with towels until it is fully supported.
2. Observe the consumer's pain response.

N The consumer with epididymitis will have decreased scrotal pain with scrotal elevation.

A P The consumer with testicular torsion will not have any change in his scrotal pain with this manoeuvre.

E Examination **N** Normal findings **A** Abnormal findings **P** Pathophysiology   Advanced Assessment

Inguinal area

E 1. With the index and middle fingers of the right hand, palpate the skin overlying the inguinal and femoral areas for lymph nodes.
2. Note size, consistency, tenderness and mobility.
3. Ask the consumer to bear down while you palpate the inguinal area.
4. Place the right index finger in the consumer's right scrotal sac above the right testicle and invaginate the scrotal skin. Follow the spermatic cord until you reach a triangular, slit-like opening (the external inguinal ring).
5. The finger is placed with the nail facing inwards and the finger pad outwards (**Figure 17.68**).
6. If the inguinal ring is large enough, continue to advance the finger along the inguinal canal and ask the consumer to turn his head and cough.
7. Note any masses felt against the finger.
8. Repeat on the left side using the left hand to perform the palpation.
9. Palpate the femoral canal. Ask the consumer to bear down.

N It is normal for there to be small (1 cm), freely mobile lymph nodes present in the inguinal area. There should not be any bulges present in the inguinal area. There should not be any palpable masses in the inguinal canal. No portions of the bowel should enter the scrotum. There should be no palpable mass at the femoral canal.

A Unilateral enlargement of the lymph nodes along with erythematous overlying skin that may contain adhesions is abnormal.

P Three of the 15 strains of *Chlamydia trachomatis*, specifically L1, L2 and L3, cause lymphogranuloma venereum (LV). These serovars are invasive and virulent and selectively infect lymphoid tissue rather than columnar epithelial cells. Firm inguinal masses result when buboes involute.

A Unilateral or bilateral enlargement of the inguinal lymph nodes is abnormal. The nodes may be tender or painless.

P Lymphadenopathy occurs when the immune system responds to bacterial infections, trauma or carcinoma. Bacterial infections commonly associated with inguinal lymphadenopathy include syphilis, chancroid and gonorrhoea.

A An **indirect inguinal hernia** palpated at the inguinal ring is abnormal (see **Figure 17.69**). An impulse may be felt on the fingertip when the consumer is asked to cough. A larger indirect inguinal hernia may feel like a mass at the inguinal canal.

P Portions of the bowel or omentum enter the inguinal canal through the internal ring and exit at the external inguinal ring. All indirect hernias are congenitally related to a patent processus vaginalis. The severity of a combination of the congenital abnormality and a condition that increases abdominal pressure (e.g. obesity, chronic obstructive pulmonary disease (COPD), hard physical labour, coughing, ascites) determines the onset and degree of the hernia.

A An oval swelling found at the pubis on inspection represents a **direct inguinal hernia** and is abnormal (see **Figure 17.70**). Coughing causes enlargement on palpation of the mass.

P In direct hernias, portions of the bowel or omentum protrude directly through the external inguinal ring. Direct hernias are acquired masses that are influenced by increases in intra-abdominal pressure and weakening of the inguinal structures as part of the normal ageing process. Other related factors include heavy lifting, obesity and COPD.

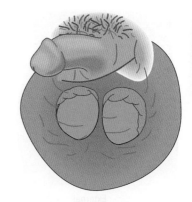

FIGURE 17.67 Scrotal oedema

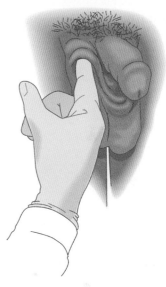

FIGURE 17.68 Palpation for an inguinal hernia

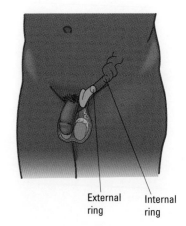

External
ring

Internal
ring

FIGURE 17.69 Indirect inguinal hernia

E Examination **N** Normal findings **A** Abnormal findings **P** Pathophysiology

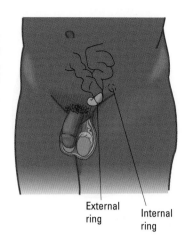

External ring   Internal ring

FIGURE 17.70 Direct inguinal hernia

REFLECTION IN PRACTICE

Teaching testicular self-examination

You are a high school nurse teaching a group of male Year 7 students the importance of performing a testicular self-examination. You proceed to demonstrate the technique on a mannequin. After the class is over, one student shyly approaches you and tells you that he is not sure he can perform testicular self-examination because 'it is masturbation'. How could you respond to the student? Reflect on any approaches you have used that worked in the past, in similar situations.

A Palpation of a mass medial to the femoral vessels and inferior to the inguinal ligament is indicative of a **femoral hernia** and is abnormal.

P A femoral hernia is caused by protrusion of the omentum or bowel through the femoral wall. Onset and size of the hernia may be affected by a congenitally large femoral ring, degradation of collagen and tissue attenuation associated with ageing, increased intra-abdominal pressure and presence of preperitoneal fat. Table 17.7 compares the different types of hernias.

TABLE 17.7 Comparison of inguinal and femoral hernias

	INDIRECT INGUINAL HERNIA	DIRECT INGUINAL HERNIA	FEMORAL HERNIA
Occurrence	More common in infants <1 year and males 16 to 25 years of age	Middle-aged and elderly men	More frequent in women
Origin of swelling	Above inguinal ligament Hernia sac enters canal at internal ring and exits at external ring Can be found in the scrotum	Above inguinal ligament Directly behind and through external ring	Below inguinal ligament
Cause	Congenital or acquired	Acquired weakness brought on by heavy lifting, obesity, COPD	Acquired, due to increased abdominal pressure and muscle weakness
Signs and symptoms	Lump or fullness in the groin that may be associated with a cough or crying	Lump or fullness in the groin area. It may cause an aching or dragging sensation	Firm or rubbery lump in the groin. Pain may be severe

HEALTH EDUCATION

Teaching testicular self-examination

Testicular self-examination (TSE) should be taught to the consumer during the scrotal examination.

> Ask the consumer if monthly testicular self-examination is performed.
> Explain the rationale for the examination. Monthly testicular examination will allow for earlier detection of testicular cancer, which occurs most often in 16- to 35-year-old males.
> Tell the consumer to pick a date to perform the exam every month. The best time to perform the examination is after a warm shower when both hands and the scrotum are warm and relaxed.
> Instruct the consumer to gently feel each testicle using the thumb and first two fingers (Figure 17.71A).
> Remind the consumer that the testicles are ovoid and movable, and that they feel firm and rubbery. The epididymis is located on top and behind the testis, is softer, and feels rope-like.

>>

E Examination   **N** Normal findings   **A** Abnormal findings   **P** Pathophysiology

>>

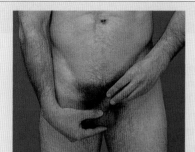
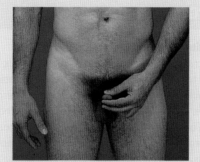

A. Palpating the testis

B. Assessing for penile discharge

FIGURE 17.71 Testicular self-examination

> Instruct the consumer to report to their general practitioner any changes from these findings, including any lumps and nodules, especially if they are nonmobile.
> Instruct the consumer to squeeze the tip of the penis and observe for any discharge (Figure 17.71B). The Testicular Cancer Society (2022) has some useful resources to assist men to remember to undertake monthly testicular self-exams.

Transillumination of the scrotum: assessing for a scrotal mass

If a scrotal mass or enlargement is detected, the scrotum should be transilluminated.

E 1. Tell the consumer what you are going to do and that it should not be painful.
2. Darken the room.
3. Using a penlight, apply the light source to the unaffected side behind the scrotum and direct it forwards.
4. Apply the light source to the side of the scrotal enlargement or mass.
5. Note whether there is transmission of a red glow (see Figure 17.72).

N A normal testicle does not transilluminate (i.e. there is no red glow).

A The transmission of a red glow indicates a serous fluid within the scrotal sac (see Figure 17.73). This can occur in hydrocoele and spermatocoele and is abnormal. Vascular structures such as a hernia and a tumour do not transilluminate.

P Refer to previous discussions of these conditions.

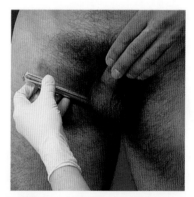

FIGURE 17.72 Transillumination of the scrotum

Auscultation

Auscultation is performed if a scrotal mass is found on inspection or palpation.

Scrotum

E 1. Place the consumer in a supine position.
2. Stand at the consumer's right side at the genitalia area.
3. Place your stethoscope over the scrotal mass.
4. Listen for the presence of bowel sounds.

N No bowel sounds are present in the scrotum.

A An indirect inguinal hernia is present if bowel sounds are present in the enlarged scrotum.

P Loops of bowel extending into the scrotum via an indirect hernia continue to produce bowel sounds unless the hernia is strangulated (lack of blood flow to bowel tissue) and bowel tissue becomes ischaemic or necrotic.

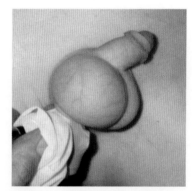

FIGURE 17.73 Transillumination of a hydrocoele. In this case a transilluminator was not available. The examiner used a penlight with a rubber glove over it to illuminate the scrotal mass, which was a hydrocoele.

E Examination **N** Normal findings **A** Abnormal findings **P** Pathophysiology Advanced Assessment

UNIT 2

Reducing a direct inguinal hernia

A strangulated hernia cannot be pushed back into the abdominal cavity. If nausea, vomiting and tenderness are present, they may indicate a strangulated hernia (no blood supply to the affected bowel), which is considered an emergency. This needs to be escalated as urgent care. How you escalate this will depend on the context of the care you are working in.

For example, if you are assessing your consumer in the community setting, the most appropriate escalation may be to the emergency department with a referral letter. If the consumer is admitted in an acute care setting, you would use internal escalation pathways to ensure the consumer receives a surgical review as a matter of urgency.

HEALTH EDUCATION

Erectile function

Many males are unwilling to explore treatment options for erectile dysfunction. You will require some level of knowledge about different treatment options. Treatment for impotence varies greatly depending on the cause, and may include any of the following:

> Patience and a relaxed atmosphere
> Oral medication: sildenafil (Viagra), other phosphodiesterase type 5 (PDE 5) inhibitors
> Penile prosthesis
> Intracavernosal injections
> Vacuum erection device
> Transurethral suppositories

To ensure this type of health education is most effective you will need to use supportive and sensitive communication approaches (refer to Chapter 2).

Examining consumers with urinary diversions

For all tubes, drains and intestinal and urinary diversions, note colour, odour, amount, consistency, and the presence of blood in any drainage. Check for an obstruction if there is no drainage. The skin around the device should be intact without excoriation.

Ileal conduit
> Stoma is pink.
> Skin barrier is used with appliance.

Ureteral stents
> Stent is secured to collection bag.
> No bleeding from insertion site.

Indwelling and suprapubic catheter
> Balloon is inflated.
> Catheter secured to consumer to prevent dislodgement.
> Urinary collecting bag is closed.
> Drainage tube is below level of bladder and without kinks

EVALUATION OF HEALTH ASSESSMENT AND PHYSICAL EXAMINATION FINDINGS

In the evaluation phase of a health assessment, the focus is on ensuring the data gathered is complete, accurate and documented appropriately (see case study as an example of the focused assessment; see Chapter 22 for a comprehensive health assessment). In evaluating the data you should:

> draw on your critical thinking and problem-solving skills to make sound clinical decisions
> act on abnormal data (include communicating findings to other health professionals)
> ensure documentation reflects the outcomes of the clinical decisions/actions taken (refer to Chapter 3, which discusses in detail why documentation is so important and how this may be undertaken in different health settings). The case study that follows steps you through this process.

THE CONSUMER WITH ENDOMETRIOSIS

This case study illustrates the application and objective documentation of the female genitalia assessment. The setting is in a Women's Health Clinic in the community.

Kaye Satino is a 34-year-old married mother who has presented to the sexual health clinic with dysmenorrhoea and menorrhagia.

HEALTH HISTORY

PATIENT PROFILE	34-year-old female	
CHIEF COMPLAINT	'Since my period returned after the birth of my twins, they are heavier and very painful.'	
HISTORY OF THE PRESENT ILLNESS	Kaye is 12 months post-partum delivery of twins via c-section. Resumed menstruation 3 months post-partum. Increased menorrhagia and dysmenorrhea over the last 9 months. Reports replacing maternity pads almost hourly and uses about 12–14 maternity pads per day. She is needing to change her clothes due to bleeding through her pads 2–3 times a day for the first 2–3 days of her period. Experiences significant pain on day preceding menstruation, during menstruation and sometimes during ovulation. Pain management strategies include self-administering over-the-counter NSAIDs, heat packs and meditation – all of which have little effect. As a result of poor pain control, patient reports unable to leave the house during first few days of her period. Menstrual cycle fluctuates from 28 to 50 days. Other symptoms include increased urinary urgency and lethargy. Patient expressed she is more tired than usual but reports that may be due to teething 12-month-old twins.	
PAST HEALTH HISTORY	**MEDICAL HISTORY**	Endometriosis, adenomyosis, polycystic ovary syndrome
	FEMALE REPRODUCTIVE HEALTH HISTORY	Menstrual history: menarche age 10; 28–50-day menstrual cycle with heavy flow lasting up to 7 days per cycle; last normal menstrual period (LNMP) 2 weeks ago
		Reproductive medical history: no sexually transmitted infections, cancer of the reproductive organs, or positive HPV tests
		Obstetric history: conceived through IVF; gravida: 2; para: 2; living child (LC): 2; caesarean section for twins at 36 weeks +3
		Premenstrual syndrome: states that she has not suffered from this
		Menopause history: N/A
		Vaginal discharge: clear
		History of uterine bleeding: describes heavier menstrual bleeding with longer cycles; states she has no midcycle bleeding
		Sexual functioning: identifies LGBTIQ (same-sex attracted), sexually active for 26 years, 1 life partner. Has been with wife for 10 years. Experiences intermittent dyspareunia
		Method of birth control: none
	SURGICAL HISTORY	Appendicectomy – 2005
		Small bowel resection – 2009
		Laparoscopy to removed adhesions – 2010
		Laparoscopy for endometriosis – stage 4 – 2019
		Caesarean – 2021
	ALLERGIES	Morphine – nausea and vomiting
	MEDICATIONS	Ponstan
		Women's multivitamin daily
		NSAIDs prn for period pain
	COMMUNICABLE DISEASES	Nil history of STI/ BBVs. Nil report of positive HPV test
	INJURIES AND ACCIDENTS	Nil identified

>>

>>

HEALTH HISTORY

	SPECIAL NEEDS	Nil identified
	BLOOD TRANSFUSIONS	Nil
	CHILDHOOD ILLNESSES	Chickenpox; asthma
	IMMUNISATIONS	Childhood immunisations up-to-date. Annual influenza vaccine. Adult diphtheria, tetanus and pertussis (Boostrix) vaccination during pregnancy
URINARY SYMPTOMS		Urgency during first three days of menstruation Frequency around time of menstruation Dysuria occasionally on first day of menstruation
FAMILY HEALTH HISTORY	Mother and maternal aunt diagnosed with endometriosis	
SOCIAL HISTORY	**ALCOHOL USE**	Drinks socially — occasional glass of wine on weekends
	TOBACCO USE	Never smoked
	DRUG USE	States she has never taken social or illegal substances
	DOMESTIC AND INTIMATE PARTNER VIOLENCE	Nil history of family or intimate-partner violence. Patient describes being in very happy and healthy relationship with her wife
	SEXUAL PRACTICE	Monogamous for 10 years
	TRAVEL HISTORY	Bali, Asia, Europe, America
	WORK ENVIRONMENT	Currently on parental leave. Prior to having children worked at local council in Early Childhood
	HOME ENVIRONMENT	Rents home with wife and twins
	HOBBIES AND LEISURE ACTIVITIES	Hiking, swimming and yoga
	STRESS	Experiences some financial stress due to becoming single-income household while she is on parental leave. Still adapting to parenthood.
	EDUCATION	Undergraduate degree in Psychology. Studying Honours in Psychology
	ECONOMIC STATUS	Wife is employed full time. Kaye is on maternity leave.
	RELIGION	Roman Catholic; active member of church; attends weekly mass services and is a member of several committees
	CULTURAL BACKGROUND	Caucasian
	ROLES AND RELATIONSHIPS	Mother, daughter, wife, employee. Spouse is supportive
	CHARACTERISTIC PATTERNS OF DAILY LIVING	Usually gets up at 5:30 a.m. with children. Breakfast is cereal (porridge). Feeds children. Tries to leave for a walk with the twins in the pram by 9:30 a.m. Home from walk and a park play with other mums at lunchtime. Lunch is usually homemade — platter of fruit and veg, or a cooked veg salad. Plays with twins in the afternoon. Begins preparing dinner at 4:30 p.m.. Dinner at 5–5:30 p.m. Bedtime between 8:30 and 9 p.m. Awakens 2–3 times overnight to tend to young twins or when in pain from endometriosis. No hobbies at the moment as too busy with young twins.

>>

>>

HEALTH HISTORY

HEALTH MAINTENANCE ACTIVITIES	SLEEP		4–6 broken hours per night due to twins. However Kaye states she was never a good sleeper. Trouble falling asleep and staying asleep. Does not sleep well when menstruating, wakes up frequently in pain.
	DIET		Tries to follow a healthy diet that includes all food groups.
	EXERCISE		Walking for an hour each day. Over the past few months this has reduced to 30 minutes due to fatigue and breathlessness.
	STRESS MANAGEMENT		Meditation and talking to friends
	USE OF SAFETY DEVICES		Does not use any form of contraception Wears seat belt in the car
	HEALTH CHECK-UPS		Last HPV test in 2020 during first trimester of pregnancy; vision and dental exams last year
EXAMINATION OF THE EXTERNAL GENITALIA	INSPECTION	PUBIC HAIR	Inverse triangle formation, no nits or lice
		SKIN COLOUR AND CONDITION	Mons pubis and vulva: well-healed low abdominal transverse scar; labia majora and labia minora nil lesions, light skin colour, moist, nil external discharge, no sign of trauma or injury
		CLITORIS	No lesions
		URETHRAL MEATUS	Midline, nil swelling or discharge
		VAGINAL INTROITUS	Pink, nil lesion, no discharge
		PERINEUM AND ANUS	Pink-brown perineum; anus skin colour
SPECULUM EXAMINATION OF THE INTERNAL GENITALIA	PALPATION	LABIA	No tenderness
		URETHRAL MEATUS AND SKENE'S GLANDS	No pain or discharge
		VAGINAL INTROITUS	Tone strong, nil bulging of pelvic contents
		PERINEUM	
		CERVIX	Colour: pink Position: slightly off midline Size: <2 cm Surface characteristics: nil signs of eversion or extropian Discharge: none Shape of the cervical os: nulliparous
EXAMINATION OF THE VAGINAL WALL	INSPECTION		Pink with rugae
BIMANUAL EXAMINATION	PALPATION	VAGINA	No masses, nontender
		CERVIX	Mobile, nontender, firm
		FORNICES	Palpable lesion about 1 cm at anterior fornix
		UTERUS	No masses, nontender
		ADNEXA	Mobile, round, nil masses or tenderness
		RECTOVAGINAL EXAMINATION	Septum intact, no masses or fissures; cervix and uterus nil lumps, lesions, strong anal sphincter tone, no occult blood

DIAGNOSTIC DATA

LABORATORY DATA	HPV test – negative
DIAGNOSTIC DATA	Transabdominal and transvaginal sonogram confirm endometriosis and adenomyosis. Endometrioma located on left ovary. Urine MSU – nil abnormalities or infection detected

EVALUATION AND CLINICAL REASONING FOR CASE STUDY

The assessment and clinical decisions you make should reflect your scope of practice. For example, advanced practice health professionals, such as nurse practitioners and remote area nurses with endorsement, may be able to make diagnostic decisions and prescribe medications without referring to a medical officer.

Fundamentally, all health professionals collect, evaluate and act on consumer-focused health information, which will at times include referral to, or collaboration with, other healthcare team members. Nurses assess consumers responses to interventions and determine when to escalate key changes in the individual's condition. The clinical reasoning cycle provides health professionals with a framework to consider all this information in a meaningful way for planning consumer care. These phases are stepped out below, and draw on information presented and collected during the health history and physical examination. We then work through the cycle components that are relevant to this case study (cycle components are bolded).

For Kaye Satino, the 34-year-old woman who has presented to the Women's Health Clinic in the community, the significant data that needs to be considered includes the following.

Collecting cues/information

Recall and Review: In the first instance you will need to reflect on what you know about endometriosis.

> Endometriosis is a chronic gynaecological condition in which tissue similar to endometrium (lining of the uterus) grows outside the uterus. Endometriosis causes a chronic inflammatory reaction that can contribute to the formation of scar tissue (adhesions, fibrosis) within the pelvis and other parts of the body (WHO, 2021).
> Endometriosis affects one in nine females (including those assigned female at birth). The cause of endometriosis is complex and multifactorial. Factors that increase the likelihood of developing endometriosis include family history, retrograde menstruation, metaplasia, advanced maternal age, menorrhagia, menstruation >5 days, early menarche <11 years, menstrual cycle 27 days or less, changes in immune cells, low body weight, and alcohol use (Hailes, 2022).
> Presenting symptoms can include dysmenorrhea; dysparaenia; lower back, abdominal and pelvis pain; irregular menstrual cycle, menorrhagia, longer periods; infertility; abdominal bloating; lethargy; mood changes – depression and anxiety; and vaginal discomfort, dysmenorrhoea, menorrhagia and fatigue. May also be accompanied by urinary symptoms including frequency, urgency, dysuria and haematuria (Hailes, 2022).
> Although there is no cure for endometriosis, pharmacotherapy and surgical intervention can assist in alleviating symptoms and improving quality of life for females living with the condition. Pharmacotherapy options aim to alter the hormonal environments that promote endometriosis by either lowering estrogen or increasing progesterone. These medical therapies include the combined oral contraceptive pill, progestins (e.g. mini-pill, implanon and IUD), and gonadotrophin releasing hormone (GnRH) analogues. Surgery may also be recommended to remove endometriosis lesions, adhesions and scar tissue. Hysterectomy may also be considered to reduce endometriosis symptoms and prevent further endometrial tissue growth elsewhere (WHO, 2021).

Chief complaint and history of present illness

> States she has been experiencing menorrhagia and dyspareunia for the past 9 months, since her periods returned 3 months after the birth of her twins
> Uses 10–14 maxi pads per day and cycles lasting up to 7 days; notes clots on many pads
> Increased urinary urgency, frequency and dysuria
> Some mild constipation

Processing information

Interpret: These symptoms and details of history outline the scope of the issue for this patient and how it is affecting her wellbeing and ability to self-manage this deviation from normal health.

Medications

> NSAIDs and Ponstan for dysmenorrhoea
> Women's multivitamin

Relate and Discriminate: At present Kaye has taken steps to relieve pain during menses. The vitamins and iron in the women's multivitamin may assist with treating some of her tiredness. It would be important at this point to find out exactly how often she takes pain medication to ensure she is maximising the effect of the analgesia.

Health maintenance activities

> Has found that she has been feeling much more tired than usual, and does not feel she has her normal level of energy
> Does not sleep well when she has her period; dysmenorrhea and menorrhagia contribute to Kaye having to get up several times overnight during menses

Interpret and Discriminate: This information indicates the significance of her present health alteration affecting her quality of life; it is important information that the nurse must acknowledge. It is also important to note that menorrhagia and raising infant twins could also contribute to tiredness. Menorrhagia can result in lowering of iron stores in the body leading to iron-deficient anaemia. A deficiency in iron may also contribute to feeling tired.

Physical assessment/diagnostic data

> Palpable 2 cm endometrioma on left ovary
> Transabdominal and transvaginal sonogram confirm endometriosis and adenomyosis
> Nil evidence of urinary tract infection despite presentation of urinary symptoms

Predict: These findings provide an accurate medical diagnosis of her condition and will form the basis of her medical care plan.

Putting it all together – synthesise information

The nurse in this case would note all of these abnormalities and hand over their findings to the Sexual and Reproductive Health Physician. Kaye may benefit from a referral to gynaecologist for further review, to consider appropriate medical treatment and evaluate the appropriateness for surgical intervention. It is likely that Kaye will be prescribed hormone therapy to control the menses flow, with consideration for surgery, pending her personal feelings/circumstances.

Actions based on assessment findings

The nurse should also provide additional education for interventions that do not require a doctor's order. These would include:

1 Provide education regarding the benefits of combined oral contraception or progestins for symptom control for menorrhagia and lethargy. It may also reduce further growth of endometriosis lesions and endometriomas. This is important to highlight other benefits of contraception; as Kaye is in a long-term same-sex relationship, she may perceive the need for contraception as low.

2 Education re correct use of NSAIDs (commence taking when menses imminent to maximise effect, correct dose 250–500 mg tds).

3 Treatment and prevention of constipation (increase water, diet high in fibre, use of laxative prn).

4 Discuss/encourage diet rich in iron to compensate for increased bleeding (will assist to improve energy levels).

5 Strategies to assist with urinary frequency/urgency (discuss incontinence devices, reassure that once she has commenced treatment this symptom should resolve).

6 Anxieties that she may have in relation to the diagnosis – encourage her to express her fears and anxieties and answer her questions honestly. A referral to counselling or a psychologist may be beneficial to help her better manage her anxiety, depression and discuss impacts of dyspareunia.

The final step in the process is accurate documentation. The nurse must document findings, referrals, interventions, and advice and education given. The patient would be advised to return to the clinic once she has seen the specialist or if symptoms do not improve.

THE MALE CONSUMER – EMERGENCY DEPARTMENT PRESENTATION, RENAL CALCULI

CASE STUDY 2

This case study illustrates the application and the objective documentation associated with male genitourinary assessment.

Peter Tamwoy is a 55-year-old man from Torres Strait Islands who presents to the emergency department with urinary symptoms, feeling tired and lacking energy.

HEALTH HISTORY

PATIENT PROFILE		55-year-old male
CHIEF COMPLAINT		Burning when he passes urine; feels tired and lacks energy
HISTORY OF THE PRESENT ILLNESS		Seven-day history of increased fatigue, reduced appetite, reduced oral intake, dysuria, night sweats, right upper back pain. Noticed reduced urine output over last few days with frequency of having to pass urine increasing.
		Dysuria: painful to stand and pass urine; experiences burning and noticed urine is odorous. Unable to prevent pain when passing urine. The pain sometimes moves from abdomen and back to groin and testicles.
		Nocturia: increase in frequency of having to pass urine during the night, resulting in disturbed sleep and increased fatigue. Drinking less during afternoon and evening helps to stop the number of times having to wake up.
		Urinary incontinence: frequency of urination results in some urinary continence as unable to get to the toilet in time. Spends a lot of time visiting the toilet.
PAST HEALTH HISTORY	MEDICAL HISTORY	He had a motor vehicle accident when he was 30, which left him with acquired brain injury and altered mobility impacting left side of the body. He has had routine health screenings and has previously been treated for trichomonas.
		Other medical conditions:
		Denies but known to have T2DM, hypertension, chronic kidney disease (CKD) – Grade 3a
	SURGICAL HISTORY	Neurosurgery following car accident
		Abdominal surgery due to splenectomy after car accident

UNIT 2

>>

HEALTH HISTORY			
		ALLERGIES	Nil known
		MEDICATIONS	Nil reported
		COMMUNICABLE DISEASES	Denies but worried about HIV
		INJURIES AND ACCIDENTS	Previous motor vehicle accident resulting in impaired mobility L > R
		SPECIAL NEEDS	Denies
		BLOOD TRANSFUSIONS	Denies
		CHILDHOOD ILLNESSES	Unknown
		IMMUNISATIONS	Up to date with flu and pneumovax, refusing COVID vaccination
FAMILY HEALTH HISTORY			Poor historian for extended family health history. Father unknown, separated from mother aged 8. Lives with sister and has a brother who lives in Cairns. No known health concerns.
SOCIAL HISTORY			On disability pension, lives with sister
		ALCOHOL USE	Denies
		TOBACCO USE	States 10 rollies per day
		DRUG USE	Denies
		DOMESTIC AND INTIMATE PARTNER VIOLENCE	Denies
		SEXUAL PRACTICE	Occasional partners for short term, doesn't wear condoms
		TRAVEL HISTORY	Remained in community for last 3 years
		WORK ENVIRONMENT	N/A
		HOME ENVIRONMENT	Lives in a 3-bedroom rental with his sister, her three children and two grandchildren
		HOBBIES AND LEISURE ACTIVITIES	Enjoys walking around the community, likes to keep active
		STRESS	No identified sources of stress
		EDUCATION	Did Diploma of Aboriginal and Torres Strait Studies in Townsville
		ECONOMIC STATUS	Low socioeconomic
		MILITARY SERVICE	Denies
		RELIGION	Christian
		CULTURAL BACKGROUND	Torres Strait Islander with connection to communities near Bamaga
		ROLES AND RELATIONSHIPS	He manages his own life – his sister and her family are very busy and give him no support
		CHARACTERISTIC PATTERNS OF DAILY LIVING	Wakes at 11–12 a.m., has noodles or meat pie for breakfast, watches TV for a few hours and then goes for a walk (about 5 km); shares evening meal with sister and her family; watches TV and goes to bed around midnight
HEALTH MAINTENANCE ACTIVITIES		**SLEEP**	8–10 hours of sleep each night; experiences disturbing dreams sometimes
		DIET	High in processed carbohydrates: rice and pasta, noodles Very little fruit and vegetables – doesn't like them Fluid intake approximately 750–1000 mL per day
		EXERCISE	Walking
		STRESS MANAGEMENT	Contact with wider community, family connections
		USE OF SAFETY DEVICES	Wears shoes when walking
		HEALTH CHECK-UPS	Annual health checks completed, not visited dentist or optometrist; does not perform testicular self-examination

>>

PHYSICAL EXAMINATION			
EXAMINATION OF THE BLADDER	**INSPECTION**	**CONTOUR SYMMETRY / RECTUS ABDOMINIS**	No altered change in contour or symmetry; rectus abdominis appears tense
		SKIN PIGMENTATION AND COLOUR / SCAR STRIAE	> Difficult to visually assess change in skin pigmentation due to dark colour of skin > No change to appearance of abdominal scar
		MASSES OR NODULES	Appearance of a distended area in groin but no observable alteration in appearance of bladder
	PALPATION	**LOCATE BLADDER**	> Bladder is painful on palpation with extreme rebound tenderness > Palpable in supra pubic region, regular smooth and oval shaped
	PERCUSSION	**NOTE ANY SOUND CHANGES**	Dullness on percussion around supra pubic region
EXAMINATION OF THE MALE GENITALIA	**INSPECTION**	**SEXUAL MATURITY RATING**	Tanner stage 5
		PUBIC HAIR DISTRIBUTION	Triangular distribution of pubic hair
		PENIS	Circumcised
		SCROTUM	Skin rugated, no erythema or oedema of the overlying skin
		URETHRAL MEATUS	Centrally located
		INGUINAL AREA	Observable lump
	PALPATION	**PENIS**	No masses; vesicles intact
		URETHRAL MEATUS	No discharge
		SCROTUM	No swelling/hydrocele
		INGUINAL AREA	Large inguinal hernia – positive cough response with hernia reducible
		BLADDER	Rebound tenderness
	AUSCULTATION	**SCROTUM**	No bowel sounds present

EVALUATION AND CLINICAL REASONING FOR CASE STUDY

The assessment and clinical decisions you make should reflect your scope of practice. For example, advanced practice health professionals such as nurse practitioners and remote area nurses with endorsement may be able to make diagnostic decisions and prescribe medications without referring to a medical officer.

Fundamentally, all health professionals collect, evaluate and act on patient-focused health information, which will at times include referral to, or collaboration with, other healthcare team members. Nurses assess patient responses to interventions and determine when to escalate key changes in a patient's condition. The clinical reasoning cycle provides health professionals with a framework to consider all this information in a meaningful way for planning patient care. These phases are stepped out below, and draw on information presented and collected during the health history and physical examination. We then work through the cycle components that are relevant to this case study (cycle components are bolded).

Peter, a 55-year-old man, attended the emergency department, has identified dysuria, severe right upper back pain, abdominal pain that moves to groin and testes, and fatigue as significant issues; the significant data that needs to be considered includes the following.

Collecting cues/information

Recall and Review: In the first instance you will need to reflect on what you know about dysuria and common causes, health screening and sexually transmitted infections.

Chief complaint and history of present illness

> Peter reports a 7-day history of dysuria and fatigue and right upper abdominal and back pain. He thinks he had this problem a year ago – he is worried he has HIV.
> Peter reports sweating at night and feeling hot.
> He has reduced appetite and taste changes.
> He thinks he has passed much urine over the last day or so.
> Peter has had acquired brain injury (ABI) for about 20 years and has episodes of psychosis.
> Peter believes the hospital has tried to kill him before and was very agitated while the examination occurred.
> Peter doesn't drink much water and eats a lot of high-salt food.

Processing information

Interpret: These symptoms and details of history outline the scope of the issue for this patient and how it affects his wellbeing and ability to self-manage this deviation from normal health.

Discriminate: The patient's wider history, including his social situation, acquired brain injury, distrust of health providers, and history of STI and unprotected sex, add to the clinical picture.

Relate: Aboriginal and Torres Strait Islander people can develop a degree of distrust with the health service through negative experiences. In addition to this, his history of acquired brain injury and paranoia or early dementia can result in poor health care and delay in accessing healthcare needs. When undertaking clinical assessments and questioning it's important to be culturally aware and undertake history taking with a relaxed conversational style such as 'yarning' (Lin, Green & Bessarab, 2016).

Infer and Predict: Obtaining and documenting a comprehensive history reduces the need for patients to retell their story to yet another health professional. However, in the situation described, the patient may prefer to discuss his symptoms and history with a male medical officer. Understanding the need for an effective therapeutic relationship and being culturally safe in this situation is essential. Thorough explanations of all procedures and any physical contact, such as taking his blood pressure, and gaining consent for the contact can assist in building trust and giving him a sense of control over the screening process. A non-judgemental empathetic approach with Peter needs to occur – considering his issues and lack of trust and current health concerns are essential to his overall wellbeing. Peter should also be offered the presence of an Aboriginal and Torres Strait Islander health worker or liaison officer to help represent him and his interest.

Allergies

> Nil known

Medications

> Nil

Discriminate and Predict: Use of medications and past allergies both need to be accurate and considered, as it will be likely that Peter will need antibiotic therapy and also good clinical assessment to determine the level of care required.

Stressors

> Ongoing disability, chronic disease especially diabetes with high blood glucose levels – place the body under stress and it can be more susceptible to infection. Poorly controlled BGLs place the individual at higher risk of skin, fungal and urinary tract infections.

Relate: Chronic disease and disability can result in a chronic inflammatory state that places the body under ongoing stress. Additionally, diabetes if untreated also increases the risk of fungal infections, and urinary tract infections.

Diet

> Highly refined carbohydrates, high salt intake and reduced daily fluid intake

Interpret, Relate and Infer: In an effort to reduce the frequency of micturition and consequently avoid pain, patients often reduce their fluid intake, so we would need to clarify if this is correct with Peter. Reducing fluid intake compounds dysuria by making urine more concentrated and increases the risk of ascending infection. High salt intake accompanied by low fluid intake can increase risk of kidney stone formation (Siener, 2021).

Putting it all together – synthesise information

The nurse in this case would note all of these abnormalities and refer to the medical officer. As it is likely antibiotics and fluid replacement will be prescribed, the nurse will need to check that any medications will have no contraindications or adverse interactions. Ensuring that Peter receives support during his time in emergency department and as an inpatient, the Aboriginal and Torres Strait Islander health worker or liaison officer should be contacted (if Peter would like this). Also acknowledging time and support needed to adapt to his new circumstances is important to address all of Peter's needs, not just his physical condition.

Actions based on assessment findings

The nurse should also provide additional education for interventions that do not require a doctor's order, such as:

1 The importance of completing the full course of antibiotic medications
2 Use of condoms to prevent any further STIs and also to protect against contracting HIV, which he is very concerned about
3 Management of diabetes and importance of medications and monitoring through undertaking BGLs
4 Education about the possible causes of pyelonephritis/urinary tract infections/kidney stones, such as diet, fluid intake, sugar management
5 Maintaining fluid intake at 1.5–2 litres per day to prevent stone formation and to dilute urine
6 Referral to a diabetes educator for ongoing follow-up and support for insulin management and monitoring of BGLs, such as the use of a libre (subcutaneous device that monitors BGL through the use of a phone scanning the device)

7 Strategies and health maintenance for Peter and his sister and their family

8 Referral for mental health to assess his psychosis and to evaluate if any treatment is needed or ongoing counselling and support.

The final step in the process is accurate documentation. The nurse must document findings, referrals, interventions, and advice and education given. The patient would then be reassessed following definitive diagnosis and medical interventions for his ongoing health maintenance.

CHAPTER RESOURCES

REVIEW QUESTIONS

For answers to these questions, see Answer section at the end of the book.

1. During the examination of the external genitalia, you notice a bulging area between the labia minora and the hymenal ring. These greater vestibular glands are known as:
   a. Skene's glands
   b. Parathyroid glands
   c. Bartholin's glands
   d. Adrenal glands

2. Menarche represents:
   a. Stage 1 of the sexual maturity rating scale
   b. Presence of human chorionic gonadotropin
   c. An increase in oestrogen production
   d. A decrease in basal body temperature

3. When advising a consumer regarding maintaining gynaecological health, which statement is incorrect?
   a. Void after coitus to prevent urinary infections.
   b. Do not leave tampons in place for more than 8 hours at a time due to risk of toxic shock syndrome.
   c. Wipe from front to back to prevent contamination of the vagina with faecal material.
   d. Douches may be used routinely to make the consumer feel refreshed.

4. Which of the following are risk factors for vaginal infections? Select all that apply.
   a. Recent antibiotic use
   b. High sugar diet
   c. Excess oestrogen
   d. Poor hygiene
   e. Tampon use
   f. Younger age

5. A 27-year-old woman has had two normal HPV tests in the last 6 years. According to the National Screening Unit in New Zealand, how often is it recommended that she have her HPV test?
   a. Yearly
   b. Every 5 years
   c. Every 3 years
   d. No longer needs HPV test

6. A woman aged 46 who has recently had a total hysterectomy should be given the following advice:
   a. There is no need for any more gynaecological check-ups.
   b. She will need to continue having regular HPV tests.
   c. She will need to maintain yearly gynaecological examinations.
   d. She will only need to see her doctor for a gynaecological check-up if she notices any problems.

7. The immunisation program for the HPV vaccine is aimed at:
   a. Girls and boys aged 12 to 13
   b. Girls and boys aged 15 to 25
   c. Girls (and boys in Australia) aged 9 to 26
   d. Girls (and boys in Australia) aged 6 to 25

8. Tom Banks, a 36-year-old man, has had a painless swelling in his left testis for the past 5 months. Physical examination reveals enlargement of the left testis. The right testis appears normal. Which of the following would you be most suspicious of?
   a. Hydrocoele
   b. Varicocele
   c. Tumour
   d. Epididymitis

9. On physical examination, a newborn has an abnormal opening of the urethra on the ventral surface of the penis. Which of the following is the most likely diagnosis?
   a. Hypospadias
   b. Phimosis
   c. Epispadias
   d. Cryptorchidism

10. A male consumer presents with the following: texture and curl of pubic hair is similar to an adult but not spread to the thighs; further growth in length, diameter and development of glans; a darkened scrotum with further growth. This male is most likely in which sexual maturity stage?
    a. Stage 1
    b. Stage 2
    c. Stage 3
    d. Stage 4

11. An indirect inguinal hernia can be differentiated from other causes of scrotal swelling by which of the following?
    a. Transillumination of the scrotum
    b. Palpating the inguinal canal and having the consumer cough
    c. Scrotal X-ray
    d. Prehn's sign

12. Cauliflower-like, pink lesions are seen on the penis. This finding is most likely which of the following conditions?
    a. Condyloma acuminatum
    b. Herpes simplex virus
    c. Syphilis
    d. Penile carcinoma
13. Which consumer would be at the highest risk for developing penile cancer?
    a. 27-year-old sexually active, circumcised male with a history of HPV type 11
    b. 38-year-old uncircumcised male who is not sexually active
    c. 50-year-old sexually active, uncircumcised male
    d. 73-year-old sexually active, circumcised male

CS CLINICAL SKILLS

The following Clinical Skill is relevant to this chapter and can be found in Tollefson & Hillman, *Clinical Psychomotor Skills,* 8th edition:

> 27 Healthcare teaching.

FURTHER RESOURCES

> Andrology Australia – Health Male: https://www.andrologyaustralia.org/
> Australian Government, Department of Health and Aged Care. Immunise Australia Program – Human papillomavirus (HPV). http://www.health.gov.au/internet/immunise/publishing.nsf/Content/immunise-hpv
> Australian Government Department of Health and Aged Care. Sexually transmitted infections: https://www.health.gov.au/topics/sexual-health
> Australian Government Department of Health and Aged Care. What we're doing about reproductive health: https://www.health.gov.au/health-topics/reproductive-health/what-we-do
> Australian Indigenous HealthInfoNet (Men): http://www.healthinfonet.ecu.edu.au/population-groups/men/reviews/our-review
> Beyond Blue: https://www.beyondblue.org.au/
> Cancer Council Australia: http://www.cancer.org.au/Home.htm
> Cancer Society of New Zealand: http://www.cancernz.org.nz/
> Canteen: https://www.canteen.org.au/
> Centers for Disease Control and Prevention: http://www.cdc.gov
> Continence Foundation of Australia: http://www.continence.org.au/
> Family Planning Alliance Australia: http://familyplanningallianceaustralia.org.au/
> Future Fertility: http://www.futurefertility.com.au/
> Health Navigator New Zealand: Men's health: https://www.healthnavigator.org.nz/healthy-living/mens-health/

> National Centre for Gynaecological Cancers: http://www.canceraustralia.gov.au/about-us/priorities-and-programs/national-centre-gynaecological-cancers
> National Cervical Screening Program (Australia): http://www.cancerscreening.gov.au/internet/screening/publishing.nsf/Content/cervical-screening-1
> National Cervical Screening Programme (New Zealand): https://www.timetoscreen.nz/cervical-screening/
> New Zealand Gynaecological Cancer Foundation: http://nzgcf.org.nz/index.cfm/PageID/75/ViewPage/Our+People
> New Zealand Ministry of Health: http://www.health.govt.nz/
> New Zealand Sexual and Health Society Incorporated: http://www.nzshs.org/guidelines.html
> Prostate Cancer Foundation of Australia: https://www.pcfa.org.au/
> Prostate Cancer Foundation of New Zealand: https://prostate.org.nz/
> Sexually transmitted infections in New Zealand: Annual surveillance report 2014 https://surv.esr.cri.nz/surveillance/annual_sti.php?we_objectID=4248
> Te Ara, The Encyclopedia of New Zealand. Men's health: https://teara.govt.nz/en/mens-health/page-1
> UNICEF: http://www.unicef.org
> Urological Society of Australia and New Zealand: http://www.usanz.org.au/
> World Health Organization: http://www.who.int

REFERENCES

Allanson, E., & Ayres, C. (2022). The epidemiology of gynaecological cancers. *O&G Magazine, 24*(3). Retrieved 13 December 2022 from: https://www.ogmagazine.org.au/24/3-24/the-epidemiology-of-gynaecological-cancers/

Australian Bureau of Statistics (ABS). (2018). Kidney disease. Retrieved 26 July 2022 from: https://www.abs.gov.au/statistics/health/health-conditions-and-risks/kidney-disease/latest-release

Australian Government Department of Health and Aged Care. (2010). National male health policy: Building on the strengths of Australian males. Canberra. Retrieved 18 April 2022 from: https://www.health. gov.au/resources/publications/national-mens-health-policy-2010?language=en

Australian Government Department of Health and Aged Care. (2019). Bladder and bowel related conditions and diseases. Retrieved 26 July 2022 from: https://www.health.gov.au/health-topics/bladder-and-bowel/bladder-and-bowel-related-conditions-and-diseases

Australian Government Department of Health and Aged Care. (2022a). About the National Cervical Screening Program. Retrieved 26 July 2022 from: https://www.health.gov.au/initiatives-and-programs/national-cervical-screening-program/about-the-national-cervical-screening-program

Australian Government Department of Health and Aged Care. (2022b). National immunisation program schedule. Retrieved 26 July 2022 from: https://www.health.gov.au/health-topics/immunisation/when-to-get-vaccinated/national-immunisation-program-schedule

Australian Government Department of Health and Aged Care. (2023). Change to single dose HPV vaccine. Retrieved 16 May 2023 from: https://www.health.gov.au/ministers/the-hon-mark-butler-mp/media/change-to-single-dose-hpv-vaccine

Australian Institute of Health and Welfare (AIHW). (2022). Chronic kidney disease. Retrieved 26 July 2022 from: https://www.aihw.gov.au/reports/chronic-kidney-disease/chronic-kidney-disease/contents/how-many-australians-have-chronic-kidney-disease

Australian Men's Shed Association (AMSA). (2019). Spanner in the Works? Retrieved 14 December 2022 from: https://malehealth.org.au/about/

Cancer Council Australia. (2022a). Gynaecological cancer in Australia statistics. Retrieved 13 December 2022 from: https://www.canceraustralia.gov.au/cancer-types/gynaecological-cancers/statistics

Cancer Council Australia. (2022b). Ovarian cancer. Retrieved 13 December 2022 from: https://www.canceraustralia.gov.au/cancer-types/ovarian-cancer/statistics

Cancer Council Australia. (2022c). HPV screening strategies for Aboriginal and Torres Strait Islander women. Retrieved 13 December 2022 from: https://www.cancer.org.au/clinical-guidelines/cervical-cancer-screening/hpv-screening-in-aboriginal-and-torres-strait-islander-women

Cancer Council Australia. (2022d). Clinical Guidelines. Retrieved 13 December 2022 from: https://wiki.cancer.org.au/australia/Guidelines:Cervical_cancer/Screening

Cancer Council. (n.d.). Types of gynaecological cancer. Retrieved 13 December 2022 from: https://www.cancer.org.au/about-us/policy-and-advocacy/prevention-policy/common-cancers/gynaecological-cancers

Centre for Men's Health. (2022). Centre for Men's Health, University of Otago. Retrieved 14 December 2022 from: https://www.otago.ac.nz/mens-health/index.html

Connory, J., & WhyHive. (2021). 'Period Pride Report: Bloody Big Survey Findings: Australia's largest survey on attitudes and experiences of periods'. Share the Dignity, Brisbane, Australia. Retrieved from: https://d1fzx274w8ulm9.cloudfront.net/05d79645459991e3a3ccd3e720166ff7.pdf

Continence Foundation of Australia (2021). Urinary incontinence. Retrieved 26 July from: https://www.continence.org.au/types-incontinence/urinary-incontinence

Family Planning Australia. (2018). Common vaginal & vulval conditions. Retrieved 13 December 2022 from: https://www.fpnsw.org.au/factsheets/individuals/gynaecological-health/common-vaginal-vulval-conditions

Hailes, J. (2022). Endometriosis, symptoms and cause. Jean Hailes Womens Health. Retrieved 14 August 2022 from: https://www.jeanhailes.org.au/health-a-z/endometriosis/symptoms-

Health Navigator New Zealand. (2022a). Sexually transmitted infections | Mate paipai. Retrieved 13 December 2022 from: https://www.healthnavigator.org.nz/health-a-z/s/sexually-transmitted-infections-stis/

Health Navigator New Zealand. (2022b). Men's health topics. Retrieved 14 December 2022 from: https://www.healthnavigator.org.nz/healthy-living/m/mens-health-topics/

HealthDirect. (2021). Chlamydia. Retrieved 13 December 2022 from: https://www.healthdirect.gov.au/chlamydia

Healthy Male. (2022). Healthy Male: Generations of healthy Australian men. Retrieved 14 December 2022 from: https://www.healthymale.org.au

Institute of Environmental Science and Research (ESR). (2021). Latest news: Reported cases of sexually transmitted infections decreased in 2021 but health inequalities remain. Retrieved 14 December 2022 from: https://www.esr.cri.nz/home/about-esr/media-releases/reported-cases-of-sexually-transmitted-infections-decreased-in-2021-but-health-inequities-remain/

Kidney Health Australia. (2022). Retrieved 26 July 2022 from: https://kidney.org.au/uploads/resources/Media-Release-New-evidence-report.pdf

Kirby Institute. (2022). HIV, viral hepatitis and sexually transmitted infections in Australia: Annual surveillance report 2022. University of New South Wales. Retrieved 14 December 2022 from: https://kirby.unsw.edu.au/sites/default/files/kirby/report/Annual-Surveillance-Report-2022_STI.pdf

Lin, I., Green, C., & Bessarab, D. (2016). 'Yarn with me': applying clinical yarning to improve clinician-patient communication in Aboriginal health care. *Australian Journal of Primary Health*, *22*(5), 377–82. https://doi.org/10.1071/PY16051

Ministry of Health/Manatù Hauora. (2017). Urinary tract infection. https://www.health.govt.nz/your-health/conditions-and-treatments/diseases-and-illnesses/urinary-problems/urinary-tract-infection

Ministry of Health/Manatù Hauora. (2021a). Sexually transmitted infections (STIs). Retrieved 14 December 2022 from: https://www.health.govt.nz/your-health/conditions-and-treatments/diseases-and-illnesses/sexually-transmitted-infections-stis

Ministry of Health/Manatù Hauora. (2021b). HPV vaccination. Retrieved 3 August from: https://www.health.govt.nz/our-work/preventative-health-wellness/immunisation/hpv-immunisation-programme/hpv-vaccine

Ministry of Health/Manatù Hauora. (2021c) Cervical Screening. Time to screen. Retrieved 26 July 2022 from: https://www.timetoscreen.nz/cervical-screening/

Ministry of Health/Manatù Hauora. (2023) Kidney disease. Retrieved 16 May 2022 from: https://www.health.govt.nz/your-health/conditions-and-treatments/diseases-and-illnesses/kidney-disease)

New Zealand Government. (2022).HPV immunisation. Health New Zealand Retrieved 13 December 2022 from: https://www.health.govt.nz/your-health/healthy-living/immunisation/immunisation-older-children-and-teenagers/human-papillomavirus-hpv/hpv-immunisation

Sheppard, C. (2020). Treatment of vulvovaginitis. *Australian Prescriber*, *43*(6),195–9. doi: 10.18773/austprescr.2020.055. Epub 2020 Dec 1. PMID: 33363301; PMCID: PMC7738700.

Siener, R. (2021). Nutrition and kidney stone disease. *Nutrients*, *13*(6), 1917. doi:https://doi.org/10.3390/nu13061917

Tanner, J. M. (1962). *Growth at adolescence* (2nd ed.). Oxford: Blackwell Scientific Publications.

Testicular Cancer Society. (2022). Testicular self-exam. Retrieved 3 August 2022 from: http://www.testicularcancersociety.org/testicular-self-exam.html

World Health Organization (WHO). (2021). Endometriosis, Key facts. Retrieved 14 August 2022 from: https://www.who.int/news-room/fact-sheets/detail/endometriosis

Xiao, H., Doolan-Noble, F., Liu, L., White, A., & Baxter, D. (2022). Men's health research in New Zealand: A scoping review. *International Journal of Men's Social and Community Health*, *5*(SP 1). https://doi.org/10.22374/ijmsch.v5iSP1.67

Your Health Link. (2022). Your health link: health information the right way. Website. Retrieved 14 December from: https://yourhealthlink.health.nsw.gov.au/resource_type/mens-health/

CHAPTER 18

ANUS, RECTUM AND PROSTATE

LEARNING OUTCOMES

By the end of this chapter you should be able to:
1   identify anatomic landmarks of the rectum and the prostate gland
2   describe the characteristics of the most common rectal and prostatic complaints
3   inspect the anus and rectum, and describe the assessment of prostate on an adult
4   explain the pathophysiological rationale for abnormal findings
5   identify health education opportunities for consumers
6   discuss the clinical reasoning in evaluating outcomes of health assessment and physical examination including documentation requirements for recording information, health education given and relevant health referral.

BACKGROUND

The anorectal examination is an important part of the physical examination, but one that many consumers are reluctant to undertake due to comfort levels and embarrassment. The level of assessment that you would undertake will depend on your scope of practice; for example, prostate palpation is appropriate for advanced practitioners (e.g. nurse practitioners) in roles that demand this level of examination. In the male consumer, this may include assessment of the anus, rectum and prostate gland; for the female consumer, assessment of the anus and rectum is performed. These assessments are usually performed last so that the consumer has a level of comfort and trust with the practitioner, but should be performed on a regular basis to screen for anorectal and prostate cancers. The practitioner whose role and scope does not include prostate palpation should still undertake a health history specific to conditions of, or indicative of, prostate issues.

Common conditions that will be discussed include:
> Pilonidal cyst or sinus
> Ulcerative colitis
> Prostatitis
> Acute bacterial prostatitis
> Anorectal abscess
> Haemorrhoids
> Faecal incontinence
> Benign prostatic hypertrophy (BPH)
> Rectal and prostate cancers.

In Australia and New Zealand, awareness and examination of anorectal problems is becoming a higher priority in general health examinations initiated by the health practitioner. Many consumers are reluctant to talk about issues to do with these body parts.

Prostate cancer is the most common cancer diagnosed in Australia, overtaking breast cancer as the country's leading cause of cancer (Prostate Cancer Foundation of Australia (PCFA), 2022a; Cancer Australia, 2022). This is largely thought to be attributed to better screening and higher levels of awareness of the need to screen those at high risk (men who have immediate family members who had a prostate cancer) (AIHW, 2022; Cancer Council, 2022; PCFA, 2022a). Another trend is the significant increase in the survival rate of men who have been diagnosed with prostate cancer (AIHW, 2022). Although prostate cancer is the second-leading cause of cancer-related deaths in men (behind lung cancer), with one in six men diagnosed before the age of 85 (Cancer Council NSW, 2022), the survival rate for men post-cancer diagnosis has improved significantly over time. Between 1989–1993 and 2014–2018, five-year relative survival for prostate cancer improved from 63% to 96% (Cancer Australia, 2022).

Improved detection and diagnosis of prostate cancer means that the number of men surviving long after diagnosis has been steadily increasing; however, the quality-of-life outcomes for these men vary. Research shows that a significant proportion of prostate-cancer survivors still suffer the consequences of their cancer diagnosis and treatment, find it difficult to talk about persistent long-term issues (particularly sexual dysfunction), and therefore don't feel they receive the right information and support they need (Mazariego et al., 2020). It is pertinent for healthcare professionals undertaking health history and physical examination to identify those who may need education and referral for follow-up care and monitoring post treatment (Cancer Council NSW, 2022).

In New Zealand, prostate cancer is the most diagnosed cancer in men (behind skin cancers), with more than 4000 men diagnosed and 700 dying from the disease each year (Prostate Cancer Foundation NZ, 2022). As in Australia, the overall number of men diagnosed in New Zealand is increasing (with higher rates of testing) and the death rate is slowly dropping (largely due to better outcomes from early diagnosis and the availability of improved treatments). Compared to the overall male population in New Zealand, Māori men have a slightly lower incidence of prostate cancer but a higher death rate (Prostate Cancer Foundation NZ, 2022). There are several reasons for the disparity in outcomes for Māori, including differences in staging and characteristics at diagnosis, differences in screening and treatment offered, and general barriers to health care that exist for Māori men in New Zealand (Egan et al., 2020).

For all cancers combined, Indigenous Australians are also more likely to be diagnosed with and die from cancer than non-Indigenous Australians (AIHW, 2018). Differences between the rates for Indigenous and non-Indigenous Australians may be related to a range of factors including the prevalence of risk and/or protective factors such as smoking, alcohol consumption, access to healthcare services and uptake of screening and diagnostics testing (AIHW, 2018). For prostate cancer in particular, incidence and mortality rates are lower than rates for non-Indigenous Australians; but in spite of this, Aboriginal and Torres Strait Islander men who are diagnosed with prostate cancer still experience comparatively poor survival outcomes (PCFA, 2022b). Indigenous Australians diagnosed with prostate cancer on average had an 86% chance of surviving for five years, as compared with a 96% chance for non-Indigenous Australians (AIHW, 2018).

Haemorrhoidal disease is the most common anorectal disorder (Fowler et al., 2019); however, incidence is difficult to identify in the population as only about 4% of most Caucasian populations require treatment for them (Ravindranath & Rahul, 2018). Some groups are more likely to experience haemorrhoids at a particular point in their lives (e.g. pregnant women) (Department of Health and Aged Care, 2019), and because of higher incident levels in such groups, it is reasonable to prioritise conducting assessments to detect these conditions. Treatments for prostate diseases and haemorrhoids have evolved quickly and are now more effective and accessible by a higher proportion of the population. Nurses should be mindful of the prevention of conditions such as haemorrhoids whenever possible. For example, if we routinely educate about the implications, it may be possible to reduce the severity of haemorrhoids or even their development altogether.

ANATOMY AND PHYSIOLOGY

Rectum

The large intestine is composed of the caecum, colon, rectum and anal canal. The caecum and colon are discussed in Chapter 15. The sigmoid colon begins at the pelvic brim. Beyond the sigmoid colon, the large intestine passes downwards in front of the sacrum. This portion is called the **rectum** (Figure 18.1). The rectum contains three transverse folds, or valves of Houston. These valves work to retain faecal material so it is not passed along with flatus.

Anus

The anus is made up of the last 3 to 4 cm of the large intestine and may also be called the **anal canal**. It also includes the muscular rings often termed the **sphincter**. The anal canal fuses with the rectum at the anorectal junction, or dentate line, and together these structures form the **anorectum**. The anal orifice is located at the seam of the gluteal folds; it serves as the exit to the gastrointestinal tract and it is marked by corrugated skin.

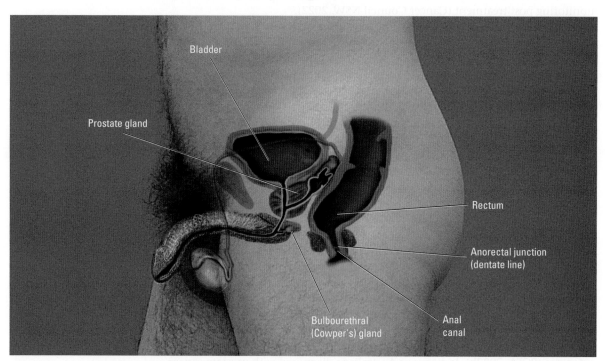

FIGURE 18.1 The anorectum and prostate

In the superior half of the anal canal are **anal columns**, which are longitudinal folds of mucosa (also called columns of Morgagni). The **anal valves** are formed by inferior joining anal columns. There are pockets located superior to the valves called the **anal sinuses** (Figure 18.2). These sinuses secrete mucus when they are compressed by faeces, providing lubrication that eases faecal passage during **defecation**.

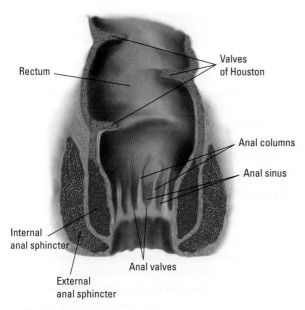

Rectum

Valves
of Houston

Anal columns

Anal sinus

Internal
anal sphincter

Anal valves

External
anal sphincter

FIGURE 18.2 Anal canal

The anal canal opens to the exterior through the anus. Internal and external anal sphincter muscles surround the anus. Smooth muscle, which is under involuntary control, forms the internal sphincter. Skeletal muscle forms the external sphincter and is under voluntary control, allowing a person to control bowel movements.

The motility of the large intestine is controlled mainly by its nerves. There are two types of nerves: those that lie within the large intestine (the intrinsic nerves) and those that lie outside it (the extrinsic nerves). The rectum has more segmental contractions than does the sigmoid colon. These contractions keep the rectum empty by retrograde movement of contents into the sigmoid colon. As faecal material is forced into the rectum by mass peristaltic movements, the stretching of the rectal wall initiates the defecation reflex. A parasympathetic reflex signals the walls of the sigmoid colon and rectum to contract and the internal anal sphincter to relax. During defecation, the musculature of the rectum contracts to expel the faeces.

Prostate

Contiguous with part of the anterior rectal wall in the male is the **prostate** gland. The prostate is an accessory male sex organ that is slightly smaller than a ping pong ball, approximately 3.5 cm long by 3 cm wide (**Figure 18.1**). It consists of glandular tissue and muscle, and its small ducts drain into the urethra. The prostate lies just below the bladder and encircles the urethra like a doughnut.

The prostate has five lobes: anterior, posterior, median and two lateral. The median sulcus is the groove between the lateral lobes. The right and left lateral lobes are accessible to palpation.

Prostatic secretions are thin, milky and alkaline. The secretions are made up of many different components. Citrate, a major component of prostatic fluid, provides a good transport medium for spermatozoa by maintaining the osmotic equilibrium of the seminal fluid. Prostatic fluid composes 15–30% of the ejaculate. Prostatic secretions have high levels of prostatic acid phosphatase (PAP) and prostate-specific antigen (PSA).

The prostate is primarily involved in reproduction, but it also provides a certain measure of protection against urinary tract infections. Semen contains high levels of zinc, which is derived from the prostate. Zinc is what provides the antibacterial properties to the prostate.

Within the prostatic cells, testosterone is converted to an androgen called dihydrotestosterone (DHT), which is the major androgen responsible for the benign enlargement of the prostate gland.

HEALTH EDUCATION

Practice update for prostate-specific antigen (PSA) for consumer education

Many consumers may not know or remember what a PSA test actually tests for and the relationship of this test to diagnosing cancer. In recent decades, PSA testing was used as a broadscale health screening tool for men. PSA testing for prostate cancer testing is widespread; however, new research has highlighted the possible harms that outweigh the benefits of broadscale testing. New guidelines state that only men with symptoms that may suggest prostate cancer be tested with a PSA test, to avoid unnecessary testing and investigations that can have significant harmful side effects (Health Direct, 2020).

Guidelines for early detection of prostate cancer

PSA testing should now be offered every 2 years for men who are at average risk of prostate cancer and aged 50–69 (and no longer includes a routine digital rectal exam in asymptomatic men in primary care), with further investigation offered if the total PSA concentration is >3 ng/mL (Prostate Cancer Foundation of Australia and Cancer Council Australia, 2016). For men who are at high risk (e.g. a brother diagnosed with prostate cancer before age 60), screening should take place commencing age 45 (Olver, 2015). For those at an even higher risk (e.g. both brother and father diagnosed with prostate cancer), screening can commence at 40 years of age (Olver, 2015).

Clinical practice guidelines approved by the National Health and Medical Research Council can be found at Prostate Cancer Foundation of Australia (http://www.prostate.org.au/awareness/for-healthcare-professionals/clinical-practice-guidelines-on-psa-testing/).

Risk factors for prostate cancer

Consumers who fit any of the following prostate cancer risk factors should be assessed for their level of risk and referred to a medical practitioner (or nurse practitioner if available for this) for a full prostate assessment:

> Over 50 years of age
> Family history of prostate cancer
> Race: prostate cancer is more common in people of African descent
> High intake of red meat, dietary fat, oil and sugar
> Low levels of exercise
> Men living in specific geographical areas (e.g. North America, North-western Europe, Australia, New Zealand and some Caribbean Islands).

ASSESSMENT: TAKING THE CONSUMER'S HEALTH HISTORY

Assessment is the first phase of the nursing process, and involves collecting subjective information about the consumer's health status in order to identify consumer problem areas to focus on.

Subjective data is most frequently collected during a health history and serves as the starting point for the health professional to base the depth of their assessment on. The sections for the health history include:

> **Consumer profile**
> **Chief complaint** (explained systematically using variations of location, quality, quantity, associated manifestations, aggravating factors, alleviating factors, setting and timing. This is a variation on the OPQRST assessment mnemonic you may use for other conditions such as pain assessment)
> **Past health history** (including medical history, surgical history, allergies, medications, injuries and accidents, special needs and childhood illnesses)
> **Family health history**
> **Social history** (including alcohol, tobacco and drug use, sexual practice, work and home environment, hobbies and leisure activities, stress and culture).

HEALTH HISTORY

CONSUMER PROFILE	The anus, rectum and prostate health history provides insight into the link between a consumer's life and lifestyle and anal, rectal and prostatic information and pathology. Diseases that are age-, sex- and race-specific for the anus, rectum and prostate are listed.		
	AGE	> Pilonidal cyst or sinus (20–35) > Crohn's disease of the anorectum (20–40) > Anal fissure (20–45) > Rectal condyloma acuminatum (20–50) > Ulcerative colitis (20–50) > Gonococcal proctitis (20–50) > Herpes proctitis (20–50) > Prostatitis (20–60) > Anal stenosis (>25) > Pruritus ani (>25) > Anal skin tags (<30) > Acute bacterial prostatitis (>30) > Anorectal abscess (30–40) > Anorectal fistula (30–40) > Haemorrhoids (40–65) > Prostatic abscess (>40) > Faecal incontinence (>40) > Benign prostatic hypertrophy (BPH) (>40) > Rectal cancer (>55) > Prostate cancer (>50) > Faecal impaction (>60) > Rectal prolapse (60–80)	
	SEX	**FEMALE**	Rectal prolapse, faecal incontinence
		MALE	Anorectal abscess, anorectal fistula, pruritus ani, rectal cancer, pilonidal cyst or sinus, haemorrhoids, gonococcal proctitis, herpes proctitis, benign prostatic hypertrophy, prostatitis, prostate abscess, prostate cancer
	CULTURAL BACKGROUND	**MĀORI, PASIFIKA AND ABORIGINAL AND TORRES STRAIT ISLANDER PEOPLES**	Prostate cancer – lower incidence than in European men but higher mortality
		CAUCASIAN	Rectal cancer, Crohn's disease of the anorectum, pilonidal cyst or sinus, BPH, prostate cancer
CHIEF COMPLAINT	Common chief complaints for the anus, rectum and prostate are defined and information on the characteristics of each sign or symptom is provided.		
	1. RECTAL BLEEDING	Discharge of blood from the rectum	
		QUALITY	Occult, melaena, haematochezia, massive haemorrhage
		QUANTITY	Scant, spotty, dripping, massive
		ASSOCIATED MANIFESTATIONS	Pain, absence of pain, malaise, fever, mass at anus
		AGGRAVATING FACTORS	Defecation, constipation, diarrhoea, minor trauma, pelvic irradiation
		ALLEVIATING FACTORS	Increased fibre diet, bulk agents, exercise, increased fluid intake, haemorrhoidectomy
		TIMING	Constant, intermittent

HEALTH HISTORY

2. RECTAL PAIN	The subjective phenomenon of a sensation indicating real or potential tissue damage in the rectum	
	QUALITY	Acute, sharp, tearing, burning, throbbing
	ASSOCIATED MANIFESTATIONS	Swelling, fever, blood, abdominal pain
	AGGRAVATING FACTORS	Defecation, sitting, movement, foreign bodies, pregnancy, anal sex
	ALLEVIATING FACTORS	High-fibre diet, bulk agents, exercise, increased fluid intake, warm sitz bath, topical emollients, surgery, removal of foreign body, lying down
	TIMING	More prominent with defecation; constant or episodic
3. ANAL AND FAECAL INCONTINENCE	The involuntary passage of stool	
	ASSOCIATED MANIFESTATIONS	Diarrhoea, urgency, rectal prolapse, prolapsed haemorrhoids, gaping anus
	AGGRAVATING FACTORS	Diarrhoea, impaction, cognitive impairment, anxiety, physical handicaps, neurological disorders, trauma
	ALLEVIATING FACTORS	Bulk fibre, constipating agents, laxatives, enemas, biofeedback, anal continence plugs
4. CONSTIPATION	The infrequent, difficult passage of stool	
	QUANTITY	Fewer than three bowel movements per week – for some consumers this may vary and be more often than this but still constipated compared to normal bowel habits for them
	ASSOCIATED MANIFESTATIONS	Pain, blood, mucus, hard stool, straining with defecation, flatulence, decreased appetite. Extreme constipation can cause abdominal pain and bloating, and hard faeces may be palpable via the abdomen
	AGGRAVATING FACTORS	Low-fibre diet, lack of exercise, drugs (e.g. narcotics, calcium channel blockers), chronic use of laxatives, ignoring urge to defecate, weak abdominal muscles, inadequate fluid intake, rectocoele, rectal prolapse, anal stenosis
	ALLEVIATING FACTORS	High-fibre diet, bulking agents, increased fluid intake, defecation schedule, exercise, laxatives, digital removal, suppositories
5. DIARRHOEA	Increased volume, fluidity, or frequency of bowel movements relative to the person's usual pattern	
	ASSOCIATED MANIFESTATIONS	Abdominal pain, blood, steatorrhoea, weight changes, appetite changes
	AGGRAVATING FACTORS	Viral infection, bacterial infection, antibiotics, laxatives, faecal impaction, Crohn's disease, ulcerative colitis, lactose intolerance, specific foods (very individualised but may include grapes, pineapple, prunes), irritable bowel syndrome, caffeine, alcohol
	ALLEVIATING FACTORS	Constipating agents, anticholinergics, fluid replacement, certain foods (bananas, rice, apples, toast), antibiotics
	SETTING	Stressful situations, recent ingestion of improperly stored or prepared food, recent travel abroad

HEALTH HISTORY

	6. PRURITUS	Itching of the anal and perianal skin	
		ASSOCIATED MANIFESTATIONS	Erythema, oedema, psoriasis, candidiasis, contact dermatitis, haemorrhoids, anal fissures, rectal carcinoma, intestinal parasites (worms) usually causes itching at night
		AGGRAVATING FACTORS	Psoriasis, eczema, contact dermatitis, infections, parasites, oral antibiotics, diabetes mellitus, liver disease, obesity, poor hygiene, tight underclothes, wet clothing
		ALLEVIATING FACTORS	Discontinuing current antibiotics and topical agents; eliminating coffee, tea, cola, milk, beer and wine; discontinuing laxatives; good rectal hygiene; loose clothing; non-medicated talcum powder; topical fungicides
	7. PALPABLE MASS	A mass at the anus, in the anal canal, or on the prostate	
		QUALITY	Firm, smooth, soft, mobile, nonmobile, nodular, fibrotic
		ASSOCIATED MANIFESTATIONS	Pain/absence of pain, blood, pus, mucus, fever, haemorrhoids, rectal prolapse
		ALLEVIATING FACTORS	Warm sitz baths, high-fibre diet, bulk agents, surgery
PAST HEALTH HISTORY	The various components of the past health history are linked to anal, rectal and prostatic pathology and anal-, rectal- and prostatic-related information.		
	MEDICAL HISTORY	**ANORECTAL-SPECIFIC**	Trauma, inflammatory bowel disease, prior history of STIs, polyps, rectal cancer, haemorrhoids, pruritus ani, constipation, diarrhoea, incontinence
		NON-ANORECTAL-SPECIFIC	Radiation, lymphogranuloma venereum, childbirth, arthritis, endocarditis, high serum testosterone, endometrial cancer, ovarian cancer, breast cancer, cervical cancer, HIV infection, penile or vaginal STIs
		PROSTATE-SPECIFIC	Prostate cancer, prostatitis, benign prostatic hypertrophy
	SURGICAL HISTORY	**ANORECTAL**	Sigmoidoscopy, colonoscopy, rubber band ligation, injection sclerotherapy, haemorrhoidectomy, drainage of fistula or abscess
		PROSTATE	Prostatectomy, transurethral resection of the prostate (TURP)
	ALLERGIES	Contact dermatitis of perianal area	
	MEDICATIONS	Laxatives, constipating agents, alpha blockers, 5-alpha-reductase inhibitors, antifungals, astringent ointments, suppositories	
	COMMUNICABLE DISEASES	HIV, *Neisseria gonorrhoeae*, *Treponema pallidum*, *Chlamydia trachomatis*, HPV, HSV	
	INJURIES AND ACCIDENTS	Rectal trauma, foreign body in rectum	
	CHILDHOOD ILLNESSES	Anal stenosis, Hirschsprung's disease (with rectal pull-through)	
FAMILY HEALTH HISTORY	Anal, rectal and prostatic diseases that are familial are listed: rectal polyps, rectal cancer, pilonidal cyst, prostate cancer For women, number of children birthed and/or carried, birthing delivery type (e.g. vaginal), birthing complications (perineal tears, fistula etc.)		

>>

HEALTH HISTORY		
SOCIAL HISTORY	The components of the social history are linked to anal, rectal and prostatic factors and pathology.	
	GEOGRAPHICAL LOCATION	In tropical and sub-tropical areas there is a higher incidence of intestinal parasite infestation in humans. Recent travel to any tropical and sub-tropical locations needs to be assessed.
	ALCOHOL USE	Excess intake of alcohol is associated with pruritus ani; increased amount of alcohol associated with rectal and prostate cancers.
	TOBACCO USE	Cigarette smoking increases the risk for anal carcinoma and exacerbates Crohn's disease.
	DRUG USE	Illicit drug use may distort the user's perception, increasing the risk for unsafe sexual practices and STI exposure.
	SEXUAL PRACTICE	Rectal penetration increases the risk for anal carcinoma and anorectal STIs. Use of foreign objects in the rectum can lead to anal valve incompetence.
	WORK ENVIRONMENT	Excessive sitting causes direct pressure and increases venous pooling, along with poor lifting techniques causing increased pressure in the bowel which can lead to haemorrhoids.
	HOBBIES AND LEISURE ACTIVITIES	Weight-lifting (haemorrhoids, rectal prolapse)

PERSON-CENTRED HEALTH EDUCATION

When conducting a health assessment, opportunities for the provision of person-centred health education will arise. This is a significant consideration in relation to the assessment process for examination of the anus, rectum and prostate. These occasions are identified as individualised education and may generate further data that can be added to the assessment. All education given should be documented so that, in future, health professionals can assess the impact of previous information provided to the consumer. (Refer to Chapter 1 for initiating health education.) Refer to the following examples.

INDIVIDUALISED HEALTH EDUCATION INTERVENTIONS	
Assessing the consumer for the following health-related activities can assist in identifying the need for education about these factors. This information provides a bridge between the health maintenance activities and anus, rectum and prostate functions.	
Exercise	Exercise promotes regular bowel evacuation.
Stress	Pruritus ani can be exacerbated by stress; diarrhoea can be caused by stress; constipation can be caused by depression.
Sleep	Nocturia secondary to an enlarged prostate
Diet	Increased amounts of dietary fats, cured and smoked meats and charcoal-broiled foods, and decreased amounts of fibre, fruits and vegetables are associated with prostate and rectal cancers. Excessive intake of milk, coffee, tea, coke/cola soft drinks, and spices is associated with pruritus ani. Decreased fluid intake, low-fibre diets in conjunction with some medications can impact on stool softness and amount of pressure needed to evacuate the bowel. These factors increase the likelihood of developing haemorrhoids. Vitamins A, C, E, and folate may protect against developing rectal cancer.
Use of safety devices	Condoms used with vaginal and anal intercourse and good lifting practices
Health check-ups	Haemoccult cards, digital rectal exam, flexible sigmoidoscopy, colonoscopy, PSA testing for those at risk or between ages 50 and 70

PLANNING FOR PHYSICAL EXAMINATION

The planning phase refers to evaluating subjective data to narrow the focus on physical examination, determining what objective data needs to be gathered, as well as considering the environment and equipment that will be required.

At this time, you will identify which of the four diagnostic techniques you will need to implement the physical examination, and how you will sequence these. For the physical examination of the anus, rectum and prostate you will include inspection and palpation.

Objective data is:

> collected during the physical examination of the consumer

> usually collected after subjective data

> information that is measured or observed by the clinician as opposed to being reported by the consumer

> vital to the overall health assessment, to enable you to make clinical decisions that are representative of the whole consumer picture.

Evaluating subjective data to focus physical examination

Before commencing the physical examination of the consumer's anus, rectum and prostate, consider what information the health history has provided. Critical consideration, linked to knowledge of anatomy and physiology, should focus the physical assessment so your examination will be more effective and efficient.

Environment

Assessment of anus and rectum needs a suitable physical environment that can provide adequate privacy. Ambient temperature levels need to be considered for consumer comfort.

Equipment

> Nonsterile gloves
> Water-soluble lubricant
> Haemoccult cards
> Gooseneck lamp

IMPLEMENTATION: CONDUCTING THE PHYSICAL EXAMINATION

Implementation of the physical examination requires you to consider your scope of practice as well. In this section, depending on your context, you may be performing foundation assessment with aspects of advanced assessment if you are practising in a specialised area.

EXAMINATION IN BRIEF: ANUS, RECTUM AND PROSTATE

Examination of the anus, rectum and prostate

Inspection

> Perineum and sacrococcygeal area
> Anal mucosa

Palpation

> Anal Pap collection

Advanced Assessment

UNIT 2

General approach to assessment of the anus, rectum and prostate

1. Greet the consumer and explain the assessment techniques that you will be using.
2. Ensure that the examination room is at a warm, comfortable temperature to prevent consumer chilling and shivering.
3. Use a quiet room that will be free from interruptions and will ensure privacy. Male practitioners often request a female chaperone if examining a female consumer.
4. Ensure that the light in the room provides sufficient brightness to adequately observe the consumer. It may be helpful to have a gooseneck lamp available for additional lighting when lesions are observed.
5. Instruct the consumer to void prior to the assessment.
6. Instruct the consumer to remove pants and underpants and to cover up with a drape sheet.
7. Assess the consumer's apprehension level about the assessment and reassure the consumer that apprehension is normal.
8. For inspection, place the consumer in the left lateral decubitus position and visualise the perianal skin (**Figure 18.3**). This position can also be used for palpation.
9. Don nonsterile gloves.
10. Use a systematic approach every time the assessment is performed. Proceed from the anus to the rectum in the female consumer (but ensure vaginal assessment is completed first if required – see Chapter 17). Proceed from the anus to the prostate in the male consumer.

Examination of the anus, rectum and prostate

Inspection

Perineum and sacrococcygeal area

E Inspect the buttocks and sacral region for lesions, swelling, inflammation and tenderness.

N This area should be smooth and free of lesions, swelling, inflammation and tenderness. There should be no evidence of faeces or mucus on the perianal skin.

A It is abnormal for one or several tiny openings to be seen in the midline over the sacral region, often with hair protruding from them (**Figure 18.4**).

P Pilonidal disease is an acquired condition of the midline coccygeal skin region induced by local stretching forces. There can be a cyst, an acute abscess, or chronic draining sinuses in the sacrococcygeal area. Small skin pits representing enlarged hair follicles precede development of the draining sinus or abscess. Lesions are often secondarily invaded by hair.

A Areas of hyperpigmentation, coupled with excoriation and thickened skin in the perianal area, are abnormal. The area may be intensely pruritic.

P Pruritis ani is caused by pinworms in children and by fungal infections in adults. The lesions are dull, greyish pink.

A Well-demarcated, erythematous, sometimes itchy exudative patches of varying size and shape rimmed with small, red-based pustules are abnormal.

P *Candida albicans* occurs in sites where heat and maceration provide a fertile environment. Susceptibility to candidiasis is increased with systemic antibacterial, corticosteroid or antimetabolic therapy; pregnancy; obesity; diabetes mellitus; blood dyscrasias and immunologic defects.

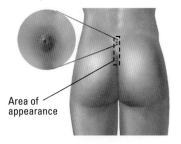

Left lateral decubitus

FIGURE 18.3 Consumer position for examination of the anus and rectum

Area of appearance

FIGURE 18.4 Pilonidal cyst

E Examination **N** Normal findings **A** Abnormal findings **P** Pathophysiology

Anal mucosa

E 1. Spread the consumer's buttocks apart with both hands, exposing the anus.
   2. Instruct the consumer to bear down as though moving the bowels.
   3. Examine the anus for colour, appearance, lesions, inflammation, rash and masses.

N The anal mucosa is deeply pigmented, coarse, moist and hairless. It should be free of lesions, inflammation, rash, masses or additional openings. The anal opening should be closed. There should not be any leakage of faeces or mucus from the anus with straining and there should not be any tissue protrusion.

A A spherical, bluish lump that appears suddenly at the anus, and that ranges in size from a few millimetres to several centimetres in diameter (Figure 18.5), is abnormal. The overlying anal skin may be tense and oedematous. Pain and pruritus may be present in the perianal region.

P **Haemorrhoids** result from dilatation of the superior and inferior haemorrhoidal veins. These haemorrhoidal veins form a haemorrhoidal plexus, or cushion, in the submucosal layer of the anorectum. An external haemorrhoid is located below the dentate line. Thrombosed external haemorrhoids (blood clots within subcutaneous haemorrhoidal veins) occur as a result of heavy lifting, childbirth, straining to defecate (which may be due to a low-fibre diet, decreased fluid intake and certain medications) or other vigorous activity. Bleeding may occur with defecation. See Table 18.1 for other reasons for rectal bleeding.

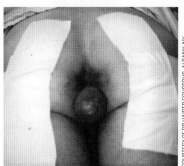

COURTESY OF DR HAIDER GOUSSOUS, ALBANY, NY

FIGURE 18.5 Thrombosed haemorrhoid

TABLE 18.1 Common stool findings and aetiologies

STOOL FINDING/DESCRIPTION	AETIOLOGY
Black, tarry (melaena)	Upper gastrointestinal bleeding
Bright red	Rectal bleeding
Black	Iron or bismuth ingestion
Grey, tan	Obstructive jaundice
Pale yellow, greasy, fatty (steatorrhoea)	Malabsorption syndromes (e.g. coeliac disease), cystic fibrosis
Mucus with blood and pus	Ulcerative colitis, acute diverticulitis
Maroon or bright red	Diverticulosis

A Excess anal or perianal tissue of varying sizes that is soft, pliable, and covered by normal skin is abnormal.

P Anal skin tags are the result of residual resolved thrombosed external haemorrhoids, pregnancy or anal operations. In some cases, there is no known cause.

A Faecal incontinence is abnormal.

P Faecal incontinence is usually a sign of an underlying acute medical problem. Some causes of faecal incontinence include faecal impaction, diarrhoea, irritable bowel syndrome, stroke, dementia, multiple sclerosis, rectal prolapse, rectal trauma and anorectal carcinoma.

A The perianal area may have erythema, excoriations, cracking and bleeding. In chronic cases the anal ring may have a shiny appearance.

P Pruritus ani is a condition in which itching around the rectum occurs. There are multiple causes of pruritus ani; however, excessive cleaning of the anal area is the most common cause. Moisture around the anus, associated with sweating or from passage of abnormal faeces, can also exacerbate or induce this problem. Other possible causes of pruritus ani include pinworms, psoriasis, eczema, dermatitis, haemorrhoids, anal fissures and sexually transmitted infections (STIs).

E Examination **N** Normal findings **A** Abnormal findings **P** Pathophysiology

UNIT 2

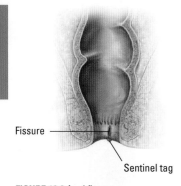

Fissure ——

Sentinel tag ——

FIGURE 18.6 Anal fissure

A Linear tears in the epidermis of the anal canal beginning below the dentate line and extending distally to the anal orifice are abnormal (**Figure 18.6**). Extreme pain, pruritus and bleeding may accompany these findings.

REFLECTION IN PRACTICE

Developing confidence in discussing sensitive topics: Anal fissures

Anal fissures are common, and may be primary or secondary. Anal fissures are most often caused by injury to the area, and the most common reason for them is passing a hard stool or a large stool. Other common causes include constipation, diarrhoea, physical injuries from objects inserted into the anus, pregnancy, childbirth and Chron's disease (Health Direct, 2022). Secondary fissures usually indicate a more serious underlying issue (e.g. malignancy). Non-surgical treatment is successful to heal fissures in half of all consumers and this treatment includes sitz bathing, high-fibre diet and medication (Steinhagen, 2018). Where this is not successful, there is a high success rate with lateral internal sphincterotomy (Steinhagen, 2018). Other aetiology of atypical fissures includes ulcerative colitis, anal cancer, tuberculosis, HIV, syphilis, herpes and leukemia.

Many health professionals may avoid discussing details of faecal habits and quality of stools, and experiences with bowel motions or sexual intercourse experiences, with consumers unless the consumer identifies an issue.

> However, considering the above information where painful anal fissures may be avoided, what level of discussion do you have about quality of faecal stools and details of habits, or even sexual intercourse experiences?

> What do you think you could do to develop this level of questioning to provide required opportunistic health education for consumers in your care?

P **Anal fissures** are the result of trauma, such as the forced passage of a large, hard stool, and anal intercourse, especially forced intercourse. Fissures occur most often in the area of the posterior coccygeal midline and less frequently in the anterior midline. This is because of weakness in the superficial external sphincter in these sectors. Predisposition to fissure is increased by perianal inflammation, which causes the **anoderm** to lose its normal elasticity. A sentinel skin tag may be visible inferior to the anal fissure and at the anal margin.

A Undrained collections of perianal pus of the tissue spaces in and adjacent to the anorectum are abnormal.

P The most common cause of **anorectal abscesses** is infection of the anal glands, usually located posteriorly and situated between the internal and the external sphincters. These glands normally drain via the internal sphincter through small ducts and into anal crypts. When these ducts are occluded by impacted faecal material or trauma, ductal stasis and abscess formation results. An indurated mass with overlying erythema displaces the anus in cases of superficial abscess.

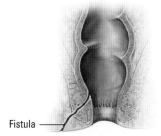

Fistula ——

Skin surface opening

FIGURE 18.7 Anorectal fistula

A An inflamed, red, raised area with purulent or serosanguineous discharge on the perianal skin is abnormal (**Figure 18.7**).

P An **anorectal fistula** is a hollow, fibrous tract lined by granulation tissue and having an opening inside the anal canal or rectum and one or more orifices in the perianal skin. Fistulas are usually the result of incomplete healing of drained anorectal abscesses; however, they may occur in the absence of an abscess history. If this is the case, other causes for the fistula must be explored. Additional predisposing factors are inflammatory bowel disease, infectious disease, malignancy, Crohn's disease, radiation therapy, chemotherapy, chlamydial infections and trauma.

A Soiling of the skin with stool and gaping of the anus are abnormal.

E Examination   **N** Normal findings   **A** Abnormal findings   **P** Pathophysiology

P **Anal or faecal incontinence** may be caused by neurological diseases, traumatic injuries or surgical damage to the puborectalis or sphincter muscles. Perineal or intestinal disorders, diarrhoea, faecal impaction and constipating agents may also cause anal/faecal incontinence.

A The protrusion of the rectal mucosa (pinkish-red doughnut with radiating folds) through the anal orifice is abnormal (**Figure 18.8**).

P **Rectal prolapse** is associated with poor tone of the pelvic musculature, chronic straining at stool, faecal incontinence and, sometimes, neurological disease or traumatic damage to the pelvis. A complete rectal prolapse involves the entire bowel wall. It is larger, red and moist looking, and has circular folds. See **Table 18.1** for common stool findings and aetiologies.

A Erythematous plaques that develop into vesicular lesions that may become pustules and ulcerate are abnormal.

P These lesions are suggestive of herpes simplex virus (HSV). Most anorectal herpes is due to HSV-2, and infections are related to anal intercourse.

A Warts or lesions that are beefy red, flesh coloured, irregular and pedunculated are abnormal findings (**Figure 18.9**). The lesions may involve the anoderm, but may also extend deep into the anal canal and involve the rectal mucosa. There may be a few scattered lesions or extensive involvement of the entire anus.

P Condylomata acuminatum are caused by human papillomavirus (HPV). Coital trauma allows entry into the anal epidermis in those in whom wart virus is latent in the anorectum. Anal warts may also develop in women via extension of genital warts along the perineum. Of the 50 strains of HPV, types 16, 18 and 31 have been associated with malignant lesions.

P Perineal chancroids (**Figure 18.10**) are caused by *Haemophilus ducreyi*. Chancroids can be seen on the genitalia as well as the perineal and perianal regions.

A Mucoid or creamy exudate, possibly blood, from the rectum is abnormal. This may be assessed by inspection of the anus and faeces, and by the practitioner who palpates the anus. A faeces sample should be obtained from the consumer, if possible, and tested for occult blood.

P Gonococcal proctitis is most often seen in homosexual men as a result of direct inoculation, but it also occurs in women through contamination by vaginal discharge.

A Multiple perianal fissures and oedematous skin tags of varying degrees are abnormal.

P Anorectal involvement occurs in the majority of consumers with Crohn's disease. Perianal disease may precede the onset of intestinal Crohn's disease by several years. Perianal disease may proceed to anal stricture and incontinence. The development of perianal Crohn's disease has no relation to other extra-intestinal manifestations of the disease.

A Foreign bodies/objects observed to be protruding from or reported by the consumer in the rectum are abnormal.

P Thermometers, enema catheters, vibrators, bottles and phallic objects may be introduced into the anus by accident, for erotic purposes, for concealment, for self-treatment or by assault. Complications may include perforation of the rectum, obstruction and pararectal infections.

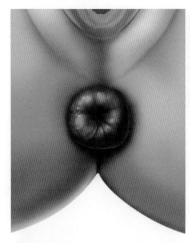

FIGURE 18.8 Rectal prolapse

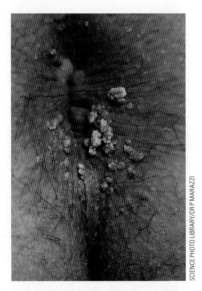

SCIENCE PHOTO LIBRARY/DR P MARAZZI

FIGURE 18.9 Human papillomavirus (HPV) in the anal region

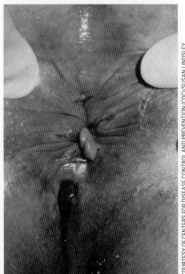

COURTESY OF CENTERS FOR DISEASE CONTROL AND PREVENTION (CDC)/SUSAN LINDSLEY

FIGURE 18.10 Perineal chancroid

E Examination N Normal findings A Abnormal findings P Pathophysiology

UNIT 2

Palpation

Anal Pap collection

Palpation of the anus, rectum and prostate is considered specialised practice, and in most areas in Australia and New Zealand is not undertaken by nurses at all. You may be asked to be an escort for the doctor and consumer while this is performed. If you are in a specialised advanced practice role that necessitates this process, or would like to understand what you are observing, refer to the Further resources list at the end of this chapter. In Australia, anal Pap collection is only carried out in a few organisations as further research is being undertaken to develop best use for screening guidelines (Australian Federation of AIDS Organisations, n.d.). Most often, a digital anorectal examination (DARE) will be conducted by the doctor to check for swelling or lumps by inserting a gloved and lubricated finger into the anus (Cancer Council, 2020).

HEALTH EDUCATION

Assessing risk through anal Pap

In Australian in 2021, 90 cases of anal cancer were diagnosed, which, although rare, have doubled in incidence in the past 20 years (Cancer Council, 2020). The anal Pap is a screening tool used to identify premalignant cytologic changes in the anal epithelium in at-risk populations. There are currently no national guidelines available that specify when the anal Pap should be performed.

Complete a comprehensive medical history with a focused anal cancer risk interview that facilitates the screening for risk factors. The interview should focus on the following areas:

> Sexual history, asking about anal intercourse and the number of sexual partners
> History of anal warts, genital warts, anal pain, anal discharge, anal dysplasia or anal cancer
> Past history of an anal Pap: if yes, why, when, and the results.
  At-risk groups that may benefit from the anal Pap include:
> HIV-infected men with any history of receptive anal intercourse
> HIV-infected men with a history of injected drug use who might benefit from aggressive treatment
> Non-HIV-infected men who participate in receptive anal intercourse or who have a history of perianal or intra-anal condylomas
> Any recipient of allograft transplantation.

CLINICAL REASONING

Practice tip: Appropriate referral and support after cancer diagnosis

Referral is an essential part of the health practitioner's role. Although anal cancer is rare, for those who do have a diagnosis of anal cancer it will be extremely important for appropriate referral for consumer support. This is due to not only the cancer diagnosis but also because most people are uncomfortable talking about this part of their bodies. Anal cancer is more common in women than men, and is usually diagnosed between ages of 50 and 60. Risk factors, while specifically unknown, do generally include previous STIs (e.g. chlamydia, genital warts, HPV, HIV/AIDS) and smoking.

Anal cancer is often referred to by its stage – also known as the 'TNM system' (tumour, nodes, metastases). The lower the number, the less advanced the cancer and more options to treat will exist. It is referred to as follows:

> T (tumour) followed by a number from 1 to 4 (number denotes how far it has spread; the higher the number the further it has spread)
> N (node) followed by a number from 1 to 3 (number denotes how many nodes it has affected nearby, scoring as above; the higher the number, the more advanced)
> M (metastases) followed by 1 denotes the cancer has spread to organs/lymph nodes not close to the anus. M following by 0 denotes no sign of cancer spreading from anus to other sites.

So that you are prepared to refer appropriately, find out in your community to whom you would refer. Identify all community/primary care support services as well as specialist acute support services.

Staging sourced from https://www.cancervic.org.au/cancer-information/types-of-cancer/anal_cancer/anal-cancer-overview.html

https://www.cancer.gov/about-cancer/diagnosis-staging/staging

>>

REFLECTION IN PRACTICE

Managing the rectal examination

The anorectal evaluation is usually reserved for the last portion of the examination after the nurse–consumer relationship has been established. A step-by-step explanation, description of expected sensations, reassurance, and a gentle technique will minimise consumer embarrassment and discomfort. It is also important for you to feel at ease about performing this examination.

How would you cope with the following situations if they occurred during the examination?
> The consumer develops an erection.
> The consumer is incontinent of faeces.
> The consumer passes flatus.

EVALUATION OF HEALTH ASSESSMENT AND PHYSICAL EXAMINATION FINDINGS

In the evaluation phase of a health assessment, the focus is on ensuring the data gathered is complete, accurate and documented appropriately (see case study as an example of the focused assessment; see Chapter 22 for a comprehensive health assessment). In evaluating the data you should:
> draw on your critical thinking and problem-solving skills to make sound clinical decisions
> act on abnormal data (include communicating findings to other health professionals)
> ensure documentation reflects the outcomes of the clinical decisions/actions taken (refer to Chapter 3, which discusses in detail why documentation is so important and how this may be undertaken in different health settings).
The case study that follows steps you through this process.

CASE STUDY

THE CONSUMER WITH HAEMORRHOIDS AND RECTAL BLEEDING

This case study illustrates the application and objective documentation of the anal, rectal and prostatic assessment.

Toby Katte is a 44-year-old male builder who presents with acutely inflamed haemorrhoids and rectal bleeding.

HEALTH HISTORY

CONSUMER PROFILE	44-year-old male builder – Caucasian
CHIEF COMPLAINT	'I have blood from my backside and it hurts when I go to the toilet. My partner says I have these red grape-like things sticking out of my backside.'
HISTORY OF THE PRESENT ILLNESS	Consumer reports that 7 days ago he started to experience some pain with defecation. The next day he noticed increased pain with defecation and blood on the surface of his stool. Yesterday the pain and bleeding worsened and they occurred without defecation and he also noted some mucopurulent anal discharge. Denies any previous history of rectal bleeding or pain. He denies any previous history of sexually transmitted diseases and has undergone recent STI screening at the start of a new relationship 8 months ago. Has not taken any medications to help him defecate or for pain relief. Has not passed faeces for past two days.

PAST HEALTH HISTORY	**MEDICAL HISTORY**	Constipation
	SURGICAL HISTORY	Nil
	ALLERGIES	Nil

>>

HEALTH HISTORY

	MEDICATIONS	> None
	COMMUNICABLE DISEASES	States that he has been tested for STIs and tests were always negative
	INJURIES AND ACCIDENTS	Nil
	SPECIAL NEEDS	Denies
	BLOOD TRANSFUSIONS	Denies
	CHILDHOOD ILLNESSES	Measles at a young age
	IMMUNISATIONS	Not sure
FAMILY HEALTH HISTORY		Father has high blood pressure and diabetes mellitus type II; mother has long history of depression; unsure of grandparents; only child
SOCIAL HISTORY	ALCOHOL USE	Drinks most nights after work, 3–6 beers per night; denies drinking then driving
	TOBACCO USE	Cigarettes pack/day × 2 years
	DRUG USE	Nil reported
	DOMESTIC AND INTIMATE PARTNER VIOLENCE	Denies
	SEXUAL PRACTICE	Sexually active at the age of 14, with 5 previous partners; 'usually' uses condoms. All female partners.
	TRAVEL HISTORY	Nil
	WORK ENVIRONMENT	Builder
	HOME ENVIRONMENT	Lives with his partner in the inner city; renting
	HOBBIES AND LEISURE ACTIVITIES	Plays rugby once a week and trains once a week; going out with friends
	STRESS	Home situation is OK. House is a bit messy; both take turns cooking and sharing chores. Irregular contact with parents.
	EDUCATION	Attended high school and completed year 12 in Melbourne
	ECONOMIC STATUS	'It's getting more expensive to live, but I am almost debt-free except for my credit card.'
	MILITARY SERVICE	Denies
	RELIGION	Was brought up Protestant but does not practise
	CULTURAL BACKGROUND	Australian and British heritage
	ROLES AND RELATIONSHIPS	Monogamous heterosexual relationship for the last 8 months with female partner who is 3 years older
	CHARACTERISTIC PATTERNS OF DAILY LIVING	Wakes at 5 a.m. 6 days a week for work. Plays sport on weekends and trains one day a week 'just social not really competitive'.

>>

HEALTH HISTORY

HEALTH MAINTENANCE ACTIVITIES	SLEEP	8 hours every night, usually sleeps well but lately wakes feeling tired
	DIET	Lots of take-away and fast food. Has fatty meals at least once a day, loves pizza, KFC and McDonald's
	EXERCISE	Rugby and work are quite physical
	STRESS MANAGEMENT	Being with partner, sports, music
	USE OF SAFETY DEVICES	Does not use safe lifting techniques when lifting heavy things
	HEALTH CHECK-UPS	Goes to GP when he has issues, but only does so when he really has to; dislikes seeking medical assistance

PHYSICAL EXAMINATION

	INSPECTION	GENERAL	Strong physical condition, particularly upper body
		PERINEUM AND SACROCOCCYGEAL AREA	1 cm fissure at posterior coccygeal midline
		ANAL MUCOSA	Deeply pigmented, coarse, moist and hairless, nil mucous discharge, anal opening closed. Prominent engorged haemorrhoids, reddened and small amount of blood present. Approximately 10 protruding from anus
	STOOL HAEMOCCULT	Consumer has been unable to pass faeces for past 2 days. Extremely painful when tries	

DIAGNOSTIC DATA

VITAL SIGNS	> T: 37.9°C > P: 89 b/min > RR: 12 b/min > BP: 128/82 mmHg > SpO$_2$: 99% on room air

EVALUATION AND CLINICAL REASONING FOR CASE STUDY

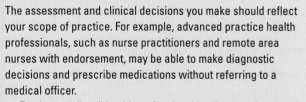

The assessment and clinical decisions you make should reflect your scope of practice. For example, advanced practice health professionals, such as nurse practitioners and remote area nurses with endorsement, may be able to make diagnostic decisions and prescribe medications without referring to a medical officer.

Fundamentally, all health professionals collect, evaluate and act on consumer-focused health information, which will at times include referral to, or collaboration with, other healthcare team members. Nurses assess consumer responses to interventions and determine when to escalate key changes in a consumer's condition. The clinical reasoning cycle provides health professionals with a framework to consider all this information in a meaningful way for planning consumer care. These phases are stepped out below, and draw on information presented and collected during the health history and physical examination. We then work through the cycle components that are relevant to this case study (cycle components are bolded).

For Toby Katte, the 44-year-old man who presents to the drop-in medical clinic with rectal bleeding, the significant data that needs to be considered includes the following.

Collecting cues/information

Recall and Review: In the first instance you will need to reflect on what you know about haemorrhoids, bleeding from the rectum, and pain.

Chief complaint and history of present illness

> Blood from anus and pain when trying to defecate
> Red grape-like protrusions coming from anus (haemorrhoids)
> 7 days ago, consumer started to experience some pain with defecation, with each day increasing pain and blood on stool and toilet paper. Yesterday the pain and bleeding worsened and they occurred without defecation. He also noted some mucopurulent (pus-like mucus) anal discharge yesterday.
> Consumer denies any previous history of rectal bleeding or pain.
> Consumer denies any previous history of sexually transmitted diseases and has undergone recent STI screening at the start of a new relationship 8 months ago.
> He has not passed stool for past 2 days.

Processing information

Interpret: These symptoms and details of history outline the scope of the issue for this consumer and how it is affecting his wellbeing and ability to self-manage this deviation from normal health. So far, he has not taken any steps in self-management.

Diet
> Poor: low in fibre, high in fat

Medical history
> Constipation

Work environment
> Builder – heavy physical work

Use of safety devices
> Not taking any precautions with lifting

Discriminate, Relate and Infer: A medical history of constipation, a heavy lifting work environment with no real understanding of safe lifting, and a poor diet predispose Toby for risk of high pressures in the anal mucosa from straining, which may lead to haemorrhoids. Without stool softeners, the haemorrhoids are likely to become acutely aggravated.

Inspection of anus
> 1 cm fissure at posterior coccygeal midline
> Deeply pigmented, coarse, moist and hairless, nil mucous discharge, anal opening closed
> Prominent engorged haemorrhoids, reddened and small amount of blood present; approximately 10 haemorrhoids protruding from anus
> T: 37.9°C

Interpret, Relate and Infer: This all shows localised signs of irritation, with possible infection. The mucus and bleeding previously described by Toby may indicate that the haemorrhoids have become infected and are discharging pus along with blood. Possible infection is supported by the appearance of the haemorrhoids being red, inflamed, engorged and painful, along with the elevated temperature.

Putting it all together – synthesise information

The nurse in this case would note all of these abnormalities and refer to the medical officer. It is likely that antibiotics and stool softeners are required, with a possible view for a surgical review if the consumer wishes to have the haemorrhoids dealt with surgically. Education about avoiding a recurrence of these symptoms is likely to be required as well, and would definitely include dietary options to support good bowel habits and stool formation.

Actions based on assessment findings

The nurse should also provide additional education for interventions that do not require a doctor's order, such as:

1 Improve diet: one that is lower in fat and higher in fibre to help soften stool so less straining is required. Straining can cause haemorrhoids to become larger and also the pressure can cause bleeding. Hard stools can also cause aggravation of the haemorrhoids and pain.
2 Practise safe lifting techniques at work, such as lifting from the knees to reduce the amount of intra-abdominal pressure asserted. This will not only improve the issues surrounding haemorrhoids but also reduces the risk of back or abdominal wall injury (such as hernia).
3 Use analgesics that do not contain codeine for analgesia, as codeine-based analgesia increases risk of constipation.
4 Practise hand hygiene to reduce the chance of introducing further infection opportunities.
5 While wiping after defecating, be gentle. If possible, shower rather than wipe using paper; this will reduce further inflammation and aggravation to the inflamed area and showering will remove any leftover faecal matter more effectively than wiping. In turn, this reduces the opportunity to introduce more infective agents from the faeces to the injured haemorrhoids.
6 Rest and sleep as much as possible until symptoms improve; this will aid the body's immune response.

The final step in the process is accurate documentation. The nurse must document findings, referrals, interventions, and advice and education given. The consumer would continue to have ongoing long-term management and follow-up by specialist medical staff in collaboration with general practitioner.

CHAPTER RESOURCES

REVIEW QUESTIONS

For answers to these questions, see Answer section at the end of the book.

1. When performing the anorectal examination on a consumer, which of the following would cause you to suspect anorectal abuse? Select all that apply.
   a. Enlarged testicles
   b. Anal fissures
   c. Haemorrhoids
   d. Anal skin tags
   e. Pain on urination
   f. Refusal by the consumer to undergo the anorectal examination

2. In caring for a consumer who has undergone surgery for repair of an anorectal fistula, the nurse would identify which of the following as additional predisposing factors?
   a. Older age
   b. Smoking
   c. inflammatory bowel disease
   d. Multiple gonorrhoea infections

3. All but one of the following are common causes of anal fissures. Which of the following conditions is not usually related to rectal bleeding?
   a. Benign polyps of the colon
   b. Inflammatory bowel disease
   c. Small bowel obstruction
   d. Forced or vigorous anal intercourse

4. A 52-year-old male presents with the complaint of rectal bleeding. Which of the following are possible causes of this bleeding? Select all that apply.
   a. Cancer of the colon
   b. Anal fissure
   c. Haemorrhoids
   d. Prostate cancer
   e. Rectal prolapse
   f. Benign prostatic hypertrophy

5. Which statement is correct in regard to performing a successful rectal examination?
   a. Provide a step-by-step explanation about the examination.
   b. Tell the consumer that you are just as nervous about this as they are.
   c. Perform the rectal examination at the beginning of the physical examination to decrease consumer anxiety.
   d. While performing the rectal examination, ask the consumer about what they enjoy doing in their spare time, to try to get their mind off the examination.

6. Which aetiology would you suspect from the consumer's complaint of black and sticky stools?
   a. Upper gastrointestinal bleeding
   b. Iron ingestion
   c. Rectal bleeding
   d. Malabsorption syndrome

7. A young man presents to the clinic with two small openings in the midline sacral region; one has a hair protruding and both are red and inflamed. What is this condition likely to be?
   a. Pilonidal cyst
   b. Anorectal disease
   c. Hyperpigmentation of the sacrum
   d. Pruritis ani

8. Anna is a 26-year-old female vet who provides animal rescue services, often flying into remote tropical areas for work. She complains of very itchy, well-demarcated patches of skin on her bottom and lower sacral region. The rims of the skin patches have small red-based pustules. What is this likely to be?
   a. Calcium deficiency
   b. Pruritis ani
   c. *Candida albicans*
   d. Ringworm (dematophytosis) infection

Questions 9 and 10 relate to the examination undertaken of Mr Craveat.

Mr Craveat is a usually fit and healthy 62-year-old man who presents with changes to urination. He states that when he goes to the toilet he has difficulty maintaining a stream, and never feels like his bladder is properly emptied. His brother was diagnosed with prostate cancer a year ago. Mr Craveat also experiences problems with constipation, lives alone, and states he likes to eat out a lot, and does not exercise. Alcohol consumption includes 8–10 standard drinks per day and he is in the obese weight range.

9. What are the risk factors Mr Craveat shows for prostate cancer?
   a. Family history of prostate cancer, obesity
   b. Family history of prostate cancer, obesity, low levels of exercise, constipation
   c. Family history of prostate cancer, low levels of exercise, over 50 years old, diet, living in Australia/New Zealand
   d. Family history of prostate cancer, low levels of exercise, over 50 years old, diet, not emptying his bladder fully when toileting

10. Mr Craveat is also concerned about his constipation, and asks for advice to improve this. Which of the following interventions would you advise he undertake?
    a. See a nutritionist to help improve diet, such as more fibre; increase gentle exercise, increase water intake, avoid codeine additive analgesics, use laxatives to help establish a bowel routine
    b. See a nutritionist to help improve diet, such as more protein; increase gentle exercise, increase water intake, avoid codeine additive analgesics, use laxatives to help establish a bowel routine
    c. See a nutritionist to help improve diet, such as more fibre; lose at least 5 kg of weight, avoid codeine additive analgesics
    d. See a nutritionist to help improve diet, such as higher fat to ease passage through the bowel; increase gentle exercise, increase water intake, avoid codeine additive analgesics, use laxatives to help establish a bowel routine

CS CLINICAL SKILLS

The following Clinical Skill is relevant to this chapter and can be found in Tollefson & Hillman, *Clinical Psychomotor Skills*, 8th edition:
> 27 Healthcare teaching.

FURTHER RESOURCES

> Anal Pap Tests – St Vincent's Hospital: https://www.svhs.org.au/our-services/list-of-services/hiv-immunology-infectious-disease/dysplasia-and-anal-cancer-services/anal-pap-tests

> Better Health Channel – Haemorrhoids: https://www.betterhealth.vic.gov.au/health/conditionsandtreatments/haemorrhoids

> Bowel Cancer Australia: http://www.bowelcanceraustralia.org
> Cancer Society of New Zealand: http://www.cancernz.org.nz/
> Colorectal Surgical Society of Australia & New Zealand: http://www.cssanz.org/
> Gastroenterological Society of Australia: http://www.gesa.org.au/
> Health Direct – Haemorrhoids: https://www.healthdirect.gov.au/haemorrhoids-piles
> Lions Australia Prostate Cancer Website – created by the Australian Prostate Cancer Collaboration: http://www.prostatehealth.org.au/
> Prostate Cancer Foundation of Australia: http://www.prostate.org.au/
> Prostate Cancer Foundation of New Zealand: http://www.prostate.org.nz/

REFERENCES

Australian Federation of AIDS Organisations. (n.d.). The bottom line: screening for anal cancer. http://www.thebottomline.org.au/site/section/show/3/screening-for-anal-cancer

Australian Institute of Health and Welfare (AIHW). (2018). Cancer in Indigenous Australians. Retrieved 7 December 2022 from: https://www.aihw.gov.au/reports/cancer/cancer-in-indigenous-australians/contents/cancer-type/prostate-cancer-c61

Australian Institute of Health and Welfare (AIHW). (2022). Cancer data in Australia, AIHW, Australian Government. Retrieved 7 December 2022 from: https://www.aihw.gov.au/reports/cancer/cancer-data-in-australia/contents/about.

Cancer Australia, (2022). Prostate cancer. Retrieved 7 December 2022 from: https://www.canceraustralia.gov.au/cancer-types/prostate-cancer/statistics

Cancer Council. (2020). Anal cancer. Retrieved from https://www.cancer.org.au/cancer-information/types-of-cancer/anal-cancer

Cancer Council NSW. (2022). A better quality of life for prostate cancer survivors. Retrieved 7 December 2022 from: https://www.cancercouncil.com.au/news/a-better-quality-of-life-for-prostate-cancer-survivors/

Department of Health and Aged Care. (2019). Pregnancy Care Guidelines: Haemorrhoids. Retrieved 7 December 2022 from: https://www.health.gov.au/resources/pregnancy-care-guidelines/part-i-common-conditions-during-pregnancy/haemorrhoids

Egan, R., Lawrenson, R., Kidd, J., Cassim, S., Black, S., Blundell, R., Bateman, J., & Broughton, J. R. (2020). Inequalities between Māori and non-Māori men with prostate cancer in Aotearoa New Zealand. *New Zealand Medical Journal, 133*(1521), 69–76. PMID: 32994638.

Fowler G. E., Siddiqui, J., Zahid, A., & Young, C. J. (2019). Treatment of hemorrhoids: A survey of surgical practice in Australia and New Zealand. *World Journal of Clinical Cases, 7*(22), 3742–50. doi: 10.12998/wjcc.v7.i22.3742. PMID: 31799299; PMCID: PMC6887603.

Health Direct. (2020). *Prostate specific antigen (PSA) test.* Australian Government. https://www.healthdirect.gov.au/prostate-specific-antigen-PSA-test

Health Direct. (2022). *Anal fissure.* Australian Government. https://www.healthdirect.gov.au/anal-fissure

Lao, C., Obertova, Z., Brown, C., Scott, N., Edlin, R., Gilling, P., Holmes, M., Tyrie, L., & Lawrenson, R. (2016). Differences in survival between Māori and New Zealand Europeans with prostate cancer. *European Journal of Cancer Care, 25,* 262–68.

Mazariego, C. G., Egger, S., King, M. T., Juraskova, I., Woo, H., Berry, M., Armstrong, B.K., & Smith D. P. (2020). Fifteen-year quality of life outcomes in men with localised prostate cancer: population based Australian prospective study. Accessed 7 December 2022 from: https://www.bmj.com/content/371/bmj.m3503

Olver, I. (2015). Highlights of PSA testing guidelines. *Cancer Forum, 39*(3), 161–3.

Prostate Cancer Foundation of Australia and Cancer Council Australia. (2016). PSA Testing Guidelines Expert Advisory Panel. Short form summary: Clinical practice guidelines for PSA testing and early management of test-detected prostate cancer. Retrieved from https://www.prostate.org.au/media/611493/PSA-Testing-Guidelines-Short-Form.pdf

Prostate Cancer Foundation of Australia (PCFA). (2022a). Prostate cancer overtakes breast cancer as Australia's most common cancer. Retrieved 7 December 2022 from: https://www.pcfa.org.au/news-media/news/prostate-cancer-overtakes-breast-cancer-as-australia-s-most-common-cancer/

Prostate Cancer Foundation of Australia (PCFA). (2022b). Prostate cancer in Australia – what do the numbers tell us? Retrieved 7 December 2022 from: https://www.pcfa.org.au/news-media/news/prostate-cancer-in-australia-what-do-the-numbers-tell-us/

Prostate Cancer Foundation NZ. (2022). Prostate cancer. Retrieved 7 December 2022 from: https://prostate.org.nz/prostate-cancer/

Ravindranath, G. G., & Rahul, B. G. (2018). Prevalence and risk factors of hemorrhoids: a study in a semi-urban centre. *International Surgery Journal, 5*(2), 469–99.

Steinhagen, E. (2018). Anal fissure. *Diseases of the Colon & Rectum, 61*(3), 293–7. doi: 10.1097/DCR.0000000000001042

UNIT 3

SPECIFIC LIFESPAN POPULATIONS

CHAPTER **19**

THE PREGNANT WOMAN

LEARNING OUTCOMES

By the end of this chapter you should be able to:

1 explain the characteristics of the most common pregnancy-related complaints
2 identify what is included in a health history obtained during a pregnant woman's first antenatal visit
3 discuss the psychosocial status of a pregnant woman
4 differentiate the normal changes of pregnancy from the pathological changes
5 explain a health assessment and physical examination of a pregnant woman
6 discuss the most common learning needs of a pregnant woman
7 identify health education opportunities for women in relation to pregnancy
8 discuss the clinical reasoning in evaluating outcomes of health assessment and physical examination including documentation, health education provision and relevant health referrals.

BACKGROUND

Pregnancy imposes many physiological, hormonal and psychological changes on a woman. The gestational period (which is considered to average 280 days or 40 weeks from the last menses) is divided into three trimesters (of approximately 13 weeks each), and each has specific changes and symptoms that can cause discomfort for the woman. You are encouraged to review Chapter 12 (Breast and regional nodes) and Chapter 17 (Genitourinary and reproductive genitalia) before beginning this chapter.

There were 309 996 births registered in Australia in 2021, an increase of 15 627 (5.3%) from 2020 (ABS, 2022). Of these births, 23 510 (7.6%) were to women who were from an Aboriginal or Torres Strait Islander background. Australia's total fertility rate is currently 1.70 births per woman, and for Aboriginal and Torres Strait Islander women it is 2.34 births per woman (ABS, 2022). The average age of women who give birth fell until the 1970s and has risen since then. In 2021, the median age of women giving birth was 31.7 years (up from 31.3 in 2017). In the Aboriginal and Torres Strait Islander population, the median age of women who give birth is also slightly increasing: from 25.6 years in 2017 to 26.5 in 2021 (ABS, 2022).

Australian maternal mortality rates are among the lowest in the world, with 16 maternal deaths occurring in 2020 (5.5 per 100 000 women giving birth) and 194 in the decade from 2011 to 2020 (a rate of 6.4 per 100 000 women giving birth) (AIHW, 2022a). The most common medical causes of mortality are obstetric haemorrhage, thromboembolism and hypertensive complications of pregnancy. Women under 20 or over 40 years of age are represented in higher numbers in maternal mortality rates: 17.2 and 11.8 respectively per 100 000 women giving birth

(AIHW, 2022a). Aboriginal and Torres Strait Islander women have a higher incidence of maternal death compared to non-Aboriginal and Torres Strait Islander women, with 16.4 deaths per 100 000 (AIHW, 2022a).

In New Zealand, there were 58 749 babies born in the 12 months to September 2022 (Stats NZ, 2022), with the majority of births occurring in a birth centre or a tertiary maternity facility; home births are more common for Māori women and women of European heritage. The median age of women giving birth is 31.0 years and the total fertility rate is 1.65 babies per woman, down slightly from 1.66 in 2020 (Stats NZ, 2022). In Māori populations, the average age of women giving birth is 27.1 years, and the fertility rate is 2.34 babies per woman (Stats NZ, 2019). The maternal mortality rate in New Zealand is 13.5 deaths per 100 000 women giving birth, and this has remained consistent since the early 2000s (PMMRC, 2017). Women aged 40 years and older and Māori and Pasifika women are at higher risk of maternal mortality in New Zealand (HQSC, 2021). More than half of the women who died during pregnancy, childbirth and in the postpartum period were overweight or obese, with 34% identified as tobacco smokers. Alcohol, substance use and family violence have contributed to 25% of these deaths (PMMRC, 2017).

A risk management approach is the focus when assessing a pregnant woman. Clinicians work in partnership with women and their families, addressing questions and providing reassurance regarding the normal physical changes associated with pregnancy. With the availability of accurate home pregnancy tests, a woman may know she is pregnant within 2 weeks of conception, affording an opportunity for early healthcare interaction. In Australia and New Zealand, the majority of care and education that is delivered in partnership with pregnant women is provided by obstetricians, midwives or general practitioners (GP). Maternity care includes antenatal, intrapartum and postnatal care for women and their babies for up to six weeks after birth. The wellbeing of the woman throughout this time is one of the most important influences on the future health of the child (AIHW, 2022b).

In Australia and New Zealand there are different models of maternity care available (Table 19.1) that, depending on what is available locally (rural or urban), women may be able to access. Each model allows for appropriate consultation, referral and transfer of care when a woman's needs escalate. A comprehensive overview of nomenclature for Australian models of maternity care is given in AIHW (2022c).

TABLE 19.1 Snapshot of models of maternity care in Australia and New Zealand

AUSTRALIA		NEW ZEALAND	
MODEL CATEGORIES	**MODEL DESCRIPTION**	**MODEL CATEGORIES**	**MODEL DESCRIPTION**
Standard care in a public hospital	Antenatal care – with midwives and/or obstetricians in the public hospital or in a community clinic Labour and birth in a public hospital	Standard care in a public hospital	Antenatal care – with midwives (employed by the District Health Boards) and/or obstetricians in the public hospital Labour and birth in a public hospital
Shared care	Regular antenatal care – with a general practitioner (GP) and some check-ups with midwives and/or obstetricians in public hospital or in a community clinic Or regular antenatal care – with midwives and/or obstetricians and check-up with public hospital clinicians Labour and birth in a public hospital	Lead maternity carer – independent/self-employed midwife (in small group practices); government funded	Antenatal care – with a midwife (chosen by the pregnant woman) Labour and birth can be at home, in small birthing centre or in a public maternity hospital (with the midwife or midwives who provided care during pregnancy)
Midwifery-led care (team or caseload midwifery)	Antenatal care – with one midwife or a small team of midwives who work in a public hospital Labour and birth in a public hospital (with the midwife or midwives who provided care during the pregnancy)	Lead maternity carer – shared care – general practitioner / midwife; government funded	Antenatal care – with a GP who has specialised in care of the pregnant woman and a community midwife (chosen by the pregnant woman) Labour and birth in a public hospital (with the community midwife/GP and/or hospital midwives)

>> **TABLE 19.1** *continued*

AUSTRALIA		NEW ZEALAND	
MODEL CATEGORIES	**MODEL DESCRIPTION**	**MODEL CATEGORIES**	**MODEL DESCRIPTION**
Birth centre care	Antenatal care – with one midwife or a small team of midwives who work in a birth centre Labour and birth in the birth centre	Lead maternity carer – private obstetrician (can be accessed free of charge if referred by GP/midwife for specialist care)	Antenatal care – with a private specialist obstetrician (chosen by the pregnant woman) Labour and birth in a private or public hospital (with the obstetrician and/or hospital midwives)
Private obstetric care	Antenatal care – with a private obstetrician (chosen by the pregnant woman) Labour and birth usually in a private hospital with care provided by the obstetrician and hospital midwives	Lead maternity carer – private obstetrician (can be accessed free of charge if referred by GP/midwife for specialist care)	Antenatal care – with a private specialist obstetrician (chosen by the pregnant woman) Labour and birth in a private or public hospital/birth centre (with the obstetrician and/or hospital midwives)
Private midwifery care	Antenatal care – at home with a private midwife (chosen by the pregnant woman) Labour and birth at home with care provided by the private midwife, or in hospital (with care provided by the private midwife or hospital midwives)		

SOURCE FROM: AIHW, 2022C; STEVENS, THOMPSON, KRUSKE, WATSON & MILLER, 2014; QLD GOVERNMENT, 2022; MINISTRY OF HEALTH/MANATŪ HAUORA, 2021

Whichever model of primary maternity care a woman has, general nurses may also be required to assist in the care of the pregnant woman or her infant; therefore, a general knowledge of pregnancy and associated healthcare issues is important. As a midwife or nurse, you may be the woman's primary contact during the pregnancy and you play a critical role in helping the woman to achieve her health goals. Using active listening and a supportive approach, you can play an important role in helping the family understand what to expect during pregnancy.

A number of common pregnancy-related health issues that may be encountered:
> Common discomforts of pregnancy including nausea and vomiting, gastro-oesophageal reflux, constipation, backache, haemorrhoids, fatigue, urinary frequency
> Urinary tract infection
> Hypertensive disorders of pregnancy/pre-eclampsia
> Gestational diabetes
> Psychosocial changes/issues; for example, antenatal depression or anxiety, tokophobia (fear of birth), birth trauma and distress, or intimate partner violence.

HEALTH EDUCATION

Obesity and pregnancy

Almost 50% of all women who become pregnant are overweight (BMI > 25–30) or obese (BMI > 30) at their first antenatal visit (AIHW, 2022d). Women who are overweight or obese face increased morbidity and mortality risks for both mother and baby. These include an increased risk of miscarriage, thromboembolism, gestational diabetes, high blood pressure, pre-eclampsia, post-partum haemorrhage and wound infection. Caesarean birth is more common. Babies of mothers who are obese have higher rates of congenital anomaly, stillbirth, neonatal death, and an increased risk of childhood obesity, compared with babies of mothers who are not obese (RANZCOG, 2022; AIHW, 2022b).

>>

>>

Guidelines for the management of pregnant women who are overweight or obese stress the importance of counselling women regarding risks and the necessity of screening for possible adverse outcomes (RANZCOG, 2022). Nurses can encourage women to lose weight before they become pregnant, by referring them for guidance on lifestyle changes that include dietary and exercise advice. The provision of non-judgemental, supportive care through pregnancy and the postnatal period is important as it encourages women who are overweight or obese to remain engaged with health care.

For further information see: Australian Government Department of Health. (2020). *Clinical practice guidelines: Pregnancy care*. Canberra: Australian Government Department of Health. https://www.health.gov.au/resources/pregnancy-care-guidelines.

ANATOMY AND PHYSIOLOGY

Physiological changes during pregnancy affect every system in the body. These changes occur to maintain maternal health and accommodate the growth of the fetus. This chapter provides an overview of these changes and is not all-inclusive.

Skin and hair

The skin is subjected to the influence of hormones during pregnancy. There is an increased subdermal fat deposit, along with thickening of the skin. Acne may either develop or improve during pregnancy. Other changes include an increase in sweat and sebaceous gland production, which, along with the increase in superficial capillaries and peripheral vasodilation, serves to dissipate heat. Existing pigmentation increases in the nipples, areolae, external genitalia, and the anal region. The face may develop **melasma** (**Figure 19.1**), known as the mask of pregnancy, which manifests as blotchy, irregular pigmentation. **Linea nigra**, or darkening of the linea alba, may present on the abdomen as a darkened vertical mid-line between the fundus and the symphysis pubis (**Figure 19.2**). Linea nigra regresses, or fades, after birth, but does not totally disappear. Naevi, circumscribed pigmented areas of skin, may be stimulated to grow; and skin tags or molluscum fibrosum gravidarum may develop from epithelial hyperplasia, especially on the upper body. With connective tissue changes of pregnancy, **striae gravidarum** (stretch marks) often develop on the abdomen, breasts and upper thighs (**Figure 19.3**); after birth, they regress or fade but do not totally disappear.

Vascular changes reflected in the skin can include the development or enlargement of spider angiomas, haemangiomas, varicosities and palmar erythema, which may become more pronounced as pregnancy progresses.

Facial hair may increase, but the scalp hair may shed and thin, especially in the postpartum period. The scalp hair may become oily.

Head and neck

The thyroid gland may increase in size after approximately 12 weeks of gestation (although studies are conflicting as to whether or not there is an increase). Human chorionic gonadotropin (the hormone that is tested for in a pregnancy test) mimics thyrotropin and stimulates both the growth of the thyroid and an increase in production of thyroid hormones, leading to a reduction in thyrotropin levels. The shifts in hormone levels are most prominent in the first trimester. Adequate dietary iodine levels are important to maintain normal thyroid function in both the pregnant woman and her fetus.

Eyes, ears, nose, mouth and throat

Corneal thickening and oedema (especially in the third trimester) may occur, causing the pregnant woman to experience visual changes that typically resolve

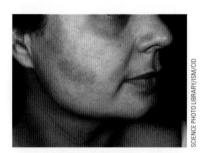

FIGURE 19.1 Melasma (left side), also known as the mask of pregnancy

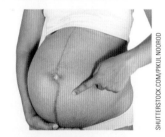

FIGURE 19.2 Linea nigra

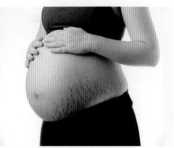

FIGURE 19.3 Striae gravidarum

shortly after birth. Contact lens wearers may also experience blurry vision secondary to increased lysozyme in tears, which may lead to an oily sensation.

Increased vascularity and increased mucus production often lead to nasal stuffiness, snoring, congestion and **epistaxis**, impaired hearing or fullness in the ears, and a decreased sense of smell. The pregnant woman should be reassured that these are normal experiences that usually resolve after birth.

Increased vascularity and hormonal changes often lead to soft, oedematous and bleeding gums, commonly noticed when brushing teeth. **Epulis**, or erythematous gingival nodules that bleed easily, can be present. Women often benefit from consultation with a dentist during pregnancy, as there is an association between periodontal disease and poor perinatal outcomes (Lachat, Solnik, Nana & Citron, 2011). **Ptyalism**, excessive secretion of saliva, may be an annoying symptom and, if marked, may require evaluation for other causes, such as goitre. Vocal changes or cough may be noted due to hormonally induced changes in the larynx.

Breasts

Early breast changes may include enlargement, tingling and tenderness secondary to hormonal changes. As the pregnancy progresses, the breasts continue to enlarge and the mammary glands prepare for lactation (alveoli increase in both number and size, Montgomery's tubercles enlarge, and lactiferous ducts proliferate). This may cause the breasts to feel more nodular on palpation than in the nonpregnant state. The areolae may darken. The nipples may become darker and more erect. **Colostrum**, a thick, yellow form of early breast milk, may be produced as early as the second trimester. Veins in the breasts may become more apparent and bluer, as they become engorged from increased vascularisation.

Thorax and lungs

The physiological changes of pregnancy lead to increased oxygen delivery and carbon dioxide excretion. This increases the availability of oxygen for the fetus and facilitates the transfer of carbon dioxide from the fetus to the maternal circulation for elimination. With advancing pregnancy, the diaphragm elevates approximately 4 cm and the movement of the diaphragm increases, so that most respiratory effort is diaphragmatic. Stimulated by progesterone, the thoracic cage relaxes and expands by 5 to 7 cm in circumference to accommodate these increased respiratory demands, and this may cause discomfort or pain as the intercostal muscles stretch. The tidal volume increases by 30–40% during pregnancy, probably due to the stimulatory effects of increased levels of progesterone. These physiological changes often lead to an increased respiratory rate, or increased awareness of breathing, especially on exertion such as climbing stairs.

Heart and blood vessels

Blood volume increases by 30–50% (largely due to rising plasma volume), thus increasing cardiac output. This process begins at 12 weeks of gestation and peaks at 28 to 34 weeks. This increase protects the mother from haemorrhage, increases oxygen transport, increases renal filtration, and dissipates fetal heat production. With cardiac dilatation (maximal by 10 weeks), the mother's heart lies more horizontally and shifts upwards and to the left along with the apical impulse. Heart rate increases by 10 to 20 beats per minute, a split first heart and S_3 sound and physiological systolic murmurs of grade 2/6 may be heard, and blood pressure varies according to maternal position and trimester. In addition, the increased breast vascularisation may lead to a continuous murmur, especially near the end of the pregnancy, known as the 'mammary souffle'. Supine hypotension, resulting from the weight of the uterus on the inferior vena cava, is common; it is recommended that pregnant women avoid a supine position after 20 weeks, unless there is a uterine tilt to the side. A lateral sleeping position alleviates the compression and can also reduce the risk of stillbirth. It is important to consider communication here, to convey the message without creating increased anxiety (Gordon et al., 2015).

HEALTH EDUCATION

Positions for sleeping or resting in late pregnancy

A side-lying position, with a pillow under the abdomen, behind the back or between the legs, may provide the most comfort (Figure 19.4).

> Educate to avoid supine sleeping positions during late pregnancy, which helps avoid supine hypotension.

> Supine sleeping in late pregnancy has been linked to a possible risk for late-pregnancy stillbirth in an already compromised fetus (Perinatal Society of Australia & New Zealand and Centre of Research Excellence Stillbirth. Position statement, 2019).

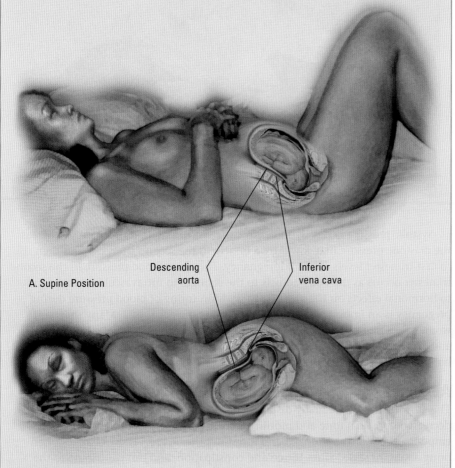

A. Supine Position

Descending aorta

Inferior vena cava

B. Right Lateral Position

FIGURE 19.4 A. Supine hypotension can occur when the woman is in the supine position. The weight of the gravid uterus may partially occlude the descending aorta and vena cava. B. Encouraging the woman to maintain a lateral sleeping position alleviates the compression.

Committed back sleepers may find comfort by placing a medium-sized pillow such as a body pillow underneath one side to displace uterine weight off the vena cava.

HEALTH EDUCATION

Managing leg oedema during pregnancy

Oedema of the lower extremities is common during late pregnancy. It is a result of hormone-induced sodium retention, and in late pregnancy it is due to the enlarged uterus putting pressure on the pelvic veins and inferior vena cava, slowing venous return. It may be especially noticeable after prolonged periods of sitting or standing. To minimise this, recommend that women:

> rest on the left side to favour venous return
> elevate the feet while sitting
> wear compression stockings
> avoid sitting for long periods – after 1 hour go for a short walk (**Figure 19.5**).

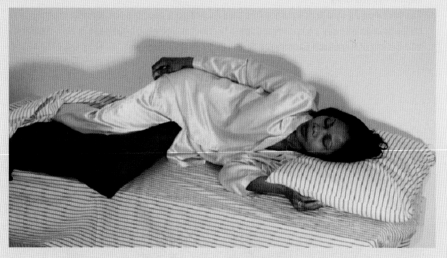

FIGURE 19.5 Resting in the lateral position helps to alleviate pooling of blood in the lower extremities.

Systolic pressure is not significantly different throughout pregnancy, whereas the diastolic pressure may lower by 5 mmHg in the second trimester and then rise to first-trimester levels after midpregnancy. The lower blood pressure in the second trimester occurs as the body adjusts to the changes in intravascular volume and to hormonal effects on the vascular walls. Monitoring of blood pressure during pregnancy is an important factor in diagnosing pre-eclampsia. Many pregnant women experience dependent oedema partially due to peripheral vasodilation and decreased vascular resistance. This swelling is most commonly seen in the feet, but can also occur in the hands and face.

Abdomen

The growing uterus gradually displaces the abdominal contents, leading to decreased intestinal tone and motility, decreased bowel sounds, and an increased emptying time for the stomach and intestines (**Figure 19.6**). These changes often bring about increased **flatulence** and constipation, and can contribute to the development of haemorrhoids.

Indigestion (heartburn) is often experienced by pregnant women due to relaxation of the oesophageal sphincter with subsequent reflux and slowed gastric emptying. Nausea and vomiting are common early in pregnancy and may lead to weight loss in the first trimester.

Increased emptying time and chemical changes in bile composition can put pregnant women at increased risk for **cholelithiasis**, the presence or formation of bilestones or calculi in the gall bladder or duct, and oestrogen may augment any tendency to develop **cholestasis** (arrest of bile excretion).

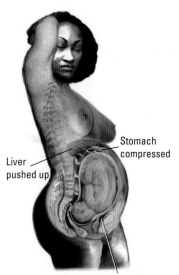

Liver pushed up

Stomach compressed

Bladder largely in pelvis therefore frequent urination

FIGURE 19.6 Crowding of abdominal contents by gravid uterus

Some women will also experience a separation of the rectus muscle of the abdominal wall, known as **diastasis recti**, which may be asymptomatic and noticed only as a vertical protrusion midline. Diastasis requires no medical intervention.

CLINICAL **REASONING**

Practice tip: Hyperemesis gravidarum

Severe nausea and vomiting in pregnancy is known as hyperemesis gravidarum. It is associated with rapid weight loss, malnutrition, dehydration and electrolyte abnormalities and may require hospitalisation. This could have potential maternal and neonatal adverse consequences; therefore, closely monitor women who are experiencing excessive nausea and vomiting, and refer as necessary (see Australian College of Midwives. (2021). *National midwifery guidelines for consultation and referral*, ACM, Canberra).

HEALTH EDUCATION

Managing gastrointestinal discomforts during pregnancy

Women may find it helpful to manage symptoms of nausea, vomiting, constipation and indigestion by:

> eating several small, frequent meals
> avoiding spicy and fatty foods and carbonated beverages
> drinking 8 to 10 glasses of water a day
> increasing dietary fibre or supplemental fibre
> exercising regularly
> getting adequate rest
> using antacids only in moderation and with healthcare provider approval.

Urinary system

Secondary to the increased intravascular volume, glomerular filtration rate (GFR) increases by approximately 50% and the reabsorption rate of various chemicals, especially sodium and water, changes. Urinary frequency usually increases in the first trimester. **Glycosuria**, glucose in the urine, is common in pregnancy. There is also an increased loss of amino acids that may show as mild **proteinuria** on a urine dipstick. Dilation of the ureters and renal pelvises, and a decrease in bladder tone place the pregnant woman at risk for urinary tract infection and asymptomatic bacteriuria. In both early and late pregnancy, the bladder is encroached upon by the enlarging uterus and fetal presenting parts. **Nocturia**, or excessive night-time urination, may disrupt the pregnant woman's sleep pattern.

HEALTH EDUCATION

Maintaining urinary health during pregnancy

Due to urinary system changes in pregnancy, urinary tract infections (UTI) can be an issue. The following strategies may assist the pregnant woman to avoid developing a UTI:

> Drink plenty of fluids, avoiding those with caffeine or sugar.
> Drink cranberry juice (particularly pure concentrated juice).
> Void frequently, especially after intercourse.
> Always wipe from front to back after voiding and having bowels open.

Musculoskeletal system

The hormones relaxin and progesterone affect all joints in the pregnant woman's body. This leads to a widening (and, occasionally, a separation) of the symphysis pubis at approximately 28 to 32 weeks, increased pelvic mobility to accommodate birth, and alteration in gait. These hormones also allow the thoracic cage to change shape, which can lead to complaints of upper back or rib pain.

Developing lordosis of the lumbar spine keeps the centre of gravity over the legs and is often associated with lower back pain. **Figure 19.7** shows the progression of lordosis in pregnancy. Sciatic nerve pain may also present as lower back pain, a shooting pain down the leg, or leg weakness. For unknown reasons, muscle cramps, particularly in the calves, thighs and buttocks, may develop, especially at night.

Shoe size may increase by as much as one full size as pregnancy progresses, due to oedema and relaxation of foot joints

HEALTH EDUCATION

Avoiding muscle cramps during pregnancy
To minimise muscle cramping, pregnant women may find it helpful to:
> perform muscle-stretching exercises
> wear low-heeled shoes
> consume adequate dietary calcium
> avoid excessive milk intake (higher phosphorus content may cause muscle cramps)
> take a calcium and/or magnesium supplement if required, and after collaboration with their healthcare provider.

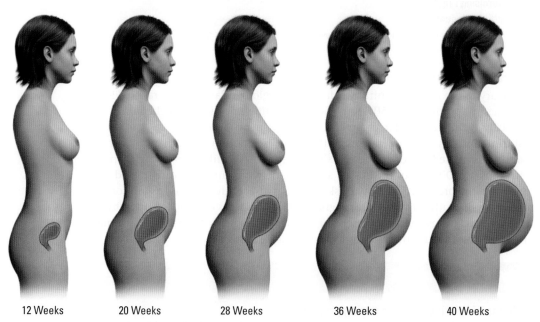

| 12 Weeks | 20 Weeks | 28 Weeks | 36 Weeks | 40 Weeks |

FIGURE 19.7 The progression of lordosis in pregnancy

HEALTH EDUCATION

Centre of balance during pregnancy (increasing awareness)
Women may be more susceptible to falls and accidents because of the change in their centre of balance. You should advise pregnant women to exercise caution when changing position, moving over uneven surfaces, ascending and descending stairs, and participating in activities such as riding a bicycle.

Neurological system

The most commonly experienced neurological changes in pregnancy include headaches, numbness and tingling. The more bothersome neuropathies include carpal tunnel syndrome, footdrop, facial palsy, fatigue and difficulty remaining asleep at night. After ruling out any underlying disorder, women can be reassured that these are temporary symptoms. Headaches may be relieved by small, frequent meals, adequate rest, and posture and work environment adjustments. Seizure activity with no prior history may indicate the development of **eclampsia**, or seizures associated with hypertensive disorders of pregnancy (HDP), also called pregnancy-induced hypertension (PIH). Dizziness and light-headedness may be due to uterine pressure on the vena cava. Lapses of memory are common, but the aetiology is poorly understood.

Female genitalia

The pelvic organs undergo vascular, hormonal and structural changes during pregnancy. Amenorrhea, secondary to the hormonal changes of pregnancy, is generally the first noticeable sign of pregnancy. Uterine vessels dilate progressively and at term can hold one-sixth of the maternal circulation, with a blood flow of 500 mL/min. With increased blood flow, a pregnant woman may note a feeling of pelvic congestion as well as vulvar oedema.

The pregnant woman's uterus begins as a pelvic organ, becoming enlarged at 6 to 7 weeks (**Figure 19.8**), and progresses to an abdominal organ at approximately 12 weeks of gestation. At 16 weeks the fundus of the uterus is midway between the symphysis pubis and the umbilicus, and at 20 weeks the fundus is typically at the umbilicus.

From 28 weeks of gestation until birth, the height of the uterine fundus above the symphysis pubis is measured in centimetres (and documented using a centile chart to plot the height) to assess fetal growth.

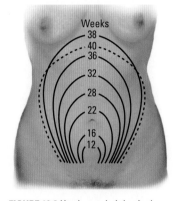

FIGURE 19.8 Uterine and abdominal enlargement of pregnancy

HEALTH EDUCATION

Reducing risk of vaginal candidiasis
During pregnancy the vaginal mucosa changes and becomes more alkaline. This increases the possibility of developing vaginal thrush (candidal) infection. Give advice on good vaginal hygiene practices that can reduce the possibility of developing vaginal thrush:
> Avoid clothing that fits tightly in the crotch.
> Choose underwear with a cotton rather than a nylon crotch.
> Remove a wet bathing suit promptly.
> Avoid vaginal douching.

The round and broad ligaments elongate to accommodate the growing fetus, and may cause the woman lower quadrant discomfort. **Lightening**, also called dropping, is a decrease in fundal height due to the descent of the presenting fetal part into the pelvis. This typically occurs in the weeks prior to the onset of labour in a nulliparous woman, and is accompanied by increased pressure in the pelvis and increased frequency of urination. In a **multiparous** woman, lightening may not occur until active labour begins. **Braxton Hicks contractions**, which are irregular and usually painless, begin as early as the first trimester.

The cervix experiences increased vascularity and increased **friability**, susceptibility to bleeding, especially following a cervical smear or intercourse. The endocervical glands increase in number and size. This causes a softening of the cervix. Mucus production occurs to form an endocervical protective plug, and the vaginal mucosa thickens secondary to hormonal changes. Throughout pregnancy, the vaginal discharge increases and is typically of a white, milky consistency, called leucorrhoea. From 36 weeks on, vaginal discharge may become noticeably thicker and clumps may be present when the mucus plug is expelled. The hormonally induced changes in the vaginal environment lead to an increased risk of candidal infection.

Anus and rectum

Decreased gastrointestinal tract tone and motility produce a sense of fullness, indigestion, constipation, bloating and flatulence. Development of haemorrhoids is common and can become very problematic. As pregnancy progresses and the uterus enlarges, mechanical pressure may aggravate constipation and haemorrhoids. Vitamin and iron supplementation may increase these symptoms and commonly darken the stool.

Haematological system

Common haematological changes include increased white blood cell (WBC) count, increased total red blood cell (RBC) volume, increased plasma volume, decreased number and increased size of platelets, and increased fibrinogen and clotting factors VII to X. The relatively larger increase in plasma volume compared to RBC volume leads to physiological anaemia of pregnancy. The coagulation changes protect against haemorrhage at birth but may also put the pregnant woman at increased risk for thromboembolic disease, such as deep vein thrombosis (DVT). The maternal immunological system is also less resistant to infection due to a decreased cellular immune response.

Endocrine system

The basal metabolic rate (BMR) increases by 15–25% due to increased oxygen consumption and to fetal metabolic demands. This can often lead to feelings of warmth and heat intolerance.

As pregnancy progresses, an increasing resistance to insulin develops, causing pregnancy to be called a 'diabetogenic state'. Causes for this phenomenon are incompletely understood but are partially related to placental manufacture of the enzyme insulinase. This process occurs to ensure adequate amounts of glucose for fetal demands. Glycosuria may be noted because the distant renal tubules cannot respond to the increased amount of glucose in the circulatory system. Pregnancy-induced glucose intolerance or diabetes can be a risk factor for future development of noninsulin-dependent diabetes mellitus.

ASSESSMENT: TAKING THE WOMAN'S HEALTH HISTORY

Assessment is the first phase of the nursing process, and involves collecting subjective information about the woman's health status in order to identify any problem areas to focus on.

Subjective data is most frequently collected during a health history and serves as the starting point for the health professional to base the depth of their assessment on. The sections for the health history include:

> **Woman's profile**
> **Current pregnancy symptoms** (explained systematically using variations of location, quality, quantity, associated manifestations, aggravating factors, alleviating factors, setting and timing. This is a variation on the OPQRST assessment mnemonic you may use for other conditions such as pain assessment)
> **Past health history** (including medical history, surgical history, allergies, medications, injuries and accidents, special needs and childhood illnesses)
> **Family health history**
> **Social history** (including alcohol, tobacco and drug use, sexual practice, work and home environment, hobbies and leisure activities, stress and culture).

HEALTH HISTORY

PROFILE		The pregnant woman's health history provides insight into her life, lifestyle and pregnancy-related information and pathology.
		The health history for the pregnant woman is generally recorded on a form designed specifically for pregnancy. These forms capture information about the woman from early pregnancy to birth, as well as for the newborn. They cover standard health history questions, any prior obstetric history, family history, current signs and symptoms, examination findings, and laboratory data. This comprehensive approach is useful for directing risk-factor assessment and developing a plan of management.
		Table 19.2 illustrates a typical maternity history. Diseases that are age- and race-specific for pregnancy are listed.
	AGE	Being under 17 or over 35 for first pregnancy can put a woman at increased risk for various pregnancy complications such as pre-eclampsia, gestational diabetes, genetic disorders, twins, miscarriage, operative delivery and preterm labour and/or delivery.
	CULTURAL BACKGROUND	A woman's cultural background should be considered to ensure that culturally safe care is provided.
CURRENT PREGNANCY SYMPTOMS		A maternity history includes questions about the woman's current pregnancy, such as fetal movements, and any vaginal discharge or bleeding, and aims to identify any concerns and/or information needs of the woman.
PAST HEALTH HISTORY		Conditions that may impact on pregnancy, or that may be impacted on by pregnancy should be sought and noted.
	MEDICAL HISTORY	Asthma, diabetes mellitus, cardiac disease, renal disease, seizure disorder, autoimmune disorders
	SURGICAL HISTORY	Uterine surgery, cone or excisional biopsy of the cervix, abdominal surgery leading to internal or external scarring or adhesions
	ALLERGIES	Symptoms may change with pregnancy. Non-prescribed medications for allergy should be reviewed as some are not advised for use in pregnancy.
	MEDICATIONS	Certain medications for chronic conditions may be continued during pregnancy, such as methyldopa and hydralazine for hypertension, and metformin for diabetes. Other medications may have a teratogenic effect on the fetus; for example, coumadin/warfarin, which should be changed to heparin. Medications for seizure disorders or psychiatric conditions should be discussed in terms of risk–benefit ratio for both the mother and the fetus, as well as any possible alternative medications for use during pregnancy and lactation. Some over-the-counter medications such as paracetamol are considered safe during pregnancy. Prescribers should always ask whether women are (or plan to become) pregnant or lactating prior to making a medication recommendation.
	COMMUNICABLE DISEASES	TORCH diseases (toxoplasmosis, rubella, cytomegalovirus, herpes), measles, varicella, mumps, human parvovirus B19, HIV, hepatitis B, a rubella titre, rapid plasma reagent (RPR) or venereal disease research laboratory (VDRL), and hepatitis B surface antigen are routinely offered to all pregnant women. HIV testing is recommended, following pre-test counselling. Rubella (German measles), especially in the first trimester, and syphilis during pregnancy can cause fetal anomalies and other complications. Other infectious diseases may affect the pregnancy, depending on their severity and the gestational age at which the disease is contracted; e.g. COVID-19 can cause increased risk of severe illness and increase risk of premature birth; varicella may present a problem to the fetus if active at the time of birth. Other infectious diseases to review include tuberculosis and sexually transmitted infections (STIs).
	INJURIES AND ACCIDENTS	Any trauma that leads to abdominal scarring or injury to the pelvic organs themselves may affect pregnancy; injuries to the back may also be of concern.
	SPECIAL NEEDS	Disabilities and handicaps do not generally interfere with pregnancy. Some neuromuscular disorders such as myasthenia gravis may affect muscle response as pregnancy progresses and during labour. Paralysis does not interfere with pregnancy other than impacting the woman's ability to note significant changes in her physical status (e.g. change in vaginal discharge or increase in uterine contractions).

HEALTH HISTORY

	CHILDHOOD ILLNESSES	Rheumatic heart disease, if mitral valve stenosis developed, may put the woman at risk for endocarditis, and prophylactic antibiotics may be advised around the time of birth. Knowledge of childhood diseases leading to immunity may decrease anxiety if exposure to those illnesses occurs during pregnancy.
	IMMUNISATIONS	Typically, immunisations, especially those containing live viruses, should be avoided during pregnancy. The COVID vaccine, hepatitis B series and tetanus toxoid are not contraindicated during pregnancy. Any unavoidable travel to an area with known infectious disease risk requires a discussion of the risk–benefit ratio of immunisation. Immune status testing should be encouraged at any preconceptual visit. If immune status is unknown or immune status testing reveals a lack of adequate titres, rubella and varicella immunisations should be given, along with instructions to avoid pregnancy for 3 months. Whooping cough and flu vaccines are recommended later in last trimester.
FAMILY HEALTH HISTORY	Pregnancy-related conditions and diseases that are familial are listed.	
	Preterm labour or birth; hypertensive disorders of pregnancy; diethylstilboestrol (DES) exposure; multiple births in female relatives of the pregnant woman's mother; chromosome abnormalities such as Down syndrome; genetic disorders such as Tay-Sachs or Gaucher diseases or sickle cell disease; inheritable diseases such as Huntington's chorea; congenital anomalies such as cleft lip or palate; neural tube defects; cardiac deformities; blood disorders; diabetes (gestational, non-insulin dependent, insulin dependent); neuromuscular diseases; psychiatric disorders; any history of abuse, neglect or substance abuse Family history of baby's father: genetic, hereditary or chromosomal disorders, abuse or neglect, substance abuse	
SOCIAL HISTORY	The components of the social history are linked to pregnancy factors and pathology.	
	ALCOHOL USE	Can lead to fetal alcohol syndrome (FAS). The absolute safe level of alcohol consumption is unknown. Women should be advised to avoid alcohol.
	TOBACCO USE	Smoking can lead to a small-for-gestational-age (SGA) infant, preterm labour, spontaneous abortion, and lower Apgar scores (refer to Table 20.3 Apgar scoring). The effects are dose-related, and tobacco use during pregnancy should be discontinued. Referral to a smoking cessation program should be offered to all women who smoke, and nicotine replacement therapy may be considered. With a history of smoking or secondary smoke exposure, smoking status should be checked frequently throughout pregnancy.
	ILLICIT DRUG USE	The effects on the fetus vary according to the drug(s) used and gestational age at the time of use. The most common complications are spontaneous abortion, preterm birth, congenital anomalies and stillbirth. Some drugs, such as cocaine and heroin, lead to withdrawal symptoms in the newborn infant. Cocaine use is associated with a high incidence of abruptio placenta and preterm birth.
	SEXUAL PRACTICE	Sexual expression or practice throughout pregnancy is not contraindicated unless there are specific reasons to do so, such as placenta praevia or prelabour rupture of the membranes. Women remain at risk during pregnancy for acquiring STIs and should be advised to use condoms if they are at risk for these.
	TRAVEL HISTORY	Ask about travel to regions at risk for infectious diseases. Air travel should be taken only in pressurised cabins. Pregnant women should move about every hour, drink plenty of liquids, and travel with enough food for small, frequent meals or snacks.
	WORK ENVIRONMENT	Prolonged sitting or standing; heavy lifting; an extremely loud, cold or wet environment; work with chemicals, lead or mercury; or a one-way commute greater than 1 hour may put the pregnant woman at risk for preterm labour or congenital anomalies in the newborn. Employers have an obligation to provide a safe workplace for their employees, and this includes during pregnancy.
	HOME ENVIRONMENT	The pregnant woman should avoid toxic chemicals; exposure to toxoplasmosis should be avoided by not cleaning cat litter boxes and by wearing gloves and washing hands after gardening. Physical work should be avoided if it either leads to excessive contractions or aggravates pregnancy discomforts.

>>

HEALTH HISTORY

	HOBBIES AND LEISURE ACTIVITIES	May be continued during the pregnancy unless they present a physical risk such as certain high-risk sports, including skiing and horseback riding.
	PSYCHOSOCIAL	Exposure to violence and susceptibility for depression can contribute significantly to maternal mortality. Antenatal care provides an opportunity to ask women about exposure to violence especially at home or in their family; she may be a victim of intimate partner violence. Women should be given an explanation of the purpose of the questions (e.g. identifying any need for psychosocial support) and asked for their permission. Asking questions should be done in a sensitive way, using open-ended questions about her perception of safety at home or can be done with the use of an assessment tool. The aim is to identify psychosocial factors without detracting from the normal experiences of pregnancy and motherhood. If there are issues, enable access to additional support and care, including community, legal and police support services. It is also an opportunity to identify the potential for depression and related disorders that can occur in the perinatal period. Ask about previous or current mental health disorders, and if a woman affirms their presence, ask whether she would like help with any of these issues. (Note: the Edinburgh Postnatal Depression Scale (EPDS) screening tool should be implemented early in the pregnancy.)

TABLE 19.2 Maternity history

PRESENT PREGNANCY HISTORY

> Last menstrual period (LMP)
> Menstrual cycles (menarche, frequency, duration)
> History since LMP (e.g. fever, rashes, disease exposures, abnormal bleeding, nausea and vomiting, medication use, toxic exposures)
> Signs and symptoms of pregnancy
> Use of fertility drugs
> Contraception
> Estimated date of birth (EDB)*

PAST PREGNANCY HISTORY

> Gravidity (number of pregnancies)
> Parity (number of births 20 weeks or greater); usually listed as term (37–42 weeks gestational age), preterm (20–37 weeks gestational age) or post-term (>42 weeks gestational age)
> Miscarriage
> Pregnancy termination
> Ectopic pregnancy
> Multiple pregnancy (more than one fetus)
> Number of living children
> Pregnancy history (see **Table 19.3**: Woman who may require additional care):
  • Complications during pregnancy
  • Duration of gestation
  • Date of birth
  • Type of birth (spontaneous vaginal, instrumental, caesarean); if not spontaneous, reason for intervention
  • Perineal trauma (episiotomy or laceration, and degree)
  • Length of labour
  • Medications and anaesthesia used
  • Complications during labour and birth
  • Postpartum complications, including depression
> Infant weight and sex, APGAR scores (Appearance, Pulse, Grimace, Activity, Respiration; see Chapter 20 on APGAR scoring)
> Infant health issues
> Type of feeding (breastfeeding versus artificial feeding)
> Breastfeeding duration

Note: To manually determine the EDB, use Naegele's rule: subtract 3 months from the first day of the LMP, then add 7 days. This is based on a 28-day cycle and may have to be adjusted for shorter or longer cycles. For example, if the LMP is 1 September:

1 September – 3 months = 1 June
1 June + 7 days = 8 June
The EDB for this woman is 8 June.

A gestation wheel may also be used (see **Figure 19.9**), but these may be inaccurate. Use of an 'app' or computer software embedded in the electronic medical records is used to calculate an accurate EDB and the current gestation.

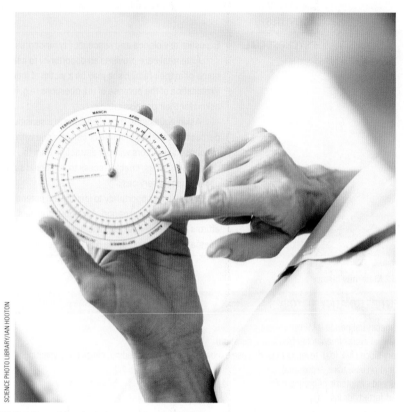

SCIENCE PHOTO LIBRARY/IAN HOOTON

FIGURE 19.9 Gestation calculation wheel used to determine EDB. 'First day of LMP' arrow is placed on that date. The other arrow, labelled 'expected birth date', shows the expected date of birth.

CLINICAL REASONING

Practice tip: Gravidity and parity abbreviations

You can summarise women's prior pregnancy history by using the following abbreviations. During the initial visit it is important to note all of the categories.

In subsequent visits, not all categories are required to be documented, just the number of pregnancies (gravida) and births (para).

> G = gravida
> P = para
> T = term
> P = preterm
> A = abortion (either therapeutic or spontaneous; may be listed separately)
> E = ectopic pregnancy
> LC = living children
   Examples:
> G 4, P 2, T 2, P 0, A 1, E 1, LC 2 = 4 pregnancies, 2 births, 2 term births, 0 preterm births, 1 abortion, 1 ectopic pregnancy, 2 living children
> G 3, P 3, T 2, P 1, A 0, E 0, LC 4 = 3 pregnancies, 3 births, 2 term births, 1 preterm birth, 0 abortions, 0 ectopic pregnancies, 4 living children (preterm birth 5, 1 set of twins)
> G 3, P 3 = 3 pregnancies, 3 births
> G 4, P 3, A 1 = 4 pregnancies, 3 births, 1 abortion
> G 4, P 3, T 2, P 1, A 1, E 0, LC 2 = 4 pregnancies, 3 births, 2 term births, 1 preterm birth, 1 abortion, 0 ectopic pregnancies, 2 living children

TABLE 19.3 Woman who may require additional care

To optimise pregnancy care in partnership with the woman, some circumstances may indicate a need for a referral for obstetric review (for more information see Australian College of Midwives (2021), *National midwifery guidelines for consultation and referral*, ACM, Canberra).

EXISTING CONDITIONS

> Cardiovascular disease (hypertension)
> Renal disease, pyelonephritis, asymptomatic bacteriuria
> Diabetes mellitus
> Sickle cell disease
> Anaemia
> Pulmonary disease
> Endocrine disorder
> Mental health disorders
> Female genital mutilation

REPRODUCTIVE HISTORY

> More than one prior termination
> More than two miscarriages
> Four or more previous births
> Ante-natal or post-natal haemorrhage
> Gestational diabetes
> Previous caesarean section
> Perinatal death
> Pre-eclampsia or eclampsia
> Preterm birth or premature labour, or both
> Delivery of infant less than 2500 g
> Delivery of infant greater than 4000 g
> Delivery of infant with congenital or perinatal disease
> Delivery of infant with isoimmunisation or ABO incompatibility
> Postpartum psychosis

PREVIOUS MAJOR SURGERY

> Bariatric (gastric bypass, lap-banding)
> Gastrointestinal (e.g. bowel resection)
> Gynaecological (e.g. myomectomy, cone biopsy, large loop excision of the transformation zone [LLETZ])
> Cardiac (including correction of congenital anomalies)

LIFE STYLE CONSIDERATIONS

> Alcohol consumption
> Recreational drug use, such as marijuana, heroin, cocaine (including crack cocaine), amphetamines (e.g. 'ice') and ecstasy

PSYCHOSOCIAL FACTORS

> Abusive relationship and other violence or family relationship stresses
> Developmental delay or other disabilities
> Vulnerability or lack of social support

ADAPTED FROM: AUSTRALIAN GOVERNMENT DEPARTMENT OF HEALTH. (2020). *CLINICAL PRACTICE GUIDELINES: PREGNANCY CARE*. CANBERRA: AUSTRALIAN GOVERNMENT DEPARTMENT OF HEALTH. HTTPS://WWW.HEALTH.GOV.AU/RESOURCES/PREGNANCY-CARE-GUIDELINES

PERSON-CENTRED HEALTH EDUCATION

When conducting a health assessment, opportunities for the provision of woman-centred health education will arise. Women should be asked at each point of contact with a health professional whether they have questions or informational needs, and education should be tailored to meet the specific needs of the individual. Often this can be provided by the clinician during the consultation. Formal childbirth classes, or education specific to particular pregnancy conditions (for example, diabetes education) are provided by professionals with specific skills in these areas. All education given should be documented so that in future, health professionals don't repeat information that has been previously provided, and can check whether women have follow-up questions. (Refer to Chapter 1 for initiating health education.) Refer to the following examples.

INDIVIDUALISED HEALTH EDUCATION INTERVENTIONS	
Assessing the pregnant woman for the following health-related activities can assist in identifying the need for education about these factors. This information provides a bridge between the health maintenance activities and pregnancy.	
Sleep	Increased demand, complicated frequently by nocturia or difficulty in finding and maintaining a comfortable position.
Diet	All meats should be well cooked and all dairy products should be pasteurised to prevent infections such as toxoplasmosis and listeria.
Exercise	Normal activities may be continued and exercise may help with some of the common complaints such as constipation. Exercise done in moderation is beneficial, but any exercise should be discontinued or modified if pain occurs. Care should be taken to avoid overheating, especially in humid weather, and water intake should be increased as needed.
Use of safety devices	Seat belts are recommended, with the lap portion worn below the pregnant abdomen.
Health check-ups	Cervical screening tests as recommended by national guidelines; avoid X-rays.

PLANNING FOR PHYSICAL EXAMINATION

The planning phase (in consultation with the woman) refers to evaluating subjective data to narrow the focus on physical examination, determining what objective data needs to be gathered, as well as considering the environment and equipment that will be required.

At this time, you will identify which of the four diagnostic techniques you will need to implement the physical examination, and how you will sequence these. For the physical examination of the pregnant woman you will include inspection, palpation, percussion and auscultation.

Objective data is:

> collected during the physical examination of the woman

> usually collected after subjective data

> information that is measured or observed by the clinician as opposed to being reported by the woman

> vital to the overall health assessment, to enable you to make clinical decisions that are representative of the whole woman's health picture.

Evaluating subjective data to focus physical assessment

Before commencing the physical examination of the pregnant woman, consider what information the health history has provided. Critical consideration, linked to knowledge of anatomy and physiology, should focus the physical assessment so your examination will be more effective and efficient.

Environment

The assessment and examination of a pregnant woman can be done in most physical environments in healthcare settings that provide the level of privacy that is required. Reassuring the pregnant woman that privacy will be maintained during the assessment by providing screens and/or closing the door will assist her to feel more at ease during the assessment.

Equipment

> For foundation assessment
  - Stethoscope
  - Doppler or **fetoscope** (Pinards stethoscope)
  - Centimetre tape measure
  - Watch with a second hand
  - Nonsterile gloves
  - Sphygmomanometer
  - Urine cup
  - Urine dipsticks
> If cervical screening is required: (as above plus following)
  - Speculum
  - Cervical screening supplies (see Chapter 17)

IMPLEMENTATION: CONDUCTING THE PHYSICAL EXAMINATION

Implementation of the physical examination requires you to consider your scope of practice and assessment skills.

EXAMINATION **IN BRIEF: THE PREGNANT WOMAN***

General approach to examination of the pregnant woman	Leopold's manoeuvres
Uterine size	> First manoeuvre
Fundal height by centimetres	> Second manoeuvre
Fetal heart rate	> Third manoeuvre
	> Fourth manoeuvre
	*Only pregnancy-specific assessments are listed.

Assessment of the pregnant woman includes a comprehensive initial examination as well as subsequent specific follow-up examinations largely focused on fetal growth. The initial assessment and examination occurs when the pregnant woman first seeks care. Encourage her to seek antenatal care by 10 weeks of gestation. Pre-conception care is not often utilised, but is recommended. This is especially important for women with pre-existing medical problems such as diabetes mellitus, cardiac disease or seizure disorders. Following the initial assessment and examination, the schedule for antenatal visits is then personalised to the individual woman (Australian Government Department of Health, 2020) depending on their needs and health history. For a woman's first pregnancy without complications, a schedule of 10 visits is sufficient; for subsequent uncomplicated pregnancies, seven visits is adequate. A woman whose pregnancy extends beyond the 40th week of gestation requires additional support and assessment. Antenatal care should be woman-focused, with each antenatal visit structured around specific content based on the woman's needs. The following examination guidelines discuss how each system examination is different for the pregnant woman than for the nonpregnant woman. See the previous chapters for the specific assessment of each system. The goal of the first consultation assessment and examination is to first confirm pregnancy and gestational age, and also to evaluate general health, so you can provide any needed intervention and education to the pregnant woman to maintain and promote her health as well as that of the fetus. See **Table 19.4** for signs and symptoms of pregnancy. In addition, antenatal care provides guidance for the labour and birth process and can be viewed as the foundation for a healthy family.

TABLE 19.4 Signs and symptoms of pregnancy

PRESUMPTIVE*	PROBABLE**	POSITIVE***
> Amenorrhea > Breast tenderness and enlargement > Fatigue > Changes in skin pigmentation > Nausea, vomiting, or both > Urinary frequency	> Abdominal enlargement > Uterine changes > Cervical changes > Braxton Hicks contractions > Ballottement > Quickening > Positive pregnancy test – HCG in blood or urine	> Fetal heart beats > Fetal movement > Fetal outline on palpation > Ultrasound

*Presumptive: Signs or symptoms that are associated with pregnancy but are not conclusive
**Probable: Signs or symptoms that are more indicative of pregnancy, including physical assessment changes
***Positive: Signs or symptoms that confirm a definite pregnancy

General approach to examination of the pregnant woman

1. Introduce yourself to the woman and explain how the assessment will proceed. Ensure that you have her specific consent before proceeding. Offer her a chaperone.
2. Ensure that the examination room is ready and supplies are at hand.
3. Use a quiet room where her privacy is ensured.
4. Ensure that there is adequate lighting, including a light that is appropriate for the pelvic assessment.
5. Offer the woman the option to void prior to the examination, both for her comfort and to facilitate uterine and adnexal evaluation (which can be impeded by a full bladder). The urine can be saved if further testing is required.
6. For the physical assessment, ask the woman to loosen her clothing to facilitate the examination and cover her lower body with a sheet.
7. Perform the initial assessment in a head-to-toe manner. Minimise the pregnant woman's time in the supine position, and use a wedge under her hip if this is not possible. Always inform her before touching her of what you will be doing and what to expect ('This may pinch', 'You may feel some pressure', and so on). Special sensitivity should be given to adolescents and the woman who is having her first pelvic examination. The woman may be dizzy upon sitting up or upon standing. It may be beneficial to assist her to a sitting position or to brace her arm. She should be cautioned not to stand or sit up abruptly.

Examination of the pregnant woman
General assessment, vital signs and weight

E 1. Conduct a general assessment, including obtaining vital signs.
While taking the pregnant woman's blood pressure:
- The woman should be seated in a comfortable position with her feet on a flat surface; a supine position should be avoided because of supine hypotension syndrome. Allow 2–3 minutes rest before taking measurement.
- Blood pressure should be taken on both arms at the initial visit, to exclude rare vascular abnormalities (such as subclavian stenosis and aortic dissection).
- It is important that the correct cuff size is used for accurate blood pressure recording, as this reduces the over-diagnosis of hypertension during pregnancy (Queensland Health, 2021).
- Palpate systolic pressure at the brachial artery, and inflate a further 20 mmHg above this.

E Examination **N** Normal findings **A** Abnormal findings **P** Pathophysiology

- Record BP using Korotkoff phase V (i.e. when sounds disappear) as this is the better estimation of true diastolic pressure (Campbell, Sultan & Pillarisetty, 2022).
2. Measure the woman's weight (**Figure 19.10**).

See Chapter 6 for normal general assessment, and the Anatomy and physiology section of this chapter for blood pressure changes that occur in pregnancy. See Chapter 15 for the recommended weight gain in pregnancy. See **Table 19.5** for common discomforts of pregnancy.

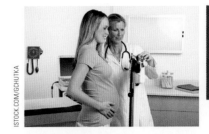

FIGURE 19.10 The pregnant woman's weight is determined at each antenatal visit.

TABLE 19.5 Common discomforts in pregnancy

ISSUE	RELIEF MEASURES
Backache, sciatic pain, femoral nerve pain	For posture, stand with abdomen pulled in and buttocks tucked in. Do cat-arch exercises and stretching exercises for legs, gluteal muscles and back. Avoid bending at waist – bend at knees to pick up objects from floor. If available, attend a pregnancy exercise class or program. Wear flat, comfortable shoes. A maternity girdle or support can be helpful, as can local heat and massage.
Bleeding gums	Maintain good dental hygiene. Use a soft toothbrush and floss regularly.
Breast soreness, tenderness or tingling	A well-fitting, supportive bra, worn as much as 24 hours a day.
Constipation	High-fibre diet and 8–10 glasses of water a day plus exercise.
Difficulty sleeping	Pillows for support, between legs, under abdomen and shoulders. Exercise, a warm bath before bed. Avoid caffeine. Go to bed at the same time every night.
Dizziness	Avoid sudden position changes or prolonged standing, especially in heat or a closed room. Eat and drink frequently.
Fatigue	Increased rest and relaxation, which may necessitate a change to less intense work at home and in employment.
Haemorrhoids	Avoid constipation. Local treatment with local anaesthetic cream will reduce burning and itching. Rest in left lateral position.
Headache	Frequent meals and increased rest. If severe, discuss with healthcare provider.
Heartburn	Eat small, frequent meals; avoid foods that aggravate heartburn (e.g. spicy or fatty foods, and carbonated drinks). If severe, discuss medication with provider.
Increased vaginal fluid	It is acceptable to wash more often with plain tepid water, or a mild, non-irritating soap and water. Douching is not safe. Panty liners may be necessary. Tell your healthcare provider if you notice an odour, itching, or unusual colour. Report any episode of bleeding.
Leg cramps	Make sure dietary calcium is sufficient (dairy products, dark, leafy vegetables), but avoid an excessive milk intake (calcium in the form of phosphate); calcium carbonate supplement may be indicated (particularly for women with lactose intolerance) and/or a magnesium supplement. Stretching exercises, flexing calf muscle; avoid hyperextending calf muscle.
Oedema	Left lateral position for rest. Drink plenty of fluids.
Shortness of breath	Extra pillows under head, shoulders or upper back may help relieve pressure on the diaphragm, especially late in pregnancy. If this persists or worsens seek advice from your healthcare provider.
Stuffy nose	Avoid allergens (cats, sleeping with window open) when possible. Saline nasal products may be helpful.
Sweating/acne/melasma/ptyalism	Dress in layers. Fans may help at home or desk. Maintain hygiene, but avoid over-cleaning, especially face so as not to irritate skin. Avoid prolonged sun exposure. Wear sunscreen when outside.
Urinary changes (increased frequency, urinary incontinence)	Maintain fluid intake. Wear a pad designed for urinary incontinence. Consult your healthcare provider if dysuria or discharge is present.
Varicose veins	Left lateral position for rest. Frequent movement of legs if work requires prolonged standing or sitting. Support stockings or even antiembolism-type stockings may be helpful.

E Examination   **N** Normal findings   **A** Abnormal findings   **P** Pathophysiology

Ⓐ Hypertension at any time in pregnancy is considered abnormal. In pregnancy, hypertension is defined as a systolic pressure greater than 140 mmHg and a diastolic pressure greater than 90 mmHg. This is assessed by taking the blood pressure twice, at least 6 hours apart. Hypertension noted prior to 20 weeks is most likely chronic hypertension. After 20 weeks, hypertension is related to hypertensive disorders of pregnancy (also referred to as pregnancy-induced hypertension (PIH)). **Table 19.6** lists additional information on hypertensive disorders during pregnancy.

TABLE 19.6 Hypertensive disorders of pregnancy

GESTATIONAL HYPERTENSION
> Blood pressure is elevated during the second half of pregnancy or 3 months postpartum without other features of pre-eclampsia. > Blood pressure returns to normal by three months, and often within 2 weeks of birth. > Gestational hypertension generally does not require treatment.

PRE-ECLAMPSIA
Hypertension: Systolic blood pressure of 140 mmHg or greater or a diastolic blood pressure of 90 mmHg or greater, when accompanied by one or more of the following: > Renal involvement – proteinuria, oliguria, elevated creatinine > Haematological involvement – thrombocytopaenia, haemolysis, disseminated intravascular coagulation > Liver involvement – raised liver function tests, liver pain > Neurological involvement – headache, hyperreflexia, visual disturbances, seizures (eclampsia) > Pulmonary oedema > Fetal growth restriction > Placental abruption

SEVERE PRE-ECLAMPSIA	
> BP of at least 160/110 on two separate occasions at least 6 hours apart > 5 g protein in 24-hour urine sample or persistent 3–4+ proteinuria on dipstick > Oliguria: <500 mL for 24 hours > Neurological symptoms: altered level of consciousness, headache, blurred vision or scotomata	> Pulmonary oedema > Epigastric or RUQ pain > Impaired liver function > Thrombocytopaenia: platelet count ≤100 000 mm³ > Elevated serum creatinine >73 mmol/L

ECLAMPSIA
> Signs or symptoms of pre-eclampsia plus > Development of seizures

CHRONIC HYPERTENSION
> Hypertension present prior to pregnancy or diagnosed <20 weeks > Hypertension persists >42 days postpartum

CHRONIC HYPERTENSION WITH SUPERIMPOSED PRE-ECLAMPSIA
> Chronic hypertension and showing signs of developing pre-eclampsia > Appearance of oedema or proteinuria

(For more information see: Australian Government Department of Health. (2020). *Clinical practice guidelines: Pregnancy care*. Canberra: Australian Government Department of Health.)

Ⓟ The pathophysiology of pre-eclampsia is still being researched.

Ⓐ A weight gain that is more than the recommended amount is abnormal.

Ⓟ Excessive weight gain may be due to increased caloric intake, multifetal pregnancy, polyhydramnios or oedema secondary to pre-eclampsia.

Ⓐ A weight gain that is less than the recommended amount is abnormal.

Ⓔ Examination Ⓝ Normal findings Ⓐ Abnormal findings Ⓟ Pathophysiology

P Weight loss or insufficient weight gain in pregnancy can be due to hyperemesis gravidarum, decreased caloric intake, and malabsorption syndromes.

Skin and hair

E Examine the skin and hair.

N See Chapter 8 and the Anatomy and physiology section of this chapter.

A **Prurigo** of pregnancy presents as excoriated papules, which are highly pruritic and usually distributed on the hands and feet, but in more severe cases may be noted on the upper trunk. They are most commonly found in mid to late pregnancy and are abnormal.

P Aetiology is poorly understood, but there is no increase in fetal mortality, and the eruptions fade after delivery.

A Papular dermatitis of pregnancy may manifest at any time during pregnancy as erythematous, pruritic, widespread, soft papules. These papules are typically 3–5 mm in size and are surmounted by smaller, firmer papules or small crusts. There tend to be several new eruptions daily, and those already present heal in 7–10 days, possibly with hyperpigmentation. Papular dermatitis is abnormal.

P The pathophysiology of these lesions is poorly understood. Papular dermatitis is associated with an increased risk for fetal loss, which may be significantly reduced by the use of oral prednisone.

A Erythematous plaques that develop into vesicular lesions that may become pustular are abnormal.

P Primary genital herpes (see Chapter 17) contracted in the first trimester places the fetus at risk for abnormalities. In the absence of a preformed immune response it is likely to cross the placental barrier, possibly leading to fetal abnormalities. Recurrent genital herpes infection carries a less severe outcome throughout the pregnancy. If herpes lesions are present at the onset of labour, caesarean section may be recommended in order to avoid transmission to the infant.

A Rashes are generally abnormal and should be further investigated.

P These should be evaluated for infectious, collagen or other disease aetiology as described in Chapter 8.

Head and neck

E N See Chapter 9 and the Anatomy and physiology section of this chapter.

A The appearance of hyperthyroidism or hypothyroidism is abnormal in pregnancy.

P Neoplastic disorders such as choriocarcinoma, ovarian teratoma and **hydatidiform mole**, as well as a single active thyroid nodule or multinodular goitre, should be considered with the diagnosis of hyperthyroidism in the pregnant woman.

Eyes, ears, nose, mouth and throat

E N See Chapters 10 and 11 and the Anatomy and physiology section of this chapter.

A Arterial constriction of retinal vessels is abnormal. This may lead to blurred vision, scotomata and, rarely, a retinal detachment.

P This can occur in pre-eclampsia.

A Any growth in the mouth is abnormal.

P Some women develop pregnancy tumours (epulis) in their mouths (**Figure 19.11**). These growths are usually benign. The vascular proliferation occurs secondary to hormonal changes. They may not resolve at the end of pregnancy.

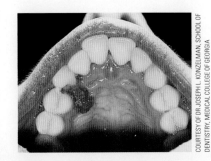

COURTESY OF DR JOSEPH L. KONZELMAN, SCHOOL OF DENTISTRY, MEDICAL COLLEGE OF GEORGIA

FIGURE 19.11 Pregnancy tumour

E Examination   **N** Normal findings   **A** Abnormal findings   **P** Pathophysiology

| Press just behind areola | Normal nipple protraction |
| Pseudo-inverted | Inverted |

FIGURE 19.12 Assessing for protractivity of the nipple

Breasts

E
1. Examine the breasts as described in Chapter 12.
2. Don gloves.
3. Assess the shape of each nipple by putting your thumb and index finger on the areola and pressing inwards to express any discharge. Note whether the nipple protracts (becomes erect) or retracts (inverts) (**Figure 19.12**).

N Refer to Chapter 12 and the Anatomy and physiology section of this chapter. Nipples normally protract when stimulated.

A Accessory breast tissue (supernumerary nipple), most commonly in the axilla, and secondary nipples on the nipple line are abnormal.

P This finding is a result of abnormal embryologic development, but does not present a problem in pregnancy. These areas may develop during the pregnancy along with the normal breast tissue.

CLINICAL **REASONING**

Nipple assessment
Assess nipples at the initial visit and again in the third trimester for any changes. The assessment may change as the breasts enlarge with advancing pregnancy. If a woman has inverted nipples this will not prevent her from breastfeeding, and referring her to a lactation consultant can reassure her.

Thorax and lungs

E See Chapter 13.

N See Chapter 13 and the Anatomy and physiology section of this chapter.

A P Pathology noted in Chapter 13 would also be considered abnormal for the pregnant woman.

Heart and blood vessels

E Assess the pregnant woman as described in Chapter 14.

N See Chapter 14 and the Anatomy and physiology section of this chapter.

A Generalised oedema, in contrast to the dependent oedema of pregnancy, is abnormal.

P The most common causes for this are standing or sitting too long and pre-eclampsia. In pregnancy there is a decrease in the colloid osmotic pressure within the vasculature, therefore allowing fluid to leak into the tissues. Other potential causes to be considered are kidney disease and cardiovascular disease such as cardiomyopathy.

Abdomen

E Assess the pregnant woman as described in Chapter 15.

N See Chapter 15 and the Anatomy and physiology section of this chapter.

A Severe nausea and vomiting (**hyperemesis gravidarum**) leading to significant weight loss in pregnancy is abnormal.

P Hyperemesis gravidarum is a disease of unknown aetiology. It usually presents in the first trimester and may continue throughout the pregnancy. This is more severe than morning sickness and may persist throughout the day, leading to nutritional deficiencies. There often is associated hyperthyroidism. Other less common causes may include cholestasis, acute fatty liver disease, hepatitis, cirrhosis, appendicitis and ulcers.

E Examination **N** Normal findings **A** Abnormal findings **P** Pathophysiology

A Epigastric or right upper quadrant pain is abnormal.

P This is usually a result of liver inflammation or necrosis from pre-eclampsia. It must be differentiated from cholecystitis or other liver disorders. It may be confused with commonly experienced pregnancy heartburn, but epigastric pain resulting from liver pathology is over the liver itself, whereas heartburn is felt more midline.

Urinary system

E 1. Obtain a complete urinalysis at the initial antenatal visit.

2. Obtain a urine culture if indicated by urinalysis or the pregnant woman's history.

3. It is common (but not proven to affect outcome) to assess urine for protein, glucose, leucocytes and nitrates at each subsequent antenatal visit.

N The urine may turn a brighter yellow as a result of antenatal vitamins. Trace amounts of protein may be noted. Glycosuria may be noted without pathology, but concern for diabetes mellitus cannot be ignored. Leucocytes (white blood cells) and nitrates are normally absent.

A Nitrates or a large number of leucocytes are abnormal.

P Nitrates, a breakdown product of bacteria, and a large number of leucocytes may indicate a urinary tract infection.

A Dysuria that presents as any of the following is abnormal: difficulty in initiating urinary flow, increased urinary frequency, or a feeling of being unable to empty the bladder.

P Dysuria results most commonly from a bacterial infection, inflammation of the bladder (cystitis), or urinary tract infection.

A Pain in the flank area (costovertebral angle tenderness) is abnormal.

P The pregnant woman is more prone than the nonpregnant woman to develop **pyelonephritis** from a lower urinary tract infection secondary to the dilation of the ureters and renal pelvises, along with decreased tone and peristalsis, which lead to stasis. This results from the physiological changes that occur during pregnancy.

A Asymptomatic bacteriuria is abnormal.

P A clean-voided urine specimen containing more than 100 000 organisms of the same species per millilitre of urine is consistent with infection. Asymptomatic bacteriuria sometimes progresses to acute symptomatic infection unless treated. Through poorly understood mechanisms, bacteriuria is associated with an increased rate of preterm labour and birth.

A Proteinuria greater than trace as shown on a urine dipstick is abnormal.

P The most common cause is pre-eclampsia. Double-check that the specimen has not been contaminated by vaginal secretions. Other possible causes are collagen disorders or kidney diseases.

Musculoskeletal system

E Assess the pregnant woman as described in Chapter 16.

N See Chapter 16 and the Anatomy and physiology section of this chapter.

P Abnormalities and pathology described in Chapter 16 are also considered abnormal for the pregnant woman.

Neurological system

E Assess the pregnant woman as described in Chapter 7.

N See Chapter 7 and the Anatomy and physiology section of this chapter.

E Examination **N** Normal findings **A** Abnormal findings **P** Pathophysiology

A Seizures are abnormal.

P Eclampsia is the most common cause of seizures in the pregnant woman. Other less common causes are stroke, tumours and epilepsy. The coagulation and vascular changes associated with pregnancy may exacerbate pre-existing conditions.

A Hyperreflexia and **clonus** are abnormal.

P Pre-eclampsia can cause these findings.

Female genitalia

E 1. For the initial antenatal visit, genital assessment is only required if the woman describes symptoms suggesting a problem, or if cervical screening is to be performed. If genital assessment is appropriate, perform the assessment as described in Chapter 17.

2. Perform cultures as indicated in **Table 19.7** with the woman's consent.

3. Routine cervical assessment is rarely indicated prior to the onset of labour.

N See Chapter 17 for normal findings of the female genitalia assessment. The multiparous vulva and vagina may appear more relaxed in tone, with a shorter perineum. There is often a visible, white, milky discharge during pregnancy, and the cervix may show more ectropion (also called eversion and friability). Ectropion is the condition in which the columnar epithelium extends from the os past the normal squamocolumnar junction, often producing a red, possibly inflamed appearance.

TABLE 19.7 Maternal screening tests (recommended/offered)

TEST	TIMING
FBC to include: > WBC (leucocytes) > Hb > Platelets	Initial visit Repeat at 26–28 weeks and 36 weeks gestation as needed.
Blood type (A, B, O, AB)	Initial visit
Rh (Rhesus factor)	Initial visit Repeat at 26 and 34 weeks gestation for women who are RhD negative.
Rubella	Initial visit
Rapid plasma regain (RPR) test for syphilis	Initial visit Repeat at 24–28 and 34–36 weeks gestation for women identified as high risk.
Hepatitis B surface antigen	Initial visit
Hepatitis C antibody	Initial visit
HIV (human immunodeficiency virus)	Initial visit; repeat based on history or exposure
HbA1c (glycated haemoglobin)	Early pregnancy for women with risk factors for hyperglycaemia (Australia)
Oral glucose tolerance test (OGTT)	Universal screening for gestational diabetes is recommended between 26–28 weeks gestation
Toxoplasma IgG (toxoplasmosis)	As indicated by any history of exposures and symptoms
Genital bacterial/group b Streptococcus (GBBS) (self-collected)	At 36 weeks gestation (at risk or universal screening; check facilities policy)
Chlamydia (first catch urine or self-applied swab)	Initial visit, only for women at risk
Gonorrhoea (first catch urine or self-applied swab)	Initial visit, only for women at risk
Urinalysis	Initial visit; repeat each trimester or as needed per symptoms and history
Urine culture	Initial visit; as needed per symptoms and history

>>

E Examination   **N** Normal findings   **A** Abnormal findings   **P** Pathophysiology

>> **TABLE 19.7** *continued*

TEST	TIMING
SCREENING FOR FETAL CHROMOSOMAL ANOMALIES	
Tests to assess risk: > Free beta-human chorionic gonadotrophin β-hCG > Pregnancy-associated plasma protein-A (PAPP-A) > Nuchal translucency (NT) scan > Non-invasive prenatal test (NIPT) or cfDNA	Universally recommended 11–14 weeks Universally recommended 9–14 weeks gestation Universally recommended 9–14 weeks gestation First trimester (if applicable – instead of or in addition to the above tests)
Increased chance of chromosomal anomaly: > Chorionic villus sampling (placental tissue from the villi of the chorion) > Amniocentesis (amniotic fluid collected for fetal skin cell sample)	11–13 weeks 16–18 weeks
ADDITIONAL SCREENING AND EVALUATION	
Ultrasound scan	At any time during pregnancy as indicated: > To determine gestational age (most accurate in early pregnancy) > To confirm or rule out placenta praevia, multiple pregnancy > Confirm presenting fetal part > Evaluate amniotic fluid volume > Evaluate fetal growth (in particular to rule out intrauterine growth restriction or discordant growth with a multiple pregnancy) > Evaluate for ectopic pregnancy or fetal demise
Cardiotocograph (CTG) (to monitor fetal heartbeat and the uterine contractions)	Later in pregnancy as indicated: > To assess fetal wellbeing – decreased fetal movement, known decreased fluid volume, history of certain maternal diseases (insulin-dependent diabetes, collagen vascular disease) > To monitor obstetric complications such as interuterine growth retardation, postdates, pre-eclampsia, discordant twin, or multiples

ADAPTED FROM AUSTRALIAN GOVERNMENT DEPARTMENT OF HEALTH. (2020). *CLINICAL PRACTICE GUIDELINES: PREGNANCY CARE.* CANBERRA: AUSTRALIAN GOVERNMENT DEPARTMENT OF HEALTH.

N Manual assessment should show uterine size appropriate for gestational age, and the uterus may be slightly more tender than in a nonpregnant woman. The **retroverted** and **retroflexed uterus** may be more difficult to assess. Palpation of the adnexa may demonstrate a slight tenderness and enlargement of the ovulatory ovary secondary to the corpus luteum of pregnancy.

A Persistent abdominal pain or tenderness is abnormal and should be evaluated.

P Either finding may indicate many underlying disorders related or unrelated to pregnancy. HDP and **abruptio placenta** are the most common causes of pain related to pregnancy. HDP pain is secondary to the hepatic involvement. Abruptio pain is due to the retroplacental bleeding of the placental separation. Disorders unrelated to pregnancy include ulcers, cholecystitis, appendicitis and pancreatitis.

A Painful adnexal masses are abnormal.

P In early pregnancy, these may indicate an **ectopic pregnancy** (pregnancy other than intrauterine, such as in the abdomen or fallopian tube), infection or cancerous growth. Pain associated with an adnexal mass may be elicited via cervical motion during bimanual assessment.

Uterine size

Uterine size is determined by internal pelvic exam prior to 12 weeks (if this information is clinically required), by palpation alone under 18 weeks, and by fundal height in centimetres for subsequent visits.

E Examination **N** Normal findings **A** Abnormal findings **P** Pathophysiology

UNIT 3

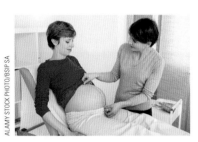

FIGURE 19.13 Measuring fundal height

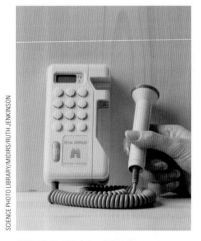

FIGURE 19.14A A fetal Doppler

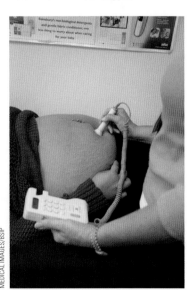

FIGURE 19.14B Using a Doppler to assess the fetal heart

URGENT FINDING ⚠

Ectopic pregnancy

An ectopic pregnancy is defined as a pregnancy that is outside of the uterus, and the majority of these (95%) occur in the fallopian tube. This can lead to rupture of the tube, and can cause maternal death. It is the ninth-highest cause of maternal death in Australia, affecting approximately 0.4 per 100 000 pregnant women (AIHW, 2022a).

The symptoms that would alert you to an ectopic pregnancy include a positive pregnancy test result, abnormal vaginal bleeding, abdominal or pelvic soreness or pain that is typically one-sided. The pain is often perceived as a cramping sensation or intense and localised.

On physical examination you may identify cervical tenderness, and blood on the cervix or in the vagina. If a tubal pregnancy has ruptured (a time-sensitive emergency), the woman may present with signs and symptoms of hypovolaemic shock.

Management of a woman who presents with symptoms of ectopic pregnancy include a thorough physical examination, quantitative serum HCGs, and an ultrasound as a priority. Any tissue passed from the vagina should be saved. If a woman has a suspected ectopic pregnancy, she should be informed of the risks of a possible rupture. In these situations, emergency surgery is strongly advised.

Some tubal pregnancies actually resolve on their own or with medical intervention such as methotrexate, but all women require close supervision.

Fundal height by centimetres

E
1. Place the pregnant woman in a supine position. Place a wedge under one hip to avoid supine hypotension.
2. Place the zero-centimetre mark of the tape measure at the symphysis pubis in the midline of the abdomen.
3. Palpate the top of the fundus and pull tape measure to the top (**Figure 19.13**).
4. Note the centimetre mark.

N A 16-week uterus is between the symphysis pubis and umbilicus, a 20-week uterus is at the umbilicus (20 cm), and from 18 to 32 weeks the size is approximately equal to the centimetre height of the uterine fundus. Plot the symphysio-fundal height on a centile chart as a means of assessing fetal growth.

A Uterine size larger than expected given LMP is abnormal.

P This may indicate hydatidiform mole or molar pregnancy (especially in the absence of fetal heart tones), multiple gestation, inaccurate dating, uterine pathology (fibroid), polyhydramnios or, later in pregnancy, macrosomia (newborn weighing greater than 4000 g).

A Uterine size smaller than expected given LMP is abnormal.

P This may indicate a nonviable pregnancy, inaccurate dating or, later in pregnancy, intrauterine growth restriction (IUGR) or transverse lie of the fetus.

Fetal heart rate

E
1. Place the pregnant woman in the supine position. Place a wedge under one hip to avoid supine hypotension.
2. Place Doppler or fetoscope (Pinards stethoscope) (see **Figure 19.14A**) on abdomen over the location of the fetal shoulder as identified on palpation (see **Figure 19.14B**). Refer to **Figure 19.15** to see the best location for auscultation based on fetal position.
3. Count the fetal heart rate (FHR) for 60 seconds to determine rate and absence of an irregularity.

N During early gestation, the fetal heart is generally heard in the midline area between the symphysis pubis and the umbilicus. It can usually be heard via Doppler by

---

E Examination   **N** Normal findings   **A** Abnormal findings   **P** Pathophysiology

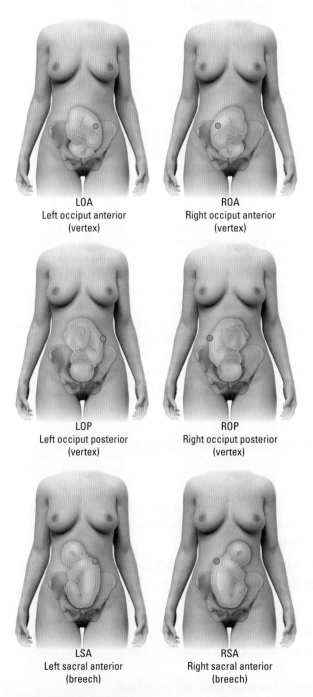

N approximately 12 weeks. Use the Doppler to auscultate the FHR prior to 20 weeks; a fetoscope can be used after 20 weeks. A Doppler is commonly used throughout pregnancy, as it is more convenient and allows the pregnant woman to hear the FHR. The normal FHR is 110–160 bpm. Check the mother's pulse rate to verify it is the FHR that you are listening to and not the mother's heart rate. Near-term FHRs are generally heard at maximum intensity in the left or right lower quadrant. If FHRs are best heard above the umbilicus, you should suspect a breech presentation. The fetal heart is best heard over fetal shoulder, which can be located by performing Leopold's manoeuvre as described in **Figure 19.16**.

LOA
Left occiput anterior
(vertex)

ROA
Right occiput anterior
(vertex)

LOP
Left occiput posterior
(vertex)

ROP
Right occiput posterior
(vertex)

LSA
Left sacral anterior
(breech)

RSA
Right sacral anterior
(breech)

FIGURE 19.15 Auscultating fetal heart rate

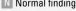

E Examination **N** Normal findings **A** Abnormal findings **P** Pathophysiology

A An FHR below 110 bpm indicates bradycardia, which is abnormal.

P Bradycardia may be a sign of fetal compromise. An FHR of 60 bpm or below may be indicative of a heart block. Heart block may be benign and convert to normal after birth, but a consultation with a perinatologist is advised for consideration of intervention with the newborn.

A Absence of fetal heart activity is abnormal.

P Absence of fetal heart tones may indicate an ectopic pregnancy, a blighted ovum, fetal demise or a molar pregnancy.

A FHR above 160 bpm indicates tachycardia, which is abnormal.

P Tachycardia may indicate a cardiac dysrhythmia, maternal fever or fetal compromise. Prior to approximately 28 weeks of gestation, tachycardia is a natural consequence of the immaturity of the fetal nervous system. In early gestation, the sympathetic system exerts a greater influence. As the fetus matures, the sympathetic and parasympathetic systems mature and the FHR should remain within the normal range of 110–160 bpm.

HEALTH EDUCATION

Fetal movement

The pregnant woman should be provided with information about fetal movement early in her pregnancy.

At approximately 18–20 weeks in a primigravida pregnancy and as early as 16–18 weeks in a subsequent pregnancy, the first fetal movements felt in utero, known as *quickening*, are noticed by most pregnant women. These are felt as fluttering or kicking, and initially may be difficult to differentiate from other pregnancy symptoms such as gas and ligament stretching. Absence of fetal movement by approximately 20 weeks should alert to the possibility of either inaccurate dating or, in the absence of FHR, a nonviable pregnancy. Beginning at approximately 28 weeks, fetal movement self-monitoring should be encouraged. The pregnant woman's sensation of fetal movement may change in the third trimester, going from 'somersaults' to rolling from side to side, to kicks or subtle shifts; however, the actual amount of fetal movement should not decrease dramatically. Any decrease in fetal movement requires same-day evaluation and investigation.

Leopold's manoeuvre

Beginning at 36 weeks, determine fetal presentation using Leopold's manoeuvre (Figure 19.16).

First manoeuvre

E 1. Ask the pregnant woman to assume a supine position with the knees bent. Place a wedge under one hip to avoid supine hypotension.

2. Stand to her right side facing her head.

3. Keeping the fingers of your hand together, palpate the uterine fundus.

4. Determine which fetal part presents at the fundus.

Second manoeuvre

E 1. Move both hands to the sides of the uterus.

2. Keep your left hand steady and palpate the woman's abdomen with your right hand.

3. Determine the positions of the fetus' back and small parts.

4. Keep your right hand steady and palpate the woman's abdomen with your left hand.

E Examination **N** Normal findings **A** Abnormal findings **P** Pathophysiology   Advanced Assessment

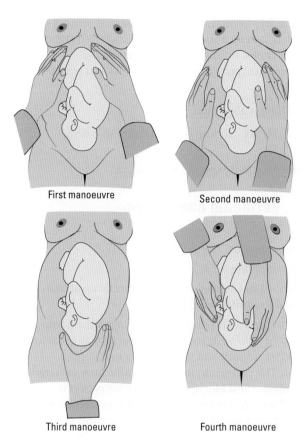

First manoeuvre

Second manoeuvre

Third manoeuvre

Fourth manoeuvre

FIGURE 19.16 Leopold's manoeuvre

Third manoeuvre

E 1. Place your right hand above the symphysis pubis with your thumb on one side of the presenting fetal part and your fingers on the other side.

2. Gently palpate the presenting fetal part.

3. Determine whether the buttocks or the head is the presenting part in the pelvis. (This should confirm the findings of the first manoeuvre.)

(Note: You may see varying practice encountered with this manoeuvre, as the technique can be painful for women. Practices are influenced by the healthcare context the practitioner is working in, so it is important to review and follow your local clinical practice guidelines).

Fourth manoeuvre

E 1. Change your position so you are facing the pregnant woman's feet.

2. Place your hands on each side of the uterus above the symphysis pubis and attempt to palpate the cephalic prominence (forehead). This will assist you in determining the fetal lie (long axis of fetus in relationship to long axis of mother) and attitude (head flexed or extended).

N The fetal head is usually the presenting part. It feels firm, round and smooth. The head can move freely when palpated. If the baby is in a breech position, the buttocks feel soft and irregular. With palpation of the breech-presenting fetus, the whole fetal body seems to move. The fetal back is firm, smooth and continuous. The limbs are bumpy and irregular. A fetus not in a vertex presentation can impact the safety of a vaginal birth; for example, a fetus in a persistent transverse or oblique lie is unlikely to birth vaginally. Breech

[N] presentation, if uncorrected (i.e. by external version – the manual turning of the fetus by the healthcare provider), can be associated with an increased risk of perinatal morbidity and mortality. Pre-birth diagnosis of non-cephalic presentation permits women and care providers time to discuss and plan the preferred mode of birth.

[A] Inability to determine fetal outline is abnormal.

[P] Polyhydramnios and maternal obesity can lead to an inability to outline the fetus.

Refer to a textbook on obstetrics for more specific information.

Examination of the anus, perineum and rectum
Inspection and palpation

[E] 1. Observe for colour and shape of anus.

2. Observe texture and colour of perineum.

3. Palpate the rectum as described in Chapter 18. A digital rectal examination may be part of the bimanual examination in pregnancy.

[N] The anus should be dark pink to brown and puckered. Skin tags are a normal variant and haemorrhoids may be seen with pregnancy, especially as the fetus enlarges. The perineum should be smooth and slightly darkened. A prior episiotomy scar may be visible. The perineum may vary significantly in length. The rectum should be free of masses and blood; however, constipation is common in early pregnancy. Discomfort is common with this examination, which is why it should only be performed when there is a clear clinical indication and with the express consent of the woman.

[A] Warty growths or abnormal lesions, fissures or tears are not normally found.

[P] Possible causes of fissures and tears are trauma, abscess or unhealed episiotomy. Warty growths can represent HPV. Abnormal lesions can represent a malignancy.

Assessment of the haematological system

[E][N] See Table 19.7.

Examination of the endocrine system

[E] See Table 19.7 for information on the glucose screen.

[N] See Table 19.7.

[A] Fasting plasma glucose (oral glucose tolerance test – OGTT) greater than 7.0 mmol/L is considered abnormal.

[P] Normal physiological changes that occur during pregnancy affect glucose metabolism. In some pregnant women, these changes accentuate and lead to gestational diabetes. These changes affect the known diabetic by altering her need for insulin throughout the pregnancy. The diabetic pregnant woman is at increased risk for pre-eclampsia, infection, macrosomia or intrauterine growth restriction, fetal demise, polyhydramnios, and postpartum haemorrhage.

Nutritional assessment
See Chapter 15.

Psychosocial assessment
The diagnosis of pregnancy can lead to mixed feelings. Not all pregnancies are planned or desired. The feelings women report can range from ambivalence to anger, fear or excitement. Early pregnancy symptoms such as nausea and fatigue may accentuate these feelings. Among the changes confronting the pregnant

[E] Examination [N] Normal findings [A] Abnormal findings [P] Pathophysiology [ ] Advanced Assessment

woman and her significant others are role expectations (e.g. lifestyle and career); relationship expectations, definitions and requirements (e.g. parent versus lover); and physiological changes. Feelings may fluctuate throughout the pregnancy depending on the trimester, and can be predicated on a change in medical status, such as the development of pregnancy complications. Early in pregnancy the woman often focuses on herself and on how these changes are affecting her physical state and her lifestyle. As pregnancy progresses, she usually shifts her focus from herself to the fetus as an individual and to the wellbeing of the fetus. The pregnant woman's age, prior history, family history, prior pregnancy experience; whether the pregnancy was planned or not; and any known risk factors all serve to affect her state of mind. Social support systems, socioeconomic status, environmental hazards and culture are also influencing factors.

CLINICAL REASONING

Practice tip: Antenatal anxiety and depression

Anxiety and depression can have a negative effect on the woman and on newborn care and development. It is important to screen and monitor for symptoms of depression and/or anxiety throughout pregnancy and the postnatal period.

Specific symptoms can include:

> inability to enjoy activities that were enjoyed prior to pregnancy or birth
> lack of concentration, difficulty making decisions or getting things done
> physical symptoms such as heart palpitations, constant headaches, sweaty hands
> feeling overwhelmed and constantly exhausted
> feeling numb and remote from family and friends
> feeling out of control, or 'crazy', even hyperactive
> inability to rest
> having thoughts of harming herself or the baby (infanticide) (RANZCOG, 2017).

The Edinburgh Postnatal Depression Scale (EPDS) screening tool should be conducted as early as practical in pregnancy and repeated at least once later in pregnancy and when clinically warranted. This tool is a 10-item self-report measure that should be utilised in conjunction with a clinical assessment.

Further screening questions may include personal or family history of depression or anxiety, prior or current use of antidepressants, difficulty dealing with life stress, lack of support, relationship problems, equivocal feelings about pregnancy and/or significant premenstrual moodiness.

The health professional should discuss these screening questions and any symptoms the woman identifies at her routine antenatal check. The results of the EPDS and the discussion should be documented and a referral organised when necessary to an appropriate health professional (psychologist, midwife, nurse practitioner or obstetrician).

For further information refer to Screening for depressive and anxiety disorders, Australian Government Department of Health (2018a).

REFLECTION IN PRACTICE

Assessing a pregnant woman's learning needs

You are teaching a childbirth preparation class for 10 women. Seven women are married with husbands, one is wearing a hijab. One woman is accompanied by her female partner. One woman is a single mother with no companion, and one woman has her sister with her (her husband is overseas). Discuss how you would assess the learning needs of such a diverse group, to ensure you are inclusive. Would this diverse group change how you would conduct the class?

Learning needs

The learning needs of the pregnant woman will change throughout pregnancy, and your assessments and teaching must change accordingly. Many communities offer pregnancy-related classes that start with early pregnancy and progress through the childbirth process, breastfeeding, infant care and sibling involvement. The pregnant woman should be informed of available childbirth education classes. The first-trimester classes typically focus on the physiological changes occurring during pregnancy and what the woman should do to develop a healthy infant; for example, nutrition, rest, exercise, and behaviours to avoid. During the second trimester, emphasis shifts to information on 'warning' signs and symptoms (Table 19.8). At 24–26 weeks, the pregnant woman should be provided verbal and written information on signs and symptoms of preterm labour.

TABLE 19.8 Warning signs in pregnancy

SIGN OR SYMPTOM	ADVICE
Vaginal bleeding*	Call healthcare provider immediately. Small amounts of bleeding may require only rest and observation at home. More significant bleeding or significant cramping, pain or fever may require intervention at a hospital. Concerns would be for miscarriage, preterm labour and placenta praevia.
Leaking or gush of watery fluid*	Call healthcare provider immediately. Nothing should be put in the vagina unless the provider inserts a sterile speculum to evaluate for rupture of membranes. A sample of the fluid can be tested to evaluate if it is amniotic fluid.
Abdominal or pelvic pain or cramping*	Call healthcare provider immediately after consideration of the normal discomforts of pregnancy (e.g. round or broad ligament pain). It is important for the pregnant woman to describe the quality of the pain, duration and location. Concerns would be for premature labour, ectopic pregnancy, placenta abruptio or urinary tract infection.
Severe headache or blurring of vision	Call healthcare provider immediately because of the concern for eclampsia. Evaluation would include blood pressure measurement and laboratory tests (blood chemistries, liver function tests, platelet count).
Persistent chills or fever greater than 38.8°C	Call healthcare provider. Associated symptoms may be helpful in determining underlying cause and its significance (e.g. infection, dehydration). Paracetamol may be used to manage any associated discomfort.
Persistent vomiting	Call healthcare provider immediately. Need is to determine underlying cause (e.g. gastritis, food poisoning) and treat symptoms before dehydration.
Decreased fetal movement or lack of fetal movement	Call healthcare provider immediately. At 20–24 weeks, lack of fetal movement could require an ultrasound to confirm dates and fetal viability. Decreased fetal movement or lack of movement later in pregnancy would require evaluation for fetal wellbeing.
Change in vaginal discharge or pelvic pressure before 36–37 weeks*	Call healthcare provider to evaluate for preterm labour.
Frequent (more than four per hour) uterine contractions or painless tightenings between 20 and 37 weeks*	Call healthcare provider. Rest, fluids or a snack may be recommended if uterine activity is not excessive or for prolonged period of time. If either is true, evaluation for preterm labour is required.

*Associated with preterm labour

Third-trimester classes focus on the preparation for childbirth and the care of a newborn infant. The topic of breastfeeding should be introduced in the first trimester and discussed throughout the pregnancy. Major community health units may offer classes designed for specific groups of women, such as young parents, women with multiple pregnancy, women who gave birth via caesarean section in the previous pregnancy, or for specific language or cultural groups. It is important to know what is available in your area so you can refer women appropriately.

Women's learning needs should be assessed on an ongoing basis so that interventions can occur at the appropriate times. A social services consultation may be helpful for certain pregnant women, such as those with a history of physical, emotional or sexual abuse, those experiencing current drug and/or alcohol abuse and those requiring help with basic housing and food needs. Appropriate written or visual information should be used to reinforce verbal discussions, and women should be given the opportunity to ask questions when they have had time to consider the material.

Any couple who suffer fetal loss, regardless of the timing of this, should be offered supportive follow-up. Many communities have support groups, or couples may seek help from a counsellor or therapist. Couples who experience early miscarriages often find that they are not allowed by society to grieve their losses; supportive follow-up should thus be offered to these couples.

Women often look to their care provider to raise a discussion about sexual activity in pregnancy and the postnatal period, as they lack the confidence and sometimes the language skills to know how to do so. Intercourse, unless specifically proscribed, is considered safe during pregnancy, although it may not always be easy or comfortable. During the first trimester, there may be no changes in libido for the woman, unless nausea and other physical changes leave her feeling miserable. During the second trimester, the pregnant woman may experience increased libido, whereas the physical and psychological changes of the third trimester may decrease the woman's interest in sexual relations. As pregnancy advances, the woman may find that she is most comfortable on her side, perhaps with a pillow under the abdomen, facing away from her partner. This position may decrease the depth of penetration of the penis. Male partners may express concern about injuring the fetus or the perceived discomfort of the pregnant woman, and it can be of value for them to discuss their concerns in a non-judgemental way with a clinician.

HEALTH EDUCATION

Overview of possible education that should be considered (related to pregnancy, childbirth and breastfeeding)

> Each laboratory, ultrasound and/or genetic test may require specific explanation and/or education; for example, the recommendation of Anti-D to rhesus-negative non-isoimmunised women at 28 and 34 weeks.
> Early in the pregnancy, encourage relevant preparation classes, which are offered by most healthcare systems and hospitals. These classes cover optimal nutrition, importance of normal weight gain, exercise and self-care during pregnancy, and warning signs of complications and preterm labour.
> At approximately 20 weeks, in addition to advising the pregnant woman to avoid sleeping on her back, you can enquire whether the woman has experienced any barriers to registering for childbirth preparation classes, and assist her to overcome these.
> At about 26 (24–28) weeks is the best time to review the signs and symptoms of preterm labour and appropriate action. There are generally handouts available. You can also discuss awareness of fetal movement.
> Some women may need encouragement to take breastfeeding classes because they perceive that it is a natural process and therefore should require no teaching. If a pregnant woman is planning to breastfeed, classes should be encouraged because they can be very beneficial in helping her understand the physical and hormonal changes she is experiencing, and the benefits to the newborn of breastfeeding.

CLINICAL REASONING

Practice tip: Fetal abnormality or miscarriage

Prior pregnancy loss, miscarriage, fetal demise, neonatal death or genetic or chromosomal abnormality in the current or a prior pregnancy often requires professional counselling with grief counsellors, support groups, therapists and genetic counsellors. A woman with a history of recurrent miscarriages may also benefit from referral to a reproductive specialist.

Each woman and family will bring to this event their own cultural beliefs and feelings. It is important to determine each woman's particular needs. What actions have already been taken? What support does the woman and her family have? Is there discord or blaming, acceptance or apathy?

>>

When seeing the woman following a loss, try to schedule her and any family members to be seen when there are no pregnant women in the waiting room. Allow plenty of time and privacy for emotions and questions. Talk with the woman and have her healthcare provider talk with her and her family in a private office before performing any physical examination.

Listen, offer empathy and, when appropriate, arrange referrals. Women often report that health professionals say things that are inappropriate. Attend education on how to support women during times of loss. Collecting mementos of the baby can be useful for families in the time after a loss. There are organisations that can provide hand-made garments or blankets for the baby, or take professional photographs to remember the baby by.

Subsequent or return antenatal visits

Return antenatal visits include measurement of vital signs, FHR, fundal height, documentation of fetal movement appropriate for gestational age, weight, assessment of any oedema, assessment of uterine activity, and assessment of any vaginal discharge or pelvic pain or pressure. Other issues discussed at return visits include concerns of the mother, weight gain, diet, childbirth preparation, breastfeeding, contraception, preparation of the home, any family issues, and blood and other tests as appropriate to the gestational age.

CLINICAL REASONING

Identifying the woman experiencing domestic violence in pregnancy

Abusive relationships (also known as intimate partner violence) are prevalent across all socioeconomic groups. An abusive situation often intensifies during a woman's pregnancy. During your encounters with the pregnant woman, you should make routine enquiries (in the absence of the partner or other family members) about this possibility with all women. In addition, be alert for undisclosed abuse if women:

> have a pattern of frequent visits, especially with vague complaints
> present with complaints inconsistent with a known injury (any unusual pattern of bruises on the head, neck, breasts, chest, abdomen and genitalia)
> frequently miss appointments
> are always accompanied by an overly solicitous partner.

If any of these issues are identified, you should assist the woman to develop a safety plan and ask her what assistance she would find helpful. Follow your institution's policy and procedures, and escalate when necessary to the appropriate support services.

For further information related to screening for domestic violence, refer to Family violence, Australian Government Department of Health (2018b).

REFLECTION IN PRACTICE

Care provision: situation

The woman experiencing intimate partner violence may be too ashamed to seek help, may have genuine fears of the consequences of reporting this, and may maintain hope that the partner will change and the abuse will end. The often-described 'cycle of violence' (a period of tension-building followed by violence then followed by remorse, calm and even kindness on the part of the perpetrator) may keep the woman feeling trapped.

What are some supportive nursing strategies you can provide for the pregnant woman that will respect her dignity and reduce the risk of harm?

EVALUATION OF HEALTH ASSESSMENT AND PHYSICAL EXAMINATION FINDINGS

In the evaluation phase of a health assessment, the focus is on ensuring the data gathered is complete, accurate and documented appropriately (see case study as an example of the focused assessment; see Chapter 22 for a comprehensive health assessment). In evaluating the data you should:

> draw on your critical thinking and problem-solving skills to make sound clinical decisions
> act on abnormal data (include communicating findings to other health professionals)
> ensure documentation reflects the outcomes of the clinical decisions/actions taken (refer to Chapter 3, which discusses in detail why documentation is so important and how this may be undertaken in different health settings). The case study that follows steps you through this process.

THE PREGNANT WOMAN

This case study illustrates the application and objective documentation of the pregnant woman's assessment.

Amina Tengku is a 27-year-old woman who is 16 weeks pregnant with her first baby. She and her husband are on student visas while they are both studying environmental science at the local university. They are Muslim, and Amina wears a hijab (head covering) and clothing that covers her arms and legs at all times. She is attending the clinic today to go through the results of the tests she had performed last month. You are working in the clinic as a registered nurse, along with a registered midwife.

HEALTH HISTORY

WOMAN'S PROFILE		27-year-old Malaysian woman
REASON FOR VISIT		Routine antenatal visit, to discuss test results
HISTORY OF THE PRESENT ILLNESS		Amina is well but a little anxious that she has not yet felt the baby move.
PAST HEALTH HISTORY	MEDICAL HISTORY	Mild asthma since childhood
	SURGICAL HISTORY	Appendicectomy at age 16
	ALLERGIES	Nil
	MEDICATIONS	Pregnancy supplement daily, salbutamol prn, budesonide prn
	COMMUNICABLE DISEASES	Was screened for TB, HIV, Hep B as part of her visa application – all negative
	INJURIES AND ACCIDENTS	Nil
	SPECIAL NEEDS	Has good everyday English but struggles with health terms; speaks Malay
	BLOOD TRANSFUSIONS	Never
	CHILDHOOD ILLNESSES	Chickenpox
	IMMUNISATIONS	All routine childhood immunisations complete, including HPV and hepatitis B
FAMILY HEALTH HISTORY		Amina's mother died from breast cancer last year. Her father and sister have alpha thalassaemia trait. Maternal grandmother has noninsulin-dependent diabetes.

>>

HEALTH HISTORY

SOCIAL HISTORY	ALCOHOL USE	Doesn't drink
	TOBACCO USE	Never
	DRUG USE	Never
	INTIMATE PARTNER VIOLENCE	Amina answered no to all questions on the screening questionnaire. Her partner was not present when she was screened.
	SEXUAL PRACTICE	Amina describes herself as heterosexual and in a monogamous marital relationship.
	TRAVEL HISTORY	Amina arrived from Malaysia 2 years ago and returns to visit her family for Eid once a year. Her visa expires in 12 months' time.
	WORK ENVIRONMENT	Full-time Master of Environmental Science student. No exposure to toxins or radiation in the workplace. Sometimes needs to be away from home for research field trips.
	HOME ENVIRONMENT	Amina and Mohamed live in a small two-bedroom apartment close to the university, which they share with another Malaysian student. They don't have a car, and she uses public transport to get to the clinic for visits.
	HOBBIES AND LEISURE ACTIVITIES	Photography
	STRESS	End of semester is approaching and she is worried because if she fails, her visa may be revoked. She misses her father and her sister who are still in Malaysia.
	EDUCATION	High school and Bachelor of Science degree in Malaysia. Currently nearing the end of semester 2 in the second year of a three-year degree.
	ECONOMIC STATUS	Mohamed's family own a large importing business in Kuala Lumpur and supports them financially. They have enough to meet their basic needs.
	RELIGION	Islam. They both attend the mosque close to the university.
	CULTURAL BACKGROUND	Malaysian
	ROLES AND RELATIONSHIPS	Amina and Mohamed are looking forward to becoming parents. They plan to defer next year's study and return to Malaysia for the birth of the baby.
	CHARACTERISTIC PATTERNS OF DAILY LIVING	Wakes at 5 a.m. for morning prayers. Attends university from 8 a.m. to 4 p.m. each weekday. Studies in the evening and goes to bed around 9 p.m. after evening prayers. Attends the mosque each week.
HEALTH MAINTENANCE ACTIVITIES	SLEEP	8 hours a night
	DIET	Amina eats traditional vegetarian Malay food that she cooks at home.
	EXERCISE	Walks 2–5 km each day.
	STRESS MANAGEMENT	Amina finds prayer very helpful.
	USE OF SAFETY DEVICES	Doesn't have access to a car.
	HEALTH CHECK-UPS	Last cervical screening test was 18 months ago – negative. Has been advised that her next screen is due 5 years after this.

PHYSICAL ASSESSMENT

GENERAL ASSESSMENT, WEIGHT AND VITAL SIGNS	Amina is well presented, wearing a green and orange head scarf, a long green jacket over a white shirt, and a long black skirt. Her weight today is 63 kg – a weight gain of 1 kg in the past month. Her BMI (calculated at her last visit) was 21.4. Her BP is 110/70 in a seated position.

>>

PHYSICAL ASSESSMENT

ABDOMINAL EXAMINATION	Prominent linea nigra, no striae or rashes. Scar from appendicectomy. Uterine fundus palpable halfway between the symphysis pubis and the umbilicus. Unable to feel fetal parts on palpation. Fetal heart rate with Doppler 145 bpm. Uterus is soft and not tender.
EXTREMITIES	Mild oedema of the feet and ankles (has just walked from university). Mild palmar erythema.

DIAGNOSTIC DATA

URINE CULTURE	No protein or glucose; no bacteria present
FULL BLOOD COUNT	Hb 95 g/L, MCV 73 fL, WCC 11×10^9/L, platelets 132×10^9/L
SEROLOGY	Hepatitis B surface antibody positive, HIV negative, Rubella immune, VDRL negative
BLOOD GROUP AND ANTIBODIES	A positive, antibody negative
FIRST TRIMESTER COMBINED SCREEN	Estimated birth date by scan is within 3 days of that calculated by LMP. Single live fetus. Increased risk of trisomy 21 (1 in 155)
VITAMIN D	29 nmol/L (test was requested as Amina receives very little sun exposure)

EVALUATION AND CLINICAL REASONING FOR CASE STUDY

The assessment and clinical decisions you make should reflect your scope of practice. For example, advanced practice health professionals such as nurse practitioners and remote area nurses with endorsement may be able to make diagnostic decisions and prescribe medications without referring to a medical officer.

Fundamentally, all health professionals collect, evaluate and act on patient-focused health information, which will at times include referral to, or collaboration with, other healthcare team members. Nurses assess patient responses to interventions and determine when to escalate key changes in a patient's condition. The clinical reasoning cycle provides health professionals with a framework to consider all this information in a meaningful way for planning patient care. These phases are stepped out below, and draw on information presented and collected during the health history and physical examination. We then work through the cycle components that are relevant to this case study (cycle components are bolded).

For Amina Tengku, the 27-year-old woman who is 16 weeks pregnant with her first baby, the significant data that needs to be considered includes the following.

Collecting cues/information

Amina is 27 years old and 16 weeks pregnant, and has attended a routine follow-up antenatal visit. She wonders if she should be feeling her baby move by now.

Recall and Review:
> English is not Amina's first language. She manages everyday conversations well, but may not understand health terminology.
> Her result of microcytic anaemia is significant, particularly in view of a family history of thalassaemia.
> A high-risk first trimester combined screen result is significant.
> A low vitamin D level is significant.

> Amina is at risk for being socially isolated as a temporary resident.
> Amina is a Malaysian Muslim and an active participant in her faith.

Chief complaint and history of present illness

Amina would like to know the results of the tests that were arranged at her last check-up.

Processing information

Interpret: A number of Amina's tests are abnormal. Her physical examination is normal for this gestation.

Infer and Relate: Amina may not be able to understand the significance of these results without the assistance of a trained Malay interpreter. She has attended the visit on her own, and is at risk for social isolation, so she may find it difficult to receive the news that further testing is recommended, which may lead to considerations of pregnancy termination. This information needs to be delivered in a culturally appropriate way.

Microcytic anaemia may indicate iron deficiency and Amina is vegetarian, so her iron intake may be low. There is also a possibility that she has alpha thalassaemia trait, a genetic condition.

A high-risk first trimester combined screen indicates that Amina's fetus is at higher risk for being affected by Down syndrome (trisomy 21). Further testing will be advisable in order to confirm or exclude this possibility.

A low vitamin D level can occur with low sun exposure, and can be exacerbated by a vegetarian diet, as many sources of vitamin D are animal based. This can lead to poor bone development in the baby and a risk of osteoporosis for Amina in later life. A supplement is recommended in pregnancy and for the infant after birth, with follow-up testing to ensure that the levels have been normalised.

Any dietary suggestions need to be made in a manner that is consistent with Amina's religious and cultural practices.

Putting it all together – synthesise information

1 Amina has no symptoms of concern and her physical examination findings were normal. It is important to reassure her that her pregnancy appears to be progressing normally. The absence of fetal movements at 16 weeks is normal in a first pregnancy.

2 Amina was hoping to be informed of the results of the tests that she had performed since her last visit, so is likely to be unprepared for abnormal findings. No arrangements were made for her to attend with her partner nor for the assistance of a trained Malay interpreter. It is important to communicate the test results to Amina in a way that she can understand, so that she can participate in making decisions about her care and understand the steps that she can take to address any dietary changes or new supplements that maybe required.

Actions based on assessment findings

The nurse plans the following actions, making sure they are documented in Amina's health record:

1 Explain the normal physical examination findings and the normal test results, as Amina is likely to be able to understand these. This assists in keeping Amina aware that most of the information about how her pregnancy is progressing is reassuring.

2 Explain that three of the tests were abnormal and that follow-up testing will be required. The nurse points out that even for women who have English as a first language these results can be difficult to understand, and answers Amina's questions, especially in relation to medical terminology, in simple language. She also writes down some of the important terms so that Amina can show them to her husband.

3 Arrange for Amina to return to the clinic tomorrow with her partner, and for a Malay translator to be present (if Amina would like). The nurse makes this appointment with a doctor who is able to order the additional tests that are required, and briefs the doctor on Amina's history prior to the visit.

4 Verify Amina's email address, offering to source information sheets about her test results in Malay and forward them to her so that she can read them before her appointment tomorrow.

5 Education is provided about when fetal movements can be expected to first be felt, and what to watch out for. The importance of being aware of fetal movement in later pregnancy is mentioned, and will be revisited in the third trimester of pregnancy.

6 Consultation with a dietitian, who is able to provide illustrated written information about a diet high in vitamin D and iron that is appropriate for a vegetarian.

CHAPTER RESOURCES

REVIEW QUESTIONS

For answers to these questions, see Answer section at the end of the book.

1. During pregnancy, the connective tissue changes and stretchmarks may form on the abdomen, breasts and upper thighs. What are the stretchmarks called?
   a. Linea nigra
   b. Naevi
   c. Melasma
   d. Striae gravidarum

2. Cassie presents to the clinic at 18 weeks gestation. The nurse takes her blood pressure and it is 148/98. When the nurse checks her urine, the dipstick is 4+ for protein. The nurse asks Cassie if she has any history of high blood pressure, to which she answers no. The nurse knows that Cassie will need close monitoring during her pregnancy because she most likely has:
   a. Gestational hypertension
   b. Chronic hypertension
   c. Pre-eclampsia
   d. Chronic hypertension with superimposed pre-eclampsia

3. Rosemary comes to the clinic at 25 weeks gestation complaining of lower back pain and painful urination. The nurse taps Rosemary's flank area, and Rosemary complains of tenderness and pain. She most likely has:
   a. Interstitial cystitis
   b. Vaginal infection
   c. Pyelonephritis
   d. Chorioamnionitis

4. Yasmin is pregnant for the sixth time. She tells you that she has four children and had one ectopic pregnancy. You also discover that three of her children were preterm. How would you most accurately describe Yasmin's obstetrical history?
   a. G 6, P 3, T 6, P 5, A 1, E 1, LC 4
   b. G 6, P 5, T 4, P 3, A 0, E 1, LC 5
   c. G 6, P 3, T 5, P 5, A 1, E 0, LC 5
   d. G 6, P 5, T 1, P 3, A 0, E 1, LC 4

5. Amelia comes to the clinic with bruises on her arms and face. She has missed her last two appointments and her husband provides the answers to the majority of your questions. You suspect abuse and want to speak to Amelia alone. Which of the following interventions will most likely provide that opportunity?
    a. Tell Amelia you need to teach her the 'clean catch' technique for collecting a urine sample in the restroom
    b. Send Amelia to the laboratory for a blood draw
    c. Tell Amelia to go to the clinic waiting room
    d. Offer childbirth education classes

6. Grace comes to her antenatal visit complaining that she must need new contacts because her vision has become blurry. The nurse explains to her that this is a common occurrence during pregnancy because of:
    a. Excessive saliva secretion
    b. Increased mucus production
    c. Corneal thickening
    d. Increased lysozyme in tears

7. Which of the following nursing actions would be appropriate if a woman describes decreased fetal movement at 35 weeks gestation?
    a. Ask her to come to the clinic for an evaluation
    b. Elicit a family history
    c. Teach labour coping techniques
    d. Query the woman on the outcome of her last vaginal culture

8. Cali's urine sample has moderate proteinuria. Which of the following conditions might explain this finding?
    a. Molar pregnancy
    b. Pre-eclampsia
    c. Gestational hypertension
    d. Gestational diabetes

9. Lilibett is 28 weeks pregnant. During her assessment you find that her symphysio-fundal height measures 31 cm and it is difficult to feel the fetus. The nurse suggests that:
    a. This is normal and no action is needed
    b. Lilibett restrict her calorie intake to prevent the baby from growing any larger
    c. If the measurement is more than her gestational age at the next visit, then she should see a doctor
    d. Referral for an ultrasound to assess the amniotic fluid index (AFI) in the next week would help to determine if polyhydramnios is present

10. Jackalin is expecting her third baby. She is 37 weeks pregnant. At her antenatal visit she explains to the nurse that she is having trouble sleeping because of leg cramps. The nurse advises Jackalin to:
    a. Book an appointment with her doctor to obtain a prescription for sleeping tablets
    b. Drink a litre of milk each day
    c. Take a supplement containing calcium and magnesium with her evening meal
    d. Drink a glass of wine each night before going to bed

CS CLINICAL SKILLS

The following Clinical Skill is relevant to this chapter and can be found in Tollefson & Hillman, *Clinical Psychomotor Skills*, 8th edition:
> 27 Healthcare teaching.

FURTHER RESOURCES

> Australian College of Midwives: http://www.midwives.org.au
> Australian Diabetes in Pregnancy Society: http://www.adips.org
> Australian Government Department of Health: Pregnancy, Birth and Baby Helpline: http://www.health.gov.au/pregnancyhelpline
> Australian Institute of Health and Welfare: http://www.aihw.gov.au/
> Everybody.co.nz. Pregnancy: http://www.everybody.co.nz/page-fecde513-88b8-4e2e-8aab-2ccc91dfd780.aspx
> HealthInsite: http://www.healthinsite.gov.au/topics/Pregnancy
> New Zealand College of Midwives: http://www.midwife.org.nz/

> New Zealand Ministry of Health. Pregnancy services: http://www.health.govt.nz/new-zealand-health-system/publicly-funded-health-and-disability-services/pregnancy-services
> Pregnancy and maternity in New Zealand: http://www.womens-health.org.nz/
> Pregnancy resources: http://www.pregnancy.com.au/resources/links/australian_links/index.shtml
> Royal Australian and New Zealand College of Obstetricians and Gynaecologists: http://www.ranzcog.edu.au/
> Women's Health Action Trust New Zealand: http://www.womens-health.org.nz/

REFERENCES

Australian Bureau of Statistics (ABS). (2022). Births, Australia. Retrieved 17 December 2022 from: https://www.abs.gov.au/statistics/people/population/births-australia/2021

Australian College of Midwives. (2021). *National midwifery guidelines for consultation and referral.* ACM, Canberra. Retrieved 14 August 2022 from: https://ranzcog.edu.au/wp-content/uploads/2022/05/National-Midwifery-Guidelines-for-Consultation-and-Referral-4th-Edition-2021.pdf

Australian Government Department of Health. (2018a). Family violence, Retrieved 14 August 2022 from: https://beta.health.gov.au/resources/pregnancy-care-guidelines/part-e-social-and-emotional-screening/family-violence

Australian Government Department of Health. (2018b). Screening for depressive and anxiety disorders. Retrieved 14 August 2022 from: https://beta.health.gov.au/resources/pregnancy-care-guidelines/part-e-social-and-emotional-screening/screening-for-depressive-and-anxiety-disorders

Australian Government Department of Health. (2020). *Clinical practice guidelines: Pregnancy care.* Canberra: Australian Government Department of Health. Retrieved 14 August 2022 from: https://www.health.gov.au/resources/pregnancy-care-guidelines

Australian Institute of Health and Welfare (AIHW). (2022a). Australian mothers and babies: Maternal deaths. Retrieved 17 December 2022 from: https://www.aihw.gov.au/reports/mothers-babies/maternal-deaths-australia

Australian Institute of Health and Welfare (AIHW). (2022b). Mothers and babies. Retrieved 17 December 2022 from: https://www.aihw.gov.au/reports-data/population-groups/mothers-babies/overview

Australian Institute of Health and Welfare (AIHW). (2022c). Maternity models of care in Australia, Retrieved 17 September 2022 from: https://www.aihw.gov.au/reports/mothers-babies/maternity-models-of-care/contents/about

Australian Institute of Health and Welfare (AIHW). (2022d). Australia's mothers and babies. Body mass index. Retrieved 17 September 2022 from: https://www.aihw.gov.au/reports/mothers-babies/australias-mothers-babies-data-visualisations/contents/antenatal-period/body-mass-index

Campbell, M., Sultan, A., & Pillarisetty, L. S. (2022). Physiology, Korotkoff sound. [Updated 25 June 2022]. In: StatPearls [Internet]. Treasure Island (FL): StatPearls Publishing; 2022, Jan. Retrieved 19 September 2022 from: https://www.ncbi.nlm.nih.gov/books/NBK539778/

Gordon, A., Raynes-Greenow, C., Bond, D., Morris, J., Rawlinson, W., & Jeffery, H. (2015). Sleep position, fetal growth restriction, and late-pregnancy stillbirth: The Sydney Stillbirth Study. *Obstetrics & Gynecology, 125*(2), 347–55.

Health Quality and Safety Commission New Zealand (HQSC). (2021). Fourteenth Annual Report of the Perinatal and Maternal Mortality Review Committee. Retrieved 17 December 2022 from: https://www.hqsc.govt.nz/assets/Our-work/Mortality-review-committee/PMMRC/Publications-resources/Maternal_mortality.pdf

Lachat, M. F., Solnik, A. L., Nana, A. D., & Citron, T. L. (2011). Periodontal disease in pregnancy: Review of the evidence and prevention strategies. *Journal of Perinatal & Neonatal Nursing, 25*(4), 312–19.

Ministry of Health/Manatū Hauora (2021). Maternity care. Ministry of Health New Zealand. Retrieved 18 September 2022 from: https://www.health.govt.nz/your-health/pregnancy-and-kids/services-and-support-during-pregnancy/maternity-care

Perinatal Society of Australia and New Zealand and Centre of Research Excellence Stillbirth. Position statement. (2019). Mothers' going-to-sleep position in late pregnancy. Centre of Research Excellence in Stillbirth, Brisbane, Australia. Retrieved 14 August 2022 from: https://sanda.psanz.com.au/assets/Uploads/Position-Statement-Side-Sleeping.pdf

PMMRC. (2017). Eleventh Annual Report of the Perinatal and Maternal Mortality Review Committee: Reporting mortality and morbidity 2015. Wellington, NZ: Health Quality & Safety Commission. Retrieved 2 July 2018 from: https://www.hqsc.govt.nz/assets/PMMRC/Publications/2017_PMMRC_Eleventh_Annual_Report.pdf

Queensland Government. (2022). Choosing an option for maternity care. RBWH Metro North Hospital and health service. Retrieved 14 August 2022 from: https://metronorth.health.qld.gov.au/rbwh/healthcare-services/maternity-services/choosing-an-option-for-maternity-care

Queensland Health. (2021). Hypertension and pregnancy. Queensland Clinical Guidelines. Retrieved from 17 September 2022 from: https://www.health.qld.gov.au/__data/assets/pdf_file/0034/139948/g-hdp.pdf

RANZCOG. (2017). Perinatal anxiety and depression. Royal Australian and New Zealand College of Obstetricians and Gynaecologists. College Statement. C-Obs 48. Retrieved 19 September 2022 from: https://www.ranzcp.org/news-policy/policy-and-advocacy/position-statements/perinatal-mental-health-services

RANZCOG. (2022). The management of obesity in pregnancy. Retrieved 16 August 2022 from: https://ranzcog.edu.au/wp-content/uploads/2022/05/Management-of-Obesity-in-Pregnancy.pdf

Stats NZ. (2019). How is Māori population growing. Retrieved 3 July 2022 from: https://www.stats.govt.nz/?_gac=1.221052138.1530245438.Cj0KCQjwjtLZBRDLARIsAKT6fXxCbEmJI3v9gGiVLtSzdR0r3N2sOKIlpw28iWjLKyRY-vKDQkT9DDIaApZvEALw_wcB

Stats NZ. (2022). Births and deaths: Year ended September 2022. Retrieved 17 December 2022 from: https://www.stats.govt.nz/information-releases/births-and-deaths-year-ended-september-2022/

Stevens, G., Thompson, R., Kruske, S., Watson, B., & Miller, Y. D. (2014). What are pregnant women told about models of maternity care in Australia? A retrospective study of women's reports, *Patient Education and Counseling.* http://dx.doi.org/10.1016/j.pec.2014.07.010

CHAPTER **20**

THE PAEDIATRIC CONSUMER

LEARNING OUTCOMES

By the end of this chapter you should be able to:

1 differentiate the structural and physiological variations between paediatric consumers and adults
2 identify personal-social, language, fine and gross motor findings when using the Denver II
3 demonstrate a complete health history from a consumer or caregiver using standard components of a paediatric health history
4 describe various techniques for approaching consumers at different developmental stages prior to initiating the physical examination
5 perform aspects of inspection, palpation, percussion and auscultation in a head-to-toe assessment of a paediatric consumer
6 discuss the clinical reasoning in evaluating outcomes of health assessment and physical examination, including documentation, health education provision and relevant health referrals.

BACKGROUND

In Australia, there are 4.8 million children aged 0–14, with boys making up a slightly higher proportion of the population than girls (51% compared with 49%) (AIHW, 2022a). The majority of children live in a two-parent/carer family (43.7%). A further 14.9% live in a single-parent/carer household (ABS, 2021). In New Zealand, there are 968 600 children aged 0–14 (Stats NZ, 2021a), with an estimated 66% of these children living in a two-parent/carer family, and 15% living in a sole-parent/carer household (Stats NZ, 2021b). Development through childhood to adolescence is a crucial period for establishing positive health and social behaviours, with a child's early years of development providing the foundation for their future health and wellbeing. A child's health and development outcomes are closely related to the social setting in which they live and the quality of their living environment. The living environment can influence participation in many aspects of life, including learning, development of relationships and recreational activities. These experiences can have a positive or negative effect on a child's social and emotional wellbeing.

The most prominent topics of public interest relating to child health and wellbeing in today's society include obesity, sleep disorders and the effects of digital screen-time use. Obesity and being overweight in particular have become a significant public health concern in Australia and New Zealand. Children who are obese or overweight are at an increased risk of morbidity and mortality as they develop into adulthood (AIHW, 2022a). The area of greatest physical health risk for children 5–14 is the development of asthma, followed by four mental health conditions: anxiety disorders, depressive disorders, conduct disorder and autism spectrum disorders (AIHW, 2022a).

In Australia, 24% (1 in 4) of children aged between 5 and 14 years are obese (7.7%) or overweight (17%) (AIHW, 2022a). A higher proportion (37%) of Aboriginal and Torres Strait Islander children aged 2–14 are obese (Wallace et al., 2022; Obesity Evidence Hub, 2021; ABS, 2019). In New Zealand, 12.7% of children (1 in 8) aged between 2 and 14 years are obese and a further 18.1% are overweight (Ministry of Health New Zealand, 2022a), with 35.3% of Pasifika children and 17.8% of Māori children identified as obese (Ministry of Health New Zealand, 2021). Australian children living in a regional and remote area were more likely to be overweight or obese (29%) than children living in major cities (23%) (AIHW, 2022a). In New Zealand, children who live in lower socioeconomic households are 2.5 times more likely to be overweight than children living in more financially stable situations (Ministry of Health New Zealand, 2021).

Children are unique individuals who undergo rapid changes from birth through to adolescence. Physical growth, motor skills, and cognitive and social development are the main areas in which to note specific changes when carrying out a child's health assessment and physical examination. During the assessment of a child, referred to as the paediatric consumer, it is important to be aware of these changes, and to continually reassess what is considered within normal limits for the child.

The common paediatric health problems that may be encountered in Australia and New Zealand are:

> Physical – Respiratory diseases (upper respiratory tract infections, asthma, hay fever, allergic rhinitis and chronic sinusitis), diseases of the eye (long and short sightedness), and diseases of the ear (specifically otitis media – middle ear infection).

> Injuries – Preventable injuries are more common in children. The most common causes are falling from a low height of 1 metre or less (falling off a bike), hitting something or being hit by something (pedestrian accident), or being bitten or stung (bees, bluebottles, wasps). All cause numerous health issues such as fractures, head injuries and skin reactions. Drowning and near-drowning are also significant.

> Mental and behavioural problems – The most frequently identified mental health problems are somatic complaints (i.e. chronic physical complaints without a known cause), anxiety disorders, depression (especially in teenagers) delinquent behaviour, attention problems and aggressive behaviour.

CLINICAL REASONING

Post pandemic considerations

The long-term effect of the COVID-19 pandemic on children's health and their development needs to be monitored to understand the impacts, and to provide healthcare interventions to assist in any identified issues. The public health measures such as lockdowns and home confinements that were implemented to limit the spread of the virus have caused significant changes to children's routines. This is particularly an issue for children who have pre-existing conditions and those from lower socioeconomic backgrounds.

It has been reported that some children who live in areas that had long periods of lockdown were exposed to increased isolation, increased abuse and neglect; decreased physical activity and increased screen time; and possible disruptions to the length and quality of sleep, impacting on their social, emotional and cognitive development (Centre for Community Child Health, 2022). This has led to increased mental health difficulties including anxiety and depression and attachment-seeking behaviours. Hence, support for children and their family's mental health will need to be even more so a priority, particularly for more vulnerable children and families, both in the short and longer term post pandemic (De Young et al., 2021; Singh et al., 2020).

PHYSICAL GROWTH

One important set of parameters required for paediatric health assessment is physical growth. The parameters of weight, length or height, head circumference, and body mass index (BMI) pending age of the child are essential in assessing serial physical growth (chest circumference is of less importance). These measurements are then used to compare with the expected parameters of children of the same age and sex, enabling health professionals to determine whether the child is growing appropriately for their age and sex. For example, by plotting a child's growth on a chart (see Figure 20.1), you are able to determine normal or abnormal growth curves according to the child's age. It is important to note here that while growth charts are a useful tool, children from specific cultural backgrounds may not track the same as their peers; hence, the important thing is that their growth is consistent.

There are several variations of growth charts (see Clinical reasoning, 'Which growth chart?') used throughout the world. Figure 20.1 compares the WHO Child Growth Standards and the Centers for Disease Control and Prevention (CDC) 2000

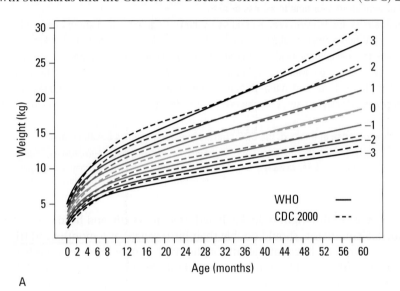

A

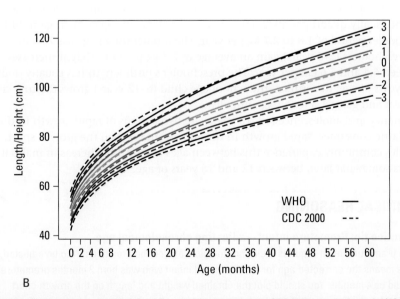

B

FIGURE 20.1 Charts compare the WHO Child Growth Standards and the CDC 2000 growth charts for (A) weight and (B) length/height for boys.

SOURCE: TWO GRAPHS SHOWING PHYSICAL GROWTH CHARTS FROM WHO CHILD GROWTH STANDARDS – METHODS & DEVELOPMENT, FIGURE16, PAGE 68 – LENGTH/HEIGHT COMPARISON, FIGURE 46, PAGE 128 WEIGHT COMPARISON, HTTPS://WWW.WHO.INT/CHILDGROWTH/STANDARDS/TECHNICAL_REPORT/EN/

growth charts. For the purpose of this text, the CDC growth charts have been used as a baseline tool. Special growth charts are available for genetic syndromes such as Down or Turner syndrome.

CLINICAL REASONING

Practice tip: Which growth chart?
The WHO infant growth charts are based on optimal (rather than average) growth of healthy, exclusively breastfed infants from six countries living in ideal health and environmental conditions. Other growth charts are the US Centers for Disease Control and Prevention (CDC) weight, height and BMI charts, which are based on data from a snapshot of weights and heights of US children. Growth patterns of breastfed and formula-fed infants in the first year of life are different. For example, healthy breastfed infants typically gain weight at a slower rate than formula-fed infants. Regardless of which growth chart is used, serial measurements of a child's weight and length (or height) should be accurately plotted on a growth chart over time to assess growth.

In Australia, the NHMRC recommend using the WHO growth chart standards for children 0–2 years. When a child reaches 24 months, the CDC growth charts are used. (In the NT and WA, refer to local guidelines about growth charts for children over 2 years.)

In New Zealand, the Ministry of Health adopts the NZ-WHO growth charts. These are based on charts developed in the UK that combine the WHO charts and data collected in the UK90 project. However, babies that have only been breastfed are assessed using the WHO growth charts.

For the purpose of this text, the CDC charts have been used as baseline tools.

Source: Royal Children's Hospital, Melbourne (2022), https://www.rch.org.au/childgrowth/about_child_growth/Growth_charts; Ministry of Health New Zealand (2015), https://www.health.govt.nz/system/files/documents/pages/factsheet-2-growth-charts-well-child.pdf

---

The average birth weight is 3.5 kg, length is 48 to 53 cm, and head circumference is 33 to 35.5 cm. Infants should double their birth weight at 6 months and triple their birth weight by 1 year of age, although it is not uncommon for infants to double their birth weight by 4 months. An infant's height increases about 2.5 cm per month for the first 6 months, and then slows to 1.3 cm per month until 12 months. Growth in the toddler period (12–24 months) begins to slow. The birth weight usually quadruples by 2.5 years of age, with an average weight gain during the toddler period of 1.8 to 2.7 kg per year. The toddler usually grows 7.6 cm.

Preschoolers (2–6 years) gain an average of 2.3 kg per year. Height increases between 6.4 and 7.6 cm per year. The preschooler's birth length has usually doubled by 4 years of age. In contrast, the school-age child (6–12 years) grows 2.5 to 5 cm per year and gains 1.3 to 2.7 kg annually.

Infancy and adolescence (13–18 years) are two periods of rapid growth in the paediatric consumer. Rapid growth in the adolescent is called the growth spurt. Females commonly experience this between ages 10 and 14, whereas in males it occurs somewhat later, between 12 and 16 years of age.

CLINICAL REASONING

Practice tip: Premature infant – adjusting chronological age
The premature infant requires their chronological age on the growth chart to be adjusted. This means the corrected age for a 6-month-old infant who was born 2 months prematurely would be 4 months. You should plot the obtained weight and length on the growth chart under the child's corrected age, and document above the measurement 'corrected'. This corrected age rule applies until the child is 18 months old.

ANATOMY AND PHYSIOLOGY

Structural and physiological variations

Children differ from adults and among themselves at various stages of development in their structural and physiological makeups. Following is a list of important variations that occur from birth through to a child's maturation.

Vital signs

Vital signs including blood pressure, pulse rate, respiration rate and temperature remain relatively constant throughout adult life. However, children are not 'small adults' and their vital signs change as they grow and develop (see **Table 20.1** for age-related paediatric vital signs).

> One notable difference in the way children and adults regulate temperature is the inability of infants aged 6 months and younger to shiver in the face of lower ambient temperature. The absence of this important protective mechanism puts infants at risk for hypothermia, bradycardia and acidosis.

> By age 4, temperature parameters are comparable to those seen in adults, and will fluctuate depending on the time of day, and normal body temperature for that individual.

> Both pulse and respiratory rates in children tend to decline with advancing age and reach levels comparable to those found in adulthood by adolescence.

> In children 1 year of age and older, there is an easy rule of thumb for determining normal systolic blood pressure: normal systolic BP (mmHg) = 80 + (2 × age in years).

> Normal diastolic blood pressure is generally two-thirds of systolic blood pressure.

TABLE 20.1 Paediatric vital signs – age related

HEART RATE			RESPIRATORY RATE	
Normal heart rate by age (beats/minute) **Reference: PALS Guidelines, 2021**			**Normal respiratory rate by age** **(breaths/minute)** **Reference: PALS Guidelines, 2021**	
Age	**Awake rate**	**Sleeping rate**	**Age**	**Normal respiratory rate**
Neonate (<28 d)	100–205	90–160	Infants (<1 y)	30–53
Infant (1–12 months)	100–190	90–160	Toddler (1–2 y)	22–37
Toddler (1–2 y)	98–140	80–120	School-age (6–11 y)	18–25
School-age (6–11 y)	75–118	58–90	Adolescent (12–15 y)	12–20
Adolescent (12–15 y)	60–100	50–90		

BLOOD PRESSURE			
Normal blood pressure by age (mmHg) **Reference: PALS Guidelines, 2021**			
Age	**Systolic pressure**	**Diastolic pressure**	**Systolic hypotension**
Birth (12 h, <1000 g)	39–59	16–36	<40–50
Birth (12 h, 3 kg)	60–76	31–45	<50
Neonate (96 h)	67–84	35–53	<60
Infant (1–12 mo)	72–104	37–56	<70
Toddler (1–2 y)	86–106	42–63	<70 + (age in years × 2)

>> **TABLE 20.1** *continued*

BLOOD PRESSURE			
Normal blood pressure by age (mmHg) **Reference: PALS Guidelines, 2021**			
Age	**Systolic pressure**	**Diastolic pressure**	**Systolic hypotension**
Preschooler (3–5 y)	89–112	46–72	<70 + (age in years × 2)
School-age (6–9 y)	97–115	57–76	<70 + (age in years × 2)
Preadolescent (10–11 y)	102–120	61–80	<90
Adolescent (12–15 y)	110–131	64–83	<90

For further information on hypertension in children and adolescents refer to The Royal Children's Hospital Melbourne (2021a), Clinical Practice Guidelines: https://www.rch.org.au/clinicalguide/guideline_index/Hypertension_in_children_and_adolescents/

TEMPERATURE	OXYGEN SATURATION

Normal temperature range by method
Reference: CPS Position Statement on
Temperature Measurement in Pediatrics, 2021

Method	Temperature (°C)
Rectal	36.6–38
Ear	35.8–38
Oral	35.5–37.5
Axillary	36.5–37.5

Temperature ranges do not vary with age. Axillary, tympanic and temporal temperatures for screening (less accurate). Rectal and oral temps for definitive measurement (unless contraindication).

Normal paediatric pulse oximetry (SpO_2) values have not yet been firmly established. SpO_2 is lower in the immediate newborn period. Beyond this period, an SpO_2 of <92% should be a cause of concern and may suggest a respiratory disease or cyanotic heart disease.

Developed by Dr Chris Novak and Dr Peter Gill for PedsCases.com.10 July 2018

Note that these variables are slightly different from those identified in Chapter 6. It is not unusual to have slightly different ranges published across the literature and as adopted by the health environment. Therefore, you should ensure that you check your health services 'normal ranges' and guidelines, so that you can respond and escalate as appropriate according to the published guidelines of your work environment.

Skin and hair

> **Lanugo**, a fine, downy hair, can be present on the skin of a newborn. The lanugo is most prominent over the temples of the forehead and on the upper arms, shoulders, back and pinna of the ears. Dark-skinned newborns have an increased amount of lanugo, which is readily evident as very dark black hair.
> **Vernix caseosa**, a thick, cheesy, protective integumentary deposit that consists of sebum and shed epithelial cells, is present on the newborn's skin.
> Relative to an adult, a child has a higher ratio of body surface area to body surface mass.

Head

> Suture ridges are palpable until approximately 6 months of age, at which time unionisation occurs.
> The posterior fontanelle, which is triangular in shape and is formed by the junction of the sagittal and lambdoidal sutures, usually closes by 3 months of age (Figure 20.2).
> The junction of the sagittal, coronal and frontal sutures forms the anterior fontanelle. It is diamond shaped. This fontanelle should close by 19 months of age.

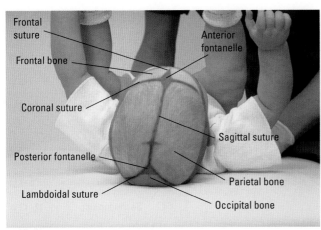

A. Superior view

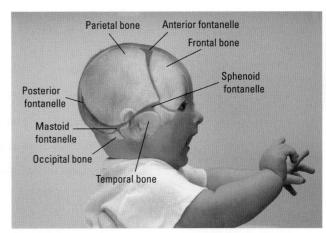

B. Lateral view

FIGURE 20.2 Infant head structures

Eyes, ears, nose, mouth and throat

> At birth, the newborn's peripheral vision is intact. Visual acuity is approximately 6/60. The child's visual acuity is usually 6/6 at 6–8 years.

> Newborns do not produce tears until their lacrimal ducts open, at around 2 to 3 months of age.

> The external auditory canal of a child is shorter than that of an adult, and it is positioned upwards.

> The eustachian tube is wider, shorter and more horizontal than that of an adult. These factors increase the likelihood of middle ear infections caused by migration of pathogens from the nasopharynx.

> Only the ethmoid and maxillary sinuses are present at birth. At approximately 7 years of age, the frontal sinuses develop. The sphenoid sinuses do not develop until after puberty.

> Eruption of the first lower central incisors occurs between 5 and 7 months of age. By 2.5 years of age, toddlers have 20 primary, or deciduous, teeth. By puberty, permanent teeth and four molars have replaced the primary teeth. Wisdom teeth normally appear between 18 and 21 years of age (see **Figure 20.3**).

> Salivation starts at about 3 months, and the infant drools until the swallowing reflex is more coordinated.

HEALTH EDUCATION

Ensuring fluoridation in children

The Australian and New Zealand Society of Paediatric Dentistry strongly supports water fluoridation to prevent tooth decay. All of Australia and most of New Zealand now has fluoridated water for this reason. Parents should be encouraged to check with their child's paediatrician or dentist if they do not live in an area with fluoridated water, as they are at high risk of developing dental caries. In these cases, fluoride supplementation is considered.

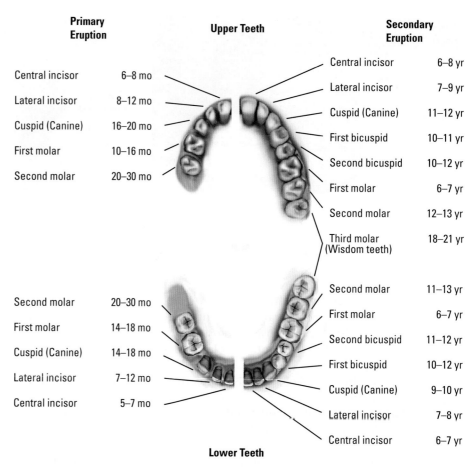

Primary Eruption		Upper Teeth		Secondary Eruption
Central incisor	6–8 mo		Central incisor	6–8 yr
Lateral incisor	8–12 mo		Lateral incisor	7–9 yr
Cuspid (Canine)	16–20 mo		Cuspid (Canine)	11–12 yr
First molar	10–16 mo		First bicuspid	10–11 yr
Second molar	20–30 mo		Second bicuspid	10–12 yr
			First molar	6–7 yr
			Second molar	12–13 yr
			Third molar (Wisdom teeth)	18–21 yr
			Second molar	11–13 yr
			First molar	6–7 yr
Second molar	20–30 mo		Second bicuspid	11–12 yr
First molar	14–18 mo		First bicuspid	10–12 yr
Cuspid (Canine)	14–18 mo		Cuspid (Canine)	9–10 yr
Lateral incisor	7–12 mo		Lateral incisor	7–8 yr
Central incisor	5–7 mo		Central incisor	6–7 yr
		Lower Teeth		

FIGURE 20.3 Deciduous and permanent teeth

CLINICAL REASONING

Practice tip: SIDS – safe sleeping recommendations

Sudden infant death syndrome (SIDS) is the sudden, unexpected and unexplained death of an otherwise healthy baby under the age of 1 year (Healthdirect, 2020).

To decrease the risk of SIDS, advise caregivers to:

> place infants on their back when sleeping
> avoid soft bedding, cover mattress with fitted sheet, and ensure no other loose bedding is present
> remove all soft toys from the cot
> exclusively breastfeed as long as possible
> encourage room sharing, not bed sharing
> encourage smoke-free environment during pregnancy and after birth
> ensure all immunisations are up to date.

Further information can be gained from Australian and New Zealand SIDS websites (http://www.sidsandkids.org and http://www.sids.org.nz).

Breasts

> Breast tissue in the female starts to develop between 8 and 10 years of age. Mature adult breast tissue is achieved between 14 and 17 years of age. Refer to **Table 12.1** for Tanner's sexual maturity rating.

Thorax and lungs

> A newborn's chest is circular because the anteroposterior and transverse diameters are approximately equal (Figure 20.4). By 6 years of age, the ratio of anteroposterior to lateral diameters reaches adult values.
> Decreased muscularity is responsible for the thin chest wall in infants.
> Ribs are displaced horizontally in infants.
> The trachea is short in the newborn. By 18 months of age, it has grown from the newborn length of 5 cm to 7.6 cm. Towards the latter part of adolescence, the trachea has grown to adult size, normally 10.2 to 12.7 cm.
> Until 3 to 4 months of age, infants are totally dependent on breathing through their noses.
> During infancy and the toddler period, abdominal breathing is always prevalent over thoracic expansion.

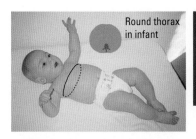

FIGURE 20.4 Infant chest configuration

Heart and blood vessels

> The heart of the infant, toddler and preschooler lies more horizontally than an adult's heart; thus the apex is higher at about the left fourth intercostal space.
> The fetal circulation changes to a pulmonary circulation when the umbilical cord is separated from the maternal circulation. Normally, the three fetal shunts (ductus venosus, foramen ovale and ductus arteriosus) close at birth or shortly thereafter. The ductus venosus allows blood to flow from the placenta into the right heart. Blood flows from the right side of the heart to the left through an opening called a foramen ovale. This opening is a flap valve located on the atrial septum between the septum secundum and septum primum. The ductus arteriosus, located between the left pulmonary artery and the descending aorta, allows blood to flow from the pulmonary artery to the aorta.
> The cardiac output of an infant is normally 1 litre/minute. Towards the end of the toddler period it increases to 1.5 litres/minute. At the age of 4 years it is 2.2 litres/minute. By 15 years of age, cardiac output has reached the adult level of 5.5 litres/minute.
> Infants have a higher circulating blood volume (normally around 85 mL/kg) than adults (65 mL/kg).

Abdomen

> At birth, the neonate's umbilical cord contains two arteries and one vein.
> The infant's liver is proportionately larger in the abdominal cavity than the liver of an adult.
> The abdomens of infants and toddlers are more protuberant, but this does not necessarily indicate pathology.

Musculoskeletal system

> Bone growth ends at age 20, when the epiphyses close.

Neurological system

> The neurological system of the infant is incompletely developed. The autonomic nervous system helps maintain homeostasis as the cerebral cortex develops.
> In the first year, the neurones become myelinated, and primitive motor reflexes are replaced by purposeful movement. The myelinisation occurs in a cephalocaudal and proximodistal manner (head and neck, trunk, and extremities).
> Myelination of neurones in the bowel and bladder allows the child to control these functions.

Urinary system

> In infancy, the urinary bladder is between the symphysis pubis and umbilicus.

Female genitalia

> Development of pubic hair in the female begins at puberty, between 8 and 12 years of age. Within about 1 year, the pubic hair becomes dark, coarse and curly but is not considered fully developed. Axillary hair follows 6 months later. After about age 13–15, pubic hair distribution approaches adult quantity and consistency. See Tanner's sexual maturity rating in Table 17.1.

Male genitalia

> The testes usually descend by the age of 1 year.
> Puberty usually starts between the ages of 9½ and 13½ and can last 2 to 5 years. Testicular enlargement is usually the first area of sexual development to occur. Within about 1 year, the pubic hair becomes dark, coarse and curly but is not fully developed. Axillary hair follows 6 months later. Facial hair follows approximately 6 months after the emergence of axillary hair. See Tanner's sexual maturity rating in Table 17.2 for additional information.

Growth and development

Refer to Chapter 2 for a summary of motor, language and sensory tasks that normal children from infancy through adolescence are able to accomplish.

CLINICAL **REASONING**

Practice tip: Attention deficit hyperactivity disorder (ADHD)

ADHD is a chronic mental health condition that is characterised by an ongoing pattern of behaviour, starting in childhood. The symptoms of ADHD include poor concentration and inattention, distractibility, hyperactivity and impulsivity. It is unknown what causes ADHD, but it has been linked to an imbalance in chemical neurotransmitters that affect the brain (ADHD Australia, 2019). ADHD can affect a child's learning and social skills, and can also impact on family dynamics and function. It is the most common mental health disorder in children aged between 4 and 17 years, with 7.4% of this population having this diagnosis (AIHW, 2022a; AIHW, 2022b).

Assessing for attention deficit hyperactivity disorder (ADHD)

Pose the following questions to the caregiver if the child is displaying inattention, impulsiveness and hyperactivity. If the caregiver answers yes to eight or more questions and the behaviours in question have been demonstrated for at least 6 months, a referral for a more comprehensive evaluation should be made to rule out ADHD.

> Does your child fidget with his or her hands or feet or squirm in his or her seat?
> Do you notice your child having difficulty remaining seated?
> Is your child easily distracted?
> Does your child have difficulty waiting for a turn?
> Does your child blurt out answers prior to questions being completed?
> Do you have to repeatedly tell your child to do a task?
> Have you observed your child having difficulty staying focused on tasks or in play activities?
> Does your child go from one uncompleted activity to another?
> Do you notice your child having difficulty playing quietly?
> Does your child talk excessively?
> Do you notice your child interrupting others?
> Does your child have difficulty listening to what is said?
> Does your child lose items necessary for school activities or home tasks?
> Does your child take part in any activity that could be detrimental to his or her physical wellbeing, such as head banging?

ASSESSMENT: TAKING THE CONSUMER'S HEALTH HISTORY

Assessment is the first phase of the nursing process, and involves collecting subjective information about the consumer's health status in order to identify consumer problem areas to focus on.

Subjective data is most frequently collected during a health history and serves as the starting point for the health professional to base the depth of their assessment on. The sections for the health history include:

> **Consumer profile**

> **Chief complaint** (explained systematically using variations of location, quality, quantity, associated manifestations, aggravating factors, alleviating factors, setting and timing. This is a variation on the OPQRST assessment mnemonic you may use for other conditions such as pain assessment)

> **Past health history** (including medical history, surgical history, allergies, medications, injuries and accidents, special needs and childhood illnesses)

> **Family health history**

> **Social history** (including alcohol, tobacco and drug use, sexual practice, work and home environment, hobbies and leisure activities, stress and culture).

CLINICAL **REASONING**

Practice tip: $H_1E_2A_3D_4S_5$ assessment

A valuable tool that is easily remembered during the adolescent's health history is the $H_1E_2A_3D_4S_5$ assessment. This tool highlights vital areas of an adolescent's daily life that can impact physical and mental wellbeing, and is designed to move from important but less threatening questions to those regarded as highly personal. The letters in HEADS represent the first letter in the subject area that is to be asked, and the subscript represents the number of assessment areas that begin with this letter. The $H_1E_2A_3D_4S_5$ acronym stands for:

> H_1
  - Home environment

> E_2
  - Education
  - Exercise

> A_3
  - Alcohol
  - Activities
  - Attitudes about life

> D_4
  - Diet
  - Drugs
  - Dentist
  - Depression

> S_5
  - Sleep
  - Safety
  - Sexual identity and activity
  - Stressors
  - Suicidal ideation

HEALTH HISTORY

BIOGRAPHICAL DATA	The same principles that apply in obtaining an adult health history, such as questioning, listening, observing and integrating, apply in obtaining the paediatric history. Because the historian in a paediatric history is less often the child and more likely the caregiver, it is very important to document the historian's relationship to the child. The following serves only to expand on the adult health history by providing information not previously discussed but relevant to the child.		
	CONSUMER NAME	In addition to the paediatric consumer's name, obtain the full name of the legal guardian. Occasionally, the caregiver is not the legal guardian; for example, when the child is a ward of the state.	
	ADDRESS AND PHONE NUMBER	Obtain the address and phone number of the caregiver if different from those of the paediatric consumer.	
	SOURCE OF INFORMATION	Other than the paediatric consumer or caregiver, information can be obtained from medical and school records, diaries, clinic notes, and health agencies such as child health services, school nurse and general practitioners. Written consent is needed to release records to a third party.	
CHIEF COMPLAINT	The caregiver is often the individual who seeks health care for the child and provides a description of the perceived problems, especially for infants, toddlers and young preschoolers whose age and mental status prevent them from offering genuine descriptions of their problem. You must frequently rely on the caregiver's intuition in such cases. The caregiver is usually acutely aware of cues to the child's illness. For instance, changes in sleeping patterns (difficulty falling asleep, reversion to night waking), regression to outgrown behaviours (bedwetting, finicky eating, thumb sucking), and unusual physical complaints in an otherwise healthy child (headaches, stomach aches) are important signs that the child may be experiencing stress or illness and warrant further investigation. The older preschooler, school-age child and adolescent are able to provide verbal descriptions of their complaints. Refer to Chapter 6 for pain rating scales that are used for children.		
PAST HEALTH HISTORY	Much of the information outlined in the past health history for an adult is applicable to a child. Additional pertinent information should be elicited regarding the birth history, including prenatal, labour and delivery, and postnatal history. If the main carer is the mother, then direct questions as follows. However, these questions would need to be reframed if the carer, for example, is the father.		
	BIRTH HISTORY	PRENATAL	1 How long was this pregnancy planned for? 2 How many weeks after thinking that you were pregnant did you go to a healthcare provider for a check-up? 3 How many children have you carried to full term? 4 Were there any pregnancies that you were not able to carry to full term? What happened? 5 Did you take any prescribed or over-the-counter medications during pregnancy? 6 Did you drink alcohol or caffeine or smoke cigarettes during pregnancy? 7 Did you take any drugs during pregnancy, such as marijuana, crack cocaine, amphetamines, or hallucinogens such as LSD and mescaline? If so, what were the amounts and frequency of use? 8 Were there any problems or illnesses that either you or your healthcare provider worried about during pregnancy (hypertensive disorders of pregnancy, preterm labour, gestational diabetes, COVID-19, group B streptococcus, TORCH infection [toxoplasmosis, rubella, cytomegalovirus, herpes], or an abnormal finding on a prenatal ultrasound)? 9 Was the pregnancy conceived naturally?
		LABOUR AND DELIVERY	1 How many weeks did you carry the baby before delivering? 2 Was the labour spontaneous or induced? 3 How many hours was the labour? 4 Was the baby delivered vaginally or by caesarean? If by caesarean, why? 5 What type of anaesthetic did you have? What type of pain relief was used? 6 Did you hold your baby immediately after delivery? (This question will provide information about the neonate's condition at delivery.) 7 What were the baby's Apgar scores at 1 and 5 minutes? (See later section on Apgar scoring in this chapter.)

>>

HEALTH HISTORY

			8 What were the birth weight and length of the baby? 9 Was the baby's father at the birth with you? 10 Where was the baby born (home, hospital, car or other location)?
		POSTNATAL	1 Did you and your baby go home together? (If answered no, inquire as to the reason for separate discharges.) 2 If hospital delivery, how long was the hospitalisation for you and the baby? 3 Did the baby have any breathing or feeding problems during the first week? 4 To your knowledge, did your baby receive any medications during the first week? 5 How would you describe the baby's colour at 1 week? (For light-skinned babies, ask if the skin was pale, pale pink, blue or yellow. For the dark-skinned baby, inquire about the colour of the sclera, oral mucosa and nail beds.) 6 Was the baby circumcised? 7 Did you start breast- or bottle-feeding your baby? 8 Were there any problems with your choice of feeding? 9 Did you or the baby have a fever after delivery? 10 How did you feel 1 to 2 weeks after delivery? 11 Did you have anyone to help you take care of the baby in the first few weeks after delivery?
MEDICAL HISTORY		Inquire about the circumstances and outcomes of any hospitalisations or emergency department visits. Keep in mind that some children's caregivers may use the emergency department for episodic health care and may not have their own general practitioner (primary care provider).	
	INJURIES AND ACCIDENTS	Determine if the child has a pattern of frequent injuries or accidents. Repeat trauma may indicate abuse.	
	CHILDHOOD ILLNESSES	Document past and current exposure to measles, mumps, rubella, pertussis, chickenpox and respiratory syncytial virus (RSV).	
	IMMUNISATIONS	Immunisations provide protection against many contagious diseases of childhood. Maternal antibodies pass through the placenta and breast milk, offering the baby limited protection from disease. **Table 20.2** lists the National Immunisation Program (NIP) schedule for Australia and New Zealand. Many healthcare providers follow the immunisation schedule as a guide for well-child check-ups. A record of immunisations is often important for childcare facilities and school admission and to avoid repeat vaccinations.	
SOCIAL HISTORY	**WORK ENVIRONMENT**	Childcare facilities and schools are the child's equivalent of a work environment. Inquire about the number of hours the child attends a care facility or school per week. Inquire about the child's academic performance. In addition, ask if the child is home alone before or after school.	
	HOME ENVIRONMENT	Ask about potential exposure to lead in paint/painted surfaces (chipping paint), because lead is harmful to the developing brain and nervous system of fetuses and young children. This group is four to five times more likely to absorb lead by ingestion than are older children (Daley, Pretorius & Ungerer, 2018).	
	CHILD'S PERSONAL HABITS	1 Determine what activities the child enjoys. 2 Ask how the child copes with stress and if a security object (blanket, stuffed toy) helps calm the child. 3 Determine if the child is prone to temper tantrums and what type of discipline is used.	
	DOMESTIC AND INTIMATE PARTNER VIOLENCE	Adolescents are not immune to intimate partner violence (IPV). Specific questions about IPV can be asked during the Home environment section. 1 Do you have a boyfriend or girlfriend? 2 What happens when one disagrees with the other? 3 Have you ever been hurt by someone you know?	

REFLECTION IN PRACTICE

Adolescent at risk for suicide

Mental health is a significant issue for adolescent youth in Australia and New Zealand, contributing to the rising rate of suicide in young adults aged 15–24 years. Suicide in this age group has been exacerbated by the social media phenomenon, cyber bullying, increased stress and pressure around school, getting a job, and body image. In Australia, Aboriginal and Torres Strait Islander youth have significantly higher rates of suicide compared to non-Indigenous youth (AIHW, 2022c). New Zealand also has a higher incidence of suicide for Māori youth compared to non-Maori youth (Ministry of Health New Zealand, 2022b). Further, higher rates of youth suicide have been found in young people who are LGBTIQ, or young people who live in rural or remote areas (Suicide Prevention Australia, 2021). Suicide occurs when someone has lost hope and sees no way forward in life. If mental health problems in adolescents are identified early, prevention and management will have a better outcome.

Consider the following scenario:

Sixteen-year-old Jason has just moved to Orewa, in the Bay of Islands, New Zealand. Before the interview, his mother confides in you that Jason has been acting differently, both socially and physically, since the family move. During your interview with Jason, he tells you he had so many friends before the family moved but has not been able to meet anyone to 'hang out with'. Jason proceeds to tell you he just mailed his cricket bat and his cricket ball to a friend in Auckland.

You summarise the information Jason has given and he replies, 'Life is not worth living and I just want to find a way to put an end to this.'

> How would you respond to Jason's last statement?
> Would you feel obligated to share this information with anyone?
> What other actions would you take to maintain Jason's safety?

URGENT FINDING

Identifying the adolescent at risk of suicide

A range of biological, psychological and social factors are associated with an increased risk of suicide. If you are concerned that a young person might be planning to take their own life, it is important to take them seriously.

Behaviours that can indicate imminent risk can include:

> verbalising, writing or drawing about death, dying and ways to commit suicide
> planning ways to kill themselves
> expressing feelings of hopelessness or worthlessness, that life is not worth living
> giving personal items away to friends and family
> withdrawing from friends, family and social activities
> increased changes in mood, such as anger and agitation
> demonstrating difficulty with accepting individual failures or disappointments
> problem behaviour and substance abuse with no concern for their safety
> exhibiting an attitude of disgust or discouragement with day-to-day living
> appearing dishevelled, not bathing and not taking care of appearance.

Note: Non-suicidal self-injury in adolescents may be different from suicidal behaviours (see Brown & Plener, 2017). If you identify a young person is at high risk of attempting suicide:

> stay with them or organise for another person to supervise them until you can organise an urgent review by an appropriately qualified health professional (such as mental health nurse, psychiatrist, GP)
> remove any objects from the environment that they could use to harm themselves (drugs, alcohol, medications, sharp objects)
> contact their next of kin, such as parent or guardian
> document contemporaneously.

Source: Headspace.org.au

TABLE 20.2 Recommended immunisation schedule

National Immunisation Program (NIP) schedule for Australia and New Zealand (medically at-risk and Indigenous children living in certain regions require extra protection against some diseases; therefore, they have some different and additional schedules [*within table in italics*]). Note: National immunisations change regularly; at the bottom of this table please see referral to access the most current information.

AUSTRALIA		NEW ZEALAND	
AGE	**DISEASES COVERED AND VACCINES**	**AGE**	**DISEASES COVERED AND VACCINES**
Birth	> Hepatitis B (HepB)		
2 months	> Hepatitis B (HepB) > Diphtheria, tetanus and pertussis (DTPa) > Haemophilus influenzae type b (Hib) > Polio (inactivated poliomyelitis IPV) > Pneumococcal conjugate > Rotavirus > *Meningococcal B (Indigenous children)*	6 weeks	> Rotavirus > Hepatitis B (HepB) > Diphtheria, tetanus, pertussis (DTPa) > Haemophilus influenzae type b (Hib) > Polio (inactivated poliomyelitis IPV) > Pneumococcal conjugate
4 months	> Hepatitis B (HepB) > Diphtheria, tetanus and pertussis (DTPa) > Haemophilus influenzae type b (Hib) > Polio (inactivated poliomyelitis IPV) > Pneumococcal conjugate (7vPCV) > Rotavirus > *Meningococcal B (Indigenous children)*	3 months	> Hepatitis B (HepB) > Diphtheria, tetanus and whooping cough (acellular pertussis DTPa) > Haemophilus influenzae type b (Hib) > Polio (inactivated poliomyelitis IPV) > Rotavirus
6 months	> Hepatitis B (HepB) > Diphtheria, tetanus and pertussis (DTPa) > Haemophilus influenzae type b (Hib) > Polio (inactivated poliomyelitis IPV) > *Pneumococcal conjugate (7vPCV) (Indigenous children NT, QLD, SA, WA)* > *Meningococcal B (Indigenous children, medically at risk)*	5 months	> Hepatitis B (HepB) > Diphtheria, tetanus and whooping cough (acellular pertussis DTPa) > Haemophilus influenzae type b (Hib) > Polio (inactivated poliomyelitis IPV) > Pneumococcal conjugate
12 months	> Meningococcal (menACWY) > Pneumococcal conjugate (7vPCV) > Measles, mumps and rubella (MMR) > *Meningococcal B (Indigenous children)*	12 months	> Measles, mumps and rubella (MMR) > Pneumococcal conjugate
18 months	> Measles, mumps, rubella, varicella (chickenpox) (MMRV) > Haemophilus influenzae type b (Hib) > Diphtheria, tetanus and pertussis (DTPa) > *Hepatitis A (Vaqta paediatric) (Indigenous children: NT, QLD, SA, WA)*	15 months	> Haemophilus influenzae type b (Hib) > Measles, mumps and rubella (MMR) > Varicella
4 years	> Diphtheria, tetanus and pertussis (DTPa) > Polio (inactivated poliomyelitis IPV) > *Pneumococcal (Indigenous Children: NT, QLD, SA, WA)* > *Hepatitis A (Indigenous Children: NT, QLD, SA, WA)*	4 years	> Diphtheria, tetanus and pertussis (DTPa) > Polio (inactivated poliomyelitis IPV)
> 5 years	> Influenza (children with specified medical risk conditions) > Influenza (Indigenous children)		
12–13 years	> Human papillomavirus (HPV) – > Diphtheria, tetanus and pertussis (dTPa booster)	11–12 years	> Diphtheria, tetanus and pertussis (dTPa booster) > Human papillomavirus (HPV): • 2 doses 6 months apart for those aged 14 years and under • 3 doses given over 6 months for those aged 15 and older
14–16 years	> Meningococcal ACWY		
All ages	> *Pneumococcal polysaccharide (23vPPV) – Indigenous peoples medically at-risk*	45 years	> Diphtheria, tetanus (ADT booster)

>>

>> **TABLE 20.2** *continued*

AUSTRALIA		NEW ZEALAND	
AGE	**DISEASES COVERED AND VACCINES**	**AGE**	**DISEASES COVERED AND VACCINES**
50 years & over	> *Pneumococcal (Indigenous adults)*		
70 years and over	> Herpes zoster > Pneumococcal	65 years	> Diphtheria, tetanus (ADT booster) > Herpes zoster > Influenza
Annual influenza vaccination	> 6 months and over with certain medical risk factors > *Aboriginal and Torres Strait Islander children 6 months to less than 5 years* > *Aboriginal and Torres Strait Islander peoples 15 years and over* > 65 and over > Pregnant women		

This schedule steps out the diseases and vaccinations, indicating the recommended ages for routine administration of currently licensed vaccines for children up to adults. These are sourced from the Australian Government Department of Health (as at 9 May 2023) and Ministry of Health New Zealand (as at 14 October 2022). Please note some of these vaccinations are administered in combination and that immunisation schedules are regularly reviewed and updated. For more comprehensive information about the Immunisation programs visit the following websites:

Australia: https://www.health.gov.au/sites/default/files/2023-03/national-immunisation-program-schedule.pd

New Zealand: https://www.health.govt.nz/our-work/preventative-health-wellness/immunisation/new-zealand-immunisation-schedule

SOURCE: AUSTRALIAN GOVERNMENT DEPARTMENT OF HEALTH (2023); MINISTRY OF HEALTH NEW ZEALAND (2018)

PERSON-CENTRED HEALTH EDUCATION

When conducting a health assessment, opportunities for the provision of person-centred health education will arise. This is a significant consideration in relation to the assessment process for examination of the paediatric consumer, as specihc health education or promotion will also need to be directed to the parents/caregivers. These occasions are identified as individualised education and may generate further data that can be added to the assessment. All education given should be documented so that in future, health professionals can assess the impact of previous information provided to the consumer and/or caregiver. (Refer to Chapter 1 for initiating health education.) Refer to the following examples.

INDIVIDUALISED HEALTH EDUCATION INTERVENTIONS	
Assessing the paediatric consumer for the following health-related activities can assist in identifying the need for education about these factors. This information provides a bridge between the health maintenance activities and the paediatric consumer.	
Sleep	1. Determine if the child takes naps and if the child shares a bedroom, because children's different sleep habits may lead to interrupted sleep. 2. Ask whether the child experiences night terrors. 3. Ask whether the child sleepwalks.
Diet	Questions concerning diet need to be tailored to the consumer's developmental level.
Safety	Childproofing the environment, especially for young children, is an essential practice. Incorporate these questions into your interview. 1. Tell me how you have childproofed your home. 2. Do you have gates at the top and bottom of the stairs? 3. Are the slats on the cot less than 8.5 cm apart? 4. Have you taken the cot mobile down and taken out the bumper pads (applies to infants who are trying to pull themselves up)? 5. Is all sleepwear flame retardant? 6. Is the hot water thermostat turned down to 50°C? 7. Do you keep curtain and blind strings out of reach? 8. Have you placed all sharp items such as razors and knives out of reach of the child? 9. Do you monitor your child's bath? Do you always drain the water in the bath after getting out?

>>

Safety	10.	Have you got bath tap covers in place?
	11.	Do you use a non-skid bath mat in the bath?
	12.	Are there power point covers on every electrical power point outlet in the house?
	13.	When you are cooking, do you keep the pot or pan handles turned in?
	14.	Have you taken tablecloths off all tables?
	15.	Do you keep the phone cord out of reach?
	16.	Is the slack taken up on all electrical appliances and lamp cords?
	17.	Are all your pot plants out of reach?
	18.	Are your deck slats covered with a mesh net?
	19.	Are there slip protectors under all rugs?
	20.	If you have a pool in the yard, are the legal and safety requirements regarding fencing correct?
	21.	Do you empty buckets that contain liquid after using them?
	22.	Are medications, cosmetics, pesticides, petrol, cleaning solutions, paint thinner and all other poisonous materials out of the child's reach?
	23.	Do you have your local poison control centre's telephone number next to each phone?
	24.	Do you have smoke detectors close to or in the child's bedroom and appropriately placed around the house?
	25.	Do you have a fire extinguisher handy?
	26.	Have you devised and practised an escape route plan in case of fire?
	27.	Have you done a basic first aid course including CPR?
	28.	What would you do in case of an emergency?
	29.	Do you have the correct and appropriately fitted child's car seat?
	30.	Does your child use protective gear such as a helmet or knee or elbow pads if participating in an activity in which injuries may occur?
	31.	Do you keep all plastic products (plastic rubbish bags, plastic shopping bags etc.) out of the child's reach?
	32.	Do you give your child nutritional supplements or herbal remedies? If so, name the type and amount given.
	33.	Do you have a dog? Is the dog child-friendly? Do you keep the dog chained on a leash when other children are visiting your home?

PLANNING FOR PHYSICAL EXAMINATION

The planning phase refers to evaluating subjective data to narrow the focus on physical examination, determining what objective data needs to be gathered, as well as considering the environment and equipment that will be required.

At this time, you will identify which of the four diagnostic techniques you will need to implement the physical examination, and how you will sequence these. For the physical examination of the paediatric consumer you will include inspection, palpation, percussion and auscultation.

Objective data is:

> collected during the physical examination of the consumer

> usually collected after subjective data

> information that is measured or observed by the clinician as opposed to being reported by the consumer

> vital to the overall health assessment, to enable you to make clinical decisions that are representative of the whole consumer picture.

Evaluating subjective data to focus physical examination

Before commencing the physical examination of the paediatric consumer, consider what information the health history has provided. Critical consideration, linked to knowledge of anatomy and physiology, should focus the physical assessment so your examination will be more effective and efficient.

Environment

The paediatric assessment can be done in most physical environments in healthcare settings that will provide the level of privacy that is required. For the paediatric consumer, ensuring they feel safe is a primary goal to reduce anxieties; hence, the main caregiver should always be present or available. The environment should be a pleasant, comfortable setting that has different items of distraction available that can be used when a consumer is uncooperative, upset or focusing on what will be done next. Distractions include small toys that easily hook onto a stethoscope, and wind-up musical, humming or whistling toys.

Equipment

> Equipment listed in Chapter 6
> Scale (infant or stand-up)
> Appropriate-sized blood pressure cuff
> Snellen E and Tumbling E charts
> Sight cards/Vision screening cards
> Colour vision charts
> Ophthalmoscope
> Otoscope, speculum (2.5 to 4 mm), pneumatic attachment
> Paediatric stethoscope
> Appropriate growth chart
> Small bell
> Brightly coloured object
> Denver II materials/PEDs
> Nonsterile gloves
> Disposable centimetre tape measure

IMPLEMENTATION: CONDUCTING THE PHYSICAL EXAMINATION

Implementation of the physical examination requires you to consider your scope of practice as well. In this section, depending on your context, you may be performing foundation assessment with aspects of advanced assessment if you are practising in a specialised area. Assessment of the paediatric consumer should always take into consideration their age and development.

EXAMINATION **IN BRIEF: THE PAEDIATRIC CONSUMER***

Developmental assessment
> Denver II/PEDs

Physical growth
Weight
Length and height
Head circumference
Apgar scoring

Head
Inspection
> Shape and symmetry
> Head control

Palpation
> Fontanelle
> Suture lines
> Surface characteristics

Eyes
General approach
Vision screening
> General approach
> Tumbling E chart

Strabismus screening
> Hirschberg test
> Cover/uncover test
> Colour vision

>>

Advanced Assessment

>>

Inspection
> Eyelids
> Lacrimal apparatus

Anterior segment structures
> Sclera
> Iris
> Pupils
> Lens

Musculoskeletal system
General approach
Inspection
> Muscles
> Joints

Palpation
> Joints
> Feet
> Hip and femur

Neurological system
General approach
Reflex mechanisms of the infant
Rooting reflex
Sucking reflex
> Palmar grasp reflex
> Tonic neck reflex
> Stepping reflex
> Plantar grasp reflex
> Babinski reflex
> Moro (startle) reflex
> Galant reflex
> Placing reflex
> Landau reflex

Cranial nerve function
> Infant (birth to 12 months)
> Toddler and preschooler (1 to 5 years)

*Only paediatric-specific tests are listed.

General approach to paediatric physical examination

1. Assess the consumer in a warm, quiet room. To prevent hypothermia, always keep infants under the age of 6 months warm during the examination.
2. Use natural lighting, if available, during the assessment. Fluorescent lighting makes assessing varying degrees of cyanosis and jaundice difficult.
3. To help reduce anxiety and uncooperativeness (especially when assessing young children), have a familiar caregiver present during the assessment.
4. Talk to the child in a soothing voice; even an infant who cannot understand your words will take comfort in a calm and supportive approach.
5. Explain all procedures and allow older infants, toddlers, preschoolers and younger school-age consumers to touch or manipulate medical equipment (see **Figure 20.5**).
6. To promote the child's feeling of security, allow the infant who cannot sit up and the younger child to sit on the caregiver's lap for as much of the examination as possible.
7. Until the infant or toddler is comfortable, maintain eye contact with the caregiver while the assessment is taking place. Maintaining eye contact with the child who experiences anxiety in the presence of strangers can interfere with completing the examination. Maintain eye contact with caregiver if other means of alleviating the fears are not successful.
8. If appropriate, interview the older school-age child or adolescent separately, without the caregiver. Talking to the individual without the caregiver present may yield important information not gained during a group interview (e.g. that the consumer is using drugs).
9. Respect the consumer's modesty.
10. Warm your equipment (e.g. stethoscope).
11. Avoid making abrupt movements because these may startle a child.
12. If the child is sleeping, take advantage of the situation by performing simple procedures (length, head circumference) and system assessments that require a quiet room (such as the cardiac and respiratory assessments) first.
13. Perform all invasive or uncomfortable procedures (ear inspection, hip palpation) last because they may cause discomfort, crying, fear, and increased heart rate.

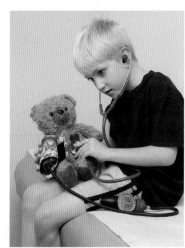

A. A preschooler listening to a teddy bear's chest will gain an understanding of the assessment that is to come.

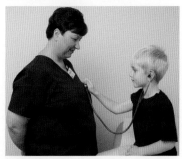

B. A child may also feel more comfortable trying his new skills on a caregiver or healthcare provider.

FIGURE 20.5 Allowing a child to touch and manipulate medical equipment may reduce fear and anxiety during the physical examination.

14. Always provide comfort measures following pain. It is especially helpful to allow the caregiver the opportunity to provide supportive measures. This shows the child that you are genuinely concerned about his or her feelings.

15. To prevent falls, always keep one hand on any infant who is placed on the examination table.

16. Prior to completing the examination, ask the caregiver and consumer what questions they have.

Developmental assessment

Human development is the progression and evolution that we go through from infancy to independent adulthood. Growth and development of the brain and central nervous system, known as psychomotor development, is a key focus of assessment in young children. Early identification of any regression or loss of previously acquired skills should prompt a referral for detailed assessment, to ensure early intervention if required. Every child health consultation is an opportunity to gauge if a child is meeting their milestones in relation to four specific areas: personal-social, fine motor-adaptive, language, and gross motor skills. A commonly used tool that assesses these four areas of development from birth through to 6 years of age is the Denver II (see **Figure 20.6**). A total of 125 items are described on the test. Some items can be accomplished easily by observing the child without commands from the observer. For instance, the child may be smiling spontaneously, saying words other than 'mama' or 'dada', or sitting with their head held steady. Certain items can be given an automatic pass mark if the caregiver indicates that the child is able to accomplish the corresponding item, such as drinking from a cup, washing and drying hands, or dressing without help

---

CLINICAL **REASONING**

Practice tip: Facilitating the paediatric assessment

When working with the paediatric consumer to undertake assessment and physical examination:

> Consider age and developmental level; observe for 'readiness' clues.

> Take time to get 'acquainted'.

> Use game playing and distraction to increase consumer cooperativeness.

> Demonstrate procedures on a doll, stuffed toy, or even the caregiver prior to performing them on the child.

Before administering the test, determine the child's chronological age and draw a straight line through the four sections intersecting the age intervals on the top and bottom of the sheet. This line indicates the items that are to be tested for the child's chronological age. Begin testing by assessing the item that is three items to the left of the age line. Documentation is reflected by using a 'P' for pass, 'F' for fail, 'R' for refuses, and 'NO' for no opportunity. Give up to three trials before documenting the score for the particular item on the Denver II. At the end, complete the five Test Behaviour questions. A normal test consists of no delays and a maximum of one caution. A caution is failure of the consumer to perform an item that has been achieved by 75% to 90% of children the same age. A delay is a failure of any item to the left of the age line. A suspect test is one with one or more delays or two or more cautions; in these instances, retest the child in 1 to 2 weeks.

Keep in mind that current illness, lack of sleep, fear and anxiety, deafness or blindness can affect a child's performance. If these or other logical rationale can explain a child's failure to successfully complete a series of Denver II items during a session, re-administer the test in one month, providing resolution of the pre-existing condition is accomplished, where appropriate. If the child does, in fact, have a developmental disability, early detection can lead to appropriate intervention and assistance.

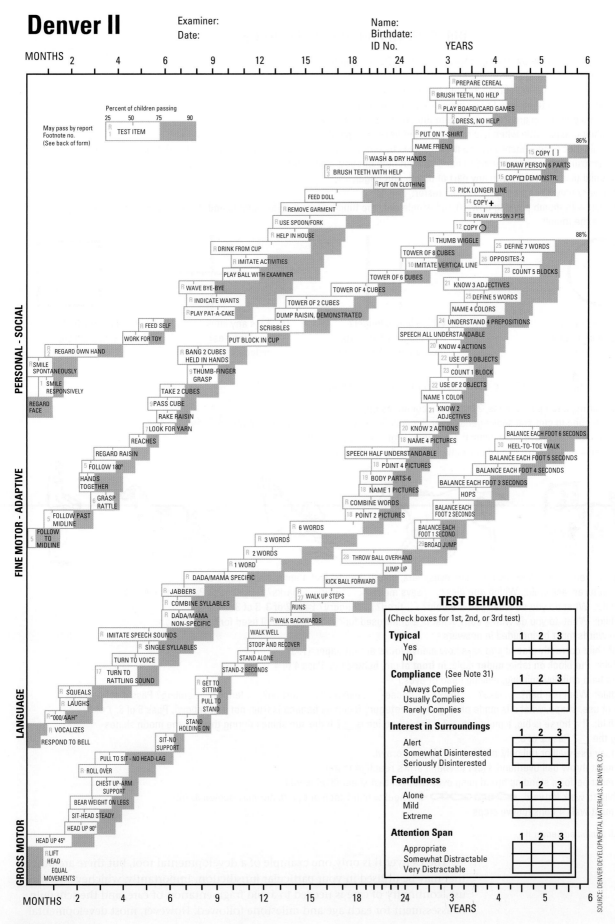

FIGURE 20.6 Denver II

SOURCE: DENVER DEVELOPMENTAL MATERIALS, DENVER, CO.

DIRECTIONS FOR ADMINISTRATION

1. Try to get child to smile by smiling, talking or waving. Do not touch him/her.
2. Child must stare at hand several seconds.
3. Parent may help guide toothbrush and put toothpaste on brush.
4. Child does not have to be able to tie shoes or button/zip in the back.
5. Move yarn slowly in an arc from one side to the other, about 20 cm above child's face.
6. Pass if child grasps rattle when it is touched to the backs or tips of fingers.
7. Pass if child tries to see where yarn went. Yarn should be dropped quickly from sight from tester's hand without arm movement.
8. Child must transfer cube from hand to hand without help of body, mouth or table.
9. Pass if child picks up raisin with any part of thumb and finger.
10. Line can vary only 30 degrees or less from testers line. $\mathcal{V}$
11. Make a fist with thumb pointing upward and wiggle only the thumb. Pass if child imitates and does not move any fingers other than the thumb.

12. Pass any enclosed form. Fail continuous round motions.

13. Which line is longer? (Not bigger.) Turn paper upside down and repeat. (Pass 3 of 3 or 5 of 6.)

14. Pass any lines crossing near midpoint.

15. Have child copy first. If failed, demonstrate.

When giving items 12, 14 and 15, do not name the forms. Do not demonstrate 12 and 14.

16. When scoring, each pair (2 arms, 2 legs, etc.) counts as one part.
17. Place one cube in cup and shake gently near the child's ear, but out of sight. Repeat for other ear.
18. Point to picture and have child name it. (No credit is given for sounds only.)
    If less than 4 pictures are named correctly, have child point to picture as each is named by tester.

 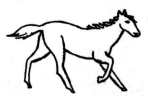 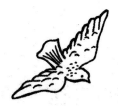 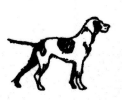 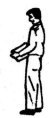

19. Using doll, tell child: Show me the nose, eyes, ears, mouth, hands, feet, tummy, hair. Pass 6 of 8.
20. Using pictures, ask child: Which one flies? . . . says meow? . . . talks? . . . barks? . . . gallops? Pass 2 of 5, 4 of 5.
21. Ask child: What do you do when you are cold? . . . tired? . . . hungry? Pass 2 of 3, 3 of 3.
22. Ask child: What do you do with a cup? What is a chair used for? What is a pencil used for?
    Action words must be included in answers.
23. Pass if child correctly placed <u>and</u> says how many blocks are on paper. (1, 5)
24. Tell child: Put block **on** table; **under** table; **in front of** me, **behind** me. Pass 4 of 4.
    (Do not help child by pointing, moving head or eyes.)
25. Ask child: What is a ball? . . . lake? . . . desk? . . . house? . . . banana? . . . curtain? . . . fence? . . . ceiling? Pass if defined in terms of use, shape, what it is made of, or general category (such as banana is fruit, not just yellow). Pass 5 of 8, 7 of 8.
26. Ask child: If a horse is big, a mouse is __? If fire is hot, ice is __? If the sun shines during the day, the moon shines during the __? Pass 2 of 3.
27. Child may use wall or rail only, not person. May not crawl.
28. Child must throw ball overhand 3 feet to within arm's reach of tester.
29. Child must perform standing broad jump over width of test sheet (8½ inches).
30. Tell child to walk forward, ⚫➤ heel within 1 inch of toe. Tester may demonstrate.
    Child must walk 4 consecutive steps.

FIGURE 20.6 *continued* Denver II

The Denver II is only one example of a developmental tool, but there are others that may be utilised in your particular jurisdiction. Importantly, whichever tool you use, continuity of care is needed to avoid fragmentation of care, and the schedule of assessment for each age and milestone followed. However, most developmental tools are often completed in isolation and do not consider a child's sociocultural environment, or take into account parents' observations or concerns. Parents or carers are generally more aware of their child achieving normal milestones, and if they are asked the right questions, they can provide accurate information about their child's strengths and weaknesses. Another screening tool that is now used (usually in conjunction with the standard development tools) is the Parents' Evaluation of Developmental Status (PEDS). An updated version, PEDS Revised (PEDS-R), was scheduled for release in late 2023. This is an evidence-based screening tool that prompts and addresses parental/carer observations and concerns about their child's development, health and wellbeing (The Royal Children's Hospital, 2018). PEDS-R is a simple questionnaire with 12 items (see revised banner in **Figure 20.7**), which the parent/carer completes, related to language, fine and gross motor skills, self-help, early academic skills, and mental health, social-emotional and behavioural risk. Implementation and application of this tool can assist in early identification of mental health, social emotional, behavioural risk and developmental delay/disorder risk and is suitable to use with infants and children up to eight years of age (The Royal Children's Hospital, 2018). Once completed by the parent or carer, it is scored in conjunction with the healthcare professional to clarify and interpret responses. If any issues are identified, further assessment and referral will be organised. For further information please visit the Centre for Community Child Health at The Royal Children's Hospital, http://www.peds.org.au.

Parents' Evaluation of Developmental Status-Revised®

PEDS-R® Directions

FIGURE 20.7 Parents' evaluation of developmental status response form banner

SOURCE: © AUTHORISED AUSTRALIAN VERSION, THE ROYAL CHILDREN'S HOSPITAL, CENTRE FOR COMMUNITY CHILD HEALTH. ADAPTED WITH PERMISSION FROM FRANCES PAGE GLASCOE AND PEDSTEST.COM LLC.

CLINICAL **REASONING**

Practice tip: Trans and gender diverse young people

Gender dysphoria is felt by individuals whose sense of being as either female or male differs from their physical body. When caring for the paediatric consumer/individual it is important that the nurse ensures a culturally responsive environment for all, acknowledging trans and gender diverse young people and their families.

Gender-affirming care is holistic care that considers diverse people's physical, mental and social health needs, including gender identity and expression in all healthcare encounters. When conducting a health assessment and physical examination with any young person, it is important that you work in a gender-affirming way. This can be achieved by:

> reflecting on your own beliefs and attitudes about gender, as this aids in understanding the experiences of trans and gender diverse young people, without imposing judgement

> providing culturally safe care – being sensitive, responsive and mindful of how gender identity influences interactions within healthcare systems, acknowledging power differentials between the consumer and the nurse

> not assuming a person's gender or pronouns – check if they use the same language and terminology, or whether there is other language that they'd prefer you to use to describe themselves, their experiences, and body. This can be done by introducing yourself and sharing your own pronouns: 'Hi, I'm Jacinta, I use they/them pronouns. How should I refer to you?'

>>

>>

> working systemically with families to support young people experiencing gender-related distress or dysphoria, to manage and alleviate distress including provision of gender-specific supports and advocacy.

(Adapted from Telfer, Tollit, Pace & Pang, 2020),

For further information and guidance on assessment, intervention, safety and other considerations for working with trans and gender diverse young people, access the *Australian Standards of Care and Treatment Guidelines for trans and gender diverse children and adolescents*, Version 1.3 at https://www.rch.org.au/uploadedFiles/Main/Content/adolescent-medicine/australian-standards-of-care-and-treatment-guidelines-for-trans-and-gender-diverse-children-and-adolescents.pdf

Paediatric pain assessment

Pain increases a child's sense of fear and vulnerability, an emotion that is already felt whenever a child is sick or injured. Thus, for children who cannot easily verbalise or communicate their experiences, pain potentially compounds the child's fear and feelings of vulnerability. Although several pain assessment tools have been developed and are available, none has been identified as the best in all situations. The individual child's age and developmental level should be taken into consideration when choosing a pain assessment tool. Two tools that have been successful in assessing children's pain are the Wong-Baker FACES Pain Rating Scale (FACES) (see **Figure 6.24**), and the Faces, Legs, Activity, Cry and Consolability (FLACC) scale (**Table 6.8**). Assessment tools should be used to assist in establishing and documenting a child's pain. However, they should be used in conjunction with nurses' observational and assessment skills (**Figure 20.8**).

Nurses should also be aware of behavioural and physiologic signs that may indicate a child is in pain; these include grimacing, posture and positioning of affected areas of the body. Parents and caregivers can also be helpful in determining whether their child's behaviour indicates discomfort or pain.

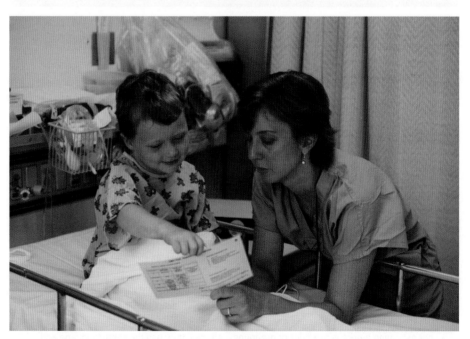

FIGURE 20.8 The nurse can use clinically validated tools to assess a child's pain.

Physical examination

Many assessment techniques for the child are similar to those for the adult. Refer to the specific system chapters for detailed explanations of assessment techniques covered in those chapters.

Techniques for approaching the paediatric consumer vary from one age group to the next. A basic principle during any physical assessment is building a trusting relationship; this can be done in a variety of ways. First, always explain what will be done prior to each portion of the assessment and answer questions honestly. Second, praise the consumer for positive behaviours, such as cooperating during assessment of the middle ear. Portraying a caring attitude will greatly influence both the consumer's and the caregiver's sense of trust. Show respect for the consumer as an individual and allow expression of feelings (whimpering, crying).

CLINICAL **REASONING**

Practice tip: Allaying childhood fears

Throughout childhood, children exhibit various fears and behaviours in response to past and present healthcare encounters. The following tips can calm fears and control behaviours children may exhibit during an examination.

Infant

The fear of parents leaving the room begins at around 6 months of age. Older infants experience a fear of strangers called stranger anxiety.

> Tip: Allow parents to be present and to hold their child during the examination. Speak in a calm, reassuring voice and allow the consumer to use security objects such as a pacifier, blanket or stuffed animal during the examination.

Toddler

Fear of strangers and parents leaving the room continues in the toddler age group. Clinginess is prevalent in toddlers. They may also become upset if their parent is feeling stressed. Additionally, fear of pain and discomfort usually begins in the toddler years.

> Tip: Allow parents to be present and to hold their child during the examination. Speak in a calm, reassuring voice. Allow use of security objects such as a pacifier, blanket or stuffed animal. Explain what is happening in simple words and allow time for the toddler to play, explore and express his or her feelings. Allowing choices will give the toddler a feeling of control.

Preschooler

This age group fears being left alone and experiencing pain. Behaviours exhibited include clinginess, temper tantrums, asking for help with things that were once done without help, baby talk, or thumb sucking (regression-type behaviours).

> Tip: Allow parents to be present and to hold their child during the examination. Speak in a calm, reassuring voice and let the child know what is going to be examined. Allow manipulation of equipment, and be honest about what is going to happen next.

School age

Behaviours once thought to be outgrown may often come back as mechanisms for coping with stress. Fears include separation from parents, pain and losing control. Some behaviours seen in school-age children include asking for help with things that were once done without help, acting out by yelling or screaming, and attention seeking.

> Tip: Allow parents to be present. Allow time for play or manipulation of examination equipment, and let the child ask questions, acknowledge feelings, allow choices, and set limits for losing control.

Adolescent

Adolescents may be sceptical concerning truth-telling and think healthcare professionals avoid telling the truth. The fear of pain and losing control may persist during adolescence. Privacy is a big factor during adolescent exams.

> Tip: Involve the adolescent in planning and decision making, allow the choice of the parent leaving during the examination, and encourage expressions of feelings.

Vital signs
General approach

1. The act of measuring vital signs is often disturbing to a young consumer. Past experiences influence the degree of cooperation you will encounter.
2. Vital signs may be obtained at the beginning of the assessment or during the assessment of a certain system. Blood pressure measurements are more threatening and should be performed towards the end of the assessment, preferably before using the otoscope.
3. If the child is particularly anxious, it is best to integrate the assessment of vital signs into the overall assessment.

CLINICAL **REASONING**

Practice tip: Obtaining blood pressure in children
It is not common practice to take blood pressure in younger children unless:
> they are seriously overweight or underweight
> they are in the ICU (intensive care unit)/critical care facility
> they have/had any known neurological, heart, lung or circulatory problems.
　If you do have to take a young paediatric consumer's blood pressure, never use the phrase 'blood pressure' because the child may equate this with venipuncture. Say instead, 'I am going to hug your arm with this cuff' or, to the older child, 'I am going to measure your pressure'.

Temperature
You need to be proficient in measuring axillary, oral and tympanic temperatures. Accurate oral temperature is difficult to obtain in most toddlers and pre-schoolers; therefore, it is more common for a tympanic or axillary temperature to be taken. Axillary temperature, although quick and painless, is often less reliable than oral or tympanic temperatures.

Axillary

E 1. When taking a child's temperature, have the child sit or lie on the caregiver's lap to free your hands for other observations or to prepare for the next area of assessment.
2. Explain to the consumer that this type of measurement does not hurt. To pass time when taking axillary or oral temperature, ask the caregiver to read the child a story.

N A P See Chapter 6.

Respiratory rate

1. Try to obtain the rate early in the assessment, when the consumer is most cooperative and not crying.
2. If the consumer is crying, the measurement will not be accurate and should be retaken.
3. Remember to observe the expansion of the abdomen in infants and toddlers.

N A P See Chapter 6.

Physical growth
Weight
Use the same scale at each visit, if possible, to prevent variations in serial weight checks.

E 1. If using an infant scale, cover it with a paper protector.
2. Balance or zero the scale.

E Examination　**N** Normal findings　**A** Abnormal findings　**P** Pathophysiology

E 3. Place infants supine and young toddlers seated on the scale (**Figure 20.9**). Always keep one hand on the child to prevent falls, and lift your hand slightly when obtaining the actual weight reading.

4. Preschoolers and young school-age children can wear street clothes to be weighed (**Figure 20.10**). Have the older child undress, don a paper or cloth gown, and step on the standard platform scale.

5. Note and record weight. (This should be plotted on a growth chart for reference, such as CDC/WHO Children's growth chart.)

N Usually, neonates lose approximately 10% of birth weight by the third or fourth day after birth, then regain it by 2 weeks of age. This expected change in weight is called **physiological weight loss**, and it is due to a loss of extracellular fluid and **meconium**, a dark green, sticky, stool-like substance excreted from the rectum within the first 24 hours after birth.

A A newborn weight less than the 10th gestational age percentile is considered abnormal.

P A newborn whose growth has been retarded in utero is referred to as small for gestational age (SGA). Potential causes include alcohol, drug or tobacco abuse by the mother, and certain genetic syndromes.

A A newborn weight greater than the 90th gestational age percentile is abnormal.

P A diabetic mother or a genetic predisposition may be responsible for producing a large for gestational age (LGA) newborn.

A A weight below the 5th or above the 95th percentiles warrants investigation, as does the consumer who falls two standard deviations below his or her own established curve. Any such finding is abnormal.

P Possible causes include organic or nonorganic failure to thrive, congenital or cyanotic heart disease, cystic fibrosis (CF), **fetal alcohol syndrome** and malabsorption diseases.

Length and height

Recumbent length is measured for children less than 2 years old.

E 1. Position the measuring board flat on the examination table.

2. Place the child's head at the top of the board and the child's heels at the foot of the board, making sure the legs are fully extended (see **Figure 20.11A**).

3. Measure and record the length.

4. If a board is not available, place the child in a supine position and mark lines on the paper at the tip of the head and at the heel, making sure the legs are fully extended.

5. Measure between the lines and record.

Height for all other age groups can be measured in the same fashion as for an adult. **Figure 20.11B** shows the height of a preschooler being measured. (These measurements should be documented on a growth chart (CDC or WHO) and compared to previous recordings.)

N Height varies widely, and normal growth is gauged by using the growth charts. Most children fall somewhere between the 5th and 97th percentile band, and consistent growth along any percentile band shows normal growth for that individual.

A A height below the 5th or above the 95th percentile warrants investigation, as does the consumer who falls two standard deviations below his or her own established curve. Any such finding is abnormal.

P Possible causes include organic or nonorganic failure to thrive, congenital or cyanotic heart disease, CF, fetal alcohol syndrome, and malabsorption diseases.

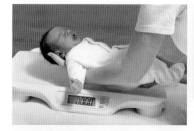

FIGURE 20.9 Measuring weight in the infant
SHUTTERSTOCK.COM/BENEDA MIROSLAV

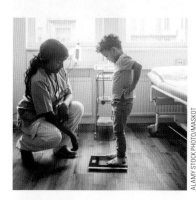

FIGURE 20.10 Measuring weight in the preschooler
ALAMY STOCK PHOTO/MASKOT

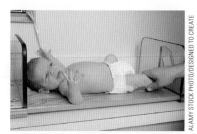

A. Recumbent length in infant
ALAMY STOCK PHOTO/DESIGNED TO CREATE

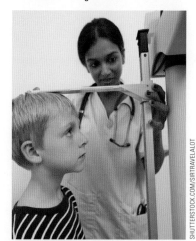

B. Height in pre-schooler
SHUTTERSTOCK.COM/SIRTRAVELALOT

FIGURE 20.11 Measuring length and height in children

E Examination **N** Normal findings **A** Abnormal findings **P** Pathophysiology

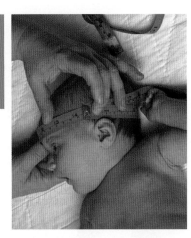

FIGURE 20.12 Measuring head circumference

Head circumference

Head circumference is measured in all children less than 2 years of age or serially in consumers with known or suspected hydrocephalus. Measuring head circumference is an invaluable tool in the infant with suspected cessation of brain growth.

E
1. Place the consumer in a sitting or supine position.
2. Using a tape measure, measure anteriorly from above the eyebrows and around posteriorly to the occipital protuberance (**Figure 20.12**). (These measurements should be documented on a growth chart (CDC or WHO) and compared to previous recordings.)

N Normal average head growth is 1 to 1.5 cm per month during the first year. Premature infants often have small head circumferences.

A **Microcephaly**, a condition characterised by a small brain with a resultant small head, is an abnormal finding.

P Microcephaly is a congenital finding associated with a mental deficit. Microcephaly can be caused by a variety of disorders including intrauterine infections, drug or alcohol ingestion (fetal alcohol syndrome) during pregnancy, and genetic defects.

A Hydrocephalus (enlarged head) is indicated when an infant's or young child's head circumference is above the 95th percentile and crosses over the consumer's established percentile lines from one serial measurement to the next. Hydrocephalus is abnormal. Note if the eyes are looking downwards ('setting sun' sign) and the sclera is visible above the iris.

P Hydrocephalus is characterised by an imbalance in cerebrospinal fluid (CSF) production and reabsorption. Hydrocephalus may result from embryological malformations of the nervous system. Congenital hydrocephalus can also be caused by syphilis, rubella, toxoplasmosis or cytomegalovirus. Bacterial meningitis and tumours are acquired causes of hydrocephalus. The setting sun sign results from progressive enlargement of the lateral and third ventricles related to excessive accumulation of CSF.

Apgar scoring

The **Apgar score** system provides a quick method to assess the need for newborn resuscitation in the delivery room. An Apgar score is given to a newborn at 1 and 5 minutes after birth. Perform steps 1–5 at 1 minute following birth; add the score in each category for the total. Repeat at 5 minutes following birth.

E
1. Auscultate the heart rate for 1 full minute.
2. Measure the degree of respiratory effort.
3. Evaluate muscle tone by attempting to straighten each extremity individually.
4. Evaluate the newborn's reflex irritability. Use a flicking motion of two fingers against the newborn's sole to rate reflex irritability.
5. Inspect the newborn's colour.

N A score of 8 to 10 demonstrates that the newborn is in good condition. **Table 20.3** outlines the scoring system for each of the five areas assessed.

TABLE 20.3 Apgar scoring

HEART RATE	RESPIRATORY RATE	TONE	REFLEX IRRITABILITY	COLOUR
Absent = 0	Apnoea = 0	Flaccid = 0	No response = 0	Cyanosis = 0
<100 = 1	Slow, irregular rate = 1	Some degree of flexion = 1	Grimace = 1	Body pink, extremities acrocyanotic = 1
>100 = 2	Crying vigorously = 2	Full flexion = 2	Crying = 2	Completely pink = 2

 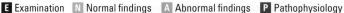

A A moderately depressed newborn earns a score of 4 to 7. A score of 0 to 3 indicates that the newborn is severely depressed and needs immediate resuscitation. Both findings are abnormal.

P A low score can be the result of one or numerous problems. Prematurity, central nervous system depression, blood or meconium in the trachea, maternal history of drug abuse, certain drugs that are given to the mother in preparation for delivery and that cross over and cause fetal depression, congenital complete heart block and congenital heart disease are some of the potential aetiologies for a low Apgar score.

CLINICAL REASONING

Practice tip: Prevalence of birth defects
Approximately one in every 31 babies born in Australia is born with a birth defect (AIHW, 2022d). The most common of these defects involve the heart (congenital heart defects), spine (spina bifida), lip/palate (cleft lip and/or palate), urinary meatus (hypospadias) and chromosomes. Taking a thorough family history of any major birth defects enables the healthcare provider to better assess potential risk factors and give advice on preventative measures for future pregnancies. For example, a mother whose baby was born with spina bifida can be counselled to take folic acid supplementation prior to conception to reduce the risk of having another child born with a neural tube defect.

CLINICAL REASONING

Practice tip: Suspected child abuse – integumentary assessment
When assessing the skin:
> Observe for injuries in a location the child cannot reach, such as the back.
> Examine for unusual markings (e.g. marks produced by irons, belts, electrical cords, cigarettes or teeth).
> Check for excessive bruising and numerous bruises in various stages of healing.
> Look for hot water scalding marks, which present as even lines across the skin (usually on the legs or buttocks).
> Check extremities for limited range of motion and tenderness, which can be related to fractures.
Note: The legal duty of nurses in reporting suspected child abuse and neglect varies across Australian and New Zealand jurisdictions. For this reason, nurses must be familiar with the legislation that exists in their area of practice.

Skin
Inspection
Colour

E Observe the colour of the body, especially at the tip of the nose, the external ear, the lips, the hands and the feet. These areas are prominent locations for detecting cyanosis or jaundice.

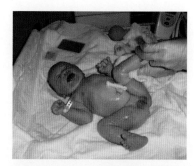
FIGURE 20.13 Acrocyanosis in a newborn

N The skin of a newborn is reddish in colour for the first 24 hours and then changes to varying shades of pale pink to pink to brown or black, depending on the child's race. It is normal for dark-skinned newborns to have a ruddy appearance and for light-skinned newborns to exhibit a bluish-purple colour of the hands and feet while the rest of the body remains pink. This is called **acrocyanosis** (Figure 20.13). It may disappear with warming. **Mongolian spots** (congenital dermal melanocytosis) (Figure 20.14), deep blue pigmentation over the lumbar and sacral areas of the spine, over the buttocks, and, sometimes, over the upper back or shoulders in newborns of African, Latino or Asian descent, are extremely common and not to be confused with ecchymosis or signs of child abuse.

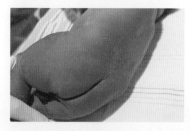
FIGURE 20.14 Mongolian spots (congenital dermal melanocytosis)

E Examination **N** Normal findings **A** Abnormal findings **P** Pathophysiology Advanced Assessment

A A blue hue is abnormal.

P Cyanosis in the newborn is often associated with a congenital heart defect secondary to abnormal mixing of arterial and venous blood. In the older child with unrepaired heart disease, cyanosis may be a sign of decreasing levels of oxygen saturation.

A A yellowing of the skin or sclera is abnormal.

P Physiological jaundice of the newborn occurs on the second or third day of life. This type of jaundice results from increased levels of serum bilirubin. The newborn's body is unable to remove the bilirubin, thus producing a yellow cast or hue to the skin of light-skinned infants and to the sclera of both light- and dark-skinned infants.

P Pathological jaundice of the newborn occurs within the first 24 hours of life. Possible causes of pathological jaundice include Rh/ABO incompatibility and maternal infections (rubella, herpes, syphilis or toxoplasmosis). The pathophysiological response occurs because there is a deficiency or inactivity of bilirubin glucuronyl transferase in the newborn.

P Breast milk jaundice occurs within the first 2 weeks of life, with the onset being 4 to 5 days after birth. The aetiology is not clear, but breast milk may contain an inhibitor of bilirubin conjugation.

A It is abnormal when the light-skinned newborn lies on one side and the dependent half becomes red or ruddy and the upper half turns pale in colour. In dark-skinned children, the dependent half becomes a ruddy colour and the upper half seems normal.

P **Harlequin colour change** is a benign condition thought to be a result of poor vasomotor control; it occurs between 48 and 96 hours after birth.

A Erythema of the palms or soles, oedema of the hands or feet, or periungual desquamation is found in consumers presenting with Kawasaki disease (mucocutaneous lymph node syndrome). In order for a practitioner to diagnose Kawasaki disease, the child must present with fever for 5 days and with four of the five diagnostic criteria. Other than the previously mentioned signs above, other signs include bilateral nonexudative conjunctival injection; at least one of the mucous membrane changes including injected or fissured lips, injected pharynx or strawberry tongue; polymorphous exanthem; and acute nonsuppurative cervical lymphadenopathy.

P The cause of Kawasaki disease is unknown. Coronary artery vasculitis is a major concern as the disease progresses.

Lesions

E N See Chapter 8.

A Lesions that are usually symmetrical, scaly, erythematous patches or plaques with possible exudation and crusting are abnormal.

P Eczema or atopic dermatitis (AD) is a common abnormal skin disorder involving inflammation of the epidermis and superficial dermis. Inhaled allergens such as pollens, moulds or dust mites, or food allergens are thought to induce mast-cell responses that cause AD.

A Small, maculopapular lesions on an erythematous base, wheals, and vesicles that erupt on the newborn are abnormal.

P Erythema toxicum is a benign rash. The cause is unknown.

A Flat, deep, irregular, localised, pink areas in light-skinned children and deeper red areas in dark-skinned children are abnormal.

E Examination   **N** Normal findings   **A** Abnormal findings   **P** Pathophysiology

P **Telangiectatic naevi**, commonly known as **stork bites**, appear on the back of the neck, lower occiput, upper eyelids and upper lip. The cause of telangiectatic naevi is capillary dilatation.

A Diffuse redness, papules, vesicles, oedema scaling and ulcerations on the area covered by a baby's nappy are abnormal.

P Possible causes of nappy rash (dermatitis) include faecal enzymes, irritated skin, stool consistency and frequency, candida, cleansing agents, sensitive skin and poor nutrition.

A Vesicles located on the palms of hands, soles of feet and in the mouth are abnormal. A papular erythematous rash may also be on the buttocks.

P Hand-foot-mouth disease is caused by coxsackievirus A16.

A A dark black tuft of hair or a dimple over the lumbosacral area is abnormal.

P The neural tube fails to fuse at about the fourth week of gestation and causes a vertebral defect known as spina bifida occulta.

A A myelomeningocoele is an open spina bifida lesion in which there is either no skin covering or neural tissue covered only by a thin membrane.

P Myelomeningocoele has been associated with maternal diabetes mellitus, obesity, fever, hyperthermia, and use of valproic acid and carbamazepine. The increased incidence of neural tube defects seen in some lower socioeconomic groups suggests that nutritional deficiencies, particularly lack of folic acid, may play a significant role in aetiology. Neural tube defects are presumably caused by failure of the neural tube to close between the third and fourth week of gestation, resulting in abnormalities of the brain and spinal cord.

REFLECTION IN PRACTICE

Suspected child abuse
A young mother of five children brings her 2-year-old child, who is wheezing and having difficulty breathing, into the emergency department. The mother tells you she was up all night with the child. On auscultation of the posterior lung fields, you note three 4 mm, rounded areas on the upper back that appear to be second-degree burns. There is erythema and tissue destruction surrounding the borders of each area.
> What would be your first reaction?
> How would you proceed with the assessment? What questions would you ask the mother?
> What is your institution's policy on reporting suspected child abuse?

Palpation
Texture

E 1. Use the finger pads to palpate the skin.
2. The technique of palpating the skin of a younger child can be accomplished by playing games. For example, use the finger pads to walk up the abdomen and touch the nose.

N Skin of the paediatric consumer normally is smooth and soft. **Milia**, plugged sebaceous glands, present as small, white papules in the newborn. Milia occur mainly on the head, especially the cheeks and nose. Preterm infants have vernix caseosa.

A An oily texture and appearance to the skin, particularly the face, chest and back, can start as early as 8 to 9 years of age as puberty is beginning.

P An oily skin during puberty is caused by a surge of sex hormones called androgens. Genetics also play a role in the amount of oil that oil glands produce.

E Examination **N** Normal findings **A** Abnormal findings **P** Pathophysiology

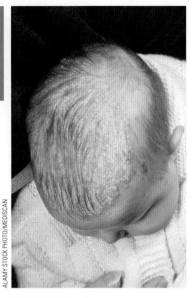

FIGURE 20.15 Cradle cap

ALAMY STOCK PHOTO/MEDISCAN

Hair
Inspection
Lesions

E **N** See Chapter 8.

A Yellow, greasy-appearing scales on the scalp of a light-skinned infant are abnormal. In dark-skinned infants, the scaling is light grey.

P Seborrheic dermatitis (**cradle cap**) is possibly related to increased epidermal tissue growth (see **Figure 20.15**).

HEALTH EDUCATION

Head lice

About one in five children is infested with head lice (*Pediculus capitis*) at any one time. These small egg-laying insects are commonly found on the human head; lice eggs (called nits) live on the hair and adhere to the hair shaft close to the scalp. These eggs hatch after 7–10 days and start to feed by sucking blood from the scalp. They then begin to lay eggs and the cycle commences again. They are spread by direct contact and children are often asymptomatic, but may complain of an itchy scalp. Lice are very contagious, so carers should be educated to frequently systematically examine their child's head and hair. If lice are found, all family members should have their hair examined and be treated at the same time. To break the cycle, medicated treatment is required (see **Figure 20.16**).

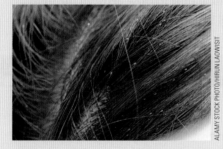 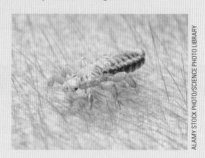

ALAMY STOCK PHOTO/HIRUN LAOWISIT

ALAMY STOCK PHOTO/SCIENCE PHOTO LIBRARY

FIGURE 20.16 Head lice

Head
Inspection
Shape and symmetry

E With the consumer sitting upright either in the caregiver's arms or on the examination table, observe the symmetry of the frontal, parietal and occipital prominences.

N The shape of a child's head is symmetrical without depressions or protrusions. The anterior fontanelle normally may pulsate with every heartbeat. The Asian infant generally has a flattened occiput, more so than infants of other races.

A A flattened occipital bone with resultant hair loss over the same area is abnormal.

P A prolonged supine position places pressure on the occipital bone.

Head control

E 1. Assess head control while the consumer is in the position used for assessing shape and symmetry.
2. With the head unsupported, observe the consumer's ability to hold the head erect.

N At 3 months of age, the infant is able to hold the head steady without lag.

E Examination **N** Normal findings **A** Abnormal findings **P** Pathophysiology

A Lack of head control is evidenced by the infant who is unable to hold the head steady while in a sitting position and is abnormal. Head lag beyond 4 to 6 months of age should be further investigated.

P Documented prematurity, hydrocephalus, and illnesses causing developmental delays are possible causes of head lag.

Palpation

Fontanelle

E 1. Place the child in an upright position.
2. Using the second or third finger pad, palpate the anterior fontanelle at the junction of the sagittal, coronal and frontal sutures.
3. Palpate the posterior fontanelle at the junction of the sagittal and lambdoidal sutures.
4. Assess for bulging, pulsations and size. To obtain accurate measurements, the consumer should not be crying. Crying will produce a distorted, full, bulging appearance.

N The anterior fontanelle is soft and flat. Size ranges from 4 to 6 cm at birth. The fontanelle gradually closes between 9 and 19 months of age. The posterior fontanelle is also soft and flat. The size ranges from 0.5 to 1.5 cm at birth. The posterior fontanelle gradually closes between 1 and 3 months of age. It is normal to feel pulsations related to the peripheral pulse.

A Palpation reveals a bulging, tense fontanelle, which is abnormal.

P Signs of increased intracranial pressure are associated with meningitis and an increased amount of CSF.

A A sunken, depressed fontanelle is abnormal.

P A sunken, depressed fontanelle is a sign of dehydration.

A A wide anterior fontanelle in a child older than 2½ years is an abnormal finding.

P An anterior fontanelle that remains open after 2½ years of age may indicate disease such as rickets, which is a bone disorder caused by deficient vitamin D, calcium or phosphate levels. Other causes of enlarged fontanelle include congenital hypothyroidism, Down syndrome and hydrocephalus.

Suture lines

E 1. With the finger pads, palpate the sagittal suture line. This runs from the anterior to the posterior portion of the skull in a midline position.
2. Palpate the coronal suture line. This runs along both sides of the head, starting at the anterior fontanelle.
3. Palpate the lambdoidal suture. The lambdoidal suture runs along both sides of the head, starting at the posterior fontanelle.
4. Ascertain if these suture lines are open, united or overlapping.

N Grooves or ridges between sections of the skull are normally palpated up to 6 months of age.

A Suture lines that overlap or override one another, giving the head an unusual shape, warrant further investigation.

P Craniosynostosis is premature ossification of suture lines, in which there is early formation and fusion of skull bones. Craniosynostosis may be caused by metabolic disorders or may be a secondary consequence of microcephaly.

Surface characteristics

E 1. With the finger pads, palpate the skull in the same manner as the fontanelles and suture lines.
2. Note surface oedema and contour of the cranium.

N The skin covering the cranium is flush against the skull and without oedema.

E Examination   N Normal findings   A Abnormal findings   P Pathophysiology

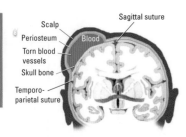

FIGURE 20.17 Cephalohaematoma (section)

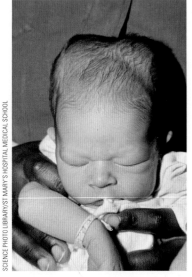

FIGURE 20.18 Cephalohaematoma

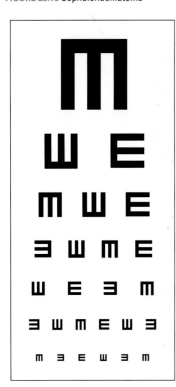

FIGURE 20.19 Tumbling E chart

A A softening of the outer layer of the cranial bones behind and above the ears combined with a ping-pong ball sensation as the area is pressed in gently with the fingers is indicative of craniotabes, an abnormal finding.

P Craniotabes is associated with rickets, syphilis, hydrocephaly or hypervitaminosis A.

A A localised, subcutaneous swelling over one of the cranial bones of a newborn is referred to as a **cephalohaematoma** (Figures 20.17 and 20.18) and is abnormal. This abnormality differs from other surface characteristics in that oedema does not cross suture lines with this condition. Varying degrees of swelling can persist up to 3 months.

P Cephalohaematomas acquired during forceps deliveries are due to subperiosteal bleeding and usually resolve within a couple of weeks, but may persist longer.

A Swelling over the occipitoparietal region of the skull is abnormal.

P **Caput succedaneum** results from pressure over the occipitoparietal region during a prolonged delivery. It usually resolves within 1 to 2 weeks after birth.

A **Moulding** can occur in conjunction with caput succedaneum.

P The parietal bone overrides the frontal bone as a result of induced pressure during delivery. It should resolve within 1 week of delivery.

Eyes
General approach

1. From infancy until about 8 to 10 years, you should assess the eyes towards the end of the assessment, with the exception of testing vision, which should be done first. Remember that the child's attention span is short, and attentiveness decreases the longer you evaluate. Children generally are not cooperative for eyes, ears and throat assessments.
2. Place the young infant, preschool, school-age or adolescent consumer on the examination table. The older infant or the toddler can be held by the caregiver.
3. Become proficient at performing fundoscopic assessments on adults prior to assessing the paediatric consumer.

Vision screening
General approach

1. The adult Snellen chart can be used on children as young as 6 years, provided they are able to read the alphabet. The E chart is used for a consumer over 3 years of age or any child who cannot read the alphabet (Figure 20.19).
2. Test every 1 to 2 years through adolescence.
3. If the child resists wearing a cover patch over the eye, make a game out of wearing the patch. For example, the young child could pretend to be a pirate exploring new territory. Use your imagination to think of a fantasy situation.

Tumbling E chart

E 1. Ask the child to point an arm in the direction the E is pointing.
2. Observe for squinting.

N Vision is 6/12 from 2 to approximately 6 years of age, when it approaches the normal 6/6 acuity. Refer the consumer to an ophthalmologist if results are 6/12 or greater in a child 3 years of age or 6/9 or greater in a child 6 years or older, or if results vary by two or more lines between eyes even if in the passing range.

A P See Chapter 10.

Strabismus screening

The Hirschberg test and the cover/uncover test screen for strabismus. The latter is the more definitive test.

Hirschberg test

E N See Chapter 10.

A It is abnormal for the light reflection to be displaced to the outer margin of the cornea as the eye deviates inwards (**Figure 20.20**).

P Esotropia is thought to be congenital. Some theories suggest that neurological factors contribute to its development.

A It is abnormal for the light reflection to be displaced to the inner margin of the cornea as the eye deviates outwards.

P Exotropia can result from eye muscle fatigue or can be congenital.

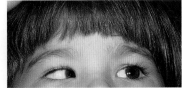

FIGURE 20.20 Infantile esotropia

COURTESY OF THE ARMED FORCES INSTITUTE OF PATHOLOGY.

Cover/uncover test

E See Chapter 10.

N Neither eye moves when the occluder is being removed. Infants less than 6 months of age display strabismus due to poor neuromuscular control of eye muscles.

A It is abnormal for one or both eyes to move to focus on the penlight during assessment. Assume strabismus is present.

P Strabismus after 6 months of age is abnormal and indicates eye muscle weakness.

Colour vision

Preschoolers aged 3–6 years old should have their ability to distinguish colours assessed during their annual check-up. The two most commonly used colour vision assessment tools are the Ishihara colour test and the Colour Vision Testing Made Easy test. The Ishihara test places numbers on a pseudoisochromatic-coloured background. The Colour Vision Testing Made Easy tool also uses a pseudoisochromatic-coloured background, but uses objects that are readily recognisable to a preschooler. Objects such as a car, boat, house and dog are used.

E 1. Show the child the colour vision test plate.
2. Have the child identify the number or object within 3 seconds.

N The child should be able to correctly identify the number or object within 3 seconds.

A If the child is unable to correctly identify the number or object within 3 seconds, a colour vision deficiency, or colour blindness, should be suspected.

P This is a congenital finding in 5–8% of males and 0.5% of females. A small number of individuals with colour blindness acquire the condition through eye, nerve or brain conditions.

Inspection

Eyelids

E 1. Sit at the consumer's eye level.
2. Observe for symmetrical palpebral fissures and position of eyelids in relation to the iris.

N The palpebral fissures of both eyes are positioned symmetrically. The upper eyelid normally covers a small portion of the iris, and the lower lid meets the iris. Epicanthal folds are normally present in Asian children.

A It is abnormal for a portion of the sclera to be seen above the iris.

E Examination **N** Normal findings **A** Abnormal findings **P** Pathophysiology   Advanced Assessment

P The sclera is exposed above the iris in hydrocephalus. As the forehead becomes prominent, the eyebrows and eyelids are drawn up, creating a setting sun appearance of the child's eyes.

A A fold of skin covering the inner canthus and lacrimal caruncle is abnormal.

P During embryonic development, the fold of skin slants in a downward direction towards the nose. This is found in a child with Down syndrome. Epicanthal folds and short palpebral fissures are seen in a child with fetal alcohol syndrome.

Lacrimal apparatus

E **N** See Chapter 10.

A The consumer's caregiver reports that the child is unable to produce tears, an abnormal finding.

P The lacrimal ducts should be patent by 3 months of age. Dacryocystitis results when the distal end of the membranous lacrimal duct fails to open or a blockage occurs elsewhere.

CLINICAL **REASONING**

Practice tip: Lid eversion in children

Lid eversion is not performed in children unless you are assessing for an infection or foreign body. This is so that children are not unnecessarily distressed. It is also a high-risk procedure in young children, because they may need to be restrained or sedated; therefore the risk of causing further injury is increased in this group. If performed, the technique is the same as for an adult.

Anterior segment structures

Sclera

E See Chapter 10.

N The newborn exhibits a bluish-tinged sclera related to thinness of the fibrous tissue. The sclera is white in light-skinned children and a slightly darker colour in some dark-skinned children.

A **P** See Chapter 10.

Iris

E Conduct the examination in the same manner as for an adult.

N Up to about 6 months of age, the colour of the iris is blue or slate grey in light-skinned infants and brownish in dark-skinned infants. Between 6 and 12 months of age, complete transition of iris colour has occurred.

A Small white flecks, called Brushfield's spots, noted around the perimeter of the iris are abnormal.

P Brushfield's spots are found on the iris of the consumer with Down syndrome. The spots develop during embryonic maturation.

Pupils

E See Chapter 10.

N When the pupils' reaction to light is assessed, a newborn will normally blink and flex the head closer to the body. This is called the optical blink reflex.

A **P** See Chapter 10.

E Examination **N** Normal findings **A** Abnormal findings **P** Pathophysiology Advanced Assessment

Lens

E Examine the paediatric consumer as you would the adult consumer.

N The lens is transparent.

A A white or pearly grey appearance is abnormal.

P This finding can be caused by a congenital or acquired cataract (**Figure 20.21**).

Ears
Auditory testing
General approach

Hearing tests are available for newborns and even mandated in some states.

1. Prior to 3 years of age, the following are a few parameters for evaluating hearing.
   a. Does the child react to a loud noise?
   b. Does the child react to the caregiver's voice by cooing, smiling or turning eyes and head towards the voice?
   c. Does the child try to imitate sounds?
   d. Can the child imitate words and sounds?
   e. Can the child follow directions?
   f. Does the child respond to sounds not directed at him or her?
2. Perform auditory testing at about 3 to 4 years of age or when the child can follow directions.

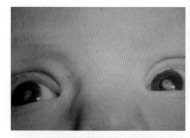

FIGURE 20.21 Paediatric cataracts
COURTESY OF THE CENTERS FOR DISEASE CONTROL AND PREVENTION (CDC)/PHIL.

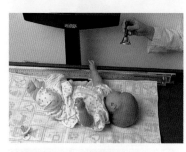

FIGURE 20.22 This 2-month-old infant is able to localise the sound of a bell.

PUTTING IT IN CONTEXT

Impact of chronic otitis media

You are the child health nurse in a remote community centre in Queensland. An Aboriginal mother brings her 21-month-old son for a health visit, stating he has been diagnosed with bilateral middle ear infections (otitis media). The mother asks you if the child's hearing will develop normally, as this is the child's fifth infection in four months. The mother starts to cry and tells the nurse that she had recurrent ear infections as a child that led to hearing impairment and subsequent language delays and speech impediments. The mother does not want her child to experience these difficulties.

In Australia, it has been reported that Aboriginal and Torres Strait Islander children experience these infections earlier, more frequently, more severely, and more persistently than other children, with rates of up to 90% in some communities (AIHW, 2022e). With this in mind, what other aspects of assessment and referral are required for this consumer?

For further information, see 'Deadly Kids | Deadly Futures (2016). Queensland's Aboriginal and Torres Strait Islander Child Ear and Hearing Health Framework 2016–2026' (Queensland Government. https://www.childrens.health.qld.gov.au/wp-content/uploads/PDF/deadly-ears/deadly-kids-futures-fw.pdf).

External ear
Inspection of pinna position

E **N** See Chapter 11.

A The top of the ear is below the imaginary line drawn from the outer canthus to the occiput.

P Kidneys and ears are formed at the same time in embryonic development. If a child's ears are low set, renal anomalies must be ruled out. Low-set ears can also occur in Down syndrome.

E Examination   **N** Normal findings   **A** Abnormal findings   **P** Pathophysiology   Advanced Assessment

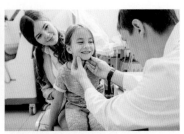

A. Preschooler in a sitting position

SHUTTERSTOCK.COM/KUZNETSOV DMITRIY

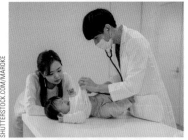

SHUTTERSTOCK.COM/MAROKE

B. Preschooler in a supine position

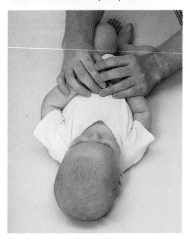

C. Infant in a supine position

FIGURE 20.23 Restraining the child for the otoscopic examination

Internal ear

Inspection

E 1. A cooperative consumer may be allowed to sit for the assessment. A young child may be held as shown in **Figure 20.23A**.

2. Restrain the uncooperative young consumer by placing him or her supine on a firm surface (**Figure 20.23B**). Instruct the caregiver or assistant to hold the consumer's arms up near the head, embracing the elbow joints on both sides of either arm. Restrain the infant by having the caregiver hold the infant's hands down (**Figure 20.23C**).

3. With your thumb and forefinger grasping the otoscope, use the lateral side of the hand to prevent the head from jerking. Your other hand can also be used to stabilise the consumer's head.

4. Pull the lower auricle down and out to straighten the canal. This technique is used in children up to about 3 years of age. Use the adult technique after age 3.

5. Insert the speculum about 0.5 cm to 1.25 cm, depending on the consumer's age.

6. Suspected otitis media must be evaluated with a pneumatic bulb attached to the side of the otoscope's light source.

7. Select a larger speculum to make a tight seal and prevent air from escaping from the canal.

8. Gently squeeze the bulb attachment to introduce air into the canal.

9. Observe the tympanic membrane for movement.

N A P See Chapter 11.

CLINICAL **REASONING**

Screening newborn babies' hearing

Hearing impairment in both ears (bilateral) is found in approximately 1 in 1000 newborns (Queensland Health, 2020). Screening is recommended for all newborns prior to discharge from hospital, to assist in identifying hearing impairments early. If a hearing impairment is present, interventions should commence as soon as possible to ameliorate speech, language and learning development challenges. The hearing test uses the automated auditory brainstem response (AABR). This is done by placing 4 to 5 separate electrodes on the head and then small earphones are placed over the baby's ears and various sounds are presented. The AABR measures the brainstem's physiological response to these sounds.

Nose

Inspection

General approach

1. Conduct the inspection of the nose utilising the same positioning used for the child ear examination.

2. Observe the mucosa, nasal septum and presence of drainage.

E 1. Gently push the consumer's nose upwards with one finger. Insert the speculum gently into the nare. Avoid touching the nasal septum with the speculum.

2. Note the colour of the mucosa, colour and consistency of drainage, presence of septal deviation, or foreign body.

N The nasal mucosa is pink or dull red. There is no evidence of polyps, foreign bodies, nasal drainage or septal deviation.

A Nasal mucosa that is pale pink, grey or blue may indicate allergic rhinitis.

E Examination   **N** Normal findings   **A** Abnormal findings   **P** Pathophysiology

P Allergic rhinitis is triggered by breathing in an allergen such as pollen or dust.

A A pearly grey-coloured grape-like growth noted within the nasal mucosa is abnormal.

P The cause of polyps is unknown but may be attributed to several factors including allergies and rhinosinusitis. Some individuals, including those with asthma, chronic rhinosinusitis or cystic fibrosis, are at greater risk for developing polyps.

A Persistent odour and unilateral nasal drainage in a child with a suspected foreign body warrants further evaluation by a trained clinician.

P A foreign body lodged in a nasal cavity may need to be removed while the paediatric consumer is under light sedation.

A A nasal septum that is not straight is abnormal. The septum may appear bowed into the nasal passage.

P Septal deviation may cause snoring, difficult nasal breathing, excessive nasal drainage, nosebleeds, rhinosinusitis and headaches.

Mouth and throat

Inspection

Lips

E 1. Follow the technique described in Chapter 11.
   2. Observe if the lip edges meet.

N The lip edges should meet.

A It is abnormal if the lip edges do not meet.

P Cleft lip is seen as a separated area of lip tissue (**Figure 20.24**). It involves the upper lip and sometimes extends into the nostril. A cleft lip is an obvious finding during a newborn assessment. It occurs mainly on the left side and is more frequently found in males. A cleft lip develops during the fifth to sixth week after fertilisation. Genetics plays a small role in aetiology.

A A thin upper lip is abnormal.

P A child with fetal alcohol syndrome exhibits this finding, as well as a flat and elongated philtrum.

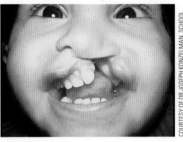

COURTESY OF DR JOSEPH KONZELMAN, SCHOOL OF DENTISTRY, MEDICAL COLLEGE OF GEORGIA

FIGURE 20.24 Cleft lip

HEALTH EDUCATION

Reducing the risk of choking in children
The airway of an infant or toddler is small and approximately the size of their 'pinky' fingers. Fresh grapes, uncut hot dogs with the skin on, popcorn and peanuts are common foods that can cause choking. These foods should not be given to young children.

For comprehensive information related to managing airway obstruction (choking) refer to ANZCOR Guideline 4 – Airway (https://resus.org.au/guidelines/).

URGENT FINDING ⚠

Stridor in children
The anatomical and physiological features of infants and young children make them more susceptible to airway obstruction when compared to adults. The upper and lower airways are smaller and more prone to occlusion due to secretions and oedema. A common presenting symptom in the paediatric population is acute stridor, which is significant and requires prompt emergency assessment and intervention. Stridor is a harsh, vibrating noise

 >>

---

that is made when air is forced through restricted or narrowed airways. An inspiratory stridor can be symptomatic of obstruction above the glottis, and an expiratory stridor suggests obstruction in the lower trachea.

Symptoms will depend on the underlying cause (e.g. croup, epiglottitis, or an inhaled foreign body) and may include tachypnoea, increased use of accessory muscles, subcostal and intercostal retraction, tracheal tug, nasal flaring, wheezing and noisy breathing. Carers may report the child has increased irritability, and may also be febrile. A sudden onset of stridor in an otherwise well child can suggest the presence of an inhaled foreign body.

To avoid further distress, initial assessment should be 'hands off' as much as possible. Treatment will depend on the cause, and should follow the healthcare facility guidelines.

Further deterioration can be indicated by increased work of breathing, hypoxia, fatigue or altered level of consciousness. In this situation, urgent intervention is required, which will include ensuring that the airway is patent. If it is not, appropriate resuscitative measures must be initiated.

Source: Royal Children's Hospital Melbourne. (2021b). Retrieved from https://www.rch.org.au/clinicalguide/guideline_index/Acute_upper_airway_obstruction/

Buccal mucosa

E Use the same technique as for an adult. If the consumer is unable to open the mouth on command, use the edge of a tongue blade to lift the upper lip and move the lower lip down.

N See Chapter 12.

A A thick, curdlike coating on the buccal mucosa or tongue is abnormal.

P Thrush can be acquired when a newborn passes through the vagina during delivery.

Teeth

E N See Chapter 11.

A A lack of visible teeth coupled with X-ray findings revealing absence of tooth buds is abnormal.

P Absence of deciduous teeth beyond 16 months of age signifies an abnormality most commonly related to genetic causes.

A It is abnormal for the teeth to turn brownish black, possibly with indentations along the surfaces of the teeth.

P Carbohydrate-rich fluid (from milk or juice) causes severe caries when a child falls asleep with a bottle in the mouth.

Hard and soft palate

E 1. Observe the palate for continuity and shape.
2. For infants, you will need to use a tongue depressor to push the tongue down. Infants usually cry in response to this action, which allows visualisation of the palates.

N The roof of the mouth is continuous and has a slight arch.

A It is abnormal if the roof of the mouth is not continuous. This anomaly is called cleft palate (**Figure 20.25**).

P Cleft palates vary greatly in size and extent of malformation. The degree of malformation is classified into two groups. A midline malformation may involve the uvula or extend through the soft or hard palates or both. If associated with cleft lip, the malformation may extend through the palates and into the nasal cavity. Cleft palates form between the sixth and tenth week of embryonic development, during fusion of the maxillary and premaxillary processes. Genetics plays a small role in aetiology.

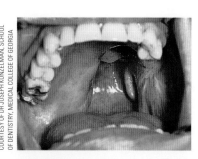

FIGURE 20.25 Cleft palate

E Examination   **N** Normal findings   **A** Abnormal findings   **P** Pathophysiology

A The roof of the mouth is abnormally arched. On inspection, the shape resembles an upside-down letter 'V'.

P High palates are usually associated with a particular syndrome. Examples include trisomy 21, trisomy 18 and Noonan syndrome.

A **Epstein pearls** in the newborn appear on the hard palate and gum margins and are abnormal. The pearls are small white cysts that feel hard when palpated.

P These cysts result from fragments of epithelial tissue trapped during palate formation.

Oropharynx

E See Chapter 11.

N Up to the age of 12 years, a tonsil grade of 2+ is considered normal. Around puberty, tonsillar tissue regresses. Tonsils should not interfere with the act of breathing.

A Excessive salivation is an early sign of a tracheoesophageal fistula (TOF). Drooling is accompanied by choking and coughing during the consumer's feeding.

P The oesophagus failed to develop as a continuous passage during embryonic formation.

A Exudative pharyngitis is present in infectious mononucleosis. Other symptoms include fever, sore throat, splenomegaly, petechiae on the palate, and cervical adenitis.

P Mononucleosis is caused by the Epstein-Barr virus.

A Hypertrophy of lymphoid tissue occurs in the posterior pharyngeal wall, causing a condition known as enlarged or hypertrophied adenoids.

P Excessive lymphoid tissue interferes with passage of air through the nose, resulting in snoring and apnoea. Obstruction of the eustachian tubes by enlarged lymphoid tissue can lead to otitis media. Sinusitis can occur when lymphoid tissue blocks the clearance of nasal mucus.

Neck

Inspection

General appearance

E 1. Observe the neck in a midline position while the consumer is sitting upright.
2. Note shortening or thickness of the neck on both right and left sides.
3. Note any swelling.

N There is a reasonable amount of skin tissue on the sides of the neck. There is no swelling.

A Additional web-like tissue found bilaterally from the ear to the shoulder is abnormal.

P Webbed necks are associated with congenital syndromes. One example is Turner syndrome, noted in female children.

A Unilateral or bilateral swelling of the neck below the angle of the jaw is abnormal (**Figure 20.26**).

P Enlargement of the parotid gland occurs in parotitis, or mumps, an inflammation of the parotid gland. There is pain and tenderness in the affected area.

A Torticollis is observed.

P Torticollis can be congenital and acquired. An infant who is always placed on the same side when supine can develop a lateral deviation at the neck with decreased range of motion.

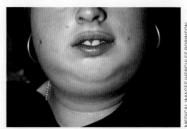

FIGURE 21.26 Parotitis (mumps)

MEDICAL IMAGES/HERCULES ROBINSON

E Examination   **N** Normal findings   **A** Abnormal findings   **P** Pathophysiology

Palpation

Thyroid

E 1. Use the same technique as for an adult with the exception of using the first two finger pads on both hands.
2. Have the younger child who is unable to swallow on command take a drink from a bottle or cup.

N A P The normal findings, abnormal findings and pathophysiology are the same as for an adult.

Lymph nodes

E 1. Because of the infant's short neck, you must extend the chin upwards with your hand before proceeding with palpation.
2. With the finger pads, palpate the submental, submandibular, tonsillar, anterior cervical chain, posterior cervical chain, supraclavicular, preauricular, posterior auricular and occipital lymph nodes.
3. Use a circular motion. Note location, size, shape, tenderness, mobility and associated skin inflammation of any swollen nodes palpated.

N Lymph nodes are generally not palpable. Children often have small, movable, cool, nontender nodes referred to as 'shotty' nodes. These benign nodes are related to environmental antigen exposure or residual effects of a prior illness and have no clinical significance.

A Enlargement of the anterior cervical chain is abnormal.

P This occurs in bacterial infections of the pharynx (strep throat) or viral infections (mononucleosis).

A Enlargement of the occipital nodes or posterior cervical chain nodes is abnormal.

P This can occur in infectious mononucleosis, tinea capitis and acute otitis externa.

Breasts

Inspection of the breasts is performed throughout childhood. Palpation is not usually performed on the consumer until puberty, unless otherwise indicated.

Sexual maturity rating (SMR)

E Using the Tanner stages in Table 12.1, assess the developmental stage of a female's breasts.

N Breast development usually starts between the ages of 8 and 10 and is finished by 14 to 17 years of age.

A An SMR that is less than expected for a female's age is abnormal.

P Pituitary pathology needs to be considered, as well as familial predisposition.

Thorax and lungs

General approach

1. Remove the consumer's clothes or gown.
2. Keep the infant warm during the assessment by placing a blanket over the chest until ready for this portion of assessment.

Inspection

Shape of thorax

E See Chapter 13.

N The infant has a barrel chest; by age 6, the chest attains the adult configuration.

A If a school-age child has an abnormal chest configuration, suspect pathology.

P In addition to the conditions discussed in Chapter 13, cystic fibrosis (CF) can lead to an altered anteroposterior–transverse diameter.

Retractions

E 1. In children, it is important to evaluate intercostal muscles for signs of increased work of breathing.
2. If at all possible, perform this examination when the consumer is quiet because forceful crying will mimic retractions.

N Retractions are not present.

A In respiratory distress, retractions are seen as an inward collapse of the chest wall. Retractions can be seen in the suprasternal, supraclavicular, subcostal and intercostal regions of the chest wall. Other signs of respiratory distress include, but are not limited to, nasal flaring, stridor, expiratory grunting and wheezing.

P Respiratory distress is a result of abnormal function or disruption of the respiratory pathway or within organs that control or influence respiration. Infants with respiratory syncytial virus (RSV) frequently present with retractions.

Palpation
Tactile fremitus
Fremitus is easily felt when a child cries. If the infant or young consumer is not crying, it is advisable to defer this procedure until later in the assessment, perhaps after the throat and ear examinations, which usually produce crying.

Percussion

E See Chapter 13.

N Normal diaphragmatic excursion in infants and young toddlers is one to two intercostal spaces.

A P See Chapter 13.

Auscultation
Breath sounds

E Use the same assessment techniques as for an adult (**Figure 20.27**). Sometimes, it is difficult to differentiate the various adventitious sounds because a child's respiratory rate is rapid; for example, differentiating expiratory wheezing from inspiratory wheezing can be difficult. Mastering the technique takes time and practice.

N Of the three types of breath sounds – bronchial, bronchovesicular and vesicular – the bronchovesicular are normally heard throughout the peripheral lung fields up to 5 to 6 years of age, because the chest wall is thin with decreased musculature. Lung fields are clear and equal bilaterally.

A Crackles are abnormal.

P Conditions such as bronchiolitis, CF and bronchopulmonary dysplasia produce crackles.

A Wheezing is abnormal.

P Consumers with CF and bronchiolitis may present with wheezing. Infants with RSV usually present with wheezing.

Heart and blood vessels
General approach

1. It is best to perform the cardiac assessment near the beginning of the examination, when the infant or young child is relatively calm (**Figure 20.28**).

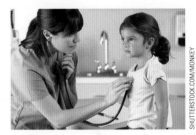
FIGURE 20.27 Auscultation of the child's thorax

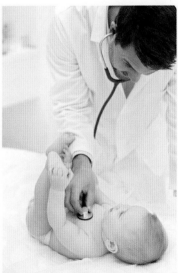
FIGURE 20.28 Heart auscultation of an infant

E Examination **N** Normal findings **A** Abnormal findings **P** Pathophysiology Advanced Assessment

2. Do not get discouraged during the assessment. The beginner nurse is not expected to identify a murmur and its location within the cardiac cycle. Be patient because skill will come only with practice.

3. During the assessment, note physical signs of a syndrome such as Down's facies in a child with trisomy 21 or Down syndrome. Many children with Down syndrome have associated atrioventricular (A-V) canal malformations. These defects each involve an atrial septal defect (ASD), ventricular septal defect (VSD) and a common A-V valve.

4. Cardiac landmarks change when a child has dextrocardia. In this condition, the apex of the heart points towards the right thoracic cavity; thus, heart sounds are auscultated primarily on the right side of the chest.

CLINICAL REASONING

Congenital heart disease (CHD)

Congenital heart disease (CHD) occurs in about 1% of live births (common CHDs include ventricular septal defects, transportation of the great vessels and hypoplastic left heart syndrome). Often, the cause of the defect is unknown, but it may be related to teratogenic, genetic or random factors. Treatment will depend on the defect, with approximately 50% of cases requiring surgery or catheter interventions. Those who have minor abnormalities, such as valve lesions, or small ventricular or atrial septal defects that have no functional impact, do not require any interventions.

Inspection

Apical impulse

E See Chapter 14.

N In both infants and toddlers, the apical impulse is located at the fourth intercostal space and just left of the midclavicular line. The apical impulse of a child 7 years or older is at the fifth intercostal space and to the right of the midclavicular line. The impulse may not be visible in all children, especially in those who have increased adipose tissue or muscle.

A **P** See Chapter 14.

Precordium

E Observe the chest wall for any movements other than the apical impulse.

N Movements other than the apical impulse are abnormal.

A Lifting of the cardiac area is abnormal.

P Heaves are associated with volume overload. A child with congenital heart disease is at risk for developing heart failure (HF) with associated volume overload. **Figure 20.29** depicts the manifestations of HF in children. Large left-to-right shunt defects, such as a VSD, cause right ventricular volume overload.

Palpation

Thrill

E 1. Palpate as for an adult or use the proximal one-third of each finger and the areas over the metacarpophalangeal joints. Many nurses feel the latter method yields greater sensitivity to the presence of thrills.

2. Place the hand vertically along the heart's apex and move the hand towards the sternum.

3. Place the hand horizontally along the sternum, moving up the sternal border about 1.25 cm to 2.5 cm each time.

E Examination **N** Normal findings **A** Abnormal findings **P** Pathophysiology ▦ Advanced Assessment

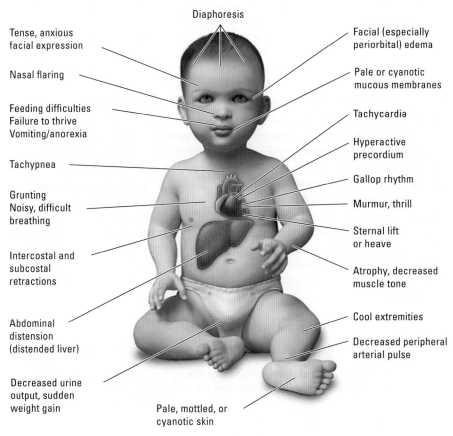

Diaphoresis

Tense, anxious
facial expression

Nasal flaring

Feeding difficulties
Failure to thrive
Vomiting/anorexia

Tachypnea

Grunting
Noisy, difficult
breathing

Intercostal and
subcostal
retractions

Abdominal
distension
(distended liver)

Decreased urine
output, sudden
weight gain

Facial (especially
periorbital) edema

Pale or cyanotic
mucous membranes

Tachycardia

Hyperactive
precordium

Gallop rhythm

Murmur, thrill

Sternal lift
or heave

Atrophy, decreased
muscle tone

Cool extremities

Decreased peripheral
arterial pulse

Pale, mottled, or
cyanotic skin

FIGURE 20.29 Infant with heart failure

E 4. When at the clavicular level, place the hand vertically and assess for a thrill
at the base of the heart.
   5. Use the finger pads to palpate a thrill at the suprasternal notch and along the
carotid arteries.

N A thrill is not found in the healthy child.

A **P** See Chapter 14.

Peripheral pulses

E 1. Use the pads of your fingers to assess each peripheral pulse. The sensation of
one finger pad versus another can be different.
   2. Use the finger pads to palpate each pair of peripheral pulses simultaneously,
except for the carotid pulse.
   3. Palpate the brachial and femoral pulses simultaneously.

N Pulse qualities are the same in the adult and the child.

A A brachial–femoral lag, when femoral pulses are weaker than brachial pulses
when palpated simultaneously, is abnormal.

P Coarctation is due to a narrowing of the aorta before, at or just beyond the
entrance of the ductus arteriosus. Thus, blood flow to the lower body is reduced.

Auscultation

Heart sounds

Auscultating the infant's or the young paediatric consumer's heart is difficult
because the heart rate is rapid and breath sounds are easily transmitted through
the chest wall.

E Examination   **N** Normal findings   **A** Abnormal findings   **P** Pathophysiology   ▨ Advanced Assessment

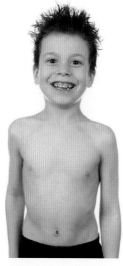

FIGURE 20.30 Z auscultation pattern for young children

E 1. Have the child lie down. If this position is not possible, the child should be held at a 45° angle in the caregiver's arms.
2. Use the 'Z' pattern to auscultate the heart. Place the stethoscope in the apical area and gradually move it towards the right lower sternal border and up the sternal border in a right diagonal line. Move gradually from the consumer's left to the right upper sternal borders (Figure 20.30).
3. Perform a second evaluation with the child in a sitting position.

N Fifty per cent of all children develop an innocent murmur at some time in their lives (see Table 20.4). Innocent murmurs are accentuated in high cardiac output states such as fever, stress or pregnancy. When the consumer is sitting, the murmurs are heard early in systole at the second or third intercostal space along the left sternal border and are softly musical in quality; they disappear when the consumer lies down. Be aware of sinus arrhythmias during auscultation of the heart's rhythm. On inspiration, the pulse rate speeds up; the pulse rate slows with expiration. To determine if the rhythm is normal, ask the child to hold his or her breath while you auscultate the heart. If the pulse stops varying with respirations, then a sinus arrhythmia is present. S_1 is best heard at the apex of the heart, left lower sternal border. S_2 is best heard at the heart base.

TABLE 20.4 Innocent heart murmurs

TYPE	AGE	INTENSITY/LOCATION	QUALITY	OTHER CHARACTERISTICS
Stills	>2 years	<III/VI midsystolic located at LMSB or between LLSB and apex	Twanging, squeaking, buzzing, musical or vibratory sound	Low frequency heard with the bell with consumer in supine position, softer when the consumer is standing
Pulmonary ejection	8–14 years	<III/VI, early midsystolic located at LUSB	Slightly grating, little radiation	Ejection-type murmur
Pulmonary flow murmur of the newborn	Low-birthweight newborn	I–II/VI with wide transmission, audible at LUSB	Rough	Disappears at 3–6 months of age
Venous hum	3–6 years	<III/VI continuous murmur, audible in right or left infraclavicular and supraclavicular areas	Humming	Originates from turbulence in jugular venous system, heard in upright position, disappears in supine position, obliterated by rotating the head or gently occluding neck veins

LLSB = left lower sternal border; LMSB = left middle sternal border; LUSB = left upper sternal border

A A split S_2 sound is abnormal.

P If the S_2 split is fixed with the act of respiration, you can suspect an atrial septal defect. In children, S_2 physiologically splits with inspiration and becomes single with expiration. This phenomenon is due to a greater negative pressure in the thoracic cavity.

A In children, S_3 often sounds like the three syllables of the word 'Kentucky', especially when accompanied by tachycardia.

P A loud third heart sound may be present in children with congestive heart failure (CHF) or VSDs. S_3 is produced by rapid filling of the ventricle.

A With tachycardia, S_4 sounds like a gallop resembling the word 'Tennessee'.

P S_4 is not normally heard in children. If detected, aortic stenosis may be present. The left ventricle's ability to pump blood through the stenotic valve produces a dilatation within the left ventricular muscle, resulting in decreased ventricular compliance.

A A systolic ejection murmur is heard between the first and second heart sounds over the aortic or pulmonic areas.

P Ejection murmurs occur in aortic and pulmonic valvular stenosis. The murmur is the result of blood passing through stenotic valves.

A Holosystolic murmurs are heard maximally at the left lower sternal border. They begin with S_1 and continue until the second heart sound, S_2, is heard.

P Holosystolic or pansystolic murmurs are heard in children with VSDs, where blood flows from a chamber of higher pressure to one of lower pressure during systole.

A Diastolic murmurs are heard between S_2 and S_1.

P Diastolic murmurs are classified into early diastolic, mid-diastolic and presystolic. Early diastolic murmurs are high-pitched and blowing. They occur in aortic regurgitation and subaortic stenosis. A mid-diastolic murmur is a low-pitched rumble. These occur in mitral stenosis or VSDs with large left-to-right shunts. A presystolic murmur is heard in consumers with mitral stenosis or tricuspid stenosis.

A Continuous murmurs heard throughout the cardiac cycle are abnormal.

P Collateral blood flow murmurs are heard radiating throughout the back, such as in pulmonary atresia.

A Continuous murmurs are present in coronary artery fistulas.

P Palliative shunt murmurs are normal and should be heard; if they are not heard, there is a possibility of a clotted shunt. These murmurs are heard over the right or left upper chest in the respective area where surgically placed. A palliative shunt is created temporarily until the consumer is ready for corrective surgery. A palliative shunt may be needed in a small infant with a combination of tetralogy of Fallot and pulmonary atresia or a hypoplastic pulmonary artery.

Abdomen
General approach

1. If possible, ask the caregiver to refrain from feeding the infant prior to the assessment because palpation of a full stomach may induce vomiting.
2. Children who are physically able should be encouraged to empty the bladder prior to the assessment.
3. The young infant, school-age child or adolescent should lie on the examination table. For the toddler or preschooler, have the caregiver hold the child supine on the lap, with the lower extremities bent at the knees and dangling.
4. If the child is crying, encourage the caregiver to help calm the child before you proceed with the assessment.
5. Observe nonverbal communication in children who are not able to verbally express feelings. During palpation, listen for a high-pitched cry and look for a change in facial expression (**Figure 20.31**) or for sudden protective movements that may indicate a painful or tender area.

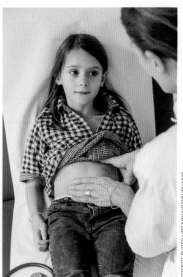

FIGURE 20.31 During palpation of the child's abdomen, the health practitioner observes for facial grimacing or other signs of discomfort.

CLINICAL **REASONING**

Practice tip: Assessing for umbilical hernias in children
If the child is upset and crying, assess the umbilicus for an outwards projection, which is indicative of an umbilical hernia. If an umbilical hernia is present, palpate the area to determine if the hernia reduces easily. If identified, refer appropriately for surgical review.

E Examination **N** Normal findings **A** Abnormal findings **P** Pathophysiology Advanced Assessment

Inspection

Contour

E See Chapter 15.

N The young child may have a 'potbelly'.

Peristaltic wave

E N See Chapter 15.

A Visible peristaltic waves seen moving across the epigastrium from left to right are abnormal.

P Obstruction at the pyloric sphincter causes a condition called pyloric stenosis. The pyloric muscle hypertrophies, causing obstruction during embryonic development.

Auscultation

After performing auscultation of the lungs, it is helpful to proceed to auscultating the abdomen because doing so allows you to complete a good portion of auscultation all at once. If the child is not cooperating, a simple distracting phrase such as 'I can hear your breakfast in there' is helpful during auscultation.

Palpation

General palpation

E N See Chapter 15.

A On palpation, an olive-shaped mass felt in the epigastric area and to the upper right of the umbilicus is abnormal.

P This is indicative of pyloric stenosis.

A Abdominal distension coupled with palpable stool over the abdomen and the absence of stool in the rectum is abnormal.

P An aganglionic segment of the colon is responsible for Hirschsprung's disease, which produces abnormal gastrointestinal findings.

A A sausage-shaped mass that produces intermittent pain when palpated in the upper abdomen is abnormal.

P Administration of the rotavirus vaccine (RotaShield) is thought to be responsible for numerous cases of **intussusception**. Most commonly, the ileocaecal region of the intestine telescopes down into the ileum itself. Classic symptoms are vomiting and currant jelly stools. RotaShield has been taken off the market. Rota has taken its place in standard paediatric immunisations.

A Bowel sounds heard in the thoracic cavity, a scaphoid abdomen, an upwardly displaced apical impulse and signs of respiratory distress are abnormal findings in the newborn.

P Approximately in the eighth week of embryonic development, the diaphragm fails to fuse, creating a **diaphragmatic hernia**. This condition results in protrusion of the intestines into the thoracic cavity.

Liver palpation

E For infants and toddlers, use the outer edge of your right thumb to press down and scoop up at the right upper quadrant. For the remaining age groups, use the same technique as for an adult.

N The liver is not normally palpated, although the liver edge can be found 1 cm below the right costal margin in a normal, healthy child. The liver edge is soft and regular.

A It is abnormal for the liver edge to be palpated more than 1 cm below the right costal margin and be full with a firm, sharp border.

P Hepatomegaly occurs in several disease states such as viral or bacterial illnesses, tumours, heart failure, and fat and glycogen storage diseases. Viral and bacterial illnesses and tumours cause liver cells to multiply in number, creating an enlarged liver. In heart failure, the hepatic veins and sinusoids enlarge from congestion, resulting in haemorrhage and fibrosis of the liver. In fat and glycogen storage diseases, fat and glycogen accumulate within the liver, and fibrosis ensues.

Musculoskeletal system

General approach

1. The extent or degree of assessment depends greatly on the consumer's or caregiver's complaints of musculoskeletal problems. Be aware that during periods of rapid growth, children complain of normal muscle aches.
2. Try to incorporate musculoskeletal assessment techniques into other system assessments. For instance, while inspecting the integument, inspect the muscles and joints.
3. Inspecting the musculoskeletal system in the ambulatory child is accomplished by allowing the child to move freely about and play in the examination room while you inquire about the health history. Your observations of the child enable you to assess posture, muscle symmetry and range of motion of muscles and joints.
4. Do not rush through the assessment. Throughout the assessment, incorporate game playing that facilitates evaluation of the musculoskeletal system.
5. Observe range of motion and joint flexibility as the child undresses.

Inspection

Muscles

E 1. Have the child disrobe down to a nappy or underwear.
2. To evaluate the small infant's shoulder muscles, place your hands under the axillae and pull the infant into a standing position. The infant should not slip through your hands. Be prepared to catch the infant if needed.
3. Evaluate the infant's leg strength in a semi-standing position. Lower the infant to the examination table so the infant's legs touch the table.
4. Place the infant older than 4 months in a prone position. Observe the infant's ability to lift the upper body off the examination table using the upper extremities.

N Degree of joint flexibility and range of motion are the same for the child as for the adult.

A Increased muscle tone (spasticity) is abnormal.

P Cerebral palsy (CP) results from a nonprogressive abnormality in the pyramidal motor tract. One of the contributing factors, perinatal asphyxia, causes abnormal posture and gross motor development and varying degrees of abnormal muscle tone.

A The inability to rise from a sitting to a standing position is abnormal. In attempting to rise from a supine position, the child first turns over onto the abdomen and raises the trunk to a crawling position. Then, with the aid of the arms, the child places the feet firmly on the floor and gradually elevates the upper part of the body by climbing up the legs with the arms.

P This is called Gower's sign. Gower's sign occurs in Duchenne muscular dystrophy (MD) early in childhood. Genetics is responsible for the abnormality in the short arm of the X chromosome.

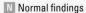
E Examination   **N** Normal findings   **A** Abnormal findings   **P** Pathophysiology   Advanced Assessment

Joints

E See Chapter 16.

N The infant's spine is C-shaped. Head control and standing create the normal S-shaped spine of the adult. Lordosis is normal as the child begins to walk. A toddler's protruding abdomen is counterbalanced by an inwards deviation of the lumbar spine.

A Extra fingers or toes are abnormal.

P Supernumerary digits, or polydactyly (**Figure 20.32**), may be found in certain congenital syndromes such as Carpenter, fetal hydantoin, orofaciodigital, Smith-Lemli-Opitz, trisomy 13 and VATER.

A A fusion between two or more digits is abnormal.

P Syndactylism is also associated with certain congenital syndromes such as Aarskog, Apert, Carpenter, orofaciodigital, Russell-Silver and acrocephalosyndactyly. Look for other physical signs of a syndrome if either syndactyly or polydactyly is present.

A It is abnormal for a young male (usually 2 to 12 years old) to present with a painless limp from the affected hip. The limp is accompanied by limited abduction and internal rotation, muscle spasm and proximal thigh atrophy.

P Legg-Calvé-Perthes disease, also called coxa plana, is caused by an interruption in the blood supply to the capital femoral epiphysis. Avascular necrosis of the femoral head results.

A The affected hip has loss of flexion. The consumer is unable to rotate the hip inwards. The affected leg turns outwards and may appear shorter than the other leg while in a standing position. The adolescent often presents with a limp.

P These findings occur in slipped capital femoral epiphysis. The ball at the upper end of the femur slips from its normal position in a backwards direction. This is due to weakness of the growth plate. It commonly develops during periods of accelerated growth, shortly after the onset of puberty. Slipped capital femoral epiphysis occurs with greater frequency in males and in children who are overweight.

A An exaggerated lumbar curvature of the spine is abnormal after 6 years of age.

P Lordosis can be attributed to bilateral developmental dislocation of the hip or postural factors such as progression of congenital kyphosis (**Figure 20.33**), or can occur secondary to contractures of hip flexors.

Palpation

Joints

E **N** See Chapter 16.

A Knee pain aggravated by any motion or activity that puts undue pressure on the joint is abnormal. Palpation of a slight elevation of the tibial tuberosity is abnormal.

P The deformed tubercle in Osgood-Schlatter disease is caused by repetitive stress on the area. A fibrocartilage microfracture may cause joint pain.

A Swollen, inflamed, painful joints are abnormal.

P Juvenile rheumatoid arthritis causes synovial inflammation and degeneration of the joint. Its cause is unknown.

Feet

E 1. Place the consumer on the examination table or caregiver's lap.
2. Stand in front of the child.
3. Hold the right heel immobile with one hand while pushing the forefoot (medial base of great toe) towards a midline position with the other hand.
4. Observe for toe and forefoot adduction and inversion.
5. Repeat on the left foot.

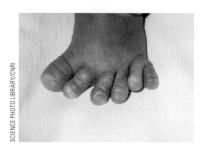

SCIENCE PHOTO LIBRARY/CNRI

FIGURE 20.32 Polydactyly

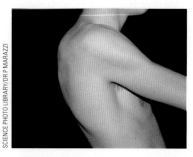

SCIENCE PHOTO LIBRARY/DR P MARAZZI

FIGURE 20.33 Child with kyphosis, in which the back below the neck is curved out and rounded, and lordosis, in which the lower back is excessively hollow

E Examination **N** Normal findings **A** Abnormal findings **P** Pathophysiology

N The toes and forefoot are not deviated.

A Toes or forefeet that are deviated are abnormal.

P **Metatarsus varus** is a medial forefoot malalignment. In **talipes equinovarus** (clubfoot), there is heel inversion, forefoot adduction, and plantar flexion of the foot. Heredity plays a role in the aetiology, as well as abnormal intrauterine position of the fetal foot.

Hip and femur

Ortolani manoeuvre is always performed at the very end of the assessment because it may produce crying. The test is performed on one hip at a time. Evaluate the hips up until 18 months of age or until the child is an established walker.

E
1. Place the infant supine on an examination table with the feet facing you.
2. Stand directly in front of the infant.
3. With the thumb, hold the inner thigh of the femur, and with the index and middle fingers, hold the greater trochanter (**Figure 20.34A**). These two fingers should rest over the hip joint.
4. Slowly press outwards and abduct until the lateral aspects of the knees nearly touch the table (**Figure 20.34B**). The tips of the fingers should palpate each femoral head as it rotates outwards.
5. Listen for an audible clunk (Ortolani sign).
6. With the fingers in the same locations, adduct the hips to elicit a palpable clunk (Ortolani sign). As each hip is adducted, it is lifted anteriorly into the acetabulum.
7. Place both of the infant's feet flat on the examination table with the knees together.
8. Observe the height of the knees. This is called Allis sign.
9. Turn the infant to a prone position and observe the levels of the gluteal folds.

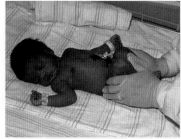

A. Hand placement

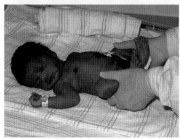

B. Hip abduction

FIGURE 20.34 Ortolani manoeuvre

N A clunk is not audible or palpated. The knees should be at the same height with the feet on the examination table. The gluteal folds are approximately at the same level.

A Abnormal findings include a positive Ortolani sign; a sudden, painful cry during the test; asymmetrical thigh skin folds; uneven knee level; and limited hip abduction.

P Epidemiology of **developmental dislocation of the hip** (DDH) is related to familial factors, maternal hormones associated with pelvic laxity, firstborn children, oligohydramnios and breech presentations.

A Knees that are not at the same level are abnormal.

P This is another technique that can potentially detect DDH.

A Unequal gluteal folds are abnormal.

P This also can lead to a finding of DDH.

Neurological system
General approach

1. Some aspects of the neurological assessment for the infant and the young child are different from those for the adult. An infant functions mainly at the subcortical level. Memory and motor coordination are about three-quarters developed by 2 years of age, when cortical functioning is acquiring dominance.
2. Incorporate findings for fine and gross motor skills previously tested during the musculoskeletal assessment. In addition, use the Denver II and PEDs to assess personal-social and language skills. Refer to normal developmental milestones (see Chapter 2) and extrapolate warning signs of neurological development lag.

E Examination   **N** Normal findings   **A** Abnormal findings   **P** Pathophysiology

UNIT 3

3. Because the infant cannot verbally express level of consciousness, assess the newborn's ability to cry, level of activity, positioning and general appearance.
4. Only reflex mechanisms and cranial nerve testing are described in this section. Refer to the adult neurological assessment for all other testing.

Reflex mechanisms of the infant

Neonatal reflexes must be lost before motor development can proceed.

Rooting reflex

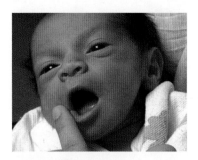

FIGURE 20.35 Rooting reflex

E 1. Place the infant supine with the head in a midline position.
2. With your forefinger, stroke the skin located at one corner of the mouth (**Figure 20.35**).
3. Observe movement of the head.

N Up until 3 or 4 months of age, the infant will turn the head towards the side that was stroked. In the sleeping infant, the rooting reflex can be present normally until 6 months of age.

A An absent rooting reflex from birth to 3 to 4 months is abnormal.

P Central nervous system disease such as frontal lobe lesions accounts for an absent rooting reflex.

Sucking reflex

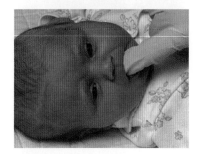

FIGURE 20.36 Sucking reflex

E 1. Place the infant in a supine position.
2. With your forefinger, touch the infant's lips to stimulate a response (**Figure 20.36**).
3. Observe for a sucking motion.

N The sucking reflex occurs up to approximately 10 months.

A Absence of the sucking reflex is abnormal.

P A premature infant or the breastfed infant of a mother who ingests barbiturates does not exhibit the reflex, secondary to CNS depression.

Palmar grasp reflex

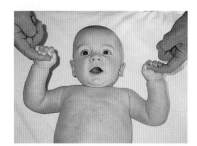

FIGURE 20.37 Palmar reflex

E 1. Place the infant supine with the head in a midline position.
2. Place the ulnar sides of both index fingers into the infant's hands while the infant's arms are in a semiflexed position (**Figure 20.37**).
3. Press your fingers into the infant's palmar surfaces.

N Normally, the infant grasps your fingers in flexion.

A Presence of the palmar grasp reflex after 4 months of age is abnormal.

P The aetiology is attributed to frontal lobe lesions.

Tonic neck reflex

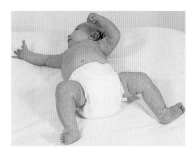

FIGURE 20.38 Tonic neck reflex

E 1. Place the infant in a supine position on the examination table.
2. Rotate the head to one side and hold the jaw area parallel to the shoulder.
3. Observe for movement of the extremities.

N The upper and lower extremities on the side to which the jaw is turned extend, and the opposite arm and leg flex (**Figure 20.38**). Sometimes, this reflex does not show up until 6 to 8 weeks of age.

A After 6 months of age, a tonic neck reflex is abnormal.

P Cerebral damage is suspected if the tonic neck reflex is seen after 6 months of age.

E Examination **N** Normal findings **A** Abnormal findings **P** Pathophysiology

Stepping reflex

E 1. Stand behind the infant, grasp the infant under the axillae, and bring the body to a standing position on a flat surface. Use the thumbs to support the back of the head if needed.
2. Push the infant's feet towards a flat surface and simultaneously lean the infant's body forwards (**Figure 20.39**).
3. Observe the legs and feet for stepping movements.

N Stepping movements are made by flexing one leg and moving the other leg forwards. This reflex disappears at about 3 months of age.

A Presence of the stepping reflex beyond 3 months of age is abnormal.

P Consumers with CP demonstrate a stepping reflex beyond 3 months of age.

Plantar grasp reflex

E 1. Position the infant supine on the examination table.
2. Elevate the foot to be examined.
3. Touch the infant's foot on the plantar surface beneath the toes (**Figure 20.40**).
4. Repeat on the other side.

N The toes curl down until 8 months of age.

A It is abnormal for the plantar grasp reflex to be absent on one or both feet.

P An obstructive lesion such as an abscess or tumour can cause the plantar grasp reflex to be absent on the affected side. Bilateral absence can occur in CP.

Babinski reflex

E 1. Position the infant supine on the examination table.
2. Elevate the foot to be examined.
3. Stroke the plantar surface of the foot from the lateral heel upwards with the tip of the thumbnail.

N A child less than 15 to 18 months of age normally fans the toes outwards and dorsiflexes the great toe (**Figure 20.41**).

A After the child masters walking, presence of the Babinski reflex is abnormal.

P Presence of the Babinski reflex after 18 months of age can be indicative of a perinatal insult such as CP.

Moro (startle) reflex

E 1. Place the infant supine on the examination table.
2. Make a sudden, loud noise such as hitting your hand on the examination table.
3. Another technique is to brace the infant's neck and back on the undersurface of your arm while holding the undersurface of the buttocks with the other hand and then mimicking a falling motion by quickly lowering the infant.

N The infant under 4 months of age quickly extends, then flexes the arms and fingers while the manoeuvre is performed. The thumb and index fingers form a C shape (see **Figure 20.42**).

A Presence of the startle reflex after 4 to 6 months of age is abnormal.

P Neurological disease such as CP can be a cause of a positive response after the normal age of disappearance.

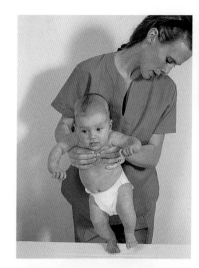
FIGURE 20.39 Stepping reflex

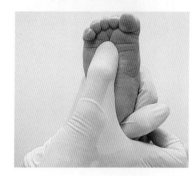
FIGURE 20.40 Plantar grasp reflex

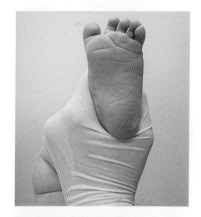
FIGURE 20.41 Babinski reflex

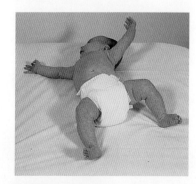
FIGURE 20.42 Moro reflex

E Examination **N** Normal findings **A** Abnormal findings **P** Pathophysiology

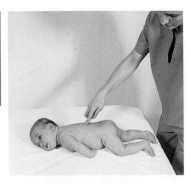

FIGURE 21.43 Galant reflex

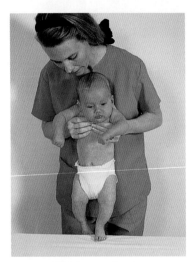

FIGURE 20.44 Placing reflex

Galant reflex

E 1. Place the infant prone, with the infant's hands under the abdomen.
2. Use your index finger to stroke the skin along the side of the spine (see **Figure 20.43**).
3. Observe the stimulated side for any movement.

N An infant less than 1 to 2 months of age will turn the pelvis and shoulders towards the stimulated side.

A Lack of response from an infant less than 2 months of age is abnormal.

P A spinal cord lesion is suspected.

Placing reflex

Do not test the placing and stepping reflexes at the same time because they are two different reflexes.

E 1. Grasp the infant under the axillae from behind and bring the body to a standing position. Use the thumbs to support the back of the head if needed.
2. Touch the dorsum of one foot to the edge of the examination table (**Figure 20.44**).
3. Observe the tested leg for movement.

N The infant's tested leg will flex and lift onto the examination table.

A Lack of response is abnormal.

P It is difficult to elicit this reflex in breech-born babies and in those with paralysis or cerebral cortex abnormalities.

Landau reflex

E 1. Carefully suspend the infant in a prone position, supporting the chest with your hand.
2. Observe for extension of the head, trunk and hips.

N The arms and legs extend during the reflex. The reflex appears at about 3 months of age.

A Presence of the Landau reflex beyond 2 years of age is abnormal. Also, it is abnormal for the infant to assume a limp position.

P An intellectual disability may account for an abnormality.

Cranial nerve function

A thorough assessment of cranial nerve function is difficult to perform on the infant less than 1 year old. Difficulty is also encountered with toddlers and preschoolers because they often cannot follow directions or are not willing to cooperate. Testing for the school-age child or the adolescent is carried out in the same manner as for an adult.

Infant (birth to 12 months)

E 1. To test cranial nerves (CNs) III, IV and VI, move a brightly coloured toy along the infant's line of vision. An infant older than 1 month responds by following the object. Also evaluate the pupillary response to a bright light in each eye.
2. CN V is tested by assessing the rooting or sucking reflexes.
3. CN VII is tested up until 2 months by assessing the sucking reflex and by observing symmetrical sucking movements. After 2 months of age, an infant will smile, allowing assessment of symmetry of facial expressions.
4. A positive Moro reflex in an infant less than 6 months old is evidence of normal functioning of CN VIII.

E 5. CNs IX and X are examined by using a tongue blade to produce a gag reflex. Do not test if a positive response was already elicited by using a tongue blade to view the posterior pharynx.

6. To test CN XI, evaluate the infant's ability to lift the head up while in a prone position.

7. CN XII is assessed by allowing the infant to suck on a pacifier or a bottle, abruptly removing the pacifier or bottle from the infant's mouth, and observing for lingering sucking movements.

N A P See Chapter 7.

Toddler and preschooler (1 to 5 years)

E 1. The older preschooler is able to identify familiar odours. Most children readily identify the smells of peanut butter and chocolate. Test CN I one side at a time by asking the child to close the eyes and to identify the smells of peanut butter and chocolate. Test each nostril with different substances while occluding the other nostril with your finger.

2. Test vision (CN II) using Allen cards.

3. CNs III, IV and VI are tested in the same fashion as for the infant.

4. CN V is tested by giving the child something to eat and evaluating chewing movements. Sensory responses to light and sharp touch are still not easily interpreted in these age groups.

5. Observe facial weakness or paralysis (CN VII) by making the child smile or laugh. An older preschooler may cooperate by raising the eyebrows, frowning, puffing the cheeks out and closing the eyes tightly on command.

6. To evaluate CN VIII, ring a small bell out of the child's vision and observe the response to unseen sounds.

7. Test CNs IX and X in the same manner as for the infant.

8. CN XII is difficult to assess in this particular age group.

N A P See Chapter 7.

Female genitalia

General approach

1. Place the up-to-preschool-age child on the caregiver's lap or examination table. Ask the caregiver to assist by holding the child's legs in a froglike position. Place the child older than 4 years on the examination table in a semilithotomy position.

2. Explain the procedure prior to the assessment. Never ask the caregiver of the infant or young school-age child to leave the room during this portion of the examination because the caregiver is a source of comfort to the child.

3. The child should be told before the genitalia exam that it is all right for the provider to touch the genitals with the parent present but not for anyone else to do so for any reason.

4. Drape the older-than-preschool-age child.

5. A vaginal and pelvic exam is not routinely performed on young females. A vaginal assessment is warranted, however, when signs of possible sexual abuse are present. See the Clinical reasoning on Signs of sexual abuse in children later in this chapter. The assessment is undertaken by a healthcare provider who is trained to perform paediatric vaginal examinations and can evaluate these problems.

6. Any female who has reached menarche needs to be evaluated for a pregnant uterus, when dictated by the health history.

E Examination   **N** Normal findings   **A** Abnormal findings   **P** Pathophysiology

Inspection

Sexual maturity rating

E 1. Using the Tanner stages in Table 17.1, assess the developmental stage of the pubic hair.
2. Determine the SMR.

N Adolescents usually start developing pubic hair by 8 to 12 years of age. Females usually reach the adult stage by age 15.

A An SMR that is less than expected for a female's age is abnormal.

P Delayed puberty may be familial, genetic or caused by chronic illnesses.

HEALTH EDUCATION

Sexually transmitted infections – education for adolescents

The following preventative guidelines are essential to discuss during your interview. To fit appropriately into the context of the interview, inquiry is preferable after questioning about sexual relationships and use of contraceptives.

> If the adolescent is sexually active, discuss his or her feelings on the subject.
> Talk about the various sexually transmitted infections (HIV, chlamydia, HSV, HPV, gonorrhoea), including their symptoms and sequelae.
> Mention that abstinence is the only certain method of preventing sexually transmitted infections and pregnancy.
> If the individual chooses to be sexually active, discuss proper condom application and use.
> Discuss healthcare services that offer confidential testing if the individual believes that he or she or a partner has contracted a sexually transmitted infection.
> Discuss the dangers of oral sex without condom use.

Perineal area

E See Chapter 17.

N The infant's labia minora are sometimes larger than the labia majora. The hymen is sometimes intact up until the point of sexual activity.

A It is abnormal for the female infant to display a rudimentary penis in the clitoral area.

P Genital ambiguity occurs during embryonic development as a consequence of genetic causes, androgens or androgen inhibitors that reverse genital characteristics.

A A bloody discharge noted at the vaginal opening or on the nappy is abnormal.

P It is not uncommon to note pseudomenstruation in an infant under 2 weeks of age. Maternal hormones such as oestrogen are the cause.

CLINICAL REASONING

Practice tip: Signs of sexual abuse in children

The following are possible signs of sexual abuse in children:

> A strong fear of the physical examination of the perineal area
> Presence of sexually transmitted infections
> Abnormal perineal discharge or odour
> Anorectal tears
> Absent or delayed anal reflex
> Persistent or recurring pain during urination or bowel movements
> Anorectal ecchymosis, pruritus, scarring, HPV or bleeding

>>

E Examination   **N** Normal findings   **A** Abnormal findings   **P** Pathophysiology

>>

> > In a female child, a broken hymen can be a sign of sexual abuse. Keep in mind that a broken hymen can also occur from foreign objects being placed into the vagina by the child, forceful use of baby wipes during a nappy change, tampon use, and strenuous exercise such as gymnastics and horseback riding.
> > Vaginal tears
> > Describes sexual acts
> > Direct or indirect disclosures
> > Age-inappropriate behaviour or persistent sexualised behaviour
> > Self-destructive behaviours
> > Unexplained behaviour changes
> > Persistent running away from home
> > Poor school concentration
> > Not wanting to go home from school
> > Anorexia or over-eating
> > Regression in development.
> > If you identify any of these possible signs of sexual abuse, and you have reason to suspect a child is experiencing harm, or is at risk of experiencing harm, you must follow your jurisdiction's legislation for reporting.
>
> Adapted from SECASA, 2015; Parents protect, 2018

Male genitalia

General approach

1. Female nurses may encounter difficulty assessing a reluctant adolescent. Be firm when explaining that this portion of the assessment is a required part of his examination. Infants and toddlers do not object to the assessment.
2. In case the infant or toddler urinates during the examination, have a nappy or disposable cloth available to catch the stream of urine.
3. The older school-age child and the adolescent should be draped in order to maintain modesty.

Inspection

Sexual maturity rating

E 1. Using the Tanner stages in **Table 17.2**, assess the developmental stage of the pubic hair, penis and scrotum.
   2. Determine the SMR.

N Males usually begin puberty between the ages of 9½ and 13½. The average male proceeds through puberty in about 3 years, with a possible range of 2 to 5 years.

A An SMR that is less than expected for a male's age is abnormal.

P Delayed puberty may be familial or caused by chronic illnesses.

A A normally formed but diminutive penis is abnormal. There is a discrepancy between the penile size and the age of the individual.

P A microphallus can result from a disorder in the hypothalamus or pituitary gland. It may be secondary to primary testicular failure due to partial androgen insensitivity. Maternal diethylstilboestrol (DES) exposure has teratogenic effects caused by defects in nonandrogen-dependent regulatory agents. Microphallus can also be idiopathic in nature.

A It is abnormal when the penis appears larger than what is generally expected for the stated age. This condition is usually evident only before the age of normal puberty.

E Examination **N** Normal findings **A** Abnormal findings **P** Pathophysiology

P Hormonal influence of tumours of the pineal gland or hypothalamus, tumours of the Leydig cells of the testes, tumours of the adrenal gland, or precocious genital maturity may cause penile hyperplasia.

A A testicle that is smaller and softer than normal (less in the fully developed male) is abnormal.

P An atrophic testicle may be the result of Klinefelter syndrome (hypogonadism), hypopituitarism, oestrogen therapy or orchitis.

Penis

E 1. Note the appearance of the penis. If you are not able to determine circumcision status, ask the caregiver if the child was circumcised.
2. Note the position of the urethral meatus.

N The meatus is normally found on the tip of the penis. A disappearing penis phenomenon occurs normally in infants with increased adipose tissue in the area surrounding the penis. Reassure the caregiver that this is normal and will resolve after adipose tissue is lost.

A It is abnormal for the urethral meatus to be located behind or along the ventral side of the penis.

P During the third month of fetal development, the urethral meatus fails to move toward the glans penis, creating a condition known as hypospadias. Children at greater risk for hypospadias are those whose mothers were on hydantoin for epilepsy during pregnancy.

A It is abnormal for the meatal opening to be on the dorsal surface of the penis.

P During the third month of fetal development, the urethral meatus fails to move towards the glans penis, causing an epispadias deformity.

Scrotum

E 1. Evaluate scrotal size and colour.
2. Note if the testes are seen in the scrotal sac.

N The scrotum appears proportionately large in size when compared to the penis. The sac colour is brown or black in dark-skinned children and pink in light-skinned children. Two testes should be present, but, in infants, they may retract into the inguinal canal or abdomen due to various stimuli, including cold and palpation.

A P See Chapter 18.

Palpation

Scrotum

E 1. Place the infant in a supine position on the examination table. Instruct the young child to sit cross-legged to inhibit the cremasteric reflex from occurring. The older child may be allowed to stand for this portion of the exam.
2. Locate each testis within the scrotal sac by using the fingers of one hand in a milking motion to cause the testes to descend.
3. Palpate and note the size, shape and mobility of each testis.

N See Chapter 18.

A It is abnormal to be unable to palpate the testes.

P Cryptorchidism is a failure of a testis to descend into the scrotal sac. One or both testes failing to descend within the inguinal canal occurs during embryonic development.

E Examination **N** Normal findings **A** Abnormal findings **P** Pathophysiology

A An enlargement of the scrotum is abnormal.

P A congenital hydrocoele results from failure of the male reproductive tract to develop properly while the fetus is in utero. This mass will transilluminate.

Hernia

E 1. For the infant who is unable to stand, place him supine on the examination table. All other children should stand during the examination.
2. Use the little finger for examination of the infant and the index finger for examination of the younger child.
3. Follow the inguinal canal as is done on an adult male.
4. If possible, perform the assessment on a crying infant.
5. Have preschoolers and early school-age children attempt to blow up a balloon while you palpate the inguinal areas.
6. Palpate the inguinal areas while the older school-age child or adolescent coughs.

N **A** **P** See Chapter 18.

Anus

As a rule, rectal assessments are not performed on children unless you detect a problem or suspect abuse; in these cases, refer children for further evaluation if you are not trained specifically for this procedure and follow your institution's guidelines.

Inspection

E 1. Ask the child to lie on the abdomen.
2. Gently separate the buttocks to allow direct visualisation of the anal opening.
3. Observe for bleeding, fissures, prolapse, skin tags, haemorrhoids, lesions and pinworms.
4. During separation of the buttocks, observe any movement of the anus.
5. Stroke the perianal area with your finger and note any movement. This is called the anal reflex or anal wink.

N No bleeding, fissures, prolapse, skin tags, haemorrhoids, lesions or pinworms should be present. An anal reflex is observed.

A An absent anal reflex is abnormal.

P Conditions such as a spinal cord lesion, trauma and tumours that interrupt nervous innervation to the anal sphincter cause this finding.

CLINICAL **REASONING**

Threadworm or pinworm
Threadworm or pinworm, is the most common worm infection and is found most often in children. Pinworm infections may not produce any symptoms, but often the eggs may cause intense itching, especially at night. Other symptoms can include:
> reduced appetite
> feeling mildly unwell
> inflammation of the vagina
> adult worms seen in the faeces, and eggs clinging to the skin around the anus
> irritability and behavioural changes.
  Treatment includes a two-dose course of medication that should be taken by all members of the affected household.

E Examination **N** Normal findings **A** Abnormal findings **P** Pathophysiology

EVALUATION OF HEALTH ASSESSMENT AND PHYSICAL EXAMINATION FINDINGS

In the evaluation phase of a health assessment, the focus is on ensuring the data gathered is complete, accurate and documented appropriately (see case study as an example of the focused assessment; see Chapter 22 for a comprehensive health assessment). In evaluating the data you should:

> draw on your critical thinking and problem-solving skills to make sound clinical decisions

> act on abnormal data (include communicating findings to other health professionals)

> ensure documentation reflects the outcomes of the clinical decisions/actions taken (refer to Chapter 3, which discusses in detail why documentation is so important and how this may be undertaken in different health settings).

The case study that follows steps you through this process.

THE PAEDIATRIC CONSUMER WITH ACUTE TONSILLITIS

This case study illustrates the application and the objective documentation of the mouth and throat assessment.

Lachlan James is a 9-year-old male who has been brought to the emergency room of a small regional hospital complaining of a sore throat and difficulty swallowing.

HEALTH HISTORY		
CONSUMER PROFILE	9-year-old Caucasian male	
CHIEF COMPLAINT	'I have had a sore throat for the last week and now I cannot swallow properly.'	
HISTORY OF THE PRESENT ILLNESS	Child was well up until about 5 days ago when he developed a sore throat. Symptoms started with generalised fatigue and a low grade fever (37.5°C) He began having difficulty swallowing approximately 2 days ago. He has experienced episodes of anorexia for the past 2 days. His mum has been giving him paracetamol – 1 tablet (500 mg) every 4 hours/prn for pain/comfort	
PAST HEALTH HISTORY	**MEDICAL HISTORY**	Has had coeliac disease since age 5
	SURGICAL HISTORY	Insertion of grommets aged 3 years
	ALLERGIES	Penicillin and gluten
	MEDICATIONS	Paracetamol prn
	COMMUNICABLE DISEASES	Denies
	INJURIES AND ACCIDENTS	Denies
	SPECIAL NEEDS	Gluten-free diet
	BLOOD TRANSFUSIONS	Denies
	CHILDHOOD ILLNESSES	Chickenpox age 6 without sequelae
	IMMUNISATIONS	All childhood vaccines up to date

>>

HEALTH HISTORY

FAMILY HEALTH HISTORY		Younger sister has asthma
SOCIAL HISTORY	ALCOHOL USE	None
	TOBACCO USE	None
	DRUG USE	None
	DOMESTIC AND INTIMATE PARTNER VIOLENCE	None
	SEXUAL PRACTICE	None
	TRAVEL HISTORY	None
	WORK ENVIRONMENT	None
	HOME ENVIRONMENT	Lives with mum and dad. Has a twin sister as well as another younger sister Lives in an urban area
	HOBBIES AND LEISURE ACTIVITIES	Swimming, soccer
	STRESS	Normal school stress
	EDUCATION	In Grade 4 at the local primary school
	ECONOMIC STATUS	Middle-class family
	MILITARY SERVICE	None
	RELIGION	Roman Catholic
	CULTURAL BACKGROUND	Father from the UK; father's family lives in the UK Mother Australian
	ROLES AND RELATIONSHIPS	Has good relationship with his siblings and parents; has a few close school friends
	CHARACTERISTIC PATTERNS OF DAILY LIVING	Wakes at 7 a.m., has shake for breakfast, goes to local pool and undertakes swimming training 2 times a week. Comes home by 8.30, has breakfast, gets ready for school. Normal school day has lunch with friends. Goes to bed between 9 and 9.30 p.m.
HEALTH MAINTENANCE ACTIVITIES	SLEEP	8–9 hours of sleep during the week; 8–9 hours on the weekends
	DIET	Gluten-free diet
	EXERCISE	Swimming training × 2 per week
	STRESS MANAGEMENT	Denies stress – states his sport keeps him occupied
	USE OF SAFETY DEVICES	Uses seat belt in car
	HEALTH CHECK-UPS	Usually once per year his parents take him and his sisters for a check-up with the local GP

>>

PHYSICAL EXAMINATION

EARS		AUDITORY SCREENING	Normal
		EXTERNAL EAR	Normal; no skin tags noted.
		OTOSCOPIC ASSESSMENT	Both tympanic membranes are shiny pink and mobile with visible light reflexes; without bulging or perforation. Both ears slightly red; no exudates or odour noted. Complained of ears feeling 'stuffy' and making it hard to hear
NOSE		EXTERNAL INSPECTION	Midline without swelling, bleeding, lesions or masses
		PATENCY	Each nare is patent
		INTERNAL INSPECTION	Slightly 'crusty' formations; no masses noted
SINUSES	INSPECTION		Normal
	PALPATION AND PERCUSSION		No discomfort noted
MOUTH AND THROAT		BREATH	Foul smell noted
		LIPS	Pale, slightly dry without lesions
		TONGUE	Midline, pale and dry, well papillated without fasciculations, lesions, swelling or bleeding
		BUCCAL MUCOSA	Pale, slightly dry without lesions
		GUMS	Pale and moist without swelling or bleeding
		TEETH	32 present, no caries; in proper alignment
		PALATE	Intact, rises with phonation
		THROAT	Erythematous with 3+ tonsils bilaterally, inflammation and excessive exudates; uvula midline; gag reflex positive

EVALUATION AND CLINICAL REASONING FOR CASE STUDY

The assessment and clinical decisions you make should reflect your scope of practice. For example, advanced practice health professionals, such as nurse practitioners and remote area nurses with endorsement, may be able to make diagnostic decisions and prescribe medications without referring to a medical officer.

Fundamentally, all health professionals collect, evaluate and act on consumer-focused health information, which will at times include referral to, or collaboration with, other healthcare team members. Nurses assess an individual's responses to interventions and determine when to escalate key changes in their condition. The clinical reasoning cycle provides health professionals with a framework to consider all this information in a meaningful way for planning an individual's care. These phases are stepped out below, and draw on information presented and collected during the health history and physical examination. We then work through the cycle components that are relevant to this case study (cycle components are bolded).

For Lachlan James, a 9-year-old Caucasian male who has been brought to the emergency room complaining of a sore throat and difficulty swallowing, the significant data that needs to be considered includes the following.

Collecting cues/information

Recall and Review: In the first instance you will need to reflect on what you know about the tonsils.

The tonsils are masses of lymphoid tissue located in the pharyngeal cavity (refer to Chapter 11).

Their role is to filter and protect the respiratory tract from invading pathogens and organisms as well as antibody formation. The difference between children and adults in relation to tonsils is that in children the tonsils are much larger in early years, as they are thought to be a protective mechanism due to the fact that younger children are more susceptible to upper respiratory infections. Tonsillitis often occurs with pharyngitis. It is also a common illness in children as a result of the abundance of lymphoid tissue and the frequency of URTIs. Tonsillitis is normally manifested by inflammation, with the causative agent being either viral or bacterial. Presenting symptoms can be difficulty breathing and swallowing, low grade temperature, sore throat and enlarged tonsils on examination. The child may begin to breathe through the mouth as a result of enlargement of the adenoids, which tend to block off the space behind the anterior nares, making it harder for air to pass from nose to throat. Medical treatment for tonsillitis will depend on the causative agent.

Chief complaint and history of present illness
> Well until about 5 days ago, when he developed a sore throat.
> Symptoms started with sore throat, bad breath.
> After 2 days began to complain of difficulty swallowing (5/10 intensity), generalised ear and neck pain, low-grade fever (37.5°C), episodes of anorexia and fatigue.

Processing information

Discrimination: Both use of medications and past allergies need to be accurate and considered as Lachlan has had a low-grade fever (37.5°C). It would be important to find out exactly how often his mother is giving him pain medication to make sure his pain is under control.

Health maintenance activities
> Lachlan has found it difficult to continue with his swimming training as he has been feeling tired and does not feel like swimming, which has limited his social connections and interactions.
> He is finding it difficult to sleep and has woken himself up 'snoring'.

Interpret: This information indicates the significance of his alteration in health that is affecting his quality of life.

Physical assessment/diagnostic data

Breath
> Foul smell noted
> Noted to be breathing through mouth

Throat
> Erythematous with 3+ tonsils bilaterally, inflamed and no exudates; uvula midline; gag reflex positive

Infer: The smell is an indicator of infection, which can often cause decreased airway patency through the nose (mouth breathing), with enlarged tonsils being an indication of the body's immune response in trying to overcome the localised throat infection.

Mouth
> Mucosa – pale pink

Infer: As a result of possible mouth breathing
> Lips – dry

Infer: From mouth breathing
> Secretions – build-up of saliva

Infer: As a result of difficulty swallowing

Putting it all together – synthesise information

The nurse in this case would note all of these abnormalities and refer to the medical officer. Throat cultures may be necessary to differentiate between viral and streptococcal infection. As most infections are viral in origin, tests can eliminate the need for unnecessary use of antibiotics. However, if it is a bacterial infection, and likely antibiotics will be prescribed, the nurse will need to check that medication prescribed is not of the penicillin family (as consumer has allergy to this) or have contraindications or adverse interactions with Lachlan's gluten allergies. Lachlan may or may not be considered for surgery at a later date to remove his tonsils – this could be a possibility.

Actions based on assessment findings

The nurse should also provide additional education for interventions that do not require a doctor's order, such as:
1 continue use of paracetamol for analgesia and comfort measures
2 rest and sleep as much as possible until symptoms improve; this will aid the body's immune response
3 oral hygiene to prevent further possibility of infection
4 increased fluid and food intake to limit possibility of dehydration. Encourage soft foods that may be easier to swallow.

The final step in the process is accurate documentation. The nurse must document findings, referrals, interventions, and advice and education given. The consumer would then be reassessed following definitive diagnosis and medical interventions for his ongoing health maintenance.

CHAPTER RESOURCES

REVIEW QUESTIONS

For answers to these questions, see Answer section at the end of the book.

1. Mohamod is a 13-year-old male consumer who is having a well-child check by the school nurse. The nurse is concerned about a weight gain of 10 kg over the past year. Which of the following pieces of information is most important?
   a. Family history of obesity
   b. BMI
   c. Vital signs
   d. School adaptation

2. Harper's mother calls the referral line of the local children's hospital stating she is concerned about her 15-year-old daughter's recent withdrawn behaviour. Which of the following behaviour warrants immediate evaluation?
   a. Wanting to be alone in her room
   b. Ignoring her siblings and parents at the dinner table
   c. Giving her friend a prized rabbit's foot
   d. Ignoring curfew rules

3. The nurse caring for Jimeoin in Room 3 suspects child abuse. Which of the following observations led the nurse to suspect abuse?
   a. Constant crying despite consoling measures
   b. Scratch mark near the ankle where the identification band is placed
   c. Bruising noted on the consumer's back near the left shoulder
   d. Circumferential erythema at the antecubital area where the previous nurse had started an IV

4. Max, a 2-year-old toddler, comes into the clinic for his yearly well-child check. He is extremely upset when approached. Which of the following measures would help Max?
   a. Allowing the mother to reschedule his appointment
   b. Allowing his mother to hold him during the examination
   c. Allowing Max's mother to step out of the room while you take his vital signs
   d. Allowing Max to take a walk outside with his mother while he calms down

5. A 7-month-old paediatric consumer is admitted to the hospital for dehydration. As the healthcare provider for this consumer, you are assessing reflex mechanisms. You note that the rooting reflex is absent. At what age does the rooting reflex disappear in the nonsleeping infant?
   a. 2 months
   b. 4 months
   c. 6 months
   d. 8 months

6. The mother of 2-week-old Mila is concerned because, 'the soft spots on her head are not going away'. The nurse's best response would be which of the following?
   a. 'How long were you in labour with Mila?'
   b. 'The soft spots are normal as long as they are less than 2 cm at birth and close when Mila is 8 months old.'
   c. 'Mila has craniosynostosis and needs to see a specialist.'
   d. 'Mila's soft spots are normal and should be closed by 19 months of age.'

7. The diphtheria, tetanus and whooping cough (acellular pertussis) (DTPa) vaccine should commence at what age?
   a. 20–24 weeks
   b. 8–10 days
   c. 12–16 weeks
   d. 6–8 weeks

8. At birth, a Caucasian infant has a heart rate of 112, a respiratory rate that is slow and irregular, and full flexion of the limbs; is crying; and has acrocyanotic limbs with a pink torso. What is the Apgar score of this infant?
   a. 7
   b. 8
   c. 9
   d. 10

9. At what age would a full-term infant be able to hold the head steady without lag?
   a. At birth
   b. 2 weeks
   c. 6 months
   d. 3 months

10. Which of the following is an expected finding in a 3-year-old toddler in a vision screening assessment?
    a. Tumbling E chart: right eye 6/12
    b. Hirschberg test: light reflection located on the inner margin of the left cornea as the eye deviates outward
    c. Cover/uncover test: both eyes move to focus on the penlight
    d. Tumbler E chart 6/15

CS CLINICAL **SKILLS**

The following Clinical Skills are relevant to this chapter and can be found in Tollefson & Hillman, *Clinical Psychomotor Skills*, 8th edition:

> 13 Pain assessment
> 27 Healthcare teaching
> 75 Non-pharmacological pain management interventions – therapeutic massage
> 76 Non-pharmacological pain management interventions – conventional transcutaneous electrical nerve stimulation.

FURTHER RESOURCES

> Asthma Australia. Children and asthma: https://www.asthmaaustralia.org.au
> Australian and New Zealand Society for Paediatric Dentistry: https://www.ada.org.au/
> Australian College of Children and Young People's Nurses (ACCYPN): http://www.accypn.org.au
> Australian Paediatric Endocrine Group, Growth & Growth Charts: https://apeg.org.au/clinical-resources-links/growth-growth-charts/
> Bright Futures Child Aid & Development Fund Australia Inc: http://brightfutures.com.au
> CDC Use of World Health Organization and CDC 0–59 months in the United States: http://www.cdc.gov/mmwr/preview/mmwrhtml/rr5909a1.htm
> Centers for Disease Control and Prevention: http://www.cdc.gov
> Children's health – Australia.gov.au: http://australia.gov.au/topics/health-and-safety/childrens-health
> Congenital Heart Information Network, The: http://www.tchin.org
> Headspace National Youth Mental Health foundation: https://headspace.org.au/

> HeartKids Australia: https://www.heartkids.org.au/
> KidsHealth: http://www.kidshealth.org
> Ministry of Health New Zealand. World Health Organization Growth Charts: http://www.health.govt.nz/our-work/life-stages/child-health/well-child-tamariki-ora-services/growth-charts
> National Association of Paediatric Nurse Practitioners: http://www.napnap.org
> National Institute on Drug Abuse (NIDA): http://www.drugabuse.gov/drugs-abuse/club-drugs
> Newborn hearing screening: http://www.deafchildrenaustralia.org.au/newborn_hearing_screening
> Paediatric Society of New Zealand: http://www.paediatrics.org.nz
> Royal Children's Hospital, Cleft lip and palate: http://www.rch.org.au/kidsinfo/factsheets.cfm?doc_id=7759
> Sids and Kids: http://www.sidsandkids.org/
> SIDS New Zealand Incorporated: http://www.sids.org.nz/
> Sudden Infant Death Syndrome (SIDS): https://www.healthdirect.gov.au/search-results/SIDS

REFERENCES

ADHD Australia. (2019). Attention deficit hyperactive disorder, Australia. Retrieved 25 September 2022 from: https://www.adhdaustralia.org.au/

Australian Bureau of Statistics (ABS). (2019). National Aboriginal and Torres Strait Islander health survey. Retrieved 8 December 2022 from: https://www.abs.gov.au/statistics/people/aboriginal-and-torres-strait-islander-peoples/national-aboriginal-and-torres-strait-islander-health-survey/latest-release

Australian Bureau of Statistics (ABS). (2021). Household and families: Census. Retrieved 8 December 2022 from: https://www.abs.gov.au/statistics/people/people-and-communities/household-and-families-census/2021

Australian Government Department of Health. (2023). National Immunisation Program schedule. Retrieved 9 May 2023 from: https://www.health.gov.au/sites/default/files/2023-03/national-immunisation-program-schedule.pdf

Australian Institute of Health and Welfare (AIHW). (2022a). Health of children. Retrieved 8 December 2022 from: https://www.aihw.gov.au/reports/children-youth/health-of-children#Profile.

Australian Institute of Health and Welfare (AIHW). (2022b). Australia's children. Children with mental illness. Retrieved 25 September 2022 from: https://www.aihw.gov.au/reports/children-youth/australias-children/contents/health/children-mental-illness

Australian Institute of Health and Welfare (AIHW). (2022c). Suicide and self-harm monitoring. Retrieved 25 September 2022 from: https://www.aihw.gov.au/suicide-self-harm-monitoring/data/populations-age-groups/suicide-indigenous-australians

Australian Institute of Health and Welfare (AIHW). (2022d). Congenital anomalies 2016, AIHW, Australian Government, Retrieved 5 October 2022 from: https://www.aihw.gov.au/getmedia/3743dd66-3aa9-4812-9bdf-db6cb6bc52ac/Congenital-anomalies-2016.pdf.aspx?inline=true

Australian Institute of Health and Welfare (AIHW). (2022e). Ear Health. Retrieved 7 October 2022 from: https://www.indigenoushpf.gov.au/measures/1-15-ear-health

Australian Research Alliance for Children and Youth (ARACY). (2018). Report Card 2018 – The wellbeing of young Australians. Retrieved 3 August from: https://www.aracy.org.au/publications-resources/command/download_file/id/361/filename/ARACY_Report_Card_2018.pdf

Brown, R. C., & Plener, P. L. (2017). Non-suicidal self-injury in adolescence. *Current Psychiatry Reports*, *19*(3), 20. http://doi.org/10.1007/s11920-017-0767-9

Centre for Community Child Health. (2022). The impact of the COVID-19 pandemic on children in Australian early childhood education and care. Rapid review prepared by the Centre for Community Child Health, Murdoch Children's Research Institute for the Commonwealth Department of Education, Skills and Employment. Retrieved 24 September 2022 from: https://www.rch.org.au/uploadedFiles/Main/Content/ccchdev/Impact%20of%20COVID-19%20pandemic%20on%20children%20in%20Australian%20ECEC%20(1).pdf

Daley, G. M., Pretorius, C. J., & Ungerer, J. P. (2018). Lead toxicity: an Australian perspective. *The Clinical biochemist. Reviews*, *39*(4), 61–98. PMID: 30828115; PMCID: PMC6372192.

Deadly Kids | Deadly Futures. (2016). Queensland's Aboriginal and Torres Strait Islander Child Ear and Hearing Health Framework 2016–2026. Queensland Government. Retrieved 17 August 2018 from: https://www.childrens.health.qld.gov.au/wp-content/uploads/PDF/deadly-ears/deadly-kids-futures-fw.pdf

De Young, A., Paterson, R., March, S., Hoehn, E., Alisic, E., Cobham, V., … Vasileva, M. (2021). COVID-19 Unmasked Young Children Report 2: Impact of the second wave in Australia on the mental health of young children and parents. Brisbane: Queensland Centre for Perinatal and Infant Mental Health, Children's Health Queensland Hospital and Health Service. Retrieved 24 September 2022 from: https://www.childrens.health.qld.gov.au/wp-content/uploads/PDF/COVID-19/COVID19-Unmasked-Survey-Progress-Report-02.pdf

Healthdirect, (2020). Sudden infant death syndrome. Retrieved 25 September 2022 from: https://www.healthdirect.gov.au/sudden-infant-death-syndrome-sids

Ministry of Health New Zealand. (2015). Growth charts. Ministry of Health, Manatu Hauora. Retrieved 23 September 2022 from: https://www.health.govt.nz/our-work/life-stages/child-health/well-child-tamariki-ora-services/growth-charts

Ministry of Health New Zealand. (2018). New Zealand Immunisation Schedule. Retrieved 10 August 2018 from: http://www.health.govt.nz/our-work/preventative-health-wellness/immunisation/new-zealand-immunisation-schedule

Ministry of Health New Zealand. (2021). Obesity statistics. Retrieved 8 December 2022 from: https://www.health.govt.nz/nz-health-statistics/health-statistics-and-data-sets/obesity-statistics

Ministry of Health New Zealand. (2022a). 021/22 New Zealand Health Survey. Retrieved 8 December 2022 from: https://www.health.govt.nz/publication/annual-update-key-results-2021-22-new-zealand-health-survey

Ministry of Health New Zealand. (2022b). Suicide data and stats. Retrieved 15 September 2022 from: https://www.health.govt.nz/nz-health-statistics/health-statistics-and-data-sets/suicide-data-and-stats

Obesity Evidence Hub. (2021). Obesity, diet and exercise in Aboriginal and Torres Strait Islander children. Retrieved 8 December 2022 from: https://www.obesityevidencehub.org.au/collections/trends/aboriginal-and-torres-strait-islander-children

Parents protect. (2018). Warning signs in children and adults. Retrieved 10 August 2018 from: https://www.parentsprotect.co.uk/warning-signs-in-children-and-adults.htm

Queensland Health. (2020). Screening Protocols and Guidelines 2016 V2. Retrieved 7 October 2022 from: https://www.childrens.health.qld.gov.au/wp-content/uploads/newborn-hearing-screening-protocols-guidelines.pdf

Royal Children's Hospital Melbourne. (2021a). Hypertension in children and adolescents – Clinical Practice Guidelines. Retrieved 17 September 2022 from: https://www.rch.org.au/clinicalguide/guideline_index/Hypertension_in_children_and_adolescents/

Royal Children's Hospital Melbourne. (2021b). Clinical guidelines. Acute upper airway management. Royal Children's Hospital Melbourne, Retrieved 7 October 2022 from: https://www.rch.org.au/clinicalguide/guideline_index/Acute_upper_airway_obstruction/

Royal Children's Hospital, The. (2022). Child growth learning resource. Royal Children's Hospital, Melbourne. Retrieved 23 September 2022 from: https://www.rch.org.au/childgrowth/Growth_Charts/

Royal Children's Hospital, The. (2018) Parent's Evaluation of Developmental Status. Royal Children's Hospital Melbourne. Retrieved 4 August 2018 from: https://www.rch.org.au/ccch/peds/For_clinicians/

SECASA. (2015). Indicators of child sexual abuse. The South Eastern Centre Against Sexual Assault and Family Violence. Retrieved 6 October 2018 from: https://www.secasa.com.au/pages/child-sexual-abuse-understanding-and-responding/indicators-of-child-sexual-abuse/

Singh, S., Roy, D., Sinha, K., Parveen, S., Sharma, G., & Joshi, G. (2020). Impact of COVID-19 and lockdown on mental health of children and adolescents: A narrative review with recommendations. *Psychiatry Research, 293*,113429. doi:10.1016/j.psychres.2020.113429.

Stats NZ. (2021a). National population estimates: At 30 June 2021. Retrieved 19 December 2022 from: https://www.stats.govt.nz/information-releases/national-population-estimates-at-30-june-2021

Stats NZ. (2021b). New data shows 1 in 9 children under the age of five lives in a multi-family household. Retrieved 18 December 2022 from: https://www.stats.govt.nz/news/new-data-shows-1-in-9-children-under-the-age-of-five-lives-in-a-multi-family-household/

Suicide Prevention Australia. (2021). Youth suicide fact sheet. Retrieved 25 September 2022 from: https://www.suicidepreventionaust.org/wp-content/uploads/2021/06/Youth-Suicide-Fact-Sheet.pdf

Telfer, M. M., Tollit, M. A., Pace, C. C., & Pang, K. C. (2020). Australian standards of care and treatment guidelines for trans and gender diverse children and adolescents Version 1.3. Melbourne: The Royal Children's Hospital. Retrieved 7 October 2022 from: https://www.rch.org.au/uploadedFiles/Main/Content/adolescent-medicine/australian-standards-of-care-and-treatment-guidelines-for-trans-and-gender-diverse-children-and-adolescents.pdf

Wallace, S., Scarcella, M., Sealy, L., Alexander, S., & Zwi, K. (2022). Aboriginal and Torres Strait Islander children with obesity: A review of programmes for children and young people aged 5–17 years. *Journal of Paediatrics and Child Health, 58*(12), December. https://doi.org/10.1111/jpc.16267

CHAPTER 21

THE OLDER ADULT

LEARNING OUTCOMES

By the end of this chapter you should be able to:

1 explain the structural and physiological variations of the older adult
2 identify techniques that facilitate the health history interview of the older adult
3 identify various tools that can be used to assess functional status and cognition in the older adult
4 discuss when to modify physical examination techniques used within the older adult population
5 discuss the clinical reasoning in evaluating outcomes of health assessment and physical examination including documentation requirements for recording information, health education given and relevant health referral.

BACKGROUND

An overview of the health assessment and physical examination of the older adult is presented in this chapter. Older adults are a unique population who experience specific changes in their bodies related to age (Figure 21.1). As a consequence, they will have different and unique presentations in their healthy, normal and disease states. With increasing age, the rate of decline related to disease is more diverse. Healthcare professionals differentiate between the normal changes of ageing and pathologic processes in order to provide appropriate care. It is essential to identify how the changes of ageing have affected the individual, so that care can be individualised. The management of aged care is a key focus for governments. Care is multifaceted with an array of health service providers in existence; for example, health professionals, hospital clinics, community-based, residential-based aged care and respite support services.

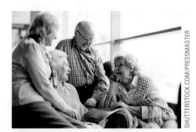

FIGURE 21.1 Older adults are unique individuals who experience specific changes related to age and other factors.

Many of the assessment techniques used are similar across age groups. Knowledge of normal ageing, and awareness of the effects of chronic diseases, heredity, environment and lifestyle on the health of older adults, is important as you conduct and interpret accurate health assessment. Older people usually present with different signs and symptoms than younger people in relation to illness. Health professionals, therefore, should have a deep understanding of the anatomical and physiological differences of the older person. Older people also have unique physical and psychosocial characteristics and needs, which should be kept in mind as individuals live to an older age, and are most likely to have one or more chronic conditions that may affect their ability to function. Although disability increases with the increased number of chronic conditions, much of the ageing population remains highly functional.

The number of older people in Australia and New Zealand continues to increase, so supporting their physical health and wellbeing is becoming even more important (AIHW, 2021a). Although the majority of people are living longer, as compared to other age groups more people over the age of 65 face health challenges due to a range of physical and mental health issues (AIHW, 2021a). In 2020, 16% of the populations of Australia and New Zealand were aged 65 years or older (ABS, 2022a; Stats NZ 2022). This accounted for 4.2 million people in Australia, which is about one in every six Australians (AIHW, 2021a). As is the case for many Indigenous populations, life expectancy is shorter for Aboriginal and Torres Strait Islander peoples and New Zealand Māori, and a range of health conditions are more prevalent. For example, in 2021 only 5.4% of Aboriginal and Torres Strait Islander peoples were aged 65 and over, compared with 16% of non-Aboriginal and Torres Strait Islander peoples (ABS, 2022b), and only 5.8% of the Māori population were over 65 years (Parr-Brownlie et al., 2020). Health conditions such as coronary heart disease, diabetes, chronic lower respiratory diseases, and cancers of the lung, bronchus and trachea are found in higher frequency in both Aboriginal and Torres Strait Islander peoples and New Zealand Māori (AIHW, 2022a; Te Whatu Ora, 2022).

KEY HEALTH CHALLENGES FOR OLDER ADULTS

Older adults reside in a variety of settings and this will depend on a number of individual factors that may include health issues. While most older people live in private dwellings (71% of women and 82% of men aged 85 years and older) and are independent (AIHW, 2021b), others require the support of a caregiver (spouse, son or daughter, other family member, or paid assistant), or reside in an aged care residential facility. These facilities range from seniors living with no assistance offered, to facilities where there are services of varying levels of assistance, including rehabilitative services post illness to long-term nursing home residence (Figure 21.2). The majority of older adults prefer to live in their own private homes and the government encourages this through policy direction and financial assistance.

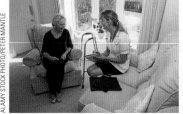

FIGURE 21.2 Care is delivered to older adults in a variety of settings.

ALAMY STOCK PHOTO/PETER MANTLE

The older population, having lived through a number of life experiences, may erroneously attribute specific health symptoms to normal ageing and delay seeking treatment. They do not typically present with all the same signs and symptoms as younger adults. The most common complaints at presentation are often nonspecific and vague, and are frequently portrayed as general lethargy, weakness or fatigue and loss of appetite. This can lead to chronic health problems and predispose the older person to a higher risk of poor health outcomes. Stoicism of the older adult and misperception of normal ageing by the person are barriers to reporting developing symptoms (e.g. pain and changes in memory), such as worrying about testing and fear of bad news and of being a burden to others. Further, fears of possible expense, physical discomfort and loss of independence are all concerns expressed by older adults. Reporting may also be hampered by cognitive impairment, inability to verbalise symptoms, concerns of not being taken seriously by healthcare providers or concerns over change.

Key Australian and New Zealand health issues for the older adult are considerable but not specific to these countries alone. As adults age, some common issues include musculoskeletal injuries due to falls (see Chapter 16); skin integumentary problems (see Chapter 8); mental health issues, particularly depression and suicide (see Chapter 7); loss of appetite and urinary incontinence (see Chapter 15); and diseases such as cancers and dementia.

In 2022, there were an estimated 487 500 Australians (Dementia Australia, 2023) and 70 000 New Zealanders (Alzheimer's New Zealand, 2023) living with dementia. More women than men will die of dementia (64.5%) and 3 out of 10 people over the age of 85 years and 1 out of 10 over 65 years will have dementia (Dementia Australia, 2023). While age is a risk fact for dementia, in 2020 it is estimated that 27 800 Australians will have younger onset dementia, meaning that they are under the age of 65 years when the diagnosis is made (Dementia Australia, 2023).With over 100 causes of dementia and no single test to confirm a diagnosis, all other treatable causes of the symptoms being experienced must first be ruled out. The diagnosis of dementia requires a comprehensive history of symptom development and a suite of assessments that involves a multidisciplinary team. The area of the brain damaged by disease will contribute to the symptoms experienced and ultimately the diagnosis given.

ANATOMY AND PHYSIOLOGY

Structural and physiological variations

Every cell, tissue, organ and organism is affected by the process of ageing. Most systems have specific changes, while a few systems have vague, deregulatory changes. These changes are due to a combination of factors, among them genetics, environment, nutrition and activity. Changes of ageing are not harmful in isolation, but physiologic resilience is compromised primarily by loss of reserves. Homeostasis becomes more difficult to maintain in times of stress such as injury, illness or surgery. These changes are more commonly seen in the very old or frail older adult. Although most changes seen in the older adult are part of the normal ageing process, many can also indicate underlying systemic or localised disease; therefore, it is important not to generalise changes as routine.

Vital signs

Respirations
As a result of ageing, reduced contractility of the breathing muscles results in reduced inspiration. To compensate for reduced oxygenation, the normal respiratory rate is between 12 and 24 breaths per minute. An elevated respiratory rate frequently precedes usual symptoms of upper respiratory infection or a developing illness.

Pulse
In the older adult, the resting heart rate remains constant but the maximum heart rate declines. Loss in strength of the heart muscle leads to a reduction in heart rate due to ageing. Reflex tachycardia is delayed due to a blunted baroreceptor reflex.

Temperature
The older adult may have an abnormally low body temperature and greater variations in temperature. Diurnal variations are not affected by age. Frail older people may present with an immune response causing absence of fever.

Blood pressure
Both diastolic and systolic blood pressure rise due to the loss of elasticity in the vasculature of the older adult. Emergence of new diastolic hypertension in an older person usually has a secondary aetiology, which should be explored. In addition, approximately 20% of older individuals exhibit postural hypotension. Postprandial hypotension is more commonly seen in older adults than in younger people. A widening of the pulse pressure also occurs.

Skin, hair and nails
The most visible signs of ageing are manifested in the skin and hair. These signs include wrinkles, sagging skin folds, greying hair and hair loss. Light-skinned individuals appear to manifest the changes of ageing more rapidly than do dark-skinned individuals, and these changes are accelerated by sun exposure. Skin disorders are also more likely to occur as a person ages.

With ageing, the epidermis thins and elastic fibres that provide support to the dermis degenerate and lead to sagging skin folds. The vascularity of the skin declines, which can lead to senile purpura, and the risk of a breakdown in skin integrity increases (i.e. skin tears, chronic leg ulcers). Because the number of sweat and sebaceous glands diminishes, a disruption in the body's thermoregulation occurs. There is also an increased incidence of hypothermia due to vasodilation and vasoconstriction of the dermal arterioles and loss of subcutaneous fat. The loss of subcutaneous tissue over bony prominences increases the risk of skin breakdown in the older adult.

A diminished inflammatory response and a diminished perception of pain increase the risk of adverse effects from noxious stimuli in the older adult; therefore, they are at a greater risk for frostbite and burns because of their diminished sensation and pain perception. Their injuries are more serious because of the thinning of the epidermis and the prolonged or delayed wound healing that increases with age. One systematic review found risk factors for delayed healing in venous ulcers were increased age, poor nutrition and decreased mobility (Parker, Finlayson & Edwards, 2015). For consumers with comorbidities such as peripheral vascular disease or peripheral neuropathy from diabetes mellitus, this healing time is greatly increased and the chance of infection is higher.

Wrinkling is the change most associated with ageing of the skin. Wrinkles are most prominent on the face and neck because these areas have the greatest sun exposure. Other factors leading to wrinkling are loss of subcutaneous fat and diminished elasticity of the skin.

Skin irritation is a common affliction in older adults. This is due to a decrease in the water content of the skin, a decrease in the number of sebaceous glands, and atrophy of the eccrine glands. The latter contributes to the risk of hyperthermia in the older adult. Depending on environments, in very cold winter areas where houses need heating (e.g. New Zealand's South Island or Tasmania), or in very dry hot areas in summer (such as the outback and in Northern Queensland), dryness and itching occur because humidity is low, indoor or outdoor temperatures are high (for those who use indoor heating, or do not have air conditioning), drying winds are present and, in some cases, water has a high mineral content (e.g. water sourced from the Great Artesian Basin). The condition is aggravated by frequent bathing in hot water, which robs the skin of moisture. Generalised itching is also associated with systemic diseases such as diabetes mellitus, atherosclerosis and liver disease.

The number and thickness of terminal hairs generally diminish, and there is a conversion of vellus hair to terminal hair in areas such as the rims of the ears and nose in men, and on the upper lip and chin in women. Decreased melanin production decreases the melanocytes at the hair follicles and leads to hair pigment loss manifested as greying hair.

The nails in the older adult may thicken, split, and become more yellow and dull. There may be an overcurvature of the toenails if tight shoes were worn for a large portion of adult life.

Head, neck and regional lymphatics

Loss of subcutaneous fat and musculoskeletal changes due to the ageing process affect the appearance and function of the head and neck. Wrinkles are more prominent. Facial symmetry may be altered because of the presence of dentures or loss of teeth. Due to reabsorption of mandibular bone, a change in facial appearance is expected. Neck veins may be more prominent due to loss of fat.

The head, neck and lower jaw may be thrust forward, especially with a kyphotic posture. A 'hump back' may appear as an accumulation of fat over the posterior cervical vertebrae. This is seen in consumers with osteoporosis. Range of motion of the head may be limited, painful, or possible only with a jerking or 'cogwheel' motion. Dizziness accompanying movement of the head may create safety problems. All of these changes may affect the older adult's ability to maintain normal activities of daily living.

Eyes

Visual impairments are among the most prevalent chronic conditions in the older adult. Sight provides information to enable people to function in the environment.

Thus, prevention of sensory impairment and resulting handicaps are challenges for the individual and the healthcare provider.

During the ageing process, the eye undergoes significant changes. Ageing changes occur in the pupil, lens, vitreous humor, macula and retro-orbital fat. This results in the eyeball receding into its socket and eyelids become droopy. There is also decreased eye lubrication and effort required to adapt to changes in light intensity, causing night vision problems. By the age of 42, the lens cortex becomes denser, compromising its ability to change shape and focus. This condition, **presbyopia**, is responsible for farsightedness and the need for bifocals. A decrease in aqueous humour secretion and increased vitreous gel debris lead to decreased cleansing of the lens and cornea as well. Next, there is a tendency for the lens to yellow and become cloudy. This change impairs a person's ability to discern colours, especially blues and greens. In addition, pupils become smaller, causing the amount of light reaching the retina to be reduced. As a consequence, older adults need more light to see and their eyes take longer to accommodate to darkness and glare. Peripheral vision is decreased and upward gaze may be limited, which can create safety issues for driving and other activities.

Externally, the older adult has a loss of pigment in the iris, decreased orbital fat, and a thinning of the eyelid tissue. Decreased corneal sensitivity and a decreased corneal reflex, in conjunction with the presence of entropion, ectropion or ptosis, can result in corneal abrasion or infection. The globe appears to be deeper in the eye socket, and the lacrimal gland may be visible because of the loss of subcutaneous fat around the eye.

Ears

Hearing loss, **presbycusis**, is a common condition among older adults. Conductive hearing loss occurs in the outer or middle ear and usually makes things sound softer. High-pitched tones are lost first. However, the more common age-related hearing loss is sensorineural, which involves the inner ear. Ossicular joint deterioration occurs, there is a degeneration of hair cells in the inner ear, and the vestibular structures, the cochlea and organ of Corti all atrophy. These bilateral ear changes can also result in an increased risk of balance and equilibrium deficits.

As we age, the pinna of the ear gets larger and becomes dry and scaly. Males tend to get increased hair growth on pinna. This growth is caused by a degeneration of hair cells and neurones in the inner ear, reduced elasticity of the tympanic membrane, and calcification of the stapes, incus and malleus, and can lead to decreased hearing and sense of balance. Externally, the pinna increases in length and width in the older adult and cerumen production decreases. This can lead to ear dryness and cerumen impaction. Otoscopic assessment may reveal more pronounced landmarks if atrophic or sclerotic changes have occurred.

Nose

Nasal hairs are coarser, and less efficient filtration occurs as a person ages. This can lead to sinus and respiratory problems. In addition, the sense of smell declines rapidly after age 50. The smaller number of smell receptors is less efficient, and smells must be more intense to be perceived. This diminished smell may result in decreased appetite. Significant loss of smell has also been identified as an early symptom of Alzheimer's disease, Parkinson's disease and various other neurological disorders, and depression.

Mouth and throat

Common alterations in the mouth of an older adult are precancerous and cancerous lesions, untreated caries (due to poor nutrition early in life, decreased saliva production, lack of funds to obtain dental care, and neglect of oral hygiene), periodontal disease (i.e. receding gum lines, gingivitis), tooth loss (which can affect closure of the mouth), worn tooth surfaces and orofacial pain. Swallowing problems increase in part due to decreased saliva production. In addition, side effects from medications (e.g. xerostomia from anticholinergic medications and antihistamines, possible oral candidiasis from inhaled steroids) can alter the normal anatomy of the mouth.

Taste may not diminish with age, but it may become less reliable due to a decreased number of taste buds and a decline in their function. Specifically, the older adult has a more difficult time discriminating the tastes of sweet, sour, salt and bitter.

The teeth and gums recede, which may lead to increased susceptibility to infection and decay. There is a higher incidence of loss of teeth and periodontal disease in the older population than in the younger age groups. Those wearing dentures may not realise that their dentures may need adjusting every year or two due to changing mandibular bone structure. Oral hygiene practices should be assessed on each comprehensive visit. Frequently heard symptoms with which the older consumer may present are foul breath and sensitivity to extremes of temperature. Periodontal disease may be the cause and should always be evaluated, as this is a major cause of tooth loss. The same symptoms, however, can be presentations of sinusitis or a pulmonary infection.

Breasts and regional nodes

The adipose tissue of the breast atrophies with age and is replaced with connective tissue. The glandular tissue gradually decreases, causing the breasts to feel granular instead of lobular. Breast tissue mass decreases with age and becomes pendulous and wrinkled. The nipples become smaller and flatter. Ductal tissue becomes more palpable, especially around the nipples, and may become firm and stringy. In addition, the musculature around the breasts tends to atrophy, which contributes to the overall droopiness of the breasts. There is an increased incidence of breast cancer after the age of 50.

Thorax and lungs

The older adult undergoes changes that involve the external and internal anatomy of the thorax and lungs. As a result, the physiology of the respiratory system becomes altered. The resulting state of the consumer depends on the extent of the changes and the presence of comorbid conditions. Variations of the respiratory system include four broad areas:

1. Anatomic changes
2. Alveolar gas exchange
3. Regulation of ventilation
4. Lung defence mechanisms.

Older adults experience degeneration of the intervertebral discs, stiffening of ligaments and joints, and calcification of the costochondral cartilage. These changes limit chest wall expansion during the respiratory cycle. Muscles atrophy and become weaker and the diaphragm flattens out, leading to decreased respiratory endurance for the older adult. Strenuous exercise is taxing, secondary to the decrease in oxygen uptake and decreased elastic recoil of the lung parenchyma. Most older adults will have some degree of a barrel chest and some kyphosis. Forced vital capacity decreases, residual volume and functional residual capacity increase, and the total lung capacity remains unchanged.

The second major change in the older adult is the alveolar gas exchange. The decreased elastic recoil of the lungs causes the closure of airways for a portion of the respiratory cycle. This occurs particularly in the lower lobes of the lungs. As a result, the apices and the bases of the lungs have a ventilation–perfusion mismatch. Other contributing factors to this loss of alveolar gas exchange are the loss of lung tissue and alveolar capillaries and pulmonary wall thickening. In essence, this creates a situation in which there is less surface area for diffusion, and this surface area is thicker. In addition, haemoglobin's affinity for oxygen decreases, which leads to a decrease in the partial pressure of oxygen.

The ageing adult experiences changes in the regulation of ventilation. The medulla is less sensitive to changes in carbon dioxide and oxygen levels, which normally trigger the respiratory drive. There is a compromised acid–base balance. Neural output to respiratory muscles is decreased. Both peripheral and central chemoreceptors are affected.

The last area of change is in lung defence mechanisms. There is less ciliary and macrophage activity, which increases susceptibility to infection. The cough reflex decreases, and the risk of aspiration increases.

Heart and blood vessels

As adults age, their cardiovascular systems undergo physiologic changes that, in many instances, are complicated by disease processes. In the older adult, the size of the cardiac muscle decreases with age. As fibrotic and sclerotic changes take place in the atria and the ventricles, cardiac output can fall by as much as 35% at rest after the age of 70. Skeletal changes such as osteoporosis, kyphosis or collapsed vertebrae can alter the position of the heart within the thoracic cavity, giving rise to changes in the electrocardiogram. Obesity leads to increased abdominal girth and diaphragm elevation, which can also displace the heart within the chest.

With the ageing process, cardiac valves may develop calcifications or fibrosis, which results in systolic or diastolic murmurs. A systolic ejection murmur commonly found at the left lower sternal border is of no diagnostic significance. The cardiovascular system has a global thickening and stiffening of the arterial walls, which leads to hypertension. If the left ventricle has thickened or enlarged, thus losing its compliance, an S_4 heart sound can be auscultated. Changes in the conduction system resulting from electrolyte imbalance, pharmacotherapy, debilitating states or thickened myocardial fibres can cause cardiac irritability, leading to a variety of dysrhythmias. The ageing adult also has a reduced beta adrenergic response.

Vascular integrity is also affected in the ageing process. The arterial system becomes increasingly rigid as the blood vessels become fibrotic. If a pathological process such as atherosclerosis is present, the insult to the vasculature becomes even greater. Elasticity is lost, the vessel lumen is narrowed, and peripheral vascular resistance is increased, thus impeding blood flow. Conditions such as smoking, which cause vascular spasm, contribute to a decrease in vascular flow. In the venous system, there is intimal thickening with dilation and loss of valve competency. Venous return to the heart is affected, and oedema or varicosities may develop. The baroreceptors located in the aortic arch and the carotid sinuses are also affected by vascular integrity. In the presence of impaired compliance, these structures are altered in their abilities to respond to blood pressure changes. A dilated aorta and cool extremities are commonly found with decreased peripheral pulses.

CLINICAL **REASONING**

Cardiac signs and symptoms in the older adult

Coronary heart disease increases rapidly with age and remains the overall leading cause of death for older adult age groups (AIHW, 2022b). It is worth noting that many older adults do not experience the more commonly described cardiac symptoms. For example, the person may not complain of experiencing severe central chest pain with an acute myocardial infarction (AMI). They may present with generalised complaints such as tiredness, weakness or generally feeling unwell and/or dyspnoea, palpitations.

It is important in these situations to focus your assessment on maintaining a person-centred approach and draw on your clinical reasoning skills to collect relevant data to determine the problems/issues and set goals to manage them. In the situation of an older person experiencing vague symptomatology, you need to determine if the situation is cardiac-related by collecting data such as vital signs, past history, ECG and oxygen saturation, and escalate for further medical management.

Abdomen

In the process of ageing, the abdominal musculature diminishes in mass and loses much of its tone. At the same time, the fat content of the body increases, leading to increased fat deposition in the abdominal area. The mucosal lining of the gastrointestinal tract becomes less elastic, and changes in gastric motility result in alterations in digestion and absorption.

Decreased oesophageal motility and lower oesophageal sphincter pressure can lead to complaints of gastro-oesophageal reflux disease (GORD) symptoms. Pancreatic, enzymatic and hormonal secretions decrease, and there is atrophy of antral cells, causing a decreased secretion of hydrochloric acid and intrinsic factor. These can cause malabsorption, altered digestion, and a cobalamin deficiency. A decrease in intestinal motility can lead to constipation, one of the most frequent complaints of the older adult.

As the intestinal wall weakens, the number of diverticuli increase. These can progress to inflammation and obstruction.

There is little evidence that liver function changes significantly with age. However, hepatic weight, blood flow and regenerative capacity decrease progressively with age. Liver mass also decreases and blood flow, leading to reduced hepatic clearance of medications and increased sensitivity of the gastrointestinal tract to medication concentrations. The result of this is a risk of reactions to medications.

CLINICAL **REASONING**

Practice tip: Gastrointestinal signs and symptoms in the older adult

Gastrointestinal complaints such as flatus, dyspepsia or heartburn constitute many of the reasons why an older adult seeks health care. Although many of these complaints may be functional in nature, other cues should be investigated. Gastric irritation can result from an increased consumption of alcohol, aspirin or nonsteroidal anti-inflammatory drugs. Occult bleeding may go undetected until a gastrointestinal bleed occurs or anaemia is detected.

In addition, constipation is a frequent complaint. Changes in bowel habits may be benign manifestations of diet, medications, a loss of sphincter tone or lack of exercise. However, in the older adult, these symptoms might signify the presence of gastric or colon malignancies.

In your assessment, if any of these signs or symptoms are noted, it is important to follow through with further focused questioning to identify specific reason/s so that you can make the appropriate clinical decisions, including documentation and referral.

CLINICAL **REASONING**

Practice tip: Assessing for polypharmacy
What is polypharmacy?

Polypharmacy is generally defined as the simultaneous use of five or more medications, however this does not consider an individual's co-morbidities; that is, the presence of two or more ongoing health conditions. Therefore, this makes it difficult for clinicians to safely and correctly clinically manage an individual's medication administration. Polypharmacy encompasses over-the-counter prescriptions as well as traditional and complementary medicines (WHO, 2019; Masoon et al., 2017).

Why should the older adult avoid polypharmacy?

The older adult should avoid inappropriate polypharmacy because of the risk of adverse effects such as drug interactions, cognitive and physical impairment that can lead to falls risk, as well as medication non-adherence (RACGP, 2019).

>>

>>

The overall goal of assessing for polypharmacy use is to ensure appropriate use of medication to minimise identified adverse effects, starting at initial treatment and continuing your assessment as an individual transitions to other healthcare contexts.

How can polypharmacy be prevented in older adults? In general, healthcare providers should minimise the number of medications prescribed for older adults. The dosage schedule should be kept as simple as possible, and medication changes should be limited.

In your assessment of an older adult's medication use, you should be mindful and consider the key steps for ensuring medication safety:

1. Appropriate prescribing and risk assessment
2. Medication review
3. Dispensing, preparation and administration
4. Communication and patient engagement
5. Medication reconciliation at care transitions.

(Refer to WHO (2019) for further information about medication safety in polypharmacy.)

Musculoskeletal system

Bone density decreases in the older adult due to an increased rate of reabsorption, which exceeds the rate of bone replenishment. Both cortical and trabecular bone mass decrease. Muscles, bones and joints have reduced density and size, which leads to increased susceptibility for fractures. Bone density loss is accentuated in the postmenopausal female due to an oestrogen deficiency. Other manifestations of the bone density loss are thoracic kyphosis and a reduction in height. Thoracic kyphosis will cause a change in the older adult's centre of gravity, making the individual more prone to loss of balance and to falls. (Refer to Chapter 16 for risk factors for osteoporosis.)

Muscles lose tone and strength, leading to changes to flexibility, co-ordination and balance. Muscle fibres deteriorate with age and are replaced by fibrous connective tissue. Muscle atrophy is accompanied by a reduction in muscle mass, a loss of muscle strength against resistance, and a reduction in overall body mass. The fat content of the body increases, with particular distribution around the waistline.

There is a decrease in the water content of cartilage, which leads to a narrowing of joint space and intervertebral discs, and may lead to pain, crepitus and decreased movement of the affected area. There is also a reduction in the ability of cartilage to repair itself following trauma or surgery. Articulating cartilage will deteriorate due to a lifetime of wear and tear.

Mental status and neurological system

Neuronal changes occur with ageing. The myelin sheath surrounding each nerve begins to degenerate, decreasing impulse transmissions and nerve conduction rates and manifesting as reduced speed of storing new information and, conversely, retrieving stored information. This can lead to a decreased reaction time manifested in slowed reaction time and decreased vibratory sense. The axons of neurones become smaller. Biochemically, the amount of neurotransmitter produced in the neurone is diminished, and the activity of the enzymes that degrade the neurotransmitter increases. Changes in neurotransmitters are known to affect sleep, temperature control and mood. Depression, for example, is associated with decreased levels of noradrenaline.

Total brain weight, the number of synapses and the number of neurones diminish with ageing, beginning at age 50. Most of the loss occurs in the cerebral cortex and the cerebellum, and less so in the brain stem. The brain atrophies, causing a widening of the sulci and gyri, especially in the frontal lobes. The tendency of the brain to atrophy increases the size of the subdural space, leaving the cortical bridging veins vulnerable to trauma, bleeding, and the formation of a chronic subdural haematoma. The ventricles increase in size, and the amount of cerebrospinal fluid increases to fill the space.

Although not a normal part of ageing, older people are at higher risk of mental illnesses and cognitive impairment such as depression, dementia, anxiety and delirium compared with young people (AIHW, 2022c). Mental health problems interact with physical function and exert a significant effect on the older person's health. Therefore, assessment of mental health is especially important when undertaking the health assessment of the older adult. Cognitive changes characteristic of ageing include a decline in mental flexibility, abstract thinking, recall and visual-spatial ability. However, recognition, attention and language skills remain unchanged. The older adult typically has an extended learning and word retrieval time. Short-term memory may decrease slightly, but this must be evaluated because it may not be due to a decline in normal neurological function. In addition, changes in affect, mood and orientation need to be investigated, as they may be signs of dementia, delirium, or acute mental confusion, especially in the older adult suffering from infection, dehydration or CNS damage. Cognitive screening should be a part of each interaction with the older consumer, and any abnormal findings investigated.

Cognitive screening is used to assess the various functions related to cognition (knowledge, memory and recall, judgement and reasoning, problem solving, decision making, comprehension and language), and can provide insight into areas of the brain responsible for these functions that may be damaged. Cognitive screening is not a test for dementia. However, when conducted regularly, the results can be used to identify early changes that may indicate dementia.

Some common tools used to assess cognition are the General Practitioner Assessment of Cognition (GPCOG) (Brodaty et al., 2004) and the Standardised Mini Mental State Exam (SMMSE) (Molloy & Standish, 1997). The Rowland Universal Dementia Assessment Scale (RUDAS) (Storey et al., 2004) was designed to minimise the effects of cultural learning and language diversity on the accuracy of the assessment. Similarly, the Kimberley Indigenous Cognitive Assessment (KICA) (LoGiudice et al., 2006) has been developed to meet the needs of the Australian Indigenous population in the Kimberly region.

CLINICAL REASONING

Practice tip: Assessing delirium

The older population is at greater risk of developing delirium. Delirium is differentiated from dementia as it presents an acute and fluctuating change in a person's cognition and has a treatable cause. The diagnosis of delirium can be challenging to detect in the older population as the signs and symptoms are diverse (hyperactivity and/or hypoactivity) and are often confused with the symptoms of dementia. As a result, delirium in the older population is underdiagnosed or misdiagnosed, and the underlying treatable cause (e.g. impaired oxygenation, pain, constipation and infection) goes untreated. Key clinical indicators of delirium are 'acute onset and fluctuating course of symptoms, inattention, impaired consciousness, and disturbance of cognition (e.g. disorientation, memory impairment, language changes)' (Inouye, Westendorp & Saczynski, 2014, p. 914). The Confusion Assessment Method (CAM) and 4AT are two tools that can be used to identify delirium. A good history and knowledge of the person's usual level of cognition is needed to detect delirium, so it is recommended that consumers over the age of 65 years are assessed using these tools on admission and throughout their hospital admission.

CLINICAL REASONING

Practice tip: Behavioural and psychological symptoms of dementia

Most people with dementia will experience at least one or more behavioural and/or psychological symptoms of dementia (BPSD) or neuropsychiatric symptoms (NPS). Although more common in the more severe stages of dementia, BPSD can be experienced at all

>>

stages of the disease trajectory and are very disturbing to the person with dementia and those caring for them. The most common BPSD include agitation, aggression, depression, apathy, wandering and vocalisations. To assess the psychological symptoms of dementia, for example depression and hallucinations, assessment tools rely on interviewing the person with dementia or an informant. The Cornell Scale for Depression in Dementia (Alexopoulos, Abrams, Young & Shamoian, 1988) is one scale frequently used to assess depression.

To accurately assess the behavioural symptoms of dementia, observation across multiple time points throughout the day, as well as the use of a validated tool, are needed to determine what is triggering the behaviour and how the behaviour impacts the person with dementia and others. Most behavioural symptoms have a validated tool available that evaluates the scope of the characteristics of the behaviour. When observing a behaviour, using the ABC approach is recommended: A – Antecedents (triggers), B – Behaviour (what occurs) and C – Consequences (what are the outcomes). Using this approach, triggers that could be eliminated to prevent the behaviour are identified, the characteristics of actions that occur are objectively described, and the impact of the behaviour is described to determine what action, if any, is needed. When considering how to respond to BPSD, the safety of the person with dementia and others must always be the first priority.

Urinary system

Please refer to Chapter 15 for specific assessment details for urinary system assessment. The following information details specific changes or considerations for the older adult.

Renal

In the older adult the kidney shrinks. Renal function can be altered due to glomerular degeneration, thickening of glomerular and tubular basement membranes, decreased length of proximal and distal tubes and decreased renal blood flow. As a result, the glomerular filtration rate decreases by 60–70% by age 75. The kidney does not respond as efficiently to vasopressin, and the ability to dilute, concentrate and acidify urine is compromised. Impaired sodium regulation can also occur.

Bladder

The bladder within the urinary tract loses elasticity and tone as the body ages. These changes result in increased urinary frequency; weakening of the pelvic floor muscles may lead to urinary incontinence. In males, the prostate may enlarge or become inflamed, causing difficulties emptying the bladder and urinary incontinence. Since the older adult has a bladder with a smaller capacity and delayed perception of voiding signals, urinary incontinence can often be the result. Also the bladder has increased detrusor muscle instability, a weakened urinary sphincter, and involuntary contractions. Increased nocturnal production of urine leads to nocturia in both men and women.

CLINICAL **REASONING**

Practice tip: Non-bladder causes for urinary incontinence
People aged 85 years and over are more than five times as likely to experience severe incontinence (bladder and bowel) (Australian Government Department of Health and Aged Care, 2019). The causes of urinary incontinence can be divided into four types: stress, urge, overflow and functional. These are defined and presented in further detail in Chapter 15 'Gastrointestinal system'.

>>

Contemplate using a system for flagging areas for additional assessment as you undertake your health assessment. The Fulmer SPICES tool is useful for assessing health in the frail older adult. Use the acronym 'SPICES' to guide your thought processes when considering non-bladder causes of urinary incontinence, especially in the older adult:

> S is for Sleep Disorders
> P is for Problems with eating or feeding
> I is for Incontinence
> C is for Confusion
> E is for Evidence of falls
> S is for Skin breakdown (Fulmer & Wallace, n.d.).

Female genitalia

The older female adult undergoes definite physical changes in her internal and external genitalia and her reproductive organs. These changes begin with menopause, which usually occurs between the ages of 45 and 55. Menopause is characterised by low oestrogen levels, which cause the cessation of menses. As ageing progresses, a generalised atrophy of the external and internal female reproductive organs evolves.

Atrophy of the internal reproductive organs causes the ovaries and fallopian tubes to diminish in size, so that they are rarely palpable. The uterus atrophies so that it may also be difficult to palpate. Also, a delayed and reduced production of vaginal secretions may cause alterations in sexual response. These changes in the vagina may cause the female to complain of dyspareunia. An increase in the pH of the vaginal secretions and a decrease in the normal vaginal flora lead to an increase in vaginal infections in older women. However, the older female experiences no change in sexual desire or pleasure or in being able to experience orgasm.

The pelvic muscles atrophy, causing a decrease in the support of the pelvic organs. These muscles are often already weakened by trauma from childbirth; thus, prolapse of the uterus and vaginal walls is common.

Male genitalia

Testicular degeneration occurs sporadically, which allows normal spermatogenesis to be present in most men until 70 years of age, when sperm count and motility decline. Sperm output may be slightly decreased.

Typically, the older male adult has no change in sexual desire or satisfaction, but the ability to obtain or maintain an erection is affected and may not be as complete. Testosterone levels decline slightly with age but are related to **impotence** in only a small minority of men who have low hormone levels. An absence or marked reduction of ejaculatory fluid emission is often seen in the older adult male. The refractory period before rearousal, after a cycle of erection and ejaculation, lengthens with age. This physiologic change in what used to be an almost automatic erection is often perceived by men as the onset of impotence. Anxiety levels rise, thus further triggering erectile dysfunction. Physiologic impotence can be caused by vascular disease, diabetes mellitus and hypogonadism.

CLINICAL REASONING

Practice tip: Sexuality and health of the older adult who identifies as LGBTIQ+
As older adults who identify as LGBTIQ+ have lived through societal reform (change in law and recent acceptance and recognition of LGBTIQ+ rights), they may have experienced trauma from early life. An older person with dementia who identifies as LGBTIQ+ and may have lost memories, such as having 'come out' and the acceptance of that, may experience unique challenges and trauma. This trauma might be the result of discrimination or incarceration, which may impact their behaviour, and is significant for those who have dementia (Dementia Support Australia, 2022).

>>

What can be done?

In 2021, the Australian Human Rights Commission released a report on medical intervention decision making that recommended reform for individuals born with variations in sex characteristics. Further, the first of the Australian Aged Care Quality Standards released in 2019 necessitate 'Consumer dignity and choice', with expectation for LGBTIQ+ individuals entering aged care contexts to be treated with dignity and respect and to maintain their identity. These individuals should be able to locate information, make an informed choice, and have control over the healthcare and support services they desire (Australian Government, My Aged Care, 2022).

Dementia Australia has numerous resources and support services available to assist older adults living with dementia who are LGBTIQ+, and their care partners, family and friends. The New Zealand Dementia Foundation (2022) has useful resources and best-practice links for gender and sexual minorities.

Healthcare providers should understand and be able to draw on current knowledge such as law, polices and services when caring for the older LGBTIQ+ consumers, so they can recognise trauma or unusual behaviour. Acknowledging and providing individualised, non-judgmental, culturally safe care is paramount.

Health professionals should encourage consumers to seek out LGBTIQ+ inclusive service providers when seeking aged care services (Dementia Australia, 2020). Some points to share with the LGBTIQ+ consumer, carer, family or friend when searching for a provider include the following:

> Review policies and costs.
> Establish how the service provider makes you feel when you ask questions or visit the facility.
> Review the service provider's discrimination policy; this should not discriminate against LGBTIQ+ individuals.
> Is there a private space where consumers and partners, family and friends can spend time alone?
> Is LGBTIQ+ inclusive language used in published and written materials about the facility? For further information refer to the following:
> National LGBTIQ+ Health Alliance is the Australian national health body that provides LGBTIQ+ and other gender and sexuality diverse health programs, services and research to people who are LGBTIQ+. See lgbtiqhealth.org.au.
> QLife is an Australian advocacy, counselling and referral service for people who are LGBTIQ+. See qlife.org.au.

Anus, rectum, and prostate

Anorectal function changes in the older adult due to the loss of muscle elasticity in the rectum. Older adults have reduced maximum tolerated volumes in the rectum, with higher rectal pressures in response to distension. Rectal prolapse is most seen in older women. Constipation commonly occurs due to a decline in large bowel transit and decreased faecal water excretion, as well as a side effect of polypharmacy.

Faecal incontinence may develop due to denervation associated with an increase in the motor unit fibre density and the afferent neurone degeneration of rectal wall. This interferes with the ability to detect changes in pressure and creates a decrease in internal sphincter tone. Faecal incontinence in the older adult is usually the result of impairment of more than one of the factors that ordinarily maintain continence.

The prostate begins to enlarge after the age of 40 and often leads to the development of benign prostatic hypertrophy. The prostate capsule may contract and prostatic urethral tone may increase, resulting in urinary obstruction. There are lower levels of zinc in the prostatic fluid of older men, which appears to reduce the amount of prostatic antibacterial factor, thereby making the older man more susceptible to urinary tract infections.

ASSESSMENT: TAKING THE CONSUMER'S HEALTH HISTORY

Assessment is the first phase of the nursing process and involves collecting subjective information about the consumer's health status in order to identify consumer problem areas to focus on.

> **Subjective data** is most frequently collected during a health history and serves as the starting point for the health professional to base the depth of the assessment on. The sections for the health history include:
>
> > **Consumer profile**
>
> > **Chief complaint** (explained systematically using variations of location, quality, quantity, associated manifestations, aggravating factors, alleviating factors, setting and timing. This is a variation on the PQRST assessment mnemonic you may use for other conditions such as pain assessment)
>
> > **Past health history** (including medical history, surgical history, allergies, medications, injuries and accidents, special needs and childhood illnesses)
>
> > **Family health history**
>
> > **Social history** (including alcohol, tobacco and drug use, sexual practice, work and home environment, hobbies and leisure activities, stress and culture).

Interview of the older adult

The older adult ranges from age 65 years onwards, with this population spanning a lengthy time period. Chronological age should not be the major factor considered in the approach to the consumer. Ability to function and interact will be as diverse as the individual regardless of age. Those young-old adults aged 65–75 will, in most cases, be highly functional, independent individuals, and the assessor's approach will need minimal modification. However, the true older adult, those 85 years and more, may have limitations that will call for modification of both the health interview and physical examination. The presence of frailty, the gradual deterioration in health status characterised by the progressive loss of cognition and physical ability that can be accelerated by illness and hospitalisation, may mandate multiple appointments in order to complete an accurate and comprehensive examination. Additional time should be incorporated into the interview to allow for accurate interpretation of the information needed and the responses.

The health history of the older adult encompasses the same major areas as the health history for a younger consumer; however, there are some basic differences. Reasons for seeking care may be a chronic condition or a new issue or problem. Issues of depression, weakness or self-care deficits may be more difficult to identify but will emerge from a thorough, skilled assessment. New pains or discomfort should never be attributed to 'getting old', and consumer education should emphasise this point. However, consumer education may be difficult if hearing has declined, and if the consumer is anxious and feeling overwhelmed by too much new information. Note that you should not assume the person has hearing difficulty and thus yell your questions to them. Past health history for the older consumer is like that for the younger adult. The length of time covered is extended, however, and therefore the interview may take more time to complete. Medication should always be carefully evaluated and, if possible, the consumer should bring all prescription medications, over-the-counter medications and complementary medicines to the appointment (**Figure 21.3**). **Table 21.1** identifies strategies to enhance the health history interview and examination of the older adult.

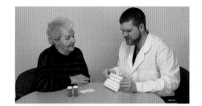

FIGURE 21.3 Older adults should be encouraged to bring all their prescription and non-prescription medications with them to each healthcare appointment.

TABLE 21.1 Guide to enhance your health interview and physical examination

POTENTIAL DEFICIT	GOAL	INTERVENTION
Vision	Maximise visual component of communication	Sit facing consumer to ensure clear view of your face. Avoid light behind you. Provide bright, indirect light without glare. Ensure consumer has clean glasses (clean as needed). Provide written material in large font with clear contrast between text and background.
Hearing	Maximise auditory component of communication and enhance information gathering	Provide quiet environment with no background noise. Ask if there is a hearing deficit and which ear is better. Speak directly to the good ear. Assist with the use of working hearing aids. If needed, use alternative mechanisms for communication, such as writing and signing. Validate that information is understood.
Mobility	Promote independence and autonomy	Explain what parts of the examination will be done. Allow extra time for the consumer to prepare for the examination. Ask if the consumer would like assistance in preparation. Ask who, if anyone, the consumer would like present during the examination.
Fatigue	Enhance quality of information and accuracy and efficacy of examination	May need to break comprehensive examination into sections and allow for rest periods as needed, or schedule on separate days. Ensure positioning is not adding to fatigue. Consumer may have less fatigue if examination is done in semi-recumbent position.
Eliciting minimal information	Enhance quality of information and accuracy and efficacy of examination	Ensure issues above are addressed adequately. Ask open-ended questions that cannot be answered yes/no.
Difficulty with focus	Enhance quality of information and accuracy and efficacy of examination	Limit questions with essential subjective information to closed-ended questions. Organise reminiscences to enhance data gathering.
Pain	Promote comfort and enhance quality of information	Allow consumer to assume position of most comfort. Provide consumer with available interventions to enhance comfort.

The psychosocial aspect of the interview is like that for the younger adult, with some areas receiving increased focus. Current living situation and the older adult's satisfaction with the living arrangements should be elicited. Engagement with friends and family should be explored, as should spousal issues that may present.

Older adults experience many life changes and these changes may accelerate with age. Their ability to cope with the stressors associated with ageing, such as retirement, moving, illness, or deaths of significant others, should be assessed. The nurse should also be assessing for depression, personality changes, or other signs of cognitive issues (**Figure 21.4**). Cognitive issues may result from medical issues that would be amenable to treatment. The normal examination findings should be emphasised, and consumer education should occur regarding commonly experienced issues of ageing.

Special assessments

Developmental assessment
Many older adults can be challenged by the ageing process, as it can be seen as a time of ineffectiveness and decline. However, older adults are a significant part of society and have their own developmental tasks to accomplish. Older adults demonstrate tremendous flexibility in their thinking, learning and adaptive ability. They have to be resilient to incorporate the ageing process into their self-image (**Figure 21.5**). Growing old is a time of enormous individual growth. Coping with the losses of spouse, family and friends through death, illness or relocation; adjusting to altered living arrangements; retiring; and adjusting to changing sexual and physical

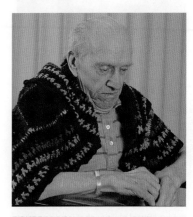

FIGURE 21.4 Assessing for cognitive changes and depression in the older adult should occur at each nursing visit.

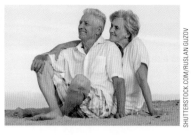

A. This couple is enjoying time together and maintaining their physical endurance.

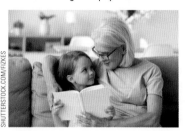

B. The oldest and youngest members of the family are enjoying their time together.

FIGURE 21.5 Developmental tasks of the older adult

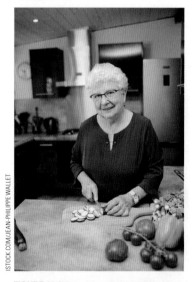

FIGURE 21.6 Preparing meals is one of the functional abilities that is assessed in older adults.

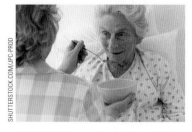

FIGURE 21.7 Assessing an older adult's nutritional status is important to helping him or her maintain a healthy lifestyle.

function are just a few examples of the developmental work that older adults accomplish. Refer to Chapter 2 for a summary of developmental tasks of the older adult.

Assessment of the older adult's functioning may allow the healthcare provider to assist the consumer in adapting to these changes or in compensating and planning for the future (see **Figure 21.6**). Assessing functionality, nutrition, sleep and caregiver strain can assist identification of issues needing intervention that will improve the quality of life and adaptation of the older consumer. Reliable and valid tools for use with the older adult include the Mental Status Assessment, Gordon's Functional Health Patterns, and the Abbey Pain Scale.

REFLECTION IN PRACTICE

Physical changes in the older adult

An 82-year-old woman is seen for management of osteoarthritis. She tells you that she can no longer knit jumpers for her grandchildren. This is very upsetting to her.

> How should you proceed with the physical examination?

> What recommendations can you make to the woman?

Cultural and spiritual assessment

Cultural background and practices are significant for older adults and these affect health practices and beliefs. There may be a link between a person's faith and health, and it is important to recognise this in caring for the older adult. When older adults are questioned, some believe in the healing power of prayer, that faith can facilitate recovery, and that their faith and religious practices are an important means of coping with illness and disability. Just as faith is an individual perception and practice at a younger age, it is relevant to many older adults.

A spiritual history is the same as for the younger adult and should include the key concepts of the older adult's idea of a higher power, the meaning of illness, the mechanisms used to maintain hope, and his or her support system. Spirituality provides personal answers about the meaning and purpose of one's life, which is usually improved with ageing. It is important to acknowledge spirituality as part of the social assessment as a powerful coping mechanism during stressful life events. There is no doubt that spirituality is closely related with mental health.

Nutritional assessment

Nutritional assessments are performed at a surface level, and consumers may need to be referred to a nutrition health professional for in-depth assessment. Specifically, important issues to assess are identified nutritional deficits, risk factors placing the individual at risk for nutritional deficiencies and weight loss. The older adult faces unique challenges in attempting to maintain good nutritional intake (**Figure 21.7**). For instance, caloric requirements decline with age, and older adults have decreased or blunted taste perception in addition to less efficient intestinal absorption. Chewing and swallowing issues are the most prevalent in this age group, and disabilities may impair actual food preparation. Financial constraints in shopping and food-buying habits are frequently seen in the older adult living on a fixed income, and loss of a partner, friends and spouse decreases the many social aspects of eating. Food and medication interactions are more common in this age group. Single living, loneliness, and loss of a spouse are major risk factors for inadequate nutrition. Refer to Chapter 15 for more comprehensive detail for nutritional assessment.

CLINICAL REASONING

Practice tip: Selecting a malnutrition screening assessment tool

There are a number of malnutrition screening assessment tools available. Queensland Health (2017), for example, published a helpful comparison guide that will assist you to select the best tool to support you to undertake a malnutrition assessment. This guide presents tools that have been validated to the population you are working with. Other considerations relate to the skill level of the tool user, implementation of the outcome and embedding with other health context practices.

When choosing a screening tool that is suitable for your facility, it is important to consider the following:

> Ensure the tool is validated to the population.
> Complexity: If the tool requires calculations (e.g. BMI, percentage weight loss) or is lengthy with many parameters, it is likely to be more time consuming and subject to error. This may also result in a low compliance with screening.
> Sensitivity: As screening is only the first step to identify those who require nutritional assessment, a screening tool needs to achieve a high sensitivity (i.e. identifies all those at risk), even if this is at the expense of high specificity (or false positives).

Other factors to consider are: Who will perform screening? How can screening be incorporated into current procedures? What action will be taken for those screened at risk?

Pain assessment

Many older people assume that pain is an inevitable part of ageing. This is one area of assessment that is not well addressed or understood by health providers. The Australian Pain Society emphasises the value of undertaking a interprofessional team approach in the management of a person's pain, and provides significant evidence-based resources to support this (Australian Pain Society, 2022). It is also worth noting that the older adult often uses other words to explain their pain, such as discomfort, soreness or achiness.

It is important that health professionals are able to accurately assess pain in older people as pain is a common problem. These are some of the most common assessment tools that are used for assessing pain in the older adult:

> Numerical rating scale (NRS) – measures pain intensity on an 11-point scale (0–10).
> Visual analogue scale (VAS) – measures pain intensity using a scale that requires the person to place a cross on the scale between 0 (no pain) and 100 (severe pain).
> Verbal rating scale (VRS) – appropriate for older adults in which they are asked to describe their pain with a verbal rating ranging from no pain to very severe pain.
> McGill Pain Questionnaire (MPQ) – multidimensional tool designed to quantitatively and qualitatively measure pain intensity and quality.
> Abbey Pain Scale – designed to assist in the assessment of pain in people who are unable to clearly articulate their needs; for example, individuals with dementia, cognition or communication issues.

Assessment of pain should include asking:

> How long has the pain been a problem?
> Is this new pain or have you had it before?
> Where is the pain? Does it radiate? Where is it the worst?
> How severe is the pain? (Ask the person to rate the pain using the Visual Analog Scale. See Chapters 3 and 6.)
> Is the pain sharp, stabbing, dull or aching?
> Is there any numbness or tingling associated with the pain?
> Has the pain interfered with any activities?
> What makes the pain worse or better?
> What have you tried to relieve the pain? Did it work?

REFLECTION IN PRACTICE

Pain assessment

Refer to the pain management content in Chapter 6. Think back to the most recent clinical situation in which you assessed pain in the older adult and work through the following questions.

> How do questions that assess the characteristics of a person's main complaint of pain guide your clinical decisions and management? Was this process followed?
> Would the consumer's outcomes have been improved had all aspects of the process been followed?
> What were the barriers to assessing the older person's pain comprehensively?

Use of a valid and reliable pain assessment instrument will improve the rating of the pain and the evaluation of the effectiveness of treatment. It should be recognised that a pain assessment instrument that can be used when an individual is not able to communicate verbally is paramount. The Abbey Pain Scale is a well-known Australian pain assessment tool that measures pain in people with dementia who are unable to verbalise (Abbey et al., 2004). Other severely cognitively impaired individuals who are also unable to communicate or describe their pain can be assessed with another well-known non-verbal pain assessment tool: the Pain Assessment in Advanced Dementia or PAINAD tool (Warden, Hurley & Volicer, 2003). Your clinical area may have a specific pain assessment instrument available for use with your older population. Most importantly, pain should be reassessed at regular intervals to evaluate the effectiveness of interventions undertaken.

PLANNING FOR PHYSICAL EXAMINATION

The planning phase refers to evaluating subjective data to narrow the focus on physical examination, determining what objective data needs to be gathered, as well as considering the environment and equipment that will be required.

Objective data is:

> collected during the physical examination of the consumer
> usually collected after subjective data
> information that is measured or observed by the clinician as opposed to being reported by the consumer
> vital to the overall health assessment, to enable you to make clinical decisions that are representative of the whole consumer picture.

Evaluating subjective data to focus physical examination

Before commencing the physical examination of the older person, consider what information the health history has provided. Critical consideration, linked to knowledge of anatomy and physiology, should focus the physical assessment so your examination will be more effective and efficient.

Environment

Assessment of the older adult requires a physical environment in the healthcare setting that has:

> an adjustable bed/table for the consumer to lie on that can be increased to a Trendelenburg position for consumers who cannot lie flat
> minimal noise for accurate auscultation of specific sounds
> adequate lighting
> adequate privacy.

Equipment

Assemble items before placing the consumer on the examination table. Materials should be arranged in order of use and within easy reach:

> Equipment as listed in Chapters 6–19
> Equipment/forms needed to conduct cognition and functional assessments.

IMPLEMENTATION: CONDUCTING THE PHYSICAL EXAMINATION

Implementation of the physical assessment requires you to consider your scope of practice. In this next section, depending on your context, you may be performing the foundation assessment or, if you are practising in an advanced practice role, you will add aspects of or all of the advanced assessment.

EXAMINATION IN BRIEF: THE OLDER ADULT

Special assessments	**Physical examination***
Developmental assessment	**Functional testing**
Cultural and spiritual assessment	**Cognition**
Nutritional assessment	* All other assessment skills are performed as described in Chapters 6–19.
Pain assessment	

The older adult population is an extremely diverse group. Life experience coupled with genetics, exposures, lifestyles, and diverse culture, diet, recreation, education, environmental influences and work types all affect an individual's health and wellness status. Significant when assessing older individuals is their functional ability within their own environment and community.

There is no specific age at which the ageing process routinely warrants screening. The older adult may have unique concerns and requirements secondary to disability, comorbid conditions, normal changes of ageing and personal coping strategies.

An essential element in the care of the older adult is incorporating the caregiver into the assessment. The older adult, however, should be respected and involved where possible in assessment and any suggestions of future care provision plans. Communication should always be directed towards the consumer while still attending to caregiver or family input.

Functional testing and cognitive testing should be conducted at each visit with the older adult. Functional status has been referred to as the 'sixth vital sign'. Functional status indicates an individual's ability to perform tasks and fulfil social roles associated with daily living across a wide range of complexity. Assessing function is important to provide indication of change in activity or ability. So, therefore, functional status serves as an important predictor for the maintenance of health and wellbeing, and indicates a need for acute or extended residential care.

A scoping review that focused on the use of functional and cognitive assessment in the emergency department concluded that there is not a consistent set of tools that can assist health professionals to undertake these decisions (Taylor, Broadbent, Wallis & Marsden, 2018). In addition, Table 21.2 offers a quick screening tool to assess the health of the older adult. Chapter 2, Table 2.6, provides further examples of developmental assessment tools that have application when assessing an older adult.

TABLE 21.2 Older adult quick health screen

ASSESSMENT	SCREEN
Function	Positive response to one or more questions, when asked, 'Do you need help with': > shopping? > doing light housework? > walking across a room? > washing in shower or bath? > doing finances?
Mobility	Note current mobility and balance. Are any aids in use?
Nutrition	Weight loss of more than 4.5 kg in the past 6 months without trying (or) body mass index <20 Malnutrition screening tool (MST) (Ferguson, Capra, Bauer & Banks, 1999): Assess and score recent weight loss and recent poor intake
Vision	Check ability to read newspaper headline and one sentence with correction. If unable, check each eye with Snellen chart.
Hearing	Unable to hear fingertip friction at 15 cm both ears
Cognition	Mental status assessment Cognition can be tested using three memory tests. First is immediate recall (recite a list of three things, and ask the consumer to repeat them immediately). Second is recent memory (ask the consumer to tell you something that occurred today that is verifiable; for example, what was eaten at the last meal. Third is long-term memory; you will need to ask the consumer about events from years ago that are verifiable. Memory can also be tested by mathematical calculation (count back from 100 in 7s without pen or paper) (Tollefson, 2022).
Depressive symptoms	Positive answer to: 'Do you often feel sad or depressed?'

General approach to older adult assessment

1. Assess the older adult in an environment that is warm and comfortable.
2. Always address questions to the older adult even in the presence of the caregiver. If the caregiver does not allow the consumer the opportunity to speak, explain to the caregiver that they will be given an opportunity to speak after the consumer has answered.
3. Use bright, indirect light and ensure a quiet environment with minimal background noise.
4. Minimise interruptions in the health assessment interview and physical examination.
5. Allow adequate time for the examination. A comprehensive examination of the frail older individual may require an extended visit with rest periods, or multiple visits.
6. Allow the older adult to maintain independence in all activities related to the examination, even if it increases the time needed.
7. Ask prior to assisting the older consumer whether they would like assistance preparing for the examination.
8. Instruct the older adult to remove all items of clothing for a full examination and provide a gown with instructions for its use. Always respect consumer modesty.
9. Provide a warmer temperature or, if unadjustable, offer blankets.
10. Ascertain that the older adult has clean glasses (clean as needed) and working hearing aids, if needed. If a hearing aid would enhance the examination, offer a temporary amplification device. If no amplification is wanted or available, ask which is the older adult's better ear. Use low-pitched, normal-volume speech. Validate that all information presented to the consumer has been heard correctly.

11. Ask if the frail older adult would like the caregiver to remain during the examination.
12. Allow the older adult to select a position of comfort. Frail older adults may be less fatigued and more comfortable if examined in a semi-recumbent position.
13. Maximise the visual cues the older adult can use by ensuring a clear view of your face without bright background glare.
14. Ask open-ended questions and avoid closed questions to ensure completeness of interview and examination.
15. At the conclusion of the examination, elicit essential subjective information related to answers to the closed-ended questions to validate findings.
16. Utilise evidence-based tools specific to the older adult to ensure accuracy of information.
17. Always conclude the examination by asking if there are other concerns that have not been addressed or if the consumer has questions about anything discussed.

Physical examination

Functional testing

Functional testing may be accomplished using valid and reliable tools. The tool selected should be specific to the older population and to the older adult's situation. If the older adult is living independently, the Lawton Instrumental Activities of Daily Living (IADL) scale should be used, as it covers all activities needed to maintain oneself at home and maintain independence safely. If the older adult resides in an institution offering assistance, or resides with and receives assistance from caregivers, the narrower focus of the Katz activities of daily living (ADL) index may be more appropriate. If the individual resides in a facility with a high level of care and the major concern is safety, then other functional assessment tools will be more appropriate. You should consult your organisation's guidelines.

Cognition

Safety is affected by cognitive function. Early identification of cognitive impairment has a significant influence on quality of life, and many causes of impairment can be treated (Figure 21.8). New developments in the treatment and delay of the progression of dementias are emerging and driving initiatives aimed at earlier recognition. Once recognition is established, the cause of the cognitive disorder must be established, as each disorder is treated differently. The major causes to be considered are depression, dementia and delirium. Their contrasting characteristics are found in Chapter 7, Table 7.8.

Cognition may be assessed using a number of reliable and valid tools specific to the older adult. For the undergraduate nurse, the most appropriate tool to use is the Mental Status Assessment described in Tollefson (2022). This assessment does not require any specific forms but relies on the nurse assessing components of mental status such as:

> general appearance
> level of consciousness (including alertness, confusion, lethargy, delirium, stupor, coma)
> orientation to person, place and time
> mood and behaviour
> knowledge and vocabulary
> judgement and abstraction
> memory
> thought process and content
> language and speech
> sensory and motor assessment.

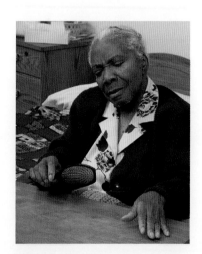

FIGURE 21.8 The nurse needs to assess the older adult's cognitive status at each encounter.

In some organisations, the use of a specific tool such as the Folstein Mini Mental State Exam is the gold standard of cognitive tests for all ages, even though it is susceptible to educational and cultural bias. However, to use this tool successfully and with the least bias, an understanding of the above concepts and assessment outlined in Tollefson (2022) is a good basis to begin from. Cognitive impairment of dementia and delirium may also be assessed using a test called the Mini-Cog, which is available at https://mini-cog.com/.

Delirium can be objectively assessed using the Confusion Assessment Method (CAM), and by referring to your organisation's guidelines. Older adults who have delirium will have a labile level of consciousness, and drift in and out during the examination. They may be able to perform cognitive testing well during lucid periods but still demonstrate impairment on testing. The cause may be infection, metabolic abnormalities, CNS damage, cranial lesions or the addition of new medications. Withdrawal from prescribed and over-the-counter medicines must also be considered. Older adults exhibiting signs of delirium should be questioned about alcohol use. A complete work-up is indicated to determine the aetiology. Secondary treatment includes assessment and maintenance of consumer safety and symptomatic treatment.

Depressive symptoms may be easily screened by using the Cornell Scale for Depression in Dementia (CSDD); depressive symptoms are suggested by a total score of eight or more and scores are determined by a combination of observation and interview of the person.

The presence of depressive symptoms necessitates that a nurse should always ask about suicidal ideation prior to the older adult's transfer or discharge. Older white males have the highest successful suicide rates of all age groups. A person diagnosed with geriatric depression responds as well to treatment as a younger person who is depressed. The consumer's safety is always paramount and must be ensured. Please refer to Chapter 7 for further information. You should note that the older adult may not express depressed mood or thoughts, but refer to a decrease in function and overall quality of life.

Vital signs

Vital signs for the older adult are assessed in the same way as for the younger adult consumer. Refer to Chapter 6 for a complete discussion of vital signs.

Pulse

The radial artery is used for assessment of heart rate. If the consumer has an irregular heart rate, accuracy of assessment will be higher if an apical pulse is assessed. Heart rate normal ranges do not change for this age.

Temperature

An older adult with severe cognitive impairment may be unable to comprehend the instruction to hold the thermometer under the tongue. An axillary or tympanic temperature may thus be easier to obtain (**Figure 21.9**).

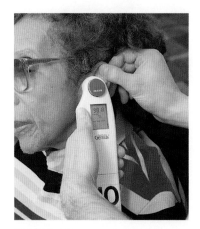

FIGURE 21.9 The tympanic thermometer can be used with ease in the older adult.

N The older adult may have a lower body temperature, down to 35.5°C, which is normal.

Blood pressure

Blood pressure should be measured in the supine and standing postures, especially if the consumer is taking antihypertensive medication.

N Increased systolic and diastolic pressures may be seen. Widening of pulse pressure is common.

A A fall in diastolic blood pressure is seen more frequently in older adults with risk factors for hypotension. Decreases may range from 20 to 40 mmHg.

E Examination **N** Normal findings **A** Abnormal findings **P** Pathophysiology

A Bilateral differences in blood pressure from each arm may be present.

A Isolated systolic hypertension is a blood pressure of greater than 160 mmHg (systolic) over less than 90 mmHg (diastolic).

P These changes can occur due to the consequences of atherosclerosis and arteriosclerosis.

Height and weight

The frail or weak older adult may require assistance with being weighed. A modified standing or sitting scale may be necessary. Height may decrease with age due to osteoporosis. Older adults may also lose weight. Weight should be assessed at each consumer interaction and carefully documented and monitored. Unexplained weight loss should be investigated.

Skin

Skin assessment in the older adult should be performed as presented in Chapter 8.

N The following changes can be observed in the skin of the older adult:

> Skin may be drier and may be accompanied by less perspiration.
> A thin, parchment-like appearance of the skin with wrinkles and sagging skin folds may be present.

Liver spots, or solar lentigo, are irregular, flat, deeply pigmented macules that appear in sun-exposed areas (**Figure 21.10**). They result from the inability of melanocytes to produce an even pigmentation of the skin. Larger areas, called lentigines, are generally seen on the backs of the hands and wrists of light-skinned people and are related to the degree of sun exposure.

Sebaceous hyperplasia are flattened papules with a central depression and are usually yellowish.

Sebaceous keratoses are characterised by overgrowth of the horny layer. Lesions are raised but flattened growths with a wart-like appearance (**Figure 21.11**). They commonly appear somewhat greasy and as though they could easily be scraped from the skin surface. They may be scaly and dry in presentation and range from pale white to brownish in colour. They are usually not premalignant.

In senile purpura, bluish-purple spots develop on the older adult's skin, especially in areas of trauma, even slight trauma.

A Actinic **keratosis**, or solar keratosis, is seen in areas of the greatest sun exposure and is premalignant to squamous cell carcinoma (SCC). These lesions are superficial, flattened papules covered by dry scales, which may be irregular in shape and pink or tan in colour.

A Basal cell carcinoma (BCC) is more common among the older adult population, but is usually not life-threatening (**Figure 21.12**). Most instances of BCC occur on the head and neck. Caucasian males are at highest risk, especially those with prolonged exposure to the sun and tanning salons, and previous therapy with ionising radiation. The lesions can be pigmented or pearly white or pink, and they frequently bleed or scab.

A Squamous cell carcinoma (**Figure 21.13**) is also more common in older adults, but is far less common than BCC. Unlike BCC, SCC tends to occur on the backs of the hands and scalp, and the top of the pinna. The SCC lesion often appears red and has an inflamed base. The lesion is mobile with well-defined borders.

P These lesions are associated with sun exposure. UVB radiation is a risk factor for SCC, as is damage from thermal burns or chronic inflammation.

Hair

Assess the hair as described in Chapter 8.

N The hair becomes thinner and coarser, possibly with some degree of alopecia, in the older adult. Facial hair may be seen on women.

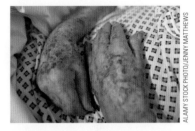
FIGURE 21.10 Senile lentigo

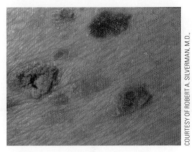
FIGURE 21.11 Seborrhoeic keratoses

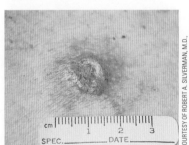
FIGURE 21.12 Basal cell carcinoma

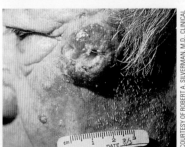
FIGURE 21.13 Squamous cell carcinoma

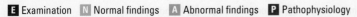
E Examination **N** Normal findings **A** Abnormal findings **P** Pathophysiology

UNIT 3

Considerations for education advice to avoid integumentary damage

Advise the older person to:

> identify hazards in the home that could cause trauma (e.g. loose rugs, sharp table edges, glass items in the bathroom, stoves and electric appliances)

> wear multiple layers of clothing in cooler temperatures, and gloves and socks to protect the distal extremities from hypothermia and frostbite

> keep electric blankets and heating pads on a medium setting to prevent burns

> apply emollient lotions to decrease xerosis and pruritus, but to avoid lotions with a high alcohol content, which can cause further drying of the skin

> protect their skin, as it will tear more easily and is prone to shearing. This is because their epidermal layers are thinner, and because the integumentary system is slower to recover from trauma, healing from such injuries will take longer. Current research shows a 50% reduction in skin tears for residents in aged care who apply moisturiser twice daily (Finch et al., 2018).

A national wound care research team has developed skin integrity resources for older adults located in residential aged care. These resources are useful to assist in the assessment of impaired or at-risk skin integrity. Refer to 'Wound care in residential aged care facilities – Creating champions for skin integrity' (National Dissemination): https://research.qut.edu.au/ccm/projects/wound-care-in-residential-aged-care-facilities-national-dissemination/.

Nails

Assess the nails as detailed in Chapter 8.

N Nails commonly become thicker, harder and yellowish in the older adult. Nails may develop ridges and split into layers.

Head and neck

Refer to Chapter 9 for complete information on assessing the head and neck.

E In the older adult, range of motion of the neck should be assessed using a single motion at a time to diminish the possibility of dizziness. Monitor for pain, crepitus and dizziness in addition to range of motion.

N There should be a full range of motion. In addition, there may be an altered appearance of the face due to tooth loss and the absence or presence of dentures.

A Range of motion may be limited. A stiff neck may indicate the presence of cervical arthritis.

P Cartilage and ligaments become less elastic and may be prone to calcification as a person ages. Tendons and muscles lose elasticity and tone. Cervical intervertebral discs lose water and disc space narrows.

Eyes

Assess the eyes as described in Chapter 10.

Inspection

N The following changes can occur in the older adult's eyes as part of the normal ageing process and may be noted on inspection:

> Greying of eyebrows and eyelashes
> Diminished tearing
> Loss of pigment in the iris
> Diminished or absent corneal reflex
> Decreased peripheral vision
> Altered colour perception; difficulty discriminating blue, green and violet colours
> Arcus senilis, a greyish or whitish arc or circle around the limbus not associated with an underlying condition.

E Examination N Normal findings A Abnormal findings P Pathophysiology

A The lower eyelid can drop away from the eye (ectropion) in the older adult.

P Genetic predisposition, lid muscle dysgenesis, trauma, infection and autoimmune causes can lead to ectropion.

A The lower lid can turn inwards (entropion) in the older adult.

P Laxity of medial and lateral muscles, CN III or VII paralysis, Bell's palsy, herpes zoster or cranial nerve lesions – in addition to trauma, infection and autoimmune disorders – are aetiologies of entropion.

A Decreased central vision can occur in the older adult. This can occur in conjunction with the older adult looking forwards when addressing someone who is standing to the side.

P Macular degeneration is commonly age-related and is a common visual problem affecting the older adult. The older adult will require significant magnification to compensate for the central loss. An altered head position maximises available vision.

Anterior chamber and lens

A The pupil may have a pearly grey appearance.

P This may indicate cataract formation.

P Acute-angle glaucoma occurs in the older adult at a higher rate than in the younger adult. It may be caused by an inhibition of the flow of fluid from the posterior to the anterior chamber or by 'plateau iris syndrome' with iris laxity. Other causes are anterior uveal displacement, posterior segment inflammation and tumours.

Pupil

N The older adult may have a decreased pupil size with slow accommodation.

A An irregularly shaped pupil, either bilaterally or unilaterally, is abnormal.

P Cataract repair will alter the shape of the surgical pupil.

Posterior segment structures

N The older adult's posterior segment structures may have the following changes:

> Pale blood vessels
> Dullness of retinal structures
> Narrower light reflex of arterioles
> Straighter and narrower retinal vessels.

CLINICAL **REASONING**

Practice tip: Awareness of visual limitations
Visual limitations have the potential to limit driving, ambulation, and safety in general. In the social setting, visual changes affect social interactions and safety in the home.

When undertaking a focused eye assessment and examination, aspects that should be included are:
> noting reports of any visual difficulties while driving or walking on stairs
> loss of peripheral vision
> loss of night vision
> difficulty distinguishing colours.

A home safety visit can facilitate remediation with lighting and hazard elimination. The older individual should be educated on the importance of regular eye examinations to preserve vision. They should also be educated about positive lighting changes that can enhance function, possible driving hazards and fall-prevention techniques.

Ears

During the examination, the older consumer's ears should be assessed for wax build-up and impaction, which can be removed by irrigation and curette. Ensure that any hearing aids are functional, with working batteries and correct placement. If impairment is noted and the consumer has not had an audiological examination, one should be encouraged. Face the older individual to whom you are speaking. Speak slowly, in a low-pitched voice, and avoid raising your voice or yelling. Eliminate as much background noise as possible. Monitor balance and equilibrium and assess the risk for falls. Arrange to have the home environment assessed, and educate the consumer and caregiver on modifications to enhance safety. Review Chapter 11 for a complete description of the ear examination.

CLINICAL **REASONING**

Practice tip: Hearing impairment

A change in auditory function is a common occurrence as a person ages; it is usually a gradual decline over time. Hearing impairment has the potential to isolate any individual. If the person is not able to use any hearing devices, the use of a portable amplifier with headphones may be of benefit.

In your communication interactions with the older person, remember that a hearing impairment is not necessarily linked to a cognitive impairment and therefore speak to them with the same respect you would give to any individual. Older adults found to have hearing loss that interferes with their functioning and quality of life should be referred for an audiology examination and fitted with hearing aids if indicated.

Auditory testing

Ask the older adult about hearing problems. Consider using standardised tools to assess the individual's perception of hearing, such as the whisper test. This is a simple hearing test designed for the older adult and detects voice at a conversation and whisper level. This serves as a screening test for referral to a hearing specialist.

A Some hearing loss or presbycusis is common in the older adult.

P Conductive hearing loss occurs in the outer ear (because of obstruction or loss of elastic tissue in the tympanic membrane) and middle ear (because of rigidity of movable bones in the inner ear) and mutes sound.

P Sensorineural loss is common in the older adult and involves the inner ear.

External ear

N Pendulous earlobes that are wrinkled can develop normally in the older adult. Wiry hair protruding from the auditory canal is normal. Cerumen is dry, which leads to an increased incidence of impaction.

A Skin lesions on the external ear may be malignant (SCC or BCC) or premalignant; they need to be evaluated.

P The external ear receives a significant amount of sun exposure, especially in men.

Internal ear

N The ageing adult's normal ear may have pronounced landmarks if atrophic or sclerotic changes have occurred (**Figure 21.14**). The tympanic membrane may appear white, opaque and thickened. It is also less resilient.

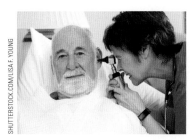

FIGURE 21.14 The nurse may find a slightly altered appearance to the tympanic membrane in the older adult.

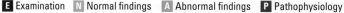

E Examination **N** Normal findings **A** Abnormal findings **P** Pathophysiology

Nose

Chapter 11 should be consulted for complete information on nasal assessment.

N The following are changes in the nose of an older adult:
> The nose increases in size due to increased cartilage formation.
> Nasal hairs are coarser.
> There is a decrease in the sense of smell because the number of sensory cells in the nasal lining decreases.

Mouth and throat

If the older adult has dentures, the mouth and oral cavity should be examined both with dentures and without. Chapter 11 provides additional information.

N The following changes occur in the older adult:
> Lip surface develops deep wrinkling, with an increase in granular lining on the lips and cheeks.
> The buccal mucosa thins, with a decrease in its vascularity.
> Gums are paler in colour with recession.
> Saliva production decreases (may be partly due to medications).
> Fissuring of the tongue increases with atrophy of papilla.
> Taste sensation diminishes due to atrophy and loss of taste buds.
> Gingival tissue has less elasticity.
> Dental roots become exposed.

A Fissures may develop at the corners of the mouth.

P This may be due to a vitamin deficiency or to yeast (due to impaired immunity).

A Lesions on the lips, especially on smokers, are abnormal and should always be investigated.

P Lips are exposed to the elements and sun damage. Tobacco use increases the risk of oral cancers.

CLINICAL REASONING

Practice tip: Diminished sense of taste

If an older person is experiencing any alteration in the sense of taste, you can suggest adding seasonings to their food such as herbs, garlic, pepper and curry. You can also suggest preparing aromatic foods that first stimulate the olfactory sense to enhance appetite. Note the avoidance of salt seasoning due to association with some disease processes, such as increased risk of cardiovascular disease.

Consider the link between early loss of taste and early signs of depression. This should prompt an assessment of the person's risk factors or symptoms for depression. Please refer to Chapter 7.

Breasts

Breast exams should continue throughout the life span. The major risk factor for breast cancer is advancing age. Refer to Chapter 12.

N The following are breast changes in the older adult female:
> Breasts may appear flattened and elongated due to relaxation of suspensory ligaments.
> The nipples may be smaller and flatter.
> Cystic breasts may feel smoother as the woman ages and glandular tissue decreases.
> The inframammary ridge thickness increases in prominence.

A Masses or lesions should be evaluated.

P Increased incidence of breast cancer occurs with advancing age.

E Examination   **N** Normal findings   **A** Abnormal findings   **P** Pathophysiology

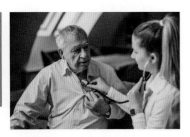

FIGURE 21.15 The nurse may need to give the older adult frequent rest periods when assessing the lungs.

ISTOCK.COM/PHOTODJO

Thorax and lungs

This examination may necessitate frequent breaks for the older adult to avoid fatigue and hyperventilation (**Figure 21.15**). Refer to Chapter 13.

N Expansion of the chest wall decreases, requiring increased inspiratory effort in the older adult.

Heart and blood vessels

The ageing heart functions without compromise under normal stress. However, it has reduced reserve and may not be able to compensate for stress, blood loss, extreme exertion or high fever. Chapter 14 provides comprehensive assessment information.

N The apical impulse may be displaced due to a decrease in the size of the heart in the older adult. A systolic ejection murmur may be auscultated at the left lower sternal border due to stiffening of the musculature and valvular leaflets.

A An S_4 heart sound is a common finding.

P Left ventricular thickening and/or enlargement resulting in loss of compliance result in the S_4.

A Decreased pulse volume may be present. Limbs may be cool.

P This can be due to atherosclerosis.

Abdomen

Chapter 15 provides comprehensive information on the abdominal assessment.

N Abdominal musculature diminishes in mass and tone in the older adult. The fat content of the body increases with age, leading to increasing deposits in the abdomen. The liver decreases in size.

A Increased incidence of urinary and faecal incontinence commonly occurs, but is not a normal change of ageing and should be evaluated.

P Incontinence is secondary to changes of ageing such as thinning of perineal tissues secondary to loss of oestrogen, damage from childbirth, surgery, prostate problems, neurological disorders and functional disability. Refer to Chapter 17, **Table 17.6** for types of urinary incontinence.

Musculoskeletal system

The health of the musculoskeletal system can impact the quality of life of the older adult dramatically. Assessment should include mobility, fine and gross motor skills, and activities of daily living (ADL). Examination should be carefully performed to ensure joint stabilisation. Slow, gentle, passive movements should be used to assess range of motion. Regular exercise should be encouraged, and information regarding the components of a program should be discussed. Maximal benefit will occur when the consumer includes aerobic exercise in addition to muscle strengthening and balance. The older consumer gains significant benefit from physiotherapy or occupational therapy consultation and information on environmental modifications to maximise function. Refer to Chapter 16 for detailed information.

Inspection

N The following changes occur in the musculoskeletal system with the ageing process:
> Posture changes to a more flexed position, which changes the centre of gravity.
> Steps tend to be shorter, with a wider base in men while women maintain a narrow standing base. The step height is reduced.

E Examination **N** Normal findings **A** Abnormal findings **P** Pathophysiology

N > The gait has a higher risk for unsteadiness due to changes in the centre of gravity and changes in the ear cochlea that result in a decreased ability to compensate.

> Transfers in and out of a sitting position will be more difficult for the older adult because of vertebral inflexibility and reduced muscle strength.

A A reduction in height occurs with the ageing adult. Kyphosis may be present.

P Intervertebral discs lose water, causing narrowing of the disc space, with a resultant loss of 3.8 to 7.6 cm in height.

A The lordotic curve of the back flattens, and both flexion and extension of the back decrease.

P Bone mass loss, bone density loss due to increased rate of bone reabsorption and slowed bone cell replacement lead to these variations.

CLINICAL REASONING

Elder abuse and neglect

There is an increased incidence of physical abuse and neglect among the older population. Abuse of the older adult or 'elder abuse' refers to any form of intentional or unintentional neglect ranging from physical, emotional, financial to sexual. It is not tolerated and complaints support is available in New Zealand and Australia (Health Navigator New Zealand, 2022; Australian Government, 2022). Abuse in community settings is scrutinised in both private (paid or unpaid) care and paid care facilities. Be aware that certain incidents of abuse and neglect need to be reported to the Aged Care Quality and Safety Commission and may require involvement of the police (Elder Abuse Prevention Unit, 2022). Elder abuse remains a topical issue for governments to address, and includes debate about mandatory reporting of abuse and analysis of the issues (AIHW, 2019). Further information to assist health professionals to assess services for those suspected of being subjected to elder abuse can be found at https://www.myagedcare.gov.au/contact-us/complaints#concernselderabuse.

In your assessment consider the contributing factors for elder abuse and neglect, which can include stress related to financial difficulties, multiple family members residing in limited space, the lack of nearby family members, and dealing with an older relative with dementia or incontinence. Possible indications of physical abuse include unexplained bruises, swelling, haematomas, burns, fractures, poor hygiene and poor nutritional status. Healthcare providers are obligated to investigate these symptoms further when they are unexplained or when the explanation is inappropriate for the location and severity of the trauma. Be familiar with your institution's policy on elder abuse and your role in supporting consumers.

REFLECTION IN PRACTICE

Restraints

Restraint use for any consumer should only be a last resort (for the safety of the consumer or others) and is ideally temporary while a care plan is developed and refined for the consumer. There are laws in place governing use of restrictive practices in aged care (Australian Government Department of Health and Aged Care, 2022; Ministry of Health, 2022).

> Have you heard or seen consumers being restrained?

> What was the reason for the restraint (e.g. protective of falls, aggressive behaviour)?

> What did you think about this in the situation you were in?

Consider contributing factors that lead clinicians to use restraints and check your state/territory's legislation and your facility's policy on use of restraints.

Restraining consumers without undertaking the correct process not only affects the consumer's dignity and rights but may also cause legal issues for the practitioner.

E Examination   **N** Normal findings   **A** Abnormal findings   **P** Pathophysiology

Muscles

N Reduced muscle mass and loss of strength, especially against resistance, occur in the muscles of the older adult.

Joints

A Decreased range of motion of individual joints and pain at rest and with range of motion can occur with the ageing process. Crepitus may be present with joint movement.

P There is a decrease in the water content of cartilage and a narrowing of joint space with age. A lifetime of wear and tear results in deterioration.

REFLECTION IN PRACTICE

Recognising possible elder abuse and neglect

A 76-year-old female with dementia is admitted through the emergency department with a diagnosis of probable aspiration pneumonia. Assessment findings include:

> chest X-ray that reveals pulmonary infiltrates consistent with the diagnosis of pneumonia as well as multiple old rib fractures
> cachexia
> poor general hygiene
> urinary and faecal incontinence
> faecal impaction
> pressure areas noted on the sacral area
> bruising of both arms in a 'grip' fashion and multiple bruises and abrasions of the buttocks and lower legs
> consumer moans in pain frequently during the physical assessment
> limb X-rays reveal an old healed fracture of the left humerus.

The consumer is a widow and has been living with her divorced daughter for the last year. The daughter is the consumer's only child and she is her primary caregiver. The daughter works full time, and the consumer is looked after by a personal carer. The caregiver informs the daughter that her mother 'falls frequently during the day'.

> What is your initial reaction to these clinical findings?
> Do the findings of the physical assessment indicate possible physical abuse or neglect? Explain.
> What would you say to the consumer's daughter?
> What questions would you ask the consumer?

Mental status and neurological techniques

Changes of ageing affect the nervous system in a gradual fashion. The changes are both structural and functional. Chapter 7 provides comprehensive information.

Mental status

Review mental status assessment clinical skills competency in Chapter 7 and explanation in Tollefson (2022).

N A slight decline in short-term memory is normal in the ageing adult. There is minimal cognitive decline in normal ageing.

A There is an increased incidence of depression in the older adult.

P Decreases in the neurotransmitters noradrenaline and serotonin caused by changes in dendrite distribution and decreased enzymatic activity can lead to depression.

E Examination **N** Normal findings **A** Abnormal findings **P** Pathophysiology

Sensory assessment

N The following changes occur in the sensory assessment of the older adult:
> Reduced sensation of vibrations
> Reduced sensation of cold/heat
> Reduced sensation of touch discrimination, especially fine touch; some older adults develop an increased sensitivity to light touch due to thinner skin
> Decline in proprioception.

Cranial nerves

For a detailed assessment, refer to Chapter 7.

Cerebellar function

N The older adult commonly has some balance impairment and may have an altered gait. There may be a decline in coordination.

A Abnormal gait accompanied by new incontinence or confusion is abnormal.

P Normal pressure hydrocephalus is more frequently seen in the older adult.

REFLECTION IN PRACTICE

Sexuality in older women
Think back to the last time you conducted a sexual history on an older woman.
> Did you ask her the same questions you would pose to a 25-year-old female?
> Did you introduce any:
  • gender bias?
  • cultural bias?
  • economic bias?
  • education bias?
> What are your personal views on sexuality in a:
  • 50-year-old female?
  • 60-year-old female?
  • 70-year-old female?
  • 80-year-old female?
  • 90-year-old female?

Female genitalia

Examination of the pelvis should not be avoided in the older adult. The focus of the examination changes to evaluation for the problems of incontinence, pelvic relaxation, irritation, dryness or rectal problems. Always screen for cancer if intact reproductive organs remain, if consistent with the goals of care. A smaller speculum may be needed. See Chapter 17.

Inspection

N The following changes may be found during inspection of the older adult female's genitalia:
> The clitoris and labia become smaller.
> The labia become flatter and lose pigmentation.
> The labial skin becomes thin, shiny, avascular and dry.
> Pubic subcutaneous fat is lost.
> Pubic hair becomes sparse and turns grey or white.

Palpation

N These changes may be found during palpation of the older adult female's genitalia:
> The ovaries and fallopian tubes may not be palpable due to shrinkage.
> The uterus atrophies and may be difficult to palpate.

E Examination   N Normal findings   A Abnormal findings   P Pathophysiology

UNIT 3

N > The cervix becomes smaller, paler and less mobile.
> The cervical os becomes smaller but remains palpable.
> The vagina shortens, narrows and thins.
> The introitus constricts due to atrophy.
> The vaginal wall loses rugae and elasticity.
> Vaginal secretions are delayed, and production is reduced.

A The risk of a prolapsed uterus and vagina increases with age.

P This is caused by the atrophy of pelvic muscles, which leads to a decrease in pelvic organ support. Ligaments and connective tissue of the pelvis also lose muscle tone.

A Uterine enlargement, nodularity, irregularity or induration should be investigated.

P Advancing age is a risk factor for malignancies such as ovarian, cervical and endometrial cancers.

Male genitalia

Inspection

See Chapter 17 for more information.

N The following changes may be found during the inspection of the older adult male's genitalia:
> The pubic hair thins and turns white or grey.
> The penis atrophies.
> The scrotal sac loses elasticity and elongates.
> The testicles may be smaller.

Palpation

N The testicles are smaller and atrophic.

REFLECTION IN PRACTICE

Dealing with changes in sexual function

You are an aged-care nurse practitioner who works in a community respite care facility. You are performing a physical examination of Mr Pakpoy, a new client. He tells you that his wife will be joining him after her discharge from the hospital. He also tells you that he and his wife are sexually active, but he voices concerns about difficulty in sustaining an erection in the past few weeks.

> What additional questions would you ask him?
> What anticipatory guidance would you provide?
> Consider what you would need to take into account if Mr Pakpoy wishes to take pharmacological assistance and the other medications he may be on (e.g. Viagra and anti-angina medication such as glyceryl trinitrate).

Anus, rectum and prostate

Chapter 18 contains additional information.

Palpation

N The older male adult typically has a smooth and rubbery prostate that is enlarged.

E Examination   **N** Normal findings   **A** Abnormal findings   **P** Pathophysiology

REFLECTION IN PRACTICE

Bowel incontinence in the older person

Richard is an 86-year-old man who has been in the hospital for 8 days and was admitted with a diagnosis of pneumonia. He was placed on intravenous antibiotics. On day five of his admission Richard developed persistent diarrhoea, passing 8 to 12 stools per day. His perianal skin is excoriated. You assist him in cleaning up after another stool, and he starts to cry. Richard tells you that this is no way for a man of his age to live. He expresses his wish to die. How would you respond to this man? You should consider broadly the reasons for his diarrhoea, but you must first address his psychosocial wellbeing.

EVALUATION OF HEALTH ASSESSMENT AND PHYSICAL EXAMINATION FINDINGS

In the evaluation phase of a health assessment, the focus is on ensuring the data gathered is complete, accurate and documented appropriately (see case study as an example of the focused assessment; see Chapter 22 for a comprehensive health assessment). In evaluating the data, you should:

> draw on your critical thinking and problem-solving skills to make sound clinical decisions
> act on abnormal data (include communicating findings to other health professionals)
> ensure documentation reflects the outcomes of the clinical decisions/actions taken (refer to Chapter 3 which discusses in detail why documentation is so important and how this may be undertaken in different health settings).
The case study that follows steps you through this process.

THE OLDER ADULT

This case study illustrates the application and the assessment of an older consumer.

Amelie Barker is an 81-year-old woman who presents to the emergency department following a fall at home.

HEALTH HISTORY

CONSUMER PROFILE	81-year-old female born in Australia	
CHIEF COMPLAINT	Pain in left hip area following a fall	
HISTORY OF THE PRESENT ILLNESS	Has been feeling 'off' for the last three days with decreased appetite, a general feeling of malaise, increased frequency and urgency of urination. Had a fall last night as she got out of bed to rush to the toilet. The fall was witnessed by her husband who saw her sway and then stagger as she stood up from the bed. She landed on the floor on her left side. There was no loss of consciousness and her husband is almost certain she did not knock her head. Her husband tried to help her up off the floor and back into bed, but Nancy was experiencing pain on movement and difficulty weight bearing through her left leg. Her husband notified the ambulance to bring her to the emergency department for review.	
PAST HEALTH HISTORY	MEDICAL HISTORY	Hypertension since age 56 Amelie has had type II diabetes for more than 10 years. It is currently managed by oral medication and diet. Macular degeneration – mild visual impairment
	SURGICAL HISTORY	Hysterectomy at age 54

>>

HEALTH HISTORY

	OBSTETRIC HISTORY	G 4, P 3
	ALLERGIES	Nil known allergies
	MEDICATIONS	Bendrofluazide 2.5 mg daily Cilazapril 5 mg daily Glipizide 5 mg daily
	COMMUNICABLE DISEASES	Denies
	INJURIES AND ACCIDENTS	Husband reports previous falls, no serious injuries, only some minor lacerations to arms and legs
	SPECIAL NEEDS	Denies
	BLOOD TRANSFUSIONS	Denies
	CHILDHOOD ILLNESSES	Does not recall
	IMMUNISATIONS	Annual flu vaccine – due in two months
FAMILY HEALTH HISTORY		Father died at age 67 from cardiac-related problems; mother died at age 75 following a stroke. Has two younger siblings, who both have hypertension and hyperlipidaemia.
SOCIAL HISTORY	**ALCOHOL USE**	Occasional sherry or glass of wine on special social occasions such as family birthdays or Christmas
	TOBACCO USE	Non-smoker
	DRUG USE	Denies the use of any drugs or medications other than those prescribed by her general practitioner
	DOMESTIC AND INTIMATE PARTNER VIOLENCE	Husband, happily married for 62 years
	SEXUAL PRACTICE	Monogamous relationship with husband
	TRAVEL HISTORY	Visits son, daughter-in-law and grandchildren in Queensland once a year (June/July) Cruise to Fiji 12 months ago
	WORK ENVIRONMENT	Retired medical receptionist Currently involved in volunteer work through the local community care agency. This work involves visiting and providing social contact to frail older people in the community, two afternoons per week.
	HOME ENVIRONMENT	Lives with husband in a single-level home townhouse. The property is owned by Amelie and her husband.
	HOBBIES AND LEISURE ACTIVITIES	Attends a tai chi class at the local community centre once a week Helps with funding-raising activities through the community centre Walking Spending time with family and friends
	STRESS	A close childhood friend has recently been diagnosed with breast cancer. Amelie has been offering support by providing meals, and attending clinic appointments with her friend at the oncology day stay unit.
	EDUCATION	Completed high school
	ECONOMIC STATUS	Financially comfortable, own home, receives superannuation

>>

HEALTH HISTORY

	MILITARY SERVICE	N/A
	RELIGION	Anglican; does not attend church regularly
	CULTURAL BACKGROUND	English ancestry
	ROLES AND RELATIONSHIPS	> Married to Richard for 62 years > Two grown children, five grandchildren > Richard is reasonably fit and active. He has a history of coronary artery disease (CAD), hyperlipidaemia and hypertension, which are managed with medications. He underwent a transurethral resection of the prostate (TURP) last year which has relieved his urinary retention problem. > Eliza lives in the same city and visits regularly with the grandchildren. > They have a son-in-law who is a builder and assists with any home maintenance issues that arise. > Alan, their son, lives interstate in Queensland; Amelie and Richard visit him annually and he visits with his family at Christmas time. Recently Alan bought his parents a webcam and they now FaceTime once a week to talk with the family.
	CHARACTERISTIC PATTERNS OF DAILY LIVING	> Wakes around 5.30 a.m., listens to the radio in bed with husband till 7.00 a.m. when she gets up and has a wash/shower. Breakfast is usually at 7.30 a.m. and consists of toast, fruit, a glass of prune juice and a cup of tea. > Amelie and her husband usually do the household chores together except for Tuesdays when Richard plays golf. > Amelie always sits down for a cup of tea and a light snack mid-morning. Lunch is usually salad, cold meat or fish. Her afternoon activities vary between tai chi, volunteer work, grocery shopping or out for a walk with her husband or a friend. Amelie and her husband like to eat their evening meal about 6.30 p.m. The evenings are spent watching television with her husband, doing a crossword, sudoku puzzle or an evening walk (in summer). Amelie has a light supper while watching the late news on television and goes to bed around 11 p.m.
FUNCTIONAL ABILITY	**ACTIVITIES OF DAILY LIVING**	Independent with washing, grooming, dressing and eating.
	INSTRUMENTAL ACTIVITIES OF DAILY LIVING	Manages household activities. Prepares meals. Husband assists with some of the activities around the house. Amelie is unable to drive a car due to decreased vision and finds the traffic unnerving. Richard is still able to drive and able to take the couple where they need to go.
	COGNITIVE FUNCTIONING	No reported changes in cognitive function.
HEALTH MAINTENANCE ACTIVITIES	**SLEEP**	Sleeps 6–7 hours per night; usually goes to the toilet during the night.
	DIET	Utilises the glycaemic index recommendations from the Diabetes Association for planning meals and snacks.
	EXERCISE	Tai chi once a week Regular walks (usually up to an hour at a time, weather permitting) Household chores
	STRESS MANAGEMENT	Supportive family and friends Tai chi and walking help Amelie feel relaxed
	USE OF SAFETY DEVICES	Amelie does have a St John Ambulance alarm pendant; however, she does not wear it, but keeps it in the top drawer beside her bed.
	HEALTH CHECK-UPS	> Regular BP and blood glucose monitoring at local GP clinic > Annual optometrist and dental checks > 6-monthly podiatry appointments > Last mammogram 12 years ago

>>

>>

PHYSICAL EXAMINATION

VITAL SIGNS		> Pulse rate: 90 bpm, thready
		> Respiration: 18 bpm, shallow, accessory muscles relaxed
		> Blood pressure:
		  • Lying – 108/74 mmHg
		  • Standing – 98/60 mmHg
		> Temp 37.4°C
		> Blood glucose level 3.7 mmol/L

NEUROLOGICAL		> GCS 13 > Pupils equal and reactive to light > Lethargic, eyes open when spoken to, follows commands, orientated to place and person, not time, some difficulty attending to assessment questions and some responses are a little muddled > Cranial nerves – intact > Bilateral reduced sensitivity to touch in feet and lower legs > Difficult to test muscle strength due to pain from injury on left side > Reflexes not tested due to consumer's pain and consumer's lethargic state
CARDIOVASCULAR		> Heart rate: regular 90 bpm > No heart murmurs detected > JVP – absent
PERIPHERAL PERFUSION	**INSPECTION**	> Both feet pale in colour > No sacral or ankle oedema
	PALPATION	> Bilateral cool skin temperature in feet, hands warm > Peripheral pulses present but dorsalis pedis weak bilaterally > Capillary refill feet and hands >3 s
RESPIRATORY SYSTEM	**INSPECTION**	20 breaths per minute, shallow and regular, accessory muscles relaxed, no evidence of difficulties
	PALPATION	No reports of pain on palpation; chest expansion symmetrical
	PERCUSSION	Bilateral resonance in all areas
	AUSCULTATION	No abnormal breath sounds noted
MUSCULOSKELETAL SYSTEM	**INSPECTION**	Blue/red coloured haematoma left hip and extends to left buttock Swelling evident No breakage in skin or evidence of bone protrusions Decreased range of movement around hip Touch weight bearing on left leg, unable to walk due to pain
	PALPATION	Tender on palpation of hip area Hip joint feels intact
SKIN	**INSPECTION**	No evidence of lacerations/skin injuries from fall Skin on lower legs shiny appearance with patches of dry scaling areas
	PALPATION	Skin texture dry, in general warm to touch, feet cold
ORAL ASSESSMENT	**INSPECTION**	Lips: dry with beginning evidence of cracks/chapping Buccal mucosa: pink but dry Tongue: mildly furrowed, dry Gums: pink Teeth: partial plate top front

>>

\>>

PHYSICAL EXAMINATION

ABDOMINAL ASSESSMENT	INSPECTION	Generalised distension Striae present over lower abdomen No dilated veins or lesions
	AUSCULTATION	Bowel sounds in all 4 quadrants No bruits
	PERCUSSION	Tympany throughout
	PALPATION	Mild tenderness in lower abdominal area and costovertebral angle tenderness No masses or bulges detected Bladder non-palpable
URINARY SYSTEM		Non-palpable bladder 3-day history of increased urinary frequency and urgency No pain on passing urine, slight discomfort in lower abdominal area when urinating Amelie had one episode of urinary incontinence that coincided with her fall Passed 100 mL of dark cloudy, malodorous urine an hour ago; urine specimen obtained for urinalysis
GASTROINTESTINAL		Normally eats and drinks well, but has been off food the last few days due to nausea No vomiting Has deliberately decreased her fluid intake to minimise the need to urinate Regular daily bowel movements (after breakfast) History of constipation but managed with glass of prune juice in the mornings Last bowel movement yesterday, formed dry stool, normal colour, a little more difficult to pass than usual No history of faecal incontinence

EVALUATION AND CLINICAL REASONING FOR CASE STUDY

The assessment and clinical decisions you make should reflect your scope of practice. For example, advanced practice health professionals, such as nurse practitioners and remote area nurses with endorsement, may be able to make diagnostic decisions and prescribe medications without referring to a medical officer.

Fundamentally, all health professionals collect, evaluate and act on consumer-focused health information, which will at times include referral to, or collaboration with, other healthcare team members. Nurses assess consumer responses to interventions and determine when to escalate key changes in a consumer's condition. The clinical reasoning cycle provides health professionals with a framework to consider all this information in a meaningful way for planning consumer care. These phases are stepped out below, and draw on information presented and collected during the health history and physical examination. We then work through the cycle components that are relevant to this case study (cycle components are bolded).

For Amelie Barker, the 81-year-old woman who presented to the emergency department following a fall, the significant data that needs to be considered includes the following.

Collecting cues/information

Recall and Review: In the first instance you will need to reflect on what you know about causes of falls and subsequent risks

to health. You will also need to be aware of the multifactorial nature of symptoms that can present in the older adult and how clustering of symptoms can assist you in identifying consumer issues. Older consumers have many physiological changes as well as issues such as comorbidities and polypharmacy that are important to consider, often making care complex.

Chief complaint and history of present illness
> Symptoms started three days ago with increased frequency, urgency and abdominal discomfort on passing urine.
> These symptoms were accompanied by a general feeling of malaise, nausea and decreased appetite.
> Amelie has not taken anything for her symptoms but has decreased her fluid intake to prevent the need to pass urine.
> She fell last night on her way to the toilet, and now has pain and difficulty weight bearing through her left leg.
> On arrival at the emergency department, Amelie is noted to be mildly disorientated and lethargic.

Processing information

Interpret: These symptoms and details of history outline the scope of the issue for this consumer and how it affects her wellbeing and ability for self-management.

Relate: The assessment data also demonstrates how, in an older adult, homeostatic balances can be easily tipped, resulting in a cascade effect of problems. In older adults, often the presentation of illness does not follow the typical signs and symptoms seen in a younger person. The older adult can present with symptoms such as delirium or falls that indicate an underlying illness.

Discriminate: Urinary frequency and urgency in an older person can often be viewed by health professionals as a normal part of ageing and therefore these symptoms can be overlooked.

Relate and Infer: Increased urinary frequency and urgency, cloudy and malodorous urine are suggestive of a urinary tract infection, even though Amelie does not have the typical symptom of dysuria. In an older person, the immune response does not always produce an elevated temperature, and core body temperature tends to be lower. A temperature of 37.4°C could be very significant in an older person and indicative of an infection.

Although urinary tract infections can often be resolved with antibiotic therapy, there is a risk of the infection spreading to the kidneys. Costovertebral angle tenderness can be an indication that this has occurred.

Relate: The risk of fracture following a fall is high in the older person due to ageing changes in bone density.
> Leg alignment normal and leg lengths equal.

Discriminate, Relate and Infer: A fractured neck of femur will often result in alterations in alignment such as external rotation and shortening of the affected leg. Amelie does not have these symptoms and it is likely she has not sustained a fracture during the fall. However, it is important that X-rays are undertaken to completely rule out the possibility of a fracture in the hip or pelvic area.
> No evidence of bone protrusions
> Swelling and haematoma

Interpret: This indicates soft tissue damage.
> Pain on movement and weight bearing

Interpret: Injury is affecting consumer's ability to function normally.

Extent of injury from fall and potential for other injuries or complications
> Pupils equal and reactive to light
> Cranial nerves intact
> GCS 13
> Disorientated to time and lethargic
> Husband does not believe Amelie knocked her head in the fall

Infer and Predict: It is likely Amelie's slight disorientation and lethargy is related more to delirium rather than a head injury; however, it is important not to rule this out and regular neurological monitoring should be part of the nursing plan.

Other significant assessment information
> No evidence of skin damage from the fall
> Skin on lower legs shiny appearance with patches of dry scaling areas
> Peripheral pulses present, dorsalis pedis weak bilaterally
> Capillary refill feet and hands >3 s
> Bilateral low skin temperature and pale colouring in feet

Relate, Infer and Predict: If these symptoms were unilateral on the left side it might indicate that the injury has resulted in blood flow and nerve function distal to the haematoma; however, the bilateral nature suggests Amelie is developing peripheral vascular disease and peripheral neuropathy (both can be related to complications of diabetes). Nevertheless, neurovascular status should continue to be monitored for any acute changes in the left leg that may indicate vascular or neural complications related to the swelling and haematoma.
> Decreased fluid intake
> Skin dry texture

Interpret and Discriminate: Tissue turgor is not always a good indication of hydration status due to normal ageing changes in the skin that decrease skin moisture and elasticity.
> Lips dry with beginning evidence of cracks/chapping, buccal mucosa pink but dry, tongue mildly furrowed, dry
> Small volume concentrated (dark) urine

Interpret and Discriminate: These are signs of dehydration. The ageing kidneys are not as able to conserve fluid and hence the risk of dehydration is greater in the older adult.
> Mildly disorientated and lethargic

Relate and Infer: Could be due to dehydration.
> JVP – absent

Interpret and Discriminate: This is a sign of hypovolaemia.

Falls risk and cause
> Heart rate regular, no cardiac abnormalities detected.

Interpret and Discriminate: Arrhythmias can decrease perfusion to the brain and result in falls.
> Orthostatic hypotension

Interpret and Discriminate: This can be associated with hypovolaemia related to dehydration and is a common risk of falls in the older adult.
> No loss of consciousness, no cranial nerve impairment.

Interpret, Discriminate and Infer: A stroke can cause a fall; Amelie is presenting as mildly disorientated; however, other assessment findings do not indicate a stroke.
> Decreased sensation in feet.

Interpret and Discriminate: Can impair a person's ability to recognise positioning and result in falls.
> Macular degeneration

Interpret and Discriminate: Impaired vision increases the risk of falling.
> Urinary urgency

Interpret and Discriminate: Can result in a person needing to rush to the toilet, increasing the risk of falling.

Relate and Infer: Falls are often multifactorial in nature. In the case of Amelie, it is likely her fall resulted from a combination of needing to rush to the toilet, poor balance related to decreased sensation in her feet, and orthostatic hypotension, which caused a temporary decrease in oxygen supply to the brain and resulted in dizziness and loss of balance.

Putting it all together – synthesise Information

The nurse in this case would note all of these abnormalities and refer to the medical officer. Immediate nursing management of Amelie will involve monitoring for any potential complications related to her injury and restoring fluid and potential electrolyte imbalances. Amelie also has the pre-existing condition of diabetes, which will need to be managed and monitored, as illness and infection can alter blood glucose levels. The possibility of neural and vascular impairment in the distal limbs needs to be documented and referred on to an appropriate medical professional for further investigation. The above assessment data suggests that Amelie is experiencing dehydration. Rehydration is important to reverse her current state of disorientation and lethargy, maintain and prevent damage to kidney function and oral mucosa, and minimise strain on her cardiac system.

Safety is another factor the nurse must consider; in particular falls risk, but also risk of pressure-related tissue damage as the pain related to her soft tissue injury will result in decreased mobility. Another risk the nurse needs to minimise is constipation related to decreased mobility and dehydration. Ongoing care of Amelie will include maintaining her level of functional ability, and education relating to safety.

Actions based on assessment findings

The nurse should also provide additional education for interventions that do not require a doctor's order:

1 Once the nurse ascertains that Amelie does not need to be 'Nil By Mouth', encourage oral fluids, alongside monitoring and administering any intravenous fluids ordered.

2 Undertake fluid balance monitoring.

3 Treatment and prevention of constipation (due to reduced mobility, dehydration and any pain following the fall – probably in conjunction with possible polypharmacy effects on bowels).

4 Strategies to assist with urinary frequency/urgency (discuss incontinence devices, reassure that once she has commenced treatment this symptom should resolve).

5 Undertake formal risk assessment of Amelie's falls; may need to refer to an allied health professional for a home assessment to identify and minimise any risks identified at home.

6 Explore any anxieties that may have arisen in relation to the diagnosis – encourage Amelie to express her fears and anxieties.

7 Consider the importance of social supports and relationship/roles for the older adult. Fortunately, Richard is independent and does not rely on Amelie to care for him. Review possible alternative support service options with Richard and family, in preparation for any future health changes.

8 Identify other health maintenance activities that Amelie can be involved in to increase her ability to live independently.

9 Plan for education before discharge, especially on wearing the emergency call pendant to reduce risk of not being able to access help at home. This might arise if Amelie fell while Richard was out; she would not be able to call for help without the pendant.

The final step in the process is accurate documentation. The nurse must document findings, referrals, interventions, and advice and education given. The consumer would then be reassessed following definitive diagnosis and medical interventions for her ongoing health maintenance.

CHAPTER RESOURCES

REVIEW QUESTIONS

For answers to these questions, see Answer section at the end of the book.

1. Which of the following changes occurs in the older male consumer?
   a. The scrotal sac constricts.
   b. Pubic hair thickens.
   c. The testicles retract into the abdomen.
   d. The penis atrophies.
2. Which of the following vital signs needs to be addressed in an 85-year-old female?
   a. Respiratory rate of 22 bpm
   b. Heart rate of 96 bpm
   c. Temperature of 36°C
   d. Blood pressure of 142/98 mmHg
3. What is a greyish halo seen in the eyes of the older adult called?
   a. Pterygium
   b. Arcus senilis
   c. Cataracts
   d. Hyphaema
4. 82-year-old Veronica complains of very dry, itchy skin during her clinic visit. What can you tell this woman about her condition? Select all that apply.
   a. Increasing the humidity level in her house may help her.
   b. Pruritus is due to a decrease in water content of the skin.
   c. Atrophy of the eccrine glands decreases the risk of hyperthermia in older adults.
   d. Xerosis and pruritus are more common in autumn and spring.
   e. Pruritus may be associated with the consumer's diabetes.
   f. Frequent bathing in hot water can worsen her symptoms.

5. Which of the following are more frequently found on the skin of the older adult than on a younger person? Select all that apply.
   a. Seborrheic keratoses
   b. Solar lentigo
   c. Squamous cell carcinoma
   d. Cellulitis
   e. Comedomes
   f. Contact dermatitis

6. Which of the following is a normal examination finding in the older adult? Select all that apply.
   a. An S_3 heart sound
   b. An S_4 heart sound
   c. Buccal mucosa thins
   d. Pectus carinatum
   e. Increased fat deposits in the abdomen
   f. Thickened buccal mucosa with increased vascularity

7. A 92-year-old consumer is admitted to the ER for evaluation after falling at home. The consumer has a history of dementia. Which of the following symptoms are consistent with dementia? Select all that apply.
   a. A stable state of consciousness
   b. A sudden onset of symptoms
   c. Impaired judgement
   d. Disorientation to time and place
   e. Rapid progression of symptoms
   f. Can occur concurrently with depression

8. Which of the following reasons best describes why the S_4 heart sound is a common finding in the older adult?
   a. The increase in the incidence of chronic heart failure
   b. Decreased compliance of the left ventricle
   c. Sclerosis of the mitral and aortic valves
   d. Due to the displaced apical impulse

9. The following items should be included in a mental status assessment:
   a. General appearance, person, place and time, serial sevens, level of consciousness, Apgar score
   b. Glasgow coma score, neurovascular measures, general appearance, memory, ability to count by 5s back from 100
   c. General appearance, orientation, mood, level of consciousness, Weber and Rhinne test, behaviour, knowledge and vocabulary, judgement and abstraction, memory, language and speech, sensory and motor assessment
   d. General appearance, orientation, mood, level of consciousness, behaviour, knowledge and vocabulary, judgement and abstraction, memory, language and speech, sensory and motor assessment.

10. Mrs Taylor is an 87-year-old aged-care resident who has been hospitalised for pneumonia. On admission she is pleasant, alert, and orientated to person, place and time. The next day Mrs Taylor awakens when her name is called but then closes her eyes during the conversation. She is distracted by voices in the hallway, and questions must be repeated. She is now slurring her words and having difficulty with word finding. Which condition best explains Mrs Taylor's symptoms?
    a. Alzheimer's disease
    b. Dementia
    c. Delirium
    d. Depression

CS CLINICAL SKILLS

The following Clinical Skills are relevant to this chapter and can be found in Tollefson & Hillman, *Clinical Psychomotor Skills,* 8th edition:
> 16 Mental status assessment
> 27 Healthcare teaching.

FURTHER RESOURCES

> Australian Government, My Aged Care: https://www.myagedcare.gov.au/for-health-professionals
> Australian Government. Aged Care Quality Standards: https://www.myagedcare.gov.au/aged-care-quality-standards
> Australian Human Rights Commission. LGBTI+: https://humanrights.gov.au/our-work/lgbti
> Australian Pain Society: www.apsoc.org.au
> Australian Psychological Society: https://www.psychology.org.au/for-members/publications
> Continence Foundation of Australia: https://www.continence.org.au/pages/key-statistics.html
> Dementia Australia. LGBTI resources: https://www.dementia.org.au/resources/LGBTI
> Elder Abuse Complaints: https://www.myagedcare.gov.au/for-health-professionals https://www.myagedcare.gov.au/contact-us/complaints#concernselderabuse
> Mini-Cog Screening for Cognitive Impairment in Older Adults: https://mini-cog.com/

> Ministry of Health/Manatū Hauora – Health of older people: http://www.health.govt.nz/our-work/life-stages/health-older-people
> The Psychogeriatric Nurses' Association Australia: http://www.pgna.org.au/
> QUT Health. Wound care in residential aged care facilities – Creating champions for skin integrity (National Dissemination): https://research.qut.edu.au/ccm/projects/wound-care-in-residential-aged-care-facilities-national-dissemination/
> Queensland Government. Elder abuse in aged care: https://eapu.com.au/elder-abuse-in-aged-care/
> World Health Organization. Celebrating sexual health for benefits throughout life: https://www.who.int/news/item/31-08-2022-celebrating-sexual-health-for-benefits-throughout-life

REFERENCES

Abbey, J., Piller, N., Bellis, A., Esterman, A., Parker, D., Giles, L., & Lowcary, B. (2004). The Abbey pain scale: a 1 minute numerical indicator for people with end stage dementia. *Palliative Nursing. 10*, 6–13.

Alexopoulos, G., Abrams, R., Young, R., & Shamoian, C. (1988). Cornell scale for depression in dementia. *Biological Psychiatry*, 23, p. 271–84. doi: 0006-3223(88)90038-8

Alzheimer's New Zealand. (2023). Facts and figures. Retrieved 5 May 2023 from: https://alzheimers.org.nz/explore/facts-and-figures/

Australian Bureau of Statistics (ABS). (2022a). National, state and territory population. Retrieved 8 December 2022 from: https://www.abs.gov.au/statistics/people/population/national-state-and-territory-population/latest-release

Australian Bureau of Statistics (ABS). (2022b). Estimates of Aboriginal and Torres Strait Islander Australians. Retrieved 8 December 2022 from: https://www.abs.gov.au/statistics/people/aboriginal-and-torres-strait-islander-peoples/estimates-aboriginal-and-torres-strait-islander-australians/latest-release

Australian Government. (2022). My Aged Care. Retrieved 8 December 2022 from: https://www.myagedcare.gov.au/contact-us/complaints#concernselderabuse

Australian Government Department of Health and Aged Care. (2019). Bladder and bowel for older Australians. Retrieved 28 October 2022 from: https://www.health.gov.au/health-topics/bladder-and-bowel/bladder-and-bowel-throughout-life/bladder-and-bowel-for-older-australians#:~:text=People%20aged%2085%20years%20are,hold%20as%20much%20wee%20(urine)

Australian Government Department of Health and Aged Care. (2022). Restrictive practices in aged care – a last resort. https://www.health.gov.au/health-topics/aged-care/providing-aged-care-services/working-in-aged-care/restrictive-practices-in-aged-care-a-last-resort

Australian Human Rights Commission (2021). Ensuring health and bodily integrity (2021). Protecting the human rights of people born with variations in sex characteristics in the context of medical interventions. Retrieved 4 November 2022 from: https://humanrights.gov.au/intersex-report-2021

Australian Institute of Health and Welfare (AIHW). (2019). Elder abuse: context, concepts and challenges. Retrieved 8 December 2022 from: https://www.aihw.gov.au/getmedia/affc65d3-22fd-41a9-9564-6d42e948e195/Australias-Welfare-Chapter-7-summary-18Sept2019.pdf.aspx

Australian Institute of Health and Welfare (AIHW). (2021a). Older People. Retrieved 9 December 2022 from: https://www.aihw.gov.au/reports/older-people/older-australians/contents/demographic-profile

Australian Institute of Health and Welfare (AIHW). (2021b). Older Australians. Retrieved 28 October 2022 from: https://www.aihw.gov.au/reports/older-people/older-australians/contents/housing-and-living-arrangements

Australian Institute of Health and Welfare (AIHW). (2022a). Indigenous health and wellbeing. Retrieved 11 December 2022 from: https://www.aihw.gov.au/reports/australias-health/indigenous-health-and-wellbeing

Australian Institute of Health and Welfare (AIHW). (2022b). Life expectancy and deaths. Retrieved 28 October 2022 from: https://www.aihw.gov.au/reports-data/health-conditions-disability-deaths/life-expectancy-deaths/overview

Australian Institute of Health and Welfare (AIHW). (2022c). Burden of disease. Retrieved 28 October 2022 from: https://www.aihw.gov.au/reports-data/health-conditions-disability-deaths/burden-of-disease/overview

Australian Pain Society. (2022). Supporting multidisciplinary pain management in Australia –Resources. Retrieved 28 October 2022 from: https://apsoc.org.au/

Brodaty, H., Pond, D., Kemp, N. M., Luscombe, G., Harding, L., Berman, K., & Huppert, F. A. (2002). The GPCOG: a new screening test for dementia designed for general practice. *Journal of the American Geriatrics Society*, *50*(3), 530–34.

Dementia Australia. (2020). LGBTI and dementia. Retrieved 4 November 2022 from: https://www.dementia.org.au/resources/lgbti-and-dementia

Dementia Support Australia. (2022). Understanding changes in behaviour. Retrieved 4 November 2022 from: https://www.dementia.com.au/understanding-behaviour-changes

Dementia Australia. (2023). Dementia statistics. Retrieved 5 May 2023 from: https://www.dementia.org.au/statistics

Elder Abuse Prevention Unit. (2022). Elder abuse in aged care. Retrieved 6 November 2022 from: https://eapu.com.au/elder-abuse-in-aged-care/

Ferguson, M., Capra, S., Bauer, J., & Banks, M. (1999). Development of a valid and reliable malnutrition screening tool for adult acute hospital consumers. *Nutrition*, *15*(6), 458–64. doi.org/10.1016/S0899-9007(99)00084-2

Finch, K., Osseiran-Moisson, R., Carville, K., Leslie, G., & Dwyer, M. (2018). Skin tear prevention in elderly consumers using twice-daily moisturiser, *Journal of Wounds Australia*, *26*(2), 99–109.

Fulmer, T. & Wallace, M. (n.d). Fulmer SPICES: An overall assessment tool for older adults. Retrieved 14 September 2022 from: https://hign.org/consultgeri/try-this-series/fulmer-spices-overall-assessment-tool-older-adults

Health Navigator New Zealand. (2022). Elder abuse. Retrieved 6 November 2022 from: https://www.healthnavigator.org.nz/health-a-z/a/abuse-elder/

Inouye, S., Westendorp, R., & Saczynski, J. (2014). Delirium in elderly people. *Lancet*, Mar 8, *383*(9920), 911–22. doi: 10.1016/S0140-6736(13)60688-1

LoGiudice, D., Smith, K., Thomas, J., Lautenschlager, N. T., Almeida, O. P., Atkinson, D., & Flicker, L. (2006). Kimberley Indigenous Cognitive Assessment tool (KICA): development of a cognitive assessment tool for older indigenous Australians. *International Psychogeriatrics*, *18*(2), 269–80.

Masnoon, N., Shakib, S., Kalisch-Ellett, L., & Caughey, G. (2017). What is polypharmacy? A systematic review of definitions. *BMC Geriatrics*, *17*. doi: 10.1186/s12877-017-0621-2

Ministry of Health/Manatù Hauora. (2022). Sector guidance for Ngā Paerewa for Health and Disability Services Standards (NZS 8134:2021) Part 6: Restraint and seclusion. https://www.health.govt.nz/our-work/regulation-health-and-disability-system/certification-health-care-services/services-standard/resources-nga-paerewa-health-and-disability-services-standard/sector-guidance-nga-paerewa-health-and-disability-services-standard-nzs-81342021/part-6

Molloy, W., & Standish, T. (1997). A guide to the Standardized Mini-mental State Examination. *Psychogeriatrics*, *9*(Suppl 1), 87–94. https://doi.org/10.1017/S1041610297004754

New Zealand Dementia Foundation. (2022). Best practice links gender and sexual minorities. Retrieved 4 November 2022 from: https://www.nzdementia.org/Best-Practice-Resources/Supporting-diverse-needs/Gender-and-sexual-minorities

Parker, C. N., Finlayson, K. J., & Edwards, H. E. (2015). Risk factors for delayed healing in venous leg ulcers: a review of the literature. *International Journal of Clinical Practice*, *69*(9), 967–77. doi: 10.1111/ijcp.12635

Parr-Brownlie, L. C., Waters, D. L., Neville, S., Neha, T., & Muramatsu, N. (2020). Aging in New Zealand: Ka haere ki te ao pakeketanga, *The Gerontologist*, *60*(5), August, https://doi.org/10.1093/geront/gnaa032

Queensland Health. (2017). Validated malnutrition screening and assessment tools: Comparison guide. Retrieved 9 September 2018 from: https://www.health.qld.gov.au/__data/assets/pdf_file/0021/152454/hphe_scrn_tools.pdf

RACGP. (2019). Silver Book – Part A Polypharmacy. Retrieved 8 December from: https://www.racgp.org.au/clinical-resources/clinical-guidelines/key-racgp-guidelines/view-all-racgp-guidelines/silver-book/part-a/polypharmacy

Stats New Zealand (NZ). (2022). One million people aged 65+ by 2028. Retrieved 8 December 2022 from: https://www.stats.govt.nz/news/one-million-people-aged-65-by-2028/

Storey, J. E., Rowland, J. T., Conforti, D. A., & Dickson, H. G. (2004). The Rowland universal dementia assessment scale (RUDAS): a multicultural cognitive assessment scale. *International Psychogeriatrics*, *16*(1), 13–31.

Taylor, A., Broadbent, M., Wallis, M., & Marsden, E. (2018). The use of functional and cognitive assessment in the emergency department to inform decision making: A scoping review. *Australasian Emergency Care*, *21*, 13–22.

Te Whatu Ora. Health New Zealand, (2022) Mortality web tool. Retrieved 11 December 2022 from: https://www.tewhatuora.govt.nz/our-health-system/data-and-statistics/mortality-web-tool

Tollefson, J. (2022). Clinical psychomotor skills: Assessment tools for nurses (8th ed.), Australia–New Zealand edn., Melbourne: Cengage Learning Australia Pty Ltd.

Warden, V., Hurley, A. C., & Volicer, L. (2003). Development and psychometric evaluation of the Pain Assessment in Advanced Dementia (PAINAD) scale. *Journal of the American Medical Directors Association*, *4*(1), 9–15.

World Health Organization (WHO). (2019). Medication safety in polypharmacy. Retrieved 11 December 2022 from: https://www.who.int/publications/i/item/WHO-UHC-SDS-2019.11

PUTTING IT ALL TOGETHER

CHAPTER 22   HEALTH ASSESSMENT AND PHYSICAL EXAMINATION IN CONTEXT

HEALTH ASSESSMENT AND PHYSICAL EXAMINATION IN CONTEXT

LEARNING OUTCOMES

By the end of this chapter you should be able to:

1 identify legal and ethical considerations for the health assessment and physical examination

2 explain the components of the health assessment and physical examination in context

3 demonstrate and document a comprehensive health assessment and physical examination on a consumer

4 demonstrate and document a focused health assessment and physical examination on a consumer.

BACKGROUND

Performing a comprehensive health assessment and physical examination is a skill that takes time and practice to develop. Accurate recognition of normal findings is crucial to differentiate abnormal and pathological findings. Learning the examination techniques, system by system, as described in this text, helps you to continue to improve and refine your skills. You should become more time efficient as you practise your skills. It is important to develop your own health assessment and physical examination approach that you are comfortable with, so that you have consistency in your practice. The consumer's physical, emotional or mental state may necessitate a change in the usual progression of the assessment. Your clinical reasoning and experience will dictate when specific steps should be omitted, deferred or repeated.

If the consumer's chief complaint is not of an urgent or critical nature, then their first visit to the healthcare facility is the ideal time to perform a comprehensive assessment. A focused assessment (indicated when the consumer has identified very specific symptoms), an interval or a follow-up visit frequently require partial assessments that document changes. An emergency assessment is even briefer (usually a primary survey assessment – ABCDE), and specifically focuses on the presenting problem and the time-related aspects of the concern. These visits require substantially less time.

Considering concepts explored in Unit 1: Laying the Foundation, as well as Chapters 6 to 21, this final chapter contextualises an example of a comprehensive and focused health assessment and physical examination of an adult consumer. This textbook has also described some advanced techniques for health assessment and physical examination and should be implemented according to your scope of practice. Your experience will guide you in determining when advanced techniques are warranted *if* they are in your scope of practice. The advanced techniques are mostly omitted from the assessment sequence used in the two examples provided. This chapter also provides a brief overview of legal and ethical considerations for health assessment and physical examination context.

CLINICAL **REASONING**

Practice tip: Enhancing consumer cooperation
Consumer cooperation is essential to complete an accurate health assessment and physical examination. This can be enhanced by using sound therapeutic communication skills. These guidelines will assist you:
> Minimise individual wait time prior to the examination; explain any delays that occur.
> Greet the consumer first and put them at ease; reassure them of confidentiality.
> Proceed in an efficient and organised manner.
> Encourage the individual to actively participate in the assessment process (e.g. provide information, ask questions).
> Use terms the individual will understand.
> Ask the consumer to demonstrate understanding of person-centred health education.
> Be honest; do not offer false reassurance or jump to conclusions.
> Arrange for the presence of a third party if requested.

LEGAL CONSIDERATIONS

The increasingly litigious nature of society has not bypassed the nursing profession. These are some specific guidelines to support health professionals and consumers:
> Document all consumer interactions (face-to-face, telephone, email, letters).
> Respect the consumer's confidentiality. Do not discuss any aspect of their case in a public area or with colleagues who are not involved in their team; always keep discussions at a strictly professional level.
> Report any disease that is considered a public health concern (according to local, state and federal regulations).
> Respect a consumer's right to privacy.
> Respect a consumer's right to refuse treatment or assessments (document thoroughly).
> When appropriate, ask the consumer for permission to perform various assessments and examinations, especially those that may be uncomfortable. If the individual refuses permission or declines to answer questions, explain the importance and reason for the assessment or examination. If they still deny permission, document refusal.
> Know your institution's policies and standards of practice, and practise within those guidelines.
> Know your Nurses' Code of Conduct/Ethics and practise within its scope.
> Consult with your line manager/supervisor and consumer safety coordinators about any other legal concerns.

ETHICAL CONSIDERATIONS

It is helpful to keep in mind the following ethical principles to guide your clinical reasoning within an ethical framework:
> **Autonomy:** A consumer's right to self-determination; the duty to respect a consumer's thoughts and actions to make their own decisions
> **Beneficence:** To do what is 'good' for the consumer
> **Nonmaleficence:** To do no harm to the consumer
> **Justice:** To be fair and impartial to the consumer
> **Advocacy:** The duty to inform consumers of their rights and to provide objective information to support them to make their own decisions
> **Veracity:** To be truthful to the consumer
> **Utilitarianism:** The duty to perform the greatest good for the greatest number of people

These principles may create challenges for you and the consumer when an ethical dilemma presents itself in the clinical setting. The principles are not failsafe, nor are they always easy to practise. Having an awareness of them helps to advocate for the rights of a consumer; ultimately, this is one of the key roles of the nurse. Your practice is bound by the professional nursing ethics statements adopted by your organisation or registration authority, to help guide nursing actions. Use these or whatever resources are available to you when presented with ethical dilemmas or questions.

APPROACH TO COMPREHENSIVE HEALTH ASSESSMENT AND PHYSICAL EXAMINATION

> Use a structured approach to preparing and undertaking the health history and physical examination (consider the APIE process and the clinical reasoning cycle [see Chapter 1]).
> Determine the type of assessment to be undertaken (comprehensive, focused or emergency (primary survey) [see Chapter 3]).
> Approach the consumer from a holistic viewpoint and try to understand their perspective; take a person-centred approach.
> Apply critical thinking, which incorporates the consideration of subjective and objective data. Always ask, 'Why?'
> Remain calm and present with the consumer.
> Act in a professional manner at all times; remember the consumer is simultaneously examining you (mannerisms, facial expressions, hesitations in speech).
> Recognise both the consumer's and your own potential stressors (work, home environment, schedules) and try to account for them.
> Acknowledge emotional reactions to illness (anger, fear, anxiety, disbelief, confusion, guilt, shame, blame, hurt, betrayal).
> Apply sensitivity to cultural and spiritual issues.

ASSESSMENT: TAKING THE CONSUMER'S HEALTH HISTORY

Conduct the health history. Depending on the consumer's reason for the visit, this can be the complete, episodic, **interval (follow-up)**, focused (brief) or emergency health history. Components of the developmental, cultural and spiritual assessments are evaluated during the course of the consumer interaction. Thorough assessments of any or all of these special assessments can be completed if indicated by the consumer's situation.

Approach to physical examination

> Ensure that the examination table is at a comfortable height for you and the consumer, with easy access.
> Respect the consumer's modesty.
> Have the consumer make as few position changes as possible (group assessment related to positioning requirements), but allow them to reposition to be comfortable.
> Ensure all equipment is accessible and arranged in a logical manner (**Figure 22.1**).
> Develop an approach that is logical but allows flexibility.
> Keep interruptions to a minimum.
> Use clinical judgement to modify the examination sequence and adapt it to circumstances.
> Teach self-assessment while the consumer is gowned or during specific system examinations.
> Advise the consumer prior to procedures about sensations and or discomforts.

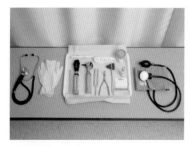

FIGURE 22.1 All equipment required for the examination should be neatly organised and readily available.

> Ask the consumer about pain or unexpected sensations during assessments and examination.
> Offer cleaning wipes or tissues to the consumer following certain examinations (e.g. the pelvic and rectal examinations).
> Provide the consumer with privacy for redressing.
> Allow time at the conclusion of the examination to discuss relevant findings and to encourage the consumer to ask questions.
> Remember to adapt the physical examination so that the time spent in undertaking this is appropriate for the age and condition of the consumer (e.g. children will not tolerate lengthy examinations in one session, and systemically unwell consumers may require frequent rest breaks).

IMPLEMENTATION: CONDUCTING THE PHYSICAL EXAMINATION

Physical examination is guided by the health history; however, in emergency presentations, physical examination usually occurs at the same time as the health history. For example, if a consumer has presented to the emergency department following a motor vehicle collision, you would be asking questions while you undertake a primary survey (ABCDE). This text has provided a head-to-toe assessment format in order to discuss body systems in their entirety. However, in practice, a head-to-toe assessment combines systems when assessing most body parts. For example, when assessing the hands, you combine components of the skin, musculoskeletal and neurological assessments. The sample case studies at the end of this chapter document a comprehensive as well as a focused health assessment and physical examination.

General appearance

The consumer's general appearance is assessed during the health history, incorporating the following into this assessment:

1. Physical status
   - Age: stated age versus apparent age
   - Body symmetry
   - Body fat
   - Body conformation and posture
   - Motor activity: gait, speed, and effort of movement; weight bearing; absence or presence of movement in different body areas
   - Body and breath odours
2. Psychological status
   - Mental status and cognitive function (level of consciousness and neurological assessment)
   - Facial expressions
   - Dress, grooming and personal hygiene
   - Mood and manner
   - Speech and communication ability
3. Distress
   - Physical
   - Psychological
   - Emotional
4. Vital signs (as may affect appearance)
   - Height and weight
5. Pain

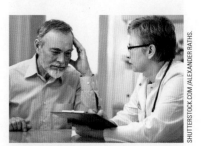

FIGURE 22.2 Observe the consumer's overall appearance and demeanour during the interview.

SHUTTERSTOCK.COM/ALEXANDER RATHS.

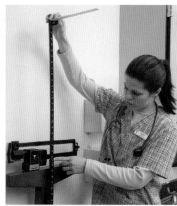

A. Measuring height

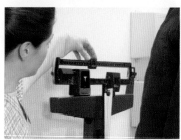

B. Weighing the consumer

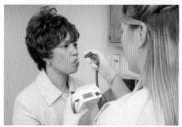

C. Taking temperature

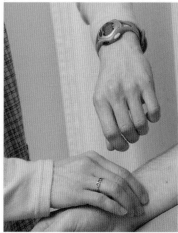

D. Pulse determination

FIGURE 22.3 General measurements

Measurements and vital signs

Record the consumer's measurements (see **Figure 22.3**):

1. Height
2. Weight
3. Temperature
4. Pulse (radial preferred site in adult)
5. Respirations
6. Blood pressure
7. Oxygen saturation
8. Pain assessment

Mental status and neurological assessment

1. Assess mental status and cognitive function: level of consciousness, physical appearance and behaviour, speech and communication, suicidal ideation, cognitive abilities and mentation (see Chapter 7).

   After the mental status examination, ask the consumer to undress and don an examination gown; underwear may be worn. Ask the person to empty their bladder prior to commencing the assessment process. The urine may be collected for a specimen. Ask the individual to sit on the examination table with the legs hanging over the front. A second drape can be provided to cover the lap and legs. Stand in front of the individual.
2. Assess light touch: face (CN V), hands, lower arms, abdomen, feet, legs.
3. Assess superficial pain (sharp and dull): face (CN V), hands, lower arms, abdomen, feet, legs.
4. Assess two-point discrimination: tongue, lips, fingers, dorsum of hand, torso, feet.
5. Assess vibration sense: fingers, toes.
6. Assess stereognosis, graphaesthesia and extinction.
7. Assess cerebellar function: finger to nose, rapid alternating hand movements, touching thumb to each finger, running heel down shin, foot tapping.
8. Assess deep tendon reflexes: biceps, triceps, brachioradialis, patellar, Achilles.
9. Assess plantar reflex and Babinski reflex.

Skin

Throughout the entire head-to-toe assessment, inspect the skin for the following characteristics (see **Figure 22.4**):

1. Colour
2. Bleeding
3. Ecchymosis
4. Vascularity
5. Lesions

Throughout the entire head-to-toe assessment, palpate the skin for these characteristics:

1. Moisture
2. Temperature
3. Texture
4. Turgor
5. Oedema

Head and face

1. Inspect the shape of the head.
2. Inspect and palpate the head and scalp.

3. Inspect the colour and distribution of the hair. Note any infestations; palpate the hair.
4. Inspect the face for expression, shape, symmetry (CN VII), symmetry of eyes, eyebrows, ears, nose and mouth.
5. Instruct the consumer to raise the eyebrows, frown, smile, wrinkle the forehead, show their teeth, purse the lips, puff the cheeks and whistle (CN VII).
6. Palpate the temporal pulses. Palpate the temporalis muscles (CN V).
7. Palpate and auscultate the temporomandibular joints.
8. Palpate the masseter muscles (CN V).

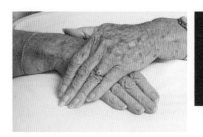

FIGURE 22.4 Inspect the characteristics of the skin such as colour, vascularity and presence of lesions.

Eyes

1. Test distance vision and near vision (**Figure 22.5**)(CN II).
2. Test colour vision.
3. Test visual fields via confrontation (CN II).
4. Assess extraocular muscle mobility: cover/uncover test, corneal light reflex, six cardinal fields of gaze (CNs III, IV, VI).
5. Assess direct and consensual light reflexes and accommodation (CN III).
6. Inspect the eyelids, eyebrows, palpebral fissures and position of eyes.
7. Inspect and palpate the lacrimal apparatus.
8. Inspect the conjunctiva, sclera, cornea, iris, pupils and lenses.
9. Assess the corneal reflex.

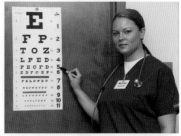

A. Test distance vision

Ears

1. Test gross hearing: voice-whisper test or watch-tick test (CN VIII).
2. Inspect and palpate the external ear.
3. Assess ear alignment.

Nose and sinuses

1. Inspect the external surface of the nose.
2. Assess nostril patency bilaterally.
3. Test olfactory sense (CN I).
4. Conduct internal assessment with nasal speculum: mucosa, turbinates, septum.
5. Inspect, percuss and palpate frontal and maxillary sinuses.

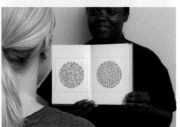

B. Test colour vision

FIGURE 22.5 Visual acuity assessment

Mouth and throat

1. Note breath odour.
2. Inspect the lips, buccal mucosa, gums, and hard and soft palates.
3. Inspect the teeth; count the teeth.
4. Inspect the tongue; ask the consumer to stick out the tongue (CN XII).
5. Inspect the uvula; note movement when the consumer says 'ah' (CNs IX, X).
6. Inspect the tonsils; note grade.
7. Inspect the oropharynx.
8. Test gag reflex (CNs IX, X).
9. Test taste (CN VII).
10. Palpate the lips and mouth, if indicated.

Neck

1. Inspect the musculature of the neck.
2. Inspect range of motion, shoulder shrug, and strength of sternocleidomastoid and trapezius muscle (CN XI).
3. Palpate the musculature of the neck.
4. Inspect and palpate the trachea.
5. Palpate the carotid arteries (one at a time).

6. Inspect the jugular veins for distension; estimate jugular venous pressure (JVP), if indicated.
7. Inspect and palpate the thyroid (use only one approach, either anterior or posterior).
8. Auscultate the thyroid and carotid arteries.
9. Inspect and palpate the lymph nodes: preauricular, postauricular, occipital, submental, submandibular, tonsillar.

Jugular veins

As the individual changes from a sitting to a supine position for the next stage of the assessment, observe the jugular veins when they are at a 45° angle. Assess again when the consumer is supine.

1. Inspect the jugular veins for distension; estimate JVP, if indicated.

Back, posterior and lateral thoraxes

Move behind the consumer. Untie the gown so that the entire back is exposed. The gown should cover the shoulders and the anterior chest.

1. Palpate the thyroid (posterior approach).
2. Inspect and palpate the spinous processes; inspect range of motion of the cervical spine.
3. Note thoracic configuration, symmetry of shoulders and position of scapula.
4. Palpate the posterior thorax and lateral thorax.
5. Perform posterior thoracic expansion.
6. Percuss the posterior thorax (Figure 22.6A) and lateral thorax.
7. Perform diaphragmatic excursion.
8. Auscultate the posterior thorax and lateral thorax; perform voice sounds if indicated (Figure 22.6B).

Anterior thorax

Move in front of the consumer and drape their gown to waist level (females may cover their breasts).

1. Inspect shape of the thorax, symmetry of the chest wall, presence of superficial veins, costal angle, angle of ribs, intercostal spaces, muscles of respiration, respirations and sputum (see Figure 22.7).
2. Palpate the anterior thorax.
3. Perform anterior thoracic expansion.
4. Percuss the anterior thorax.
5. Auscultate the anterior thorax; perform voice sounds if indicated.

Heart

1. Auscultate cardiac landmarks: aortic, pulmonic, mitral and tricuspid areas, and midprecordial (Erb's point) (Figure 22.8).
2. Inspect cardiac landmarks for pulsations.
3. Palpate cardiac landmarks for pulsations, thrills and heaves.
4. Palpate the apical impulse.
5. With the diaphragm of the stethoscope, auscultate the cardiac landmarks; count the apical pulse.
6. With the bell of the stethoscope, auscultate the cardiac landmarks.
7. Turn the consumer on the left side and repeat auscultation of cardiac landmarks.

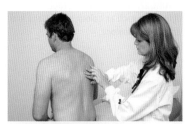
A. Percuss the posterior thorax

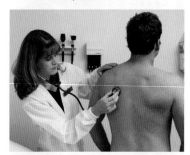
B. Auscultate the posterior thorax

FIGURE 22.6 Posterior thorax assessment

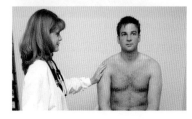
FIGURE 22.7 Inspect the anterior thorax for shape and symmetry.

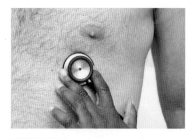
FIGURE 22.8 Auscultate the cardiac landmarks.

Female and male breasts

1. Ask the consumer to uncover the breasts.
2. Palpate each breast. The arm on the same side of the assessed breast should be raised over the head.
3. Compress the nipple to express any discharge.

Abdomen

With the consumer in the supine position, cover their anterior thorax with the gown. Uncover the abdomen from the symphysis pubis to the costal margin.

1. Inspect contour, symmetry, pigmentation and colour.
2. Note scars, striae, visible peristalsis, masses and pulsations.
3. Inspect the rectus abdominis muscles (supine and with head raised) and respiratory movement of the abdomen.
4. Inspect the umbilicus.
5. Auscultate bowel sounds.
6. Auscultate for bruits, venous hum and friction rub.
7. Percuss all four quadrants.
8. Lightly palpate all four quadrants.
9. Note any muscle guarding.

Inguinal area

1. Inspect and palpate the inguinal lymph nodes.
2. Inspect for inguinal hernias.
3. Palpate the femoral pulses.
4. Auscultate the femoral pulses for bruits.

Musculoskeletal system

Ask the consumer to stand barefoot on the floor. If the person is unsteady, use caution when performing the next few tests and remain physically close to them at all times.

1. Assess mobility: casual walk, heel walk, toe walk, tandem walk, backwards walk, stepping to the right and left, deep knee bends (one knee at a time). Note any indications of discomfort.
   Stand behind the consumer.
2. Assess range of motion of the spine.
   Open the individual's gown to expose the back and then ask them to bend forward at the waist.
3. Inspect the spine for scoliosis.
   Close the consumer's gown.

Upper extremities

1. Inspect nail bed colour, shape and configuration (**Figure 22.10**); palpate nail bed texture.
2. Assess capillary refill on nail bed.
3. Inspect muscle size and palpate muscle tone of hands, arms and shoulders.
4. Palpate the joints of fingers, wrists, elbows and shoulders.
5. Assess range of motion and strength of fingers, wrists, elbows and shoulders.
6. Test position sense.
7. Palpate radial and brachial pulses.

Lower extremities

Cover the exposed abdomen with the gown. Lift the drape from the bottom to expose the lower extremities.

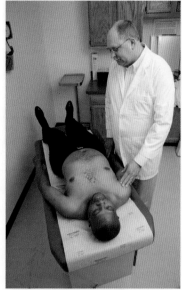

A. Inspect the abdomen

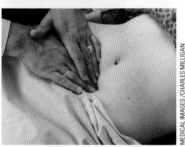

B. Palpate the abdominal quadrants

MEDICAL IMAGES/CHARLES MILLIGAN

FIGURE 22.9 Inspection and palpation of the abdomen

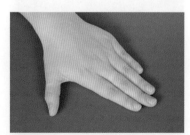

A. Inspect the nail beds

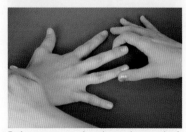

B. Assess range of motion and strength of the fingers

FIGURE 22.10 Upper extremity assessment

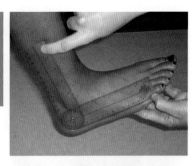

FIGURE 22.11 Inspect the lower extremities and determine range of movement (a goniometer can be used to measure dorsiflexion).

1. Inspect for colour, capillary refill, oedema, ulcerations, hair distribution and varicose veins.
2. Palpate for temperature, oedema and texture.
3. Palpate the popliteal, dorsalis pedis and posterior tibial pulses.
4. Inspect muscle size and palpate muscle tone of the legs and feet.
5. Palpate the joints of the hips, knees, ankles and feet.
6. Assess range of motion (**Figure 22.11**) and strength of the hips, knees, ankles and feet.

Female genitourinary, reproductive, anus and rectum

1. Inspect the abdomen (contour, symmetry and skin pigmentation).
2. Palpate and percuss the bladder.
3. Inspect pubic hair and skin colour and condition: mons pubis, vulva, clitoris, urethral meatus, vaginal introitus, sacrococcygeal area, perineum and anal mucosa.
4. Palpate the labia, urethral meatus, Skene's glands, vaginal introitus and perineum.
   Assist the consumer to a sitting position and offer tissues to wipe the perineal area. Ask the individual to redress.

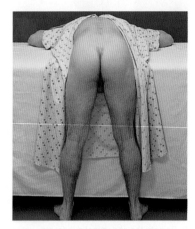

FIGURE 22.12 Ask the male consumer to bend over the examination table for the rectal exam.

Male genitourinary, reproductive, anus, rectum and prostate

Ask the male consumer to stand. Sit on a stool in front of the consumer. Have the consumer lift the gown to expose the genitalia.

1. Inspect the abdomen (contour, symmetry and skin pigmentation).
2. Palpate and percuss the bladder.
3. Inspect pubic hair distribution, penis, scrotum and urethral meatus.
4. Palpate the penis, urethral meatus and scrotum.
5. Palpate the inguinal area for hernias.

Ask the consumer to bend over the examination table (**Figure 22.12**). If the consumer is bedridden, the knee-chest or left lateral position may be used. Expose the buttocks. Stand behind the individual.

6. Inspect the perineum, sacrococcygeal area, and anal mucosa.
7. Palpate the anus and rectum (advanced practice).
8. Palpate the prostate (advanced practice).
9. If stool is on the glove, save it to test for occult blood (advanced practice).

Re-cover the individual's buttocks, offer tissues to wipe the rectal area. Ask the person to stand up and redress.

When completing the assessment, ensure that you leave the consumer comfortable and safe. For example, for the bedridden consumer, ensure that the side rails are up (if appropriate) and that the call bell is readily accessible.

Now that you have all of this information, what do you do with it and how do you make sense of it (**Figure 22.13**)? Refer back to Chapter 1, which discusses how to use clinical reasoning based on assessment data to formulate an action plan to address each identified concern.

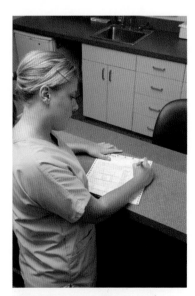

FIGURE 22.13 Be certain to carefully document all assessment findings and consumer responses.

LABORATORY AND DIAGNOSTIC DATA

Review any laboratory and diagnostic data such as X-ray reports, CT scans and blood pathology obtained and consider the significance of these results in your clinical reasoning. Remember that technology should not replace advanced listening skills, so ensure that you have heard and understood the consumer.

THE PROCESS OF PULLING IT TOGETHER

The health assessment, physical examination, and laboratory and diagnostic data provide the basis for your clinical reasoning and action planning. By using the APIE framework, the nurse is able to systematically collect data, identify actual and potential problems and issues, and plan and evaluate care. Using a structured framework enables you to identify similar signs, symptoms and findings that are then clustered together in a meaningful way (see Chapters 1–3 for detailed process).

TECHNOLOGY AND DOCUMENTATION

Technology is changing the way we work in the healthcare context. For example, in many areas computers are used at the bedside to document assessment findings and consumer care. Consumers provide health history, schedule appointments, obtain test results, and question their healthcare providers about treatment issues online. Technology can readily put the consumer in direct contact with a healthcare provider, but the privacy and legal issues are complex and still evolving. Regardless of the use of technology or paper-based documentation, the principles behind why, when and what to document remain the same regardless of *how* the consumer assessment, examination and care is recorded.

THE CONSUMER WITH UNSTABLE ANGINA

This case study illustrates the application and objective documentation of a comprehensive health and physical assessment. The setting is in an emergency department.

Catherine Windsor has presented with chest pain. She is subsequently diagnosed with unstable angina, an acute coronary syndrome (ACS).

HEALTH HISTORY

TODAY'S DATE	29 November 2022	
BIOGRAPHICAL DATA	**CONSUMER NAME**	Catherine Windsor
	DATE OF BIRTH	9 March 1954
	BIRTHPLACE	Adelaide, Australia
	OCCUPATION	Retired (was an early childhood teacher)
	EMERGENCY CONTACT	William Windsor (husband)
CONSUMER PROFILE	68-year-old married Caucasian female	
REASON FOR SEEKING HEALTH CARE	'I have been feeling a bit nauseous and short of breath for the last 3 days, and my back has been aching. I am feeling more tired than usual and not feeling I can undertake gardening anymore.'	
PRESENT HEALTH	Consumer states that she has had good health most of her life and continues to be fairly active. She attends a GP health check-up twice a year and also sees a dermatologist twice a year due to history of skin carcinoma. Consumer states she is concerned at feeling so tired, even though she has slowed down her activities in the past 3 weeks.	
PAST HEALTH HISTORY	**MEDICAL HISTORY**	Osteoarthritis Diabetes mellitus type II (diet controlled)
	SURGICAL HISTORY	Hysterectomy at age 45 Left total knee replacement at age 63

>>

>>

HEALTH HISTORY		
	ALLERGIES	Nil known to meds; denies allergies to foods, insect bites/bee stings, environmental/seasonal allergens
	MEDICATIONS	Paracetamol PRN Caltrate +D plus
	COMMUNICABLE DISEASES	Malaria from travel to East Timor
	INJURIES AND ACCIDENTS	Fractured right arm at age 37
	SPECIAL NEEDS	Nil requirements
	BLOOD TRANSFUSIONS	Denies any
	CHILDHOOD ILLNESSES	Recalls measles and mumps as a child
	IMMUNISATIONS	Has annual flu vaccination (had this 6 months ago)
FAMILY HEALTH HISTORY		Sister has had breast cancer. Parents both died in their 80s, mother and brother – cardiovascular disease.
SOCIAL HISTORY	**ALCOHOL USE**	Glass of sherry in the evening and one glass of wine with meals occasionally
	TOBACCO USE	Denies current use but was a smoker in late teens for about 5 years
	DRUG USE	Denies
	DOMESTIC AND INTIMATE PARTNER VIOLENCE	Denies any history
	SEXUAL PRACTICE	Monogamous relationship for 45 years
	TRAVEL HISTORY	Has travelled extensively with family on holidays.
	WORK ENVIRONMENT	Retired
	HOME ENVIRONMENT	Single-storey home, comfortable; has two cocker spaniel dogs
	HOBBIES AND LEISURE ACTIVITIES	Active, enjoys bushwalking, gardens extensively, goes to a female gym
	STRESS	States she has been stressed lately as worried about her son (38), who has just separated from his wife due to an extramarital affair, and about his young son's distress at the separation
	EDUCATION	Completed degree in social sciences
	ECONOMIC STATUS	'We're comfortable.'
	RELIGION	Church of England, is active participant in her parish church. Volunteers and helps when she can; does the flowers in the church for weddings etc.
	ETHNIC BACKGROUND	Caucasian
	ROLES AND RELATIONSHIPS	Husband is very supportive; she enjoys being a grandmother
	CHARACTERISTIC PATTERNS OF DAILY LIVING	Wakes at 6 a.m., takes the dogs for an early morning walk, breakfast, then gardening in their 1 acre garden (with husband). Most Sundays will go for a bushwalk with a group of friends, leaving at around 8 a.m. for a couple of hours. Attends the gym three times a week. 12.30 lunch. Usually has an afternoon nap at about 2 p.m. Saturday evenings attends church at 6 p.m. Dinner at 6.30 p.m. all other days. Bedtime is around 10 p.m.

HEALTH HISTORY		
HEALTH MAINTENANCE ACTIVITIES	**SLEEP**	Approximately 8 hours each night, but has been feeling very tired much of the day for past 3 weeks; has a nap most afternoons for 30 minutes
	DIET	Manages a strict diabetic diet, low sodium
	EXERCISE	Gym classes × 3 per week, bushwalk weekly, gardening
	STRESS MANAGEMENT	Her husband/friends very supportive. Sees her daughter weekly and talks things over with her. Feels that being active helps her cope with her everyday stresses
	USE OF SAFETY DEVICES	No special devices required; uses seat belt in car, has smoke alarms in house
	HEALTH CHECK-UPS	Sees GP twice per year (saw GP 6 weeks ago). Sees dermatologist twice a year
REVIEW OF SYSTEMS	**GENERAL**	'At the moment I feel I have no energy, I feel lousy … I am a mess!'
	SKIN	Denies rashes, itching, no changes in skin pigmentation, ecchymoses, skin texture, sores, lumps, odours, sweating, acne, denies sunbathing, uses sunscreen and wears a hat when outdoors
	HAIR	Nil issues
	NAILS	Denies changes in texture, splitting, breaking, onychomycosis
	EYES	Wears glasses; denies diplopia, eye pain, and halos around objects; had sight checked 2 months ago
	EARS	Denies discharge, vertigo, otalgia, tinnitus, hearing aid, hearing problems
	NOSE AND SINUSES	Denies epistaxis, no changes in sense of smell, allergies, sinusitis, admits to snoring
	MOUTH	States good oral hygiene, brushes teeth × 2 daily. Denies halitosis, toothache, tooth abscess, bleeding/swollen gums, difficulty chewing, no change in taste
	THROAT AND NECK	Denies hoarseness, dysphagia, goitre; no changes in voice
	BREASTS	Denies pain, tenderness, discharge, lumps, dimpling; had regular biannual mammograms up until 2 years ago (age 66)
	RESPIRATORY	Recent SOB over last 3 days, denies asthma or any respiratory health problems
	CARDIAC	Denies experiencing chest pain recently and does not have any at the moment. Denies orthopnoea, palpitations and heart murmur
	BLOOD VESSELS (PERIPHERAL VASCULATURE)	Denies feet/ankle oedema, cyanosis, syncope, cold or discoloured hands/feet, leg cramps, DVT, thrombophlebitis, varicose veins, intermittent claudication
	GASTROINTESTINAL	Regular bowel movements, denies GORD, abdominal pain
	MUSCULOSKELETAL	Back has ached over last 3 days, complains of tiredness and unable to maintain normal physical activities
	NEUROLOGICAL	Denies tremors, involuntary movements, no changes in consciousness
	PSYCHOLOGICAL	Denies depression, irritability, suicidal ideation; has occasional sleep disturbances
	URINARY	Denies incontinence or history of UTI
	FEMALE REPRODUCTIVE	Had last Pap smear 2 years ago; all Pap smears have been normal
	NUTRITION	As stated previously, maintains strict diabetic and low sodium diet; consumer complains of feeling nauseous, but has been able to maintain a light diet over last 3 days
	ENDOCRINE	Well-managed type II diabetes mellitus; denies exophthalmos, heat/cold intolerance
	LYMPH NODES	Denies enlargement, tenderness
	HAEMATOLOGICAL	History of malaria, no recurrences for 25 years; no history of anaemia, or bleeding disorders

HEALTH HISTORY

PHYSICAL EXAMINATION	GENERAL SURVEY AND VITAL SIGNS	> Facial pallor noted, otherwise a reasonably healthy looking 68-year-old Caucasian female > Pain assessment: denies any at present > HT: 165 cm > WT: 69 kg > T: 37°C > P: 88 BPM regular > R: 24 RPM > BP: 148/85 mmHg (arm sitting) > SpO_2 – 98% RA
	SKIN, HAIR AND NAILS	No lesions, rashes, ecchymoses, bleeding or diaphoresis, smooth texture, turgor normal; hair no infestations; patches of scattered seborrhoea; nail beds pink, firm with 1 sec capillary refill, no clubbing; old suture line on L knee
	HEAD	Normocephalic, no lesions, masses, depressions or tenderness; face symmetrical, no involuntary movement or swelling; scalp shiny and intact, no lesions or masses
	EYES	Acuity by Snellen chart with glasses: right eye: 6/12, left eye 6/12; has difficulty reading magazine; eyebrows full and symmetrical, eyelashes evenly distributed and no inflammation or lid lag; lacrimal apparatus, no inflammation or discharge; corneal light reflex symmetrical; no strabismus
	EARS	Gross hearing intact by whisper test; pinna, no masses, lesions, nodules, inflammation or tenderness; EAC clear, no inflammation
	NOSE AND SINUSES	No deformities, bleeding, lesions, masses, swelling; nares patent, nontender; septum midline, no perforation; mucosa pink; sinuses nontender, resonant
	MOUTH AND THROAT	No halitosis; lips pink, no swelling or lesions; gums and mucosa pink and moist; 30 teeth in good repair; tongue midline, well papillated, and no fasciculations, lesions, swelling or bleeding; hard and soft palates intact, no lesions or masses; pharynx erythematous; uvula midline and rises, no phonation; tonsils normal; gag reflex, normal
	NECK	Supple, no masses or spasms, neck symmetrical, no masses or tenderness or lymphadenopathy; trachea midline, thyroid nontender, no enlargement/mass/goitre, bruits, JVP, no elevation
	BREASTS	No thickening, oedema, vascularity, erosion, fissures, lesions, masses, retraction, discharge; areola and nipples dark in pigmentation; nonpalpable lymph nodes
	THORAX AND LUNGS	AP: transverse diameter = 1:2, chest wall symmetrical, no bulging of intercostal spaces or retractions, no use of accessory muscles, respirations regular, thoracic expansion 3 cm ant and 3 cm post, lungs resonant, diaphragmatic excursion 2 cm bilateral, clear breath sounds; no adventitious breath sounds
	HEART	Precordium: no pulsations/heaves/thrills, apical pulse 88 beats per minute, apical impulse 2 cm at 5th intercostal space, S_1 and S_2 present, no other abnormalities detected
	ABDOMEN	No dilated veins, scars, incisions; bowel sounds in 4 quads, no bruits, abdomen soft, no masses/tenderness to light/deep palpation; liver nontender
	BLOOD VESSELS	No pitting oedema in feet and ankles, no ulcerations, pulse regular and strong, no pulsus paradoxus, no bruits

	CAROTID	BRACHIAL	RADIAL	FEMORAL	POPLITEAL	DORSALIS PEDIS	POSTERIOR TIBIAL
R	2+	2+	2+	2+	2+	2+	2+
L	2+	2+	2+	2+	2+	2+	2+
SCALE: 0–4+							

>>

HEALTH HISTORY

	MUSCULOSKELETAL	Female sitting in chair, able to stand without any difficulty; mild kyphosis; gait is normal; joints, no erythema, swelling, bruising, nodules, masses, crepitus; arthritic change deformities noted in hands with ulnar drift, also bilateral hallux valgus; muscle strength equal bilaterally; no involuntary movement; ROM reduced in knees and hips (arthritis). No tenderness, lumps, redness or swelling in lower back where consumer complains of backache. Aching in right knee and previous break site in right arm
	NEUROLOGICAL	Mental status: consumer is alert and orientated; she is cognisant of her surroundings
	GENITALIA AND RECTUM	No abnormal bleeding, discharge, haemorrhoid or abnormal lesions noted

FURTHER DIAGNOSTIC DATA THAT HAS BEEN COLLECTED	LABORATORY DATA DIAGNOSTIC	(TODAY'S RESULTS)		
			CONSUMER'S VALUES	NORMAL VALUES
		Sodium	142 mmol/L	(135–145 mmol/L)
		Potassium	4.4 mmol/L	(3.5–4.5 (plasma) mmol/L)
		Chloride	105 mmol/L	(100–110 mmol/L)
		Bicarbonate (total CO_2)	28 mmol/L	(22–32 mmol/L)
		Anion gap	9 mmol/L	(4–13 mmol/L)
		Osmolality (calc)	291 mmol/L	(275–295 mmol/kg)
		Glucose (not fasting)	4.2 mmol/L	(3.0–7.8 mmol/L not fasting)
		Urea	6.8 mmol/L	(2.9–8.2 mmol/L age >60)
		Creatinine	69 mmol/L	(46–99 mmol/L female age 60–90)
		Protein (total)	69 g/L	(60–83 g/L)
		Albumin	40 g/L	(35–50 g/L)
		Globulin	35 g/L	(25–45 g/L)
		Bilirubin (total)	11 µmol/L	(<20 µmol/L)
		Alkaline phosphatase	73 µ/L	(53–141 µ/L female age >60)
		Total cholesterol	8.4 mmol/L	(<4 mmol/L)
		Calcium (total)	2.19 mmol/L	(2.15–2.55 mmol/L)
		Phosphate	0.86 mmol/L	(0.81–1.45 mmol/L)
		Urate	0.36 mmol/L	(0.15–0.50 mmol/L)
		Troponin I	0.6 n/mL	(0–0.9 n/mL)
		CXR – Lungs clear, no cardiomegaly		
		ECG – Sinus rhythm, nil abnormalities noted		

EVALUATION AND CLINICAL REASONING FOR CASE STUDY

The assessment and clinical decisions you make should reflect your scope of practice. For example, advanced practice health professionals, such as nurse practitioners and remote area nurses with endorsement, may be able to make diagnostic decisions and prescribe medications without referring to a medical officer.

Fundamentally, all health professionals collect, evaluate and act on consumer-focused health information, which will at times include referral to, or collaboration with, other healthcare team members. Nurses assess consumer responses to interventions and determine when to escalate key changes in a consumer's condition. The clinical reasoning cycle provides health professionals with a framework to consider all this information in a meaningful way for planning consumer care. These phases are stepped out below, and draw on information presented and collected during the health history and physical examination. We then work through the cycle components that are relevant to this case study (cycle components are bolded).

For Catherine Windsor, the 68-year-old woman who has presented with a history of chest pain, the significant data that needs to be considered includes the following.

Collecting cues/information

Recall and Review: In the first instance you will need to reflect on the assessment data collected thus far and Catherine's presenting symptoms, and how these relate to her subsequent diagnosis of unstable angina, an acute coronary syndrome (ACS). ACS is a range of acute myocardial ischaemic states, encompassing unstable angina, non-ST segment elevation myocardial infarction (NSTACS – ST segment elevation generally absent on ECG), and ST segment elevation infarction (STACS – persistent ST segment elevation usually present on ECG). Angina itself is chest discomfort caused by poor blood flow through the coronary vessels of the myocardium. In unstable angina, symptoms occur in a more random and unpredictable fashion; it is 'unstable' because, as with all forms of ACS, it is most often caused by the actual rupture of a plaque in a coronary artery. Consumers presenting as typical presentations describe the chest discomfort as pressure-like chest pain that may radiate to the jaw or shoulder. However, cardiac symptoms can be quite different in women and men, especially for those with diabetes mellitus, and this difference can present a hazard to women and diabetic consumers. Women with angina will often report a hot or burning sensation, or even tenderness to touch; this may be located in the back, shoulders, arms or jaw. Shortness of breath, nausea and fatigue may also be apparent. Often, they have no actual chest discomfort at all, as is the situation with Catherine in this case scenario. Catherine's immediate care would be dealing with any discomforts, ruling out any heart damage, investigating history of malaria for recurrence, then follow up with other investigations.

Chief complaint and history of present illness
> 'Feeling nauseous, and short of breath over past 3 days'
> Complains of back aching, and being more tired, not being able to do normal activities
> Report of some stress – related to son's recent marriage breakdown

Processing information

Interpret: These symptoms and details outline the scope of the issue for this consumer and how it will now affect her present deviation from normal health.

Family health history
> History of mother and brother with heart disease

Relate and Match: There is an increased risk of developing heart disease if there is a family member, specifically a parent, with a history of heart disease.

Social history
> Stress, lately worried about son (38) who has just separated from his wife

Discriminate and Relate: This is noteworthy as uncontrolled stress is known risk factor for coronary heart disease.

Review of the systems
> General – feeling she 'has no energy … I am a mess'
> Shortness of breath over past 3 days
> Musculoskeletal – backache over past 3 days, unable to do normal activities
> Nutrition – feeling nauseous – only eating a light diet

Relate, Infer and Discriminate: As women with angina usually do not present with 'typical' symptoms of an ACS and often present late (with atypical symptoms), an awareness of these subjective symptoms needs to be acknowledged as possibly cardiac related, and investigated further.

Physical assessment/further diagnostic data
> B/P 148/85 mmHg
> ECG – NAD
> CXR – Clear
> Laboratory data
> Cholesterol & Troponin I

Interpret and Discriminate: The significance of these findings indicates that Catherine's cholesterol levels are elevated, and this is also a known risk factor for coronary artery disease.

Putting it all together – synthesise information

To gain a definitive diagnosis for unstable angina, the doctor would request further investigations, specifically, a series of biochemical analysis of serum troponin levels, and RDT (rapid diagnostic test) for malaria detection. If the results are negative, then an exercise stress test and possibly a coronary angiogram would be undertaken. This is undertaken to investigate the location of atherosclerosis lesions in the coronary arteries. The role of the nurse in this case is to continue close observation for any deviations from normal, to ensure that if Catherine has another episode of angina, interventions can be implemented immediately. Continuous primary survey – ABCDE (see Chapter 8) and Glasgow Coma Scale (GCS) would need to be done.

Actions based on assessment findings

The nurse should also provide support and additional information/education for interventions that do not require a doctor's order.

The nurse should consider the following:

1 Medication: Catherine is likely to be prescribed an anti-angina medication, such as nitroglycerine (spray or sublingual tablets), to use when she experiences these 'cardiac-related' symptoms. She will need to be educated on how to use this medication (use as soon as she feels symptoms, sit quietly for 10 minutes after use; if symptoms persist seek medical assistance).

2 Medication: Catherine most likely will be commenced on statin medications to assist in reducing her cholesterol levels. Education on the importance of this medication to aid in compliance will need to be given.

3 Risk factor modification education: In particular, diet, stress reduction, exercise, and continued close monitoring of her diabetes mellitus will need to be discussed.

4 Catherine may require a referral for a stress management course, especially since she has had increased stress of late, due to her son's recent marriage breakdown.

5 Catherine will need to be referred back to her general practitioner for follow-up and management, but also to organise an emergency chest pain management plan. Discuss with consumer and other family members about pain and discomfort management (signs and symptoms) and what to do when it occurs (i.e. do not wait if pain persists, call an ambulance; ensure other family members are aware of the plan and provide resources).

The final step in the process is accurate documentation as displayed above. The nurse must document findings, referrals, interventions, and advice and education given. The consumer would then be reassessed following definitive diagnosis and medical interventions.

THE CONSUMER WITH A COLLES FRACTURE

This case study illustrates the application and objective documentation of a focused musculoskeletal assessment.

David Attenborough is a 16-year-old teenager who had a fall off his skateboard and has presented to the emergency department with pain in his L wrist; he is accompanied by his guardian.

HEALTH HISTORY

TODAY'S DATE	29 November 2022	
CONSUMER PROFILE	16-year-old, male	
CHIEF COMPLAINT	'My wrist hurts, I cannot move it and it is all swollen.'	
HISTORY OF PRESENT ILLNESS	Consumer reports that he was skateboarding with his friends when he fell off. To break his fall, he said he put both arms out, landing mainly on his left hand. He felt something crack.	
PAST HEALTH HISTORY	**MEDICAL HISTORY**	Denies any history of any health issues
	SURGICAL HISTORY	Nil
	ALLERGIES	Nil known
	MEDICATIONS	Does not take any medication
	INJURIES AND ACCIDENTS	No other accidents or injuries
SOCIAL HISTORY	**HOME ENVIRONMENT**	Lives at his boarding school, returns home to his family's cattle station in the Northern Territory during school holidays
	RELIGION	Says nil
	ETHNIC BACKGROUND	English descent
HEALTH MAINTENANCE ACTIVITIES	**SLEEP**	Sleeps approximately 8 hours per night
	DIET	'Boarding school food is horrible.'
	EXERCISE	Plays rugby and is a member of the state quidditch team
	USE OF SAFETY DEVICES	Does not use a helmet, wrist guards or knee pads when he rides his skateboard or plays quidditch

>>

>>

HEALTH HISTORY		
FOCUSED PHYSICAL ASSESSMENT (MUSCULOSKELETAL – KEY CONSUMER SYMPTOM IDENTIFICATION)	L ARM	L arm: elbow, upper arm and shoulder, nil tenderness or pain, normal movement
	L WRIST	L wrist: swollen, with some bruising on the thumb side of the wrist. Painful when attempting to move wrist. Deformity of the arm just above the wrist (increased angulation); skin intact
FOCUSED NEUROVASCULAR ASSESSMENT	PAIN	R arm: nil pain L arm: Consumer states that he has a considerable amount of pain in his left wrist area, rating it 8/10. Some relief is gained from holding it in position, with hand up on chest
	COLOUR	R arm: pink L arm: very swollen with ecchymosis on the thumb side, nail beds pink
	TEMPERATURE	R arm: warm to touch L arm: warm to touch
	PULSES	R arm: radial and ulnar pulses – rate and volume normal L arm: due to swelling difficult to feel radial pulse, ulnar pulse – rate and volume normal. Capillary refill <2 seconds
	SENSATION	R arm: no numbness, tingling and has sensation in each digit L arm: denies numbness, tingling: has sensation in each digit
	MOTOR FUNCTION	R arm: normal ROM L arm: some reduction in range of moment (pain and swelling), able to flex and extend each digit
	DIAGNOSTIC DATA	X-ray: Distal radius fracture; a Colles fracture that is extra-articular, uncomplicated and stable

EVALUATION AND CLINICAL REASONING FOR CASE STUDY

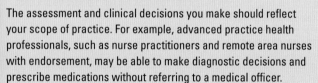

The assessment and clinical decisions you make should reflect your scope of practice. For example, advanced practice health professionals, such as nurse practitioners and remote area nurses with endorsement, may be able to make diagnostic decisions and prescribe medications without referring to a medical officer.

Fundamentally, all health professionals collect, evaluate and act on consumer-focused health information, which will at times include referral to, or collaboration with, other healthcare team members. Nurses assess consumer responses to interventions and determine when to escalate key changes in a consumer's condition. The clinical reasoning cycle provides health professionals with a framework to consider all this information in a meaningful way for planning consumer care. These phases are stepped out below, and draw on information presented and collected during the health history and physical examination. We then work through the cycle components that are relevant to this case study (cycle components are bolded).

For David Attenborough, the 16-year-old male who has presented to the emergency department following a fall off his skateboard, the significant data that needs to be considered includes the following.

Collecting cues/information

Recall and Review: In the first instance you will need to reflect on what you know about musculoskeletal systems, in particular, skeletal fractures. From the assessment data, David has a distal Colles fracture of his L wrist. Now you will need to consider what you know about Colles fractures. Fractures are classified by **type**; for example, compound (when broken bone protrudes through skin) or simple (closed); and **location**. In David's case, the Colles fracture is distal to the shaft of the radius. This injury commonly occurs when a person attempts to break a fall by throwing their hands and arms out in front of them. The hands take the weight of the body, causing the radius and ulna to buckle or break. Neurovascular assessment is integral when assessing these types of injuries to detect early signs of possible nerve or circulation problems and possible onset of compartment syndrome. An X-ray will be required to provide definitive diagnosis by a medical officer and then treatment will be based on this. Closed Colles fractures that are not displaced are usually treated with a short-arm cast or splint, if the fracture is stable. Closed fractures with fragments out of position will require reduction, either closed with local or regional anaesthesia, or during surgery (open reduction).

Chief complaint and history of present illness
> Fell from skateboard, breaking fall with his left hand
> 'My wrist hurts, I cannot move it and it is all swollen.'

Processing Information

Interpret: These symptoms and details outline the scope of the issue for this consumer and how it will now affect his present deviation from normal health.

Health maintenance activities
> Use of safety devices: David does not use a helmet, wrist guards or knee pads while riding his skateboard or playing quidditch.

Infer and Predict: The significance of these findings indicates that David and his guardian will need some health education in relation to using safety equipment to prevent injuries when using his skateboard.

Focused physical assessment (musculoskeletal – key consumer symptom identification)
> L wrist is swollen, with some bruising on the thumb side of the wrist. Painful when attempting to move wrist. Deformity of the arm just above the wrist (increased angulation). Skin intact.

Interpret and Infer: This objective data, with the history of a fall, strongly indicates that David has a possible Colles fracture.

Focused neurovascular assessment
> L arm: Consumer states that he has a considerable amount of pain in his left wrist area, rating it 8/10. Some relief is gained from holding it in position, with hand up on chest.
> All other neurovascular assessment data at this stage indicates that there are no signs of possible nerve or circulation problems or compartment syndrome.

Interpret, Infer and Predict: The significance of these findings is the pain that David has in his left wrist, further indicating a probable Colles fracture. His pain will need to be addressed as soon as possible.

Diagnostic data
> X-ray

Interpret: Provides a definitive diagnosis of a Colles fracture.

Putting it all together – synthesise information

The role of the nurse in this case is primarily education and monitoring David closely until a plaster cast is placed on his L wrist.

Actions based on assessment findings

The nurse should provide additional information/education for interventions that do not require a doctor's order. The nurse should consider the following:

1 Neurovascular assessment: Regularly undertaken to detect nerve or circulation problems or compartment syndrome.
2 Pain assessment and management: Alleviating discomfort is a paramount intervention for trauma cases. The nurse should administer prescribed medication as ordered, and evaluate using pain assessment scales. Pain management will not always require pharmacological intervention alone, as position, casting/splinting and application of ice to the swelling will also assist in decreasing pain, and reducing further tissue trauma.
3 Immobilise and support the L wrist: This will prevent further damage and assist in reducing pain.
4 Provide education/information to David, his guardian and his school nurse in relation to cast care, pain management and follow-up appointments.
5 Education for safety: For both David and the school, provide information/pamphlets and stress the importance of using safety devices (helmet/wrist guards/knee pads), to reduce the risk of further injuries when riding his skateboard and playing quidditch.

The final step in the process is accurate documentation as shown above. The nurse must document findings, referrals, interventions, and advice and education given. The consumer would continue to be assessed following the application of the cast, until discharge.

CONCLUSION

Nurses see consumers across many health settings and at different development stages. Consumers will require different levels of assessment, care, teaching and support. As care is planned on the basis of consumer assessment, all nurses should possess expert clinical assessment skills. This textbook has provided the information to assist the beginner to advanced clinician in acquiring, refining and applying health history and physical examination skills. The type of health assessment required is dependent on the individual's situation and healthcare context, as well as the nurse's scope of practice. The process to guide decision making about which approach to employ for individual consumers (comprehensive versus focused assessment) has been presented and applied to case studies. The use of a structured approach in considering consumer needs, environment and other impacting factors, when undertaking health assessment and physical examination, centres on the APIE framework. The clinical reasoning process is used to organise and interpret data generated from the health assessment and physical examination to guide care planning.

CHAPTER RESOURCES

CS CLINICAL **SKILLS**

The following Clinical Skills are relevant to this chapter and can be found in Tollefson & Hillman, *Clinical Psychomotor Skills,* 8th edition:

> 5 Hand hygiene
> 6 Personal protective equipment
> 10 Temperature, pulse and respiration measurement
> 11 Blood pressure measurement
> 12 Monitoring pulse oximetry
> 13 Pain assessment
> 14 Blood glucose measurement
> 15 Physical assessment
> 16 Mental status assessment
> 17 Focused cardiovascular health history and physical assessment
> 18 12-lead electrocardiogram
> 19 Focused respiratory health history assessment and physical assessment
> 20 Focused neurological health history and physical assessment
> 21 Neurovascular observations
> 22 Focused gastrointestinal health history and abdominal physical assessment
> 23 Height, weight and waist circumference measurement
> 24 Focused musculoskeletal health history and physical assessment and range of motion exercises
> 27 Healthcare teaching
> 75 Non-pharmacological pain management interventions – therapeutic massage
> 76 Non-pharmacological pain management interventions – conventional transcutaneous electrical nerve stimulation.

FURTHER RESOURCES

> Australian Chronic Disease Prevention Alliance: https://www.cvdcheck.org.au/
> Centers for Disease Control and Prevention: http://www.cdc.gov
> HealthyPeople 2020: http://www.healthypeople.gov
> Heart Foundation: http://www.heartfoundation.org.au

> National Heart Foundation of Australia, Heart Attack Action Plan: http://www.heartattackfacts.org.au/Action-plan.aspx
> Nursing and Midwifery Board of Australia: http://www.nursingmidwiferyboard.gov.au/
> Nursing Council of New Zealand: http://www.nursingcouncil.org.nz/

APPENDIX: FUNCTIONAL ASSESSMENTS

INSTRUMENTAL ACTIVITIES OF DAILY LIVING (IADL) AND PHYSICAL SELF-MAINTENANCE ACTIVITIES

I **Instrumental activities of daily living (IADL)**

  A **Ability to use telephone**
1. Operates telephone independently – looks up and dials numbers
2. Dials a few well-known numbers
3. Answers phone but does not dial or use touch tone
4. Does not use telephone at all

  B **Housekeeping**
1. Maintains house independently or with occasional assistance for 'heavy work'
2. Performs light tasks such as bedmaking and dishwashing
3. Performs light daily tasks but cannot maintain adequate level of cleanliness
4. Needs assistance with all home maintenance tasks
5. Does not participate in any tasks

  C **Laundry**
1. Does personal laundry completely
2. Launders small items such as socks and stockings
3. All laundry must be done by others

  D **Mode of transportation**
1. Independently drives own car or uses public transportation
2. Arranges own travel via taxi or special transportation services, but does not use public transportation and does not drive
3. Travels on public transportation when assisted or with others
4. Travel limited to taxi or special transportation services with assistance
5. Does not travel at all

  E **Responsibility for medications**
1. Takes medication in correct dosages at correct time independently
2. Takes medication if medication is prepared in advance in separate doses
3. Not capable of dispensing own medications

  F **Ability to handle finances**
1. Independently manages finances – pays bills, keeps track of income
2. Manages own finances with assistance
3. Not capable of managing own finances

  G **Shopping**
1. Does all of the shopping independently
2. Shops for small purchases independently
3. Not able to go shopping without assistance
4. Unable to shop for any purchase

  H **Food preparation**
1. Able to prepare and serve food without assistance
2. Prepares adequate meals if supplied with food
3. Able to heat and serve prepared meals
4. Unable to prepare and serve meals

II **Physical self-maintenance activities**
A **Feeding**
1 Eats without assistance
2 Eats with minor assistance at meal times and helps in cleaning up
3 Feeds self with moderate assistance
4 Requires extensive assistance – all meals
5 Does not feed self at all and resists efforts of others to feed him or her
B **Toilet**
1 Cares for self completely, no incontinence
2 Needs to be reminded or needs help in cleaning self
3 Soils the bed while asleep – more than once a week
4 Soils clothing while awake – more than once a week
5 No control of bladder or bowel
C **Grooming (hair, nails, hands, face)**
1 Able to care for self
2 Occasional minor assistance needed (e.g. with shaving)
3 Moderate and regular assistance needed
4 Needs total grooming care, but accepts some
5 Actively negates efforts of others to maintain grooming
D **Bathing**
1 Bathes self without help
2 Bathes self with help into and out of bath or shower
3 Can wash face and hands only
4 Does not wash self but is cooperative
5 Does not try to wash self and resists efforts of others to help
E **Dressing**
1 Dresses, undresses, and selects clothes from wardrobe
2 Dresses and undresses with minor assistance
3 Needs moderate assistance in dressing or selection of clothes
4 Needs major assistance
5 Completely unable to dress self and resists efforts of others to help
F **Ambulation**
1 Ambulates about grounds or city without assistance
2 Ambulates within residence or nearby
3 Ambulates with assistance of:
    a another person
    b a railing
    c cane
    d walker
    e wheelchair
4 Sits unsupported in chair or wheelchair but cannot propel self
5 Bedridden more than half the time

ADAPTED FROM: *ASSESSMENT OF OLDER PEOPLE: SELF-MAINTAINING AND INSTRUMENTAL ACTIVITIES OF DAILY LIVING* BY M. LAWTON AND E. BRODY, 1969, *THE GERONTOLOGIST, 9,* PP. 179–86.

ANSWERS TO REVIEW QUESTIONS

CHAPTER 2
1(b) 2(c) 3(a, b, e, f) 4(c) 5(d) 6(d) 7(b) 8(b)
9(d) 10(a)

CHAPTER 3
1(a) 2(d) 3(c) 4(d) 5(a, b, c, d, f) 6(b) 7(c)
8(a, c, d, e, f) 9(b, c, e) 10(d)

CHAPTER 4
As these are reflective questions, there are no
set answers to these questions.

CHAPTER 5
1(a, c, d, e, f) 2(a) 3(c) 4(c) 5(a, b, c, e) 6(a) 7(d)
8(d) 9(c) 10(c)

CHAPTER 6
1(c) 2(d) 3(d) 4(a) 5(b) 6(d) 7(b) 8(a) 9(c) 10(d)
11(d) 12(b)

CHAPTER 7
1(a, c, d, f) 2(a) 3(b, c, d, f) 4(c) 5(a) 6(a, b, d, f)
7(c) 8(a) 9(c) 10(b, d, e) 11(b) 12(a, c, e)

CHAPTER 8
1(a, c, d, f) 2(b, c, d) 3(a) 4(c) 5(c, e, f) 6(c) 7(d)
8(c) 9(b) 10(a)

CHAPTER 9
1(a, c) 2(d) 3(e, f) 4(d) 5(c) 6(a) 7(d) 8(b) 9(a) 10(b)

CHAPTER 10
1(d) 2(a, b, d, f) 3(c) 4(b) 5(a, b, e) 6(b) 7(a)
8(a, b, c) 9(a)

CHAPTER 11
1(a) 2(b) 3(d) 4(b) 5(b, c, e, f) 6(c) 7(b) 8(b)
9(c) 10(a)

CHAPTER 12
1(c) 2(a) 3(c) 4(b) 5(d) 6(a) 7(a, b, d) 8(c) 9(b) 10(b)

CHAPTER 13
1(c, d, f) 2(c) 3(d) 4(b) 5(c) 6(a) 7(d) 8(c) 9(c) 10(a)

CHAPTER 14
1(d) 2(d) 3(d) 4(a) 5(b) 6(d) 7(b) 8(c) 9(b) 10(c)

CHAPTER 15
1 (a, b, f) 2(c) 3(d) 4(c) 5(b, d, f) 6(d) 7(a) 8(b)
9(b) 10(b)

CHAPTER 16
1(c) 2(d) 3(b) 4(d) 5(c) 6(a) 7(d) 8(b) 9(a) 10(b)

CHAPTER 17
1(c) 2(c) 3(d) 4(a, b, d) 5(b) 6(c) 7(a) 8(c) 9(a) 10(d)
11(b) 12(a) 13(c)

CHAPTER 18
1(b, f) 2(c) 3(c) 4(a, b, c) 5(a) 6(a) 7(a) 8(c) 9(c) 10(a)

CHAPTER 19
1(d) 2(a, b, d) 3(d) 4(c) 5(d) 6(a) 7(a) 8(b) 9(d) 10(c)

CHAPTER 20
1(b) 2(c) 3(c) 4(b) 5(b) 6(d) 7(d) 8(b) 9(d) 10(a)

CHAPTER 21
1(d) 2(d) 3(b) 4(a, b, e, f) 5(a, b, c) 6(b, c, e)
7(a, c, d, f) 8(b) 9(d) 10(c)

GLOSSARY

A

Aboriginal and Torres Strait Islander peoples the diverse cultures, languages and nations of the First Peoples of this land we know as Australia

abruptio placenta separation of the placenta from the uterine wall, which may cause significant internal (and perhaps external) bleeding, pain and fetal compromise

accommodation visual focusing from a far to a near point as pupils constrict and eyes converge

acini *See* **alveoli (of the breast)**

acknowledgement of Country an opportunity to introduce yourself and show your respect for Country and the waters that you are on, and pay respects to Traditional Custodians of the peoples who have a continuing connection to Country and have had so for over 60 000 years

acrocyanosis normal phenomenon in light-skinned newborns whereby the hands and feet are blue and the rest of the body is pink

acromegaly abnormal enlargement of the skull, bony facial structures, and bones of the extremities, caused by excessive secretion of growth hormone

action response attempt to stimulate consumers to make some change in their thinking and behaviour

active listening act of perceiving what is said both verbally and nonverbally

adnexa fallopian tubes, ovaries and their supporting ligaments

adventitious breath sound added breath sound that is superimposed on normal breath sounds

afterload initial resistance that the ventricles must overcome in order to open the semilunar valves to propel the blood into both the systemic and the pulmonary circulation

age-related macular degeneration (ARMD) a degenerative eye condition caused by changes to the macular region of the retina; results in loss of central vision

ages and stages developmental theory belief that individuals experience much the same sequential physical, cognitive, socioemotional and moral changes during the same age periods, each of which is termed a developmental stage

ageusia loss of the sense of taste

aggravating factors events that worsen the severity of the consumer's chief complaint

agnosia inability to recognise the form and nature of objects or persons

agonal respirations irregularly irregular respirations that signal impending death

agraphia loss of the ability to write

air trapping abnormal respiratory pattern with rapid, shallow respirations and forced expirations; the lungs have insufficient time to fully exhale and air becomes trapped, leading to overexpansion of the lungs

albinism a generalised whiteness of the skin, hair and eyebrows, which is caused by a congenital inability to form melanin

albumin substance that transports nutrients, blood and hormones and helps maintain osmotic pressure

alexia loss of the ability to grasp the meaning of written words and sentences; also known as word blindness

alleviating factors events that decrease the severity of the consumer's chief complaint

alogia inability to express oneself through speech

alopecia partial or complete loss of hair

alveoli (of the breast) milk-producing glands located in the lobules; also called acini

alveoli (of the lung) smallest functional unit of the respiratory system; where gas exchange occurs

amblyopia permanent loss of visual acuity resulting from certain uncorrected medical conditions

amenorrhoea absence of menses

anaemia decreased number of red blood cells

anaesthesia absence of touch sensation

anal canal terminal 3 to 4 cm of the large intestine

anal columns longitudinal folds of mucosa in the superior portion of the anal canal

anal fissure linear tear in the epidermis of the anal canal

anal (or faecal) incontinence involuntary release of rectal contents

anal orifice exit to the gastrointestinal tract; located at the seam of the gluteal folds

anal sinuses pockets in the anal canal that lie superior to the anal valves; they secrete mucus when compressed by faeces

anal valves folds in the anal canal that are formed by joining anal columns

aneroid manometer blood pressure measurement equipment with a calibrated dial and indicator that points to numbers representing blood pressure

angina myocardial ischaemia that manifests as chest, neck or arm pain

angle of Louis (manubriosternal junction or sternal angle) junction of the manubrium and the sternum

anisocoria difference in pupil sizes

anoderm epithelial tissue that lies in the lower 2 cm of the anal canal

anorectal abscess undrained collection of perianal pus of the tissue spaces in and adjacent to the anorectum

anorectal fistula hollow, fibrous tract lined by granulation tissue and filled with purulent or serosanguineous discharge; it has an opening inside the anal canal or rectum, and one or more orifices in the perianal skin

anorectum area where the anal canal fuses with the rectum

anosmia loss of the sense of smell

anterior axillary line vertical line drawn from the origin of the anterior axillary fold along the anterolateral aspect of the thorax

anterior chamber space anterior to the pupil and iris

anterior triangle area of the neck formed by the mandible, the trachea and the sternocleidomastoid muscle; contains the anterior cervical lymph nodes, the trachea and the thyroid gland

anthropometric measurements measurements of the human body, including height, weight and body proportions

anticipatory guidance approach covering health promotion and education; designed to inform at-risk individuals of physical, cognitive, psychological and social changes that occur and what their nutritional needs are

antigen skin testing test of immune function

apex (of the heart) lower portion of the heart

apex (of the lung) top of the lung

Apgar score a system for evaluating the newborn at 1 and 5 minutes of age, giving 0–2 points for each of heart rate, respiratory effort, muscle tone, reflex irritability, and colour

aphasia impairment or absence of language function

aphonia total loss of voice

apneustic respirations prolonged gasping in inspiration followed by a very short, inefficient pause that can last 30 to 60 seconds

apnoea lack of spontaneous respirations for 10 or more seconds

apocrine glands sweat glands that are associated with hair follicles

appendicular skeleton peripheral skeleton including the limbs, pelvis, scapula and clavicle

apraxia inability to convert intended speech into the motor act of speech; inability to perform purposeful acts or to manipulate objects

arcus senilis hazy, grey ring about 2 mm in size and located just inside the limbus; most commonly found in older individuals

areola pigmented area approximately 2.5 to 10 cm in diameter that surrounds the nipple

arrector pili muscle muscle that causes contraction of the skin and hair, resulting in 'goose bumps'

arrhythmia irregular heart rhythm; also known as dysrhythmia

ascites excess accumulation of fluid in the abdominal cavity

aspiration may mean a procedure in which a doctor draws fluid out of an area that should not have fluid, or when a person inhales fluid or an object into their lungs (i.e. aspirate stomach contents into lungs)

assessment first step of the nursing process; the orderly collection of objective and subjective data on the consumer's health status

associated manifestations signs and symptoms that accompany a consumer's chief complaint

asystole absence of cardiac activity, flat line on ECG

ataxic respirations *See* Biot's respirations

atheist person who believes that God does not exist

atherosclerosis development of lipid plaques along the coronary arteries

atlas first cervical vertebra

atrial kick final phase of ventricular diastole, when the atria contract to complete the final 20–30% of ventricular filling

atrioventricular (A-V) node one of the heart's pacemakers that delays the impulse from the atria before it goes to the ventricles; inherent rate is 40 to 60 beats per minute

atrioventricular (A-V) valves valves that prevent blood from entering the ventricles until diastole and prevent retrograde blood flow during systole; composed of the tricuspid and mitral valves

atrophy reduction in muscle size

augmentation mammoplasty surgical breast augmentation

auricle external flap of the ear; also called the pinna

auscultation process of active listening to sounds within the body to gather information on a consumer's health status

auscultatory gap a silent interval that may be heard between the systolic and diastolic blood pressures that can occur in hypertensive consumers; this can lead to a falsely elevated high diastolic or falsely low systolic blood pressure measurement

avolition lack of motivation for work or other goal-directed activity

axial skeleton central skeleton, including the facial bones, skull, auditory ossicles, hyoid bone, ribs, sternum and vertebrae

axillary nodes nodes composed of four groups: brachial (lateral), central axillary (mid axillary), pectoral (anterior), subscapular (posterior)

axis second cervical vertebra

B

balanitis inflammation of the glans penis

baroreceptors receptors located in the walls of most of the great arteries that sense hypotension and initiate reflex vasoconstriction and tachycardia to bring the blood pressure back to normal

barrel chest abnormal thorax configuration in which the ratio of the anteroposterior diameter to the transverse diameter of the chest is approximately 1:1

Bartholin's glands (greater vestibular glands) located in the cleft between the labia minora and the hymenal ring; these glands secrete a clear, viscid, odourless, alkaline mucus that improves the viability and motility of sperm along the female reproductive tract

basal metabolic rate (BMR) the amount of kJ burned at rest – basically the amount of energy needed by the body to maintain itself

base (of the heart) uppermost portion of the heart

base (of the lung) bottom of the lung

Bell's palsy idiopathic facial palsy of CN VII resulting in asymmetry of the palpebral fissures, nasolabial folds, mouth, and facial expression on the affected side

Biot's (or ataxic) respirations irregularly irregular respiratory pattern caused by damage to the medulla

blepharitis inflamed, scaly, red-rimmed eyelids, sometimes with loss of the eyelashes

blood pressure vital sign collected to assess cardiac output and vascular resistance; it measures the force exerted by the flow of blood pumped into the large arteries

body mass index (BMI) measurement that indicates body composition based on a person's height and weight; an increased BMI indicates obesity and a decreased BMI indicates possible malnutrition

borborygmi loud, audible, gurgling bowel sounds

Bouchard's node bony enlargement of the proximal interphalangeal joint of the finger

bradycardia pulse rate under 60 beats per minute in a resting adult

bradypnoea respiratory rate under 12 breaths per minute in a resting adult

Braxton Hicks contractions a pattern of intermittent, painless uterine contractions that occurs more frequently at the end of pregnancy (every 10–20 minutes or even more frequently); these are not true labour pains

breasts pair of mammary glands located on the anterior chest wall and extending vertically from the second to the sixth rib and laterally from the sternal border to the axillae

bregma junction of the coronal and sagittal sutures

bronchial (or tubular) breath sound breath sound that is high in pitch and loud in intensity and that is heard best over the trachea; has a blowing or hollow quality; heard longer in expiration than inspiration

bronchophony voice sound where the consumer says the words 'ninety-nine' or 'one, two, three' to determine if the lung is filled with air, fluid or a solid

bronchovesicular breath sound breath sound that is moderate in pitch and intensity and that is heard best between the scapula and the first and second intercostal spaces lateral to the sternum; its quality is a combination of bronchial and vesicular breath sounds; heard equally in inspiration and expiration

bruit blowing sound that can be auscultated when the blood flow becomes turbulent because blood is rushing past an obstruction

Brushfield's spots small, white flecks located around the perimeter of the iris, associated with Down syndrome

bulbar conjunctiva covering of the anterior surface of the sclera

bulbourethral glands pea-sized glands located below the prostate; secretions are emptied from here at the time of ejaculation

bursae sacs filled with fluids

C

cachexia extreme malnutrition in which the consumer exhibits wasting

callus thickening of the skin due to prolonged pressure

canthus nasal or temporal angle where the eyelids meet

caput medusae venous pattern of congested veins around the umbilicus; attributed to obstruction of the portal vein and seen in liver dysfunction

caput succedaneum swelling over the occipitoparietal region of the skull that occurs during delivery of the newborn

carbohydrate major source of energy for various functions of the body; supplies fibre and assists in the utilisation of fat

cardiomegaly enlargement of the heart

carpal tunnel syndrome pressure on the median nerve at the carpal tunnel of the wrist, causing numbness, tingling, weakness and pain

caruncle round, red structure in the inner canthus; contains sebaceous glands

cataract opacity in the lens of the eye that gives the pupil a pearly grey appearance

cephalocaudal head-to-toe approach

cephalohaematoma localised subcutaneous swelling over one cranial bone that occurs during delivery of the newborn

cerebrospinal fluid (CSF) a clear, watery fluid that fills the space between the arachnoid mater and the pia mater

cerumen waxlike substance produced in the ear canal

cervix inferior aspect of the uterus

Chadwick's sign a blue, soft cervix, normally during pregnancy

chalazion chronic inflammation of the meibomian gland in the upper or lower eyelid

chancre reddish, round ulcer or small papular lesion with a depressed centre and raised, indurated edges

chancroid tender, ulcerated, exudative, papular lesion with an erythematous halo, surrounding oedema, and a friable base

characteristic patterns of daily living consumer's normal daily routines; includes meals, work and sleeping schedules and patterns of social interactions

cherry angioma bright red, circumscribed area that may be flat or raised and that darkens with age

Cheyne-Stokes respirations crescendo or decrescendo respiratory pattern interspersed between periods of apnoea

chief complaint symptom or problem that causes the consumer to seek health care

cholelithiasis presence or formation of bile stone or calculi in the gallbladder or duct

cholestasis arrest of bile excretion

cholesterol lipid found only in animal products; it is transported in the body by high-density lipoproteins (HDLs) and low-density lipoproteins (LDLs)

choroid vascular tissue of the posterior uveal tract lining the inner surface of the globe of the eye, beneath the retina; provides nutrition to the retina and helps absorb excess light

ciliary body extension of the uveal tract that produces aqueous humour

circadian rhythm normal fluctuation of body temperature, pulse and blood pressure during a 24-hour period

click extrasystolic heart sound that is high-pitched and can radiate in the chest wall

clinical pathways pathways or maps show the outcome of predetermined consumer goals over a period of time; that is, they state what activity the consumer should be capable of performing daily, on the basis of the consumer's diagnostic-related grouping (DRG)

clinical reasoning a disciplined, creative and reflective thinking used with critical thinking to establish potential strategies for consumers to reach their health goals

clinical yarning foregrounds First Nations cultural communication preferences with the important aspects of healthcare conversations. It is a way of communicating that is culturally secure and encourages deep listening, and helps to build a trusting relationship

clitoris cylindrical, erectile body located at the superior aspect of the vulva, between the labia minora; it contains erectile tissue and has a significant supply of nerve endings

clonus rhythmic oscillation of involuntary muscle contraction

clustering placing similar or related data into meaningful groups

cochlea snail-shaped structure in the bony labyrinth of the inner ear

collaborative consumer problem consumer problem for which the nurse works jointly with the physician and other healthcare workers to monitor, plan, and implement treatment

colloquialism word or phrase particular to a community and used in informal conversation and writing

colostrum a thin, milky secretion expressed by the breast during pregnancy and for a few days after parturition; it is rich in antibodies and colostrum corpuscles

complete health history (CHH) comprehensive history of the consumer's past and present health status; includes physical, emotional, psychological, developmental, cultural and spiritual data

condyloma acuminatum genital wart

cones retinal structures in the macular region that are responsible for colour vision

confabulation fabrication of answers, experiences or situations unrelated to facts

conservation the understanding that altering the physical state of an object does not change the basic properties of that object

constructional apraxia inability to reproduce figures on paper

consumer acuity the amount of care needed by a consumer; this will depend on both the physical and psychological need/demand of the consumer

consumer health goal broad, unmeasurable statement directed toward removal of related factors or consumer response to an adverse condition

consumer profile demographics that may be linked to health status

Cooper's ligaments ligaments that extend vertically from the deep fascia through the breast to the inner layer of the skin; they provide support for the breast tissue

corn conical area of thickened skin

cornea transparent covering of the iris

costal angle angle formed by the intersection of the costal margins at the sternum

costal margin medial border created by the articulation of the false ribs

cradle cap seborrheic dermatitis manifesting as greasy-appearing scales on an infant's scalp

craniosynostosis abnormal shape of the skull due to premature ossification of one or more suture lines before brain growth is complete

craniotabes softening of the skull

crepitus subcutaneous emphysema; beads of air escape from the lungs and create a crackling sound when palpated; a grating or crackling sound that can be felt/heard with joint movement

crescendo heart murmur configuration that proceeds from soft to loud

critical thinking a purposeful, goal-directed thinking process that strives to problem-solve consumer care issues through clinical reasoning

cryptorchidism condition in which a testicle has not descended into the scrotum

Cullen's sign bluish discolouration encircling the umbilicus and indicative of blood in the peritoneal cavity

cultural competence a system-level set of policies, expected behaviours and views that promotes safe and effective cross-cultural interactions for professional staff

cultural safety the provision of a safe environment that is free from assault and challenge, and accepts an individual's identity and needs

culture learned and socially transmitted orientation and way of life of a group of people that is based on shared values, beliefs, customs and norms of behaviour, and that determines how members of the group think, act, and relate to and with others as well as how they perceive and respond to all aspects of their lives

cyanosis/cyanotic blue colouration of the skin or nails that occurs when more than 5 g/dL of haemoglobin is deoxygenated in the blood

cystitis an inflammation (swelling) of the bladder, usually caused by an infection

cystocoele bulging of the anterior vaginal wall

D

dacryoadenitis acute inflammation of the lacrimal gland

dacryocystitis inflammation of the lacrimal duct

decerebrate rigidity rigidity and sustained contraction of the extensor muscle

decorticate rigidity hyperflexion of the arms, hyperextension and internal rotation of the legs, and plantar flexion

decrescendo heart murmur configuration that proceeds from loud to soft

deep palpation palpating the body's internal structures to a depth of 4 to 5 cm to elicit information on organs and masses, including position, size, shape, mobility, consistency, and areas of discomfort

defecation expulsion of faeces from the rectum

dehydration lack of fluid in the tissues

dermatome skin area innervated by afferent spinal nerves from a specific nerve root

dermis (or corium) the second layer of the skin

desquamation shedding of old skin cells as new cells are pushed up from the lower layers of the epidermis

development patterned and predictable increases in the physical, cognitive, socioemotional and moral capacities of individuals that enable them to successfully adapt to their environment

developmental dislocation of the hip dislocated hip found in newborns and young infants and related to familial factors, maternal hormones, firstborn children and breech presentations

developmental stage one of multiple sequential age periods during which individuals experience the same physical, cognitive, socioemotional and moral changes

developmental task specific physical or psychosocial skill that must be achieved during each developmental stage

diaphragmatic excursion technique used to assess the consumer's depth of ventilation

diaphragmatic hernia protrusion of intestines into the thoracic cavity

diaphysis central shaft of the long bone

diastasis recti separation of the rectus muscle of the abdominal wall

diastole phase in the cardiac cycle when the heart is at rest

direct (or immediate) auscultation active listening to body sounds via the unaided ear

direct (or immediate) percussion striking of an area of the body directly with the index or middle finger pad or fist to elicit sound

direct fist percussion using the ulnar aspect of a closed fist to strike the consumer's body to elicit tenderness over specific body areas

direct inguinal hernia protrusion of the bowel and/or omentum directly through the external inguinal ring

dislocation complete dislodgement of a bone from its joint cavity

distress negative stress that is harmful and unpleasant

disuse atrophy decrease in muscle mass and strength as a result of immobility

Doppler device that emits ultrasound waves and senses shifts in frequency as the ultrasound waves are reflected from fetal heart valves

Down syndrome congenital chromosomal aberration marked by slanted eyes with inner epicanthal folds; a short, flat nose; a protruding, thick tongue; and mental retardation

ductus (vas) deferens tube that permits sperm to exit from the epididymis and pass from the scrotal sac upwards into the abdominal cavity

dullness descriptor for a percussible sound that is moderate in intensity and duration, of high pitch, thudlike, and normally located over organs

duration (of percussion) time period over which a sound is heard

dysarthria disturbance in muscular control of speech

dyscalculia inability to perform calculations

dysdiadochokinesia inability to perform rapid alternating movements

dysmenorrhoea pain or cramping during menses

dysmetria impairment of judgement of distance, range, speed and force of movement

dyspareunia painful sexual intercourse

dysphagia difficulty swallowing

dysphasia partial or complete impairment of communication

dysphonia a voice disorder resulting from involuntary movements (spasms) of the voice box muscles. The voice may sound strained or strangled, or have breathy notes of missing sound for some words depending on the parts of the vocal chords that are affected

dyspnoea subjective feeling of shortness of breath

dysrhythmia *See* **arrhythmia**

dyssynergy lack of coordinated action of the muscle groups

E

ecchymosis a red-purple discolouration of varying size caused by extravasation of blood into the skin; a black-and-blue mark

eccrine glands sweat glands that are not associated with hair follicles

echolalia involuntary repetition of a word or sentence that was uttered by another person

eclampsia seizure associated with hypertensive disorder of pregnancy

ectodermal galactic band *See* **milk line**

ectopic pregnancy pregnancy that occurs outside of the uterus

ectropion (of the eye) turning outward or eversion of the eyelid, usually the lower

ectropion (or eversion, of the cervix) a red, inflamed appearance of the cervix as the columnar epithelium extends from the os past the normal squamocolumnar junction

egophony voice sound where the consumer says the sound 'ee' to determine if the lungs are filled with air, fluid or a solid

ejaculatory ducts ducts located posterior to the urinary bladder; they eject sperm into the prostatic urethra prior to ejaculation

electrocardiogram (ECG or EKG in US) a recording of the electrical activity of the heart

electronic medical records (EMRs) create a paperless system that can reduce charting/documentation time once the clinician is familiar with the system. EMRs enable the nurse to use voice recognition, narrative writing and/or check boxes with drop-down menus to record consumers' histories and assessment findings; other advantages of EMRs are their legibility, easy accessibility, ability to be accessed by multiple users simultaneously at different work stations in different areas in real time, and capability of accessing real-time laboratory and diagnostic studies

emergency health history history taken from the consumer or other sources when the consumer is experiencing a life-threatening state

entropion turning inward or inversion of the eyelid, usually the lower

epidermis multilayered outer covering of the skin, consisting of four layers throughout the body, except for the palms of the hands and soles of the feet, where there are five layers

epididymis comma-shaped organ that lies along the posterior border of each testis; consists of a tightly coiled tube in which sperm maturation occurs

epimysium connective tissue sheath covering the muscle belly

epiphyses ends of the long bone

epispadias congenital abnormality in which the urethral meatus lies on the dorsal surface of the penis

epistaxis nosebleed

Epstein's pearls small, hard, white cysts found on a newborn's hard palate and gum margins

epulis any tumour-like enlargement (i.e. lump) situated on the gingival or alveolar mucosa

eructation belching

erythematous redness caused by increased blood flow to the superficial capillaries

escutcheon characteristic triangular pattern of coarse curly hair that develops over the mons pubis at puberty

esophoria latent misalignment of the eye; nasal, or inward, drift

esotropia inward deviation of the eye

ethnocentrism judging another on the basis of your own personal cultural experiences

eupnoea normal breathing; respirations are 12 to 20 per minute for the resting adult

eustachian tube auditory tube that serves as an air channel connecting the middle ear to the nasopharynx to allow equalisation between the air pressure in the ear and in the atmosphere

eustress positive stress that challenges, provides motivation, and prevents stagnation

evaluation last step of the nursing process; the consumer's progress in achieving the outcomes is determined

evidence-based practice uses the outcomes of well-designed and executed scientific studies to guide clinical decision making and clinical care

exophoria latent misalignment of the eye; temporal, or outward, drift

exophthalmos abnormal protrusion of the globe of the eye

exotropia outward deviation of the eye

F

fallopian tubes site of fertilisation; they extend from the cornu of the uterus to the ovaries and are supported by the broad ligaments

false ribs rib pairs 8–10

fats substances that supply essential fatty acids that form a part of the structure of all cells

fat-soluble vitamins vitamins stored in dietary fat and absorbed in the fat portions of the body's cells

femoral hernia protrusion of the omentum or bowel through the femoral wall

fetoscope special stethoscope for hearing fetal heart beats

fibroma fibrous, encapsulated tumour of connective tissue, often called fibroid or myoma

First Nations *See* **Aboriginal and Torres Strait Islander peoples**

fissure groove separating the different lobes of the lungs

flatness descriptor for a percussible sound that is soft in intensity, short in duration, of high pitch, and normally located over muscle or bone

flatulence passage of excess gas via the rectum

floating ribs rib pairs 11 and 12; they do not articulate at their anterior ends

focused history shorter than the complete health history and is specific to the consumer's current reason for seeking health care

fetal alcohol syndrome (FAS) a pattern of craniofacial, cardiovascular and limb defects, with prenatal and postnatal growth retardation associated with maternal alcohol use

fornices pouchlike recesses around the cervix

fourchette transverse fold of skin of the posterior aspect of the labia minora; also known as a fraenulum

fovea centralis centre of the macula; the area of sharpest vision

fraenulum (of the mouth) tissue that connects the tongue to the floor of the mouth

friability susceptibility to bleeding from the cervix

functional health assessment documents a person's ability to perform instrumental activities of daily living and physical self-maintenance activities

functional health patterns groups of human behaviour that facilitate nursing care; there are 11 patterns

fundus superior aspect of the uterus

G

gallop extra heart sound; an S_3 is a ventricular gallop, whereas an S_4 is an atrial gallop

ganglion benign, cystic growth

genu valgum inward deviation toward the midline at the level of the knees; also known as knock-knees

genu varum outward deviation away from the midline at the level of the knees; also known as bow legs

glans penis bulbous end of the penis

Glasgow Coma Scale (GCS) international scale used in grading neurological response

glaucoma disease in which intraocular pressure is elevated

glycosuria glucose in the urine

goitre enlargement of the thyroid gland

goniometer device used to measure the angle of the skeletal joint during range of motion; it is a protractor with two movable arms

granulation tissue inflamed tissue, new vessels, and white blood cells at the base of a wound in the process of healing

granulomatous reaction (in the breast) development of small, nodular, inflammatory lesions and capsular membranes over the breasts

graphaesthesia ability to identify numbers, letters or shapes drawn on the skin

growth increase in body size and function to the point of optimum maturity

gynaecomastia enlargement of male breast tissue; may occur normally in adolescent and elderly males

H

haematemesis vomiting of blood

haematocrit measurement to determine the percentage of red blood cells in the volume of whole blood

haemoglobin measurement of the iron component that transports oxygen in the blood

haemorrhoids dilatation of haemorrhoidal veins in the anorectum

hallux valgus lateral deviation of the big toe and medial deviation of the first metatarsal; also known as a bunion

hammer toe flexion of the proximal interphalangeal joint and hyperextension of the distal metatarsophalangeal joint

harlequin colour change condition in which one-half of a newborn's body is red or ruddy and the other half appears pale

health education activities any activity that engages people in learning about health, health promotion and health management, and symptom prevention

health maintenance activities practices that a person incorporates into a lifestyle that can promote healthy living

health outcome measurable statement of the expected change in consumer behaviour

heave lifting of the cardiac area secondary to an increased workload and force of left ventricular contraction; also known as a lift

Heberden's node bony enlargement of the distal interphalangeal joint of the finger

hemiparesis unilateral weakness or paralysis; also known as hemiplegia

hemiplegia *See* **hemiparesis**

high-density lipoprotein (HDL) substance that carries cholesterol away from the heart and arteries and toward the liver

hirsutism excessive body hair

history of the present illness chronological account of the consumer's chief complaint and the events surrounding it

holistic nursing a form of nursing that addresses all aspects of a consumer's health and wellbeing, including spirituality and religion

holosystolic murmur that is heard throughout all of systole; also known as pansystolic

Homan's sign pain in the calf when the foot is dorsiflexed; sign of venous thrombosis of the deep veins of the calf

hordeolum infection of a sebaceous gland in the eyelid

hydatidiform mole molar or trophoblastic pregnancy; often requires careful monitoring of HCG after dilation and curettage of the uterus; if HCG remains elevated, chemotherapy may be indicated

hydrocephalus enlargement of the head without enlargement of the facial structures; it is due to increased accumulation of cerebrospinal fluid within the ventricles of the brain

hydrocoele fluid collection within the tunica vaginalis of the testis

hymen avascular, thin fold of connective tissue surrounding the vaginal introitus; it may be annular or crescentic in shape

hyperemesis gravidarum excessive nausea and vomiting during pregnancy

hyperglycaemia increase in serum glucose

hyperkinetic increased movement

hyperopia farsightedness

hyperpnoea breath that is greater in volume than the resting tidal volume

hyperresonance descriptor for a percussible sound that is very loud in intensity, long in duration, of very low pitch, boomlike, and normally not found in the healthy adult

hypertelorism abnormal width between the eyes

hypertension blood pressure remaining consistently above 140 mmHg systolic or 90 mmHg diastolic in an adult

hyperthermia generalised or localised excessive warming of the skin; body temperature that exceeds 38.58°C

hypertrophy increase in muscle size due to an increase in the bulk of muscle fibres

hyphaema condition in which there is blood in the anterior chamber of the eye

hypogeusia diminution of taste

hypoglycaemia decrease in serum glucose

hypokinetic decreased movement

hypospadias congenital abnormality in which the urethral meatus lies on the ventral surface of the penis

hypotension blood pressure that is lower than what is needed to maintain adequate tissue perfusion and oxygenation

hypothermia generalised or localised cooling of the skin; body temperature that is below 34.8°C

hypotonicity decrease in normal muscle tone (flaccidity)

hypovolaemic shock shock state caused by lack of circulating blood volume

hypoxaemia an abnormally low concentration of oxygen in the blood

I

immediate auscultation *See* **direct auscultation**

immediate percussion *See* **direct percussion**

implementation fifth step of the nursing process; the execution of the nursing interventions that were devised during the planning stage to help the consumer meet predetermined outcomes

impotence inability to achieve or maintain an erection

indirect (or mediate) auscultation active listening to body sounds via some amplification or mechanical device, such as a stethoscope or Doppler transducer

indirect (or mediate) percussion using the plexor to strike the pleximeter to elicit sound

indirect fist percussion using the closed ulnar aspect of the fist of the dominant hand to strike the nondominant hand to elicit tenderness over specific body areas

indirect inguinal hernia portions of the bowel or omentum that enter the inguinal canal through the internal inguinal ring and exit at the external inguinal ring

infarction (myocardial) necrosis of cardiac muscle due to decreased blood supply

injection redness around the cornea

inspection use of one's senses to consciously observe the consumer; in physical assessment, vision, hearing, smell and touch are used

insufficiency *See* **regurgitation**

integumentary system skin, or cutaneous tissue

intensity (of percussion) relative loudness or softness of sound; amplitude

intercostal space area between the ribs

intermediary individual who serves to assist with communication between the consumer and another individual, usually a member of the healthcare team

interpleural space *See* **mediastinum**

intervention nursing action designed to achieve consumer outcomes

intimate partner violence (IPV) involves more than physical abuse; it includes psychological, emotional, sexual and financial abuse or coercion

intussusception formation of a sausage-shaped mass in the upper abdomen that results when the ileocaecal region of the intestine telescopes into the ileum

iris most anterior portion of the uveal tract; provides a distinctive colour for the eye

ischaemia (myocardial) local and temporary lack of blood supply to the heart; may progress to an infarction if left untreated

isoelectric line electrical resting period after the T-wave on the ECG

isthmus (of the thyroid) narrow portion of the thyroid gland that connects the two lobes and lies over the tracheal rings

isthmus (of the uterus) constricted area between the body of the uterus and the cervix

J

jaundice yellow-green to orange cast or colouration of skin, sclera or mucous membranes; caused by an elevated bilirubin level

joining stage introduction or first stage of the interview process, during which the nurse and consumer establish rapport

joint union between two bones

K

keratosis lesions on the epidermis characterised by overgrowth of the horny layer

Kinship establishes where a person fits in their community, and it helps determine a personal relationship as well as a responsibility towards other people, the universe and Country

Korotkoff sounds sounds generated when the flow of blood through an artery is altered by the inflation of a blood pressure cuff around an extremity

Kussmaul's respirations respirations characterised by extreme increased rate and depth, as in diabetic ketoacidosis

kyphosis excessive convexity of the thoracic spine; known as 'humpback'

L

labia majora two longitudinal folds of adipose and connective tissue that extend from the clitoris anteriorly and gradually narrow to merge and form the commissure of the perineum posteriorly

labia minora two thin folds of skin that enclose the vulval vestibule and extend to form the prepuce, or hood, of the clitoris anteriorly and a transverse fold of skin that forms the fourchette posteriorly

labyrinth bony and membranous system of interconnecting tubes in the inner ear; essential for hearing and equilibrium

lacrimal apparatus lacrimal gland and ducts

lactiferous ducts openings at the nipple through which milk and colostrum are excreted

lagophthalmos condition in which the consumer is unable to completely close the eyelid

lanugo fine, downy hair present during gestational life and that gradually disappears toward the end of pregnancy; it remains in smaller quantities over the temples, back, shoulders and upper arms after birth

lens crystalline structure of the eye that changes shape to refract light from various focusing distances

lentigo areas of hyperpigmentation resulting from the inability of melanocytes to produce even pigmentation of the skin; known as 'liver spots'

lesion circumscribed, pathological change in tissue

lichenification localised thickening, hardening and roughness of the skin; can be a result of chronic pruritus

life event or transitional developmental theory belief that development occurs in response to specific events, such as new roles (e.g. parenthood) and life transitions (e.g. career changes)

ligament strong, fibrous, connective tissue that connects bones to each other at a joint

light palpation superficial palpation; depressing the skin 1 cm to elicit information on skin texture and moisture, masses, fluid, muscle guarding, and tenderness

lightening descent of the presenting fetal part into the pelvis

limbus junction of the sclera and cornea

linea alba tendinous tissue that extends from the sternum to the symphysis pubis in the middle of the abdomen

linea nigra darkening of the abdominal linea alba during pregnancy

linear raphe linear ridge in the middle of the hard palate

lipoma nonmobile, fatty mass with a smooth, circular edge

list leaning of the spine

listening response attempt made by the nurse to accurately receive, process and respond to the consumer's messages

lobes (of the breast) glandular breast tissue arranged radially in the form of 12 to 20 spokes

lobules (of the breast) grapelike bunches that are clustered around several lactiferous ducts; each lobe is composed of 20 to 40 lobules that contain milk-producing glands called alveoli or acini

location (of a sound) refers to the area where the sound is produced and heard

lordosis excessive concavity of the lumbar spine

low-density lipoprotein (LDL) substance that carries cholesterol toward the heart

lunula white, crescent-shaped area at the proximal end of each nail

lymphatic drainage yellow, alkaline drainage originating in the lymph vessels and composed primarily of lymphocytes

M

macromineral major mineral needed by the body in large amounts

macrosomia newborn weighing more than 4000 g

macula tiny, darker area in the temporal area of the retina

manubrium upper bone of the sternum; it articulates with the clavicles and the first pair of ribs

mast cells body's major source of tissue histamine, which triggers the body's reaction to invasive allergens

mastectomy excision, or surgical removal, of the breast

matrix undifferentiated epithelial tissue from which keratinised cells arise to form the nail plate

McBurney's point anatomic location that is approximately at the normal location of the appendix in the right lower quadrant; point of increased tenderness in appendicitis

meconium dark green, sticky, stool-like material excreted from the rectum of the newborn within the first 24 hours after birth

mediastinum (interpleural space) area between the lungs

mediate auscultation *See* indirect **auscultation**

mediate percussion *See* indirect **percussion**

medullary cavity interior of the diaphysis; contains the bone marrow

melaena black, tarry stool

melanocytes cells that produce pigmented substances that provide colour to the hair, skin and choroid of the eye

melasma irregular pigmentation on the face due to pregnancy; also known as chloasma

menarche onset of menstruation

menopause cessation of menstruation

menorrhagia heavy menses

metatarsus varus medial forefoot misalignment

microcephaly small brain with a resultant small head

micromineral trace mineral needed by the body in small amounts

microphallus small penis for developmental stage

midaxillary line vertical line drawn from the apex of the axilla; it lies midway between the anterior and the posterior axillary lines

midclavicular line vertical line drawn from the midpoint of the clavicle

midspinal (vertebral) line vertical line drawn from the midpoint of the spinous processes

midsternal line vertical line drawn from the midpoint of the sternum

milia plugged sebaceous glands manifesting as small, white papules and appearing on the infant's head, especially on the cheeks and nose

milk line ectodermal galactic band that develops from the axilla to the groin during the fifth week of fetal development

mineral inorganic element that regulates body processes and builds body tissue; classified into macrominerals and microminerals

Mongolian spots various irregularly sized areas of deep bluish pigmentation on the upper back, shoulders, buttocks and lumbosacral area of newborns of African, Latino and Asian descent

monounsaturated fat a 'good' fat that is sourced mainly from vegetables, nuts, seeds and fish. It has fewer hydrogen atoms bonded to their carbon frames than the saturated fats

mons pubis pad of subcutaneous fatty tissue lying over the anterior symphysis pubis

Montgomery's tubercles sebaceous glands present on the surface of the areola

moulding condition in which the newborn's parietal bone overrides the frontal bone as a result of increased pressure during delivery

multiparous any number of prior deliveries

myopia nearsightedness

N

naevi pigmented moles that may be flat or elevated

nail bed vascular bed located beneath the nail plate

nail plate tissue that covers and protects the distal portion of the fingers and toes

nail root nail portion that is posterior to the cuticle and attached to the matrix

neologism word coined by a consumer that is meaningful only to the consumer

nipple a round, hairless, pigmented protrusion of erectile tissue approximately 0.5 to 1.5 cm in diameter located in the centre of the breast

nociception a multistep process that involves the nervous system and other body systems in perceiving pain

nociceptors receptive neurons of pain sensation that are located in the skin and various viscera

nocturia excessive urination at night

nonverbal communication communicating a message without using words

nulliparous descriptor for a woman who has not given birth

nursing process dynamic, six-step process that incorporates information in a meaningful way in the use of problem-solving strategies to place the consumer, family or community in an optimal health state; includes assessment, nursing diagnosis, planning, outcome identification, implementation and evaluation

nursing-related consumer problem consumer-focused problems that the nurse and consumer can work on together to improve

nutrient substance found in food that is nourishing or useful to the body

nutrition processes of the human body that metabolise and utilise nutrients

nystagmus involuntary oscillation of the eye

O

obesity weight greater than 120% of ideal body weight

object permanence ability to form a mental image of an object and to recognise that, although removed from view, the object still exists

objective data data that is tangible or visible and can be corroborated by others; unbiased data not based on opinion or feeling

oculomotor nerve damage affects the third cranial nerve and damage may cause diplopia, ptosis and pupil mydriasis (dilated pupil)

oedema accumulation of fluid in the intercellular spaces, leading to swelling of the extremities, usually the feet and hands

oogenesis development and formation of an ovum

optic disc round area on the nasal side of the retina, where retinal fibres join to form the optic nerve

orchitis acute onset of testicular swelling

orthopnoea difficulty breathing except in an upright position

orthostatic hypotension hypotension that occurs when changing from a supine to an upright position

ossicles three tiny bones in the middle ear that play a crucial role in the transmission of sound: the malleus, the incus and the stapes

osteoporosis disease characterised by reduced bone mass

otitis media inflammation or infection of the middle ear

ovaries pair of almond-shaped glands, approximately 3 to 4 cm in length, in the upper pelvic cavity; oogenesis and hormonal production are their principal functions

P

Paget's disease malignant breast neoplasm that is usually unilateral in its involvement and presents as persistent eczematous dermatitis of the areola and nipple

pain an unpleasant sensory or emotional experience associated with actual or potential tissue damage, or described in terms of such damage

pain assessment a systematic approach to assessing a consumer's level and impact of pain

pallor lack of colour

palpation touching the consumer in a diagnostic manner to elicit specific information

palpebral conjunctiva mucous membrane covering the interior surface of the eyelid

palpebral fissure opening between the eyelids

palpitation irregular and rapid heartbeat, or sensation of fluttering of the heart

pansystolic *See* **holosystolic**

papilla/papillae small projection on the dorsal surface of the tongue and containing openings to taste buds

papillary layer upper layer of the dermis; composed primarily of loose connective tissue, small elastic fibres, and an extensive network of capillaries that serve to nourish the epidermis

papule red, solid, circumscribed, elevated area of the skin

paraesthesia an abnormal sensation such as numbness, pricking or tingling

paranasal sinuses air-filled cavities in the cranial bones that are lined with mucous membranes

paraphimosis condition in which the retracted foreskin develops a fixed constriction proximal to the glans penis

parietal pericardium pericardial layer that lies close to the fibrous tissues

parietal pleura lining of the chest wall and the superior surface of the lungs

parous descriptor for a woman who has given birth to one or more neonates

past health history (PHH) history that covers the consumer's health from birth to the present

past medical history (PMH) history that covers the consumer's health from birth to the present

peau d'orange thickening or oedema of the breast tissue or nipple; may present itself as enlarged skin pores that give the appearance of orange rind

pectus carinatum abnormal thorax configuration in which there is a marked protrusion of the sternum; known as 'pigeon chest'

pectus excavatum abnormal thorax configuration in which there is a depression in the lower body of the sternum; known as 'funnel chest'

penis cylindrical male organ of copulation and urination

percussion striking one object against another to cause vibrations that produce sound

pericarditis inflammation of the pericardium

perineum external surface located between the fourchette and the anus

periungual tissue tissue that surrounds the nail plate and the free edge of the nail

pertinent negatives manifestations that are expected in the consumer with a suspected pathology but that are denied or absent

pes cavus foot with an exaggerated height to the arch

pes planus foot with a low, longitudinal arch; also known as 'flatfoot'

pes valgus foot that is turned laterally away from the midline

pes varus foot that is turned inward toward the midline

petechiae reddish-purple skin discolouration that is less than 0.5 cm in diameter and does not blanch

phimosis constriction of the distal penile foreskin that prevents normal retraction over the glans

physiologic cup pale, central area of the optic disc

physiological weight loss tendency of a neonate to lose approximately 10% of birth weight within a few days after birth and regain it by 2 weeks of age

pinguecula yellow nodule on the nasal, or temporal, side of the bulbar conjunctiva

pinna external flap of the ear; also called the auricle

pitch (of percussion) highness or lowness of a sound

planning fourth step of the nursing process; involves the prioritisation of nursing diagnoses and selection of nursing interventions

pleura serous sac that encases the lung

pleural friction fremitus palpable grating that feels more pronounced on inspiration when there is an inflammatory process between the pleura

pleural friction rub continuous adventitious breath sound caused by inflamed parietal and visceral pleura; it resembles a creaking or grating sound

pleximeter stationary finger of the nondominant hand used in indirect percussion

plexor middle finger of the dominant hand used to strike the pleximeter to elicit sound in indirect percussion

polycythaemia elevated number of red blood cells

polydactyly extra digits on the hand or foot

positive findings those associated manifestations that the consumer has experienced along with the primary complaint

posterior axillary line vertical line drawn from the posterior axillary fold

posterior chamber space immediately posterior to the iris

posterior triangle area of the neck between the sternocleidomastoid and the trapezius muscles, with the clavicle at the base; contains the posterior cervical lymph nodes

prealbumin (also called thyroxine-binding prealbumin) the transport protein for thyroxine and retinol-binding protein

precordium anterior area of the body that lies over the heart, its great vessels, the pericardium, and some pulmonary tissue

preload resting force on the myocardium as determined by the pressure in the ventricles at the end of diastole

prepuce foreskin covering the glans penis

presbycusis hearing loss commonly found in older individuals

presbyopia/presbyopic impaired near vision occurring in middle-aged or older individuals

priapism abnormal prolonged penile erection unrelated to sexual desire

primary open angle glaucoma predominant subtype of glaucoma in which the anterior chamber angle appears open but has raised intraocular pressure with no other underlying disease. This is a progressive condition and is the most common cause of blindness

prioritise ranking the consumer's nursing diagnoses; the most critical concerns should be dealt with first

proprioception position sense

prostate glandular organ that lies anterior to the wall of the rectum and encircles the urethra; an accessory male sex organ

protein group of complex nitrogenous compounds, each containing amino acids

proteinuria presence of protein in the urine

prurigo itchy skin eruptions of unknown cause

pruritus severe itching

pterygium triangular, yellow thickening of the bulbar conjunctiva, extending from the nasal side of the cornea to the pupil

ptosis drooping of the eyelid

ptyalism excessive secretion of saliva

pulse palpable expansion of an artery in response to cardiac functioning; used to determine heart rate, rhythm, and estimated volume of blood being pumped by the heart

pulse deficit apical pulse rate greater than radial pulse rate; occurs when some heart contractions are too weak to produce a palpable pulse at the radial site

pulse pressure difference between systolic and diastolic blood pressures

pulsus paradoxus pathological decrease in systolic blood pressure by 10 mmHg or more on inspiration

puncta opening at the inner canthus of the eye through which tears drain

pupil opening in the centre of the iris; regulates the amount of light entering the eye

purpura condition characterised by the presence of confluent petechiae or confluent ecchymosis over any part of the body

pyelonephritis kidney infection or inflammation

Q

qualifier adjective that describes or qualifies the human response

quality (of percussion) timbre; how a sound is perceived musically

quickening first fetal movements felt by a pregnant woman

R

race classification of individuals based on shared inherited biological traits such as skin colour, facial features and body build

racial bias bias based on a person's racial background

rash cutaneous skin eruption that may be localised or generalised

reason for seeking health care problem or healthcare need that brought the consumer to seek health care

rebound tenderness pain elicited during deep palpation, frequently associated with peritoneal inflammation or appendicitis

rectal prolapse protrusion of the rectum through the anal orifice

rectouterine pouch deep recess formed by the outer layer of the peritoneum; the lowest point in the pelvic cavity, encompassing the lower posterior wall of the uterus, the upper portion of the vagina, and the intestinal surface of the rectum

rectovaginal septum surface that separates the rectum from the posterior aspect of the vagina

rectum lower portion of the large intestine; passes downwards in front of the sacrum

re-epithelialisation reformation of epithelium over denuded skin

regurgitation backwards flow of blood through a diseased heart valve; also known as insufficiency

resonance descriptor for a percussible sound that is loud in intensity, moderate to long in duration, low in pitch, hollow, and normally located in healthy lungs

respiration breathing act that supplies oxygen to the body and occurs in response to changes in the concentration of oxygen, carbon dioxide and hydrogen in the arterial blood

reticular layer lower layer of the dermis that is formed by a dense bed of vascular connective tissue; it also includes nerves and lymphatic tissue

retina innermost layer of the eye

retroflexed uterus a condition in which the main body of the uterus is tipped back at the cervix

retromammary adipose tissue tissue that composes the bulk of the breast

retroverted uterus a uterus that is displaced backwards, with the cervix pointing upwards toward the symphysis pubis

reversibility the understanding that an action does not need to be experienced before one can anticipate the results or consequences of the action

review of systems (ROS) the consumer's subjective responses to a series of questions related to body systems; serves as a double-check that vital information is not overlooked

rhonchal fremitus coarse, palpable vibration produced by the passage of air through thick exudate in the large bronchi or the trachea

Rinne test method of evaluating hearing loss by comparing air and bone conduction of tuning fork vibrations

rod retinal structure responsible for peripheral vision and dark or light discrimination

Rovsing's sign technique to elicit referred pain indicative of peritoneal inflammation

S

saturated fats lipids derived from animal or vegetable sources in which the fatty acid chains have only single bonds

scapular line vertical line drawn from the inferior angle of the scapula

sclera opaque covering of the eye; appears white

scoliosis lateral curvature of the thoracic or lumbar vertebrae

scrotum pouchlike supporting structure of the testes

sebaceous glands sebum-producing glands that are found almost everywhere in the dermis except the palmar and plantar surfaces

sebum oily secretion that is thought to retard evaporation and water loss from the epidermal surface

seizure transient disturbance of cerebral function caused by an excessive discharge of neurons

self-regulation via reflective practice it is a key component of the critical-thinking process

semicircular canals anterior, posterior and lateral canals in the bony labyrinth of the inner ear that provide balance and equilibrium

seminal vesicles paired pouches located posteriorly to and at the base of the bladder; fluid from here forms 60% of the volume of semen

septum/septa (of the heart) wall that divides the left side of the heart from the right side

sequelae aftermath

shifting dullness a sign that may be seen during physical examination of the abdomen for ascites. This test checks for fluid in the peritoneal cavity by percussing the abdomen when the patient is in different positions. The practitioner is listening for changes in tympany sounds when moving across the abdomen, and where fluid is encountered, a dullness is heard compared to normal tympany sounds. When the patient is then moved to a lateral position, if there is ascites present, the dullness will move to a different section of the abdomen when percussing, hence the term 'shifting dullness'.

sighing normal respiration interrupted by a deep inspiration and followed by a deep expiration

sign objective finding

sinoatrial (S-A) node normal pacemaker of the heart; intrinsic adult rate is approximately 70 beats per minute

Skene's glands (paraurethral glands) glands that open in a posterolateral position to the urethral meatus and provide lubrication to protect the skin

skinfold thickness anthropometric measurement to determine body fat stores and nutritional status

smegma white, cottage cheese-like substance sometimes found under the female labia minora or the male foreskin

snap high-pitched sound that is heard in early diastole; usually occurs in mitral stenosis

Snellen chart used for testing distance vision; contains letters of various sizes with standardised visual acuity numbers at the end of each line of letters

social history information related to the consumer's lifestyle that can have an impact on their health

spasticity increase in muscle tension on passive stretching, especially rapid or forced stretching of a muscle

spermatic cord connective tissue sheath made up of arteries, nerves, veins, lymphatic vessels and the cremaster muscle

spermatocoele well-defined cystic mass on the superior testes

spermatogenesis production of sperm

sphincter a circular muscle that opens or closes an orifice or passage

sphygmomanometer gauge used to measure blood pressure; consists of a blood pressure cuff with an inflatable bladder, connecting tubes, bulb air pump, and a manometer

spider angioma bright red, star-shaped vascular marking that often has a central pulsation; it blanches in the extensions when pressure is applied

spinnbarkeit test test used to determine elasticity of cervical mucus during ovulation

spiritual relating to religious belief as it affects a person's spirit/soul rather than physical affect

sputum substance that is produced by the respiratory tract and can be expectorated or swallowed; it is composed of mucus, blood, purulent material, microorganisms, cellular debris and, occasionally, foreign objects

squamocolumnar junction cervical area between the squamous epithelial surface and the columnar epithelial surface

standard precautions practices healthcare providers use to prevent the exchange of blood and body fluids when coming into contact with a consumer; outlined by the Centers for Disease Control and Prevention (CDC)

steatorrhoea pale yellow, greasy, fatty stool

stenosis narrowing or constriction (e.g. diseased heart valve)

Stensen's ducts openings from the parotid glands; located just opposite the upper second molars

stereognosis ability to identify objects by manipulating and touching them

sternal angle *See* **angle of Louis**

stork bites *See* **telangiectatic naevi**

strabismus true deviation of gaze due to extraocular muscle dysfunction

stratum corneum horny layer, or outer layer of the epidermis

stress physiologically defined response to changes that disrupt the resting equilibrium of an individual

striae atrophic lines or scars commonly found on the abdomen, breasts, thighs or buttocks

striae gravidarum stretch marks that occur in pregnancy

stroke a term relating to a brain condition in which oxygen to brain tissue is interrupted either due to a blockage or haemorrhage; this interruption can cause ischaemia or cell death

subcutaneous tissue superficial fascia composed of loose areolar connective tissue or adipose tissue, depending on its location in the body; it lies below the dermis

subjective data information perceived by the consumer to be real; such data cannot always be verified by an independent observer

subluxation partial dislodgement of a bone from its place in the joint cavity

sulcus terminalis midline depression separating the anterior two-thirds from the posterior one-third of the tongue

supernumerary nipples extra nipples or breast tissue along the milk line resulting from incomplete atrophy of the galactic band

suprasternal notch visible and palpable depression in the midsternal line superior to the manubrium

sutures immovable joints connecting the cranial bones

sweat glands glands that produce perspiration; composed of two types: eccrine and apocrine glands

symptom subjective finding

syncope fainting; transient loss of consciousness due to decreased oxygen or glucose supply to the brain

syndactyly fusion between two or more digits on the hand or foot

synovial effusion excessive synovial joint fluid

systemic vascular resistance (SVR) the amount of resistance the heart must overcome to open the aortic valve and push the blood volume out into the systemic circulation

systole phase in the cardiac cycle during which the myocardial fibres contract and tighten to eject blood from the ventricles; correlates with the first Korotkoff sound

T

tachycardia pulse rate greater than 100 beats per minute in an adult

tachypnoea respiratory rate greater than 20 breaths per minute in an adult

tactile (or vocal) fremitus palpable vibration of the chest wall that is produced by the spoken word

tail of Spence upper outer quadrant of the breast that extends into the axilla

talipes equinovarus (clubfoot) medially adducted and inverted toes and forefoot

tangential lighting light that is shone at an angle on the consumer to accentuate shadows and highlight subtle findings

tarsal plates connective tissue that gives shape to the upper eyelid

telangiectatic naevi marks appearing on the back of the neck, lower occiput, upper eyelids and upper lip of the newborn that are flat, deep, irregular, and pink in light-skinned children and deep red in dark-skinned children; also known as 'stork bites'

temperature vital sign collected to assess core body heat

tendons a flexible and inelastic cord or fibrous collagen tissue that connects bone to muscle

terminal hair coarse body hair in the axillary and pubic areas as well as the eyebrows, eyelashes, scalp and, in men, the chest and face

termination stage last segment of the interview process, during which information is summarised and validated

testes pair of ovoid glands located in the scrotum

the nursing process is described in different ways, for example as a four-, five- or six-phased process: APIE – Assessment, Planning, Implementation and Evaluation; ADPIE – Assessment, Diagnosis, Planning, Implementation and Evaluation; APOPIE – Assessment, Patient problem, Outcomes identification, Planning, Implementation and Evaluation

thenar eminence rounded prominence at the base of the thumb

thoracic expansion the extent and symmetry of chest wall expansion

thrill vibrations related to turbulent blood flow that feel similar to what one feels when a hand is placed on a purring cat

tilts set of blood pressures taken in supine, sitting and standing positions

torticollis lateral deviation of the neck; intermittent or sustained dystonic contraction of the muscles on one side of the neck

transitional developmental theories based on the premise that development occurs in response to specific events, such as new roles (e.g. parenthood) and life transitions (e.g. career changes)

transmission-based precautions infection-control practices involving contact, droplet and airborne transmission of microorganisms that are known to exist in a consumer or are suspected in a consumer; they are practised in conjunction with Standard Precautions

traumatic brain injury (TBI) an injury caused to the brain from trauma of some kind – usually by external force; e.g. blunt or penetrating force

triglyceride substance that accounts for most of the fat stored in the body's tissues

true ribs *See* **vertebrosternal ribs**

tubular breath sound *See* **bronchovesicular breath sound**

turbinate (or concha) projection from the lateral wall of the nose and covered with mucous membranes that greatly increase the surface area within the nose

turgor elasticity of the skin; it reflects the skin's state of hydration

tussive fremitus palpable vibration produced by coughing

tympany descriptor for a percussible sound that is loud in intensity, long in duration, of high pitch, drumlike, and normally located over a gastric air bubble

U

urethra duct from the urinary bladder to the urethral meatus; carries urine and, in the male, semen

uterus inverted, pear-shaped, hollow, muscular organ in which the impregnated ovum develops into a fetus

uvula fingerlike projection hanging down from the centre of the soft palate

V

vagina pink, hollow, muscular tube extending from the cervix to the vulva, located posterior to the bladder and anterior to the rectum

vaginal introitus entrance to the vagina, situated at the inferior aspect of the vulval vestibule

varicocele bluish mass resulting from abnormal dilatation of the veins of the pampiniform plexus of the spermatic cord

vellus hair fine, faint hair that covers most of the body

venous hum continuous, medium-pitched sound originating in the inferior vena cava and associated with obstructed portal circulation

venous star linear or irregularly shaped, blue vascular pattern on the skin; does not blanch when pressure is applied

vernix caseosa protective integumentary mechanism of the newborn; consists of sebum and shed epithelial cells

vertebra prominens the long spinous process of the seventh cervical vertebra

vertebrosternal (or true) ribs rib pairs 1–7; they articulate via the costal cartilage to the sternum

vertigo dizziness or lightheadedness

vesicular breath sound breath sound that is low in pitch and soft in intensity and is heard best over the peripheral lung; has a breezy, gentle, rustling quality; heard longer on inspiration than expiration

vestibule boat-shaped area between the labia minora and containing the urethral meatus, the openings of Skene's glands, the hymen, the openings of Bartholin's glands, and the vaginal introitus

vestibule (of the ear) part of the inner ear located between the cochlea and the semicircular canals

visceral pericardium pericardial layer that lies against the actual heart muscle

visceral pleura lining of the external surface of the lungs

visual analog scale numerical scale used to rate pain from 0 to 10

vital signs measurements, including temperature, pulse, respiration and blood pressure, that provide an index of a consumer's physiological status

vitamin organic substance needed to maintain the function of the body

vitiligo patchy, symmetrical areas of white on the skin

vitreous humour gelatinous material that fills the centre cavity of the eye and helps maintain the shape of the eye and the position of the internal structures

vocal fremitus *See* **tactile fremitus**

voice sounds techniques used to assess whether the lungs are filled with air, fluid or a solid

W

water-soluble vitamin vitamin that is soluble in water; is not stored in the body but is excreted in the urine

Weber test tuning fork test to evaluate hearing loss and determine whether the loss is conductive or sensorineural

welcome to Country a ceremony performed by Traditional Custodians to welcome visitors to ancestral land

Wharton's ducts openings from the submaxillary glands; located on either side of the frenulum

whispered pectoriloquy voice sound where the consumer whispers the words 'ninety-nine' or 'one, two, three' to determine if the lungs are filled with air, fluid or a solid

word salad a confused or unintelligible mixture of seemingly random words and phrases

working stage that segment of the interview process during which the majority of data is collected

X

xanthelasma creamy, yellow plaque on the eyelid and secondary to hypercholesterolaemia

xerosis excessive dryness of the skin

xiphoid process cartilaginous process at the base of the sternum; it does not articulate with the ribs

Y

yarning a free-flowing, reciprocal conversation that involves deep listening (dadirri) to storytelling that creates new knowledge and understanding in an environment where all participants feel safe and respected

INDEX

Printed in the United States
By Bookmasters